Surgery of the Pancreas

*This book is dedicated
to our beloved wives,
Ursula and Ilske.*

For Churchill Livingstone

Publisher: Peter Richardson
Project Editor: Lucy Gardner
Production Controller: Neil Dickson
Sales Promotion Executive: Caroline Boyd

Surgery of the Pancreas

Edited by

Michael Trede BA BChir MD HonFRCS(Eng and Irel) HonFRCPS(Glas)

Professor and Chairman, Chirurgische Klinik, Klinikum Mannheim,
Universität Heidelberg, Mannheim, Germany

David C. Carter MD FRCS(Ed) FRCS(Glas) FRCP(Ed)

Regius Professor of Clinical Surgery, Royal Infirmary, Edinburgh, UK

Foreword by
W. P. Longmire Jr MD FACS

Professor of Surgery Emeritus, UCLA School of Medicine, Los Angeles, California, USA

Illustrations by Gillian Lee

CHURCHILL LIVINGSTONE
EDINBURGH LONDON MADRID MELBOURNE NEW YORK AND TOKYO 1993

CHURCHILL LIVINGSTONE
Medical Division of Longman Group UK Limited

Distributed in the United States of America by
Churchill Livingstone Inc., 650 Avenue of the Americas,
New York, N.Y. 10011, and by associated companies,
branches and representatives throughout the world.

First published 1993

ISBN 0-443-04427-9

British Library of Cataloguing in Publication Data
A catalogue record for this book is available from the
British Library.

Library of Congress Cataloging in Publication Data
Surgery of the pancreas/edited by Michael Trede, David C. Carter;
  foreword by W.P. Longmire, Jr; illustrations by Gillian Lee.
    p.   cm.
  Includes index.
  ISBN 0-443-04427-9
  1. Pancreas---Surgery. 2. Pancreas---Diseases. I. Trede, M.
II. Carter, David C. (David Craig)
    [DNLM: 1. Pancreatic Diseases-diagnosis. 2. Pancreatic Diseases---
surgery. 3. Pancreas---surgery. WI 800 S9605 1993]
  RD546.S5329 1993
  617.5'57059---dc20
  DNLM/DLC
  for Library of Congress   93-12700

The
publisher's
policy is to use
**paper manufactured
from sustainable forests**

Printed and bound in Great Britain by
William Clowes Limited, Beccles and London

Contents

Foreword   ix
Acknowledgements   xi
Contributors   xiii

SECTION 1
Introduction: History of pancreatic surgery
Anatomy and physiology

1. History of pancreatic surgery   3
   R. C. Praderi

2. Embryology and surgical anatomy of the pancreas
   17
   M. Trede

3. Physiology of the pancreas   29
   D. C. Carter

SECTION 2
Preoperative diagnosis of pancreatic disease

4. Conventional radiography   51
   P. C. Freeny

5. Ultrasonography   55
   P. C. Freeny

6. Computed tomography   61
   P. C. Freeny

7. Magnetic resonance imaging   73
   P. C. Freeny

8. Percutaneous transhepatic cholangiography   77
   P. C. Freeny

9. Angiography   81
   P. C. Freeny

10. Endoscopic retrograde cholangiopancreatography   87
    P. J. Connors, D. L. Carr-Locke

11. Endoscopic ultrasonography   111
    T. L. Tio

12. Percutaneous fine-needle aspiration cytology   121
    I. Ihse, Å. Andrén-Sandberg

13. Laboratory evaluation of pancreatic function and
    disease   127
    R. Klapdor

SECTION 3
Intraoperative diagnostic procedures

14. Approaches to the pancreas and abdominal
    exploration   141
    M. Trede

15. Intraoperative ultrasonography   147
    J. Machi, B. Sigel

16. Intraoperative needle aspiration and biopsy   153
    E. Bodner, K. Glaser

SECTION 4
Acute pancreatitis

17. Definition and classification of pancreatitis   161
    D. C. Carter

18. Aetiology and pathogenesis of acute pancreatitis   165
    J. L. Cameron, J. A. Clemens

19. Diagnostic assessment and prognostication in acute
    pancreatitis   193
    D. C. Carter

20. Non-operative management of acute
    pancreatitis   209
    J. H. C. Ranson

21. Special aspects of gallstone pancreatitis   221
    D. C. Carter

22. Operative management of acute pancreatitis   233
    H. G. Beger, W. Uhl

23. Complications of acute pancreatitis and their
    management   245
    E. L. Bradley, K. A. Allen

SECTION 5
Chronic pancreatitis

24. Aetiology and pathogenesis of chronic
    pancreatitis   263
    M. K. Müller, M. V. Singer

25. Conservative management of chronic
    pancreatitis   273
    D. C. Carter, M. Trede

26. Preoperative assessment and indications for operation
    in chronic pancreatitis   283
    M. Trede, D. C. Carter

27. Endoscopic interventional techniques in chronic
    pancreatitis   299
    A. Maydeo, H. Grimm, N. Soehendra

28. Surgical drainage procedures in chronic
    pancreatitis   309
    D. C. Carter

29. Distal pancreatectomy in chronic pancreatitis   321
    C. F. Frey

30. Partial pancreatoduodenectomy for chronic
    pancreatitis   329
    J. W. Braasch, R. L. Rossi

31. Total pancreatoduodenectomy   339
    R. C. G. Russell

32. Pain-relieving procedures in chronic pancreatitis   349
    L. F. Hollender, B. Laugner

33. Late results of surgical treatment of chronic
    pancreatitis   359
    J. Horn

SECTION 6
Congenital anomalies of the pancreas

34. Congenital anomalies of the pancreas   369
    F. G. Moody, J. R. Potts

SECTION 7
Tumours of the exocrine pancreas and periampullary region

35. Aetiology and epidemiology of pancreatic and
    periampullary cancer   383
    D. C. Carter

36. Pathology and classification of tumours of the
    pancreas   399
    V. Becker, P. Stömmer

37. Clinical evaluation and preoperative
    assessment   423
    M. Trede, D. C. Carter

38. The surgical options   433
    M. Trede

39. Local excision for tumours of the papilla   443
    M. Trede

40. Technique of Whipple pancreatoduodenectomy   447
    M. Trede

41. Total pancreatectomy   461
    M. Trede

42. Vascular problems and techniques associated with
    pancreatectomy   465
    M. Trede

43. Left hemipancreatectomy   477
    M. Trede

44. Palliative management by endoscopic
    procedures   481
    B. C. Manegold

45. Palliative management with percutaneous and
    rendezvous techniques   487
    W. R. Jaschke, B. C. Manegold

46. Surgical palliation of pancreatic and periampullary
    tumours   497
    P. C. Bornman, J. E. J. Krige

47. Chemotherapy and radiotherapy in the treatment of
    pancreatic cancer   515
    J. Jeekel

SECTION 8
Endocrine tumours of the pancreas

48. Endocrine tumours of the pancreas: clinical picture,
    diagnosis and therapy   521
    W. Creutzfeldt, R. Arnold

49. Islet cell tumours of the pancreas   545
    J. A. van Heerden, G. B. Thompson

SECTION 9
Injuries to the pancreas

50. Injuries to the pancreas   565
    C. F. Frey, J. W. Wardell

SECTION 10
Pancreatic transplantation

51. Pancreatic transplantation   593
   K. L. Brayman, D. E. R. Sutherland, J. S. Najarian

SECTION 11
Pancreatic surgery: anaesthesia and complications

52. Anaesthesia in pancreatic surgery   623
   K. van Ackern, D. M. Albrecht

53. The complications of pancreatoduodenectomy and
   their management   629
   M. Trede, D. C. Carter

Index   645

Foreword

The pancreas, more than any other abdominal organ, continues to provide fascinating surgical frontiers in both the basic sciences as well as in clinical medicine as the structure and functions of ductal, acinar and islet cell components undergo further amazing detailed analysis. Such basic studies have contributed to our further understanding of the clinical behaviour of the various neoplastic, inflammatory, traumatic and congenital abnormalities of the pancreas and have provided a more rational and reasoned basis for clinical management.

This volume presents an unparalleled compendium of information ranging from the historical aspects of the organ and its diseases to the current status of such frontiers as transplantation and the adjunctive therapy of malignancies. New and refined diagnostic procedures, some of which are continuing to evolve as we learn how they may be best utilized, aid in the evaluation of pancreatic diseases and provide more detailed information upon which treatment may be based. A dozen or so such diagnostic aids are herein discussed in the two excellent sections on preoperative and intraoperative diagnostic procedures.

The varied clinical presentations and current therapies of both acute and chronic inflammatory diseases of the pancreas, which are of increasing clinical importance, are discussed in detail by an international array of surgeons with an extensive experience in the management of these difficult clinical problems.

Although pessimism prevails in many quarters regarding the current effectiveness of surgical treatment of malignancies of the exocrine pancreas, the methods of management presented by the authors have produced results that are considerably more encouraging. Indeed, a discussion of their techniques and the results so produced, which rank with the best in the world, form a major section of the book.

Other sections include coverage of the fascinating field of endocrine tumours as the advantages and benefits of conservative and surgical management are discussed, and authoritative discussion of great practical importance concerning the management of injuries of the pancreas. The volume is completed with discussions of congenital anomalies, transplantation and anaesthesia, and ends with one of the most important practical sections, namely the management of the complications of pancreatectomy.

The editors have sought their contributions from nine different countries and have recruited some of the most experienced and widely recognized authorities in the field of pancreatic surgery, all of whom have made important contributions to advance our knowledge of the physiology, pathology and/or clinical management of this intriguing organ. This volume presents information that will serve the student, the investigator and, most importantly, those physicians and surgeons who come face to face with the difficult diagnostic and therapeutic problems of pancreatic diseases in their clinical practice.

W. P. L.

Acknowledgements

The authors gratefully acknowledge the continuing support provided by their long-suffering wives during the countless hours needed to write and edit this book. The skilled assistance of Ilske Carter in translating and editing was of enormous assistance. We are grateful to our colleagues who provided such excellent chapters for this work, some of whom managed the rare feat of actually sending in their manuscripts on time. The excellence of Gillian Lee's illustrations has been a source of great pleasure and we are grateful for her prompt service and meticulous attention to detail. We acknowledge the skilled secretarial assistance of Anne McKellar and Susan Rowley (Edinburgh), and Gesine Schilling (Mannheim), assistance without which the book would have been stillborn.

We wish to acknowledge the debt that we both feel to our teachers, paying particular homage to Dr William P. Longmire Jr, with whom we both had the privilege to work at the University of California in Los Angeles, and to the late Dr Morton Grossman who inspired a generation of surgeons in the field of gastrointestinal and pancreatic physiology as it relates to surgery. We pay tribute to our colleagues in the University Surgical Clinic at Mannheim and the Royal Infirmary of Edinburgh without whom our experience of pancreatic disease and its surgery would have been greatly diminished. The international community devoted to the study of the pancreas and its surgery has been a constant source of encouragement and has given us a strong incentive to finish this task. We owe specific debts to Dr Calum Muir (for advice on the aetiology of pancreatic cancer) and to Dr Skandalakis (for his kindness in allowing us to draw heavily on his classic studies of pancreatic anatomy).

Finally, we are grateful to our publishers, Churchill Livingstone, for their continued support and forbearance. We acknowledge a special debt of gratitude to Mr Peter Richardson for initiating the project, to Miss Lucy Gardner (Senior Project Editor) for her kindly but no-nonsense dealings with ourselves and our more recalcitrant colleagues, and to Teresa Brady and Nicky Carrodus for their meticulous sub-editing and preparation of the material.

1993   M. T.
                                                        D. C. C.

Contributors

D. M. Albrecht MD
Professor, Leitender Oberarzt des Instituts für Anästhesiologie und Operative Intensivmedizin, Klinikum der Stadt Mannheim, Mannheim, Germany

K. L. Allen MD
Department of Surgery, Emory University School of Medicine, Atlanta, Georgia, USA

Åke Andrén-Sandberg MD PhD
Associate Professor, Department of Surgery, Lund University, Lund, Sweden

R. Arnold MD
Medizinische Klinik and Poliklinik, Georg-August-Universität, Göttingen, Germany

Volker Becker MD
Emeritus Professor, Pathologisches Institut der Universität Erlangen-Nürnberg, Erlangen, Germany

Hans G. Beger MD FACS
Professor of Surgery and Head, Department of General Surgery, University of Ulm, Surgical University Hospital, Ulm, Germany

Ernst Bodner MD
Professor and Head of II. Department for Surgery, University of Innsbruck, Innsbruck, Austria

P. C. Bornman FRCS(Ed) MMed(Surg)
Professor of Surgery, University of Cape Town; Head, Surgical Gastroenterology, Groote Schuur Hospital, Observatory, Cape Town, South Africa

John W. Braasch MD PhD
Senior Consultant, Department of General Surgery, Lahey Clinic Medical Center, Burlington; Assistant Clinical Professor of Surgery, Harvard Medical School, Boston, Massachusetts, USA

Edward L. Bradley III MD
William G. Whittaker Jr Professor of Surgery, Emory University School of Medicine, Atlanta, Georgia, USA

Kenneth L. Brayman MD PhD
Assistant Professor of Surgery and Director, Pancreas and Human Islet Transplant Program, University of Pennsylvania Medical Center, Philadelphia, Pennsylvania, USA

John L. Cameron MD BA FACS FRCSI
Professor and Chairman, Department of Surgery, The Johns Hopkins University School of Medicine; Chief of Surgery, The Johns Hopkins Hospital, Baltimore, Maryland, USA

David L. Carr-Locke MA MB BChir DRCOG FRCP FACG
Director of Endoscopy, Brigham and Women's Hospital; Associate Professor, Harvard Medical School; Boston, Massachusetts, USA

David C. Carter MD FRCS(Ed) FRCS(Glas)
Regius Professor of Clinical Surgery, Royal Infirmary, Edinburgh, UK

J. Clemens MD
Johns Hopkins Hospital, Baltimore, Maryland, USA

Pamela J. Connors MD
Assistant Professor of Medicine, Jefferson Medical College, Philadelphia; Director of Endoscopy, Thomas Jefferson University Hospital, Philadelphia, Pennsylvania, USA

Werner Creutzfeldt MD FRCP
Emeritus Professor of Medicine, Former Chairman, Department of Medicine and Director, Division of Gastroenterology and Endocrinology, University of Göttingen, Germany

P. C. Freeny MD
Clinical Professor of Radiology, Virginia Mason Clinic, University of Washington School of Medicine, Department of Radiology, Washington, USA

Charles F. Frey MD
Professor and Vice Chairman, Department of Surgery, University of California, Davis Medical Center, Sacramento, California, USA

K. Glaser MD
II. Universitätsklinik für Chirurgie, Innsbruck, Austria

Horst Grimm MD
Department of Endoscopic Surgery, University Hospital Hamburg, Hamburg, Germany

Louis F. Hollender MD FACS(Hon) FRCS(Hon)
Emeritus Professor of Surgery, University Louis Pasteur, Strasbourg; Honorary Surgeon in Chief, Department of General and Digestive Surgery, University Hospitals, Strasbourg, France

J. Horn MD
Chefarzt der Chirurgischen Abteilung, Stadt Krankenhaus Mu-Harlaching, Munich, Germany

Ingemar Ihse MD PhD
Professor and Chairman, Department of Surgery, Lund University, Lund, Sweden

Werner R. Jaschke MD
Professor and Clinical Radiologist, Klinikum Mannheim, Universität Heidelberg, Heidelberg, Germany

J. Jeekel MD
Chief, Department of Surgery, University Hospital Dÿkzigt, Rotterdam, The Netherlands

Rainer Klapdor MD
Professor of Internal Medicine, Department of Medicine, University Hospital Hamburg, Hamburg, Germany

J. E. J. Krige MB ChB FRCS FCS(SA)
Associate Professor of Surgery, University of Cape Town and Groote Schuur Hospital, Observatory, Cape Town, South Africa

B. Laugner MD
Anaesthesiologist, Pain Clinic, Hopitaux Universitaires, Strasbourg, France

Junji Machi MD PhD
Research Assistant Professor, Department of Surgery, Medical College of Pennsylvania, Philadelphia, Pennsylvania, USA

Bernd C. Manegold MD
Professor, Department of Endoscopy, Chirurgische Klinik, Klinikum Mannheim, University of Heidelberg, Mannheim, Germany

Amit Maydeo MD
Department of Endoscopic Surgery, University Hospital of Hamburg, Hamburg, Germany

Frank G. Moody MD
Denton A. Cooley Professor and Chairman, Department of Surgery, The University of Texas Medical School, Houston, Texas, USA

M. K. Müller MD
Senior Lecturer, Medizinische Klinik IV (Gastroenterology), Klinikum Mannheim, University of Heidelberg, Mannheim, Germany

John S. Najarian MD FACS FRCS(Hon)
Chairman, Regents' Professor and Jay Phillips Distinguished Chair, Surgery Department, University of Minnesota, Minneapolis, Minnesota, USA

John R. Potts III MD
Associate Professor, Department of Surgery, University of Texas Medical School, Houston, Texas, USA

Raul C. Praderi MD
Professor of Surgery, Republic University School of Medicine, Maciel Hospital, Montevideo, Uruguay

John H. C. Ranson MD MA BM BCh
S. A. Localio Professor of Surgery, New York University School of Medicine; Director, Division of General Surgery, New York University Medical Center; Attending Surgeon, Bellevue Hospital and Manhattan VA Medical Center, New York, USA

Ricardo L. Rossi MD
Associate Clinical Professor of Surgery, Harvard Medical School; Chairman, Department of Surgery, Lahey Clinic Medical Center, Burlington, Massachusetts, USA

R. C. G. Russell MS FRCS
Consultant Surgeon, The Middlesex Hospital, London, UK

Bernard Sigel MD
Professor of Surgery, Department of Surgery, Medical College of Pennsylvania, Philadelphia, Pennsylvania, USA

Manfred V. Singer MD
Professor of Medicine and Chairman, Department of Medicine IV (Gastroenterology), Klinikum Mannheim, University of Heidelberg, Mannheim, Germany

Nib Soehendra MD
Professor of Surgery and Director, Department of Endoscopic Surgery, University Hospital of Hamburg, Hamburg, Germany

Peter E. Stömmer PrivDoz DrMed DrMedHabil
Lecturer in General Pathology and Pathologic Anatomy, University of Erlangen-Nürnberg; Head, Private Institute of Pathology, Augsburg, Germany

David E. R. Sutherland MD PhD
Professor of Surgery, University of Minnesota, Minneapolis, Minnesota, USA

Geoffrey B. Thompson MD FACS
Assistant Professor of Surgery, Mayo Medical School;

Consultant, St Mary's Hospital and Rochester Methodist Hospital, Mayo Clinic, Rochester, Minnesota, USA

Lok T. Tio MD
Professor of Medicine, Georgetown University Hospital, Reservoir, Washington DC, USA

Michael Trede BA BChir MD HonFRCS(Eng and Irel) HonFRCPS(Glas)
Professor and Chairman, Chirurgische Klinik, Klinikum Mannheim, Universität Heidelberg, Mannheim, Germany

Waldemar Uhl MD
Department of General Surgery, University of Ulm, Ulm, Germany

K. van Ackern MD
Institut für Anästhesiologie und Operative Intensivmedizin, Klinikum Mannheim der Universität Heidelberg, Mannheim, Germany

Jon A. van Heerden MB ChB(Cape Town) FACS FRCS(C) FRCS(Edin)(Hon) FRCPS(Glas)(Hon) MS(Surg)(Minn)
Fred C. Andersen Professor of Surgery, Mayo Clinic and Mayo Foundation, Rochester, Minnesota, USA

Jonathan W. Wardell MD
Assistant Clinical Professor of Surgery, Department of Surgery, University of California, Davis Medical Center, Sacramento, California, USA

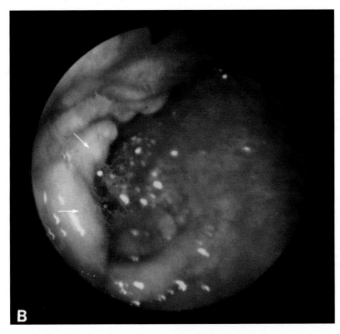

Fig. 11.7B See page 117 for caption.

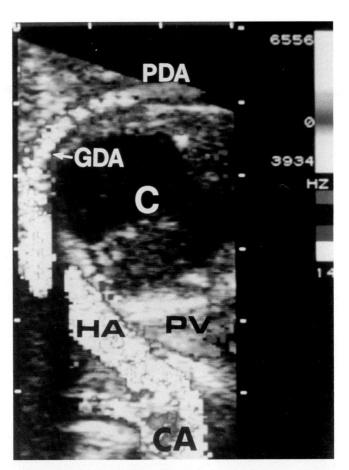

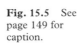

Fig. 15.5 See page 149 for caption.

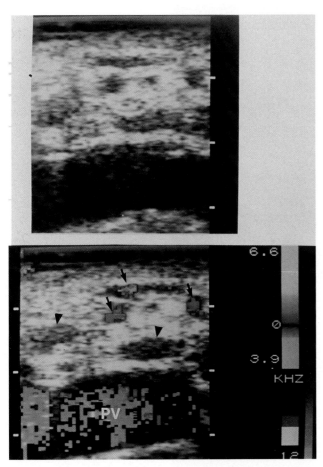

Fig. 15.6 See page 149 for caption.

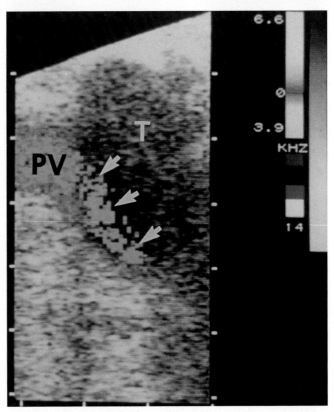

Fig. 15.7 See page 150 for caption.

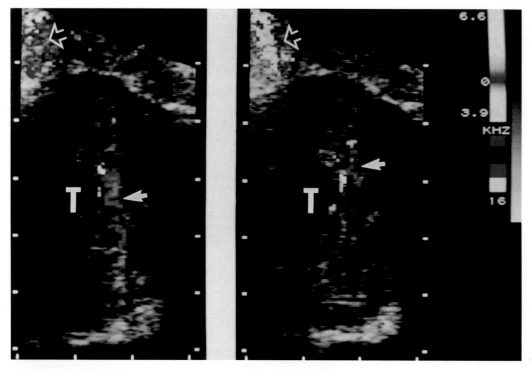

Fig. 15.8 See page 150 for caption.

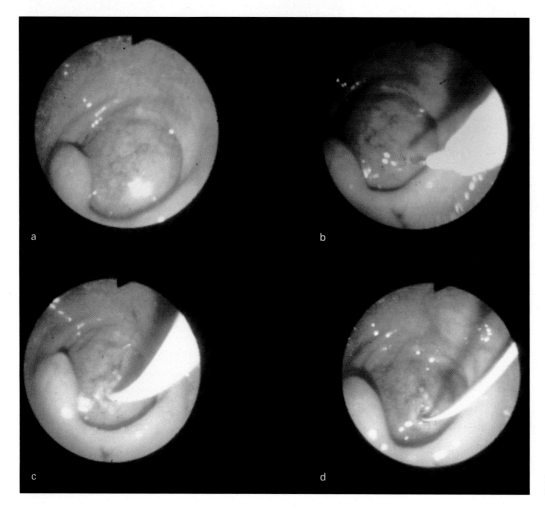

Fig. 27.5A, B, C, D
See page 304 for caption.

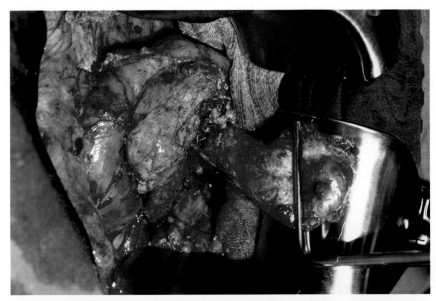

Fig. 31.4 See page 344 for caption.

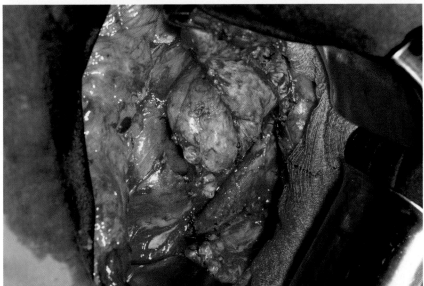

Fig. 31.5 See page 344 for caption.

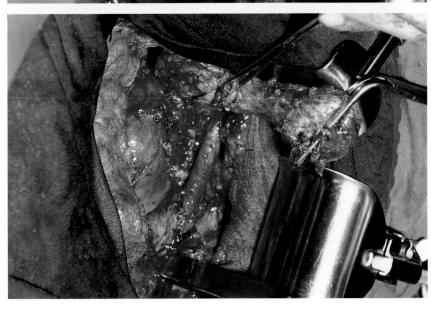

Fig. 31.6 See page 344 for caption.

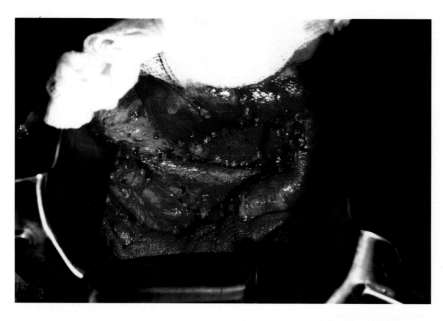

Fig. 31.7 See page 345.

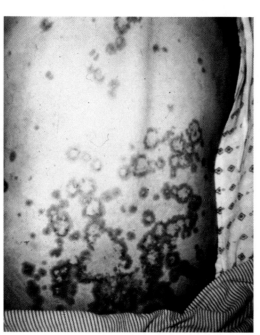

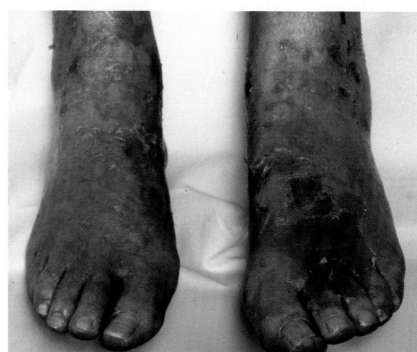

Fig. 49.10 See page 556 for caption.

Introduction: History of pancreatic surgery
Anatomy and physiology

1. History of pancreatic surgery

R. C. Praderi

This chapter is dedicated to Dr Robert Zollinger (Fig. 1.1) who passed away in 1992. Ironically, this doctor who devoted his entire life to the study of pancreatic pathology, himself suffered from a pancreatic tumour.

Pancreatic surgery is surgery of the twentieth century. The pancreas is a deep-seated organ which is difficult to manipulate: little was known of its physiology prior to 1900 and, given its 'dangerous irritability', surgeons feared to approach it. Pancreatic surgery, like biliary surgery, had to wait for the advent of anaesthesia, antisepsis and im-

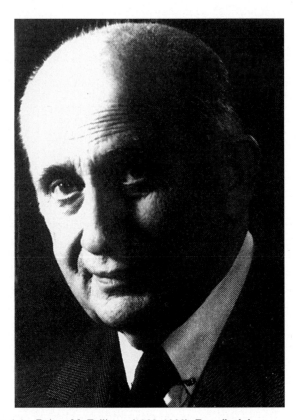

Fig. 1.1 Robert M. Zollinger (1903–1992). Described the Zollinger–Ellison syndrome and founder member of the American Board of Surgery.

proved haemostasis before it could develop. A key event ushering in the era of pancreatic surgery was the isolation of the 'vitaminic factor' in coagulation by Dam, a factor which Quick had studied before him (Quick 1935, Dam 1939). The isolation of vitamin K and determination of its formula (Dam 1940) led to its use as medication to prevent bleeding due to hypoprothrombinaemia in jaundiced patients, thus opening the door to major hepatobiliary and pancreatic operations.

The history of pancreatic surgery is often dealt with cursorily as an opening chapter in books such as this. In such chapters, reference is frequently confined to mention of key anatomical discoveries during the Renaissance; to the physiological research initiated by Claude Bernard in the nineteenth century; to key developments in endocrinology in this century, and to the recent expansion in clinical and pathopysiological knowledge relating to the pancreas. In order to concentrate on matters relating to pancreatic surgery without ignoring these discoveries, Tables 1.1 and 1.2 have been prepared so that the reader can establish the historical context in which the various surgical techniques were developed and applied.

A number of descriptions of the history of pancreatic surgery have particular importance. Towards the middle of the last century two books on diseases of the pancreas pancreas were published, one by Classen (1842) in Germany and the other by Ancelet (1866) in France, each describing the clinical experience with pancreatic cancer in Europe at that time. Meanwhile in 1858 in the United States, Da Costa from Philadelphia reviewed 35 cases of carcinoma which had been reported previously by various authors. Nicolas Senn, a native of Switzerland who settled in Milwaukee and acceded to the Chair of Surgery in Chicago, presented a seminal paper to the American Surgical Association at its sixth meeting in 1886. In this extensive paper, Senn analysed his experimental work on the pancreas and reviewed the available international literature.

Two articles appearing around the turn of the century in France reviewed all pancreatic operations which had

Table 1.1 Landmarks in the discovery and understanding of pancreatic anatomy and physiology in the years up to 1926

Year	Name	Place	Nature of discovery/advance
c. 300 BC	Herophilus	Chalcedon	Discovery of the pancreas
c. 100 AD	Aretaeus (81–138 AD)	Cappadocia	Use of the term 'diabetes'
c. 100 AD	Rufus (98–117 AD)	Ephesus	Use of the term 'pan-kreas' ('all flesh')
1541	Andreas Vesalius (1515–1564) (Professor, of Padua)	Brussels	First illustration of pancreas
1641	Johann Veslingus (1598–1649) (Professor, of Padua)	Augsburg	New description of pancreas
1642	Johann Wirsung (1600–1643) (Prosector, of Padua)	Miden	Discovered the pancreatic duct
1654	Francis Glisson (1597–1677)	Cambridge	Defined a sphincteric mechanism in the common duct
1664	Reinier De Graaf (1641–1673)	Leyden	Description of pancreatic juice, pancreatic fistula and lithiasis
1674	Thomas Willis (1621–1675)	Oxford	Discovery of sweet urine in diabetics. Named 'diabetes mellitus'
1682	Johann C Brunner (1653–1727)	Switzerland	Described polydipsia in pancreatectomized dogs
1720	Abraham Vater (1684–1751) (Professor of Anatomy)	Wittenberg	Described the duodenal papilla
1732	Jakob Winslow (1669–1760) (Professor of Anatomy, Paris)	Odense	Described foramen of Winslow
1742	Giovanni P Santorini (1681–1737)	Venice	Described the accessory pancreatic duct
1791/96	Samuel T Soemmering (1755–1830)		Named the pancreas 'Bauchspeicheldrüse' (abdominal salivary gland)
1849	Claude Bernard (1813–1874) (Professor of Physiology)	Paris	Defined exocrine function of pancreas
1853	Wenzel Treitz (1819–1872)		Description of retropancreatic fascia and Treitz' band
1862	A Eckert (1841–1850)		Described and named 'annular pancreas'
1869	Paul Langerhans (1847–1888)	Berlin	Description of pancreatic islets
1872	Alexander Danilevsky		Discovery of trypsin
1874	Willie Kühne (1837–1900) (Professor, of Amsterdam)	Heidelberg	Isolation of trypsin
1887	Ruggiero Oddi (1864–1913)	Perugia	Description of choledochus sphincter
1889	Carl Toldt (1840–1920) (Professor of Anatomy)	Vienna	Description of Toldt fascia
1889	Oskar Minkowski (1849–1908) Joseph Von Mering (1851–1931)	Strasbourg	Described diabetes in pancreatectomized dogs
1893	M E Laguesse	Paris	Discovered that the islets of Langerhans produced hormone
1900	Eugene L Opie (1873–1971)	Baltimore	Described relationship between interstitial pancreatitis and diabetes mellitus
1902	Leonid W Ssobelow (1876–1919)		Discovered that ligation of pancreatic duct produces atrophy of acinar tissue while islets of Langerhans remain intact
1902	Sir William M Bayliss (1860–1924) Ernest H Starling (1866–1927)	London	Discovery of the first pancreatic hormone (secretin)
1903	Theodore Kocher (1841–1915)	Berne	Described Kocher's manoeuvre, (described earlier by Jourdan 1895, Vautrin 1896, Wiart 1899)
1908	Ludwig G Svelzer (1870–1949)		Isolated pancreatic extract capable of provoking hypoglycaemia
1914	Pierre Fredet	Paris	The most complete anatomical description of pancreatic fascias
1920	Moses Barron (1883–1961)		Confirmed the experience of Ssobelow
1922	Sir Frederick C Banting (1891–1941) (Charles H Best (1899–)	Toronto	Isolated isletin, later named insulin
1926	John Jacob Abel (1857–1938)		Crystallization of insulin

been carried out in Europe (Nimier 1893, Villar 1905). In most cases the pancreatic surgery had been incidental and secondary to wounds inflicted in wars such as the Franco-Prussian war of 1870–1871, amounting in most instances to drainage of haematomas or abscesses. In Germany in the closing years of the same century, Körte (1898) also wrote a book on surgical diseases of the pancreas.

During the Thirteenth International Congress of Medicine held in Paris in 1900, the growing European experience of pancreatic surgery was the subject of reports by Mayo Robson from Leeds, Andrea Ceccherelli from Parma and Jules Boeckel from Strasbourg. In 1908, Sauvé reviewed practically all of the surgical experience on the subject, an article which is frequently referred to in the literature on pancreatic surgery. Another key review of the related area of biliary surgery became available in 1923 when Henry Hartmann, a surgeon from Strasbourg (a town which passed from Germany to France after World War I) wrote a remarkable book demonstrating his acquaintance with the available German, French and English bibliography. This book contains a detailed account of patients in whom resection of papillary cancers had been undertaken.

In the first edition of Howard & Jordan's book on pancreatic surgery published in 1969, Allen O. Whipple, the first surgeon to perform a pancreatic resection with survival in North America, contributed a chapter on the history of such surgery. With exemplary honesty, Whipple refers to the operations performed by the Europeans

Table 1.2 Landmarks in pancreatic pathology 1865–1977

Year	Name	Nature of discovery/advance
1865	Carl Rokitanksy	Description of necrotic haemorrhagic pancreatitis
1883	Hans Chiari	Enzymatic pathogenesis of pancreatitis
1886	Nicolas Senn	'The Surgery of the Pancreas'
1888	M Prince	Gallstone-associated pancreatitis
1888	L Bard, A Pic	Gallbladder dilated in periampullary cancer
1889	R H Fitz	Different forms of pancreatitis
1890	Ludwig Courvoisier	Courvoisier's law in relation to malignant obstructive jaundice
1896	Bernard Riedel	Classic description of chronic pancreatitis
1898	Werner Körte	'Surgical Diseases and Wounds of the Pancreas'
1900	A Mayo Robson, A Ceccherelli, J Boeckel	'Surgery of the Pancreas'
1901	Eugene L Opie	Described the common channel theory
1902	A G Nicholls	Described the first adenoma of islet tissue
1908	M A Lane	Differentiated alpha and beta cells
1922	Frederick G Banting, Charles H Best	Isolated and named insulin
1926	Shields Warren	Collected 20 cases of islet cell adenomas
1927	R M Wilder, F N Allan, M H Power	Hyperinsulinism described in carcinoma of pancreatic islets
1927	R Elman, J McCaughan	Serum amylase test
1938	A. O Whipple	Whipple's triad in insulinoma
1944	Sidney Farber	Relation of pancreatic achylia to meconium ileus in mucoviscidosis
1954	F Wermer	Multiple adenomatosis of endocrine glands
1955	R M Zollinger, E H Ellison	Gastrinoma
1958	J V Verner, A B Morrison	Islet cell tumour with diarrhoea and hypokalaemia
1964	R A Gregory, H J Tracy	Isolated gastrin from Zollinger–Ellison tumours
1966	M G McGavran, R H Unger, L Recant	Described glucagon-secreting pancreatic tumour
1974	A G E Pearse, J M Polak	Development of apudoma/apud concept
1977	O P Ganda, G C Weir, J S Soeldner	Somatostatinoma defined by radioimmunoassay
1977	L Larsson, J Holst, J. Kuhl	Somatostatinoma defined by immunocytochemistry
1977	S R Bloom, A M West, J M Polak	Islet cell tumours shown to secrete multiple hormones

Kausch (1909, 1912) and Tenani (1922) who had preceded him in this type of surgery. In the latest edition of this same book, Rhoads & Folin (1987) have updated the history of pancreatic surgery in the light of modern developments.

The first chapter of Patrick J. Fitzgerald's book, 'The Pancreas' (1980) also merits reading, dealing as its title suggests with 'Medical Anecdotes Concerning some Diseases of the Pancreas'. There we learn that St. Pancreas, the patron saint of those suffering from diabetes mellitus lies buried in a small chapel under the site now occupied by St. Pancras' railway station in London.

THE BEGINNINGS OF PANCREATIC SURGERY

Direct pancreatic surgery started in 1879 when Thiersch drained, in two stages, a fluctuating tumour of the abdomen, evacuating 3 litres of chocolate-coloured liquid. The resulting pancreatic fistula closed spontaneously (Thiersch 1881). In 1882, Bozeman resected a 20 lb cyst which he had initially diagnosed as ovarian, while in 1883 Capparelli drained a pancreatic cyst with subsequent formation of an external fistula. This last patient, a baroness, passed over 100 stones over a period extending for 6 years. In the same year, Gussenbauer (1883), a pupil of Billroth, first marsupialized a pancreatic pseudocyst with survival. There soon followed other descriptions including those of Senn (1886), Springfield & Wolfer in 1886, Tremaine in 1886 and Parkes & Lindner in 1889, all of whom performed this same operation with survival.

Their case histories were cited by Nimier in his review published in 1893.

Another key development took place in 1909 when Coffey anastomosed the tail of the pancreas to an omega loop of small bowel. In 1911, Ombredanne anastomosed a pancreatic cyst to the duodenum, while 10 years later Jedlicka successfully anastomosed a pancreatic cyst to the back of the stomach (Jedlicka 1923). Anastomosis of such cysts to the gallbladder was attempted in 1926 by Walzel (Walzel 1934) and in 1932 by Neuffer in the hope that the cyst content would be absorbed by the biliary tree or drain through it into the intestine. Despite technical feasibility and patient survival, the procedure was not thought to be successful and was abandoned. However more success attended the first performance of cysto-jejunostomy (Chesterman 1943) and shortly thereafter, König (1946) performed the same operation, this time using a Roux loop of jejunum.

Surgery for pancreatic neoplasia also began towards the end of the last century. Although a few pedunculated tumours of the pancreas had been operated upon earlier, Trendelenburg in 1882 (cited by Ceccherelli 1900) undertook one of the first major resections, removing a tumour classified as a sarcoma in an operation which included resection of the tail of the pancreas and the spleen. Unfortunately, the patient did not survive the procedure. In 1889, Ruggi resected a solid tumour weighing over half a kilogram and located in the tail of the pancreas, the lesion being classified as an adenosarcoma (Ruggi 1890), while Briggs (1890) in St Louis, resected another such tumour with success. In Italy, in 1884, Biondi removed a tumour arising from the lower two-thirds of the head of the pancreas; a biliary and pancreatic fistula developed but healed in 25 days, and a year-and-a-half later the patient was still well (Biondi 1897). Other early resections of tumours of the tail of pancreas include those undertaken by Malthe in 1894 (cited by Ceccherelli 1900) and by Tricomi in 1897 (Tricomi 1898). In this last case, the tumour was adherent to the body of the stomach, an experience also reported a few years later by Franke (1901).

BILIARY–DIGESTIVE ANASTOMOSIS AND PANCREATIC TUMOURS

As was soon well-recognized, obstructive jaundice due to pancreatic cancer gives rise to intolerable itch and bleeding, often in association with severe intractable pain. Absence of bile from the intestine and, as is now appreciated, consequent failure to absorb vitamin K, had such central importance that operations were developed to restore the flow of bile to the intestine and so reduce the coagulopathy. From the outset, surgeons were aware of the problem posed by biliary peritonitis following this type of surgery, and both Bernhard Riedel of Jena in 1880 and Herman Kümmell of Breslau in 1884 successfully removed calculi from the common bile duct only to have their patients succumb following bile leakage from the suture line into the peritoneal cavity (Riedel 1892, Kümmell 1890).

Alexander von Winiwarter (Fig. 1.2) one of Billroth's disciples who later became Professor of Surgery in Liège, operated in 1882 on a female patient suffering from obstructive jaundice due to a cancer of the head of the pancreas. In order to connect the gallbladder with the intestine, he performed a cholecystostomy along with a colostomy, thinking that the fistulas would communicate spontaneously. This did not occur as the colostomy closed prematurely, and the patient required five further operations until eventually a cholecystojejunostomy was performed and proved to be effective. The procedure had originally been planned as a two-stage procedure but turned out to be so complicated that it was never repeated.

Early attempts to anastomose the gallbladder of experimental animals to the intestine had not been uniformly successful, although in 1887 Ruggiero Oddi successfully anastomosed the gallbladder to the stomach in three dogs following ligation of the common bile duct. The animals had no digestive problems and all gained weight. During the following year these experiments were translated from the physiology laboratory to surgical practice and in 1888 Bard & Pic published their landmark paper on the clinical pathology of pancreatic tumours. At the same time, Kappeler (1889) in Musterlingen and Socin in Basel performed lateral anastomosis of the gallbladder to the

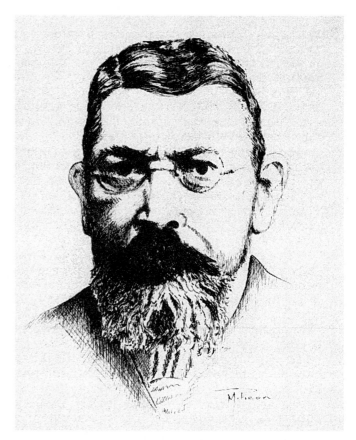

Fig. 1.2 Alexander von Winiwater (1848–1917). Disciple of Billroth, later Professor of Surgery in Liège, Belgium. Performed the first biliodigestive anastomosis.

jejunum; both patients survived. Also in 1888, Monastyrski in Russia anastomosed the gallbladder to the duodenum in a patient suffering from pancreatic cancer, an operation repeated successfully by Bardenheuer in the same year. Incidentally, it was also in 1888 that Mayo Robson in Leeds, faced with a patient who had developed a complete biliary fistula following cholecystostomy, performed a cholecystoduodenostomy with good results (Mayo Robson & Dobson 1904). In the following year, the French surgeon Terrier described a patient with pancreatic cancer and gallbladder enlargement who was treated by the same procedure. His article predated by one year the book in which Ludwig Courvoisier (Fig. 1.3) described his autopsy experience of numerous patients who had died with jaundice (Courvoisier 1890). This explains why in the French literature the law set down by the Swiss surgeon Courvoisier is known as the law of Courvoisier–Terrier.

In 1892 Murphy in Chicago had successfully performed three cholecystoduodenostomies using his metallic button to facilitate anastomosis. Meanwhile, in Vienna another of Billroth's students, Robert Gersuny (1882) performed a cholecystogastrostomy because the duodenum and jejunum were blocked by pancreatic tumour. The patient did well in that her jaundice quickly disappeared. This

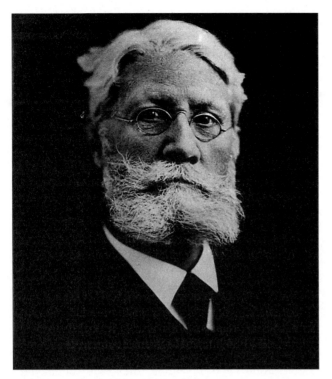

Fig. 1.3 Ludwig Courvoisier (1846–1901). Surgeon in Basel. Performed the first choledochotomy and described Courvoisier's law.

operation was repeated successfully by Terrier in Paris (1894) and Jaboulay in Lyons (1898) in several patients, and thus established a place in the surgical repertoire which it held throughout the first four decades of the present century, largely because of its simplicity. In general, a gastroenterostomy was performed at the same time to diminish gastric distension, to prevent food from refluxing into the biliary tract, and to allow food to bypass the obstructed duodenum. Later on Whipple also employed this technique in patients undergoing pancreatic resection.

The manoeuvre of duodenal mobilization employed by Kocher (1903) of Berne in the course of gastrectomy was later applied to biliary surgery to facilitate exploration of the duodenal papilla. Shortly thereafter another manoeuvre described by Kocher's disciple, César Roux (1897) of Lausanne, was also used in biliary surgery, although it had originally been developed for use following subtotal gastrectomy. Monprofit, in 1904, first employed a 'Roux-en-Y' procedure in biliary surgery, using the Roux loop for cholecystojejunostomy. Later in a contribution to the French Congress of Surgery in 1908, he proposed that the technique should be used for hepaticojejunostomy. Dahl was the first to use a Roux loop successfully in biliary surgery in 1909, although Maragliano had earlier, in 1903, performed a cholecystojejunostomy using a Braun loop. Cholangitis had been an ever-present hazard following biliary–enteric anastomosis and so the new technique safeguarded patients from infection caused by reflux of gut contents, particularly when the anastomosis was of small calibre. The Roux-en-Y technique has proved to be one of the most significant contributions to biliary and pancreatic surgery, and in this respect matches the Braun loop and its modifications as used by surgeons such as Warren, Hivet and the present author (Praderi et al 1973). In my view it is regrettable that there are some surgeons who still employ the duodenum for biliary–digestive bypass in the palliation of pancreatic cancer.

THE FIRST OPERATIONS ON THE PAPILLA

Before the turn of the century some surgeons such as Pozzi and Czerny who had accidentally opened the duodenum, were able to extract papillary calculi through the duodenotomy, while others such as Charles MacBurney (1878) had successfully performed elective duodenotomy and papillotomy to deal with embedded calculi. In 1895, Theodore Kocher published his description of the use of choledochoduodenostomy following the removal of supra-ampullary and choledochal calculi. By 1899 he had already performed 20 duodenotomies for this purpose and surgeons soon began to appreciate the possibility of operating on periampullary tumours.

William Halsted of Johns Hopkins Hospital was well acquainted with the progress of European surgery. In 1898 he operated on a 60-year-old woman suffering from obstructive jaundice, diarrhoea, coagulopathy and an enlarged gallbladder. He resected a portion of the duodenum, tumour included, reimplanted the common duct into the duodenum, and also removed the gallbladder. Later that year he reoperated, removing the gallbladder and implanting the cystic duct into the duodenum. The patient survived for 7 months before dying with carcinomatosis.

Another North American surgeon, William Mayo (Fig. 1.4), operated in 1900 upon a 49-year-old man afflicted with papillary cancer who had previously undergone a cholecystostomy. He opened the duodenum, removed the tumour, reimplanted the common bile duct, and closed the duodenotomy. When jaundice recurred one-and-a-half years later, he performed a cholecystoduodenostomy, the patient's third operation. Removal of the papilla (or ampullectomy as it was sometimes called) proved to be a swift and elegant procedure which was not too difficult technically, and which soon became the procedure of choice in an era where hypocoagulability made major surgery a formidable undertaking in such jaundiced patients.

In Uruguay in 1908, Alfredo Navarro performed a papillectomy on a patient who survived for 30 years, while Kausch (1912) and Hartmann (1923) also give accounts of transduodenal resection of periampullary tumours at the beginning of the century, many of which operations

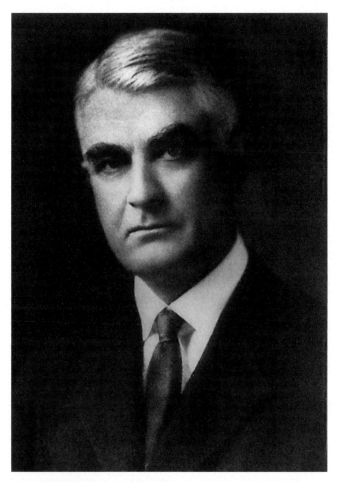

Fig. 1.4 William James Mayo (1861–1939). Founder of the Mayo Clinic in Rochester, USA. Resected a periampullary tumour with survival of the patient in 1900.

were successful. Cordua (1906) and Hirschel (1914) described the use of gastroenterostomy as a precautionary measure when undertaking transduodenal papillary resection. There is no doubt that transduodenal excision of the papilla is still a useful operation today in selected patients, given that fibre optic duodenoscopy allows periodic surveillance for follow-up purposes.

PANCREATICODUODENECTOMY

The first successful removal of a periampullary carcinoma with a sleeve of duodenum was undertaken by William Halsted in 1898. It was however his only successful case and Mayo Robson (1900) and Körte (1905) repeated the operation with poor results. In 1898 the Italian surgeon Alessandro Codivilla (Fig. 1.5) surged ahead of his contemporaries by performing the first pancreaticoduodenectomy for a lesion in the head of the pancreas. Codivilla operated on a jaundiced patient with pancreatic cancer in Imola, a town near Bologna, and resected the duodenum, head of pancreas and pylorus, closed the duodenal stump, cut and ligated the common bile

duct above the pancreas, and performed a cholecystojejunostomy (with Murphy's button) and a gastroenterostomy-en-Y. The patient survived for only 24 days but had he lived for 30 days he would have passed the arbitrary period which we surgeons have set for 'operative mortality'.

Once it had been demonstrated that resection of the head of the pancreas should be accompanied by resection of the duodenum (at least of its first and second portion), other surgeons began to follow Codivilla's example. In 1907 Desjardins explored the feasibility of carrying out the operation in two stages by demonstrations in a cadaver, while Sauvé (1908) carried out the operation in one stage. However, it was to be Kausch (1909, 1912) who first performed a successful pancreaticoduodenectomy. Kausch (Fig. 1.6) was a brilliant disciple of Mikulicz and worked in the Augusta Viktoria Hospital in Berlin between 1906 and 1928. It was there on June 15,1909, that he operated upon a jaundiced 49-year-old man with a periampullary tumour, first performing a cholecystojejunostomy using a Braun loop. Six weeks later he reoperated, performing a posterior side-to-side gastroenterostomy and resecting the head of pancreas, pylorus and first and second parts of the duodenum,

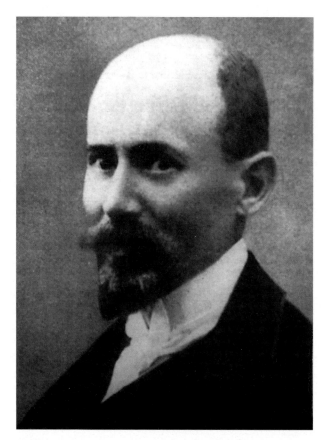

Fig. 1.5 Alessandro Codivilla (1861–1912). Professor of Surgery in Bologna. Performed the first pancreaticoduodenectomy in 1898.

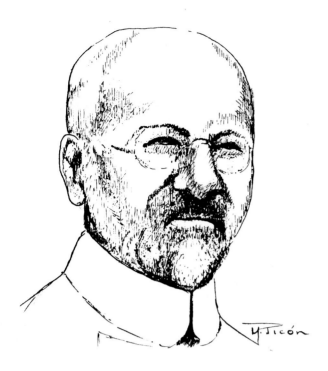

Fig. 1.6 Walter Kausch (1967–1928). Performed the first successful pancreaticoduodenectomy in 1909 in Berlin.

operation in one stage, but by 1941, 41 such cases had been reported with an operative mortality of 27% and thereafter the technique was gradually perfected. As one of the first refinements, the cholecystogastric anastomosis was abandoned in favour of cholecystojejunostomy (Brunschwig 1937). Then the common bile duct rather than the gallbladder was sutured to the jejunum, and the pancreas was connected to the jejunum rather than the duodenum (Hunt 1941). Finally, a more extensive gastric resection was undertaken so that the operation began to resemble its modern counterpart with an attendant lowering of operative mortality. It is clear that although surgeons in English-speaking countries call pancreatico-duodenectomy the 'Whipple operation', the procedure has a history dating back for many years before the description by Whipple and his colleagues in 1935.

No less than 68 combinations of the various possible anastomoses between bile duct, pancreas, stomach and jejunum have been described (Leger & Bréhant 1956). The majority of these variations have historical value only but some are still employed. For example, surgeons such as Goldsmith (1971) and Estefan and colleagues (1980) do not perform an anastomosis between the pancreatic remnant and the intestine. Many variations designed to

anastomosing the third part of the duodenum to the pancreatic remnant. The operation lasted for 4 hours and the patient lived for 9 months before dying in May 1910. In 1912 Kausch wrote an article entitled 'Cancer of the duodenal papilla and its treatment' in which he reviewed all of the published cases, including those papillectomies already mentioned.

Two years later, Hirschel (1914) performed a one-stage pancreaticoduodenectomy, bridging the gap between bile duct and duodenum with a rubber tube. His patient's jaundice was relieved, with survival for one year. Kausch's operation was repeated with success in 1922 by Tenani who also performed it in two stages but with one important difference in that choledochojejunostomy and gastroenterostomy were performed during the first operation. A month later the duodenum and head of pancreas were resected and the pancreatic remnant was implanted into the distal duodenum as described by Kausch. As already indicated, these must have been formidable undertakings in deeply jaundiced patients with profound coagulopathy in the days before vitamin K (Dam 1939) and blood banks became available.

In North America, Whipple (Fig. 1.7), Parsons and Mullins (1935) had also published a description of two cases of pancreaticoduodenectomy carried out for cancer of the periampullary region, and performed in two stages in the Columbia Presbyterian Hospital in New York. It was not until 1940 that it became possible to perform this

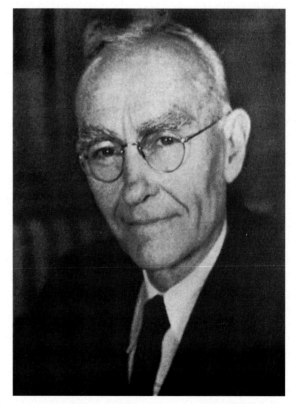

Fig. 1.7 Allen Oldfather Whipple (1885–1963). The father of modern pancreatic surgery. Professor of Surgery at Columbia University, New York.

prevent breakdown of the pancreaticojejunal anastomosis have also been described. For example, Machado (1976) in Brazil described the use of a 'double Roux-en-Y', one loop being anastomosed to the pancreas and the other to the common bile duct. Another Brazilian surgeon, Pereyra Lima (1978) proposed an ingenious technique in which a ligature is placed on an omega loop so that it separates the biliary and pancreatic anastomoses for some 2 months before falling off spontaneously to restore continuity.

When dealing with selected periampullary and duodenal tumours as well as certain benign lesions, some surgeons prefer to divide the third part of the duodenum behind the root of the mesentery (Praderi & Estefan 1990). As this technique leaves no jejunal stump for anastomosis to the pancreas, the pancreatic remnant is implanted into the stomach as described by Dill & Russell (1952) and Ingesbigtsen & Langfeldt(1952).

There has also been renewed interest in preservation of the pylorus when operating on papillary tumours and chronic pancreatitis (Flautner et al 1985). The procedure of pylorus-preserving pancreaticoduodenectomy was popularised by Traverso & Longmire (1978) and entails division of the duodenum some 2 cm distal to the pylorus, preserving the blood supply of the proximal duodenum through the pyloric and right gastroepiploic arteries. The proximal duodenal stump is anastomosed in end-to-side manner to the jejunal loop used for implantation of the hepatic duct. This innovation has met with considerable success during the past decade. Other surgeons have introduced other modifications in which the first and third portions of the duodenum are anastomosed in end-to-end fashion following resection of the head of the pancreas (Jordan 1987).

OTHER FORMS OF PANCREATIC RESECTION FOR NEOPLASIAS

At the time of its introduction, pancreaticoduodenectomy was regarded as an operation to deal with periampullary cancer and cancer of the head of the pancreas. Resection was later extended to deal with cancers of the common bile duct and duodenum, and in time to the management of various endocrine tumours of the pancreas. The first operation to deal with an islet cell tumour of the pancreas was described by Whipple in 1960 as follows;

In 1927 came the first dramatic report of a case of hyperinsulinism with a tumor of islet cells. Wilder and his associates reported a case of islet cell carcinoma in a physician who had suffered with attacks of unconsciousness and a blood sugar of 25 mg per cent during the attack. Dr Will Mayo explored the patient finding a tumor of the pancreas with metastases to the liver, the lymph nodes and the mesentery. An extract from one of the metastases acted like insulin when injected into a rabbit.

The first operation for a functioning adenoma was performed by Roscoe Graham (1929) in Toronto. The patient had been diagnosed by W.L. Robinson and was cured in that there was no recurrence. The first successful total pancreatectomy was performed by J. T. Priestley in a patient who had hyperinsulinism but no palpable adenoma of the pancreas (Priestley et al 1944). The tumour was eventually found by the pathologist and measured 1.5 cm in diameter; the patient was cured by the operation. In fact the first total pancreatectomy had been performed a year earlier by Rockey (1943) but the patient died of biliary peritonitis on the 15th postoperative day.

The first successful total pancreatectomy for pancreatic cancer was carried out in 1944 by Fallis & Szilagyi (1948) and, in 1954, Ross advocated total pancreatectomy for cancer of the head of the pancreas in order to eliminate residual or multicentric cancer. It was hoped that total extirpation would reduce operative morbidity and mortality by avoiding a pancreaticojejunal anastomosis with its attendant risk of leakage. ReMine (1970) and Brooks (1976) were amongst those who adopted this technique but its promise has remained largely unfulfilled.

Cancers of the body and tail of the pancreas were particularly difficult to diagnose before imaging methods such as CT scanning became available, and most patients coming to surgery did so with advanced and unresectable disease. Successful cure of such lesions is still rare, and Jordan, writing in 1987, considered that only three such cases had been described in the world literature, one of them by Gordon Taylor (1934) who reported a patient who had survived for 7 years. Distal pancreatic resections are much more frequently indicated in the treatment of chronic pancreatitis than in the treatment of cancer.

In view of the poor results obtained in the surgical treatment of pancreatic cancer, Fortner in 1973 proposed the operation of regional pancreatectomy, an operation which he described further in 1984. The operation includes total pancreatectomy, resection of the pancreatic segment of the portal vein, subtotal gastrectomy and regional lymph node dissection (type I regional pancreatectomy) and may be extended further to include resection of the hepatic and superior mesenteric arteries if these vessels appear to be invaded by tumour (type II regional pancreatectomy). Resected portions of these major arteries are replaced by grafts. The operation is technically most demanding and it is convenient to alternate with a team of vascular surgeons during its performance. It should only be undertaken by highly trained surgeons and its role remains controversial (Praderi 1986).

SURGERY OF ACUTE PANCREATITIS

As indicated above, the earlier operations on the pancreas were undertaken to drain abscesses, haematomas or cysts, lesions which in the majority of cases were the complications of acute pancreatitis. During the period 1880 to 1938, the surgery of acute pancreatitis was of an aggressive nature. In the words of Ockinczyc (1933), 'Go right to the target, expose, drain .... and Hope!'

During the German Congress held in 1938, Nordman supported the opinion being expressed at about that time by several European and North American surgeons (Walzel 1934, Mikkelsen 1934, Demel 1936, Trasoff & Scarf 1937, Pratt 1939, Fallis 1939), namely that the approach to acute pancreatitis should once again be conservative given that the mortality rate of emergency surgery was 50–78%. Even though his proposal was generally accepted, some patients with acute pancreatitis still came to surgery as a result of diagnostic error or uncertainty, or in the course of treatment of acute gallstone pancreatitis, or because of the need to deal with complications such as abscesses and pseudocysts (Cattell & Warren 1953).

Although Theron Claggett from the Mayo Clinic had performed total pancreatectomy for chronic pancreatitis in 1944 (Claggett 1946, 1947), the first successful total pancreatectomy for acute fulminant pancreatitis was undertaken by Watts in England in 1963. There can be no doubt that the pioneering contributions of individuals such as Francis Moore (1959), Thomas Shires (Shires et al 1964) and Shoemaker (Shoemaker & Walker 1970) led to better metabolic management of ill patients with acute pancreatitis and as a result, fewer patients died from shock. The advent of intensive care units also made a major contribution, so that patients began to survive their initial attack only to fall prey to complications such as necrosis, sequestra formation and abscess.

Groups of surgeons including Hollender et al (1972), Boutelier & Edelmann (1972), Fagniez et al (1974), Kümmerle et al (1975), Schönborn et al (1975) and Alexandre et al (1977) next proposed surgical resection to remove necrosed parts of the pancreas at an earlier stage. It became possible to save some patients who might otherwise have died, although it soon became clear that viable pancreas was often removed in the course of resection and that the death rate remained unacceptably high in the postoperative period. During the decade that followed, rules for the evaluation of the severity of the attack were established (Ranson et al, 1976) and the surgical treatment of sequestra, abscesses and peritonitis was systematized. Surgical opinion began to move away from formal pancreatic resection in favour of blunt necrosectomy in the treatment of necrotizing pancreatitis, a subject that will be dealt with elsewhere (Ch. 22).

All that remains to be mentioned is the improvement in our understanding of the pathogenesis of acute gallstone pancreatitis and its treatment (Carter 1989). Much of this development has followed the studies of Acosta and Ledesma (1974) from Rosario, Argentina which drew attention to the importance of transient impaction of gallstones at the ampulla of Vater. As an alternative to early surgery to eradicate gallstones, a new procedure has been added to the therapeutic armamentarium, namely early endoscopic papillotomy to extract calculi impacted at the papilla (Safrany et al 1980).

SURGERY OF CHRONIC PANCREATITIS

The first procedure aimed at the treatment of this disease consisted of an anastomosis between the tail of the pancreas and an omega loop of jejunum (Coffey 1909). In 1953, Link established external drainage of the Wirsung duct in a young female who lived for 30 years expelling calculi periodically. Eventually, autopsy revealed a left subphrenic abscess and atrophy of the pancreas so that only a small portion of the gland remained. Roget (1958) collected 50 cases treated in this way but only 13 were 'cured' by drainage. Slightly earlier, pancreatography had been introduced with drainage of the duct of Wirsung by sphincterotomy (Doubilet & Mulholland 1948), the sphincterotomy being performed transcholedochally although a transduodenal approach was subsequently adopted.

In view of the success of cystojejunostomy in the treatment of pancreatic pseudocysts (König 1946, Griesmann 1948), Richard Cattell (1947) used a side-to-side anastomosis between a vertical loop of jejunum and the pancreatic duct in patients suffering from carcinoma of the head of the pancreas with distended pancreatic ducts. Subsequently, Longmire in 1951 (Longmire et al 1956) performed an end-to-end pancreaticojejunostomy making use of a Roux loop, but this was not successful when applied to the treatment of chronic pancreatitis. Merlin Du Val (1957) also described resection of the tip of the tail of the pancreas after duct exploration and pancreatography, but again, attempts to drain the pancreatic duct into a loop of jejunum was not successful.

The main driving force behind the use of pancreatic ductal drainage in chronic pancreatitis eventually proved to be Leger & Bréhant (1956) in France. Subsequently, Puestow & Gillesby (1958) demonstrated that chronic pancreatitis frequently gave rise to a 'chain of lakes' appearance of the main pancreatic duct with multiple strictures and areas of dilatation. Consequently, they unroofed the pancreatic duct, a method which allowed better decompression of the duct system after anastomosis to a jejunal loop. Mercadier (1964) developed a similar technique in France and there followed a further variation in which decompression of the pancreatic duct was achieved without the need for splenectomy. During the last decade, further technical variations have been proposed by Prinz & Greenlee (1981) and Frey & Smith (1987).

In 1952, Mallet Guy advocated resection of the left half of the pancreas for chronic pancreatitis. Still later, Mercadier (1964) and Fry & Child (1965) extended the left-sided resection so that only a small portion of the head was preserved alongside the duodenum. The more modern resection techniques for chronic pancreatitis such as those used by Warren et al (1984), Beger et al (1985) and Rossi et al (1987) will be described later in this book.

PANCREATIC TRANSPLANTATION

Homografting of pancreatic tissue in man was first attempted in Boston by Brooks and Gifford (1959). Minced fragments of pancreas from stillborn infants were implanted into the quadriceps muscles of their diabetic mothers but without success. Subsequent use of diffusion chambers by the same group allowed transient reduction in insulin requirements in two diabetic patients following transplantation of insulinoma tissue. Vascularized whole organ (pancreaticoduodenal) allotransplantation was first undertaken by Lillehei's group in Minnesota in 1966 (Kelly et al 1967) and at least 3200 vascularized pancreas

transplants have now been performed in some 115 institutions (London & Bell 1992). Although technical success and effective immunosuppression now means that the recipient may be rendered normoglycaemic, it is still debatable whether the procedure avoids the complications of diabetes such as retinopathy and nephropathy.

Transplantation of pancreatic islets has been attempted by a number of centres in the years following 1970, but until recently the results have been poor, largely because of problems with islet purification and viability. However, these difficulties are being overcome and longer periods of independence from insulin are now being reported. It is hoped that with improved immunomodulation, rejection will be preventable and that islet transplantation will prevent the long-term sequelae of diabetes mellitus (London & Bell 1992). Pancreatic surgery has come a long way from its humble beginnings and continues to evolve.

REFERENCES

Abel J J 1926 Crystalline insulin. Proceedings of the National Academy of Sciences 12: 132

Acosta J, Ledesma C 1974 Gallstone migration as a cause of acute pancreatitis. New England Journal of Medicine 270: 484

Acosta J M, Pellegrini C A, Skinner D B 1980 Etiology and pathogenesis of acute biliary pancreatitis. Surgery 88: 118

Alexandre J H, Camilleri J P, Assan R, Guerrieri M T, Bonan A 1977 Indications et résultats de la pancréatectomie totale dans le traitement des pancréatites aigues nécrosantes. Chirurgie 103: 858

Ancelet E 1866 Étude sur les maladies du pancréas. Savy, Paris

Aretaeus Cappadocianus 1856 The extant works of Aretaeus the Cappadocian. Sydenham Society, London

Badouin M 1908 M. le Pr. Nicolas Senn de Chicago. Revue de Chirurgie 37: 279

Bard L, Pic A 1888 Contribution a l'étude clinique et anatomopathologique du cancer primitif du pancréas. Revue de Médecine de Paris 8: 257–282

Bardenheurer R 1888 Anlegung einer Gallenblasen-Dünndarmfistel. Berliner Klinische Wochenschrift 25: 877

Barron M 1920 The relation of the islet of Langerhans to diabetes with special reference to cases of pancreatic lithiasis. Surgery. Gynecology and Obstetrics 31: 437

Bayliss W M, Starling E H 1902 The mechanism of pancreatic secretion. Journal of Physiology 28: 325

Beger H G, Krautzberger W, Bittner R et al 1985 Duodenum-preserving resection of the head of the pancreas in patients with severe chronic pancreatitis. Surgery 97: 467

Belloni L 1965 Ruggiero Oddi e la scoperta dello sfintere del coledoco. Simposi Clinici 2: 17

Bernard C 1856 Mémoire sur le pancreas et sur le rôle du suc pancréatique dans les phénomènes digestifs particulièrement dans la digestion des matières grasses neutres. Baillière, Paris

Biondi G 1897 Contributo clinico e sperimentale alla chirurgia del pancreas. Clinica Chirurgica 5: 132

Bloom S R, Polak J M, West A M 1978 Somatostatin content of pancreatic endocrine tumors. Metabolism 27: 1235

Boeckel J 1900 La chirurgie du pancréas. XIIIme Congrès International de Médecine, Paris 10: 207

Boutelier P, Edelmann G 1972 Tactique chirurgicale dans les

pancréatites aigues nécrosantes. Plaidoyer en faveur des sequestrectomies. Annales de Chirurgie 26: 249

Bozeman N 1882 Removal of cyst of the pancreas weighing $20\frac{1}{2}$ pounds. Medical Record 21: 46

Briggs E 1890 Tumor of the pancreas, laparotomy, recovery. St Louis Medical and Surgical Journal 58: 154

Brooks J R, Gifford G H 1959 Pancreatic homotransplantation. Transplantation Bulletin 6: 103

Brooks J R, Culebras J M 1976 Cancer of the pancreas: palliative operation, Whipple procedure or total pancreatectomy. American Journal of Surgery 131: 516

Brunner J C A 1683 Experimenta nova circa pancreas. Apud Wetstenium, Amstelaedami

Brunschwig A 1937 Resection of the head of the pancreas and duodenum for carcinoma. Pancreatoduodenectomy. Surgery, Gynecology and Obstetrics 65: 681–684

Capparelli 1883 In Giudice A Il Policlinico 1896: 42. *Cited by Villar 1905*

Carter D C 1989 Gallstone pancreatitis. In: Carter D, Warshaw A (eds) Pancreatitis. Churchill Livingstone, Edinburgh

Cattell R B 1947 Anastomosis of the duct of Wirsung; its use in palliative operations for cancer of the head of the pancreas. Surgical Clinics of North America 27: 636–643

Cattell R B, Warren W 1953 Surgery of the pancreas. W B Saunders, Philadelphia

Ceccherelli A 1900 La chirurgie du pancréas. XIIIme Congrès International de Médecine, Paris 10: 159

Chesterman J T 1943 Treatment of pancreatic cysts. British Journal of Surgery 30: 234

Clagett O T 1946 Total pancreatectomy: symposium presenting 4 successful cases and report on metabolic observations. Proceedings of the Mayo Clinc 21: 25

Clagett O T 1947 Surgery of the pancreas. Texas Journal of Medicine 43: 12

Claessen F 1842 Krankheiten der Bauchspeicheldrüse. Schauberg, Cologne

Codivilla A 1898 Rendiconto statistico della sezione chirurgica dell'ospedale di Imola

Coffey R C 1909 Pancreato-enterostomy and pancreatectomy; a preliminary report. Annals of Surgery 50: 1238

Cordua 1906 Carcinom der Papilla duodenalis. Münchener Medizinische Wochenschrift 53: 2324

Courvoisier L G 1890 Casuistisch-Statistische Beitrage zur Pathologie und Chirurgie der Gallenwege. Vogel, Leipzig

Da Costa J M 1858 Cancer of the pancreas. North American Medico-chirurgical Review 2: 883

Dahl R 1909 Eine neue Operation der Gallenwege. Zentralblatt für Chirurgie 36: 266

Dam C P 1939 Isolierung des Vitamins K in hochgereinigter Form. Helvetica Chirurgica Acta 22: 310

Dam C P 1940 The constitution of vitamin K_2. Journal of Biologic Chemistry 133: 721

Danilevsky A 1862 Ueber specifisch wirkende Körper des natürlichen und künstlichen pancreatischen Saftes. Virchows Archiv Pathologie Anatomie 25: 279

De Graaf R 1664 Disputatio medica de natura et usu succi pancreatici. Ex officina Hackiana, Lugduni Batavorum

Demel R 1936 Umstrittene Fragen bei akuter Pankreasnekrose. (Aktuelles zur Aetiologie. Diagnose und Behandlung der akuten Pankreasnekrose) Wiener Klinische Wochenschrift 49: 1273, 1309

Dill Russell A S 1952 Pancreaticogastrostomy, Lancet i: 589

Doublet H, Mulholland J H 1948 The surgical treatment of recurrent acute pancreatitis. Surgery, Gynecology and Obstetrics 86: 295

Du Val M K 1957 Pancreaticojejunostomy for chronic relapsing pancreatitis. Surgery 41: 1019

Ecker F 1862 Zeitschrift Rationale Medizin 16: 354 *Cited by Howard and Jordan 1960*

Elman R 1942 Surgical aspects of acute pancreatitis, with special reference to its frequency as revealed by serum amylase test. Journal of the American Medical Association 118: 1265

Estefan A, Estrugo R, Rompani O et al 1980 La exclusión del páncreas residual después de duodenopancreatectomía cefálica. Cirugia del Uruguay 50: 366

Fagniez P L, Julien M, Vellet M, German A 1974 Sur le traitement chirurgical des pancréatites aigues necrosantes. A propos de 47 cas. Chirurgie 100: 816

Fallis L S 1939 Acute pancreatitis. American Journal of Surgery 46: 593

Fallis L S, Szilagyi D E 1948 Observations on some metabolic changes after total pancreatoduodenectomy. Annals of Surgery 128: 639–667

Farber S 1944 The relation of pancreatic achilia to meconium ileus. Pediatrics 24: 387

Fink A S, De Souza L R, Mayer E A et al 1988 Long-term evaluation of pylorus preservation during pancreatico-duodenectomy. World Journal of Surgery 12: 663

Fitz R H 1889 Acute pancreatitis: a consideration of pancreatic hemorrhage, hemorrhagic, suppurative and gangrenous pancreatitis, and of disseminated fat-necrosis. Boston Medical and Surgical Journal 120: 181, 205: 229

Fitzgerald P J 1980 Medical anecdotes concerning some diseases of the pancreas. In: Fitzgerald P J, Morrison A B (eds) The pancreas. Williams and Wilkins, Baltimore, p 1–29

Flautner L, Tihangi T, Szecseny A 1985 Pancreatogastrostomy: an ideal complement to pancreatic head resection with preservation of the pylorus in the treatment of chronic pancreatitis. American Journal of Surgery 150: 608

Fortner J G 1973 Regional resection of cancer of the pancreas: A new surgical approach. Surgery 73: 307

Fortner J G 1984 Regional pancreatectomy for cancer of the pancreas, ampulla and other related sites. Tumor staging and results. Annals of Surgery 199: 418

Franke H 1901 Über die Extirpation der krebsigen Bauchspeicheldrüse. Archiv für Klinische Chirurgie 64: 364

Fredet P 1914 Le péritoine. In: Poirier P, Charpy A, Nicholas A (eds) Traité d'anatomie humaine, vol 4: 321 Masson – Paris

Frey C F, Smith G J 1987 Description and rationale of a new operation for chronic pancreatitis. Pancreas 2: 701

Fry W J, Child C G 1965 Ninety-five per cent distal pancreatectomy for chronic pancreatitis. Annals of Surgery 162: 543

Ganda O P, Stuart J 1977 Somatostatinoma, follow-up studies. New England Journal of Medicine 297: 1352

Gillesby W J, Puestow C B 1949 Pancreaticojejunostomy for chronic relapsing pancreatitis: an evaluation. Surgery 50: 859

Goldsmith H S, Ghos B C, Huvos A G 1971 Ligature versus implantation of the pancreatic duct after pancreatoduodenectomy. Surgery, Gynecology and Obstetrics 132: 87

Gregory R A, Tracy H J 1964 A note on the nature of the gastrin-like stimulant present in Zollinger-Ellison tumours. Gut 5: 115

Griesmann H 1948 Zur Behandlung der Pankreascysten. Der Chirurg 19: 302

Gussenbauer G 1883 Zur operativen Behandlung der Pancreascysten. Archiv für Klinische Chirurgie 29: 355

Hall D P 1962 Our surgical heritage: Theodore Kocher. American Journal of Surgery 104: 126

Halpert B 1932 Carl Langenbuch: Master surgeon of the biliary system. Archives of Surgery 25: 178

Halsted W S 1899 Contributions to the surgery of the bile passages, especially of the common bile-duct. Boston Medical and Surgical Journal 141: 645–654

Hartmann H 1923 Chirurgie des voies biliaires. Masson, Paris

Hartmann H, Navarro A 1910 Cancer de l'ampoule de Vater. Extirpation. Guérison. Bulletin et Mémoires de la Société de Chirurgiens de Paris 2: 1340

Hirschel C 1914 Die Resektion des Duodenums mit der Papille wegen Karzinoms. Münchener Medizinische Wochenschrift 61: 1728

Hollender L F 1979 Resection of the pancreas for acute hemorrhagic and necrotizing pancreatitis. World Journal of Surgery 3: 637

Hollender L F, Kohler J J, Klein A 1972 Zur chirurgischen Behandlung der akuten nekrotischen Pankreatitis. Der Chirurg 43: 256

Hollender L F, Starlinger M, Meyer C 1977 Die Chirurgie der akuten Pankreatitis. Aktuelle Chirurgie 12: 43

Howard J M, Jordan G H (eds) 1960 Surgery of the pancreas. J B Lippincott, Philadelphia, p 1–8

Howland G, Campbell W, Maltby E, Robinson W 1929 Dysinsulinism: convulsions and coma due to islet cell tumor of pancreas with operation and cure. Journal of the American Medical Association 93: 674

Hunt V C 1941 Surgical management of carcinoma of the ampulla of Vater and of the periampullary portion of the duodenum. Annals of Surgery 114: 570–602

Ingesbigtsen R, Langfeldt E 1952 Pancreaticogastrostomy. Lancet 2: 270

Jaboulay M 1898 La cholécystogastrostomie pour les tumeurs de la tête du pancréas. Lyon Medical 89: 365

Jedlicka R 1923 Eine neue Operations methode der Pankreascysten. Zentralblatt für Chirurgie 50: 132

Jordan G L 1987 Pancreatic resection for pancreatic cancer. In: Howard J M, Jordan G L, Reber H A (eds) Surgical diseases of the pancreas. Lea and Febiger. Philadelphia

Jourdan M 1895 De la cholédocotomie. G Steinheil, Paris

Kappeler A 1889 Die einzeitige Cholecystenterostomie. Korrespondenzblatt für Schweizerische Ärtze 17: 513

Kausch W 1909 Die Resektion des mittleren Duodenums – eine typische Operation. Vorläufige Mitteilung. Zentralblatt für Chirurgie 39: 1350

Kausch W 1912 Das Carcinom der Papilla duodeni und seine radikale Entfernung. Beitrage zur Klinischen Chirurgie 78: 29

Kehr H 1913 Chirurgie der Gallenwege. Enke, Stuttgart

Kelly W D, Lillehei R C, Merbel F K et al 1967 Allotransplantation of the pancreas and duodenum along with the kidney in diabetic nephropathy. Surgery 61: 827

Kocher T 1887 Korrespondenzblatt für Schweizerische Ärzte 279. *Cited by Nimier 1893*

Kocher T 1895 Ein Fall von Choledochoduodenostomia interna wegen Gallenstein. Korrespondenzblatt für Schweizerische Ärzte 1: 193

Kocher T 1903 Mobilisierung des Duodenum und Gastroduodenostomie. Zentralblatt für Chirurgie 30: 34

König E 1946 Die innere Anastomose in der Behandlung der Pankreascysten. Der Chirurg 17–24

Körte W 1898 Die chirurgischen Krankheiten und die Verletzungen des Pankreas. Enke, Stuttgart

Körte W 1905 Beitrage zur Chirurgie der Gallenwege und der Leber. Hirschwald, Berlin

Kroenlein R U 1895 Über Pankreas-Chirurgie. Berliner Klinische Wochenschrift 12: 489

Kümmell H 1890 Zur Chirurgie der Gallenblase. Deutsche Medinizische Wochenschrift 12: 237

Kümmerle F, Neher M, Schonborn H, Mangold G 1975 Vorzeitige

Operation bei akuter hämorrhagisch-nekrotisierender Pankreatitis. Deutsche Medizinische Wochenschrift 100: 2241

Küster 1884 Berliner Klinische Wochenschrift 9: 154. *Cited by Villar 1905*

Laguesse M E 1893 Sur la formation des îlots de Langerhans dans le pancréas. Comptes Rendus de la Société de la Biologie 45: 819–820

Lameris H J 1912 Hepato-cholangio-enterostomia. Zentralblatt für Chirurgie. 49: 1665

Lane M A 1908 The cytological characteristics of the areas of Langerhans. American Journal of Anatomy 7: 409

Langerhans P 1869 Beitrage zur mikroskopischen Anatomie der Bauchspeicheldrüse. Inaugural Dissertation. G Lange, Berlin

Larsson L L, Holst J, Kuhl J 1977 Pancreatic somatostatinoma: clinical features and physiological implications. Lancet 1: 666

Lindner 1889 Zentralblatt für Klinische Medizin 475. *Cited by Nimier 1893*

Leger L, Bréhant J 1956 Chirurgie du pancréas. Masson, Paris

Link G 1953 Pancreatostomy for chronic pancreatitis with calculi in the duct of Wirsung and diffuse calcinosis of the pancreatic parenchyma. Annals of Surgery 138: 287

London N J M, Bell P R F 1992 Pancreas and islet transplantation. British Journal of Surgery 79: 6–7

Longmire W P, Jordan P H, Briggs J D 1956 Experience with resection of the pancreas in treatment of chronic relapsing pancreatitis. Annals of Surgery 14: 681

MacBurney C H 1878 Removal of biliary calculi from the common duct by the duodenal route. Annals of Surgery 28: 481

McGavran M H et al 1966 A glucagon secreting alpha-cell carcinoma of the pancreas. New England Journal of Medicine 274: 1408

Machado M C, Monteiro J E, Bacchella T, Raia A 1976 A modified technique for the reconstruction of the alimentary tract after pancreatoduodenectomy. Surgery, Gynecology and Obstetrics 143: 271

Major R H 1941 Johann Conrad Brunner and his experiments on the pancreas. Annals of Medical History 3:91

Major R H 1978 Classic descriptions of disease. C Thomas, Springfield

Malthe 1894. *Cited by Ceccherelli 1900*

Mallet Guy P 1952 Pancréatectomie gauche pour pancréatite chronique recidivante. Lyon Chirurgical 47: 385

Marx K 1838 Beitrag zur Geschichte der Medizin. R Marx, Karlsruhe

Mayo W 1901 Cancer of the common bile duct. Report of a case of carcinoma of the duodenal end of the common duct with successful excision. St Paul Medical Journal 3: 374

Mayo Robson A W 1900 La chirurgie du pancréas. XIIIme Congrès International de Médecine Paris 10: 140

Mayo Robson A, Dobson J 1904 Diseases of the gall bladder and bile ducts including gall stones. Wood, New York

Mering J, Minkowski O 1889–1890 Diabetes mellitus nach Pankreasextirpation. Archiv für Experimentelle Pathologie und Pharmakologie 26: 371

Mercadier M 1964 Les pancréatectomies presque totales de gauche à droite: nouvelle tentative de traitement chirurgical de la pancréatite. Mémoires de l'Academie de Chirurgie 90: 84

Mikkelsen O 1934 Pancreatitis acuta: schwere Fälle, besonders hinsichtlich ihrer konservativen Behandlung. Acta Chirurgica Scandinavica 75: 373

Mirizzi P 1932 La colangiografia durante las operaciones de las vias biliares. Boletin de la Sociedad de Cirugia de Buenos Aires 16: 1133

Monastyrski N D 1888 Zur Frage der chirurgischen Behandlung der vollständigen Undurchgängigkeit des Ductus choledochus. Zentralblatt für Chirurgie 15: 778

Moore F 1959 Metabolic care of the surgical patient. W B Saunders, Philadelphia

Morian R 1909 Über das Choledochuscarcinom an der Papilla Vateri. Deutsche Zeitschrift für Chirurgie 98: 366

Murphy J B 1892 Cholecysto-intestinal, gastro-intestinal, entero-intestinal anastomosis and approximation without sutures. Medical Record 42: 665

Neuffer H 1932 Zur Operativen Behandlung der Pankreascysten. Archiv für Klinische Chirurgie 170: 488

Nicholl A G 1902 Simple adenoma of the pancreas arising from an island of Langerhans. Journal of Medical Research 8: 385–395

Nimier H 1893 Notes sur la chirurgie du pancréas. Revue de Chirurgie 13: 41, 757, 1007

Nordmann O 1936 Neue Anschauungen über die akute Pankreasnekrose und ihre Behandlung. Archiv für Klinische Chirurgie 193: 370

Ockinczyc P 1933 Technique operatoire du pancréas et de la rate. Doin, Paris

Oddi R 1887 D'une disposition à sphincter spéciale de l'ouverture du canal cholédoque. Archivio Italiano Biologia 8: 317

Oddi R 1888 Effetti dell'estirpazione della cistifela. Archivio Italiano Biologia 10: 425

Ombredanne L 1911 Kysto duodenostomie pancréatique. Bulletin de la Société Nationale de la Chirurgie 37: 977

Opie E L 1901 Relation of diabetes mellitus to lesions of the pancreas, hyaline degeneration of the islands of Langerhans. Journal of Experimental Medicine 5: 527

Opie E L 1903 Disease of the pancreas: its cause and nature. J B Lippincott, Philadelphia

Parkes and Lindner 1889. *Cited by Nimier 1893*

Pearse A G 1977 The diffuse neuroendocrine system and the APUD concept: related 'endocrine' peptides in brain, intestine, pituitary, placenta and cutaneous glands. Medical Biology 55: 115

Pereyra Lima L 1978 A technique for reconstructing the digestive tract after pancreatoduodenectomy. American Journal of Surgery 136: 408

Praderi R, Estefan A, Gomez Fossatti C, Mazza M 1973 Dérivations bilio-jéjunales sur anses exclués. Modifications techniques du procédé de Hivet-Warren. Lyon Chirurgical 69: 459

Praderi R 1982 One hundred years of biliary surgery. Surgical Gastroenterology 1: 269

Praderi R 1986 Geschichte der Gallenwege und Pankreatische Chirurgie. In: Hess W, Rohner A, Cirenei A, Akovbiantz A (eds) Biliopankreatische Chirurgie. Piccin, Padua

Praderi R, Estefan A 1990 Tratamiento quirúrgico del cancer biliar. Clinicas quirúrgicas. Facultad de Medicina Uruguay 8: 3

Pratt J H 1939 Diseases of the pancreas. Oxford Medicine 3: 473

Priestley J T, Comfort M W, Radcliffe J J 1944 Total pancreatectomy for hyperinsulinism due to islet cell adenoma: survival and cure at 16 months after operation; presentation of metabolic studies. Annals of Surgery 119: 221

Prinz R A, Greenlee H B 1981 Pancreatic duct drainage in 100 patients with chronic pancreatitis. Annals of Surgery 194: 313

Puestow C B, Gillesby W J 1958 Management of pancreatic cysts and pancreatic lithiasis. American Surgeon 20: 355

Quick A J 1935 The prothrombin in hemophilia and in obstructive jaundice. Journal of Biology and Chemistry 109: 73

Ranson J H C, Rifkind K M, Turner J W 1976 Prognostic signs and non-operative peritoneal lavage in acute pancreatitis. Surgery, Gynecology and Obstetrics 143: 209

ReMine W, Priestley J, Judd E, King J 1970 Total pancreatectomy. Annals of Surgery 172: 595

Rhoads J E, Folin L S 1987 The history of surgery of the pancreas. In: Howard J M, Jordan G L, Reber H A (eds) Surgical disease of the pancreas. Lea and Febiger. Philadelphia p 3–10

Riedel B 1892 Erfahrungen über die Gallensteinkrankheit mit und ohne Ikterus. Hirschwald, Berlin

Riedel B 1896 Über die entzündliche der Rückbildung fähige Vergrösserung des Pankreaskopfes. Berliner Klinische Wochenschrift 1:31

Rockey E W 1943 Total pancreatectomy for carcinoma: case report. Annals of Surgery 118: 603

Roget C 1958 La pancréatectomie gauche d'amont dans la traitement de la lithiase du canal de Wirsung. Thesis, Lyon

Rokitansky C 1842–1846 Handbuch der pathologischen Anatomie. Braumuller und Seidel, Wien

Rossi R L, Soeldener J S, Braasch J W et al 1986 Segmental pancreatic autotransplantation with pancreatic ductal occlusion after near total or total pancreatic resection for chronic pancreatitis: results at 5- to 54-month follow-up evaluation. Annals of Surgery 203: 626

Rossi R L, Rothschild J, Braasch J W et al 1987 Pancreaticoduodenectomy in the management of chronic pancreatitis. Archives of Surgery 122: 416

Roux C 1897 De la gastro-enterostomie. Revue de Gynécologie et Chirurgie Abdominale 1: 67

Ruggi 1890 Intorno ad un caso di carcinoma primitivo del pancreas, curato e guarito con l'asportazione del tumore. Giornale Internazionale della Scienza Medica 12: 81

Santorini G D 1724 Observationes Anatomicae, Venice

Safrany L, Neuhaus B, Krause S, Portocarrero G, Schott B 1989 Endoskopische Papillotomie bei akuter, biliär bedingter Pankreatitis. Deutsche Medizinische Wochenschrift 105: 115

Sauvé L 1908 Des pancréatectomies et spécialement de la pancréatectomie céphalique. Revue de Chirurgie de Paris 37: 335

Schönborn H, Pross E, Olbermann M 1975 Neuere Vorstellungen zur konservativen und operativen Therapie der akuten Pankreatitis. Internist 16: 108

Senn N 1886 Surgery of the pancreas as based upon experiments and clinical researches. Transactions of the American Surgical Association. Philadelphia 4: 99

Shires T, Coln D, Carrico J et al 1964 Fluid therapy in hemorrhagic shock. Archives of Surgery 88: 688

Shoemaker W, Walker W 1970 Fluid electrolyte therapy in acute illness. Year Book Medical Publishers, Chicago

Sprengel O 1891 Über einen Fall von Extirpation der Gallenblase mit Anlegung einer Communication zwischen Ductus choledochus und Duodenum. Archiv für Klinische Chirurgie 42: 550

Springfield and Wolfer 1886. Cited by Nimier 1893

Ssobelow L W 1902 Zur normalen und pathologischen Morphologie der inneren Secretion der Bauchspeicheldrüse. Virchow's Archiv für Pathologische Anatomie und Physiologie 168: 91

Taylor G 1934 The radical surgery of cancer of the pancreas. Annals of Surgery 100: 206

Tenani O 1922 Contributo alla Chirurgia della papilla di Vater. Policlinico 29: 291

Terrier V, in Nimier H 1894 Note sur la chirurgie du pancréas. Revue de Chirurgie 43: 215

Thiersch A 1881 Operative Drainage einer Cyste des Pankreas. Berliner Klinische Wochenschrift 18: 591

Trasoff A, Scarf M 1937 Acute pancreatitis: Medical problem. American Journal of Medical Sciences 194: 470

Traverso L W, Longmire W P 1978 Preservation of the pylorus in pancreatico-duodenectomy. Surgery, Gynecology and Obstetrics 146: 959

Treitz W 1853 Ueber einem neuen Muskel am Duodenum. Vierteljahrschrift für Practische Heilkunde 37: 113

Tremaine 1886 Transactions of the American Surgical Association 557. Cited by Nimier 1893

Tricomi E 1898 Contributo clinico alla chirurgia del pancreas. Riforma Medica 4: 483

Vater A 1720 Dissertatio Anatomica qua Novum Bilis Diverticulum circa Orificium Ductus Choledochi. Gerdisianus,Wittenberg

Vautrin A 1896 De l'obstruction calculeuse du choledoque. Revue de Chirurgie 16: 446

Verner J V, Morrison A B 1958 Islet cell tumor and a syndrome of refractory water diarrhea and hypocalcemia. American Journal of Medicine 25: 374

Vesalius 1959 Compendium Totius Anatomie Delineatro. Davisons, London

Veslingus J 1653 The anatomy of the body of man. P Cole, London

Villar F 1905 La chirurgie du pancreas. 18me Congrès Français de la Chirurgie. Paris

Von Winiwarter A 1882 Ein Fall von Gallenretention bedingt durch Impermeabilität des Ductus choledochus, Anlegung einer Gallenblasen-Darmfistel, Heilung. Prager Medizinische Wochenschrift 7: 201

Walker R M 1966 Francis Glisson and his capsule. Annals of the Royal College of Surgeons of England 38: 71

Walzel P 1934 Akute Pankreasnekrose bzw. Pankreatitis. Mediziner Klinische 30: 1518

Warren S 1926 Adenomas of the islands of Langerhans. American Journal of Pathology 2: 335

Warren W D, Millikan W J, Henderson J M et al 1984 A denervated pancreatic flap for control of chronic pain in pancreatitis. Surgery, Gynecology and Obstetrics 159: 581

Watts J T 1963 Total pancreatectomy for fulminant pancreatitis. Lancet 2: 384

Welton T S 1931 Foramen of Winslow. American Journal of Surgery 11: 133

Wermer F 1954 Genetic aspects of adenomatosis of endocrine glands. American Journal of Medicine 16: 353

Whipple A O 1941 Rationale of radical surgery of cancer of the pancreas and ampullary region. Annals of Surgery 114: 612

Whipple A O 1960 A historical sketch of the pancreas. In: Howard J M, Jordan G H (eds) Surgery of the pancreas. J B Lippincott, Philadelphia, p 1–8

Whipple A O, Parsons N, Mullins C 1935 Treatment of carcinoma of tbe ampulla of Vater. Annals of Surgery 102: 765

Wiart P 1899 Recherches sur l'anatomie chirurgicales e voie d'accés du choledoque. Revue de Gynécologie et Chirurgie 3: 149

Wilder R M, Allen R N, Power M H, Robertson H E 1927 Carcinoma of the islands of the pancreas, hyperinsulinism and hypoglycemia. Journal of the American Medical Association 89: 348–355

Willis T 1679 Pharmaceutice rationalis or an exercitation of the operations of medicines in human bodies. Dring, Harper and Leigh, London

Wirsung J, See Choulant J L 1952 Geschichte und Bibliographie der Anatomischen Abbildung. Weigel, Leipzig

Wölfler 1888 Zeitschrifte fur Heilkunde 9: 179. Cited by Nimier 1893

Wood M 1979 Eponyms in biliary tract surgery. American Journal of Surgery 138: 746

Zollinger R M, Ellison E H 1955 Primary peptic ulcerations of the jejunum associated with islet cell tumors of the pancreas. Annals of Surgery 142: 709–728

Zuelzer G L 1908 Ueber Versuche einer specifischen Fermenttherapie des Diabetes. Zeitschrift Experimental Pathologie und Therapeutik 5: 307

2. Embryology and surgical anatomy of the pancreas

M. Trede

EMBRYOLOGICAL DEVELOPMENT

In order to understand the anatomical variations and congenital anomalies of the pancreas – many of which have practical surgical implications – it is important to realize that this organ originates from two separate embryonic anlagen: a ventral and a dorsal primordium. On or about the 24th day of gestation the hepatic diverticulum begins to bud from the ventral surface of that part of the primitive digestive tube which later on is destined to become the duodenum. This hepatic anlage invades the ventral mesentery and later develops into the liver, bile ducts and gall-bladder. Some 2 days later (26th day of gestation) a similar diverticulum emanates from the dorsal surface of the digestive tube. This develops into the dorsal anlage of the pancreas, growing rapidly within the dorsal mesentery. The smaller ventral pancreatic anlage buds a little later from the hepatic diverticulum (on the 32nd day) (O'Rahilly 1978) (Fig. 2.1).

A series of rapid developments – elongation of the hepatic anlage (to form the bile duct), disappearance of the ventral mesentery, rapid growth of the left wall of the duodenum – leads to a rotation of the common bile duct, together with the ventral pancreatic anlage, into a dorsal position behind the primitive superior mesenteric vessels (Fig. 2.2).

Thus, dorsal and ventral portions of the pancreas come into close contact by the 37th day of gestation. Whilst these two and their draining ducts begin to amalgamate, the right leaf of the dorsal mesentery fuses with the posterior abdominal wall thus determining the retroperitoneal position of the pancreas and three-quarters of the duodenum. This avascular plane, the fascia of Treitz, separates the posterior aspect of the pancreas from the abdominal wall. It is this plane that facilitates the mobilization manoeuvre described by Kocher.

By the end of the seventh week of gestation with the embryo only about 13 mm long, gross morphological development of the pancreas is largely complete. The ventral

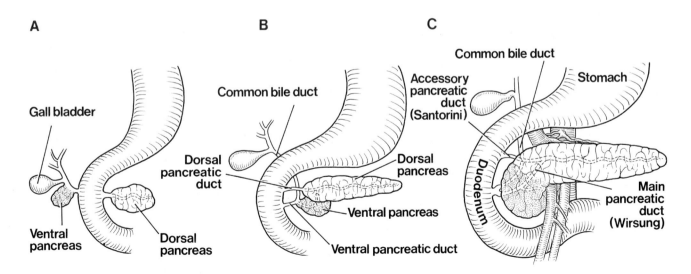

Fig. 2.1 Schematic drawing of the embryological development of the pancreas from the foregut (see text). (After Skandalakis et al 1979 Anatomical complications of pancreatic surgery. Contemporary Surgery 15: 17.)

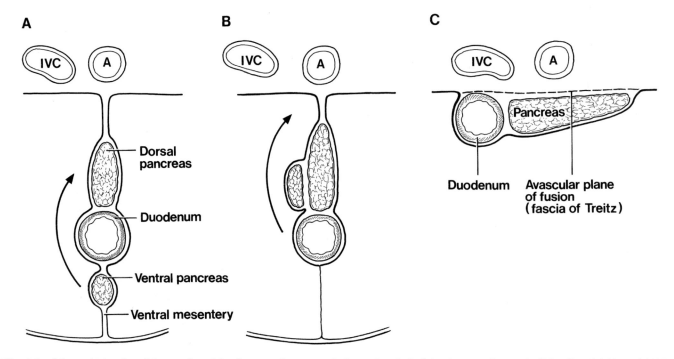

Fig. 2.2 Schematic drawing of the rotation of duodenum and pancreas during embryological development (see text). (After Skandalakis et al 1979 Anatomical complications of pancreatic surgery. Contemporary Surgery 15: 17.)

anlage now constitutes the uncinate process and most of the pancreatic head. Its duct (the duct of Wirsung) fuses with the duct of the dorsal anlage and drains into the duodenum together with the common bile duct.

The dorsal anlage constitutes the body and tail of the pancreas and the cranial part of the head. The distal part of its duct joins that draining the ventral anlage whereas its proximal portion (the duct of Santorini) either drains into the duodenum via a minor papilla or drains retrogradely into the duct of Wirsung; in some cases it may degenerate completely.

The functional development of the pancreas into an exocrine and endocrine gland occurs much later. Secretory acini first appear at the end of the ducts in the third gestational month. Trypsin is formed at about 22 weeks but full exocrine function is not present before 6 months after birth (Becker 1973).

Primary islet cells, which probably originate from the neural crest (as do other cells of the APUD system) appear at 8 weeks but are gradually replaced by secondary islets from the third gestational month onwards. Insulin may be detected at the end of the third month but full endocrine function is not established until after birth.

CONGENITAL ANOMALIES AND ANATOMICAL VARIATIONS

Congenital anomalies, including anatomical variants, and their surgical implications have their roots in the embryological development of the pancreas as just outlined.

Pancreatic aplasia

Total aplasia of the pancreas is rare and leads to death from growth retardation.

Partial aplasia, usually of the 'dorsal' pancreas (i.e. the body and tail), is equally rare and may be discovered in the course of an operation, as in the course of a Whipple resection when no pancreatic remnant is found as did occur once in the author's experience.

Aplasia of islet tissue causes serious retardation of fetal growth since maternal insulin cannot cross the placental barrier.

Aplasia of exocrine acinar tissue with a normal duct system is associated with other (usually fatal) congenital defects (Dodge & Laurence 1977) that lead to early death even though the exocrine insufficiency can be alleviated by enzyme substitution.

Ectopic pancreatic tissue

This is most frequently found in the stomach and duodenal wall and is readily explained by the presence there of glandular tissue with pancreatic potential. In fact, heterotopic pancreatic tissue has been found in the duodenal wall in 13.7% of 410 autopsy cases (Feldman & Weinberg 1952).

Ectopic pancreatic tissue is found less frequently in the mesentery, omentum, colon, appendix, gallbladder, Meckel's diverticulum and even in an anomalous broncho-oesophageal fistula. Here, too, the only explanation so far appears to lie in the metaplasia of pluripotent endodermal cells of the embryonic foregut (Fig. 2.3).

Pancreatic heterotopia usually remains asymptomatic. Symptoms may, however, be produced by ulceration, bleeding or pain due to pancreatitis in the ectopic tissue. Various diseases can be mimicked depending on the localization of the ectopia, e.g. duodenal ulcer, cholecystitis, and appendicitis. Other symptoms may be due to obstruction (pyloric or intestinal) caused by protruberant ectopic tissue. The treatment of symptomatic ectopic pancreatic tissue relies on simple surgical resection of the gastrointestinal segment involved.

Annular pancreas

This may occur as a band of pancreatic tissue including ducts, completely encircling the second part of the duodenum or as an intramural invasion of the duodenal wall by pancreatic tissue (Fig. 2.4). The former is best explained by fixation of part of the ventral pancreatic anlage to the duodenal wall before rotation to the dorsal position occurs, whereas the latter probably represents a variant of ectopic pancreatic tissue. It is surprising that more than half of those afflicted do not become symptomatic before the age of 50 (Lloyd-Jones et al 1972).

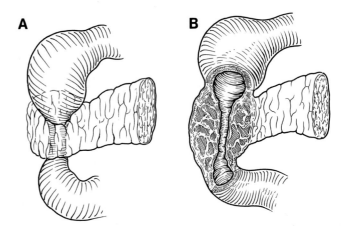

Fig. 2.4   Annular Pancreas. **A** shows extramural pancreatic ring. **B** shows intramural pancreas. (See text.)

Variations of pancreatic ducts and pancreas divisum

In the normal configuration (60% of subjects) the main pancreatic duct (duct of Wirsung) drains tail and body of the pancreas before turning downwards into the head where it opens into the duodenum at the major papilla in close association to the common bile duct.

The smaller accessory duct of Santorini runs as a continuation of the line of the main duct to drain into the duodenum some 2 cm proximally at the minor papilla (Fig. 2.5).

Becker points out that the junction of the ducts of Wirsung and Santorini represents a weak point in the pancreatic drainage system particularly prone to obstruction. Not only is there a bend or kink in the main duct, but at this same point the accessory duct of Santorini (if it has no direct opening into the duodenum) empties pancreatic juice in a retrograde fashion and against the direction of flow in the main duct of Wirsung (Becker 1973).

As for the dimensions of the main pancreatic duct, these have been perfectly summarized by Skandalakis et al using information gained largely from endoscopic retrograde cholangiopancreatography (ERCP) examinations (Kasugai et al 1972). Its length varies from 175 to 275 mm. The diameter in the tail varies from 1 to 2 mm, in the body from 2 to 3 mm and in the head from 3 to 4 mm; 2–3 ml of contrast medium fill the main duct in the normal living subject (Kasugai et al 1972), but following a Whipple resection for chronic pancreatitis, 3–6 ml of Ethibloc have been needed to obliterate the duct remaining towards the left, given that it is usually dilated (Gebhardt & Stolte 1978). Such a dilated duct can be palpated as a soft groove or ballotted as a tense tube through the anterior surface of the gland.

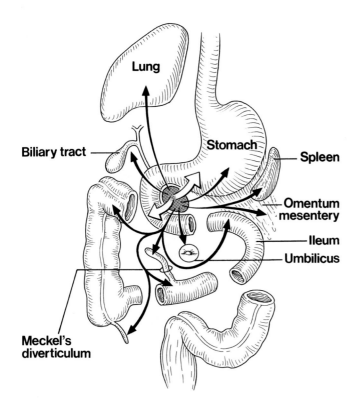

Fig. 2.3   Potential sites of heterotopic pancreatic tissue (see text). (After Skandalakis et al 1979 Anatomical complications of pancreatic surgery. Contemporary Surgery 15: 17.)

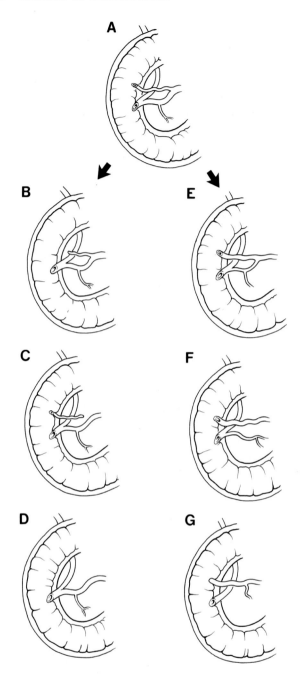

(see Fig. 2.5). Pancreas divisum is the commonest congenital anomaly of the pancreas, occurring in between 4 and 14% of subjects. Here, a long dorsal duct persists which drains via the minor papilla, whereas a short central duct opens into the major papilla together with the common bile duct.

The term 'divisum' applies to the ductal system only. There is no discernible division between the parenchyma of the ventral and dorsal anlagen. The clinical significance of this anomaly is still controversial, even though stenosis of the minor papilla might well explain bouts of recurrent pancreatitis (see Ch. 34).

Variations of the retropancreatic segment of the common bile duct

Since the common duct and ventral portion of the pancreas develop from the same anlage it is not surprising that there is a close relationship between them. Thus, Smanio (1954) describes five patterns of which the commonest are partial coverage of the duct by pancreatic tissue from behind (42.5%), total coverage of the duct which then runs within the pancreas (30%), and a duct running completely free behind the pancreas without any pancreatic coverage at all (16.5%) (Fig. 2.6). During the Kocher manoeuvre, the surgeon should attempt to palpate this portion of the

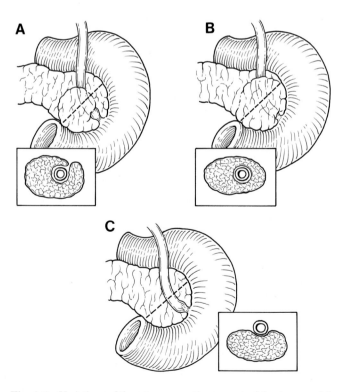

Fig. 2.6 Variations of the retropancreatic segment of the common bile duct. **A** The duct is partially covered by pancreatic tissue. **B** The duct is completely covered by pancreas. **C** The duct runs freely behind the pancreas.

Fig. 2.5 The chief variations of the pancreatic ducts. (After Skandalakis et al 1979 Anatomical complications of pancreatic surgery. Contemporary Surgery 15: 17.) **A** Normal configuration. **B–D** Progressive suppression of the accessory duct (Santorini). **D** Complete absence of accessory duct. **E–G** Progressive suppression of main duct (Wirsung). **F** Pancreas divisum. **G** Complete absence of main duct.

Skandalakis and colleagues (1979) divide the possible duct variations into two groups: those involving progressive suppression of the accessory duct (30% of subjects) and those in which there is progressive suppression of the main duct (10% of subjects).

Failure of fusion of the primitive dorsal and ventral ducts results in the configuration known as pancreas divisum common duct particularly if it is dilated and possibly obstructed by an impacted stone.

Rare anomalies with surgical implications include a prepancreatic course of the common duct and its opening into the third part of the duodenum (Doty et al 1985).

Variations of the ampulla and intramural segment of the common bile duct

In its terminal 1–2 cm the common duct pierces the duodenal wall obliquely and at the same time halves its diameter from 10 to 5 mm. It is joined by the duct of Wirsung running caudally which also is reduced in diameter from about 3 to 1.4 mm within the duodenal wall (Dowdy 1969). These two ducts normally open at the major papilla, situated on the posteromedial wall of the second part of the duodenum some 7–10 cm from the pylorus. In ERCP radiographs this papilla lies to the right of the second or third lumbar vertebra.

Since the ventral pancreatic duct develops as a branch of the bile duct, a common channel might be expected to persist. Actually, growth of the duodenal wall 'resorbs' more or less of the common bile duct leading to three types of pancreatobiliary duct opening at the papilla (Skandalakis, et al 1979). Minimal resorption leaves a common channel which forms the so-called ampulla of Vater (85% of subjects); while maximal resorption leaves the biliary and pancreatic duct with separate openings into the duodenum (Fig. 2.7).

For surgeons undertaking 95%, or duodenum-pre-serving, pancreatectomies, it is important to realize that small additional pancreatic ducts entering the intramural portion of the common bile duct or the duodenum directly, may cause leakage.

As for the sphincter of Oddi, surgeons and endoscopists are aware of the fact that its length may vary from 6 to 30 mm. Depending on the obliquity of the common bile duct's course through the duodenal wall, a proximal portion of the sphincter may well extend outside this wall into the intrapancreatic portion of the duct. Thus, sphincterotomy is always begun anterolaterally and not extended beyond 10 mm so as to avoid pancreatic injury.

SURGICAL ANATOMY

Structure and topography of the pancreas

The pancreas is between 18 and 28 cm long and weighs some 80–100 g. It lies transversely and somewhat obliquely in the retroperitoneum reaching from the head which nestles within the curve of the duodenum just to the right of the second lumbar vertebra, up to the tail which reaches the splenic hilum at the level of the twelfth thoracic vertebra.

The anterior surface is covered by the posterior peritoneal leaf of the lesser sac, but the gland lacks a firm capsule. Instead it is covered by tenuous connective tissue strands which extend between the lobules of the gland. It is this soft and friable texture of the normal pancreas that causes such technical difficulties when it comes to suturing it. In fact, the healthier the pancreas, the more do sutures tend to 'cut out', whereas the same needle may have difficulty in traversing the organ calcified by chronic pancreatitis.

The pancreas is divided into head (including the uncinate process), neck, body and tail (Fig. 2.8). The head is flattened, 1–2 cm thick and firmly fixed on the right to the second and third part of the duodenum. To the left it merges into the neck along an arbitrary line marked by the gastroduodenal artery above and the superior mesenteric and portal veins behind.

Its anterior surface is covered by the pylorus above and the transverse colon below. Together with the second part

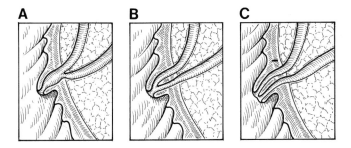

Fig. 2.7 Variations of the ampulla and intramural segment of the common bile duct. (After Skandalakis et al 1979 Anatomical complications of pancreatic surgery. Contemporary Surgery 15: 17.) **A** A long common channel of bile and pancreatic ducts forms the ampulla. **B** A short common channel. **C** The bile and pancreatic ducts open separately into the duodenum.

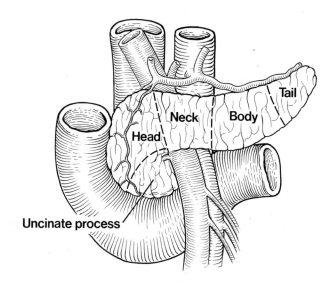

Fig. 2.8 Diagram of the main subdivisions of the pancreas.

of the duodenum it is traversed by the attachment of the transverse mesocolon which may be quite short here. Indeed some tumours of the pancreatic head may invade the mesocolon and transverse colon in such a manner that their radical removal requires right hemicolectomy as well. Similarly full mobilization of the pancreatic head is incomplete without 'taking down' the hepatic flexure of the colon (see Ch. 14).

The posterior surface of the head is separated by the avascular fascia of Treitz from the following retroperitoneal structures which lie exposed at the completion of the Kocher manoeuvre (from above downwards): the hilum and vessels of the right kidney, the inferior vena cava, left renal vein and the right spermatic or ovarian vein.

The uncinate process extends as a blunt hook from the inferior left margin of the head. It is derived from the ventral pancreatic anlage (see above) reaching behind the superior mesenteric vein and sometimes even behind the accompanying artery (Fig. 2.9). In the sagittal view it is seen to lie between the mesenteric vessels in front and the aorta and vena cava behind. The left renal vein lies cranial, the third part of the duodenum caudal to this process (Fig. 2.10). When not directly involved by disease it is fairly easy to dissect the tip of the uncinate process together with the duodenum from behind the mesenteric vessels. Care must, however, be taken at its base, where short arterial and venous branches enter it (see Fig. 2.9). Because of these relationships, malignancy involving the uncinate process is usually incurable due to early involvement of the mesenteric root. In resections performed for chronic pancreatitis the danger of damage to the adjacent vessels has led some to recommend leaving the uncinate process behind altogether (Leger 1969).

The neck of the pancreas (or isthmus) is a narrow segment reaching from the right margin of the superior mesenteric vein to the left border of the accompanying artery. It is related above to the coeliac axis, the hepatic artery to the right and the splenic artery to the left; the superior mesenteric vessels emerge from the lower border of the neck. It is covered by the lesser sac in front. Behind, it is closely related to the mesenteric vessels and the confluence of superior mesenteric and splenic veins forming the portal vein. Since venous tributaries to the anterior aspect of these veins from the neck are rare, the neck can usually be lifted off these veins with impunity. However, malignant invasion or the fibrotic changes of chronic pancreatitis can turn this into a hazardous manoeuvre (see Chs 14, 42). In the course of a Whipple procedure the neck is always removed along with the head.

The body resembles an elongated flat prism, with sizeable anterior and posterior surfaces and only a narrow inferior surface, reaching from the first lumbar vertebra towards the left. The lesser sac separates its anterior surface from the stomach. The posterior surface is related to the aorta, to the left crus of the diaphragm, the left adrenal gland, the left renal vessels and the upper third of the left kidney. The splenic vein runs firmly embedded in the posterior surface and is fixed to it by some dozen short tributaries.

The absence of any other larger vessels behind the pancreatic body facilitates its dissection from the retroperitoneum in an avascular plane. Care must, however, be taken not to damage the soft left adrenal gland with its tenous vessels–unless its removal en bloc with the pancreas as dictated by oncological necessity.

The inferior surface of the body is covered by the peritoneum of the transverse mesocolon. Apart from the middle colic artery entering between the leaves of the mesocolon at the inferior border of the pancreas and several minor epiploic branches to the greater omentum, the mesocolic attachment to the pancreatic body is avascular. That is why there is easy access to the body of the pancreas from below. Thus, in acute haemorrhagic pancreatitis, digital necrosectomy can be performed via this approach having first

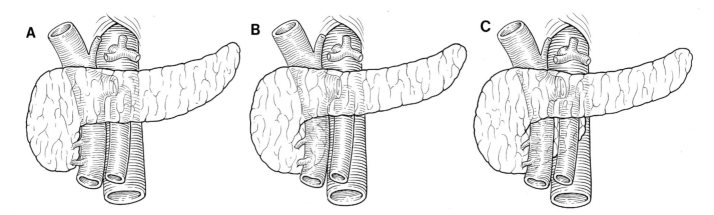

Fig. 2.9 Variations in the size of the uncinate process and its relationship to the superior mesenteric vessels (see text). (After Skandalakis et al 1979 Anatomical complications of pancreatic surgery. Contemporary Surgery 15: 17.)

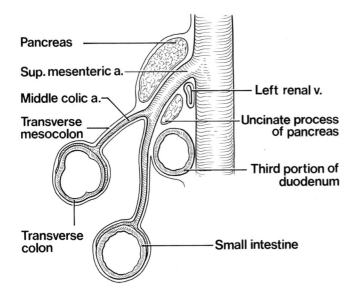

Fig. 2.10 Sagittal section through the pancreas at the level of the superior mesenteric artery (see text). (After Skandalakis et al 1979 Anatomical complications of pancreatic surgery. Contemporary Surgery 15: 17.)

lifted the transverse colon upwards. And in total pancreatectomy the inferior surface of the pancreas can be freed by dividing the mesocolic attachment without any fear of compromising the blood supply to the transverse colon.

The upper border of the body is related to the snake-like course of the splenic artery.

The tail of the pancreas lies at the level of the twelfth thoracic vertebra. It is a relatively mobile short segment of the gland reaching up to the splenic hilum. Injury to this part in the course of splenectomy may lead to a postoperative pancreatic fistula.

Blood supply of the pancreas

Arteries

The pancreas, and in particular its head, has an abundant blood supply derived basically from the coeliac axis and superior mesenteric artery. In fact, collateral pathways between these two are so efficient that the cut surface of the pancreas removed en bloc by a Whipple procedure will often continue to bleed until the very last jejunal branch (and the proximal jejunum itself) has been divided. The general pattern of the arterial blood supply is depicted in Figure 2.11 (A and B).

The pancreatic head and uncinate process receive arterial blood from two pairs of pancreatoduodenal arcades. The superior pancreatoduodenal arteries, anterior and posterior, arise from the gastroduodenal artery (either separately or from a common trunk). The inferior pair of pancreatoduodenal arteries arise from the superior mesenteric artery, either separately or together with one of the

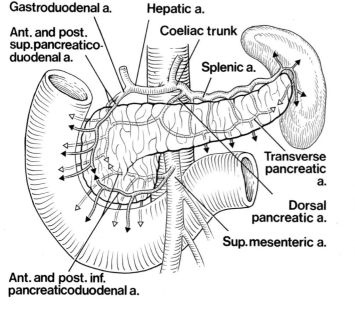

A

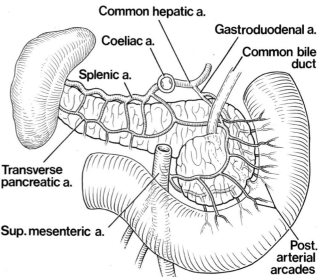

B

Fig. 2.11 **A** Arterial blood supply to the pancreas (anterior view). **B** Arterial blood supply to the pancreas as seen from behind. (After Skandalakis et al 1979 Anatomical complications of pancreatic surgery. Contemporary Surgery 15: 17.)

proximal jejunal arteries. If the latter is accidentally ligated with an inferior pancreatoduodenal artery, ischaemia of a proximal segment of jejunum may follow and necessitate removal of more jejunum (e.g. in the course of Whipple's procedure) than is normally the case.

Both pairs of arcades supply the pancreatic head as well as the duodenal wall and communicate freely with one another. Whereas the anterior pancreatoduodenal arcade runs close to the inner curve of the duodenum, the posterior arcade passes posterior to the intrapancreatic portion of the common bile duct keeping a greater distance from the duodenum.

The rule stated in most textbooks, that the close inter-relationship of duodenum and pancreas regarding blood supply prevents removal of one without the other, has been largely refuted in actual practice. Thus, duodenum-preserving total pancreatectomy has been performed successfully, provided the duodenal branch of the gastro-duodenal artery (supplying the first part of the duodenum) and the first 3 cm of the anterior inferior pancreato-duodenal artery (supplying the fourth part of the duodenum) are preserved (see Ch. 31) (Russell 1990). However, the tenuous blood supply of the remaining duodenum in some cases and oncological requirements of most other situations, makes this procedure the exception that proves the rule.

Variations of this pattern are numerous and described in detail by Michels (1955). The arcades may be doubled or even tripled; intercommunication between superior and inferior arcades is rarely incomplete; superior pancreato-duodenal arteries may arise from the right gastroepiploic artery and both superior and inferior arteries can arise from an aberrant right hepatic artery. The latter situation increases the difficulty of dissecting such an aberrant artery behind the pancreatic head.

Branches of the splenic artery supply the body and tail of the pancreas. These include multiple small branches to the upper border of the gland and the dorsal pancreatic artery. The latter arises from the proximal 2 cm of the splenic artery, but it may also originate from the gastro-duodenal or an aberrant right hepatic artery. Apart from giving branches to the head and uncinate process, this artery sends off a large but variable inferior or transverse pancreatic artery to supply the body and tail of the gland from below. Its branches usually communicate with those of the splenic artery coming from above. The inferior pancreatic artery gives off some epiploic branches to the greater omentum, which may communicate with the left colic artery.

Arterial anomalies as they relate to pancreatic surgery are discussed in Chapter 42. Most of these involve the common hepatic artery and its branches. We distinguish between totally aberrant vessels that provide blood supply to the liver (or parts of it) to the exclusion of all others, and accessory vessels that provide additional but not exclusive arterialization. Whereas the former must always be preserved, the latter are usually dispensable.

An aberrant common hepatic artery arises from the superior mesenteric artery in 4.5% of subjects (Michels 1951). An accessory right hepatic artery (also arising from the superior mesenteric) occurs in as many as 25% of subjects (Fig. 2.12).

Both of these anomalous arteries usually pass behind the pancreatic neck and head and require meticulous dissection especially if they communicate with the posterior pancreatoduodenal arcade. Rarely, they pose an even bigger surgical problem by coursing through the gland or passing in front of it (see Ch. 42).

Their course within the hepatoduodenal ligament is almost always to the right of the common duct. Careful palpation of this region gives early warning of an anomalous hepatic artery and usually makes preoperative angiography unnecessary.

An aberrant left hepatic artery may rarely arise from the superior mesenteric, or more frequently from the left gastric artery (14% of subjects). Both may be injured during dissection of the pancreatic head or during the partial gastrectomy that goes with the Whipple procedure–with possibly dire consequences for the left hepatic lobe.

Veins

The veins draining the pancreas, largely run parallel to the arteries. They drain into the portal vein or its two main tributaries the superior mesenteric and splenic veins (Fig. 2.13).

The following points should be noted by the pancreatic surgeon:

1. The anterior superior pancreatoduodenal vein drains into the right gastroepiploic vein.

2. The posterior superior pancreatoduodenal vein is that constant tributary entering the portal vein from the right, just behind the upper border of the pancreas.

3. As mentioned before, tributaries entering the anterior surface of the superior mesenteric or portal veins are very rare, but even so dissection between the pancreatic neck and the great veins must be done with great care.

4. The inferior pancreatoduodenal veins usually terminate as a common trunk draining into the superior mesenteric vein. This trunk is short and in underrunning what appears to be just one anterior vein, the posterior branch is easily perforated. The resulting torrential bleeding can be easily stopped by pressure from behind (see Ch. 42).

5. The inferior mesenteric vein enters the splenic vein in 38% of subjects (Douglass et al 1950), in another one-third it drains into the splenomesenteric confluence and in the remainder it terminates in the superior mesenteric vein. This vein need not be preserved if for technical or oncological reasons its division is inevitable.

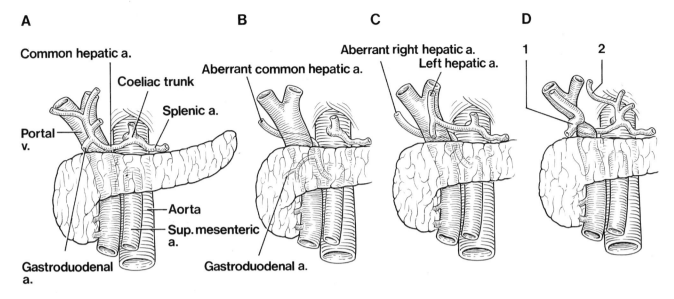

Fig. 2.12 Some variations of the hepatic arteries in relation to the pancreas: **A** Normal configuration. **B** Aberrant common hepatic artery. **C** Aberrant right hepatic artery. **D** 1, Common hepatic artery looping around the portal vein from behind (causing compression of the vein); 2, Aberrant left hepatic artery arising from left gastric artery.

6. The left gastric or coronary vein enters the portal vein in three-quarters and the splenic vein in one-quarter of subjects (Skandalakis et al 1987). This vein must be preserved in total pancreatectomy since here it is the only vessel remaining to drain the proximal gastric segment.

7. There are a number of rare anomalies of the portal vein. It may run in front of the duodenum and it may drain into the superior vena cava. Total anomalous pulmonary venous drainage may occur into the portal vein and present as a congenital 'cardiac' defect (Skandalakis et al 1979). Finally, congenital strictures of the portal vein can suggest tumourous infiltration in patients whose tumours are not really inoperable at all (see Ch. 42).

Lymphatic drainage of the pancreas

The retroperitoneal position of the pancreas, its rich vasculature and close relationship to the large retroperitoneal vessels make for a complicated lymphatic drainage, practically in all directions. This usually prevents meaningful oncological en bloc resections.

Cubilla et al (1978) dissecting regional pancreatectomy specimens resected by Fortner found some 50 nodes loosely associated with five lymph node groups. Hermanek & Giedl (1986) similarly described five groups of the first order, i.e. in close relation to the superior, inferior, anterior posterior and splenic parts of the pancreas. In addition, they described four groups of the second order at some distance from the gland: portal (along the hepatoduodenal ligament), coeliac (around the coeliac axis), mesenteric (at the root of the superior mesenteric artery) and para-aortic (which are found in the space between the inferior vena cava and aorta, caudal to the crossing left renal vein. Furthermore the mediastinal and even the supraclavicular (Virchow) nodes may be involved by metastatic spread of pancreatic carcinoma.

In recent years, several Japanese workers have counted up to 150 nodes divided among 11 groups (Fig. 2.14) (Nagai et al 1986, Deki & Sato 1988). In actual practice, when dissecting the hepatoduodenal ligament and coeliac

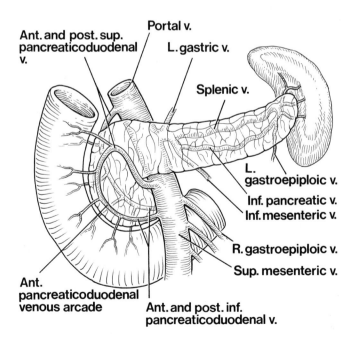

Fig. 2.13 Diagram of the veins draining the pancreas as seen from the front.

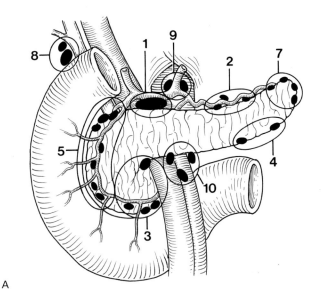

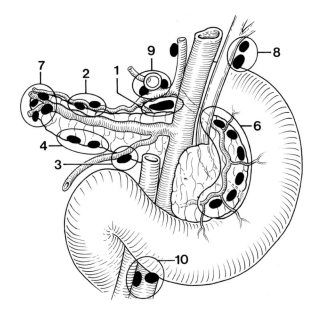

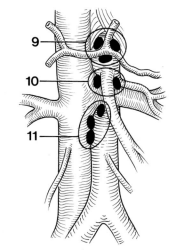

Fig. 2.14 **A** Lymphatic drainage of the pancreas as seen from the front. **B** Posterior view of lymphatic drainage. **C** Lymph nodes along retropancreatic portions of the aorta and inferior vena cava. Lymph node groups (Hermanek & Giedl 1986): 1, superior head; 2, superior body; 3, inferior head; 4, inferior body; 5, anterior pancreatoduodenal; 6, posterior pancreatoduodenal; 7, splenic; 8, portal; 9, coeliac; 10, mesenteric; 11, para-aortic.

axis one is impressed that one is not dealing so much with macroscopically separate nodes but rather with coalescing sheets of lymphoid tissue.

Hermanek & Giedl (1986) found metastases in regional lymph nodes of the second order in one-third of specimens resected for pancreatic carcinoma and in only half that number in periampullary carcinoma.

While there is no doubt that lymph node metastases imply a poor long-term prognosis (Cameron et al 1991, Nagakawa et al 1991), there are two good reasons for clearing lymph nodes of the first and second order. First, accurate staging of the tumour depends on a wide lymphadenectomy and secondly there is the occasional long-term survivor in spite of lymph node involvement (Trede et al 1990).

There are four groups of lymph nodes that are of special surgical significance.

1. A large lymph node overlies the superior border of the pancreatic head and neck and the common hepatic artery (group 1 in Fig. 2.14). Although rarely involved macroscopically in operable cases, this node is removed with the pancreatic head in the Whipple operation so as to leave a clean pancreatic cross-section free of lymphoid tissue for anastomosis.

2. The portal group lies to the right of the common bile duct, with one larger and constant lymph node in the angle between the common duct and upper border of the duodenum (group 8 in Fig. 2.14). It is this lymphoid strand that may cover an aberrant right hepatic artery.

3. The nodes found at the root of the superior mesenteric artery and its branches (group 10 in Fig. 2.14). Macroscopic involvement here is detected during mobilization of the pancreatic head in the Kocher manoeuvre. It is also palpable in the root of the mesentery at the lower pancreatic border and such involvement is a certain sign of incurability.

4. The same applies to metastases in the para-aortic nodes (group 11 in Fig. 2.14.) also exposed by the Kocher manoeuvre.

Finally, it is common experience that metastases often elude intraoperative frozen section examination of lymph nodes. The final histological work-up of the specimen, however, then reveals microscopic deposits and the ominous invasion of perineural lymphatics in 80% of cases of ductal pancreatic carcinoma (Hermanek & Giedl 1986).

REFERENCES

Becker V 1973 Bauchspeicheldrüse. In: Doerr W, Seifert G, Vehlinger E (eds) Spezielle pathologische Anatomie. Springer-Verlag, Berlin, Bd 6, p 38–57

Cameron J L, Crist D W, Sitzmann J V, Hruban R H, Boitnott J K, Seidler A J, Coleman J 1991 Factors influencing survival after pancreaticoduodenectomy for pancreatic cancer. American Journal of Surgery 161:120–125

Cubilla A L, Fortner J, Fitzgerald P J 1978 Lymph node involvement in carcinoma of the head of the pancreas area. Cancer 41:880

Deki H, Sato T 1988 An anatomic study of the peripancreatic lymphatics. Surgical and Radiological Anatomy 10:121–135

Dodge J A, Laurence K M 1977 Congenital absence of islets of Langerhans. Archives of Disease in Childhood 52: 411

Doty J, Hassall E, Fonkalsrud E W 1985 Anomalous drainage of the common bile duct into the fourth portion of the duodenum. Clinical sequelae. Archives of Surgery 120:1077–1079

Douglass T C, Lounsbury B F, Cutter W W, Wetzel N 1950 An experimental study of healing in the common bile duct. Surgery, Gynecology and Obstetrics 91: 301

Dowdy G S Jr 1969 The biliary tract. Lea and Febiger, Philadelphia

Feldman M, Weinberg T 1952 Aberrant pancreas: cause of duodenal syndrome. Journal of the American Medical Association 148: 893

Gebhardt C, Stolte M 1978 Pankreasgang-Okklusion durch Injektion einer schnellhärtenden Aminosäurenlösung. Experimentelle Studie. Langenbecks Archiv für Chirurgie 346: 149–166

Hermanek P, Giedl J 1986 Lymphogene Metastasierung des Pankreas- und periampullären Karzinoms-Häufigkeit, Topographie. In: Beger H G, Bittner R (eds) Das Pankreaskarzinom. Springer–Verlag, Berlin, p 114–119

Kasugai T, Kuno N, Kobayashi S, Hattori K 1972 Endoscopic pancreatocholangiography. I. The normal endoscopic pancreatocholangiogram. Gastroenterology 63: 217

Leger L 1969 Chirurgie du pancréas. In: Patel J, Patel J C, Leger L (eds) Nouveau traité de technique chirurgicale. Masson, Paris, tome XII, p 567–570

Lloyd-Jones W, Mountain J C, Warren K W 1972 Annular pancreas in the adult. Annals of Surgery 176:163

Michels N A 1951 The hepatic, cystic, and retro-duodenal arteries and their relations to the biliary ducts. Annals of Surgery 133: 503

Michels N A 1955 Blood supply and anatomy of the upper abdominal organs. J B Lippincott, Philadelphia

Nagai H, Kuroda A, Morioka Y 1986 Lymphatic and local spread of T1 and T2 pancreatic cancer. A study of autopsy material. Annals of Surgery 204: 65–71

Nagakawa T, Konishi I, Ueno K, Ohta T, Akiyama T, Kanno M, Kayahara M, Miyazaki I 1991 The results and problems of extensive radical surgery for carcinoma of the head of the pancreas. Japanese Journal of Surgery 21: 262–267

O'Rahilly R 1978 The timing and sequence of events in the development of the human digestive system and associated structures during the embryonic period proper. Anatomy and Embryology 153: 123

Russell R C G 1990 Duodenum-preserving total pancreatectomy for chronic pancreatitis. In: Trede M, Saeger H D (eds) Aktuelle Pankreaschirurgie. Springer-Verlag, Berlin, p 181–193

Skandalakis J E, Rowe J S Jr, Gray S W, Skandalakis L J 1979 Anatomical complications of pancreatic surgery. Contemporary Surgery 15 (5, 6): 17

Skandalakis J E, Gray S W, Skandalakis L J 1987 Surgical anatomy of the pancreas. In: Howard J M, Jordan G L Jr, Reber H A (eds) Surgical diseases of the pancreas. Lea and Febiger, Philadelphia, p 11–36

Smanio T 1954 Varying relations of the common bile duct with the posterior face of the pancreas in negroes and white persons. Journal of the International College of Surgeons 150: 22

Trede M, Schwall G, Saeger H D 1990 Survival after pancreatoduodenectomy. 118 consecutive resections without an operative mortality. Annals of Surgery 211: 447–458

3. Physiology of the pancreas

D. C. Carter

INTRODUCTION

The adult pancreas weighs only some 100 g yet secretes 5–20 g of protein zymogen per day in approximately 2.5 l of alkaline fluid. The zymogens are produced by acinar cells which make up the bulk (80%) of the pancreas while the bicarbonate-rich fluid is secreted by the cells of the duct system which make up less than 5% of the weight of the organ. It has been estimated that each ductal cell can secrete its own volume of fluid in some 2 minutes. In addition to its importance as an exocrine organ the pancreas fulfils vital endocrine functions by virtue of hormones secreted by the islets of Langerhans. The islets make up no more than 2% of pancreatic weight and are dispersed throughout the exocrine tissue. At one time the intimate anatomical relationship of exocrine and endocrine pancreas was assumed to be a chance association having little functional significance. However, it is now apparent that dispersal of the islets through the exocrine tissue may serve an important purpose, the close contact facilitating interaction between exocrine and endocrine cells.

At its simplest the physiology of the pancreas can be described as follows. Secretion of enzymes by the acinar cells is stimulated by cholecystokinin (CCK) and the vagus, while secretin stimulates secretion of HCO_3^- -rich fluid by the duct system. The islets of Langerhans contain four types of hormone secreting cells: A cells which produce glucagon; B cells which produce insulin; D cells which produce somatostatin, and PP cells which produce pancreatic polypeptide.

In reality the situation is infinitely more complicated and a number of factors combine to cloud our understanding of the function of the pancreas and mechanisms that control it. We now appreciate that both the parasympathetic (vagal) and sympathetic divisions of the autonomic nervous system influence pancreatic function and that in addition to extrinsic neural control, the pancreas possesses its own intrinsic nervous system. A host of potential chemical messengers are now identified that might influence pancreatic function. In addition to classical circulating hormones such as CCK, secretin and gastrin, a number of other messengers such as somatostatin, pancreatic polypeptide (PP), vasoactive intestinal peptide (VIP), gastrin-releasing peptide (GRP), pancreastatin and peptide YY may serve as paracrine messengers (i.e. messengers acting on local rather than distant target cells) and/or as neurotransmitters. As mentioned above, the exocrine and endocrine pancreas can no longer be regarded as functionally separate entities, and our recognition of the existence of an islet–acinar portal system has led to the realization that levels of hormones circulating in the peripheral blood may have little relevance to local physiological concentrations of the messenger concerned.

This said, our ability to unravel the complex mechanisms controlling pancreatic function has been strengthened by the development of specific radioimmunoassays for the various chemical messengers, and by advances in immunohistochemistry which allow their tissue and cellular localization. We have become aware that the various hormones influencing the pancreas exist in different molecular forms (e.g. CCK-58, CCK-39, CCK-33, CCK-8), and that a number of different hormones share common amino acid sequences (e.g. secretin and VIP) which may lead to overlap in their function and assay cross-reactivity.

Studies in experimental animals have allowed great advances in pancreatic physiology but great species variation prevents ready extrapolation of such findings to man. Nevertheless, the use of animal preparations involving gastro-enteric and/or pancreatic diversion (with or without extrinsic denervation), isolated–perfused organ systems, tissue explants and dispersed cell and cell culture preparations has allowed dissection of neurohormonal controlling mechanisms and elucidation of cellular secretory mechanisms. More recently, endoscopic cannulation of the pancreatic duct system has added to our ability to study pancreatic physiology in man. Each experimental system has its own disadvantages and the overlap between controlling mechanisms means that as soon as one mechanism is eliminated or bypassed experimentally, another may take its place.

EXOCRINE PANCREATIC SECRETION

Electrolyte content

Pancreatic juice is a watery, colourless, thin fluid which is clear or slightly opalescent. It is alkaline, ranging in pH from 7.5 to an extreme of 8.8 and its HCO_3^- concentration ranges from 25 mmol/l at low flow rates to 130–150 mmol/l at high flow rates. The juice is roughly isotonic with serum and there is an inverse relationship between its Cl^- and HCO_3^- concentrations, the sum of the two concentrations remaining constant at around 154 mmol/l. The Na^+ and K^+ concentrations roughly parallel those of serum while Ca^{2+} and Mg^{2+} concentrations are normally about one-third as high as those of serum. Calcium enters pancreatic juice by a combination of secretion by acinar cells and paracellular diffusion. CCK increases permeability to Ca^{2+} and the juice concentration of Ca^{2+} increases as flow rate decreases. These patterns may have significance in the pathogenesis of chronic pancreatitis.

Enzyme content

Pancreatic juice contains large amounts of enzymes and their precursors (or zymogens) secreted by the acinar cells and capable of digesting ingested carbohydrate (amylase), fat (lipase) and protein (trypsin, chymotrypsin etc). As indicated in Table 3.1, almost all of these enzymes are optimally active at neutral or alkaline pH, underlining the importance of HCO_3^- secretion as a means of achieving rapid neutralization of the acid chyme entering the duodenum.

Proteolytic enzymes

Enzymes such as trypsin, chymotrypsin, elastase and kallikrein (see Table 3.1) are known as serine proteases or endopeptidases in that they have a reactive serine residue which cleaves peptide bonds of the substrate. Enzymes

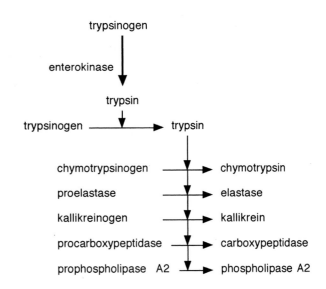

Fig. 3.1 The trypsin cascade in which activation of trypsin by duodenal enterokinase leads to activation of other pancreatic zymogens.

such as the carboxypeptidases are known as exopeptidases in that they cleave carboxyl- or amino-terminal amino acid residues from proteins or peptides.

Trypsin is the key proteolytic enzyme which triggers the activity of all other pancreatic zymogens in a cascade manner (Fig. 3.1). It is secreted from the acinar cell in the form of trypsinogens, of which there are at least three immunologically distinct forms with differing molecular weights, each producing a distinct form of trypsin. Although trypsinogens have a weak ability to activate themselves in vitro, pancreatic juice entering the duodenum usually has no proteolytic activity. However, the brush border of the duodenal mucosa produces an enzyme called enterokinase which converts trypsinogen to trypsin and in the process releases a trypsinogen activation peptide (TAP). Enterokinase activity is optimal at pH 6–9. Optimal yields of trypsin depend on the concentrations of trypsinogen present and high concentrations may be partly 'autodigested' by liberated trypsin. Small amounts of trypsin are normally secreted into the bloodstream; in acute pancreatitis serum trypsin levels may rise markedly

Table. 3.1 Pancreatic enzymes and their function

Enzyme/zymogen	Function	pH optimum
Trypsin(ogen) 1–3	Hydrolysis of proteins	7.5–8.5
Chymotrypsin(ogen)	Hydrolysis of proteins	8.0
(Pro)elastase 1–2	Cleavage of peptide bonds	7.5–10.5
Kallikrein(ogen)	Cleavage of kininogen to kinin	8.0
(Pro)carboxypeptidase A, B	Cleavage of C-terminal residues	7.5–8.0
Lipase	Hydrolysis of C_1 and C_3 bonds	8.0–9.0
Colipase I and II	Cofactor for lipase	
(Pro)phospholipase A_2	Hydrolysis of fatty acid esters	6.0
Carboxylesterase	Hydrolysis of esters	7.4
Amylase	Hydrolysis of α-1,4 glycoside bonds	7.5–8.0

and urinary excretion levels of TAP have been used recently as an index of the severity of an attack (Gudgeon et al 1990). Once trypsin has been liberated it catalyses the activation of the other zymogens with chymotrypsin being released from chymotrypsinogen, elastase (1 and 2) from proelastase (1 and 2), kallikrein from kallikreinogen, and carboxypeptidase (A and B) from procarboxypeptidase (A and B). The important functions of these activated proteolytic enzymes are summarized in Table 3.1.

Lipolytic enzymes

Although lipases are produced by the stomach and intestine, pancreatic lipase is of paramount importance in the digestion of dietary fat. The enzyme rapidly hydrolyses the C_1 and C_3 bonds of triglyceride to produce free fatty acids and a monoglyceride. The enzyme is optimally active above neutral pH and is permanently inactivated when pH falls beneath 3.0. Lipase is only active at an oil–water (hydrophobic–hydrophilic) interface so that its substrate must be presented in an emulsified or micellar form. The role of conjugated bile acids in fat digestion is complex in that while the bile acids promote emulsion of dietary fat, hydrolysis of triglycerides by lipase is actually inhibited by their presence. However, another enzyme secreted by the pancreas, colipase, overcomes this inhibition, probably by forming a complex with bile salts and lipase.

Carboxylesterase is another pancreatic enzyme which differs from lipase in that it can hydrolyse water-soluble esters as well as emulsions and its activity is greatly increased by bile salts. The enzyme may hydrolyse cholesterol and fat-soluble vitamin esters.

Amylase

Alpha-amylase activity is present in saliva but the pancreas is by far the most important source of amylase production. Pancreatic amylase and salivary amylase are chemically distinct from each other. Pancreatic amylase digests starch by breaking $\alpha 1{:}4$ glycoside links to liberate short chain polysaccharides which are digested further by intestinal maltase and glucosidase. A number of pancreatic isoamylases have been described.

Other enzymes

Phospholipase A_2 is produced by activation of the zymogen, prophospholipase A_2, by trypsin. It hydrolyses fatty acid esters and may have an important role in the pathogenesis of acute pancreatitis as it can attack membrane phospholipids. It may also generate cytotoxic lysocompounds such as lysolecithin during hydrolysis of fatty acid esters and these compounds act as detergents with further disruption of cell membranes.

Ribonuclease (RNase) and deoxyribonuclease (DNase) are both present in pancreatic juice but their physiological significance is uncertain.

The pancreatic acinar cells produce large quantities of lysosomal enzymes which like the zymogens, are synthesized on ribosomes attached to the rough endoplasmic reticulum. Although the release of lysosomal enzymes may parallel that of zymogens, they are unstable at alkaline pH and seem unlikely to play a physiological role in luminal digestion of food. It is much more likely that in addition to digesting and disposing of cell constituents, they protect the cells from accumulation of enzymes and zymogens. In this context it is possible that lysosomal enzymes may be involved in the pathogenesis of acute pancreatitis.

Protective mechanisms

The pancreas is protected from the destructive potential of its own secretions by a number of mechanisms, failure of which may result in life-threatening pancreatic inflammation. Under normal circumstances, small amounts of pancreatic zymogens and enzymes also enter the blood stream during secretion and plasma protease inhibitors prevent deleterious consequences. In acute pancreatitis the protective capacity of the protease inhibitors may be exceeded as large amounts of potent digestive enzymes enter the circulation.

Delayed activation of trypsin

Pancreatic enzymes are synthesized from amino acids, the process taking place on ribosomes attached to the rough endoplasmic reticulum. The nascent proteins are then translocated into the cisternal spaces of the Golgi complex and packaged into condensing vacuoles which mature into zymogen granules. When secretion is stimulated by agencies such as CCK, increased enzyme synthesis is accompanied by the migration of granules and discharge of their contents into the acinar lumen by a process of exocytosis. In exocytosis the lipoprotein membrane of the granule fuses with the apical cell membrane, and fusion of a number of granules may allow them to discharge through one site. Storage of potentially dangerous enzymes as inactive precursors in zymogen granules is an important self-protective mechanism for the acinar cell. If there is inadvertent admixture of zymogens and lysosomal hydrolases, intracellular activation of trypsin may in turn allow activation of the zymogen cascade and cell injury.

Under normal circumstances trypsinogen is not catalysed to trypsin until it reaches the duodenal lumen and is exposed to the brush border enzyme, enterokinase. Reflux of duodenal content into the pancreatic duct may allow this process to take place within the pancreas with potentially dangerous consequences. Bile alone does not activate trypsin so that reflux of bile into the pancreatic duct system may not in itself precipitate acute pancreatitis. Damage to the pancreatic duct mucosal barrier (see p. 35) could allow extravasation of digestive enzymes into the pancreatic parenchyma, but no mechanism for extracellular enzyme activation has yet been defined.

Trypsin inhibitors

Pancreatic tissue and juice contains a polypeptide called pancreatic secretory trypsin inhibitor (PSTI) which forms an inactive complex with trypsin and its percursor, trypsinogen. The inhibitor is sometimes named Kazal pancreatic secretory inhibitor after its discoverer. It is a small protein containing 56 amino acid residues, and is now known to be present in gastric juice and throughout the gastrointestinal tract, suggesting that it offers widespread protection against the destructive activity of luminal proteases (Freeman et al 1990).

Plasma protease inhibitors

Normal plasma contains a number of protease inhibitors which can bind and inactivate circulating proteases. It is now known that α_1-antitrypsin inactivates a number of proteases other than trypsin so that it should be called α_1-protease inhibitor. Enzymes inactivated in this way include chymotrypsin and elastase. Although the main function of α_1-protease inhibitor may be inactivation of elastase released from neutrophils, it has an important protective role in acute pancreatitis, inactivating precursors such as chymotrypsinogen as well as their active enzymes. Endopeptidases are irreversibly inhibited by α_2-macroglobulin, forming complexes which are cleared rapidly from the blood stream by the reticuloendothelial system. In contrast to the complexes between trypsin and α_1-protease inhibitor (which are completely inactive), α_2-macroglobulin–trypsin complexes retain some proteolytic activity and can activate enzymes such as chymotrypsin and trypsin. It follows that in acute pancreatitis much depends on the ability of the reticuloendothelial system to clear complexes rapidly from the circulation.

A number of other protease inhibitors have been described (e.g. α_1-antichymotrypsin) but they are of doubtful significance in pancreatic disease. It is probable that their principal function is to inhibit proteolytic enzymes released from circulating white blood cells.

Pancreatic secretory patterns (see Di Magno 1986)

Pancreatic exocrine secretion can be regarded as occurring in three phases, each being coordinated with upper gastrointestinal secretion and motility, and with entry of bile into the duodenum. A *cephalic phase* is probably present in man and may be vagally mediated; it is triggered by mastication of food, is short-lived, and results in much less enzyme secretion than that evoked by CCK. It is followed by a *postprandial digestive phase* which is triggered by eating and which is hormonally and neurally mediated. The digestive pattern may persist for 5–7 hours after eating so that in many individuals it persists throughout the day and during the initial hours of sleep. Once the upper gastrointestinal tract is cleared of food, an *interdigestive phase* persists until feeding once again triggers digestive activity. Four phases of interdigestive activity are recognized: phase 1 is characterized by minimal secretory activity; phase 2 by a burst of motor and secretory activity; phase 3 by diminution of secretion, and phase 4 by a short period of irregular contractile activity. The phasic cycle is repeated every 60–90 minutes as long as food is not ingested.

PANCREATIC DUCTAL SYSTEM

Structure

The terminal or intercalated ducts (ductules) of the pancreatic duct system are surrounded by the acinar cells responsible for enzyme secretion. These terminal ducts are lined by irregular flat or cuboidal centroacinar cells which are wedged between the larger acinar cells. The terminal ducts lead to progressively larger intralobular and interlobular ducts which drain to the main pancreatic duct. The centroacinar cells and cells lining the intralobular ducts have a smooth luminal surface (in contrast to the numerous microvilli of the acinar cells) but have a relatively poorly formed Golgi complex and rough endoplasmic reticulum. The centroacinar and intralobular duct cells have elaborate interdigitations of their lateral and basal plasma membranes, a feature shared by other cells engaged in fluid and ion transport such as the cells of the proximal convoluted tubule of the kidney. Many of the cells lining the smaller ducts and ductules possess a single cilium which projects into the lumen (Fig. 3.2). The function of these cilia is uncertain but they may have a sensory role or facilitate the flow of viscous pancreatic juice into the larger calibre ducts.

The interlobular ducts are lined by pyramidal cells which possess microvilli on their luminal surface and contain more numerous secretory granules. The granules may contain mucoprotein, some of which could remain as a protective coating or barrier on the luminal surface of the major branches of the ductal system. The main pancreatic duct is lined by columnar cells which also possess microvilli and contain secretory granules (Fig. 3.3). These cells undergo rapid turnover with exfoliation and replacement, and are interspersed with mucin-producing goblet cells and endocrine cells which do not appear to communicate with the duct lumen. The main ducts also possess branching tubular glands which protrude into the

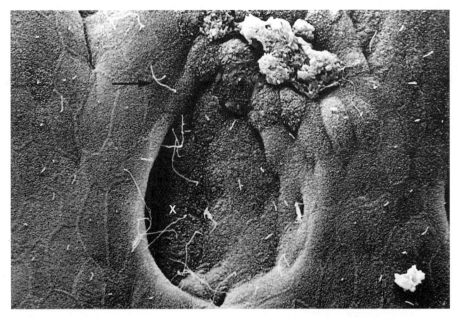

Fig. 3.2 Scanning electron micrograph of cat pancreatic duct showing surface contours of individual ephithelial cells some of which possess a solitary cilium (arrowed example) which protrudes into the lumen of the duct. The point of entry of a tributary duct is shown at X (× 520).

surrounding connective tissue. In contrast to many other exocrine glands, the duct system of the pancreas does not possess myoepithelial cells, opening the possibility that ductal distention could more easily produce rupture of the ducts (Case & Argent 1986).

At their termination, the common bile duct and main pancreatic duct are encircled by a small smooth muscle sphincter, the sphincter of Oddi (Fig. 3.4). The two ducts form a common channel prior to opening into the duodenal lumen in some 80% of individuals (Hand 1963). In addition to regulating the flow of bile and

pancreatic juice into the duodenum, the sphincter of Oddi may prevent reflux of duodenal content. Additional factors which may help to reduce reflux include the oblique passage of the ducts through the duodenal wall and the presence of mucosal 'valvules' within their lumen.

Functional studies in man show that activity of the sphincter of Oddi is characterized by phasic contractions superimposed on a modest basal pressure (see Toouli 1990). The phasic contractions are present at all times and throughout interdigestive motor activity, but they are

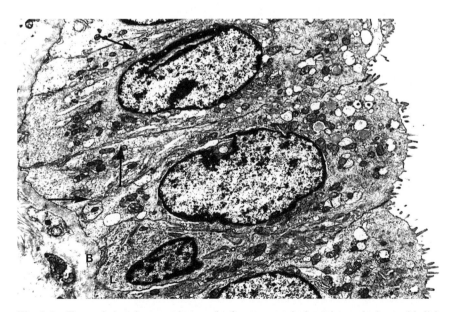

Fig. 3.3 Transmission electron micrograph of cat pancreatic duct system. An intraepithelial lymphocyte (L) is shown just above the basal lamina (B). The arrows point to the intercellular boundaries which are separated by a minimal intercellular space. Note the surface microvilli (× 3500).

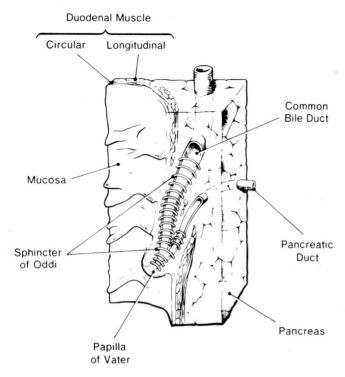

Duodenal Muscle

Circular   Longitudinal

Mucosa

Sphincter
of Oddi

Common
Bile Duct

Pancreatic
Duct

Pancreas

Papilla
of Vater

Fig. 3.4 Schematic representation of the sphincter of Oddi in man showing the circular smooth muscle sphincter which surrounds the termination of the common bile duct and the pancreatic duct. The pancreatic duct has a shorter length of sphincter than the bile duct. Most of the sphincter lies within the wall of the duodenum (Toouli 1984). Reproduced from The British Journal of Surgery 71: 251, by permission of the publishers, Butterworth–Heinemann Ltd.

independent of duodenal motor activity. The phasic contractions are thought to propel small volumes of fluid into the duodenum, but in conjunction with the basal sphincter tone they provide a small resistance to flow of bile and pancreatic juice. Feeding results in a fall in wave amplitude and duration (but not contraction frequency) with a lowering of basal sphincter pressure (Worthley et al 1989). Intravenous injection of CCK-8 inhibits the phasic contractions of the sphincter of Oddi (Geenen et al 1980, Toouli et al 1982), an effect thought to be mediated by the non-adrenergic, non-cholinergic nerves supplying the sphincter muscle (Behar & Biancani 1980). It is tempting to assume that CCK released by a meal allows sphincter relaxation while at the same time contracting the gallbladder and stimulating pancreatic secretion. However, there is still debate as to whether the observed effects of CCK-8 are pharmacological or physiological (Worthley et al 1989). Increased intraluminal pressure in the proximal biliary tree and gallbladder also reduces resistance to flow across the feline sphincter (Thune et al 1986), and neural control of the sphincter appears to involve both an excitatory and an inhibitory pathway (Behar & Biancani 1984). In man, the termination of the pancreatic duct may also be encircled by a distinct short pancreatic duct sphincter (Fig. 3.4);

there is evidence that secretin relaxes this sphincter thus facilitating the flow of pancreatic juice (Carr-Locke et al 1985).

Disturbances of the sphincter of Oddi such as sphincter stenosis and dyskinesia may be clinically important causes of biliary and pancreatic disease. Forms of sphincter dyskinesia which have been suggested include increased phasic contraction, elevated basal pressure, excessive retrograde contraction and a paradoxical response (contraction) to CCK (Toouli 1990). Morphine and other opioids are known to cause 'spasm' of the sphincter of Oddi, a factor which may have relevance in the conservative treatment of acute pancreatitis. The mechanisms involved are complex and appear to involve more than one type of opioid receptor; although cholinergic nerves do not mediate the effects of morphine they may modulate spontaneous motor activity in the sphincter (Helm et al 1988).

Pancreatic ductal function

Hollander and Birnbaum (1952) elaborated the concept that pancreatic juice contains four components:

1. mucus produced by cells lining the major ducts
2. enzymes produced by the acinar cells
3. a chloride-containing fluid (which is now known to be secreted predominantly by acinar cells rather than derived from interstitial extracellular fluid)
4. bicarbonate secreted by the centroacinar and duct cells (and produced predominantly by the cells of the small interlobular ducts).

We now appreciate that the variations in anion composition of pancreatic juice are due to secondary exchange of secreted HCO_3^- for Cl^- in the duct system, rather than the mixing of different proportions of the primary secretions of the acini and ducts. Secretin (and perhaps VIP acting as a neurotransmitter) is the stimulus to ductal HCO_3^- secretion and although its action may be potentiated by CCK and vagal stimulation, these agencies acting singly have little or no effect on HCO_3^- production by the ducts. As in so many areas of pancreatic physiology there are major species differences. For example, in the rat the ductal response to secretin is minimal whereas CCK causes the acinar cells to secrete Cl^--rich juice in amounts which are at least as large as the ductal component of secretion. In contrast, the hamster resembles man in that there is little spontaneous secretion, secretin evokes secretion rich in HCO_3^-, and CCK has little effect on electrolyte secretion (Ali et al 1990).

Ductal secretory mechanisms

Our understanding of the process of duct secretion has been based largely on studies involving perfused pancreas preparations, with more recent clarification from studies using cultured duct cells and isolated duct fragments. A number of models for HCO_3^- secretion have been proposed. In one of the most recent, it is proposed that the number of Cl^- channels in the luminal plasma membrane is increased by elevation of intracellular cyclic AMP concentration in response to secretin (Gray et al 1988). In addition, the cell membranes possess both $Cl^- : HCO_3^-$ and $Na^+ : H^+$ exchange proteins (Novak & Greger 1988, Stuenkel et al 1988), allowing transfer of bicarbonate to the duct lumen. Given that the acini produce Cl^--containing fluid, plentiful amounts of Cl^- are available within the lumen for apical exchange (Fig. 3.5). The model embraces a pump for active HCO_3^- transport and a shunt whereby cations pass through the intercellular junctional complexes. In this and similar models, pancreatic HCO_3^- secretion requires the presence of carbonic anhydrase and Na^+, K^+-adenosine triphosphatase (ATPase) activity. Carbonic anhydrase activity in the pancreas is localized specifically to ductal epithelium (Kumpulainen & Jalovaara 1981, Buanes et al 1986) and in various animals studied, Na^+,K^+-ATPase activity is confined to or highest in the centroacinar and duct cells (Buanes et al 1986, Smith et al 1987). The importance of Na^+,K^+-ATPase rests on its ability to maintain a low intracellular Na^+ concentration so that the Na^+ gradient across the basolateral plasma membranes can provide energy for the movement of other ions. Charge balance during secretion is maintained by K^+ leaving the cell through channels in the basolateral membrane. The importance of species differences cannot be overemphasized and while further work is needed to refine our understanding of secretory mechanisms in man, Cl^- channels have been described recently in human fetal pancreatic ductal epithelium (Gray et al 1989).

Secretin receptors

Studies in acinar cells have revealed two types of secretin receptor, one 'secretin-preferring' and the other 'VIP-preferring', but comparable studies in pancreatic duct cells are lacking. It is presumed that secretin acts on high affinity receptors in the plasma cell membrane of the ductal epithelium with internalization of the hormone-receptor complex and activation of adenyl cyclase to release cyclic AMP. In contrast to the situation in some species, effects of VIP on human pancreatic function have been difficult to discern.

The pancreatic duct mucosal barrier

In this concept, the pancreatic ductal epithelium represents a barrier to back diffusion of HCO_3^- ions in a manner comparable to the ability of the gastric mucosal barrier to resist back-diffusion of H^+ (Reber et al 1979). The duct does allow some movement of HCO_3^- down its concentration gradient from the duct lumen when tested at low perfusion rates but under physiological circumstances, little HCO_3^- is lost from the lumen. The mucosa is normally impermeable to macromolecules but when damaged by agents such as aspirin, ethanol or bile salts (Figs. 3.6, 3.7), marked anion flux and movement of larger molecules takes place (Harvey et al 1989, Simpson et al 1983). Such damage to the pancreatic duct mucosal barrier may be implicated in acute pancreatitis.

HORMONAL CONTROL OF PANCREATIC SECRETION

Cholecystokinin

In 1928 Ivy & Oldberg reported that food (and especially fat) liberated a hormone from the duodenal mucosa which caused the gallbladder to contract and empty; accordingly they named the hormone 'cholecystokinin' (CCK). Subsequently, Harper & Vass (1941) found that intraduodenal peptone stimulated pancreatic enzyme secretion in anaesthetized cats, even after all neural connections had been divided. Further study (Harper & Raper 1943) revealed that a hormone other than secretin

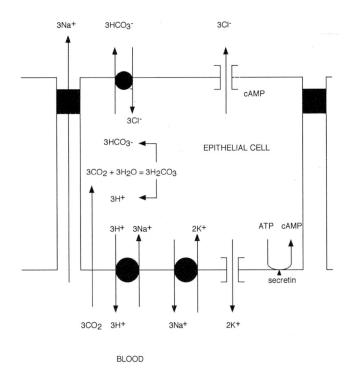

Fig. 3.5 Model for the electrogenic secretion of bicarbonate by the pancreatic ductal epithelium based on patch clamp studies in rat epithelium as described by Gray et al (1988). The activity of the chloride channel is modulated by secretin and the release of cyclic AMP (cAMP). The intercellular junctional complexes are represented as solid blocks between adjacent epithelial cells.

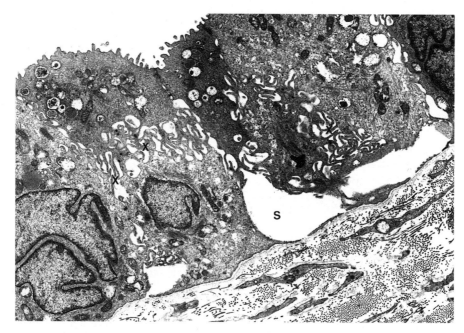

Fig. 3.6 Transmission electron micrograph of cat pancreatic duct after perfusion with 40 mmol/l sodium taurocholate solution at a pressure of 5 mmHg. No cellular damage is apparent but the lateral contact surfaces (X) are more elaborate than normal and basal intercellular spaces (S) are present (× 4300).

(see below) was responsible and that this hormone, named 'pancreozymin' (PZ), stimulated pancreatic enzyme secretion in a manner similar to vagal excitation (which until that time had been regarded as the only mechanism for enzyme release). Jorpes and Mutt (1966) working with porcine duodenal extracts, eventually concluded that the cholecystokinin and pancreozymin activity both resided in a single basic peptide having 33 amino acid residues (CCK 33) and which they called cholecystokinin-pancreozymin (CCK-PZ). Since then the hormone has come to be known simply as cholecystokinin (CCK). CCK has homology with gastrin in that the C-terminal pentapeptide sequence of the two hormones is identical, explaining the overlap in their biological activities and their cross-reactivity in immunoassay.

Like gastrin, CCK may exist in a number of different molecular forms. The primary translational product of CCK messenger RNA comprises 115 amino acids but a shorter form, CCK-58, now appears to be the major stored form of the hormone in man and may also represent its major circulating form (Eysselein et al 1990). In addition to CCK-33 other variants which may have physiological significance include CCK-39, CCK-33, CCK-22 and CCK-8. The biological activity of CCK residues in the C-terminal part of the molecule and the C-terminal octapeptide (CCK-8) appears to be at least as potent on a molar basis as larger molecular forms such as CCK-33 and CCK-39. On the other hand, larger molecules may have a longer circulating half-life and it is conceivable that extension of the N-terminal end of the

molecule makes it resistant to degradation (Dale et al 1989).

Pancreatic acinar cells appear to have two types of CCK receptor, one with high affinity but low capacity, the other with low affinity but high capacity (Matozaki et al 1989, Yu et al 1990). It is also possible that CCK may bind to a third pancreatic gastrin receptor in some species (Yu et al 1990), but the functional significance of these different binding sites remains unclear.

Our understanding of the signal transduction mechanisms involved in CCK stimulation of the pancreatic acinar cell remains incomplete (for discussion of recent advances, see Case 1989, 1990a, b). Occupation of the CCK receptor appears to lead to activation of phospholipase C with production of two intracellular messengers, namely inositol 1,4,5-triphosphate (IP_3) and diacylglycerol (DAG). Each of these messengers is capable of stimulating enzyme secretion; IP_3 does so by mobilizing Ca^{2+} while DAG activates protein kinase C. Occupation of muscarinic (cholinergic) receptors by acetylcholine appears to trigger acinar secretion by the same transduction pathway. Activation of phospholipase C involves a guanine nucleotide-binding protein (G-protein) which in addition to coupling the occupied receptor to phospholipase C also couples it to phospholipase A_2. This latter enzyme liberates arachidonic acid which in turn could serve as a negative feedback regulator; although arachidonic acid could become involved in eicosanoid synthesis, there is no firm evidence that prostaglandins have a physiological role in controlling pancreatic enzyme secretion.

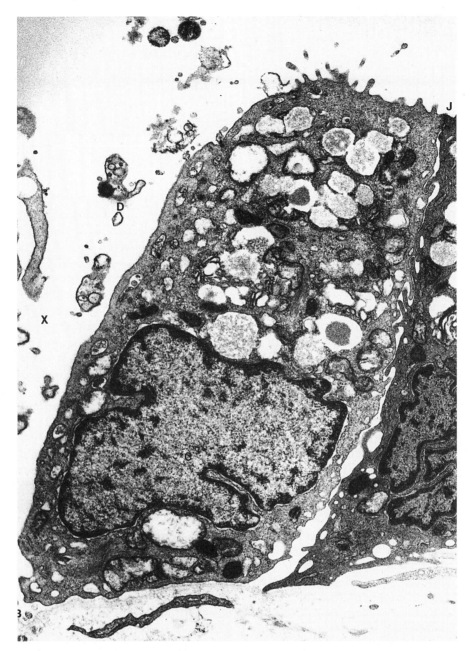

Fig. 3.7 Transmission electron micrograph from cat pancreatic duct showing effect of perfusion with 40 mmol/l sodium taurocholate solution at a pressure of 30 mmHg. Disintegrated epithelial cells have left debris (D) and wide gaps (X) down to the basal lamina (B). Cells adjacent to the gap show reactive change but are intact and remain firmly attached to their neighbours with normal junctional complexes (J) (× 6000).

CCK release and pancreatic secretion

Only insignificant amounts of CCK are released during the cephalic and gastric phases of pancreatic secretion (Anagnostides et al 1984); it is the presence of secretagogues in the duodenum that stimulates the release of CCK and consequent release of pancreatic enzymes. Products of fat and protein digestion serve as the major secretagogues, and fatty acids (such as oleic acid) and amino acids (such as tryptophan and phenylalanine) are equipotent in this regard (Dale et al 1989). Studies in dogs and man have shown that:

1. neutral fat does not stimulate CCK release and has first to be digested to fatty acids by pancreatic enzymes (Watanabe et al 1988)
2. the degree of emulsification of the fatty acid is as important as the dose (Olsen et al 1989)
3. unsaturated fatty acids such as oleic acid evoke much greater CCK release than saturated fatty acids such as stearic acid (Beardshall et al 1989).

In contrast to earlier views, hydrochloric acid is no longer thought to stimulate CCK release (Dale et al 1989). In the rat, tetrodotoxin does not block CCK release, implying that in this species at least, mural nerves are not involved in its release by luminal secretagogues (Cuber et al 1989).

In a study in human volunteers, Fried and colleagues (1989) examined the pancreatic (trypsin) and biliary (bile salt) secretory response to a variety of meals instilled intragastrically. An elemental diet (amino acids 7 g % with dextrose 21 g %) proved as effective a stimulant as a polymeric diet (albumin 7 g % with dextrose 21 g %) but the response to either meal was less than that induced by a maximal intravenous dose of CCK 8. A carbohydrate meal (dextrose 21 g % alone) produced a similar pancreaticobiliary secretory response but this was accompanied by lower circulating CCK levels than were observed with protein or amino acid meals. These observations question the contention that elemental diets may 'rest' the pancreas and call into doubt the belief that trypsin secretion is the exclusive property of CCK. Intragastric distension with normal saline is also known to stimulate pancreatic secretion, and the observed response to dextrose alone in these studies suggests that a neural reflex (mediated in all probability by cholinergic vagal pathways) is responsible.

Fried and colleagues (1988) have also studied the relationship between gastric emptying of a mixed meal, the release of various hormones including CCK, and the stimulation of pancreatico-biliary secretion. Plasma CCK levels and pancreaticobiliary secretion rose to a maximum 30–60 minutes after ingestion of the meal and thereafter declined gradually, despite continuing entry of fat and protein into the duodenum. This decline could not be explained on the basis of 'exhaustion' of the exocrine secretory capacity of the pancreas, and the authors suggest that the high levels of plasma PP and peptide YY observed in the later stages of the experiment might have inhibited pancreatic secretion and/or CCK release.

The role of vagal influences on CCK release remains controversial. Earlier reports suggested that the plasma CCK response to a Lundh meal in man was not affected by atropine whereas the pancreatic response was markedly reduced (Bozkurt et al 1988). However, electrical vagal stimulation has been shown to double circulating CCK levels in dogs by a mechanism at least partly sensitive to atropine (Kim et al 1989). Studies in dispersed canine CCK-containing intestinal cells have shown that L-amino acids have a direct stimulatory effect but that this effect can be blocked by carbachol (Barber et al 1986), supporting the concept of a tonic vagal inhibitory influence on the CCK cell. Further study is also needed to clarify the interrelationship between CCK and vagal mechanisms in controlling pancreatic enzyme secretion. Kim and colleagues (1989) have shown that CCK receptor antagonists reduce vagally-stimulated pancreatic secretion in dogs, suggesting that CCK release contributes to observed vagal effects. As will be discussed later, Adler and colleagues (1991) have produced evidence from studies in

volunteers that human pancreatic enzyme secretion may be dependent upon cholinergic tone, with CCK exercising a modulatory role in the secretory response.

The problem of interaction between neural and hormonal mechanisms is complicated further by the presence in the digestive system of potential neurotransmitters other than acetylcholine. For example, gastrin-releasing peptide (GRP) may prove to be a peptidergic neurotransmitter acting not only on CCK release but as a direct stimulant of the acinar cell. Similarly, vasoactive intestinal peptide (VIP) may be released by vagal stimulation and could also be responsible for the atropine-insensitive component of vagally-induced CCK release (Case 1990a).

While there is general agreement that CCK has a major role in the regulation of pancreatic exocrine secretion, recent studies with the potent CCK antagonist, loxiglumide, have shown that enzyme production is not abolished by such antagonism (Schwarzendrube et al 1991). Meal-stimulated output of amylase, trypsin and chymotrypsin in human volunteers was decreased by 55–70% relative to control values, and only minor reductions in duodenal volume were noted. It was concluded that CCK is probably not involved in the regulation of pancreatic fluid or bicarbonate secretion, although the latter could not be measured directly in the test meal experiments. In these studies, loxiglumide also failed to alter the increase in circulating levels of glucose, insulin and C-peptide produced by the test meal, calling into question any role for CCK as an important stimulant of insulin secretion in man.

There is abundant evidence from animal experiments that exogenous CCK in addition to stimulating pancreatic secretion, also evokes pancreatic hypertrophy and hyperplasia (Solomon 1981, Howatson & Carter 1985). The trypsin inhibitor, camostate, produces pancreatic hypertrophy and hyperplasia when given chronically to rats (Goke et al 1986, Otsuki et al 1987) an effect which is probably mediated by increased circulating levels of CCK (see below). Camostate-induced pancreatic growth can be abolished by CCK antagonists (Wisner et al 1988), supporting further the concept that CCK is important in the maintenance of pancreatic growth.

Inhibition of CCK release

In the rat, pancreatic enzyme secretion was shown to be inhibited by intraduodenal instillation of trypsin alone or bile in conjunction with pancreatic juice; on the other hand, pancreatic secretion was stimulated by infusing trypsin inhibitors or by diversion of bile and pancreatic juice (Green & Lyman 1972). The concept developed that feedback control of pancreatic secretion by intraluminal trypsin was mediated by a humoral agent originating in the duodenum–jejunum. CCK has now been confirmed as the humoral agent responsible (Louie et al

1986) and interest has centred recently on the mechanism(s) whereby intraluminal trypsin might suppress CCK release.

There is now evidence that CCK secretion in the rat is regulated by a trypsin-sensitive CCK-releasing factor with a molecular weight of between 1000 and 5000 which is secreted by the proximal small intestine (Lu et al 1989, Miyasaka et al 1989b). Rapid intestinal wash-through with phosphate-buffered saline inhibited plasma CCK release (and pancreatic enzyme secretion), although CCK levels rose with reinfusion of concentrated intestinal wash-out fluid. The stimulatory action of the concentrated perfusate was unaffected by boiling but abolished by incubation with trypsin. Diversion of bile and pancreatic juice increased plasma CCK levels and pancreatic enzyme secretion under basal conditions in fasted rats, suggesting that the factor responsible for CCK release might be tonically secreted into the proximal small bowel. There is debate regarding whether secretion of this CCK-releasing peptide is dependent on cholinergic input (Levan & Green 1986, Lu et al 1989, Guan et al 1990).

A further putative trypsin-sensitive CCK-releasing peptide has been isolated, purified and sequenced in rat bile-pancreatic juice (see Iwai et al 1988). This 61-amino acid peptide, or 'monitor peptide' is thought to compete with food for intraluminal trypsin. In this concept, dietary protein acts as a substrate for trypsin, allowing the monitor peptide to survive to release CCK and so stimulate pancreatic secretion. In the presence of excess intraluminal trypsin, the monitor peptide is hydrolysed to an inactive form, so removing the stimulus to CCK release. To make matters even more complex there is now evidence that secretin as well as CCK is involved in negative feedback regulation of pancreatic secretion by intraluminal protease in the rat (Li et al 1990a, and see below).

It must be stressed that while inhibition of CCK release by intraluminal trypsin has been demonstrated in the rat, other species may not share this mechanism for feedback regulation. For example, diversion of pancreatic juice does not increase plasma CCK levels in dogs (Kogire et al 1989). Similarly, CCK release induced by luminal oleic acid in dogs is not affected by trypsin infusion although pancreatic secretion is inhibited (Shiratori et al 1989).

In man, the existence of feedback inhibition remains controversial. In human volunteers, inhibition of intraduodenal trypsin did not stimulate pancreatic secretion (Dlugosz et al 1983, Hotz et al 1983). On the other hand, Slaff and colleagues (1984) found that duodenal perfusion of pharmacological amounts of proteases (but not amlyase or lipase) suppressed pancreatic secretion in patients with chronic pancreatitis and that pancreatic extract also decreased abdominal pain. Isaksson & Ihse (1983) also reported reduction in the pain of chronic pancreatitis following pancreatic enzyme administration

in a controlled study. However, these indirect demonstrations of feedback inhibition in man have required pharmacological amounts of intraluminal trypsin (i.e. 10–100 times greater than those achieved physiologically), and others have even reported that pancreatic extracts actually increase pancreatic enzyme secretion (Mössner et al 1989). With the advent of CCK radioimmunoassay, Olsen and colleagues (1988) failed to demonstrate inhibition of oleate-induced release of CCK, secretin or pancreatic enzymes by trypsin in healthy volunteers. Similarly, while Adler and colleagues (1988, 1989) showed an increase in pancreatic enzyme output in healthy volunteers following duodenal instillation of trypsin inhibitor (camostate), the effect was not associated with rises in plasma CCK concentration nor could it be blocked by CCK receptor antagonist (loxiglumide). However, the effect of camostate could be blocked by atropine, implying that feedback inhibition in man involves a cholinergic mechanism. Further study is clearly needed to confirm the presence of a trypsin-sensitive negative feedback mechanism controlling CCK release in man. Of interest, bile salt sequestration by cholestryramine enhances the CCK response to luminal nutrients in both dog and man (Gomez et al 1988) offering an additional potential means of feedback control involving luminal bile salts.

As mentioned above, plasma CCK levels fall approximately 1 hour after ingestion of a meal, despite continued gastric emptying of fat and protein, and it has been suggested that hormones such as PP, peptide YY, glucagon or somatostatin could also function as inhibitors of CCK release and so reduce pancreatic exocrine secretion (Fried et al 1988).

Secretin

Pavlov and his co-workers were aware that the presence of various substances, notably acids, in the duodenum stimulated pancreatic exocrine secretion. However, this was attributed to a neural reflex until Bayliss and Starling (1902) showed that intraduodenal acid still stimulated the pancreas after all accessible nervous connections had been divided. Intravenous acid was not effective, whereas intravenous administration of acidified duodenal extract caused a copious flow of pancreatic juice, an effect attributed by Bayliss and Starling to a chemical messenger or hormone, which we now know as secretin. In 1962, Jorpes and colleagues announced the isolation of secretin from hog duodenal mucosa in the form of a strongly basic peptide containing 27 amino acid residues, and Bodanszky and co-workers (1966) were subsequently able to synthesize the secretin molecule.

In contrast to CCK, the amino-terminal end of the secretin molecule appears to be important in its biological activity but to date there appears to be only one molecular form of secretin. Secretin precursors or active fragments of the parent molecule have not been reported. However, as mentioned above, secretin has sequence homology with VIP and with some other non-gastro-intestinal peptides such as growth hormone-releasing factor. Immunocytochemical studies suggest that secretin immunoreactivity in man is confined to mucosal endocrine cells found within the crypts and villi of the proximal small intestine (Usellini et al 1990).

Stimulation of secretin release

There appear to be three mechanisms for secretin release:

1. Intraduodenal acidification is the major stimulant of secretin release and the consequent flow of bicarbonate-rich juice from the pancreatic ductal system. Recent studies indicate that release of secretin in rats may be mediated by a secretin-releasing factor which appears in the intestinal lumen after acid perfusion and which loses its activity when exposed to trypsin (Li et al 1990a). The intraluminal threshold for secretin release is pH 4.5, and the amount released depends on the acid load entering the duodenum. In turn there is a linear relationship between plasma secretin concentrations and pancreatic HCO_3^- secretion.

2. Intraduodenal fatty acids, such as oleic acid, also stimulate secretin release even when infused at pH 6 (Schaffalitzky de Muckadell et al 1986). The threshold for secretin release by fatty acids is higher than that for CCK and the degree of emulsification of the fatty acid is important (Olsen et al 1989).

3. Intraduodenal bile salts stimulate pancreatic bicarbonate secretion by a mechanism which appears to involve secretin release (Riepl et al 1990).

Secretin release by fatty acids and by HCl does not appear to be under cholinergic control, and vagal stimulation does not in itself cause the release of secretin. Indeed, there is no significant direct cephalic or gastric phase of secretin release or pancreatic bicarbonate secretion. However, infusion of exogenous secretion in physiological doses in dogs does not stimulate as much HCO_3^- secretion as a meat meal (Kim et al 1979), and other factors such as vagal stimulation, CCK and peptidergic neurotransmitters, may augment or potentiate the physiological effect of secretin on pancreatic duct function (see below).

Inhibition of secretin release

As mentioned earlier, there have been recent suggestions that secretin release may be subject to 'feedback inhibition' in a manner similar to that postulated for CCK.

In dogs, oleate-induced rises in plasma secretin are attenuated by simultaneous perfusion of the duodenum with trypsin or pancreatic juice (Shiratori et al 1989), while in rats, plasma secretin levels rise after diversion of pancreatic juice from the duodenum (Sun et al 1989). However, in human volunteers trypsin failed to inhibit the release of secretin by intraduodenal oleic acid (Olsen et al 1988) and the existence of feedback inhibition remains in doubt.

Interaction between CCK and secretin

Neither CCK nor secretin given alone in physiological doses can call forth the output of pancreatic juice produced by a meal. However, at least in terms of bicarbonate secretion, CCK-8 is known to potentiate the actions of secretin (You et al 1983, Olsen et al 1986), and endogenous CCK release is thought to be as important as secretin as a stimulant of pancreatic bicarbonate secretion in response to feeding in dogs (Jo et al 1991). The two hormones thus appear to interact in the control of pancreatic secretion following a meal and the potentiation can be reduced by atropine, implying interaction of hormonal and neural mechanisms (see below). Similarly, secretin has been shown to potentiate the effect of low doses of CCK on rat pancreatic protein secretion (Haarstad & Petersen 1988).

Other potential hormonal/chemical stimulants

Insulin

The effect of insulin on pancreatic exocrine secretion will be considered in the section on islet–acinar relationships (p. 44).

Gastrin-releasing peptide

Bombesin is a tetradecapeptide first isolated form the skin of the frog Bombina bombina. It is a potent stimulant of pancreatic enzyme secretion in a number of species with a variable effect on fluid and electrolyte secretion. Its mammalian counterpart, gastrin-releasing peptide (GRP), shares with bombesin the ability to release CCK, gastrin and pancreatic polypeptide in dogs (Konturek et al 1989), opening the possibility that GRP is an indirect pancreatic stimulant. However, the acinar cells possess GRP/bombesin receptors and in man, the CCK antagonist loxiglumide does not inhibit the stimulation of pancreatic bicarbonate or enzyme secretion by bombesin (Hildebrand et al 1990), suggesting that GRP may also act directly on the pancreas. In dogs, CCK antagonists reduce but do not abolish the stimulation of pancreatic enzyme and fluid secretion by GRP (Hosotani et al

1989), indicating that GRP may have both a direct and indirect effect in this species. It remains uncertain whether GRP is a physiological stimulant of pancreatic secretion and it may yet prove to be a neurotransmitter.

Neurotensin

Neurotensin is a tridecapeptide which is present in endocrine cells in ileal mucosa and in nerve bodies of cerebral nuclei. It is a stimulant of pancreatic acini which could prove to be involved in the intestinal phase of pancreatic exocrine secretion (Feurle & Niestroj 1991).

Thyroxine

It is well recognized experimentally that thyroidectomy retards pancreatic growth and decreases enzyme synthesis and secretion, effects which can be countered by administration of thyroxine (see Gullo et al 1991). Tri-iodothyronine nuclear receptors have been demonstrated in rat pancreas (Lee et al 1989), suggesting that the gland is a target for this hormone. Gullo and colleagues (1991) have now shown that pancreatic exocrine function in man is reduced in hypothyroidism but returns to normal following treatment with thyroxine. The mechanisms responsible for pancreatic insufficiency in hypothyroidism are uncertain but thyroxine could act by stimulating enzyme synthesis, by stimulating amino acid transport, and by exerting a trophic effect akin to that exerted by CCK. An additional factor may be inhibition of pancreatic amino acid uptake, enzyme synthesis and secretion by the high circulating levels of thyrotropin-releasing hormone which occur in hypothyroidism (Wolf et al 1984, Gullo 1991). Gullo and his co-workers (1982) have also shown that pancreatic function also depends on intact adrenocortical function.

Calcium

Acute hypercalcaemia is a potent stimulus of pancreatic enzyme secretion (Goebell et al 1973) and may be implicated in the pathogenesis of pancreatitis. The mechanisms involved are uncertain but release of stimulatory gastrointestinal peptides or cholinergic excitation cannot fully explain the observed effects of hypercalcaemia (see Layer et al 1987). Studies in isolated cat pancreatic lobules have now shown that increasing calcium concentration (5 or 10 mmol/l) increases the discharge of protein, amylase and chymotrypsin (Layer et al 1987). The effect of increasing calcium concentration was similar to the maximal effect of caerulein or carbachol, and could not be blocked by atropine. Thus it appears that rises in extracellular calcium concentration can stimulate pancreatic secretion and this may have both physiological and pathophysiological significance.

Inhibition of pancreatic secretion

Somatostatin

Somatostatin is a polypeptide containing 14 amino acid residues. It is produced by pancreatic D cells which are present in all islets and it is also distributed widely throughout the digestive system. Infusion of somatostatin suppresses secretion induced in man by exogenous secretin, duodenal acidification and feeding (Hanssen et al 1977) while its analogue somatostatin 201–995 reduces pancreatic secretion induced in dogs by CCK-8 plus secretin and also reduces plasma concentrations of CCK, secretin, motilin and PP (Misumi et al 1988). On the other hand, while somatostatin inhibits rat pancreatic endocrine secretion in vitro it does not block exocrine secretion (Muller et al 1988) despite the fact that acinar cells appear to possess somatostatin receptors (Knuhtsen et al 1988, Matozaki et al 1988). Gullo and colleagues (1987) have also reported that low-dose infusion of somatostatin does not inhibit exocrine secretion induced by caerulein and secretin in man, whereas higher doses inhibit both protein and bicarbonate secretion. The physiological significance of this high-dose inhibition is uncertain. It seems unlikely that somatostatin is a circulating regulator of pancreatic function, but it may influence the pancreas indirectly by decreasing blood flow (Conway et al 1988), modulating neural activity, or regulating the release of other gut hormones such as CCK or secretin.

Pancreatic polypeptide (PP)

This 36-amino acid polypeptide is produced by PP cells located peripherally in the islets of Langerhans, particularly those situated in the middle and inferior portions of the head of the pancreas. PP concentrations in plasma increase after a meal and are greatly enhanced by vagal stimulation, so much so that PP release has been suggested as a test of the completeness of truncal vagotomy if not parietal cell vagotomy (see Konturek et al 1987). Other factors known to evoke PP release include bile salts (Riepl et al 1990) and hormones including CCK and GRP (Miyasaka et al 1989b). The physiological role of PP remains uncertain. Infusion of exogenous PP inhibits enzyme secretion in some species (e.g. Miyasaka et al 1989a) and decreases the uptake of plasma amino acids during pancreatic stimulation with caerulein in man (Gullo 1991). However, despite using doses of PP which achieve plasma concentrations similar to those observed postprandially, it is still not clear whether PP has a physiological role in the feedback regulation of pancreatic exocrine function. Acinar cells do not appear to possess PP receptors and any physiological effects may prove to be indirect or extrapancreatic.

Glucagon

The A cells which produce glucagon are also found peripherally in the islets of Langerhans, and these cells are confined to the superior portion of the head and to the body and tail of the gland. Thus A cells are found exclusively in tissue derived from the embryonic dorsal pancreatic bud whereas PP cells are found in tissue derived principally from the embryonic ventral bud. Glucagon infusion was shown to decrease pancreatic exocrine secretion in intact animals and man in earlier studies (Dyck et al 1969, Konturek et al 1974), but in vitro studies and studies of perfused pancreatic preparations have generally not shown inhibition. More recent studies in anaesthetized dogs have revealed that native glucagon first causes a transient increase in pancreatic juice output followed by inhibition (Itoh et al 1989). The fragment glucagon-(1-21)-peptide produced only inhibition. This may indicate that glucagon has a dual effect on pancreatic function, the intact molecule causing transient stimulation by an effect on blood flow while blockade of the secretin receptor by glucagon or one of its active fragments could produce inhibition. It remains doubtful whether glucagon has a significant physiological role as an inhibitor of pancreatic exocrine secretion, and decreases in plasma amino acid concentration during glucagon infusion in man are probably due to altered hepatic and renal uptake rather than a reflection of pancreatic acinar function (Gullo 1991).

Pancreastatin

Pancreastatin is a 49-amino acid polypeptide first isolated from porcine pancreas. Pancreastatin-like immunoreactivity is present throughout the gastrointestinal tract (including the secretory granules of the B and D cells of the pancreatic islets) and the peptide is known to have an inhibitory effect on insulin release (Tatemoto et al 1986). Pancreastatin has also been shown to inhibit pancreatic exocrine secretion induced by CCK-8 in conscious rats, but its failure to affect enzyme release in vitro (see Miyasaka et al 1990) suggests that any effect on exocrine function is indirect. Subsequent studies in the rat (Miyasaka et al 1990) have shown that pancreastatin inhibits pancreatic exocrine secretion induced by central vagal stimulation (2-deoxy-D-glucose) but not by peripheral cholinergic stimulation (bethanecol, cisapride). Bilateral truncal vagotomy abolished the ability of pancreastatin to inhibit pancreatic exocrine secretion in response to CCK-8. The significance of pancreastatin in pancreatic regulation remains uncertain.

Peptide YY

Peptide YY is structurally related to pancreatic polypeptide and may be responsible for the well-recognized inhibition of pancreatic secretion by food in the distal gut. The peptide has its highest concentrations in the ileum and colon, and its plasma concentrations do not rise until 120 minutes after ingestion of food (Aponte et al 1989). Peptide YY release can be triggered by perfusion of the ileum or colon with oleic acid or oleate, and infusion of exogenous peptide YY inhibits CCK-stimulated flow of biliary and pancreatic secretion (Aponte et al 1989). Like PP, peptide YY inhibits rat pancreatic exocrine secretion in vivo but not in vitro (De Mar et al 1991) and while both agents inhibit both central vagal and peripheral stimulation of pancreatic secretion, central neural stimulation is inhibited preferentially (Putnam et al 1989).

Neuropeptide Y (NPY), a 36-animo acid polypeptide, has strong sequence homology with PP and peptide YY, and NPY-positive neurons are distributed throughout the gastrointestinal tract and pancreas. NPY is a potent inhibitor of pancreatic exocrine secretion in the rat in vivo and in pancreatic lobules in vitro (Mulholland et al 1991) and the peptide may have a physiological role as an inhibitor of pancreatic neurotransmission.

Oxyntomodulin is another potential inhibitor of pancreatic secretion which like peptide YY, is distributed in the ileum and colon.

Calcitonin gene-related peptide (CGRP)

This widely distributed 37-amino acid peptide, which is encoded by the calcitonin gene, has been localized immunohistochemically in nerve terminals of the islets of Langerhans and in islet cells. The exocrine pancreas has few CGRP fibres but CGRP receptors may be present in acinar tissue. Studies in human volunteers indicate that infusion of CGRP, like calcitonin, inhibits pancreatic enzyme output but has no discernible effect on islet hormone release (Beglinger et al 1988). Further study is needed to determine the physiological significance of these findings.

NEURAL CONTROL OF PANCREATIC SECRETION

Extrinsic nerve supply

The main sources of extrinsic nerve supply to the pancreas are the vagus nerves and splanchnic nerves. The anterior and posterior vagi both send branches which may pass directly to the gland or first traverse the preaortic ganglia without interruption. The preganglionic parasympathetic nerve fibres which travel in the vagus nerve are now thought to be derived from the dorsal motor nuclei of the vagi. The nerve fibres enter the gland by passing through the 'capsule' on its upper and lower borders, often in association with the pancreatic blood supply. The fibres terminate in intrapancreatic ganglia scattered throughout the gland. From these ganglia, postganglionic fibres pass directly to the acini and ducts, and to a lesser extent to the islets. The nerve endings on the acinar cells are principally cholinergic, although in some species such as the pig, the vagus contains peptidergic fibres which release VIP (Buanes et al 1986).

The splanchnic nerves innervate the islets of Langerhans, the pancreatic ganglia and the blood vessels. Adrenergic innervation of the pancreas is derived from the fifth to tenth thoracic segments of the spinal cord and the nerve fibres travel in the splanchnic nerves, with or without synapsing in the preaortic ganglia. The splanchnic nerves carry both adrenergic and cholinergic fibres, and it is now appreciated that other neurotransmitters such as VIP, GRP, and substance P may be involved. Most of the adrenergic nerve fibres are distributed to blood vessels; very few end in association with ducts or acini.

It is clear that the conventional division of pancreatic innervation into a cholinergic (parasympathetic) and adrenergic (sympathetic) system is now obsolete, and that we still have much to learn about the role of neuropeptides and peptidergic nerve fibres in the regulation of pancreatic function.

Intrinsic nerve supply

It is now appreciated that like the gut, the pancreas has an intrinsic nervous system which although closely linked to the central nervous system, exerts significant intrinsic control of pancreatic activity. This 'intrapancreatic nervous system' is complex and can generate true reflexes and control important tonic activity. The intrapancreatic system contains intrinsic cholinergic, catecholaminergic and peptidergic neurones, the cholinergic neurones appearing to predominate. Although catecholaminergic cell bodies have not yet been observed in the pancreas, removal of the coeliac and superior mesenteric ganglia still leaves 10% of the catecholaminergic neurones, suggesting that they are part of the intrinsic system or that they are extrinsic nerves which reach the gland by alternative pathways (Anglade et al 1987). Of the various peptidergic neurones described, VIP and GRP neurones seem to be particularly common. Both of these peptides are released during vagal stimulation in pigs and presumably are involved in the control of pancreatic secretion (Knuhtsen et al 1987, Holst et al 1987).

Neural mechanisms and pancreatic secretion

Electrical stimulation of the vagus stimulates pancreatic secretion in a number of species and it seems likely that there are excitatory and inhibitory centres in the hypothalamus and/or brain stem. Studies in dogs (Furukawa

& Okada 1989) have shown that excitatory responses can be blocked by atropine or vagotomy indicating that they are mediated by vagal cholinergic fibres. As mentioned above, electrical vagal stimulation also releases GRP from isolated pig pancreas, and blocking the actions of GRP reduces vagal stimulation of enzyme secretion (Holst et al 1989). Central vagal stimulation (by 2-deoxy-D-glucose) of pancreatic exocrine secretion in rats can be inhibited by pancreastatin (Miyasaka et al 1990).

In dogs, total extrinsic denervation of the pancreas reduces protein secretion in response to intraduodenal amino acid, presumably by interrupting long vagovagal reflexes or short duodenopancreatic reflexes (Kohler et al 1987). Some HCO_3^- and enzyme secretion is still evoked by intraluminal fat or amino acids after truncal vagotomy and coeliac ganglionectomy (Barzilai et al 1987), reinforcing the contention that short duodenopancreatic reflexes are involved. In more recent dog experiments, Singer and colleagues (1989) found that total extrinsic denervation (i.e. truncal vagotomy plus removal of the coeliac and superior mesenteric ganglia) did not affect the pancreatic protein response to CCK (caerulein). Atropine was also without effect, supporting earlier contentions that neither intrinsic nor extrinsic cholinergic pathways modulate the secretory response to CCK. In these studies, truncal vagotomy alone significantly decreased the pancreatic protein secretory response to low loads of intraduodenal amino acid, again suggesting that long cholinergic vagovagal reflexes are involved in the intestinal phase of pancreatic enzyme secretion. Studies in the same dog model suggest that vagal cholinergic fibres are also involved in the HCO_3^- secretory response to intraduodenal acid; these fibres do not appear to be concerned with the regulation of secretin or CCK release, although in the case of CCK this remains controversial (Schafmayer el al 1988; also see earlier discussion).

The existence of a cholinergic pathway which stimulates pancreatic enzyme secretion and augments the response to exogenous secretin and CCK in man is not in dispute (Valenzuela et al 1986). Cholinergic blockade with atropine markedly reduces the pancreatic secretory response to intraluminal nutrients in man without diminishing plasma CCK levels (Bozkurt et al 1988, Brugge et al 1987). Similarly, the stimulation of pancreatic enzyme release by activation of duodenal volume and osmoreceptors, can be abolished by atropine (Owyang et al 1986). There is now good evidence that there is significant interaction between CCK and the cholinergic system in regulation of human pancreatic enzyme secretion. Adler and co-workers (1991) have shown that the pancreatic secretory response to a meal can be blocked completely by atropine whereas loxiglumide produced 60% inhibition (Table 3.2). Each agent significantly inhibited the enzyme response to graded doses of exogenous CCK (caerulein); whereas plasma levels of CCK were unaltered by atropine they

Table 3.2 Pancreatic enzyme output in response to duodenal perfusion of a high calorie meal in man for 120 minutes during intravenous infusion of saline, atropine or the CCK antagonist loxiglumide (Adler et al 1991)

Infusion (i.v.)	Amylase (kIU)	Lipase (kIU)	Trypsin (kIU)
Saline	39 ± 3	708 ± 174	23 ± 4
Loxiglumide	26 ± 2	262 ± 43	9 ± 1
Atropine	0.1 ± 1	41 ± 15	1 ± 1

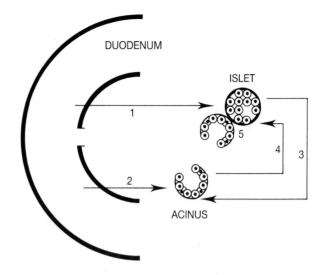

Fig. 3.8 Diagrammatic representation of the various pathways by which chemical messages may be relayed from the duodenum to the pancreatic islets (1) and acini (2), from the islets to the acini through the portal system (3), from the acini to the islets (4), and by direct diffusion from the islets into adjacent acini (5).

were increased by loxiglumide. Thus the study suggests that pancreatic enzyme secretion may be predominantly under cholinergic control, with CCK serving to modulate the secretory response.

Catecholamines inhibit pancreatic HCO_3^- secretion in a number of species including man (Joehl et al 1981) and in part, this appears due to vasoconstriction mediated by adrenergic receptors. In some species, catecholamines may also exert a direct inhibitory effect on ductal cells, the effect again being mediated by adrenergic receptors (Elisha et al 1984, Hubel 1970). However, there is great species variation and in some animals there is evidence for direct stimulation of ductal bicarbonate secretion by β-adrenoreceptors (rat) or dopamine receptors (dog) (see Case & Argent 1986). There is also evidence that humoral agents such as peptide YY may inhibit ductal function, although in the case of agents such as somatostatin and PP, this could be mediated by changes in blood flow or secretin release.

ISLET–ACINAR RELATIONSHIPS

It is now clear that the close anatomical relationship between the islet cells and the acinar cells of the pancreas has important functional significance. Acinar cells in the immediate vicinity of the islets (peri-insular region) may be in direct contact with islet cells so that peptide hormones secreted by the latter can simply diffuse across the adjoining plasma cell membranes. Furthermore, blood draining from the extensive insular capillary network is carried by an islet–acinar portal system to join the capillary network surrounding acinar cells (Fig. 3.8). Although the islets make up only 2% of the weight of the pancreas, their functional importance is reflected in the fact that they receive some 20% of the blood flow to the organ (Lifson et al 1980). The portal system ensures that the acinar cells are exposed to much higher concentrations of peptide messengers produced by the islets than any other cells of the body.

Acinar cells in the peri-insular region are about twice the size of those found in the more distant teleinsular region. Despite this size difference, the cells possess identical organelles and have the same secretory products, although the peri-insular cells contain many more zymogen granules. All acinar cells have high affinity receptors for islet hormones such as insulin and somatostatin (but not

for PP) on their plasma cell membranes (Williams & Goldfine 1985, Garry et al 1989) and the peri-insular cells have many more insulin-binding sites than their teleinsular counterparts. The relationship between islet cells and the exocrine pancreas has been underlined by the observation that in children dying with recent onset type I (insulin-dependent) diabetes, severe acinar cell atrophy surrounds insulin-deficient islets whereas acinar tissue around insulin-containing islets is normal (Foulis & Stewart 1984).

Exogenous or endogenous insulin potentiates the secretory response to CCK in intact animals and in perfused pancreatic preparations, and increases glucose uptake and protein synthesis (Saito et al 1980, Garry et al 1989, Adler & Kern 1975). Insulin appears to influence amylase gene expression and experimental induction of diabetes is accompanied by marked reduction in amylase-specific mRNA; amylase production falls markedly although production of other enzymes is affected more variably (Korc et al 1981). Acini isolated from diabetic rats also show reduced responsiveness to CCK so that insulin may also control expression of the CCK receptor or the membrane proteins involved in signal transduction (Otsuki & Williams, 1983). While overt pancreatic exocrine insufficiency is rare in human type 1 diabetes, the secretory response to CCK and secretin has been shown to be impaired (Lankisch et al 1982).

At one time it was considered that the observed differences between peri-insular and teleinsular cells were attributable solely to exposure to different concentrations of insulin. However, the differences may be even more marked in insulinopenic diabetes, indicating that other hormones may be involved. It is of interest that vagal stimulation rapidly depletes teleinsular cells of their secretory granules while discharge from the peri-insular cells is much slower (see Bendayan 1990).

It is also recognized that the acinar cells may affect islet cells. For example, patients with chronic pancreatitis may develop glucose intolerance because of insufficient insulin release rather than islet destruction by inflammation. Furthermore, hormones such as CCK and secretin which are normally regarded as regulators of exocrine function are known to have an insulinotropic effect. Finally, islet hormones may have feedback regulatory effects on their own rate of production and the production of other hormones. For example insulin exerts negative feedback on insulin production, glucagon may stimulate secretion of somatostatin and insulin, and somatostatin may inhibit production of other islet hormones.

REFERENCES

Adler G, Kern H F 1975 Regulation of exocrine pancreatic secretory process by insulin in vivo. Hormone and Metabolism Research 7: 290–296

Adler G, Mullenhoff A, Bozkurt T, Goke B, Koop L, Arnold R 1988 Comparison of the effect of single and repeated administrations of a protease inhibitor (camostate) on pancreatic secretion in man. Scandinavian Journal of Gastroenterology 23: 158–162

Adler G, Reinhagen M, Koop I, Goke B, Schafmayer A, Royati L C, Arnold R 1989 Differential effects of atropine and a cholecystokinin receptor antagonist on pancreatic secretion. Gastroenterology 96: 1158–1164

Adler G, Beglinger C, Braun U et al 1991 Interaction of the cholinergic system and cholecystokinin in the regulation of endogenous and exogenous stimulation of pancreatic secretion in humans. Gastroenterology 100: 537–543

Ali A E, Rutishauser S C B, Case R M 1990 Pancreatic and biliary secretion in the anaesthetized Syrian golden hamster in response to secretin, cholecystokinin-octapeptide, bombesin and carbachol. Pancreas 5: 314–322

Anagnostides A, Chadwick V S, Selden A C, Matos P N 1984 Sham feeding and pancreatic secretion. Gastroenterology 87: 109–114

Anglade P, Michel C, Roze C 1987 Intrinsic nerves of the pancreas after celiac and superior mesenteric ganglionectomy in rats: a morphologic study of acetylcholinesterase activity and catecholamine histofluorescence. Pancreas 2: 568–577

Aponte G W, Park K, Hess R, Garcia R, Taylor I L 1989 Meal induced peptide tyrosine inhibition of pancreatic secretion in rat. FASEB Journal 3: 1949–1955

Barber D I, Walsh J H, Soll A H 1986 Release and characterisation of cholecystokinin from isolated canine jejunal cells. Gastroenterology 91: 627–636

Barzilai A, Medina J A, Toth L, Konturek S J, Dreiling D A 1987 Effect of partial versus complete pancreatic denervation on pancreatic secretion. Pancreas 2: 159–163

Bayliss W M, Starling E H 1902 The mechanism of pancreatic secretion. Journal of Physiology 28: 325–333

Beardshall K, Frost G, Moraiyi Y et al 1989 Saturation of fat and cholecystokinin release: implications for pancreatic carcinogenesis. Lancet 2: 1008–1010

Beglinger C, Koehler E, Born W 1988 Effect of calcitonin and calcitonin gene-related peptide on pancreatic functions in man. Gut 29: 243–248

Behar J, Biancani P 1980 Effect of cholecystokinin and the octapeptide of cholecystokinin on the feline sphincter of Oddi and gallbladder. Mechanism of action. Journal of Clinical Investigation 66: 1231–1239

Behar J, Biancani P 1984 Neural control of the sphincter of Oddi. Gastroenterology 86: 134–141

Bendayan M 1990 Anatomic basis of islet–acinar interaction in the pancreas. Regulatory Peptide Letter 3: 1–7

Bodanszky M, Ondetti M A, Levine S D et al 1966 Synthesis of a heptacosapeptide amide with the hormonal activity of secretin. Chemistry and Industry (London) 42: 1757–1758

Bozkurt T, Adler G, Koop I, Arnold R 1988 Effect of atropine on intestinal phase of pancreatic secretin in man. Digestion 41: 108–115

Brugge W R, Burke C A, Izzo R S, Piaissman M 1987 Role of cholecystokinin in intestinal phase of human pancreatic secretion. Digestive Diseases and Sciences 32: 155–163

Buanes T, Grotmal T, Landsverk T, Ridderstiale Y, Raeder M G 1986 Histochemical localisation of carbonic anhydrase in the pig's exocrine pancreas. Acta Physiologica Scandinavica 128: 437–444

Carr-Locke D L, Gregg J A, Chey W Y 1985 Effects of exogenous secretin on pancreatic and biliary ductal and sphincteric pressures in man demonstrated by endoscopic manometry and correlation with plasma secretin levels. Digestive Diseases and Sciences 30: 909–917

Case R M 1989 Physiology and biochemistry of pancreatic exocrine secretion. Current Opinion in Gastroenterology 5: 665–681

Case R M 1990a Cellular mechanisms of control and secretion in exocrine pancreas. Current Opinion in Gastroenterology 6: 713–738

Case R M 1990b Physiological control of pancreatic exocrine secretion. Current Opinion in Gastroenterology 6: 724–730

Case R M, Argent B E 1986 Bicarbonate secretion by pancreatic duct cells: mechanisms and control. In: Go V L W et al (eds) The exocrine pancreas: biology, pathobiology and diseases. Raven Press, New York, p 214

Conway D R, Djuricin G, Prinz R A 1988 The effect of somatostatin analogue (SMS 201–995) on pancreatic blood flow. Surgery 104: 1024–1030

Cuber J C, Vilas F, Charles N, Bernard C, Chayvialle J A 1989 Bombesin and nutrients stimulate release of CCK through distinct pathways in the rat. American Journal of Physiology 256: G989–G996

Dale W E, Turkelson C M, Solomon T E 1989 Role of cholecystokinin in intestinal phase and meal-induced pancreatic secretion. American Journal of Physiology 257: G782–G790

De Mar A R, Taylor I L, Fink A S 1991 Pancreatic polypeptide and peptide YY inhibit the denervated canine pancreas. Pancreas 6: 419–426

Di Magno E P 1986 Human pancreatic exocrine secretion. In: Go V L W et al (eds) The exocrine pancreas: biology, pathobiology and diseases. Raven Press, New York, 193–197

Dlugosz J, Folsch U R, Creutzfeldt W 1983 Inhibition of intraduodenal trypsin does not stimulate exocrine pancreatic secretion in man. Digestion 26: 197–204

Dyck W P, Rudick J, Hoexter B, Janowitz H D 1969 Influence of glucagon on exocrine pancreatic secretion. Gastroenterology 56: 531–537

Elisha E E, Hutson D, Scratchard T 1984 The direct inhibition of pancreatic electrolyte secretion by noradrenaline in the isolated perfused cat pancreas. Journal of Physiology 351: 77–85

Eysselein V E, Eberlein G A, Hesse W E, Schaeffer M, Grandt D, Williams R, Goebell H, Reeve J R 1990 Molecular variants of cholecystokinin after endogenous stimulation in humans: a time study. American Journal Physiology 258: G951–G957

Feurle G E, Niestroj S 1991 The site of action of neurotensin in the rat pancreas. Pancreas 6: 202–207

Foulis A K, Stewart J A 1984 The pancreas in recent-onset type 1 (insulin-dependent) diabetes mellitus: insulin content of islets, insulitis and associated changes in the exocrine acinar tissue. Diabetologia 26: 456–461

Freeman T C, Playford R J, Quinn C, Beardshall K, Poulter L, Young J, Calam J 1990 Pancreatic secretory trypsin inhibitor in gastrointestinal mucosa and gastric juice. Gut 31: 1318–1323

Fried M, Jansen J B, Harpole T el al 1989 Pancreatobiliary responses to an intragastric amino acid meal: comparison to albumin, dextrose, and a maximal cholecystokinin stimulus. Gastroenterology 97: 1554–1559

Fried M, Mayer E A, Jansen J B M J et al 1988 Temporal relationships of cholecystokinin release, pancreatobiliary secretion and gastric emptying of a mixed meal. Gastroenterology 95: 1344–1450

Furukawa N, Okada H 1989 Effect of stimulation of the hypothalamic area on pancreatic exocrine secretion in dogs. Gastroenterology 97: 1534–1543

Garry D J, Garry M G, Williams J A, Mahoney W C, Sorenson R L 1989 Effects of islet hormones on amylase secretion and localization of somatostatin binding sites. American Journal of Physiology 256: G897–G904

Geenen J E, Hogan W, Dodds W J, Stewart E T, Arndorfer R C 1980 Intraluminal pressure recordings from the human sphincter of Oddi. Gastroenterology 17: 317–324

Goebell H, Steffen C, Baltzer G, Bode C 1973 Stimulation of pancreatic secretin of enzymes by acute hypercalcaemia in man. European Journal of Clinical Investigation 3: 98–104

Goke B, Printz H, Koop I, Rausch U, Richter G, Arnold R, Adler G 1986 Endogenous CCK release and pancreatic growth in rats after feeding a proteinase inhibitor (camostate). Pancreas 1: 509–515

Gray M A, Greenwell J R, Argent B E 1988 Secretin-regulated chloride channel on the apical plasma membrane of pancreatic duct cells. Journal of Membrane Biology 105: 131–142

Gray M A, Harris A, Coleman L, Greenwell J R, Argent B E 1989 Two types of chloride channel on duct cells cultured from human fetal pancreas. American Journal of Physiology 257: C240–C251

Green G M, Lyman R L 1972 Feedback regulation of pancreatic enzyme secretion as a mechanism for trypsin inhibitor-induced hyposecretion in rats. Proceedings of the Society of Experimental and Biological Medicine 140: 6–12

Guan D, Ohta H, Tawil T, Spannagel A W, Liddle R A, Green G M 1990 Lack of cholinergic control in feedback regulation of pancreatic secretion in the rat. Gastroenterology 98: 437–443

Gudgeon A M, Heath D I, Hurley P et al 1990 Trypsinogen activation peptide assay in the early prediction of severity of acute pancreatitis. Lancet 335: 4–8

Gullo L, Priori P, Labo G 1982 Influence of adrenal cortex on exocrine pancreatic function. Gastroenterology 83: 92–96

Gullo L, Priori P, Scarpignato C, Baldoni F, Mattioli G, Barbara L 1987 Effect of somatostatin-14 on pure human pancreatic secretion. Digestive Diseases and Sciences 32: 1065–1099

Gullo L, 1991 Effect of pancreatic polypeptide, thryotropin-releasing hormone, and glucagon on plasma amino acid uptake by human pancreas. Gastroenterology 100: 1095–1099

Gullo L, Pezzilli R, Bellanova B, D'Ambrosi A, Alvisi V, Barbara L 1991 Influence of the thyroid on exocrine pancreatic function. Gastroenterology 100: 1392–1396

Haarstad H, Peterssen H 1988 Interaction between secretin and a cholecystokinin-like peptide on pancreatic protein secretion and synthesis in the rat. Pancreas 3: 543–550

Hand B H 1963 An anatomical study of the choledochoduodenal area. British Journal of Surgery 50: 486–494

Hanssen L E, Hanssen K F, Myren J 1977 Inhibition of secretin release and pancreatic bicarbonate secretion by somatostatin infusion in man. Scandinavian Journal of Gastroenterology 12: 391–394

Harper A A, Raper H S 1943 Pancreozymin, a stimulant of the secretion of pancreatic enzymes in extracts of small intestine. Journal of Physiology (London) 102: 115–125

Harper A A, Vass C C H 1941 The control of the extremal secretion of the pancreas in cats. Journal of Physiology (London) 99: 415–435

Harvey M H, Wedgwood K R, Austin J A, Reber H A 1989 Pancreatic duct pressure, duct permeability and acute pancreatitis. British Journal of Surgery 76: 859–862

Helm J F, Venu R P, Geenen J E et al 1988 Effects of morphine on the human sphincter of Oddi. Gut 29: 1402–1407

Hildebrand P, Beglinger C, Gyr K et al 1990 Effects of cholecystokinin receptor antagonist on intestinal phase of pancreatic and biliary responses in man. Journal of Clinical Investigation 85: 640–646

Holst J J, Fahrenkrug J, Knuhtsen S et al 1987 VIP and PHI in the pig pancreas: coexistence, corelease and co-operative effects. American Journal of Physiology 252: G182–G189

Holst J J, Knuhtsen S, Nielsen O V 1989 Role of gastrin-releasing peptide in neural control of pancreatic exocrine secretion. Pancreas 4: 581–586

Hollander F, Birnbaum D 1952 The role of carbonic anhydrase in pancreatic secretion. Transactions of New York Academy of Science 15: 56–58

Hosotani R, Chowdhury P, Huang Y-S, McKay D, Yajima H, Rayford P L 1989 Effect of L-364, 718 on GRP-stimulated pancreatic and gastric secretions and GI peptides in conscious dogs. Pancreas 4: 550–555

Hotz J, Ho S B, Go V L W, Di Magno E P 1983 Short-term inhibition of duodenal tryptic activity does not affect human pancreatic, biliary or gastric function. Journal of Laboratory and Clinical Medicine 101: 488–495

Howatson A G, Carter D C 1985 Pancreatic carcinogenesis: enhancement by cholecystokinin in the hamster-nitrosamine model. British Journal of Cancer 51: 107–114

Hubel K A 1970 Response of rabbit pancreas in vitro to adrenergic agonists and antagonists. American Journal of Physiology 219: 1590–1594

Isaksson G, Ihse I 1983 Pain reduction by an oral pancreatic enzyme preparation in chronic pancreatitis. Digestive Diseases and Sciences 28: 97–102

Itoh H, Matsuyama T, Namba M et al 1989 Effect of glucagon- (1–21)-peptide on secretin-stimulated pancreatic exocrine secretion in anesthetized dogs. Life Science 44: 819–825

Ivy A C, Oldberg E 1928 A hormone mechanism for gallbladder contraction and evacuation. American Journal of Physiology 85: 599–613

Iwai K, Fushiki T, Fukuoka S 1988 Pancreatic enzyme secretion mediated by novel peptide: monitor peptide hypothesis. Pancreas 3: 720–728

Jo Y H, Lee K Y, Chang T-M, Chey W Y 1991 Role of cholecystokinin in pancreatic bicarbonate secretion in dogs. Pancreas 6: 197–201

Joehl R J, Kelly G A, Nahrwold D 1981 Terbutaline inhibits pancreatic secretion. Journal of Surgical Research 30: 236–240

Jorpes J E, Mutt V, Magnusson S, Steele B B 1962 Amino acid composition and N-terminal amino acid sequence of porcine secretin. Biochemical and Biophysiological Research Communication 9 275–279

Jorpes J E, Mutt V E 1966 Cholecystokinin and pancreozymin one single hormone? Acta Physiologica Scandinavica 66: 196–202

Kim M S, Lee K Y, Chey W Y 1979 Plasma secretin concentrations in fasting and postprandial states in dog. American Journal of Physiology 236: E539–E544

Kim C K, Lee K Y, Wang T, Sun G, Chang T M, Chey W Y 1989 Role of endogenous cholecystokinin on vagally stimulated pancreatic secretion in dogs. American Journal of Physiology 257: G944–G949

Knuhtsen S, Holst J J, Baldissera F G A et al 1987 Gastrin-releasing peptide in the porcine pancreas. Gastroenterology 92: 1153–1158

Knuhtsen S, Esteve J P, Bernadet B, Vaysse N, Susini C 1988 Molecular characterization of the solubilized receptors of somatostatin from rat pancreatic acinar membranes. Biochemical Journal 254: 641–647

Kogire M, Inoue K, Hosotani R, Huang Y S, Thompson J C, Tobe T 1989 Pancreatic secretion and the release of cholecystokinin after a meal in dogs with and without exclusion of pancreatic juice. Scandinavian Journal of Gastroenterology 24: 507–512

Kohler H, Nustede R, Barthel M, Schafmayer M 1987 Exocrine pancreatic function in dogs with denervated pancreas. Pancreas 2: 676–683

Konturek S J, Tasler V, Obtulowicz W 1974 Characteristics of inhibition of pancreatic secretion by glucagon. Digestion 10: 138–149

Konturek S J, Popiela T, Slowiaczek M, Bielanski W 1987 Gastric acid and pancreatic polypeptide responses to modified sham feeding. Effects of truncal and parietal cell vagotomy. Gut 28: 280–286

Konturek S J, Tasler J, Konturek J W et al 1989 Effects of non-peptide CCK receptor antagonist (L-364,718) on pancreatic responses to cholecystokinin, gastrin, bombesin, and meat feeding in dogs. Gut 30: 110–117

Korc M, Owerbach D, Quinto C, Rutter W J 1981 Pancreatic islet–acinar cell interaction. Amylase messenger RNA levels are determined by insulin. Science 213: 351–353

Kumpulainen T, Jalovaara P 1981 Immunohistochemical localisation of carbonic anhydrase isoenzymes in the human pancreas. Gastroenterology 80: 796–799

Lankisch P G, Manthey G, Otto J el al 1982 Exocrine pancreatic function in insulin-dependent diabetes mellitus. Digestion 25: 211–216

Layer P, Hotz J, Cherian L, Goebell H 1987 In vitro stimulation of pancreatic enzyme discharge by calcium. Gut 28: 1215–1220

Lee J T, Lebcthal E, Lee P C 1989 Rat pancreatic nuclear thyroid hormone receptor: characterization and postnatal development. Gastroenterology 96: 1151–1157

Levan V H, Green G M 1986 Effect of atropine on rat pancreatic response to trypsin inhibitors and protein. American Journal of Physiology 251: G64–G69

Li P, Lee K Y, Chang T M, Chey W Y 1990a Mechanism of acid induced release of secretin in rats: presence of a secretin-releasing peptide. Journal of Clinical Investigation 86: 1474–1479

Li P, Lee K Y, Ren X S, Chang T-M, Chey W Y 1990b Effect of pancreatic proteases on plasma cholecystokinin, secretin and pancreatic exocrine secretion in response to sodium oleate.Gastroenterology 98: 1642–1648

Lifson N, Kramlinger K G, Mayraun R R, Lander E J 1980 Blood flow to the rabbit pancreas with special reference to the islets of Langerhans. Gastroenterology 79: 446–473

Louie D S, May D, Miller P, Owyang C 1986 Cholecystokinin mediates feedback regulation of pancreatic enzyme secretion in rats. American Journal of Physiology 250: G252–G259

Lu L, Louie D, Owyang C 1989 A cholecystokinin releasing peptide mediates feedback regulation of pancreatic secretion. American Journal of Physiology 256: G430–G435

Matozaki T, Sakamoto C, Nagao M, Baba S 1988 Pancreatic secretagogues regulate somatostatin binding to acinar cell membranes via two functionally distinct pathways. Hormone and Metabolism Research 20: 141–144

Matozaki T, Martinez J, Williams J A 1989 A new CCK analogue differentiates two functionally distinct CCK receptors in rat and mouse pancreatic acini. American Journal of Physiology 257: G594–G600

Meehan C J, Davidson P M, Young D G, Foulis A K 1987 The partially diabetic pancreas: a histological study of a new animal model. Pancreas 2: 91–98

Misumi A, Shiratori K, Lee K Y, Barkin J S, Chey W Y 1988 Effects of SMS 201–995, a somatostatin analogue, on the exocrine pancreatic secretion and gut hormone release in dogs. Surgery 103: 450–455

Miyasaka K, Funakoshi A, Nakamura R, Kitani K, Shimizu F, Tatemoto K 1989a Effects of porcine pancreastatin on postprandial pancreatic exocrine secretion and endocrine functions in the conscious rat. Digestion 43: 204–211

Miyasaka K, Guan D, Liddle R A, Green G M 1989b Feedback regulation by trypsin: evidence for intraluminal CCK-releasing peptide. American Journal of Physiology 257: G175–G181

Miyasaka K, Funakoshi A, Kitani K, Tamamura H, Funakoshi S, Fujii N 1990 Inhibitory effect of pancreastatin on pancreatic exocrine secretions. Gastroenterology 99: 1751–1756

Mössner J, Wresky H P, Kestel W, Zeeh J, Regner U, Fischbach W 1989 Influence of treatment with pancreatic extracts on pancreatic enzyme secretion. Gut 30: 1143–1149

Mulholland M W, Lally K, Taborsky G J 1991 Inhibition of rat pancreatic exocrine secretion by neuropeptide Y: studies in vivo and in vitro. Pancreas 6: 433–440

Muller M K, Kessel B, Hutt T, Kath R, Layer P, Goebell H 1988 Effects of somatostatin-14 on gastric and pancreatic responses to hormonal and neural stimulation using an isolated perfused rat stomach and pancreas preparation. Pancreas 3: 303–310

Novak I, Greger R 1988 Properties of the luminal membrane of isolated perfused rat pancreatic ducts. Effect of cyclic AMP and blockers of chloride transport. Pflugers Archives 411: 546–553

Olsen O, Schaffalitzky de Muckadell O B, Cantor P 1986 The significance of plasma CCK and secretin in the oleate-stimulated pancreatico-biliary secretion in man. International Journal of Pancreatology 1: 363–372

Olsen O, Schaffalitzky De Muckadell O B, Cantor P et al 1988 Effect of trypsin on the hormonal regulation of the fat-stimulated human exocrine pancreas. Scandinavian Journal of Gastroenterology 23: 875–881

Olsen O, Schaffalitzky De Muckadell O B, Cantor P 1989 Fat and pancreatic secretion. Scandinavian Journal of Gastroenterology 24: 74–80

Otsuki M, Williams J A 1983 Direct modulation of pancreatic CCK receptors and enzyme secretion by insulin in isolated pancreatic acini from diabetic rats. Diabetes 32: 241–246

Otsuki M, Ohki A, Okabayashi Y, Suehiro I, Baba S 1987 Effect of synthetic protease inhibitor camostate on pancreatic exocrine function in rats. Pancreas 2: 164–169

Owyang C, May D, Louie D 1986 Trypsin suppression of pancreatic enzyme secretion. Differential effect on cholecystokinin release and the enteropancreatic reflex. Gastroenterology 91: 637–643

Putnam W S, Liddle P A, Williams J A 1989 Inhibitory regulation of rat exocrine pancreas by peptide YY and pancreatic polypeptide. American Journal of Physiology 25: G698–G703

Reber H A, Roberts C, Way L 1979 The pancreatic duct mucosal barrier. American Journal of Surgery 137: 128–134

Riepl R L, Lehnert P, Schari A et al 1990 Effect of intraduodenal bile and Na-taurodeoxy-cholate on exocrine pancreatic secretion and on plasma levels of secretin, pancreatic polypeptide, and gastrin in man. Scandinavian Journal of Gastroenterology 25: 45–53

Saito A, Williams J A, Kano T 1980 Potentiation of cholecystokinin induced exocrine secretion by both exogenous and endogenous insulin in isolated and perfused rat pancreata. Journal of Clinical Investigation 65: 777–782

Schaffalitzky de Muckadell O B, Olsen O, Cantor P, Magid E 1986 Concentration of secretin and CCK in plasma and pancreaticobiliary secretion in response to intraduodenal acid and fat. Pancreas 1: 536–543

Schafmayer A, Nustede R, Pompino A, Kohler H 1988 Vagal influence on cholecystokinin and neurotensin release in conscious dogs. Scandinavian Journal of Gastroenterology 23: 315–320

Schwarzendrube J, Nederau M, Luthen R, Niederau C 1991 Effects of cholecystokinin-receptor blockade on pancreatic and biliary function in healthy volunteers. Gastroenterology 100: 1683–1690

Shiratori K, Jo Y H, Lee K Y, Chang T M, Chey W Y 1989 Effect of pancreatic juice and trypsin on oleic acid-stimulated pancreatic secretion and plasma secretin in dogs. Gastroenterology 96: 1330–1336

Simpson C J, Toner P G, Carr K E, Anderson J D, Carter D C 1983 Effect of bile salt perfusion and intraduct pressure on ionic flux and mucosal ultrastructure in the pancreatic duct of the cat. Virchows Archiv für Cell Pathologie 42: 327–342

Singer M V, Niebel W, Jansen J B M J et al 1989 Pancreatic secretory response to intravenous caerulein and intraduodenal tryptophan studies: before and after stepwise removal of the extrinsic nerves of the pancreas in dogs. Gastroenterology 96: 925–934

Smith Z D J, Caplan M J, Forbush B III, Jamieson J D 1987 Monoclonal antibody localisation of Na^+-K^+-ATPase in the exocrine pancreas and parotid of the dog. American Journal of Physiology 253: G99–G109

Solomon T E 1981 Regulation of exocrine pancreatic cell proliferation and enzyme synthesis. In: Johnson L R (ed) Physiology of the gastrointestinal tract. Raven Press, New York, p 837–892

Slaff J, Jacobson D, Tillman C R, Curington C, Toskes P 1984 Protease-specific suppression of pancreatic exocrine secretion. Gastroenterology 87: 44–45

Stuenkel E L, Machen T E, Williams J A 1988 pH regulatory mechanisms in rat pancreatic ductal cells. American Journal of Physiology 254: G925–G930

Sun G, Lee K Y, Chang T-M, Chey W Y 1989 Effect of pancreatic juice diversion on secretin release in rats. Gastroenterology 96: 1173–1179

Tatemoto K, Efendic S, Mutt V, Makk G, Feistner G J, Barchas J D 1986 Pancreastatin, a novel pancreatic peptide that inhibits insulin secretion. Nature 324: 476–478

Thune A, Thornell E, Svanvik J 1986 Reflex regulation of flow resistance in the feline sphincter of Oddi by hydrostatic pressure in the biliary tract. Gastroenterology 91: 1364–1369

Toouli J 1984 Sphincter of Oddi motility. British Journal of Surgery 71: 251

Toouli J 1990 Clinical relevance of sphincter of Oddi dysfunction. British Journal of Surgery 77: 723–724

Toouli J, Hogan W, Geenen J W, Dodds W J, Arndorfer R C 1982 Action of cholecystokinin-octapeptide on sphincter of Oddi pressure and phasic wave activity in man. Surgery 92: 497–503

Usellini L, Finzi G, Riva C et al 1990 Ultrastructural identification of human secretin cells by the immunogold technique: their co-storage of chromogranin A and serotonin. Histochemistry 94: 113–120

Valenzuela J E, Weiner K, Saad C 1986 Cholinergic stimulation of human pancreatic secretion. Digestive Diseases and Sciences 31: 615–619

Watanabe S, Lee K Y, Chang T-M, Berger-Ornstein L, Chey W Y 1988 Role of pancreatic enzymes on release of cholecystokinin-pancreozymin in response to fat. American Journal of Physiology 254: G837–G842

Williams J A, Goldfine I D 1985 The insulin-pancreatic acinar axis. Diabetes 34: 980–986

Wisner J R, McLaughlin R E, Rich K A, Osawa S, Renner I G 1988 Effects of L-364,718, a new cholecystokinin receptor antagonist, on camostate-induced growth of the rat pancreas. Gastroenterology 94: 109–113

Wolf B, Aratan-Spire S, Czernichow P 1984 Hypothyroidism increases pancreatic thyrotropin-releasing hormone concentrations in adult rats. Endocrinology 114: 1334–1337

Worthley C S, Baker R A, Iannos J, Saccone G T P and Toouli J 1989 Human fasting and postprandial sphincter of Oddi motility. British Journal of Surgery 76: 709–714

You C H, Rominger J M, Chey W Y 1983 Potentiation effect of cholecystokinin-octapeptide on pancreatic bicarbonate secretion stimulated by a physiologic dose of secretin in humans. Gastroenterology 85: 40–45

Yu D-H, Huang S C, Wank S A, Mantey S, Gardner J D, Jensen R T 1990 Pancreatic receptors for cholecystokinin: evidence for three receptor classes. American Journal of Physiology 258: G86–G95

Preoperative diagnosis of pancreatic disease

4. Conventional radiography

P. C. Freeny

PLAIN FILMS

Conventional roentgenograms of the chest and abdomen continue to play an important but diminished role in pancreatic radiology.

Patients presenting with symptoms of abdominal pain are often evaluated first with an abdominal roentgenogram. If their symptoms are caused by acute pancreatitis, one might expect to see changes in the pancreatic bed and peripancreatic tissues, and in the gas patterns of the gastrointestinal tract.

Fat necrosis and gas-containing pancreatic abscesses can be diagnosed by abdominal roentgenograms. Fat necrosis is manifested by areas of mottled fat and water density, known as the 'abdominal fat necrosis sign' (Berenson et al 1971). Gas-containing pancreatic abscesses are seen as abnormal collections of gas and water density

in the pancreatic bed (Fig. 4.1). They usually assume one of two appearances: a focal collection of small gas bubbles, or a large, homogeneous gas collection (Freeny & Lawson 1982). The differential diagnosis includes a peripancreatic abscess unrelated to the pancreas, most often caused by a perforated duodenal or gastric ulcer, or by diverticulitis of the transverse colon or splenic flexure.

Abnormalities of the bowel gas pattern are common manifestations of acute pancreatitis. These include generalized ileus, or a focal ileus of the duodenum (Fig. 4.2) or colon (Fig. 4.3). In the latter case, this is known as the 'colon cut-off sign' and is manifested by dilatation of the colon to the splenic flexure, with minimal or no gas seen within the descending and sigmoid colon (Price 1968).

Conventional abdominal roentgenograms may show pancreatic ductal calcifications in 40–60% of patients with chronic pancreatitis (Freeny & Lawson 1982). The

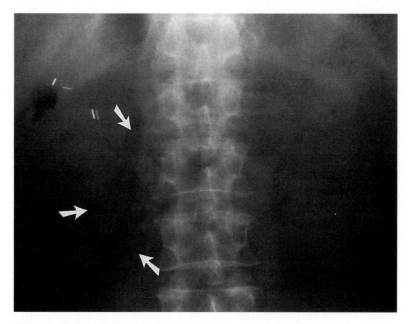

Fig. 4.1 Pancreatic abscess. Abdominal roentgenogram shows a focal, extraluminal gas collection in the region of the head of the pancreas (arrows), later shown to be an abscess.

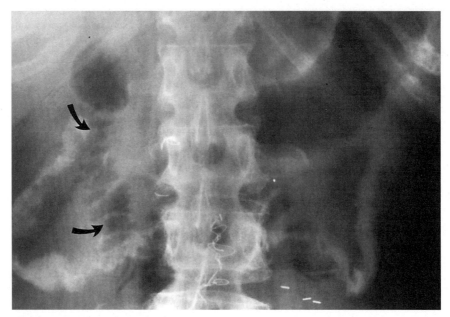

Fig. 4.2 Duodenal ileus. Abdominal roentgenogram shows gas within the duodenum (arrows) in a patient with acute pancreatitis.

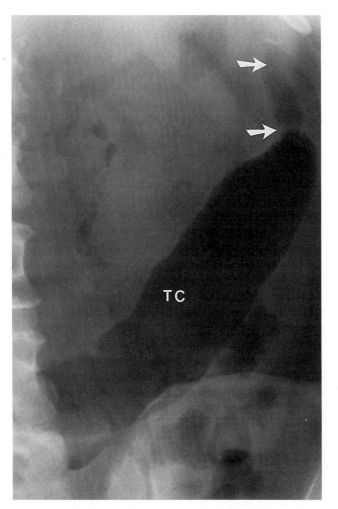

Fig. 4.3 Colon 'cut-off' sign. Abdominal roentgenogram shows a dilated transverse colon (TC) with abrupt narrowing and cut-off at the splenic flexure (arrows) caused by acute pancreatitis.

presence of multiple calcifications aligned in the pattern of the main pancreatic duct and lateral side branches is diagnostic of this disease (Fig. 4.4)

Pancreatic cancer has only a few manifestations which can be observed on an abdominal roentgenogram. These include an oval or rounded soft tissue mass in the right upper abdomen, corresponding to a dilated gallbladder in a patient with obstructive jaundice caused by a pancreatic carcinoma (Fig. 4.5), an enlarged spleen caused by obstruction of the splenic vein by tumour, ascites caused by peritoneal carcinomatosis, and rarely osteoblastic meta-stases to bone. Ductal carcinoma rarely calcifies, but a sunburst pattern of calcification has been described in about 10% of patients with benign cystic neoplasms of the pancreas (Haukohl & Melamed 1950).

BARIUM CONTRAST STUDIES

Barium studies of the gastrointestinal tract are rarely used for initial diagnosis of patients with suspected pancreatic disease. However, in patients with non-specific abdominal symptoms, or symptoms suggesting peptic ulcer disease, a barium study may be obtained and may indicate the presence of pancreatic disease.

The inflammatory process of pancreatitis can spread to involve any segment of the gastrointestinal tract (Freeny & Lawson 1982). However, the duodenum is the most frequently involved segment owing to its proximity to the head of the pancreas. Duodenal changes produced by pancreatitis include partial or complete obstruction, caused by enlargement of the head of the pancreas or by spasm caused by the contiguous inflammatory process, effacement of spiculation of the medial wall of the C-loop, and mucosal oedema with widened folds (Fig. 4.6). If the inflammatory

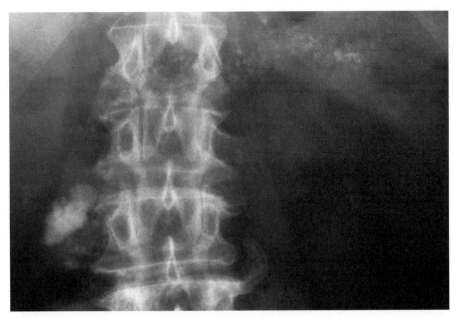

Fig. 4.4 Pancreatic calcifications. Abdominal roentgenogram shows multiple calcifications throughout the pancreas caused by chronic calcific pancreatitis.

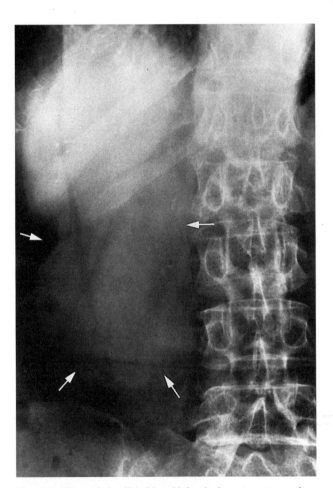

Fig. 4.5 Distended gallbladder. Abdominal roentgenogram shows a pear-shaped structure (arrows) in the right upper abdomen in a patient with pancreatic cancer and obstructive jaundice. Subsequent cholangiogram confirmed a markedly dilated gallbladder.

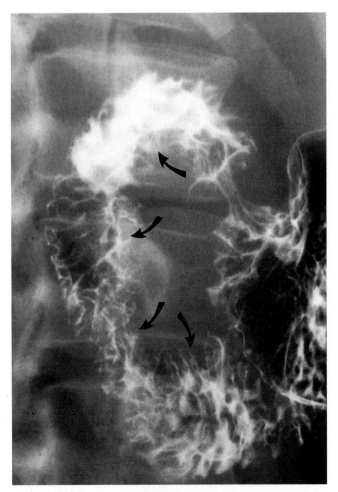

Fig. 4.6 Acute pancreatitis. Barium examination shows narrowing of the duodenal C-loop and spiculation of the medial wall (arrows) by contiguous pancreatic inflammation.

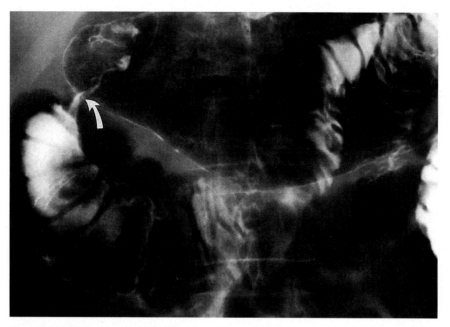

Fig. 4.7 Chronic pancreatitis. Barium examination shows focal stenosis of the duodenum (arrow) in a patient with long standing chronic pancreatitis.

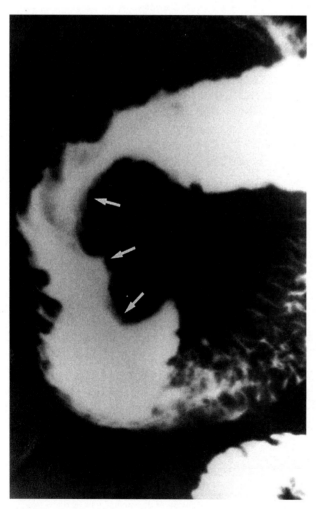

Fig. 4.8 Pancreatic cancer. Barium examination shows nodular compression of the medial wall of the duodenum by pancreatic cancer, producing a 'reversed 3' configuration (arrows).

process is severe or prolonged, as with chronic pancreatitis, a duodenal stenosis can result (Fig. 4.7).

Pancreatic carcinoma also causes changes in the duodenum which can suggest the correct diagnosis. The most frequently observed findings include extrinsic pressure (double-contour image), displacement, or encasement of the C-loop, mucosal invasion (nodularity or spiculation), Frostberg's reversed '3' sign (Fig. 4.8), barium reflux into the pancreatic or bile duct, and a tubular impression on the duodenum caused by a dilated common bile duct (Freeny & Lawson 1982)

Pancreatitis and pancreatic carcinoma also can involve the stomach, small intestine, and colon. However, barium studies are rarely performed to evaluate these organs unless clinically evident disease is present, and the precise location of an obstruction or fistula is required prior to treatment.

REFERENCES

Berenson J E, Spitz H B, Felson B 1971 The abdominal fat necrosis sign. Radiology 100: 567–571

Freeny P C, Lawson T L, 1982 Radiology of the pancreas. Springer-Verlag, New York

Haukohl R S, Melamed A 1950 Cystadenoma of the pancreas. A report of two cases showing calcification. American Journal of Radiology 63: 234–245

Price C W R 1968 The 'colon cut-off' sign in acute pancreatitis. Medical Journal of Australia 1: 313–314

5. Ultrasonography

P. C. Freeny

INTRODUCTION

Pancreatic ultrasonography is currently performed using high-resolution real-time linear array or sector scanners. These instruments can produce very detailed anatomical images of the pancreas and surrounding structures in a variety of planes. Gas within the stomach or duodenum can interfere with ultrasound imaging of the pancreas, but this can usually be prevented by oral ingestion of 300–600 ml of water prior to scanning.

The normal pancreas has smooth or slightly lobulated margins and an echo texture pattern which is usually equivalent to or slightly greater than that of normal liver (Fig. 5.1) (Freeny & Lawson 1982). The head of the gland is usually about 2.5 cm in anteroposterior diameter, and the body about 1.5 cm, measured in the axial or sagittal planes (De Graff et al 1978).

The normal pancreatic duct is seen in over 50% of cases (Lawson et al 1982). It appears as a thin, fluid-filled tube with thin, parallel, echogenic walls (Fig. 5.1). The internal diameter of the normal pancreatic duct in the body of the gland rarely exceeds 2 mm (Freeny & Lawson 1982).

The major peripancreatic vessels, superior mesenteric artery and vein, portal vein, coeliac axis, hepatic and splenic arteries and splenic vein, aorta, and inferior vena cava and renal veins, are commonly seen and are important landmarks for identifying the normal or abnormal pancreas (Fig. 5.1) (Freeny & Lawson 1982).

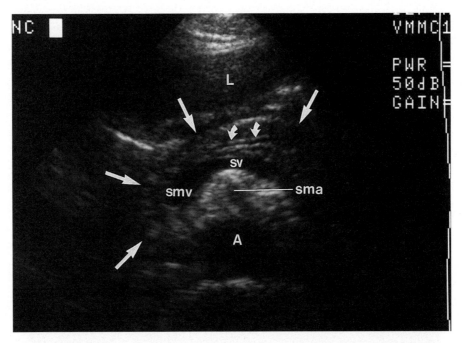

Fig. 5.1 Normal pancreas. Axial ultrasonogram shows normal pancreas (large arrows) with echo texture slightly greater than the adjacent liver (L). A normal pancreatic duct (small curved arrows) is seen; sma, superior mesenteric artery; smv, superior mesenteric vein; sv, splenic vein; A, aorta.

The common bile duct can often be seen as it passes through or behind the head of the pancreas. It usually measures about 5–7 mm in diameter (Freeny & Lawson 1982). Ultrasonography can also be used to evaluate the intrahepatic biliary ducts and gallbladder.

ULTRASONOGRAPHY AND PANCREATIC DISEASE

Pancreatitis

The ultrasonographic findings in *acute pancreatitis* include an increase in gland size, generalized decrease in

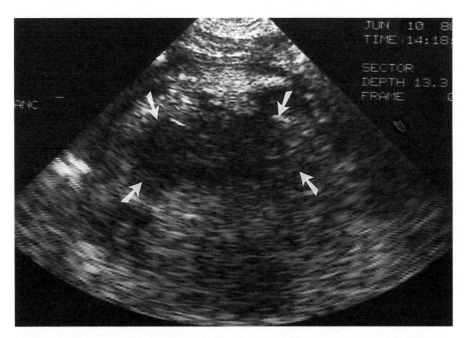

Fig. 5.2 Acute pancreatitis. Axial ultrasonography shows diffuse enlargement of the pancreas with diminished echo texture (arrows). Normal pancreatic margins and peripancreatic vessels are obscured by the inflammatory process.

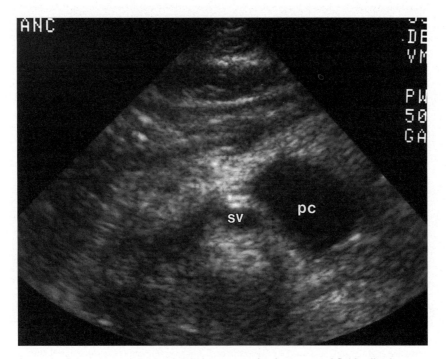

Fig. 5.3 Pancreatic pseudocyst. Axial ultrasonography shows an oval fluid collection (pseudocyst, pc) in the tail of the pancreas; sv. splenic vein.

parenchymal echogenicity, ill-defined gland margins, and the presence of fluid collections (Fig. 5.2). If the inflammatory process is severe, parenchymal echogenicity can be increased owing to the presence of haemorrhage and necrosis. Cotton and colleagues noted normal (32%), increased (16%), decreased (19%), and heterogeneous (30%) echo patterns in a series of patients with acute pancreatitis (Cotton et al 1980).

Ultrasonography is a reliable screening method for detection of some of the complications of acute pancreatitis, such as fluid collections (Fig. 5.3) and biliary duct obstruction due to compression of the intrapancreatic segment of the common bile duct (Freeny & Lawson 1982).

The ultrasonographic finding in *chronic pancreatitis* include alterations in gland size and echo texture pattern, pancreatic and biliary duct dilatation, pancreatic ductal calculi, and fluid collections (Fig. 5.4).

The size of the gland may be normal, increased (focal or diffuse), or decreased (gland atrophy), depending on the severity, activity, and duration of the disease (Lees 1984, Bolondi et al 1989). The margins of the gland also may become more lobulated. The echo texture pattern is often heterogeneously increased owing to parenchymal fibrosis (Bolondi et al 1989). However, areas of acute pancreatitis during the relapsing phase may show decreased echogenicity owing to oedema and accumulation of fluid.

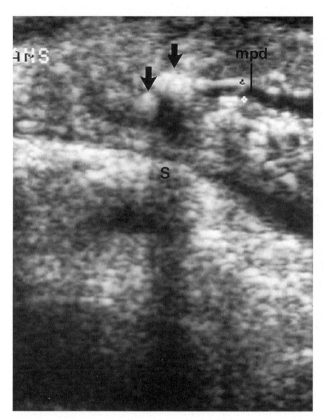

A

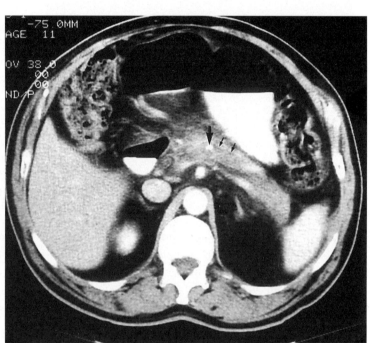

B

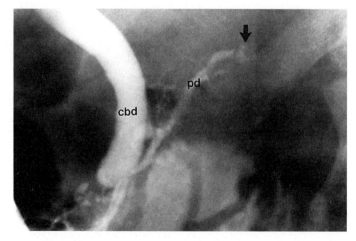

C

Fig. 5.4 Chronic calcific pancreatitis. **A** Axial ultrasonography (linear transducer) shows several echogenic foci (arrows) with posterior acoustic shadows (S), typical of stones, in the body of the pancreas. The upstream main pancreatic duct (mpd) is dilated. **B** CT at the same level as the ultrasound examination shows the calcification in the pancreatic duct (large arrow) and dilatation of the upstream duct (small arrows). **C** Endoscopic retrograde cholangiopancreatography (ERCP) shows obstruction of the pancreatic duct (pd) by a calculus (arrow); cbd, common bile duct.

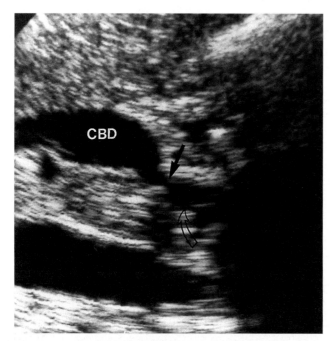

Fig. 5.5   Chronic pancreatitis. Sagittal ultrasound examination shows typical hourglass deformity of the common bile duct (CBD) caused by chronic pancreatitis. The closed arrow indicates the stenotic segment and the open arrow the normal calibre distal CBD. (From Rohrmann CA Jr & Baron RL 1989 Biliary complications of pancreatitis. Radiologic Clinics of North America 27: 93–104.)

Pancreatic duct dilatation is a common finding in chronic pancreatitis (Fig. 5.4). The walls of the dilated duct may be thickened and irregular and focal strictures with alternating segments of dilatation ('chain-of-lakes') are frequently identified (Bolondi et al 1989). Pancreatic duct calculi are seen as focal, highly echogenic intraductal masses with posterior acoustic shadowing (Fig. 5.4). Calculi have been found in as many as 57% of patients with chronic pancreatitis (Bolondi et al 1989).

Biliary duct dilatation also is commonly found in chronic pancreatitis (Rohrmann & Baron 1989). The intrapancreatic segment of the duct typically shows a long, tapered stenosis, but an 'hour-glass' deformity can be seen in up to 25% of patients (Fig. 5.5). Fluid collections or pseudocysts can be found in as many as 10% of patients with chronic pancreatitis and usually indicate the presence of severe disease if they are greater than 10 mm in diameter (Fig. 5.3) (Lees 1984).

Other findings that can be demonstrated by ultrasonography include the presence of arterial pseudoaneurysms and obstruction of the splenic or portal veins with corresponding varices (Bolondi et al 1989, Lees 1984).

Pancreatic carcinoma

Pancreatic carcinoma occurs in the head of the gland in about 60% of cases, usually causing biliary obstruction. Ultrasonography is very accurate in detecting the presence of biliary obstruction and often can define the cause when it is due to pancreatic carcinoma (Lees 1984). Thus, the reported sensitivity of ultrasonography in pancreatic carcinoma is as high as 80–95% (Lawson 1978, Cotton et al 1980, Taylor et al 1981). However, ultrasonography fails to provide an adequate evaluation of the entire gland in 14% of cases, resulting in an overall decrease in its sensitivity (Freeny & Lawson 1982). In particular, tumours arising in the body and tail of the gland are difficult to detect with ultrasound. In addition, the ability to correctly stage pancreatic carcinoma using ultrasound is significantly inferior to that of computed tomography (CT). Thus, while ultrasonography can be used efficaciously for evaluation of patients with obstructive jaundice, often correctly defining the cause, CT outperforms ultrasonography, both for tumour detection and staging (Fig. 5.6). Thus, ultrasonography is not recommended for screening patients if a diagnosis of pancreatic carcinoma is strongly suspected. However, ultrasonography continues to be an important method for evaluating patients with jaundice of unknown aetiology.

The ultrasonographic findings in pancreatic carcinoma include the presence of a hypoechoic pancreatic mass, dilatation of the upstream pancreatic and/or common bile duct, atrophy of the pancreatic parenchyma surrounding the obstructed upstream pancreatic duct, and the presence of enlarged peripancreatic lymph nodes and hepatic metastases (Fig. 5.6) (Freeny & Lawson 1982, Lees 1984). Although tumour involvement of the peripancreatic vessels, such as splenic or superior mesenteric vein obstruction, can be detected by ultrasound, overall detection of vascular involvement is poor relative to contrast-enhanced CT (Fig. 5.6).

Pancreatic endocrine tumours

Islet cell tumours account for only a small fraction of pancreatic neoplasms, but they are important because of their clinical syndromes and their high cure rate following surgical resection. Preoperative localization is often difficult and may require multiple procedures. Ultrasonography has been shown to have an accuracy as high as 72% (Thompson et al 1988). Insulinomas are most readily detected by ultrasound, with a sensitivity of 61% (see Fig. 6.15) (Galiber et al 1988). In a series of patients with gastrinomas, ultrasonography CT scanning, magnetic resonance imaging (MRI), and angiography were compared; ultrasonography had a sensitivity of only 20%, while a combination of CT, ultrasound, and angiography resulted in a sensitivity of 86% (Frucht et al 1989).

Islet cell tumours are seen by ultrasound as focal masses with diminished echogenicity relative to the contiguous or surrounding normal pancreas (see Figs 6.15, 9.5). Most functioning tumours are small, ranging from 1 to 3 cm in diameter. Nonfunctioning tumours are usually larger,

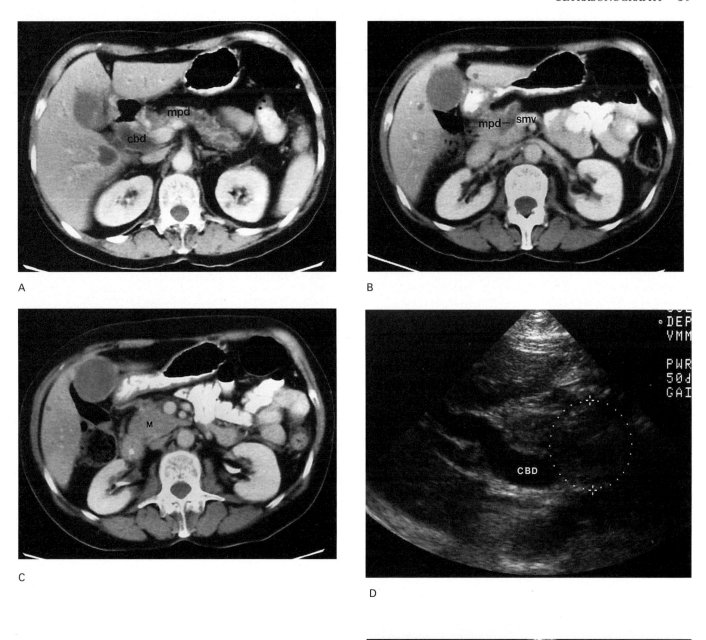

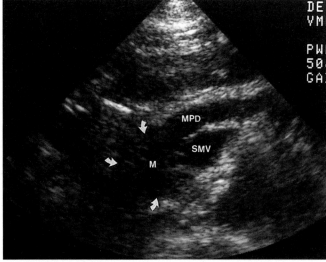

Fig. 5.6 Pancreatic cancer: Computerized tomography (CT) and ultrasonography. **A** CT shows a dilated main pancreatic duct (mpd) with atrophy of the surrounding parenchyma and dilatation of the common bile duct (cbd). **B** CT at a more caudal level shows a dilated main pancreatic duct (mpd) adjacent to the superior mesenteric vein (smv). **C** More caudal scan of the pancreas shows a mass (M) in the head of the gland caused by pancreatic carcinoma. **D** Sagittal ultrasound examination shows a dilated common bile duct (CBD) abruptly terminating at the cranial margin of a focal mass (dotted circle) in the pancreatic head. **E** Axial ultrasound examination shows the focal hypoechoic mass (M) in the pancreatic head (arrows). The upstream main pancreatic duct (MPD) is dilated. SMV, superior mesenteric vein.

about 5–10 cm in diameter. These tumours have a heterogeneous echo pattern and are difficult to distinguish from ductal carcinoma.

Intraoperative ultrasonography has a much higher sensitivity for detection of small islet cell tumours than transcutaneous ultrasonography owing to the very high resolution that can be obtained by using a high frequency transducer (7.5–10 MHz) applied directly to the surface of the pancreas (see Fig. 9.5). In one series, a sensitivity of 84% was achieved with intraoperative ultrasonography in patients with insulinomas (Galiber et al 1988). The techniques and results of intraoperative ultrasonography are discussed in more detail in Chapter 15.

Cystic pancreatic neoplasms

There are three types of cystic pancreatic neoplasms: serous cystadenomas, mucinous cystadenomas or carcinomas, and papillary-cystic tumours. They can be detected with ultrasound and their cystic components are easily defined (see Figs 6.12, 6.13) (Johnson et al 1988, Mathieu et al 1989). These tumours are discussed in more detail in the following chapter on CT.

REFERENCES

Bolondi L, Bassi S L, Gaiani S, Barbara L 1989 Sonography of chronic pancreatitis. Radiologic Clinics of North America 27: 815–833
Cotton P B, Lees W R, Vallon A G et al 1980 Gray-scale ultrasonography and endoscopic pancreatography in pancreatic diagnosis. Radiology 134: 453–459
De Graff C S, Taylor K J W, Simonds B D, Rosenfield A J 1978 Gray-scale echography of the pancreas. Reevaluation of normal size. Radiology 129: 157–161
Freeny P C, Lawson T L 1982 Radiology of the pancreas. Springer-Verlag, New York
Frucht H, Doppman J L, Norton J A et al 1989 Gastrinomas: comparison of MR imaging with CT, angiography, and US. Radiology 171: 713–717
Galiber A K, Reading C C, Charboneau J W et al 1988 Localization of pancreatic insulinoma: comparison of pre- and intraoperative US with CT and angiography. Radiology 166: 405–408
Johnson C D, Stephens D H, Charboneau J W, Carpenter H A, Welch

T J 1988 Cystic pancreatic tumours: CT and sonographic assessment. American Journal of Radiology 151: 1133–1138
Lawson T L 1978 Sensitivity of pancreatic ultrasonography in the detection of pancreatic disease. Radiology 128: 733–736
Lawson T L, Berland L L, Foley W D 1982 Ultrasonic visualization of the pancreatic duct. Radiology 144: 865–871
Lees W R 1984 Pancreatic ultrasonography. Clinics in Gastroenterology 13: 763–789
Mathieu D, Guigui B, Valette P J, Dao T H, Bruneton J N, Bruel J M, Pringot J, Vasile N 1989 Pancreatic cystic neoplasms. Radiologic Clinics of North America. 27: 163–176
Rohrmann C A, Baron R L 1989 Biliary complications of pancreatitis. Radiologic Clinics of North America 27: 93–104
Taylor K J W, Buchin P J, Viscomi G N, Rosenfield A T 1981 Ultrasonographic scanning of the pancreas prospective study of clinical results. Radiology 138: 211–213
Thompson G B, Van Heerden J A, Grant C S, Carney J A, Ilstrup D M 1988 Islet cell carcinoma of the pancreas: a twenty-year experience. Surgery 104: 1011–1017

6. Computed tomography

P. C. Freeny

Accurate pancreatic computed tomography (CT) scanning requires the use of current generation CT scanners capable of dynamic scanning at speeds of 2 s/scan or less, 5–8 mm thin-slice collimation, and the use of a simultaneous bolus injection of 150–180 ml of a 60% contrast agent (Freeny & Lawson 1982). These techniques result in highly detailed images of the pancreas, the pancreatic and biliary ducts, the peripancreatic vasculature and soft tissues, and the organs surrounding the pancreas (Fig. 6.1) (Freeny 1988).

PANCREATITIS

Acute pancreatitis

The CT findings in acute pancreatitis are characterized by a spectrum of changes which reflect the severity of the parenchymal and extraparenchymal inflammatory process. Balthazar and colleagues (Balthazar et al 1985, Balthazar 1989) have classified the CT changes of acute pancreatitis into 5 grades; grade A, normal pancreas; grade B, focal or

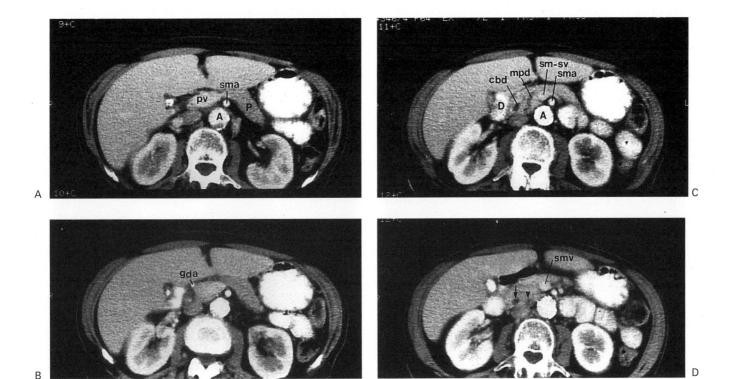

Fig. 6.1 Normal bolus dynamic pancreatic computerized tomography (CT). **A, B** Scans at the level of the tail of the pancreas (P) show the superior mesenteric artery (sma) and gastroduodenal artery (gda); A, aorta; pv, portal vein. **C, D** Scans at the level of the body and head of the pancreas show the main pancreatic duct (mpd, arrowhead) and common bile duct (cbd, arrow) and the confluence of the superior mesenteric (sm) and splenic vein (sv), posterior to the junction of the head and body.

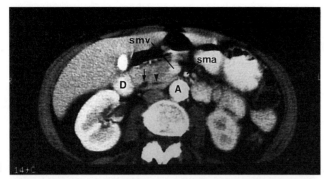

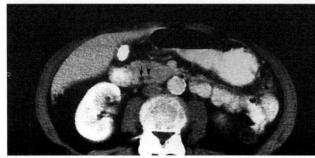

Fig. 6.1 (*continued*)   **E, F** Scans at the level of the head show the main pancreatic duct (arrowhead) and common bile duct (arrow) moving together as they enter the duodenum (D).

diffuse gland enlargement; grade C, intrinsic gland abnormalities associated with haziness and streaky densities representing inflammatory changes in the peripancreatic fat; grade D, single, ill-defined fluid collection or phlegmon, and grade E, two or more poorly defined fluid collections

or the presence of gas in or adjacent to the pancreas (Figs 6.2–6.5).

A normal CT scan may be found in 14–28% of patients with very mild forms of acute oedematous pancreatitis (Balthazar 1989). In general, virtually all other patients will have CT abnormalities if high quality, dynamic bolus CT is performed.

Necrosis of pancreatic parenchyma occurs in about 23% of patients with Balthazar grades B–E acute pancreatitis (Balthazar 1989). Necrosis is seen by dynamic CT as a zone of non-contrast-enhancing pancreatic parenchyma (Fig. 6.6). The significance of this CT finding has been established by excellent radiological-surgical correlation (Maier 1986, Büchler et al 1986). The grades of pancreatitis and the presence of associated necrosis are important indicators of prognosis (see Fig. 6.7) (Balthazar et al 1990, Beger et al 1986).

Chronic pancreatitis

The CT findings in chronic pancreatitis consist of a broad spectrum of changes which depend on the severity of the chronic inflammatory process. These include alterations in size and shape of the gland, changes in parenchymal attenuation, calculi, pancreatic and bile duct dilatation, fluid collections, and vascular involvement, such as portal venous obstruction and arterial pseudoaneurysms (Figs 6.8, 6.9) (Freeny & Lawson 1982, Freeny 1984).

There is considerable variation in the reported sensitivity of CT in the diagnosis of chronic pancreatitis, ranging from 50 to 90%. However, most of the studies appeared

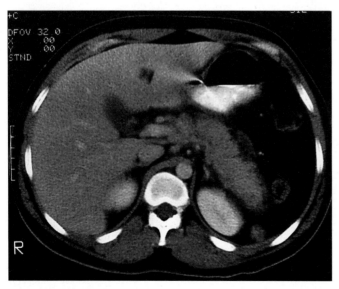

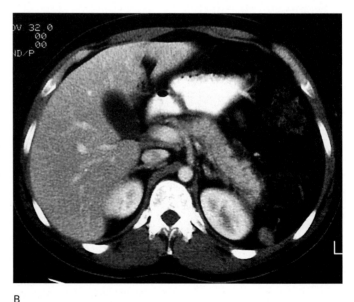

Fig. 6.2   Acute pancreatitis (Balthazar grade B). **A** CT scan of the pancreas shows mild, diffuse enlargement of the gland due to acute pancreatitis. **B** Scan 15 days later shows the gland to have returned to normal size.

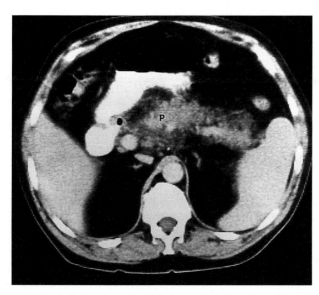

Fig. 6.3 Acute pancreatitis (Balthazar grade C). CT of the pancreas (P) shows diffuse gland enlargement, slightly heterogeneous parenchyma, and ill-defined margins owing to peripancreatic inflammation.

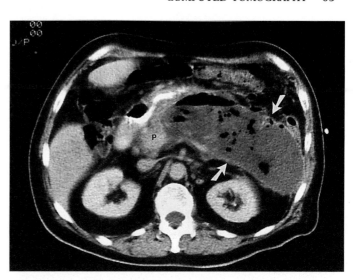

Fig. 6.5 Acute pancreatitis (Balthazar grade E). CT of the pancreas (P) shows a large gas-containing abscess (arrows) involving the entire body and tail of the gland.

prior to the introduction of the current generation of scanners and the use of 5 mm collimated scans and the dynamic incremental bolus contrast enhancement technique (Savarino 1980, Ferrucci et al 1981). A more recent paper by Luetmer and co-workers (1989), utilizing modern CT, reports a false negative rate of only 7% (4 of 56 patients) in CT detection of chronic pancreatitis. However, neither the clinical nor the functional severity of the disease in their patients was reported.

The severity of chronic pancreatitis can be staged on the basis of clinical symptoms (notably pain), diminished exocrine and/or endocrine function, and morphological changes in or around the gland as depicted by imaging studies.

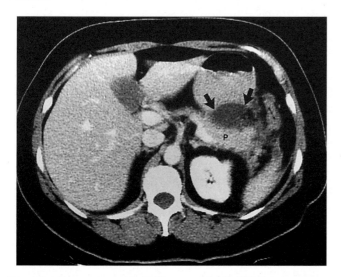

Fig. 6.4 Acute pancreatitis (Balthazar grade D). CT of the pancreas (P) shows a peripancreatic fluid collection (arrows).

A variety of reports have appeared over the last decade comparing morphological changes of chronic pancreatitis depicted by ultrasonography, CT, and endoscopic retrograde cholangiopancreatography (ERCP) with clinical symptoms (pain) and functional changes (as measured by various pancreatic function tests) (Elsborg et al 1981, Valentini et al 1981, Malfertheiner & Büchler 1989). In general, in patients with advanced chronic pancreatitis, there has been good correlation between the severity of clinical symptoms and functional impairment and the severity of morphological changes. However, in patients with mild or moderate symptoms and functional impairment, correlation with morphological changes has been poor. For example, Lankisch showed that 50% of patients with chronic pancreatitis and ductal calcifications (Cambridge classification: severe morphological changes) had only slight or moderate functional impairment (Lankisch et al 1986, Freeny 1989a). Malfertheiner & Büchler (1989) also showed that in patients with severe clinical/functional changes, morphological abnormalities depicted by CT or ERCP were mild in 14% and 20% of patients, respectively. Virtually all investigators have concluded that in general the severity of clinical/functional impairment cannot be predicted by the degree of morphological changes, and vice versa (Elsborg et al 1981, Valentini et al 1981, Malfertheiner & Büchler 1989).

Complications of pancreatitis

The complications of acute pancreatitis increase as the grade or severity of the inflammatory process increases or persists for long periods. The complications are detected readily by CT and include fluid collections and pseudocyst formation (infected and non-infected), frank pancreatic abscess, pleural and peritoneal collections of pancreatic

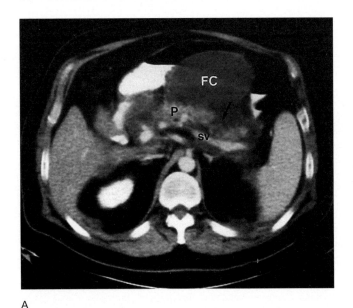
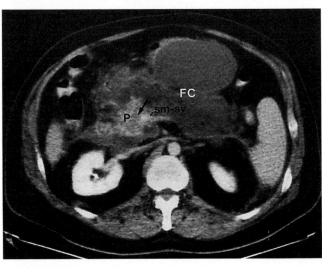

A   B

Fig. 6.6   Acute pancreatitis (necrosis). **A** Bolus dynamic CT shows contrast enhancement of the pancreas (P) with a focal area of necrosis (arrow) without enhancement. Large peripancreatic fluid collection (FC) is present. **B** Scan at the level of the pancreatic head (P) shows focal necrosis with patchy lack of contrast enhancement (arrow); sv, splenic vein; sm-sv, superior mesenteric–splenic vein confluence.

enzyme-rich fluid (pancreatic ascites), and involvement of the biliary tract, vascular system, and gastrointestinal tract.

Fluid collections (pseudocyst)

While fluid collections occur in at least 50–60% of patients with acute pancreatitis, they resolve spontaneously within 6 weeks in about 50% of patients (see Fig. 6.4) (Clavien et al 1988). Those that persist for longer than 6 weeks rarely show subsequent resolution and have a high inci-

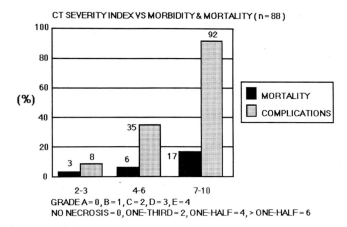

Fig. 6.7   CT severity index. Note that the patients with a severity index of 0 or 1 had no morbidity or mortality; those with an index of 2–3 had 8% morbidity and 3% mortality, while those with an index of 7–10 had 17% mortality and 92% morbidity. (From Balthazar E J, Robinson D L, Megibow A J, Ranson J H C 1990 Acute pancreatitis: value of CT in establishing prognosis. Radiology 174: 331–336.)

dence of complications, such as rupture, perforation into adjacent organs, and infection. Thus, careful observation is essential and early percutaneous catheter drainage is advocated at the first sign of infection or other complication.

Pancreatic abscess

Pancreatic abscess complicates acute pancreatitis in about 10% of cases. It can develop de novo from secondary infection of necrotic pancreatic parenchyma or as a secondary complication of a pre-existing fluid collection or pseudocyst. Clinical evaluation usually suggests the presence of infection, and this can be confirmed by CT and CT-guided fine-needle aspiration (see Fig. 6.5) (Banks & Gerzof 1987).

Percutaneous catheter drainage can be used to treat pancreatic abscesses which are loculated and composed of liquid pus, but those that contain large amounts of necrotic debris and solid material, such as infected necrosis or phlegmon, can only be temporarily relieved by catheter drainage (Freeny et al 1988a).

Pancreatic ascites and pleural effusion

Pancreatic ascites occurs if there is disruption of the pancreatic duct or rupture of a pancreatic fluid collection/pseudocyst and leakage of pancreatic juice into the peritoneal cavity (Freeny & Lawson 1982). CT can be helpful in identifying the source of the leak, but ERCP is the most useful technique.

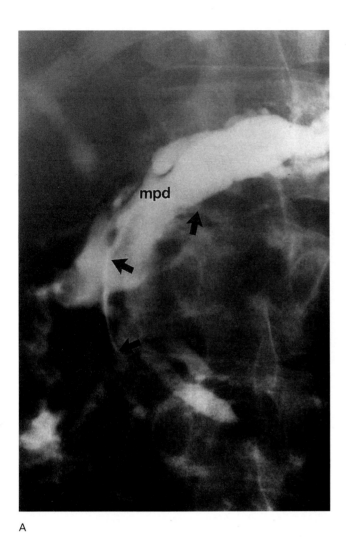

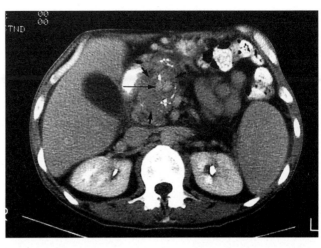

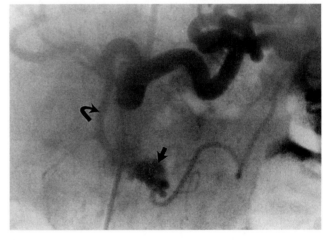

A

B

C

Fig. 6.8 Chronic pancreatitis. **A** Endoscopic retrograde cholangiopancreatography (ERCP) shows displacement (arrows) of the dilated main pancreatic duct (mpd) by a mass in the head of the pancreas. **B** CT at the level of the pancreatic head shows a focal mass (short arrows), calcifications, and a central, lobulated, contrast-enhancing mass (long arrow, pseudoaneurysm). **C** Coeliac arteriogram confirms arterial pseudoaneurysm (straight arrow) arising from the gastroduodenal artery (curved arrow).

Pleural effusions are common in acute pancreatitis. They most commonly are due to reactive exudate from a contiguous inflammatory process in the subdiaphragmatic space, but can be caused by direct extension of a pancreatic fluid collection or fistula into the pleural space.

Biliary tract involvement

The inflammatory process of acute pancreatitis often involves the intrapancreatic segment of the common bile duct. The involvement may be transient and characterized by displacement or narrowing of the duct with a return to normality as the inflammation subsides. Alternatively it may be permanent, and manifested by a focal stricture or long, tapered segmental narrowing (Rohrmann & Baron 1989).

Rarely, a biliary fistula can develop from a contiguous pseudocyst or abscess.

Transient abnormalities of liver function are common in patients with acute pancreatitis. Evaluation of the biliary tract usually proceeds only if the function tests remain abnormal or if associated complications, such as cholangitis or evidence of near or complete obstruction, are present.

Ultrasonography and CT are best used for initial evaluation of the biliary tract. They can identify ductal obstruction as well as evaluate contiguous inflammatory processes, such as an abscess or pseudocyst. Direct cholangiography is useful for more precise evaluation of the biliary ducts to plan percutaneous, endoscopic, or surgical treatment.

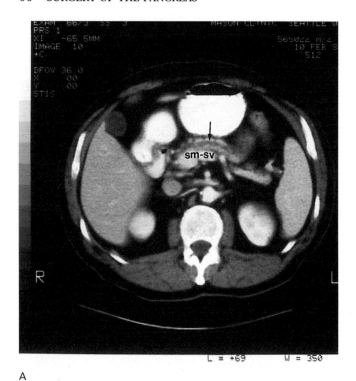 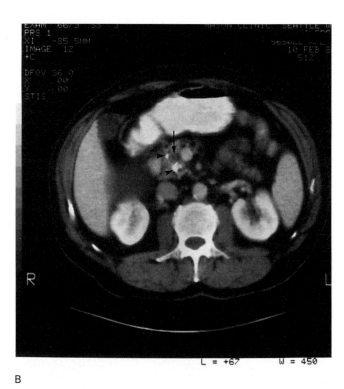

A   B

Fig. 6.9   Chronic calcific pancreatitis. **A** Scan at the level of the body of the pancreas shows a dilated main pancreatic duct (arrow); sm-sv, confluence of the superior mesenteric and splenic vein. **B** Scan at the level of the head shows a small intrapancreatic cyst and calcifications (arrowheads). ERCP (not illustrated) showed a focal stricture of the pancreatic duct in the head.

Gastrointestinal tract involvement

Acute pancreatitis can involve virtually any segment of the gastrointestinal tract from the oesophagus to the colon (Safrit & Rice 1989). CT can demonstrate spread of the inflammatory process to contiguous or remote segments of the gastrointestinal tract. In addition, it can show communications or fistulas between a fluid collection or pseudocyst and a contiguous segment of the stomach or bowel, and can identify potential sites of gastrointestinal tract involvement during the early stages of the disease. Contrast studies (barium or water soluble media) also may be useful for demonstration of suspected fistula or stenosis.

Vascular involvement

When pancreatic enzymes leak into the parenchyma of the gland or into surrounding tissues, they can cause direct erosion of pancreatic or peripancreatic vessels with resulting haemorrhage, formation of pseudoaneurysms, or thrombosis of the splenic or superior mesenteric veins followed by development of varices. Bolus-dynamic CT produces excellent opacification of the arteries and veins surrounding the pancreas and thus is an excellent method for identifying these vascular complications (see Fig. 6.8) (Freeny & Lawson 1982, Vujic 1989).

Acute pancreatic haemorrhage can be suspected by CT if one can identify a focal collection of fluid (blood) with increased attenuation or recognize an interim increase in the attenuation values of the fluid within a previously demonstrated pseudocyst or fluid collection.

Arterial pseudoaneurysms can develop within the pancreatic parenchyma, adjacent to the gland, or within a pseudocyst. They can be diagnosed by angiography or CT by demonstrating a contrast-enhancing mass (see Fig. 6.8). Venous occlusion can be seen directly by angiography as an abrupt cutoff of the contrast-filled vein, or indirectly by CT or angiography as collateral vessels enlarge and perigastric or mesenteric varices develop.

PANCREATIC CARCINOMA

Dynamic CT is the most accurate method for diagnosis and staging of pancreatic carcinoma. The primary CT findings of pancreatic carcinoma include a focal or diffuse mass, usually of diminished attenuation relative to the normally contrast-enhancing pancreatic parenchyma, and pancreatic and bile duct obstruction, either upstream from a mass, or as isolated findings in the absence of a mass (Figs 5.6, 6.10–6.12) (Freeny 1989b). The accuracy of CT in the diagnosis of pancreatic carcinoma is 91% (Freeny et al 1989b).

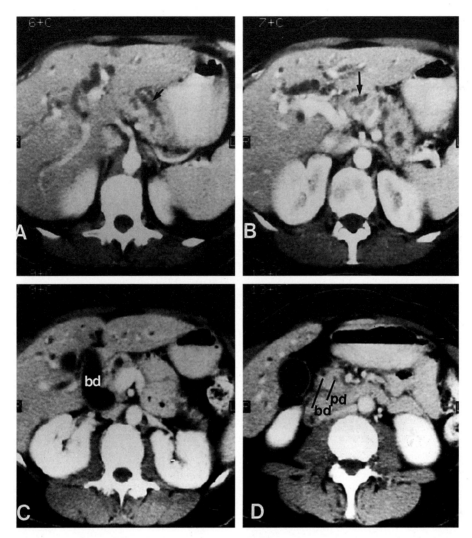

Fig. 6.10 Resectable pancreatic carcinoma. **A–D** CT scans of the pancreas show marked dilatation of the intra- and extrahepatic bile ducts (bd) and main pancreatic duct (pd, arrows) ('double duct' sign). **D** Most caudal scan shows the narrowed common bile duct (bd) and main pancreatic duct (pd) with no discernible mass in the head of the pancreas. Surgery confirmed a 2 cm carcinoma of the pancreatic head.

The CT criteria for staging of patients with pancreatic carcinoma into surgically resectable or non-resectable groups include local extension of tumour, invasion of contiguous organs, vascular involvement and hepatic, lymph node, or other distant metastases (Figs 6.11, 6.12) (Freeny et al 1988b, Freeny 1988b). In the series of 159 cases reported by this author, local extension of tumour was present in 68% of cases; contiguous organ invasion (duodenum, stomach, spleen, root of the small bowel mesentery, and left adrenal gland) in 42%; vascular involvement (encasement or obstruction of major extrapancreatic arteries and/or veins) in 84%; hepatic metastases in 36%, and lymph node metastases in 28% (Freeny et al 1988b). Correlation of CT findings with surgical exploration confirmed the accuracy of CT in defining tumour non-resectability; none of the tumours in the 42 patients with CT-unresectable tumours could be resected at the time of surgery.

It is important to realize that the CT findings of pancreatic carcinoma can be mimicked by other disease processes. These include focal pancreatitis and other tumours which have a better response to surgery or to medical or radiation therapy, such as islet cell carcinoma and lymphoma (Freeny 1989b). Therefore, it is important to confirm the CT diagnosis by a guided fine-needle aspiration biopsy, especially if no palliative treatment will be recommended to the patient (see Fig. 6.11).

CYSTIC PANCREATIC NEOPLASMS

Microcystic neoplasms (serous cystadenomas) are benign and have not been reported to become malignant, while macrocystic tumours (mucinous cystadenomas) are considered to be premalignant lesions. Thus, non-operative differentiation of these tumours is critical for appropriate patient management.

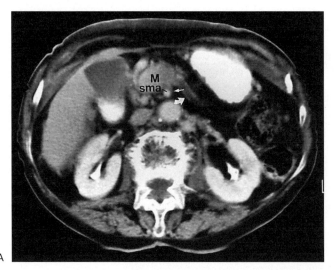
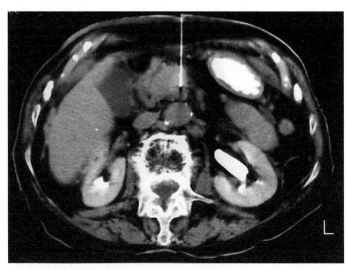

A   B

Fig. 6.11 Unresectable pancreatic carcinoma. **A** CT shows a focal mass (M) in the head of the pancreas with a dilated upstream pancreatic duct (curved arrow) surrounded by atrophic parenchyma. The tumour has grown posteriorly (small white arrow) to invade the superior mesenteric artery (sma). The superior mesenteric vein is not seen because it is occluded. **B** CT-guided fine-needle aspiration biopsy confirmed the diagnosis of pancreatic carcinoma.

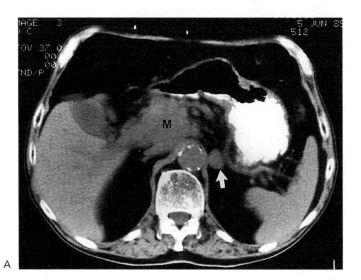
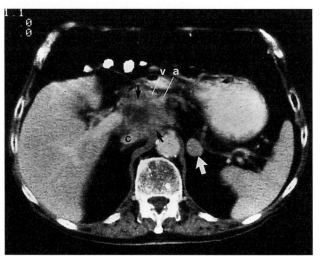

A   B

C

Fig. 6.12 Unresectable pancreatic carcinoma. **A** CT scan without contrast shows a focal mass (M) in the head of the pancreas and a right adrenal mass (arrow). **B** Bolus dynamic CT at the same level as **A** shows the mass to be hypodense (arrows). The mass has invaded around the superior mesenteric artery (a) and vein (v) and inferior vena cava (c). **C** Scan at a more caudal level shows the hypodense tumour mass contiguous with the superior mesenteric artery (arrow), aorta (A), and inferior vena cava (c).

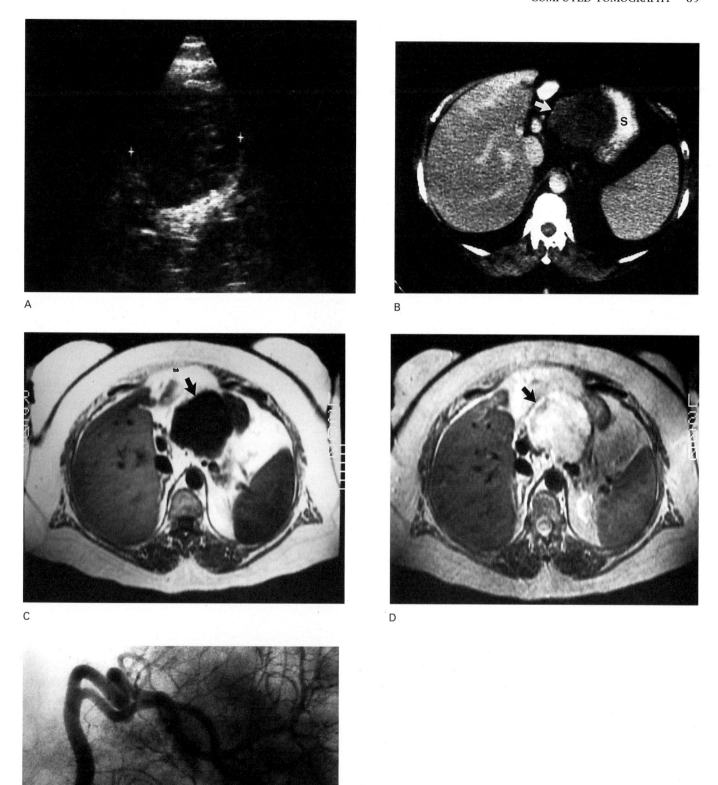

Fig. 6.13 Serous cystadenoma. **A** Axial ultrasonography shows a hypoechoic mass (cursors) in the tail of the pancreas. The mass appears to be cystic. **B** CT shows a homogeneous hypodense mass (arrow) in the tail of the pancreas. S, stomach. **C** MR scan (1.5 T, T1-weighted scan) shows the mass to have diminished signal (arrow). **D** MR scan (1.5 T, T2-weighted scan) shows the mass to have increased signal (arrow), confirming its cystic nature. **E** Selective splenic arteriogram shows the mass to be hypervascular (arrows).

The most useful imaging tests for the specific diagnosis of cystic pancreatic neoplasms are CT and ultrasonography. The number of cysts within the tumours and the diameter of the cysts are the most reliable criteria for differentiating the two types. Microcystic adenomas tend to have multiple cysts (more than 6) which are small (less than 2 cm in diameter) while macrocystic tumours usually have fewer cysts (less than 6) which are larger in size (greater than 2 cm) (Figs 6.13, 6.14) (Johnson et al 1988, Mathieu et al 1989). A central scar with radiating septae and central sunburst calcification have also been described as characteristic of microcystic tumours. However, in the series reported by Johnson et al (1988), a central scar was seen in only 2 of 16 cases (13%), while calcifications were present in 38% of microcystic tumours, 18% of macrocystic adenomas, and in 8% of macrocystic adenocarcinomas.

A number of authors have emphasized the value of fine-needle aspiration biopsy in the differentiation of these tumours (Fond et al 1984, Emmert & Bewtra 1986, Vellet et al 1988, Mathieu et al 1989). Macrocystic neoplasms contain abundant mucin, which can be identified by Giemsa staining, and columnar cells. The cytological diagnosis of carcinoma is based on changes in the cell nuclei. Microcystic tumours are lined by cuboidal cells and electron microscopy can identify intracytoplasmic glycogen granules, which are not found in macrocystic tumours.

Minami has compared CT and magnetic resonance imaging (MR) of cystic neoplasms (Minami et al 1989). MR shows that microcystic tumours are externally lobulated and contain septae and multiple cysts with decreased signal on T1-weighted images, and increased signal on T2 images. Macrocystic tumours showed thicker septae, larger cysts, and considerable variation in signal intensity on both T1 and T2-weighted images (see Fig. 6.14). MR was equal to CT in demonstration of septae, but superior in demonstrating the external shape and lobulation of the tumours. The cystic nature of the tumours was more readily apparent on MR, but calcifications seen on CT were not demonstrated by MR. Additional series need to be described to reach a conclusion about the value of MR in differentiation of the two types of cystic tumours.

ISLET CELL TUMOURS

Functioning islet cell tumours

These are usually diagnosed on the basis of clinical findings and appropriate hormonal immunoassay techniques. The role of imaging is preoperative localization and assessment of the extent of the tumour. These roles can be accomplished with a combination of ultrasonography, CT, MR, angiography, and portal venous sampling.

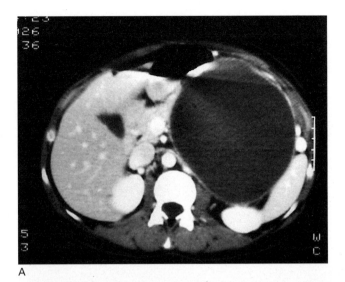

A

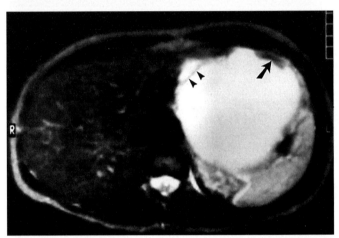

B

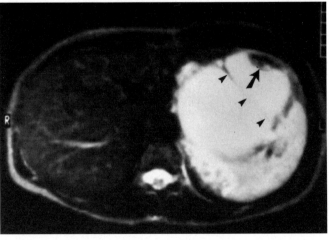

C

Fig. 6.14 Mucinous cystadenocarcinoma. **A** CT shows a large cystic mass with a thin capsule. **B, C** MR (0.5 T, T2 spin echo sequence) shows the cystic mass with high signal, internal mural nodules (arrows) and septations (arrowheads), indicating a mucinous cystic neoplasm. (Courtesy of Didier Mathieu, M.D., Centre Hospitalier Universitaire Henri Mondor, Cretiel, France.)

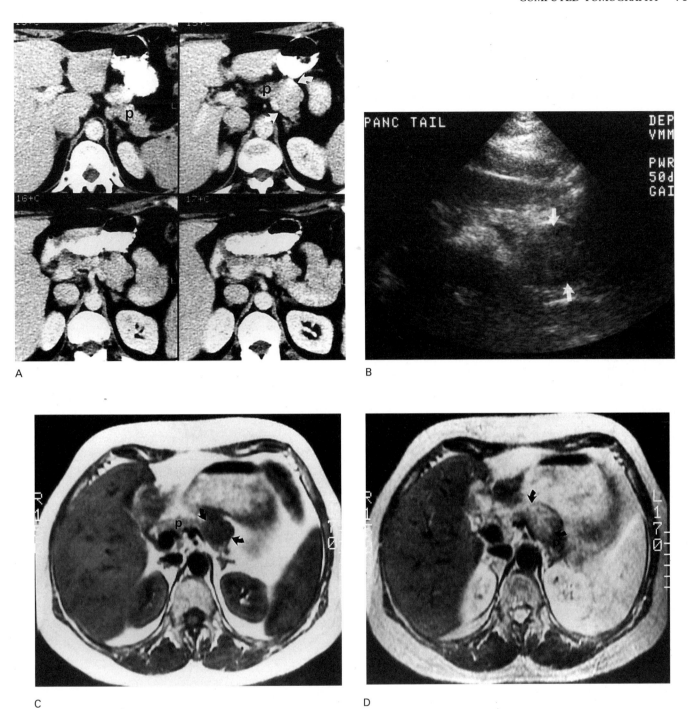

Fig. 6.15 Insulinoma. **A** Consecutive CT scans of the pancreas (p) show a focal, contrast-enhancing mass (curved arrows). **B** Axial ultrasonography confirms the presence of a pancreatic mass (arrows). **C** MR scan (1.5 T, T1-weighted scan) shows the pancreas (p) and a low-signal mass (curved arrows). **D** MR scan (1.5 T, T2-weighted scan) shows increased signal in the mass.

On CT functioning islet cell tumours usually appear as small, contrast-enhancing lesions within the pancreas, or adjacent to the gland in the case of extrapancreatic tumours, notably gastrinomas (Fig. 6.15). Malignant tumours also may be associated with hepatic and lymph node metastases.

The overall accuracy of CT in localization of functioning islet cell tumours is between 82% and 96%, with specific accuracy for insulinomas of 79%, gastrinomas 83%, and for miscellaneous cell types, 100% (Thompson et al 1988, Rossi et al 1989).

Nonfunctioning islet cell tumours

These are usually large, ranging from 5–20 cm in diameter. They have often invaded contiguous structures and organs or have metastasized to the liver or to regional lymph nodes at the time of initial evaluation (Freeny & Lawson 1982). Thus, they can be readily detected and resectability can be assessed by CT. CT usually reveals large tumours which generally show some degree of contrast enhancement, in distinction to ductal carcinomas which do not enhance and are seen as low attenuation masses (Eelkema et al 1984). The tumours may contain nodular foci of calcification and often involve contiguous organs or have metastasized to the liver.

REFERENCES

Balthazar E J 1989 CT diagnosis and staging of acute pancreatitis. Radiologic Clinics of North America 27: 19–37

Balthazar E J, Ranson J H C, Naidich D H P, Megibow A J, Caccavale R, Cooper M M 1985 Acute pancreatitis: prognostic value of CT. Radiology 156: 767–772

Balthazar E J, Robinson D L, Megibow A J, Ranson J H C 1990 Acute pancreatitis: value of CT in establishing prognosis. Radiology 174: 331–336

Banks P A, Gerzof S G 1987 Indications and results of fine needle aspiration of pancreatic exudate. In: Beger H G, Büchler M (eds) Acute pancreatitis. Research and clinical management. Springer-Verlag, Berlin, p 171–174

Beger H G, Maier W, Block S, Büchler M 1986 How do imaging methods influence the surgical strategy in acute pancreatitis? In: Malfertheiner P, Ditschuneit H (eds) Diagnostic procedures in pancreatic disease. Springer-Verlag, Berlin, p 54–60

Büchler M, Malfertheiner P, Beger H G 1986 Correlation of imaging procedures, biological parameters, and clinical stage in acute pancreatitis. In: Malfertheiner P, Ditschuneit H (eds) Diagnostic procedures in pancreatic disease. Springer-Verlag, Berlin, p 123–129

Clavien P A, Hauser H, Meyer P, Rohner A 1988 Value of contrast-enhanced computerized tomography in the early diagnosis and prognosis of acute pancreatitis. A prospective study of 202 patients. American Journal of Surgery 155: 457

Eelkema E A, Stephens D H, Ward E M, Sheedy P F II 1984 CT features of nonfunctioning islet cell carcinoma. American Journal of Radiology 143: 943–948

Elsborg L, Bruusgard L, Strandgaard L et al 1981 Endoscopic retrograde pancreatography and the exocrine pancreatic function chronic alcoholism. Scandinavian journal of Gastroenterology 16: 941–944

Emmert G M, Bewtra C 1986 Fine needle aspiration biopsy of mucinous cystic tumours of the pancreas: a case study. Diagnostic Cytopathology 2: 69–71

Ferrucci J T Jr, Wittenberg J, Black E B, Kirkpatrick R H, Hall D A 1981 Computed body tomography in chronic pancreatitis. Radiology 130: 175–182

Fond A, Bret P M, Bretagnolle M et al 1984 Ultrasound and fine needle biopsy of cystic tumours of the pancreas. Journal Belge de Radiologie 67: 277–284

Freeny P C 1984 Computed tomography of the pancreas. In: Creutzfeldt W (ed) The exocrine pancreas. Clinics in Gastroenterology 13: 791–818

Freeny P C 1988 Commentary. Radiology of the pancreas: two decades of progress in imaging and intervention. American Journal of Radiology 150: 975–981

Freeny P C 1989a Classification of pancreatitis. Radiologic Clinics of North America 27: 1–3

Freeny P C 1989b Radiologic diagnosis and staging of pancreatic ductal adenocarcinoma. Radiologic Clinics of North America 27: 121–128

Freeny P C, Lawson L 1982 Radiology of the pancreas. Springer-Verlag, New York

Freeny P C, Marks W M, Ryan J A, Traverso L W 1988a Pancreatic ductal adenocarcinoma: diagnosis and staging with dynamic CT. Radiology 166: 125–133

Freeny P C, Lewis G P, Traverso L W et al 1988b Infected pancreatic fluid collections: percutaneous catheter drainage. Radiology 167: 435–441

Johnson C D, Stephens D H, Charboneau J W, Carpenter H A, Welch T J 1988 Cystic pancreatic tumors: CT and sonographic assessment. American Journal of Radiology 151: 1133–1138

Lankisch P G, Otto J, Erkelenz I, Lembeke B 1986 Pancreatic calcifications: no indicator of severe exocrine pancreatic insufficiency. Gastroenterology 90: 617–621

Luetmer P H, Stephens D H, Ward E M 1989 Chronic pancreatitis: reassessment with current CT. Radiology 171: 353–357

Maier W 1986 Experimentelle und klinische Untersuchungen zur Rolle der Computertomographie in der Stadieneinteilung der acuten Pankreatitis. Universität Ulm

Malfertheiner P, Büchler M 1989 Correlation of imaging and function in chronic pancreatitis. Radiologic Clinics of North America 27: 51–64

Mathieu D, Guigui B, Valette P J, Dao T H, Bruneton J N, Bruel J M, Pringot J, Vasile N 1989 Pancreatic cystic neoplasms. Radiologic Clinics of North America 27: 163–176

Minami M, Itaiy Y, Ohtomo K, Yoshida H, Yoshikawa K, Iio M 1989 Cystic neoplasms of the pancreas: comparison of MR imaging with CT. Radiology 171: 53–56

Rohrmann C A, Baron R L 1989 Biliary complications of pancreatitis. Radiologic Clinics of North America 27: 93–104

Rossi P, Allison D J, Bezzi M, Kennedy A, Maccioni F, Wynick D, Maradei A, Bloom S R 1989 Endocrine tumors of the pancreas. Radiologic Clinics of North America 27: 129–161

Safrit H D, Rice R P 1989 Gastrointestinal complications of pancreatitis. Radiologic Clinics of North America 27: 73–79

Savarino V 1980 Computed tomography in the diagnosis of pancreatic disease. Italian Journal of Gastroenterology 12: 265–269

Thompson G B, Van Heerden J A, Grant C S, Carney J A, Ilstrup D M 1988 Islet cell carcinoma of the pancreas: a twenty-year experience. Surgery 104: 1011–1017

Valentini M, Cavallini G, Vantini I et al 1981 A comparative evaluation of endoscopic retrograde cholangiopancreatography and the secretin-cholecystokinin test in the diagnosis of chronic pancreatitis: a multicentre study in 124 patients. Endoscopy 13: 64–67

Vellet D, Leiman G, Mair S et al 1988 Fine needle aspiration cytology of mucinous cystadenocarcinoma of the pancreas. Further observations. Acta Cytologica 32: 43–48

Vujic I 1989 Vascular complications of pancreatitis. Radiologic Clinics of North America 27: 81–91

7. Magnetic resonance imaging

P. C. Freeny

Magnetic resonance (MR) imaging of the pancreas has been used only to a limited extent. MR can produce images of the gland at both of the commonly used magnetic field strengths of 0.5 T and 1.5 T (Stark et al 1984, Simeone et al 1985). The normal pancreas has a low signal intensity compared to the high signal intensity of the surrounding peripancreatic fat (Fig. 7.1). The major peripancreatic vessels are void of signal owing to flowing blood and thus are seen as black tubular structures without the necessity for intravenous contrast administration (Fig. 7.2). The pancreatic duct and the intrapancreatic segment of the common bile duct are rarely seen unless they are dilated.

MR has not found a definite place in pancreatic imaging. It has been used to detect pancreatic neoplasms and in imaging pancreatitis, but it has not been found to have as high an overall accuracy as CT, nor to offer any significant advantage over CT (see Figs 6.13, 6.14) (Steiner et al 1989). Occasionally, MR may be an aid in problem-solving when ultrasonography or CT are equivocal (see Fig. 6.15). However, MR technology is in a state of rapid evolution and the ability to perform fast MR scans, opacify the bowel, improve detection of hepatic metastases with contrast agents, and increase spatial resolution and signal-to-noise ratio, may lead to a significant role for MR imaging within the next few years.

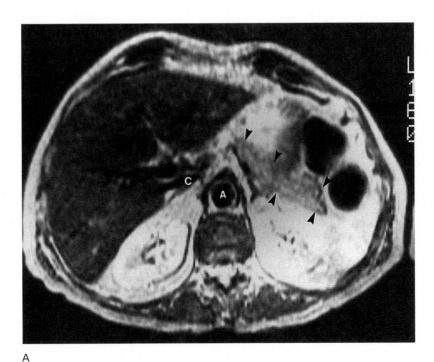

A

Fig. 7.1 Normal pancreatic MR scan (1.5 T, T2-weighted spin echo). **A** MR at the level of the pancreatic tail (arrowheads); aorta (A), interior vena cava (c).

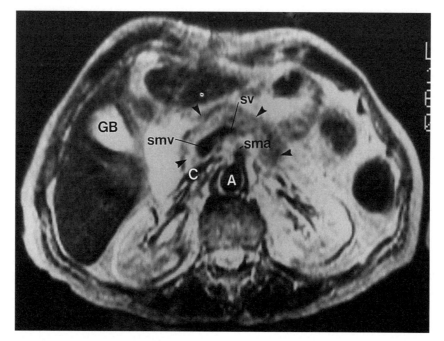

B

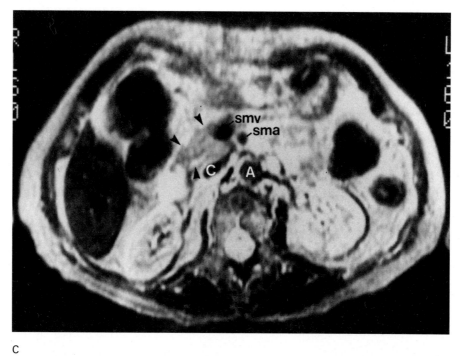

C

Fig. 7.1 (*continued*)   **B** Scan at the level of the body (arrowheads). **C** Scan at the level of the head (arrowheads); gallbladder (GB), superior mesenteric vein (smv), superior mesenteric artery (sma), splenic vein (sv).

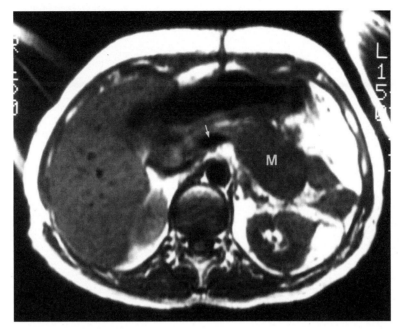

A

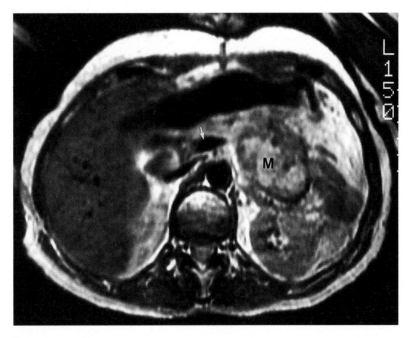

B

Fig. 7.2 Pancreatic cancer. **A** T1-weighted MR image of the pancreas shows a focal mass (M) in the tail with decreased signal intensity. **B** T2-weighted image shows heterogeneously increased signal intensity within the mass (M). Note signal void in blood vessels (superior mesenteric vein, arrow).

REFERENCES

Simeone J F, Edelman R R, Stark D D, Wittenberg J, White E M, Butch R J 1985 Surface coil MR imaging of abdominal viscera: Part III. The pancreas. Radiology 157: 437–441

Stark D D, Moss A A, Goldberg H I, Davis P L, Federle M P 1984 Magnetic resonance and CT of the normal and diseased pancreas: a comparative study. Radiology 150: 153–162

Steiner E, Stark D D, Haha P F, Saini S, Simeone J F, Mueller P R, Wittenberg J, Ferrucci J T 1989 Imaging pancreatic neoplasms: comparison of MR and CT. Radiology 152: 487–491

8. Percutaneous transhepatic cholangiography

P. C. Freeny

Endoscopic retrograde cholangiopancreatography (ERCP) has superseded percutaneous transhepatic cholangiography (PTC) for evaluation and treatment of patients with pancreatic diseases involving the biliary tract in most medical centres. However, when ERCP or endoscopic placement of biliary stents fail, PTC can be used. Thus, the current indications for PTC include cholangiography if ERCP is unavailable or fails, and percutaneous biliary stent placement if endoscopic stent placement fails or is not possible owing to gastroduodenal anatomy.

PTC is performed via a right intercostal or left subcostal approach using local anaesthesia and a 22–23 gauge needle (Freeny & Lawson 1982). Once a peripheral bile duct is opacified, further contrast medium can be injected to obtain a cholangiogram, or a 0.018 inch guide-wire can be placed through the needle to gain catheter access to the bile ducts for permanent or temporary drainage of an obstructed system.

The rendezvous procedure (combined transhepatic-endoscopic access to the biliary tract) can be used to facilitate endoscopic stent placement (Shovorn et al 1985). In this procedure, a 5 French catheter is placed into the intrahepatic ductal system via a left or right percutaneous approach and then advanced into the duodenum (Fig. 8.1). An endoscope is then introduced to the level of the papilla and a 200 cm guide-wire is passed through the

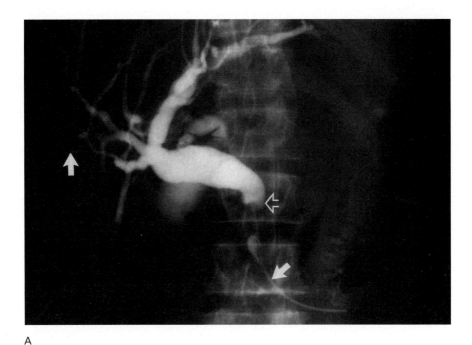

A

Fig. 8.1 Pancreatic cancer. Combined transhepatic-endoscopic (rendezvous procedure) biliary stent placement. **A** Percutaneous transhepatic cholangiography (PTC) shows dilated, obstructed common bile duct (open arrow). A 5 French catheter has been placed transhepatically into the duodenum (closed arrows).

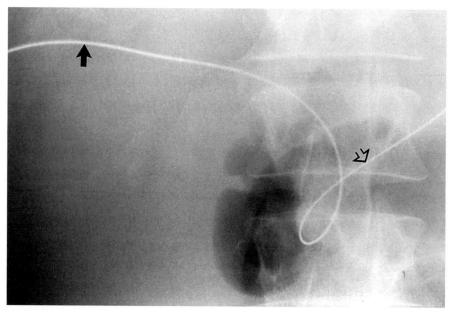

B

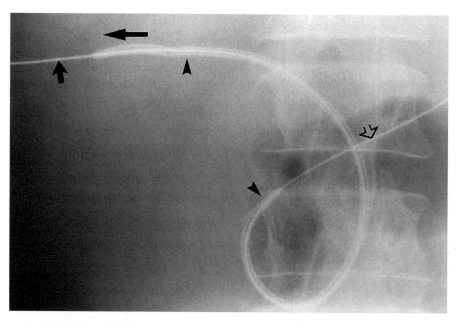

C

Fig. 8.1 (*continued*)   **B** A 200 cm guide-wire has been passed through the transhepatic catheter (closed arrow) and withdrawn through the endoscope (open arrow). **C** A 10 French stent (arrowheads) has been pushed retrogradely over the guide-wire from the duodenum (open arrow) into the intrahepatic ducts. (Short closed arrow, transhepatic segment of guide-wire.)

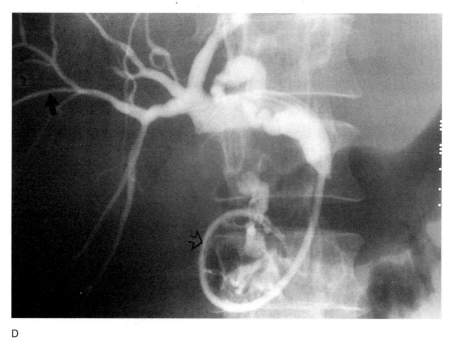

D

Fig. 8.1 (*continued*)   **D** Final cholangiogram via the transhepatic catheter (closed arrow) shows a patent biliary stent (open arrow).

catheter. A wire snare fed through the channel of the endoscope is then used to capture the guide wire and pull it back through the endoscope. A papillotome or biliary stent can then be passed retrogradely over the guide-wire and placed in the biliary duct (Fig. 8.1). The transhepatic catheter is removed when the stent is seen to function normally.

REFERENCES

Freeny P C, Lawson T L 1982 Radiology of the pancreas. Springer-Verlag, New York
Shovorn P J, Cotton P B, Mason R R, Siegel J H, Hatfield A R W 1985 Percutaneous transhepatic assistance for duodenoscopic sphincterotomy. Gut 26: 1373–1376

9. Angiography

P. C. Freeny

The role of pancreatic angiography has diminished with the introduction of cross-sectional imaging techniques and endoscopic retrograde cholangiopancreatography (ERCP). However, it continues to play several important, well-defined roles in evaluation of patients with pancreatic disease (Freeny et al 1982).

TECHNIQUES

Pancreatic angiography begins with selective coeliac and superior mesenteric injections. Superselective injections are then performed if needed for diagnosis. Accurate diagnostic pancreatic angiography often requires selective (hepatic, splenic arteries) and superselective (gastroduodenal, dorsal pancreatic, inferior pancreaticoduodenal arteries) injections so that all of the small vessels of the gland are opacified (Fig. 9.1). Opacification of the portal venous system, including the splenic, superior mesenteric and portal veins, is also important. The splenic vein is usually well-opacified on coeliac or selective splenic artery injections, but good opacification of the superior mesenteric vein and portal vein is often best accomplished by a selective injection into the superior mesenteric artery, following injection of 25–50 mg of the vasodilator tolazoline (Freeny & Lawson 1982).

INDICATIONS FOR ANGIOGRAPHY

The current indications for pancreatic angiography include investigation of patients with known pancreatitis and pancreatic neoplasms. Specifically, angiography can be used for the following indications:

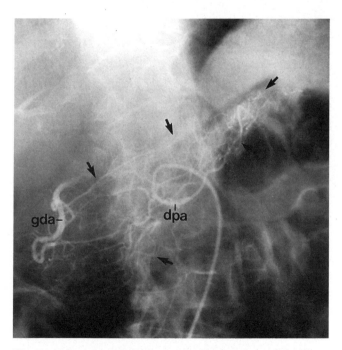

Fig. 9.1 Normal superselective pancreatic arteriogram. Selective dorsal pancreatic artery (dpa) injection shows filling of the intrapancreatic arteries (arrows) and retrograde filling of the gastroduodenal artery (gda).

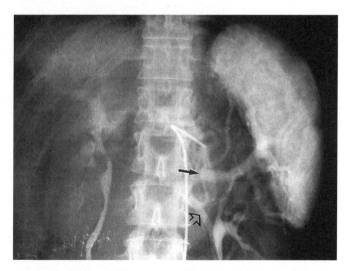

Fig. 9.2 Pancreatitis. Venous phase of selective splenic arteriogram, in a patient with acute pancreatitis and a large pseudocyst, shows occlusion of the splenic vein (closed arrow) and retrograde filling of the inferior mesenteric vein (open arrow).

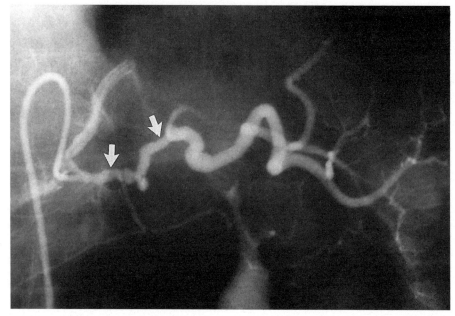

A

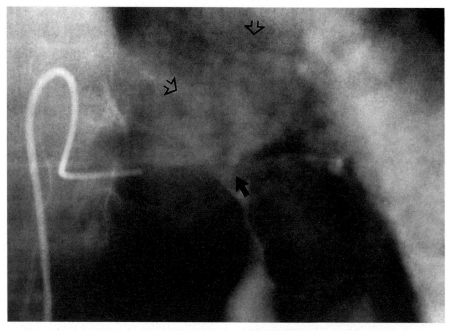

B

Fig. 9.3 Pancreatic cancer. **A** Arterial phase of selective splenic arteriogram shows a long
segment of tumour encasement of the splenic artery (arrows). **B** Venous phase shows splenic vein
obstruction (closed arrow) and perigastric varices (open arrows).

1. Precise identification of vascular involvement in
   patients with severe pancreatitis
2. Transcatheter control of haemorrhage caused by
   inflammatory or neoplastic involvement of pancreatic
   vessels
3. Preoperative definition of vascular anatomy and
   identification of vascular involvement in patients who
   are candidates for pancreatic resection for both benign
   and malignant disease
4. Localization of pancreatic islet cell tumours with
   angiography or portal venous sampling
5. Problem-solving when diagnosis by cross-sectional
   imaging or ERCP is equivocal.

Pancreatitis

Pancreatitis can cause splenic or superior mesenteric/portal venous obstruction and formation of varices; arterial erosion with massive haemorrhage or formation of pseudo-aneurysms, or arterial obstruction. Many of these complications can be demonstrated by ultrasonography, computerized tomography (CT) or magnetic resonance (MR) imaging, but precise identification of the vessels involved is often necessary prior to surgery, or for transcatheter embolization for control of haemorrhage (see Figs 6.8, 9.2) (Vujic et al 1980, Hofer et al 1987, Vujic 1989).

It is occasionally difficult to differentiate focal pancreatic inflammatory disease from pancreatic neoplasm by cross-sectional imaging with ultrasonography or CT. ERCP can often aid in this differentiation, but sometimes the diagnosis remains in doubt. Because the angiographic findings of pancreatitis and pancreatic neoplasms are quite different, superselective pancreatic angiography often provides valuable information which can assist precise diagnosis (Freeny & Lawson 1982). Equally important for problem solving is fine-needle aspiration biopsy. This is discussed in more detail in following sections.

Pancreatic neoplasms

Pancreatic carcinoma

CT is quite accurate for staging pancreatic ductal adeno-carcinoma. However, prior to pancreatic resection, angiography can be used to detect vascular involvement which may have been missed by CT and to define the peripancreatic vascular anatomy for the surgeon.

The primary angiographic findings in pancreatic carcinoma include a hypovascular mass with encasement of small intrapancreatic vessels and encasement or obstruction of major extrapancreatic arteries and veins. The latter findings indicate tumour invasion beyond the margins of the gland and reliably indicate tumour unresectability (Fig. 9.3) (Freeny & Lawson 1982).

Preoperative definition of vascular anatomy is important to the surgeon prior to performing a pancreatic resection (Freeny & Lawson 1982; Hofer et al 1987). Angiography can identify vascular anomalies, such as origin of the hepatic artery from the superior mesenteric artery, or non-tumorous obstruction of major arteries which could complicate pancreatic resection (Fig. 9.4).

Islet cell tumours

CT, ultrasonography and MR are the initial methods used for localization of pancreatic islet cell tumours. When the findings are normal or equivocal, angiography and transhepatic portal venous sampling can be used. Most islet cell tumours are hypervascular and can be identified when superselective angiography is performed (Fig. 9.5). However, some islet cell tumours are hypo-

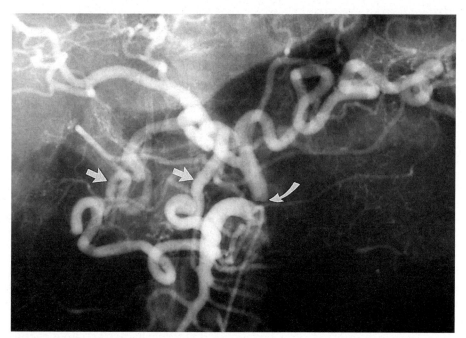

Fig. 9.4 Pancreatic cancer. Arterial phase of selective superior mesenteric arteriogram shows occlusion of the coeliac artery (curved arrow) with retrograde filling via enlarged pancreaticoduodenal arcades (straight arrows). Planned resection of the head of the pancreas was altered to first include reconstruction of the coeliac artery, since removal of the pancreaticoduodenal arcades would have caused ischaemia in the coeliac artery distribution.

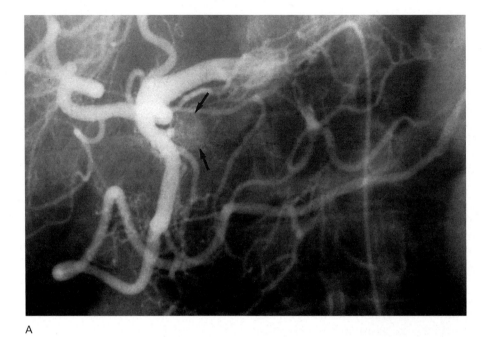

A

B

Fig. 9.5 Insulinoma. **A** Arterial phase of selective hepatic arteriogram shows a small, contrast-enhancing mass in the head of the pancreas (arrows), typical of islet cell tumour. **B** Late arterial phase shows small mass (arrows).

vascular, particularly gastrinomas. In this case, portal venous sampling with radioimmunoassay for the appropriate hormone can be used for localization (Fig. 9.6) (Freeny & Lawson 1982, Krudy et al 1984, Norton et al 1986).

The accuracy of angiographic localization of islet cell tumours varies considerably from series to series. In general, localization of hypervascular tumours, particularly insulinomas, is quite high (about 84%) while it is generally lower (about 60%) for those tumours such as gastrinomas which are usually hypovascular, although accuracy as high as 86% has been reported (Norton et al 1986, Rossi et al 1989).

Transhepatic portal venous sampling has been reported to have an accuracy of 80–85% in localization of various types of islet cell tumours (Roche 1982, Krudy et al 1984, Rossi et al 1989). However, a recent report, summarizing the world literature and reporting considerable experience

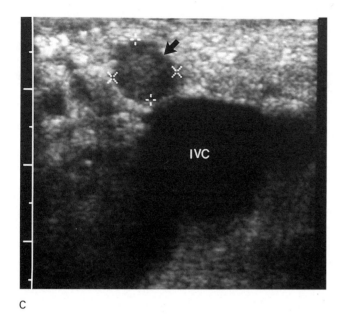

C

Fig. 9.5 (*continued*)   **C** Intraoperative ultrasonography shows small, hypoechoic mass (arrow) in the head of the pancreas anterior to the inferior vena cava (IVC). A small insulinoma was resected.

from the UK and Italy, stated that while venous sampling may help to localize tumours where other tests have failed, it is highly invasive, has significant potential complications, and failed to localized any tumours that were not identified by careful superselective arteriography (Rossi et al 1989).

Current experience suggests that preoperative imaging using current generation, high-resolution ultrasonography, CT, or MR, combined with superselective angiography, will result in correct localization of islet cell tumours in the vast majority of cases. Only when these fail should venous sampling be employed. However, intraoperative ultra-sonography performed at the time of laparotomy may be even more precise. More studies need to be performed to gather sufficient data to assess the precise role of each of these techniques.

Cystic pancreatic neoplasms

Angiography can be employed to evaluate cystic tumours of the pancreas (see Figs 6.13, 6.14). Cystic tumours contain areas of neovascularity and often show arteriovenous shunting. The degree of tumour vascularity depends upon the ratio of cystic to solid tissue within the neoplasm. Thus, vascularity cannot differentiate benign or serous cystic tumours from malignant or mucinous cystic tumours (Freeny & Lawson 1982). However, the presence of neovascularity within the wall of a pancreatic cyst can differentiate between a pseudocyst, which does not show neovascularity, and a cystic neoplasm. This differ-entiation is a not uncommon clinical problem and angiography thus can play an important role in evaluation of cystic pancreatic masses (Freeny et al 1978, Warshaw & Rutledge 1987).

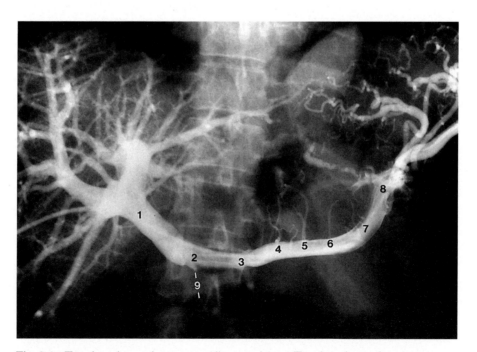

Fig. 9.6   Transhepatic portal venous sampling: gastrinoma. Transhepatic portal venogram outlines the small pancreatic veins. Venous samples were drawn selectively from each vein at the numbered sites. Focally increased levels of gastrin were found in the tail of the pancreas (site 7) and a small gastrinoma was confirmed at surgery.

REFERENCES

Freeny P C, Weinstein C J, Taft D A, Allen F H 1978 Cystic neoplasms of the pancreas: new angiographic and ultrasonographic findings. American Journal of Radiology 131: 795–802

Freeny P C, Marks W M, Ball T J 1982 Impact of high-resolution CT of the pancreas on utilization of endoscopic retrograde cholangiopancreatography and angiography. Radiology 142: 35–39

Freeny P C, Lawson T L 1982 Radiology of the pancreas. Springer-Verlag, New York

Hofer B O, Ryan J A, Freeny P C 1987 Surgical significance of vascular changes in chronic pancreatitis. Surgery, Gynecology and Obstetrics 164: 499–405

Krudy A G, Doppman J L, Jensen R T et al 1984 Localization of islet cell tumours by dynamic CT; comparison with plain CT, arteriography, sonography, and venous sampling. American Journal of Radiology 143: 585–589

Norton J A, Doppman J L, Collen M J, Harmon J W, Maton P N, Gardner J D, Jensen R T 1986 Prospective study of gastrinoma localization and resection in patients with Zollinger-Ellison syndrome. Annals of Surgery 204: 468–479

Roche A, Raissonier A, Gillon-Savouret M C 1982 Pancreatic venous sampling and arteriography in localising insulinomas and gastrinomas: procedure and results in 55 cases. Radiology 145: 621–627

Rossi P, Allison D J, Bezzi M, Kennedy A, Maccioni F, Wynick D, Maradei A, Bloom S R 1989 Endocrine tumors of the pancreas. Radiologic Clinics of North America 27: 73–79

Vujic I, Seymour E Q, Meredith H C 1980 Vascular complications associated with sonographically demonstrated cystic epigastric lesions: an important indication for angiography. Journal of Cardiovascular and Interventional Radiology 3: 75–79

Vujic I 1989 Vascular complications of pancreatitis. Radiologic Clinics of North America 27: 81–91

Warshaw A L, Rutledge P L 1987 Cystic tumours mistaken for pancreatic pseudocysts. Annals of Surgery 205: 393–398

10. Endoscopic retrograde cholangiopancreatography

P. J. Connors   D. L. Carr-Locke

INTRODUCTION

Since the first successful cannulation of the ampulla of Vater reported by McCune (McCune et al 1968), and the first successful endoscopic sphincterotomy (ES) by Classen & Demling (1974) and Kawai et al (1974), application of endoscopic retrograde cholangiopancreatography (ERCP) to the diagnosis and management of patients with pancreaticobiliary disorders has gained support and acceptance (Oi et al 1969, Cotton 1977, Safrany 1978, Cotton 1984a, b). Until recently there has been reluctance to extend these techniques to the 'emergency' situation or the 'unstable' patient, as an alternative or adjunct to surgical intervention. Resistance was primarily due to early experience, when unacceptably high complication rates were reported (Pitt 1984, Johnson & Hosking 1987, Roberts-Thomson 1987). Experience and familiarity with techniques and instrumentation have led to reduced complication rates, and the use of ERCP and ES as the initial, and sometimes sole, treatment of critically ill patients (Seifert 1978, Carr-Locke & Cotton 1986, Rosseland & Osnes 1989).

While endoscopic diagnosis in pancreatic disease was recognized as a major advance from the outset, therapeutic intervention took second place to the treatment of biliary disease for many years. As the 1980s were undoubtedly the decade for establishing endoscopic management in biliary disease, on the basis of well conducted retrospective and prospective studies, so the 1990s may be seen as the decade of development of endoscopic pancreatic therapy. Despite the difficulties of mounting randomized trials in pancreatic disease, it is essential that all new therapies promoted for benign or malignant conditions should be scientifically compared with traditional medical or surgical approaches.

ACUTE PANCREATITIS

In 1901, Opie reported a patient who died of fatal pancreatitis in whom postmortem examination showed a small stone impacted at the ampulla of Vater. The stone was small enough to lie in a common channel communicating with the common bile duct and the pancreatic duct. He reasoned that this might have allowed reflux of bile into the pancreatic duct and in subsequent experiments he produced haemorrhagic pancreatitis by injecting bile into the pancreatic duct. The pressure exerted with the injection of the bile into the pancreatic duct may have been equally responsible for the production of the pancreatitis. This observation gave rise to the 'obstructive' theory for pancreatitis.

The 'obstructive' theory has been supported by review of operative cholangiograms in patients with a history of pancreatitis, where reflux of contrast into the pancreatic duct is apparent in about 60% of such patients compared to 15% of controls who have not had pancreatitis. A common channel of 5 mm or more was found in 72% of the pancreatitis patients compared with only 20% of the control subjects (Cuschieri & Hughes 1973, Armstrong et al 1985). Gallstones can be recovered in the faeces of 85–95% of cases of acute pancreatitis, as compared to a 10% recovery rate in patients with symptomatic cholelithiasis who have not had pancreatitis (Acosta & Ledesma 1974). Review of patients with acute pancreatitis who were undergoing urgent operative intervention revealed common bile duct (CBD) stones in as many as 63–78% of cases, compared to a 3–33% incidence of CBD stones in patients undergoing delayed biliary surgery (Dixon & Hillam 1970, Acosta & Ledesma 1974, Paloyan et al 1975, Ranson 1979, Kelly 1980, Stone et al 1981).

It has been postulated that an incompetent or lax sphincter of Oddi might facilitate the reflux of activated duodenal contents, containing lysolecithin, bacterial toxin and enterokinase, into the pancreatic duct in patients prone to acute pancreatitis. This laxity could be explained by the previous passage of a gallstone, which can sometimes be identified at the time of ERCP by the presence of a patulous papilla (Cuschieri et al 1983). Components of both the obstructive and reflux theories seem plausible and both obstruction and reflux may be the consequence of stone passage through the sphincter of Oddi. There remain, however, many unanswered questions in the pathophysiology of gallstone-related pancreatitis.

The majority of patients with acute pancreatitis fully recover within a week or so of the attack, with conservative management alone. A mortality of about 10% is reported in unselected series but this figure is doubled if those cases diagnosed at postmortem are included (MRC Multicentre Trial 1977, De Bolla & Obeid 1984, Mayer et al 1984, Corfield et al 1985, Goodman et al 1985).

Stratifying patients into mild and severe categories is helpful in directing appropriate management. This stratification also allows direct comparison between groups studied at different institutions and comparison between different treatment modalities. Ranson (1982) developed an 11 factor system to predict severity, whereas the Glasgow group proposed a simpler eight factor system (Imrie et al 1978, Osborne et al 1981). The Modified Glasgow System is now widely used. It includes 'age greater than 55 years', but not 'serum transaminases greater than 200 iu/l'. This change was made because several recent reports, including one from Glasgow (Blamey et al 1984) and an independent study from Leicester (Leese & Shaw 1988), confirmed the statistical significance of age in relation to outcome but not the level of transaminases. The validity of these systems is now accepted and they are widely applied to stratify patients (Williamson 1984).

Urgent surgical intervention for acute gallstone pancreatitis was advocated at one time to prevent progression of the severity of the attack and reduce the chance of a recurrence; however, this approach has been challenged due to the high surgical morbidity and mortality. Initially, ERCP was thought to be too risky in the circumstance of ongoing pancreatitis because of the associated risk of exacerbating the attack, and fears that it would make the situation worse rather than better.

The majority of cases of acute pancreatitis fall into the mild category and respond to conservative management (Tondelli et al 1982, Neoptolemos et al 1984, Fan et al 1988, Ranson 1990). Those cases predicted to be severe by either Ranson's criteria or the Modified Glasgow criteria cause the greatest amount of controversy. Common bile duct stones are found in 30–60% of the patients who die from gallstone-associated pancreatitis and these stones are not always impacted in the ampulla or sitting in the common channel (De Bolla & Obeid 1984, Corfield et al 1985). Evaluation of the surgical literature on the treatment of gallstone-associated pancreatitis is difficult because patients are not stratified into mild or severe cases and historical controls are used to compare results. Acosta et al (1978) reported only one death in 46 patients (2.9%) in a group treated by urgent surgical intervention, as compared with 14 in 86 patients deaths (16%) in a historical control group. There was no differentiation between mild and severe cases.

Ranson (1979) urged non-operative treatment during the acute phase of gallstone pancreatitis. In his series, although he stratified his groups by severity, the comparison was not appropriate as the mean prognostic score was 5.4 in those who underwent urgent surgery, compared with 3.5 in those treated conservatively. Those who died after surgery had a higher initial severity score than those who survived surgery. This problem has been seen in other studies (Kelly 1980, Osborne et al 1981, Tondelli et al 1982).

Identification of those patients who actually have gallstones is one of the most difficult problems. Ultrasonography during the acute phase of an attack can detect only about 60% of cases of acute pancreatitis that are subsequently shown to involve gallstones (Williamson 1984). CT scanning has a low sensitivity and specificity for the detection of choledocholithiasis. Radionuclide biliary scanning is of no value in distinguishing those patients with and without gallstones during the acute phase of pancreatitis (Neoptolemos et al 1983, 1984). The risk of percutaneous transhepatic cholangiography outweighs its benefit in the diagnosis of choledocholithiasis unless there is intrahepatic ductal dilatation (Coppa et al 1981).

The initial application of ERCP and ES in acute gallstone-associated pancreatitis was reported sporadically from various centres around the world (Classen et al 1978, Van Spuy 1981, Kautz et al 1982, Roesch & Demling 1982, Safrany 1982, Schott et al 1982, Riemann & Lux 1984, Rosseland & Solhaug 1984, Neoptolemos et al 1986). The initial anxieties regarding complications related to endoscopic sphincterotomy including exacerbation of pancreatitis, cholangitis, haemorrhage, and perforation were not realized, and all authors commented on how rapidly some patients improved with establishment of effective pancreatic drainage and normalization of laboratory values. Although encouraging, these reports were deficient in terms of methods, patient selection, timing of ES in relationship to attack, stratification of patients and standardization of reporting complications.

The Leicester group published the first, and to date only, prospective randomized controlled trial of urgent ERCP and ES versus conservative treatment for acute pancreatitis due to gallstone (Neoptolemos et al 1988a). They randomized 121 patients with gallstone pancreatitis to receive either conventional conservative treatment or to undergo urgent (within 72 hours) ERCP with ES and stone extraction, only if stones were found in the common bile duct at the time of ERCP (Fig. 10.1). From a total of 223 consecutive patients admitted, the 121 were selected on the basis of urgent ultrasonography (within 24 hours) and/or biochemical prediction. Patient stratification was based on the Modified Glasgow criteria. There were 59 patients randomized to ERCP with successful cholangiography in 80% of the predicted severe group and 94% in the predicted mild group. An effort was made to not inject

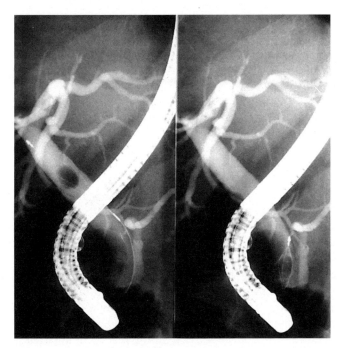

Fig. 10.1   Endoscopic retrograde cholangiogram showing common bile duct stone with basket extraction. Common bile duct stones are a frequent cause of pancreatitis.

contrast into the pancreatic duct, and if the pancreatic duct was outlined, the injection was immediately stopped. Pancreatic duct filling (often incomplete) occurred in 50% of the severe group and 90% of the mild group. Undue manipulation of the ampulla was avoided. Common bile duct stones were found in 63% of the 'predicted severe' group and in only 26% of those with 'predicted mild' attacks. Notably, the common bile duct diameter was greater in those patients within the 'predicted severe' category.

This study produced four important findings:

1   ERCP can be performed safely in acute pancreatitis, provided it is undertaken by an experienced endoscopist.

2   There was a significant reduction in major complications following ERCP–ES and stone extraction. (A total of 61% of patients developed complications in the conventional group and 12% in the ERCP group.)

3   A significant reduction in morbidity was apparent in those with 'predicted severe' attacks.

4   A significant reduction in hospital stay was seen in those with severe attacks following urgent sphincterotomy (median 9.5 days vs. 17 days).

A statistically significant difference in mortality was not demonstrated in this trial, although none was anticipated given the size of the group studied. It is notable that of the three patients in the conventional group with confirmed gallstones who died, one was found at postmortem to have a stone impacted at the ampulla of Vater. This study provides a rational basis for the application of ERCP–ES and stone extraction in cases of acute pancreatitis associated with gallstones. The increasing evidence of coexistent cholangitis may give added reason for rapid improvement after endoscopic bile duct clearance (Neoptolemos et al 1988b). The differing morbidity and mortality resulting from ERCP–ES as compared to surgical decompression may reflect the fact that outcome following ES is independent of associated medical risk factors whereas outcome after general anaesthesia and surgery is not (Neoptolemos et al 1987a, 1988b, Neoptolemos 1988).

The place of ERCP and endoscopic therapy in non-gallstone-associated acute pancreatitis during an acute attack is not yet established, other than for the purposes of identifying aetiological factors in cases of unexplained attacks.

CHRONIC PANCREATITIS

Chronic pancreatitis is characterized clinically by recurrent or continuous abdominal pain and progressive and irreversible pancreatic glandular destruction (Sarner & Cotton 1984). Patients with chronic pancreatitis may have acute exacerbations, but the condition may be painless with the only evidence of an inflammatory process being fibrosis due to previous inflammation.

Abdominal pain is the presenting complaint in approximately 75% of cases, while steatorrhoea may be the presenting complaint in 10–20% (Amman et al 1984). The inflammatory process eventually leads to both exocrine and endocrine insufficiency. The endocrine insufficiency is variable and increases as these patients are followed for longer periods. Morphologically, the pancreatic parenchyma shows varying degrees of segmental dilatation of the ductal system with strictures, calcification and/or pancreatic calculi (Freeny 1989a).

Increasingly, with the more liberal use of ERCP in the evaluation of known or suspected cases of pancreatitis, established changes of chronic disease are being found in patients seeming to present with acute attacks only. These apparent confusions have given rise to a number of different classifications, based either on clinical approaches or morphology, but all have in common the concept that the final resulting disorder that we label 'pancreatitis' is a spectrum of disease, ranging from an acute reversible condition secondary to an identifiable cause, through to a chronic irreversible destructive condition irrespective of primary cause. There are many intermediary stages ranged between these extremes (Axon et al 1984, Sarner & Cotton 1984, Singer et al 1985).

Our understanding of the mechanisms that lead to progressive organ atrophy and the symptom of pain remain limited. Therapeutic interventions, whether medical, endoscopic or surgical, are directed toward symptomatic relief of pain control and control of maldigestion with enzyme supplementation.

Diagnostic studies in chronic pancreatitis involve functional testing and imaging. Both exocrine and endocrine functional tests have been used to investigate chronic pancreatitis. Secretory stimulation tests, which involve duodenal intubation and sampling of duodenal aspirates following exogenous direct or indirect hormonal stimulation of the pancreas, are considered to be the most valuable. Direct stimulations with secretin, secretin-cholecystokinin and secretin-caerulein are most often used to investigate pancreatic function (Gyr et al 1975, Gullo et al 1976, Di Magno 1982, Lankisch 1982).

However the use of these tests should probably be restricted to specialized centres with an active interest in this area. Their sensitivity ranges from 80–90% and they have a specificity of greater than 90% for detecting abnormal exocrine function (Gyr et al 1975, Gullo et al 1976, Di Magno 1982, Lankisch 1982, Malfertheiner & Büchler 1989). Their use as tools for the diagnosis of chronic pancreatitis in the absence of exocrine impairment remains limited.

Oral function tests including the pancreolauryl test (Lankisch et al 1983, 1986) and the N-benzoyl-L-tyrosyl-P-aminobenzoic acid (NBT-PABA) test (Lang et al 1981, 1984) can detect moderate and severe pancreatic exocrine insufficiency. The attraction of avoiding intubation must be balanced by the lower sensitivity and specificity of these forms of pancreatic assessment, and they have limited application in the identification of chronic pancreatic disease (Lankisch et al 1983, 1986, Lang et al 1981, 1984).

Imaging of the pancreas includes plain film radiographs of the abdomen, ultrasound, computerized axial tomography (CT), magnetic resonance (MR) imaging and endoscopic retrograde cholangiopancreatography (ECRP). The use of imaging methods other than ECRP has been discussed elsewhere (Chs 4–9).

The widespread use of ERCP did not develop until the early seventies. Endoscopic retrograde pancreatography permitted for the first time direct, non-surgical imaging of the pancreatic ductal system. The two systems applied to the classification of pancreatitis are based on workshops in March, 1983 in Cambridge, England (Sarner & Cotton 1984) and March, 1984 in Marseilles, France (Singer et al 1985). Standardization of criteria allows improved communication and understanding of pancreatic disease among those involved in patient care and research into the natural history of pancreatitis. Both systems agree that the histological changes in chronic pancreatitis are irreversible and may be progressive but the Marseilles conference also defined a distinct morphological form of chronic pancreatitis which they labelled 'obstructive chronic pancreatitis'. The difference is that structural and functional changes tend to improve in this form of chronic pancreatitis if ductal obstruction is treated (Axon et al 1984, Banks et al 1985, Singer et al 1985).

The Cambridge classification uses terminology to describe the main pancreatic duct, side branches, parenchyma, and cavities if present (see Ch. 17). The main pancreatic duct provides the major drainage for the gland. If pancreas divisum is present, the ducts are described as dorsal or ventral. The terms upstream (towards the tail) and downstream (towards the head) are less confusing than proximal or distal duct changes.

The normal main pancreatic duct tapers smoothly from the head, through the body to the tail. There may be a normal narrowing in the head of the gland near the point of embryonic fusion of the ventral and dorsal parts. Autopsy studies have shown that the width of the main pancreatic duct increases with age and this has been confirmed by further endoscopic evaluation (Kreel & Sandin 1973, Macarty et al 1975, Anand et al 1989, Axon 1989). Collected series have defined average diameters of 3.6 mm, 2.7 mm, and 1.6 mm for the head, body and tail respectively. The main pancreatic duct is regarded as dilated when these dimensions are exceeded, or when one section of the duct is wider than the rest of an apparently normal calibre duct. When duct diameter exceeds 1 cm, it can be said to be severely dilated. The contour of the main pancreatic duct should be described, noting strictures and narrowings with upstream dilatation (Axon 1989).

The definition of normal limits for side branches is somewhat subjective with the length of side branches being regarded as normal or shortened with their calibre described as normal, dilated or narrowed with a smooth or irregular contour. The Cambridge classification defines the pancreatogram as normal when the main pancreatic duct is normal with no abnormal side branches (Fig. 10.2). The pancreatogram is regarded as equivocal when

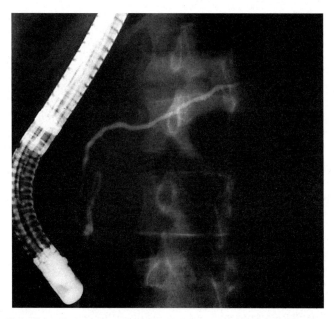

Fig. 10.2 Endoscopic retrograde pancreatogram (ERP) showing a normal pancreatic duct.

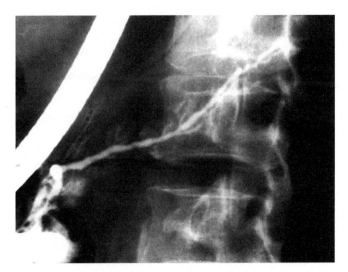

Fig. 10.3 ERP showing mild chronic pancreatitis.

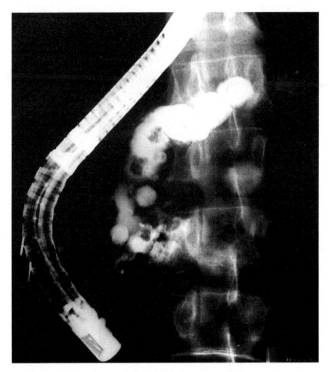

Fig. 10.5 ERP showing severe chronic pancreatitis.

there is a normal main pancreatic duct with fewer than three abnormal side branches. Mild chronic pancreatitis is present when there is a normal main pancreatic duct and three or more abnormal side branches (Fig. 10.3); moderate chronic pancreatitis if there is an abnormal main pancreatic duct with more than three abnormal side branches (Fig. 10.4), and marked chronic pancreatitis is present when there is an abnormal main pancreatic duct with more than three abnormal side branches, with either one or more additional features of large cavity (greater than 1 cm) filling defect, severe ductal dilatation, or severe ductal irregularity (Figs 10.5, 10.6).

Descriptive modifiers include local ductal changes limited to one-third of the gland or less and designated as involving the head, body or tail, while diffuse ductal changes involve more than one-third of the gland (Di Magno 1982, Axon et al 1984, Banks et al 1985, Axon 1989, Burdick & Hogan 1991).

Such classifications can never be comprehensive enough to include all manifestations of chronic pancreatic disease and, for example, focal disease such as a single pancreatic duct stricture, is not classified (Axon et al 1984, Banks et al 1985, Burdick & Hogan 1991). A further problem with classifications based on morphology

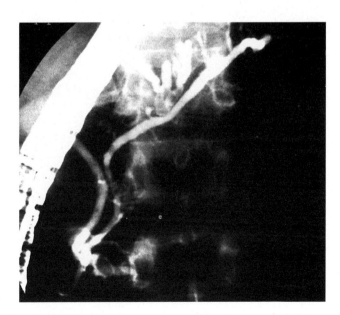

Fig. 10.6 ERP showing chronic pancreatitis with strictures and dilated side branches. Pancreatic stones are also seen within the dilated side branches.

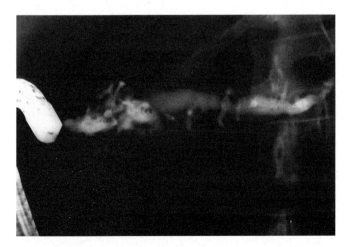

Fig. 10.4 ERP showing moderately severe chronic pancreatitis.

of the ductal system, is that the pancreatogram may be abnormal in patients without symptoms or it may be normal in patients with symptoms. The frequency of this is unknown, but may be as high as 30% (Caletti et al 1982). Pancreatography does not distinguish between the different causes of chronic pancreatitis (Axon 1989), but is helpful for surgical planning, and therapeutic endoscopic pancreatic interventions are now being investigated.

Biliary tract disease can develop as a complication of chronic pancreatitis due to the anatomical proximity of the bile duct as it passes through or behind the head of the pancreas. Jaundice is observed in approximately one-third of patients with chronic calcific pancreatitis. It is often transient and rarely accompanied by cholangitis. In collected reviews the endoscopic retrograde cholangiogram has been reported to be abnormal in 60% of patients with chronic pancreatitis (Carter 1988).

The most common radiological form of stenosis is a long, smooth, narrow stenosis of the lower common bile duct due to peripancreatic inflammation (Fig. 10.7). Occasionally, the common bile duct may be narrowed and displaced laterally by a cyst or pseudocyst of the head of the pancreas (Carter 1988, Pereyra-Lima et al 1989).

Endoscopic and/or surgical intervention is required in cases where there is persistent elevation of the alkaline phosphatase (a marker considered to be valuable as an indicator of biliary obstruction) or overt cholangitis, in order to relieve the acute problem and avoid the development of secondary biliary cirrhosis (Eckhauser et al 1983, Carter 1988, Pereyra-Lima et al 1989, Wilson et al 1989).

Pancreatic stones

Stones in the pancreas are formed primarily from calcium carbonate, proteins and polysaccharides. It was previously thought that there were two primary patterns of calcification in the pancreas: an intraductal pattern, representing true stones, and a parenchymal calcific pattern, representing calcification (Mayo 1936, Langergren 1962). The current consensus based on careful dissection and detailed histological examination of the pancreas, which have revealed remnants of duct wall around calcium deposits in every instance, is that the only type of calcification in the exocrine pancreas is the formation of intraductal calculi (Edmondson et al 1950, Stobbe et al 1970, Sarles & Sahel 1976).

Pancreatic stones occur in chronic pancreatitis and become radiologically discernible in the later stages of the disease. They may be single or multiple and range from microscopic calculi to minute, sand-like particles, to solitary or multiple stones of 1–2 cm in diameter. An abdominal film showing pancreatic calcification is virtually pathognomonic of chronic pancreatitis and is seen in up to 60% of the patients with the disease (Amman et al 1984, 1988).

The mechanism of pain in chronic pancreatitis is not well defined. The hypothesis that pancreatic juice under pressure could be responsible for at least some of the pain has led to the use of operative and endoscopic procedures designed to relieve intraductal pressure. Endoscopic sphincterotomy of the pancreatic orifice with basket extraction of pancreatic stones and/or placement of endoprosthesis (Fig. 10.8) has been applied in a limited number of cases. Fuji et al (1985) reported their experience with nonoperative treatment of chronic pancreatitis. Pancreatic sphincterotomy was successfully performed in 10 out of 13 patients with improvement in symptoms in nine. Pancreatic calculi were extracted by basket in two cases. Three patients also had a pancreatic endoprosthesis inserted to improve pancreatic drainage, although one had to be removed 3 days later because of severe abdominal pain.

Techniques such as extracorporeal shock wave lithotripsy (ESWL) and laser lithotripsy have been used to break up large concretions and allow extraction of the fragments through the ductal strictures that are frequently seen in chronic pancreatitis. Sauerbruch et al (1987) used extracorporeal shock wave lithotripsy in eight patients with pancreatic stones 5–20 mm in diameter and with dilated ductal systems. All the patients had prior endoscopic pancreatic sphincterotomy. Stone clearance was accomplished in all eight patients, and four patients had marked improvement in the intensity and frequency of their pain while four had no improvement in their

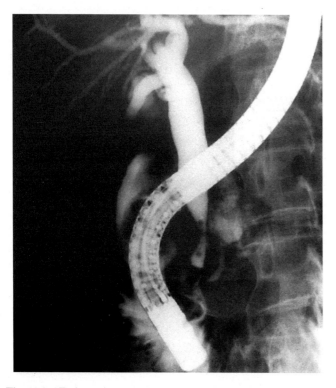

Fig. 10.7 Endoscopic retrograde cholangiopancreatogram showing smooth narrowing of the bile duct with ductal dilatation due to chronic pancreatitis.

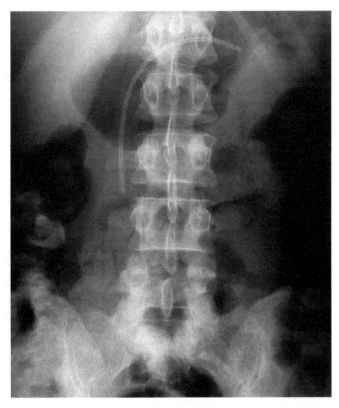

Fig. 10.8 Plain film of the abdomen with pancreatic stent in the main pancreatic duct.

symptoms. One patient who had successful clearance of pancreatic calculi had no change in his pain. The authors did not feel that successful ESWL necessarily led to pain relief.

The role of endoscopic pancreatic sphincterotomy and stone extraction have yet to be determined. The techniques for pancreatic duct clearance and drainage will have to be tested in a randomized, prospective manner to determine their efficacy.

PANCREATIC CARCINOMA AND OTHER NEOPLASMS

Operative resection provides the only potential for cure of pancreatic cancer. Early, accurate diagnosis with careful, precise staging is imperative to select appropriate candidates for operation given the postoperative morbidity and mortality of pancreatoduodenectomy. Radiological imaging used in the diagnosis of pancreatic cancer includes ultrasonography, CT scanning, MR imaging and ERCP.

Ultrasonography

As most patients present with jaundice, ultrasonography is usually the first procedure to be performed. The delineation of obstructive as opposed to non-obstructive jaundice by the detection of extrahepatic and intrahepatic duct dilatation is imperative. Ultrasonography is not accurate in differentiating the level of obstruction, or the cause if it is due to a small lesion. Ultrasound examination of a pancreatic mass may be compromised by the presence of overlying bowel gas, but the size and contour of the gland and increased or decreased echogenicity of the tumour in relation to the rest of the glandular parenchyma, can often be determined. Dilatation of the pancreatic duct may be seen, but in some cases even mass lesions may not be visualized. The real sensitivity of ultrasonography in the diagnosis of pancreatic cancer is about 70%. Visualization of the body and tail of the pancreas is difficult due to their anatomical location and they may be obscured by obesity, ascites, or overlying bowel gas (Honickman et al 1983, Kalser et al 1985, Fernandez-del Castillo & Warshaw 1990).

CT scanning

CT scanning is the single most important non-invasive imaging method in the evaluation of suspected carcinoma of the body or tail of the pancreas. Computed tomography provides cross-sectional images which allow appraisal of the size of the gland. Findings suggestive of malignancy include the presence of a focal mass with low attenuation, dilatation of the main pancreatic duct distal to the tumour, local tumour extension, contiguous organ invasion, dilatation of the biliary tree, vascular encasement, hepatic or nodal metastasis, and ascites (Wittenberg et al 1984, Freeny et al 1988, Freeny 1989).

CT has better definition than US and is not hampered by bowel gas. Furthermore, the use of intravenous contrast and dynamic imaging allows better definition of the pancreas, while percutaneous aspiration biopsy can be undertaken with CT guidance (Wittenberg et al 1984, Freeny et al 1988, Freeny 1989). The sensitivity and specificity of CT in the diagnosis of pancreatic adenocarcinoma in one series was 99% and 92% respectively. Many of the false positive results were in patients with pancreatitis or with a normal pancreas, or with malignant neoplasms other than pancreatic cancer (Freeny et al 1988, Freeny 1989).

MR imaging

The use of MR imaging in the diagnosis of pancreatic neoplasms has been hampered by motion artifacts including respiratory movements, vascular pulsation and bowel peristalsis. Thus far, MR has offered no significant advantage over CT to justify its use in the initial evaluation of suspected pancreatic disease (Steiner et al 1989).

ECRP

Accurate diagnosis in patients with obstructive jaundice and evidence of focal enlargement in the region of the head or dilatation of the pancreatic and bile ducts is crucial. The role of ERCP in differential diagnosis in this setting has expanded. The procedure allows endoscopic observation and radiological assessment with a potential for tissue sampling and treatment of the obstructive process. The reported sensitivity of ERCP in the detection of pancreatic adenocarcinoma is in excess of 90% in most series (Kaufman et al 1988).

The endoscopic features of pancreatic cancer include a mass bulging into the stomach or duodenum with compression or stenosis, and direct visualization of a mass eroding into the gut lumen. Duodenal and other periampullary lesions may also be visualized (Wittenberg et al 1984, Freeny et al 1988, Freeny 1989). Endoscopic pancreatographic features include complete obstruction of the main pancreatic duct; disruption or stenosis of the duct, with or without prestenotic ectasia; displacement of the duct with alteration of secondary branches including fragmentation and cystic destruction; acinar or field defects, and extravasation or pooling of contrast material in irregular pockets, due to duct necrosis with tumour cavitation.

In some patients, failure of ERCP may result from tumour in the head of the gland (Wittenberg et al 1984, Kaufman et al 1988, Freeny 1989). Obstruction due to tumour must be distinguished from pancreas divisum, so that if ERCP fails an attempt must be made to inject contrast into the minor papilla. The distal bile duct is frequently involved by local invasion from pancreatic cancer. The cholangiographic appearance of the so-called 'double-duct' sign, that is, stricture of the bile and pancreatic ducts at the same level with upstream dilatation (Fig. 10.9), is a very reliable sign of pancreatic malignancy, although not pathognomonic of carcinoma.

Other cholangiographic features include bile duct displacement, stenosis with irregular shouldering, and complete obstruction (Wittenberg et al 1984, Kaufman et al 1988, Freeny 1989, Soehendra et al 1989).

These abnormalities of the pancreatic duct and bile duct are not exclusive to pancreatic cancer, and in fact many of the findings resemble those of chronic pancreatitis.

Tissue sampling can be performed at the time of ERCP, using brush cytology, direct biopsy and endoscopic needle aspiration, and pancreatic juice and bile have also been collected during ERCP for cytological examination (Rustgi et al 1989, Soehendra et al 1989, Scudera et al 1990, Venu et al 1990, Foutch et al 1991, Ryan 1991). The overall diagnostic yield has been disappointing, with positive confirmation rates ranging from 18 to 56% depending on the technique used.

The new brush cytology technique reported by the Racine, Wisconsin group offers the distinct advantage of positioning the cytology brush precisely within the stricture zone (Fig. 10.9), thereby greatly increasing the yield of cytological diagnosis. In a series of 53 patients with pan-

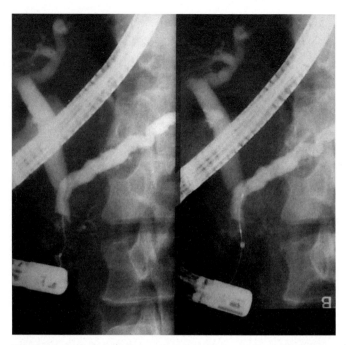

Fig. 10.9 Endoscopic retrograde cholangiopancreatogram showing slightly dilated bile duct due to mass in the head of the pancreas. A Geenen brush cytology sample is being taken from the strictured segment of the pancreatic duct.

creaticobiliary malignancy, this group reported a significant improvement in the rate of cytological confirmation with a diagnostic sensitivity of 70% and specificity of 100% (Venu et al 1990).

Endoscopic ultrasonography

The role of endoscopic ultrasonography (Ch. 11) in the diagnosis and staging of pancreatic malignancies is in its infancy. It is unclear whether this technique will provide additional information regarding local and vascular invasion to help determine tumour resectability (Yasuda et al 1988b, Hayashi et al 1989, Boyce & Sivak 1990).

CYSTIC NEOPLASMS OF THE PANCREAS

The majority of cystic lesions of the pancreas are pseudocysts which have resulted from inflammation or trauma and which are composed of a collection of pancreatic secretions surrounded by a fibrous wall without any epithelial lining. True cystic neoplasms of the pancreas have an epithelial lining and never resorb spontaneously. They comprise about 10–13% of pancreatic cysts (benign and malignant) and 1% of all pancreatic malignancies (Becker et al 1965, Warshaw & Rutledge 1987, Yamaguchi & Enjoji 1987b, Lack 1989, Warshaw et al 1990).

Two distinctive types of cystic neoplasms have emerged from the comprehensive clinicopathological review by Compagno and Oertel (1987a, b). Microcystic or serous cystic neoplasms are composed of grape-like clusters of small cysts with glycogen-rich low cuboidal epithelium. They usually follow a benign clinical course and may be a component of the von Hippel–Lindau syndrome. The macrocystic or mucinous type of cystic neoplasms are all frankly malignant or premalignant and typically they are lined by a mucin-producing columnar epithelium which may not completely line the cyst.

Other cystic neoplasms of the pancreas include papillary cystic tumours (Sanfey et al 1983, Bombi et al 1984, Rustin et al 1986); mucinous ductal ectasia (MDE) or intraductal mucin-hypersecreting neoplasms (Sachs et al 1989, Dabezies et al 1990, Bastid et al 1991, Nickl et al 1991, Rickaert et al 1991); some ductal adenocarcinomas (Lack 1989, Sachs et al 1989), and endocrine tumours of the pancreas with secondary cystic changes or degeneration (Kent et al 1981, Prinz et al 1983, Kaufman et al 1988, Warshaw et al 1990). Other cystic neoplasms include congenital cysts such as lymphangiomas and haemangiomas, fibrocystic disease of the pancreas and retention cysts and teratomas (dermoid cysts) (Mullens et al 1983, Warshaw et al 1990).

With the wider application of ultrasonography, CT scanning, and MR imaging, cystic neoplasms of the pancreas are being found incidentally, as well as in patients undergoing investigation of abdominal pain, weight loss, pancreatitis, and jaundice. The clinician must be aware of the different types of cystic tumours and of the diagnostic and therapeutic options available. Misdiagnosing a cystic neoplasm as a pseudocyst and treating it surgically as such may eliminate the possibility of surgical cure despite the slow-growing nature of these neoplasms (Warshaw & Rutledge 1987, Warshaw et al 1990).

Ultrasonography, CT scanning and other investigations

Characteristic findings of cystic neoplasia on ultrasonography and CT scanning include loculation within the cyst with delicate septae, coalescence of cysts or irregular locules, or the presence of a solid component. However, these changes are not always present radiologically (Friedman et al 1983, Itai et al 1988, Johnson et al 1988, Minami et al 1989). The multiple cystic structure of these neoplasms can make it difficult to evaluate fully the surrounding parenchyma, and identification of the particular tumour type is difficult because of the overlapping of clinical characteristics. Most cystic neoplasms occur in middle-aged women, have a mean diameter of 5–6 cm and have a variable presentation (Compagno & Oertel 1978a, Sachs et al 1989). Calcification is common in cystic tumours but rare in the wall of pseudocysts, although calcification in the pancreas itself may present in chronic pancreatitis. Calcification of the rim of the cyst wall, either partial or complete, may be reflect the long natural history of these neoplasms. In Warshaw's series of

cystic neoplasms (1990), seven cysts were calcified and all were malignant. The central 'sunburst' calcification of some serous cystadenomas is characteristic and strongly suggests that diagnosis (Friedman et al 1983, Itai et al 1988); it was seen in 11% of Warshaw's series.

Angiography is helpful if it shows hypervascularity, but is not helpful in delineating cyst type. Even if invasive disease is suggested by vascular encasement, most fit patients should go to surgery with a view to resection, given the favourable prognosis of these neoplasms (Uflacker et al 1980, Taft & Freeny 1981). Transpapillary biopsies, fine-needle aspiration, and open surgical biopsy may fail to differentiate pseudocysts from neoplastic cysts because they are often lined with a discontinuous epithelium and surgical resection is the only definitive intervention (Warshaw et al 1990).

ERCP and other endoscopic methods

Endoscopic retrograde cholangiopancreatography (ERCP) can be very useful in the evaluation of cystic neoplasms of the pancreas. It has been reported that 60–70% of pancreatic pseudocysts communicate with the pancreatic duct (Warshaw & Rattner 1985, O'Connor et al 1986), but that neoplastic cysts should not (Warshaw et al 1990). In Warshaw's series (1990), 39 pancreatograms were performed in 67 patients with cystic neoplasms of the pancreas. In 50% of cases the pancreatogram was normal while in 33% there was non-specific bowing around the mass. However, of the 17 mucinous cystadenocarcinomas 18% showed stenosis and 24% occlusion of the duct, with no instance of communication of the pancreatic duct with the cyst. There are anecdotal reports of opacification of a cystic tumour at ERCP (Lumsden & Bradley 1989, Sachs 1989, Nickl et al 1991) (Fig. 10.10). It has been suggested that an occasional neoplastic cyst may communicate with the pancreatic duct; or that, the cavity which fills may be an associated pseudocyst caused by the obstructive pancreatitis due to the underlying cystic tumour; or that the lesion was an example of mucinous ductal ectasia rather than a cystadenoma (Warshaw et al 1990, Nickl et al 1991).

Mucinous ductal ectasia is a newly-recognized entity 'distinct' from mucinous cystadenoma or cystadenocarcinoma. It is an intraductal lesion rather than an extraductal lesion, and is characterized by papillary hyperplasia involving part or all of the pancreatic duct system. The lesion secretes large quantities of thick mucus into the lumen of the pancreatic duct causing dilatation and obstruction which can lead to obstructive pancreatitis. At ERCP, viscous mucus may be seen extruding from the ampulla while pancreatography may reveal packing of dilated 'cystified' ducts with intraluminal mucus globules causing filling defects. These amorphous, radiolucent filling defects change shape when probed with a catheter and occasionally can be extracted with a balloon catheter

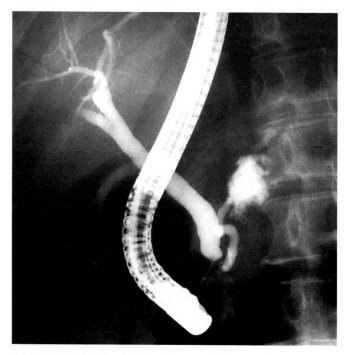

Fig. 10.10 Endoscopic retrograde cholangiopancreatogram showing normal cholangiogram with pancreatogram showing a cystic tumour of the pancreas in the neck and body of the gland.

to allow confirmation that they are mucus globules. This lesion is regarded as a curable premalignant or malignant tumour, as well as a cause of recurrent obstructive pancreatitis. It may be difficult to distinguish from chronic pancreatitis with a dilated, ectatic main pancreatic duct. The endoscopist must be aware of the importance of the appearance of the papilla and look for intraluminal evidence of mucin globules. Mucinous ductal ectasia often involves the head of the gland and therefore requires a pancreatoduodenectomy, but in some cases total pancreatectomy may be required (Lumsden & Bradley 1989, Warshaw et al 1990, 1991, Bastid et al 1991, Nickl et al 1991, Rickaert et al 1991).

Newer endoscopic modalities including endoscopic ultrasonography, endoscopic ultrasound probes and pancreatoscopy have not been widely applied in the assessment of pancreatic cystic neoplasms. They may prove to be helpful in difficult cases where there remains a question of differentiation between a pseudocyst and a cystic neoplasm, yet do not appear to change the surgical approach.

TUMOURS OF THE DUODENAL PAPILLA

The periampullary area is anatomically complex and tumours of epithelial origin may arise from the mucosa of the papilla of Vater, the pancreatic duct, the distal common bile duct or the periampullary duodenum. Tumours arising from each of these sites exhibit different growth patterns and different natural histories. Periampullary tumours are of particular interest because they represent a potentially curable lesion if the correct diagnosis is made at an early stage (Hayes et al 1987, Yamaguchi & Enjoji 1987a, Huibregste & Tytgat 1988, Sivak 1988). Other malignant neoplasms include primary carcinoid tumours of the ampulla of Vater and carcinomas which have metastasized to the ampulla of Vater, including malignant melanoma, hypernephroma, or lymphoma. There is an increased incidence of periampullary neoplasms in patients with Gardner's syndrome or familial polyposis (Huibregste & Tytgat 1988).

Benign neoplasms of the ampulla of Vater include adenoma, lipoma, fibroma, neurofibroma, granular cell tumour, leiomyoma and hamartoma (Hayes et al 1987, Yamaguchi & Enjoji 1987a, Huibregste & Tytgat 1988, Sivak 1988). Adenomas of the papilla of Vater are considered to be premalignant lesions. The evidence for this is based on common findings of elements of benign adenoma within malignant tumours, and the presence of carcinoma in situ within resected adenomas. Yamaguchi and Enjoji (1987a) found definite evidence of adenoma at the margins of the periampullary adenocarcinomas reported in their series.

The favourable prognosis of periampullary adenocarcinoma may be attributed to earlier patient presentation (due to jaundice secondary to occlusion of the distal common bile duct) and in part to the fact that periampullary adenocarcinomas tend to be more differentiated than adenocarcinomas of the head of the pancreas (Huibregste & Tytgat 1988). The peak incidence is during the sixth decade of life with jaundice being the most common presenting symptom (Sivak 1988). Other symptoms include abdominal pain, weight loss, anorexia, anaemia, occult blood positive stools and pruritus (Schlippert et al 1978, Anderson et al 1985, Knox & Kingston 1986, Hayes et al 1987, Yamaguchi & Enjoji 1987a Robertson et al 1987).

Most patients have non-specific complaints and few physical findings until jaundice occurs. A relatively large number of patients have coexistent cholelithiasis and choledocholithiasis. This increases the risk of erroneous diagnosis if the clinical manifestations of the tumour are attributed to the calculus disease. Many patients may have undergone cholecystectomy and common bile duct exploration before the presence of the periampullary neoplasm is detected (Sivak 1988, Huibregste & Tytgat 1988). In radiological evaluation, standard barium studies (and hypotonic duodenography in the past) may demonstrate a mass lesion in the medial wall of the descending duodenum; CT scan and ultrasonography usually confirm the presence of obstructive jaundice, but cannot make the diagnosis of small periampullary lesions.

Angiography has no role in the diagnostic work-up (Sivak 1988).

Endoscopy is the most accurate means of diagnosing neoplasms of the papilla of Vater and adjacent areas. The use of endoscopic ultrasonography has allowed assessment of the local extent of tumour spread and of metastatic spread to lymph nodes (Tio & Tytgat 1986, Yasuda et al 1988a). The main duodenal papilla cannot be completely visualized with a forward viewing endoscope. The side-viewing endoscope has greatly improved inspection of the papilla of Vater. There is a spectrum of periampullary abnormalities, and some of these lesions are small and difficult to recognize (Nakao et al 1982, Leese et al 1986, Shemesh et al 1989). The spectrum includes minor enlargement of the papilla, mass lesion behind the papilla covered by normal mucosa, polypoid lesions, exophytic friable growths, and frankly malignant tumours with ulceration and obvious infiltration (Hayes et al 1987, Yamaguchi & Enjoji 1987a, Huibregste & Tytgat 1988, Sivak 1988, Ponchon et al 1989). Leese et al (1986) reviewed 49 patients with an endoscopic diagnosis of periampullary tumour, 11 of whom were found to have pseudotumours which had an endoscopic appearance resembling polypoid, non-ulcerative periampullary carcinoma. These patients had clinical symptoms and biochemical abnormalities similar to those of patients with true neoplasms.

Tissue sampling is a vital component of the evaluation, and endoscopic biopsies should always be obtained. However, there is a significant number of false negative biopsies and every effort must be made to improve the diagnostic yield. In the case of large, ulcerative, exophytic lesions, a forceps biopsy may only retrieve superficial mucosa showing benign adenomatous or villous adenomatous components. To improve sampling of the periampullary mucosa various techniques have been used: the biopsy forceps can be inserted directly into the ampulla (Nakao et al 1982); large particle biopsy can be taken using a snare polypectomy technique (Sivak 1988, Ponchon et al 1989, Shemesh et al 1989), or endoscopic sphincterotomy (ES) can be performed before biopsy (Bourgeois et al 1984).

Obtaining biopsies of the ampulla of Vater post-sphincterotomy can be made difficult by bile flow from an obstructed system, by increased duodenal peristalsis which can be poorly responsive to pharmacological manipulation, by excessive bleeding which can occur when these neoplasms are cut, despite appropriate cautery, and by the necrotic fragments of tissue from the cautery itself (Bourgeois et al 1984, Blackman & Nash 1985, Leese et al 1986, Neoptolemos et al 1987b, Huibregste & Tytgat 1988, Sivak 1988, Bickerstaff et al 1990, Yamaguchi et al 1990). Bourgeois et al (1984) reviewed 25 biopsies from the ampulla of Vater after sphincterotomy in 22 patients undergoing endoscopic sphincterotomy for choledo-cholithiasis (Huibregste et al 1986) and benign stricture of the papilla (Sivak 1988). The tissue samples were taken at the inner edge of the biliary orifice with a 5 French biopsy forceps. Of the 6 biopsies from 'hypertrophic papillas', performed immediately after ES, 2 showed mild histological atypia, while 4 of the 7 biopsies done 48 hours after ES showed atypia and 2 were not interpretable. Of the 12 biopsies from 'normal papillas' taken 48 hours after ES, 3 showed atypia and 2 were not interpretable. The authors concluded there was less chance of misinterpreting epithelial atypism for neoplasm if biopsy samples were taken immediately after ES or at least 1 week after ES.

Ponchon et al (1989) corroborated these findings, demonstrating improved biopsy interpretation when biopsies were taken 10 days after ES. In their experience, ES in patients with a prominent infundibulum or obvious common bile duct dilatation, but no obvious tumour on ERCP, revealed tumour in 42% of their cases. Adenomas are considered to be premalignant conditions and resection must be considered.

Cannulation of large, exophytic, ulcerated lesions may be difficult. The area should first be examined for an opening or any remaining papillary tissue prior to probing. Probing will cause the tumour to bleed and obscure the view and chance for cannulation. In less obvious neoplastic lesions, the orifice of the bulging papilla is usually located distally, making cannulation difficult. The bulging papilla can be opened safely by the experienced endoscopist using the precut needle knife (Huibregste et al 1986). Cholangiography commonly reveals dilatation of the bile duct with a narrowing at the site of the papilla. Malignant tumours produce an irregular filling defect, while benign tumors have a more regular, smooth narrowing. Pancreatography likewise reveals ductal dilatation with distal narrowing. If Santorini's duct is patent, there may not be marked dilatation of the main pancreatic duct. If both ductal systems are dilated, a lesion of the ampulla should be suspected (Leese et al 1986).

Surgical resection has remained the optimal treatment for periampullary carcinomas. Endoscopic palliation should be considered for those patients in poor general condition with a short life expectancy, who present with advanced disease and obstructive jaundice. Endoscopic sphincterotomy alone can relieve the obstruction of the common bile duct, but the procedure has an increased risk of haemorrhage and cholangitis and a higher mortality (of up to 5%) when compared to sphincterotomy performed for choledocholithiasis (Huibregste & Tytgat 1988). Endoscopic placement of biliary endoprostheses can be accomplished without sphincterotomy.

Huibregste et al 1987 reported their experience in endoprosthesis placement in 71 patients with advanced disease or major surgical contraindications. Twenty-two patients went on to elective surgery, and 49 were followed after stent placement. Duodenal obstruction occurred in 23% of patients, necessitating gastroenterostomy in some patients and the endoprostheses clogged in 36%, after a mean interval of 312 days.

Ponchon et al (1989) reported three patients, including one with a carcinomatous focus, in whom diathermic snare resection alone was judged complete. Laser photo-destruction was performed in three patients in whom diathermic snare resections were incomplete. One patient had recurrence of villous adenoma at 24 months. Laser destruction was successfully performed without previous snare resection in five of their patients. They recommended the use of the Nd-Yag laser to ensure complete destruction. The above treatments were used as palliation in eight of their patients who were not candidates for radical resection. Tumour destruction was always incomplete.

Shemesh et al (1989) reported five patients presenting with obstructive jaundice who initially were treated with ES as a drainage procedure. Four then went on to local surgical excision. All four developed recurrent adenomas which were eradicated by diathermic fulguration through the endoscope. This was carried out with the hot biopsy forceps or the tip of a polypectomy snare. Follow-up of 12–24 months showed no recurrent adenomatous tissue. The fifth patient refused surgery and underwent snare polypectomy of a broad-based adenoma with incomplete resection. The patient had one endoscopic fulguration and then was lost to follow-up until developing adenocarcinoma of the head of the pancreas 40 months later.

Lambert et al (1988) reported their experience which included 16 patients treated by laser (mainly Nd-YAG). Altogether 7 of 8 adenomas were completely destroyed with follow-up from 14–53 months. The argon laser had been used in the first three patients, with complete destruction in only one, so that the Nd-YAG laser was then used. Three of the patients had undergone incomplete snare polypectomy.

Palliative treatment was undertaken in eight patients in very poor general condition with periampullary adenocarcinomas that were non-operable. Laser photodestruction was used in conjunction with ES and endoprosthesis placement for drainage. There was no clear influence on the duration of survival in this group. The authors emphasized the need for careful follow-up in adenoma patients due to the possibility of recurrence, even after a period with negative biopsies.

PANCREATIC PSEUDOCYSTS

Pancreatic pseudocysts occur when there is ductal disruption and formation of a localized collection of pancreatic secretions, encased by a wall of granulation tissue and lacking an epithelial lining. With the development of ultrasonography and computed tomography as many as 50% of patients who have experienced severe bouts of pancreatitis have been shown to develop pseudocysts (Siegelman 1980). The approach to a pancreatic pseudocyst depends on whether it is acute (present for less than 6 weeks) or chronic (present for more than 6 weeks), sterile or infected, and whether it is symptomatic. Acute pancreatic pseudocysts may resolve in up to 40% of cases, however chronic pseudocysts rarely resolve and have a higher complication rate (Bradley et al 1979).

The role of ERCP in the management of pancreatic pseudocysts is controversial and still evolving. In acute pancreatitis, diagnostic ERCP should be used cautiously for fear of aggravating inflammation or introducing infection; if ERCP is used at all in this context it should probably be regarded as a preoperative evaluation, being followed within 24–48 hours by surgery. Diagnostic ERCP is more valuable in patients with chronic pseudocysts and can be used to demonstrate strictures and stones in the bile ducts and pancreatic ducts, and to show communication between the pseudocyst and the pancreatic ductal system (Fig. 10.11) (Laxson et al 1985, O'Connor et al 1986).

An endoscopic approach has been used to drain pancreatic pseudocysts in some centres (Fig. 10.12, see Ch. 27). The cyst must be compressing the duodenal wall or gastric wall if it is to be punctured safely. The technique of endoscopic cystoduodenostomy (ECD) or endoscopic cystgastrostomy (EGD) involves creating a fistula through the gastric or duodenal wall. This may be done either electrosurgically (using a diathermic needle to puncture the cyst, and enlarging the cystenterostomy with a needle-knife sphincterotome), or using a Nd-Yag laser to make

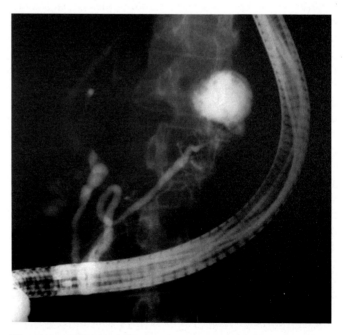

Fig. 10.11 ERP showing leak into a pancreatic pseudocyst that had developed after an episode of acute pancreatitis.

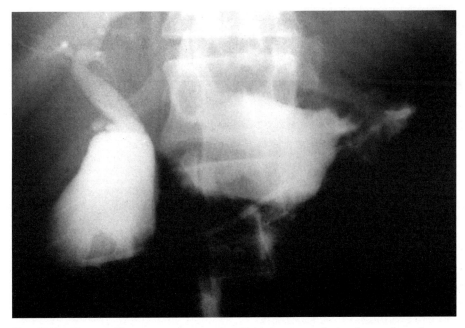

Fig. 10.12 Transpapillary pancreatic stent placed into the pancreatic pseudocyst, shown in Figure 10.11, for drainage.

the incision (Kozarek et al 1985, 1991, Sahel et al 1987, Buchi et al 1988, Heyder et al 1988, Spinetti et al 1988, Barkin & Hyder 1989, Cremer et al 1989, Kolars et al 1989). The results of these methods of management are discussed elsewhere (Ch. 23).

Kozarek et al (1991) have recently reported their experience with endoscopic transpapillary treatment of disrupted pancreatic ducts and peripancreatic fluid collections, an experience which is discussed elsewhere (Ch. 23).

PANCREAS DIVISUM

The first descriptions of anatomical variations of the major (principal) and minor (accessory) duodenal papillae and pancreatic ductal system date back to the seventeenth century (Stern 1986). The pancreas arises from two outpouchings of the endodermal lining of the duodenum, giving rise to the ventral pancreas and the dorsal pancreas at approximately the fourth week of gestation. These outpouches grow disproportionately, with the dorsal bud growing more rapidly, becoming an elongated structure extending into the dorsal mesentery. The ventral pancreas is connected to the common bile duct and is carried away from the duodenum as the biliary tree is developing. By the seventh week, the two primordia normally fuse, with the tail, body and part of the head of the pancreas formed by the dorsal segment and the remainder of the head and uncinate process formed from the ventral pancreas.

Each segment contains a duct, with the dorsal duct arising directly from the duodenal wall, and the ventral duct arising from the common bile duct. With fusion of the dorsal and ventral segments, anastomosis of the ductal systems normally occurs. The ventral duct fuses with the dorsal duct forming the main pancreatic duct. The proximal end of the dorsal duct (duct of Santorini) becomes the accessory duct, which is patent in 70% of the adult population and drains via the accessory duodenal papilla. The ventral duct (duct of Wirsung) shares the common outlet of the common bile duct, the major duodenal papilla (Sigfusson et al 1983, Stern 1986, Agha & Williams 1987, Parker 1987, Brenner et al 1990).

Pancreas divisum results from failure of the dorsal and ventral pancreatic tissue to fuse in utero (see Ch. 34). Pancreas divisum is the commonest congenital variant of the pancreas and it is only with the advent of ERCP that this variant has been recognized on a regular basis. The true incidence in the population is probably around 6% and no ethnic or geographical differences have been demonstrated so far (Cotton & Kizu 1977, Gregg 1977, Cotton 1980, 1985, Tulassay & Papp 1980, Richter et al 1981, Keith et al 1982, Delhaye et al 1985, Hayawakas et al 1989, Bernard et al 1990).

No reliable non-invasive diagnostic characteristics have been reported for CT scanning or ultrasound (Zeman et al 1988, Lindstrom & Ihse 1989, Silverman 1989, Soulen et al 1989, Seto et al 1990), but pancreas divisum may give rise to a false impression of a pancreatic head mass or 'pseudomass' with both imaging methods, requiring differentiation from benign and malignant mass-producing conditions (Silverman et al 1989, Moreira et al 1991).

The typical ERCP appearance of pancreas divisum includes a ventral duct (duct of Wirsung) that fills via a major papilla, that is short and tapered with prompt

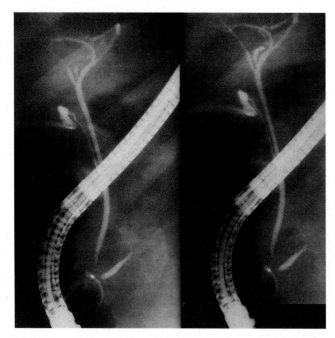

Fig. 10.13 Endoscopic retrograde cholangiopancreatogram showing the classical appearance of the ventral pancreatic segment of pancreas divisum with terminal arborization of the main duct.

arborization into fine side branches without communication with the body and tail (Fig. 10.13). Injection of the minor papilla demonstrates the long dorsal pancreatic duct running through the head, body and tail of the pancreas (duct of Santorini) (Fig. 10.14) (Stern 1986). Incomplete or partial pancreas divisum is seen when injection via the major papilla demonstrates a typical ventral pancreas, but further filling (and frequently acinization of the ventral portion) shows communication with a dominant dorsal system via small, thin rudimentary ducts, or secondary branches. Partial pancreas divisum is reported to have an

incidence of 0.13–0.9%, but its true frequency may not be appreciated due to insufficient contrast injection, tenuous communication, injection of only the major papilla, or mistaken diagnosis of pathological stenosis produced by a lesion encroaching on what is assumed to be a normal ductal system (Tulassay et al 1986, Moreira et al 1991).

A range of techniques and accessories have been invented to facilitate dorsal pancreatography so that the success rate should now be at least 80–90% in experienced hands (Schleintz & Katon 1984, O'Connor & Lehman 1985, McCarthy et al 1987, Benage et al 1990). Cannulation of the minor papilla requires meticulous attention to technique. The minor papilla is generally located approximately 2 cm cephalad and slightly anterior to the major papilla, but it is smaller and lacks a longitudinal fold. In some instances it may be very inconspicuous, appearing as a tiny dimple or papule with almost no elevation or orifice. The optimal position of the duodenoscope is in the long scope position with the endoscope bowed along the greater curve of the stomach with approximately 100 cm of scope inserted. Secretin (1 unit per kg body weight) can be injected intravenously to induce flow of pancreatic secretions and make the minor papilla orifice more evident. However, rapid and more forceful injection of contrast is required to fill the pancreatic tail during active flow of pancreatic juice and this may increase the risk of pancreatitis (Schleintz & Katon 1984, O'Connor & Lehman 1985, McCarthy et al 1987, Benage et al 1990). Needle-tipped catheters can traumatize the tissue and obscure the orifice more easily than a standard or tapered tip catheter. The potential for submucosal injection is greater with needle-tip catheters. When a pancreatogram cannot be obtained via the major papilla or a ventral pancreas is demonstrated, injection of the minor papilla for dorsal ductography is required for complete evaluation of the pancreas.

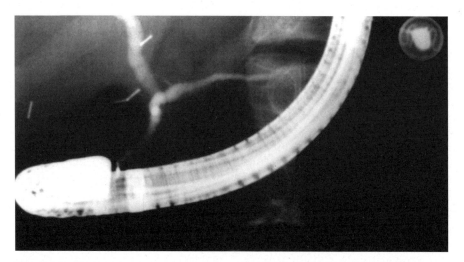

Fig. 10.14 ERP with injection via the minor papilla, demonstrating the dorsal duct in pancreas divisum.

Clinical significance of pancreas divisum

What is the clinical relevance of the anomaly of pancreas divisum? Since the first suggestions by Gregg, and Cotton & Kizu, in 1977, that pancreas divisum may be aetiologically related to recurrent pancreatitis or pancreatic pain, over 100 articles have appeared in the world literature supporting or refuting this contention. Arguments for pancreas divisum being involved in the pathogenesis of pancreatitis or pancreatic pain are based on four inter-related factors:

1. An increased incidence of pancreas divisum is reported at ERCP in cases of idiopathic acute relapsing pancreatitis, compared with other causes of pancreatitis and other pathological states (Cotton & Kizu 1977, Cotton 1980, Richter et al 1981, Sahel et al 1982, Gregg et al 1983, Bernard et al 1990, Brenner et al 1990).

2. Relative outflow obstruction of pancreatic juice through a minor papilla which is too small to accept such a volume of secretion from the greater part of the gland (Marshall & Eckhauser 1985, Saltzberg et al 1990, Warshaw et al 1990) offers a logical explanation for pancreatitis and pain. This concept is supported by clinical observations including delayed drainage from the dorsal duct after ECRP (Rusnak et al 1988); and the results of provocative tests such as the secretin-ultrasound test (Warshaw 1988, Lindstrom & Ihse 1990), the secretin-dynamic CT test (Lowes et al 1989) and the morphine-prostigmine test (Madura et al 1985, Madura 1986). There is also evidence of increased dorsal ductal pressures relative to normal controls on endoscopic manometry (Satterfield et al 1988, Staritz et al 1988), although the results from the minor papilla of normal controls have not been recorded systematically.

3. The presence of morphological (Blair et al 1984) and functional (Yvergeneaux et al 1985) changes in the duct has been recorded.

4. Improvement has been seen after endoscopic or surgical procedures which open the minor papilla in selected patients (Richter et al 1981, Keith et al 1982, 1989, Britt et al 1983, Warshaw et al 1983, 1990, Madura et al 1985, Liguory et al 1986, Madura 1986, Soehendra et al 1986, McCarthy et al 1988, Warshaw 1988, Barkun et al 1990, Brenner et al 1990, Lindstrom et al 1990, Sherman et al 1990, Lans et al 1991).

The counter-arguments that question the aetiological and clinical association between pancreas divisum and pancreatitis are:

1. There is no truly increased incidence of pancreatitis in pancreas divisum since
   a. single case reports in adults and children merely reflect coincidence of disease and the presence of an anatomical variant without proving causation (Yedlin et al 1984, Marshall & Eckhauser 1985, Agha Williams 1987, Browder et al 1987, Reshef et al 1987, Wagner & Golladay 1988, Saltzberg et al 1990)
   b. ERCP series reflect referral populations which vary from centre to centre, and many fail to find a difference in the incidence of pancreas divisum in different patient groups (Delhaye et al 1985, Hayakawas et al 1989)
   c. there may be unexpected and undocumented variations in other causes of unexplained pancreatitis which will falsely affect the proportions of those with divisum in the 'idiopathic' group.

2. There is little direct evidence for outflow obstruction from the dorsal duct during physiological pancreatic secretion and even the unphysiological secretin-ultrasound test has failed to give consistent results (Lowes et al 1989, Warshaw 1988).

3. Dorsal pancreatic changes shown by non-invasive imaging or ductal changes on ECRP are not the rule (Cotton 1980, Richter et al 1981, Sahel et al 1982, Liguory et al 1986, Hayakawas et al 1989, Brenner et al 1990).

4. The response to endoscopic and surgical management is variable (Gregg et al 1983, Jacocks et al 1984, Russell et al 1984, Harig & Hogan 1988, Adzick et al 1989, Jurcovich & Carrico 1990).

The use of endoscopic management of pancreas divisum has included endoscopic dilatation, endoscopic sphincterotomy, and stenting of the minor papilla (Fig. 10.15). When confronted with a patient who has had documented acute recurrent pancreatitis, or attacks suggestive of pancreatitis which cannot be substantiated and for which an extensive search for alternative diagnosis has been made, it seems reasonable to consider the finding of pancreas divisum as a putative factor. Proving the association is problematic unless clear dorsal pancreatographic abnormalities are demonstrated at ECRP. Several provocation tests have been reported (including the morphine-prostigmine test, secretin-ultrasound test and the secretin-CT test) and direct measurement of dorsal duct pressure can be obtained by endoscopic manometry. Theoretically, these are all attractive methods of defining an abnormality of pancreatic outflow dynamics. However, limitations including problems of standardization and technical difficulties in performance detract from their universal application. These patients have often seen many physicians and have undergone multiple investigations. Once the specialist is convinced that other causes of unexplained upper abdominal pain or recurrent pancreatitis have been ruled out, there is reason for intervention. Unfortunately, reports clearly indicate that neither endoscopic nor surgical minor or dual sphincterotomy or sphincteroplasty have much effect in those patients who experience pain only without

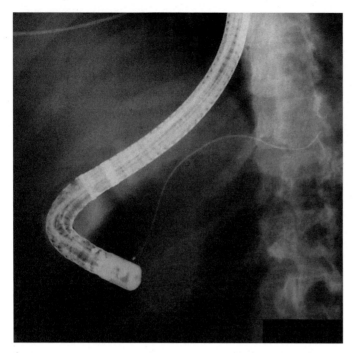

A

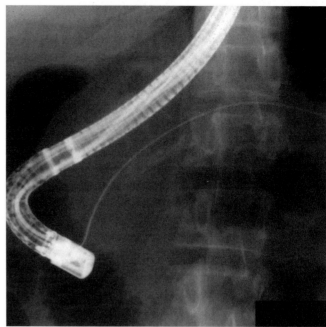

B

pancreatitis (Britt et al 1983, Warshaw et al 1983, 1990, Madura 1986, Rusnak et al 1984, Staritz et al 1988, Keith et al 1989, Lowes et al 1989, Brenner et al 1990, Siegel et al 1990, Richter et al 1981). The question is discussed further in Chapter 34.

PANCREATIC TRAUMA

Pancreatic trauma has become more frequent in recent years as a result of more severe deceleration forces in transportation accidents and the destructive effects of high velocity missiles. Compulsory seat belt laws may actually lead to pancreatic injury because the pancreas can be ruptured by compression against the spine at high velocity. Cases in children are often related to bicycle accidents, sledging injuries, or child abuse. The location of the pancreas within the retroperitoneal space, in close proximity to the vertebral column, affords some protection. However once the organ is injured its retroperitoneal location becomes a disadvantage as the signs and symptoms of injury may evolve slowly and become apparent at a much later stage (Fig. 10.16) than similar injuries in the peritoneal cavity (Taxier et al 1980, Hall et al 1986, Barkin et al 1988, Sugawa & Lucas 1988, Hayward et al 1989, Whittwell et al 1989, Jurkovich & Carrico 1990).

Preoperative diagnosis of pancreatic injury is often made difficult by the vague clinical presentation. At emergency laparotomy, the retroperitoneum may be too traumatized and obscured by haematoma to allow ready

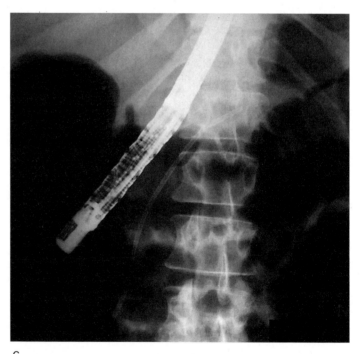

C

Fig. 10.15   A Guide-wire in place for insertion of pancreatic stent into the dorsal duct, for recurrent pancreatitis in a patient with pancreas divisum. **B** Pancreatic stent being passed into the dorsal pancreatic duct over the guide-wire. **C** Plain film taken at completion of placement of long pancreatic stent in the dorsal pancreatic duct.

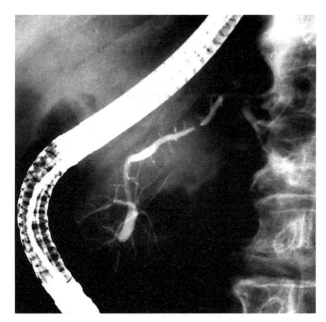

Fig. 10.16   ERP showing a tight stricture due to trauma many years ago.

identification of a pancreatic capsular laceration or pancreatic ductal rupture. A lacerated pancreatic duct may be concealed within an intact pancreatic capsule out of the view of the trauma surgeon. The preoperative diagnosis of ductal disruption could prevent serious long-term morbidity and laparotomy may be avoided if the duct is shown to be intact at ECRP. The vague clinical presentation in the non-emergency blunt abdominal trauma setting may delay the diagnosis of pancreatic trauma and ductal disruption for several hours.

Measurement of serum amylase levels, peritoneal lavage (with measurement of the number of red and white blood cells) detection of bile and debris, and ultrasonography and CT scan have all been used to make an early diagnosis of pancreatic injury, with variable results. The finding on CT scan, the best non-invasive cross-sectional imaging technique of the pancreas, is often a non-specific enlargement of the gland, with or without obliteration of the margins. This finding suggests acute inflammation and pancreatitis, but does not indicate pancreatic rupture or ductal rupture (Barkin et al 1988, Sugawa & Lucas 1988, Jurkovich & Carrico 1990).

Barkin and his group (1988) reported their experience with ERCP in 14 haemodynamically stable patients with abdominal trauma, abdominal pain, and elevated serum amylase levels. All 14 underwent ERCP within 72 hours of admission, 12 had CT scans, and seven underwent peritoneal lavage. Four patients had ductal rupture which was confirmed at laparotomy, while three others were taken to laparotomy with one having a capsular laceration. ERCP was 100% sensitive and specific in the diagnosis of pancreatic ductal rupture.

Questions that remain to be answered concern the selection of patients who would benefit and the timing of early ERCP. A delay in diagnosis of pancreatic ductal injury for more than 18–24 hours causes a precipitous rise in morbidity and mortality. This would argue that the procedure should be done on an urgent basis in the stable patient. The patient with abdominal trauma who is taken urgently to the operating room may also benefit from skilled endoscopy.

Once the patient has been stabilized, bleeding has been controlled and intraperitoneal injuries and hollow visceral injuries have been repaired, the challenge of the retroperitoneum may be addressed jointly. Operative visualization and adequate assessment of the retroperitoneum may require duodenotomy and intraoperative pancreatography. Locating the papilla of Vater may be difficult even with the use of intravenous secretin. Intraoperative ERCP may avoid much of this difficulty in the injured patient, and provide vital information to guide the therapeutic approach to the retroperitoneum (Sugawa & Lucas 1988).

PANCREATIC FISTULAS

Pancreatic fistulas may occur after blunt or penetrating trauma to the abdomen, as a complication of acute or chronic pancreatitis, or as a post-operative complication after surgery on or around the pancreas (Prinz et al 1988, Fielding et al 1989, Izbicki et al 1989, Semba et al 1990). Pancreatic fistulas may drain spontaneously into adjacent hollow viscera or communicate with the body surface externally (Prinz et al 1988, Semba et al 1990). Rarely, duct disruption or rupture of a communicating pseudocyst occurs into the peritoneal cavity leading to pancreatic ascites. If duct disruption or rupture of a pseudocyst occurs posteriorly, fluid tracks into the mediastinum alongside the oesophagus or aorta, and can then rupture into the pleural space resulting in formation of unilateral or bilateral pleural effusions. Rarely, the lung becomes involved with the formation of a pancreaticobronchial fistula (Fielding et al 1989).

Conservative treatment of cutaneous and internal fistulae is recommended in the first instance and includes nil by mouth, hyperalimentation/intravenous hydration and adequate drainage and control of sepsis. Multiple pharmacological approaches have been used, with indifferent results, including anticholinergics, beta receptor agonists and glucagon, and low-dose external radiation has also been attempted (Prinz et al 1988, Fielding et al 1989, Izbicki et al 1989, Semba et al 1990). The somatostatin analogue SMS 201-995, has shown more promising results in the management of pancreatic fistulae (Prinz et al 1988).

ERCP has been widely used to define the anatomy and location of the fistula tract/communication, to determine the presence of pseudocysts or ongoing duct disruption, and to localize a stenosis, stricture or obstruction. This aids operative planning (Prinz et al 1988, Fielding et al 1989, Izbicki et al 1989, Semba et al 1990). Placement of pancreatic stents and nasopancreatic drains as a non-surgical option for the treatment of pancreatic fistulae has been used with some success. Further investigation will be necessary to determine the value of this approach in the treatment of this complication of pancreatic disease.

AIDS-RELATED PANCREATIC DISORDERS

Patients with acquired immunodeficiency syndrome (AIDS) frequently develop hepatobiliary complications of their disease. The pancreatic manifestations of this syndrome have been less well described or defined. The disorders of the pancreas related to AIDS include: drug-induced inflammation, systemic infections involving the pancreas, and neoplastic involvement (Cello 1989, Cappell 1991). Drug-induced pancreatitis, related to the sulpha moiety of trimethoprim-sulphamethoxazole and to pentamidine, the two drugs used to treat pneumocystis carinii, is well known (Cello 1989, Schwartz & Brandt 1989, Cappell 1991). Hyperamylasaemia has been seen in opportunistic infections which have been shown at autopsy to involve the pancreas and include infection with cytomegalovirus (CMV), *Cryptococcus*, *Toxoplasma*

gondii, *Mycobacterium tuberculosis*, *Mycobacterium avium intracellulare* and candida (Cello 1989, Schwartz & Brandt 1989, Cappell 1991). Neoplastic involvement of the pancreas with Kaposi's sarcoma and lymphoma may be seen on CT scan or ultrasonography. The role of ERCP in the diagnosis of these pancreatic disorders has yet to be clearly defined.

CONCLUSIONS

ERCP has come to play a major role in the diagnosis of pancreatic disease when it is suspected on the basis of presumed pancreatic pain, unexplained steatorrhoea, detection of a pancreatic mass on other imaging studies, unexplained ascites, suspected pancreatic cancer and a history of acute pancreatitis. It remains the most important modality for the evaluation of acute recurrent pancreatitis and chronic pancreatitis, especially when non-medical therapy is contemplated. We are now entering an era of optimism concerning minimally invasive endoscopic therapy in many acute and chronic pancreatic disorders. Well-conducted prospective studies of new endoscopic treatments are essential if we are to understand the manner in which we may help patients with pancreatic conditions. Concurrently, such studies may shed further light on the mechanisms of pathogenesis of so many aspects of pancreatic disease.

REFERENCES

Acosta J M, Ledesma C L 1974 Gallstone migration as a cause of acute pancreatitis New England Journal of Medicine 290: 484–487

Acosta J M, Rossi R, Galli O M R et al 1978 Early surgery for acute gallstone pancreatitis: evaluation of a systematic approach. Surgery 83: 367–370

Adzick N S, Shamberger R C, Winter H S et al 1989 Surgical treatment of pancreas divisum causing pancreatitis in children. Journal of Pediatric Surgery 24: 54–58

Agha F P, Williams K D 1987 Pancreas divisum: incidence, detection and clinical significance. American Journal of Gastroenterology 82: 315–320

Amman R W, Akovbiantz A, Largiader F, Schueler G 1984 Course and outcome of chronic pancreatitis. Gastroenterology 86: 820–828

Amman R W, Muench R, Otto A et al 1988 Evolution and regression of pancreatic calcification. Gastroenterology 95: 1018–1028

Anand B S, Vij J C, Mac H S et al 1989 Effect of aging on the pancreatic ducts: a study based on endoscopic retrograde pancreatography. Gastrointestinal Endoscopy 35: 210–213

Anderson J B, Cooper M J, Williamson R C N 1985 Adenocarcinoma of the hepatic biliary tree. Annals of the Royal College of Surgeons of England 67: 139–143

Armstrong C P, Taylor T V, Jacock et al 1985 The biliary tract in patients with acute gallstone pancreatitis. British Journal of Surgery 72: 551–555

Axon A T R 1989 Endoscopic retrograde cholangiopancreatography in chronic pancreatitis Radiologic Clinics of North America 27: 39–50

Axon A T R, Classen M, Cotton P B et al 1984 Pancreatography in chronic pancreatitis. International definitions. Gut 25: 1107–1112

Banks P A, Bradley E L, Dreiling D A et al 1985 Classification of pancreatitis–Cambridge and Marseille. Gastroenterology 89: 928–930

Barkin J S, Hyder S A 1989 Changing concepts in the management of pancreatic pseudocysts. Gastrointestinal Endoscopy 35: 62–63

Barkin J S, Ferstenberg R M, Panullo W et al 1988 Endoscopic retrograde cholangiopancreatography in pancreatic trauma. Gastrointestinal Endoscopy 34: 102–105

Barkun A N, Jones S, Baillie J et al 1990 Endoscopic treatment of patients with pancreas divisum and pancreatitis. Gastrointestinal Endoscopy 36: 206A

Bastid C, Bernard J P, Sarles H et al 1991 Mucinous ductal ectasia of the pancreas: a premalignant disease and a cause of obstructive pancreatitis. Pancreas 6: 15–22

Becker W F, Welsh R A, Pratt H S 1965 Cystadenoma and cystadenocarcinoma of the pancreas. Annals of Surgery 161: 845–863

Benage D, McHenry R, Hawes R H et al 1990 Minor papilla cannulation and dorsal ductography in pancreas divisum. Gastrointesinal Endoscopy 36: 553–557

Bernard J P, Sahel J, Giovannini et al 1990 Pancreas divisum is a probable cause of acute pancreatitis: a report of 137 cases. Pancreas 5: 248–254

Bickerstaff K I, Berry A R, Chapman R W et al 1990 Endoscopic sphincterotomy for palliation of ampullary carcinoma. British Journal of Surgery 77: 160–162

Blackman E, Nash S V 1985 Diagnosis of duodenal and ampullary epithelial neoplasms by endoscopic biopsy: a clinicopathologic and immunohistochemical study. Human Pathology 16: 901–910

Blair A J, Russell C G, Cotton P B 1984 Resection for pancreatitis in patients with pancreas divisum. Annals of Surgery 200: 590–594

Blamey S L, Imrie C W, O'Neill J et al 1984 Prognostic factors in acute pancreatitis. Gut 25: 1340–1346

Bombi J A, Milla A, Badal M et al 1984 Papillary-cystic neoplasm of the pancreas. Report of two cases and review of the literature. Cancer 54: 780–784

Bourgeois N, Dunham F, Verhest A et al 1984 Endoscopic biopsies of the papilla of Vater at the time of endoscopic sphincterotomy: difficulties in interpretation. Gastrointestinal Endoscopy 30: 163–166

Boyce G, Sivak M 1990 Endoscopic ultrasonography in the diagnosis of pancreatic tumours. Gastrointestinal Endoscopy 36(2): S28–S32

Bradley E L, Clements J L, Gonzalez A 1979 The natural history of pancreatic pseudocysts: A unified concept of management. American Journal of Surgery 137: 135–140

Brenner P, Duncombe V, Ham J M 1990 Pancreatitis and pancreas divisum: aetiological and surgical considerations. Australia and New Zealand Journal of Surgery 60: 899–903

Britt L G, Samules A D, Johnson J W 1983 Pancreas divisum: is it a surgical disease? Annals of Surgery 197: 654–662

Browder W, Gravois E, Vega P et al 1987 Obstructing pseudocyst of the duct of Santorini in pancreas divisum. American Journal of Gastroenterology 82: 258–261

Buchi K N, Boweres J H, Dixon J A 1988 Endoscopic cystogastrostomy using the Nd:Yag laser. Gastrointestinal Endoscopy 32: 112–114

Burdick J S, Hogan W J 1991 Chronic pancreatitis: selection of patients for endoscopic therapy. Endoscopy 23: 155–160

Caletti G, Brocchi E, Agostini D et al 1982 Sensitivity of endoscopic retrograde pancreatography in chronic pancreatitis. British Journal of Surgery 69: 507–509

Cantrell B B, Bubilla A L, Erlandson R A et al 1981 Acinar cell cystadenocarcinoma of human pancreas. Cancer 47: 410–416

Cappell M S 1991 Hepatobiliary manifestations of the acquired immunodeficiency syndrome. American Journal of Gastroenterology 86: 1–15

Carr-Locke D L, Cotton P B 1986 Biliary tract and pancreas. British Medical Bulletin 42: 257–264

Carter D C 1988 Pancreatitis and the biliary tree: the continuing problem. American Journal of Surgery 155: 10–17

Cello J P 1989 Acquired immunodeficiency syndrome cholangiopathy: spectrum of disease. American Journal of Medicine 86: 539–546

Classen M, Demling L 1974 Endoskopische Sphincterotomie der Papilla Vateri und Steinextraktion aus dem ductus choledocus. Deutsche Medizinische Wochenschrift 99: 469–476

Classen M, Ossenberg W, Wurbs D et al 1978 Pancreatitis: an indication for endoscopic papillotomy? Endoscopy 10: 223 (abstract)

Compagno J, Oertel J E 1978a Microcystic adenomas of the pancreas (glycogen-rich cystadenomas). A clinicopathologic study of 34 cases. American Journal of Clinical Pathology 69: 289–298

Compagno J, Oertel J E 1978b Mucinous cystic neoplasms of the pancreas with overt and latent malignancy (cystadenocarcinoma and cystadenoma). A clinicopathologic study of 41 cases. American Journal of Clinical Pathology 69: 573–580

Cooperman M, Ferrara J J, Fromkes J J, Carey L C 1982 Surgical management of pancreas divisum. American Journal of Surgery 143: 107–112

Coppa J F, Le Fleur R, Ranson J H C 1981 The role of Chiba needle cholangiography in the diagnosis of possible acute pancreatis with cholelithiasis. Annals of Surgery 193: 393–398

Corfield A P, Cooper M J, Williamson R C N 1985 Acute pancreatitis: a lethal disease of increasing incidence. Gut 26: 724–729

Cotton P B 1977 Progress report: ERCP. Gut 18: 316–341

Cotton P B 1980 Congenital anomaly of pancreas divisum as cause of obstructive pain and pancreatitis. Gut 21: 105–114

Cotton P B 1984a Endoscopic management of bile duct stones (apples and oranges). Gut 25: 587–597

Cotton P B 1984b Endoscopic methods for relief of malignant obstructive jaundice. World Journal of Surgery 8: 854–861

Cotton P B 1985 Pancreas divisum – curiosity or culprit? Gastroenterology 89: 1431–1435

Cotton P B, Kizu M 1977 Malfusion of dorsal and ventral pancreas: a cause of pancreatitis. Gut 18: 340 (abstract)

Cremer M, Deviere J, Engelholm L 1989 Endoscopic management of cysts and pseudocysts in chronic pancreatitis: long-term follow-up after seven years' experience. Gastrointestinal Endoscopy 35: 1–9

Cuschieri A, Hughes J H 1973 Pancreatic reflux during operative choledochography. British Journal of Surgery 60: 933–936

Cuschieri A, Cumming J G R, Wood R A B et al 1983 Evidence for sphincter dysfunction in patients with gallstone associated pancreatitis. Effect of ceruletide in patients undergoing cholecystectomy for gallbladder disease and gallstone associated pancreatitis. British Journal of Surgery 71: 885–888

Dabezies M A, Campana Y, Freidman A C 1990 ERCP in the diagnosis of duct ectatic mucinous cystadenocarcinoma of the pancreas. Gastrointestinal Endoscopy 36: 410–411

De Bolla A R, Obeid M L 1984 Mortality in acute pancreatitis. Annals of the Royal College of Surgeons of England 66: 184–186

Delcenserie R, Dupas J-L, Joly J P et al 1988, Microcystic adenoma of the pancreas demonstrated by endoscopic retrograde cholangiopancreatography. Gastrointestinal Endoscopy 34: 52–54

Delhaye M, Engelholm L, Cremer M 1985 Pancreas divisum: congenital anatomic variant or anomaly? Contribution of endoscopic retrograde dorsal pancreatography. Gastroenterology 89: 1431–1435

Di Magno E P 1982 Diagnosis of chronic pancreatitis: are noninvasive tests of exocrine pancreatic function sensitive and specific? Gastroenterology 83: 143–146

Dixon J A, Hillam J D 1970 Surgical treatment of biliary tract disease associated with acute pancreatitis. American Journal of Surgery 120: 371–375

Eckhauser F E, Knol J A, Strodel W E et al 1983 Common bile duct strictures associated with chronic pancreatitis. American Surgeon 7: 350–358

Edmondson H A, Bullock W K, Mehl J W 1950 Chronic pancreatitis and lithiasis. II Pathology and pathogenesis of pancreatic lithiasis. American Journal of Pathology 26: 37–55

Fan S T, Choi T K, Lai C S et al 1988 Influence of age on the mortality from acute pancreatitis. British Journal of Surgery 75: 463–466

Fernandez-del Castillo C, Warshaw A 1990 Diagnosis and preoperative evaluation of pancreatic cancer, with implications for management. Gastroenterologic Clinics of North America 19(4): 915–933

Fielding G A, McLatchie G R, Wilson C et al 1989 Acute pancreatitis and pancreatic fistula formation. British Journal of Surgery 76: 1126–1128

Foutch P G, Kerr D M, Harlan J R et al 1991 A prospective controlled analysis of endoscopic cytotechniques for diagnosis of malignant biliary strictures. American Journal of Gastroenterology 86(5): 577–580

Freeny P C 1989a Classification of pancreatitis. Radiologic Clinics of North America 27(1): 1–3

Freeny P C 1989b Radiologic diagnosis and staging of pancreatic ductal adenocarcinoma. Radiologic Clinics of North America 27(1): 121–128

Freeny P C, Marks W, Ryan J et al 1988 Pancreatic ductal adenocarcinoma: Diagnosis and staging with dynamic CT. Radiology 166: 125–133

Friedman A C, Lichtenstein J E, Dachman A H 1983 Cystic neoplasms of the pancreas. Radiological-pathological correlation. Radiology 149: 45–50

Fuji T, Amano K, Harima T et al 1985 Pancreatic sphincterotomy and pancreatic endoprosthesis. Endoscopy 17: 69–72

Goodman A J, Neoptolemos J P, Carr-Locke D L et al 1985 Detection of gallstones after acute pancreatitis. Gut 26: 125–132

Gregg J A 1977 Pancreas divisum: its association with pancreatitis. American Journal of Surgery 134: 539–543

Gregg J A, Monaco A P, McDermott W V 1983 Pancreas divisum: results of surgical intervention. American Journal of Surgery 145: 488–492

Gregg J A, Solomon J, Clark G 1984 Pancreas divisum and its association with choledochal sphincter stenosis. Diagnosis by endoscopic retrograde cholangiopancreatography and endoscopic biliary manometry. American Journal of Surgery 147: 367–371

Gullo L, Costa P L, Gontana G et al 1976 Investigation of exocrine pancreatic function by continuous infusion of caerulein and secretin in normal subjects and in chronic pancreatitis. Digestion 14: 97–107

Gyr H, Agrawal N M, Gelsenfeld O et al 1975 Comparative study of secretin and Lundh tests. American Journal of Digestive Diseases 20: 506–512

Hall R I, Lavelle C W, Venables C W 1986 Use of ERCP to identify the site of traumatic injuries of the main pancreatic duct in children. British Journal of Surgery 73: 411–412

Harig J M, Hogan W J 1988 Pancreas divisum: a case against surgical treatment. Advances in Surgery 21: 111–126

Hayakawas T, Kondo T, Sibata Y et al 1989 Pancreas divisum, a predisposing factor to pancreatitis? International Journal of Pancreatology 5: 317–326

Hayashi Y, Nakasawa S, Kimoto E et al 1989 Clinicopathologic analysis of endoscopic ultrasonograms in pancreatic mass lesions. Endoscopy 21: 121–125

Hayes D H, Bolton J S, Gladden W W et al 1987 Carcinoma of the ampulla of Vater. Annals of Surgery 206: 572–577

Hayward S R, Lucas M R, Sugawa C, Ledgerwood A M 1989 Emergent endoscopic retrograde cholangiopancreatography. Archives of Surgery 124: 745–746

Heyder N, Flugel H, Domschke W 1988 Catheter drainage of pancreatic pseudocysts into the stomach. Endoscopy 20: 75–77

Honickman S, Mueller P, Wittenberg J et al 1983 Ultrasound in obstructive jaundice: prospective evaluation of site and cause. Radiology 147: 511–515

Huibregtse K, Tytgat G N J 1988 Carcinoma of the ampulla of Vater: the endoscopic approach. Endoscopy 20: 223–226

Huibregtse K, Katon R M, Tytgat N J 1986 Precut papillotomy via fine-needle papillotome: a safe and effective technique. Gastrointestinal Endoscopy 32: 403

Huibregtse K, Schneider B, Rauws E et al 1987 Carcinoma of the ampulla of Vater. The role of endoscopic drainage. Surgical Endoscopy 1: 79–84

Imrie C W, Benjamin I S, Ferguson J C 1978 A single centre double-blind trial of Trasylol therapy in primary acute pancreatitis. British Journal of Surgery 65: 337–641

Itai Y, Ohhashi K, Furui S et al 1988 Microcystic adenoma of the pancreas: spectrum of computed tomographic finds. Journal of Computer Assisted Tomography 12: 797–803

Izbicki J R, Wilker D K, Waldner H et al 1989 Thoracic manifestations of internal pancreatic fistulas: report of five cases. American Journal of Gastroenterology 84: 265–271

Jacocks M, ReMine S G, Carmichael D H 1984 Difficulties in the diagnosis and treatment of pancreas divisum. Archives of Surgery 119: 1088–1091

Johnson A G, Hosking S W 1987 Appraisal of the management of bile duct stones. British Journal of Surgery 74: 555–560

Johnson C D, Stephens D H, Charbonneau J W et al 1988 Cystic pancreatic tumours: CT and sonographic assessment. American Journal of Radiology 1133–1138

Jurkovich G J, Carrico C J 1990 Pancreatic trauma. Surgical Clinics of North America 70(3): 575–593

Kalser M, Barkin J, MacIntyre J 1985 Pancreatic cancer assessment of prognosis by clinical presentation. Cancer 56: 397–402

Kaufman A, Sivak M, Ferguson D 1988 Endoscopic retrograde cholangiopancreatography in pancreatic islet cell tumors. Gastrointestinal Endoscopy 34(1): 47–52

Kautz G, Kohaus H, Keferstein R-D et al 1982 Zur Pathogenese und endoskopischen Therapie der akuten bilaren Pankreatitis. Klinikarzt 11: 1202–1212

Kawai K, Akasaka Y, Murakami I, Tada M, Kohli Y, Nakajima M 1974 Endoscopic sphincterotomy of the ampulla of Vater. Gastrointestinal Endoscopy 20: 148–151

Keith R G, Shapero T F, Saibil F G 1982 Treatment of pancreatitis associated with pancreas divisum by dorsal duct sphincterotomy. Canadian Journal of Surgery 25: 622–626

Keith R G, Shapero T F, Saibil F G et al 1989 Dorsal duct sphincterotomy is effective long-term treatment of acute pancreatitis associated with pancreas divisum. Surgery 106: 660–666

Kelly T R 1976 Gallstone pancreatitis: pathophysiology. Surgery 80: 488–492

Kelly T R 1980 Gallstone pancreatitis. The timing of surgery. Surgery 88: 345–349

Kent R B, Van Heerden J A, Weiland L H 1981 Nonfunctioning islet cell tumors. Annals of Surgery 19: 185–190

Knox R A, Kingston R D 1986 Carcinoma of the ampulla of Vater. British Journal of Surgery 73: 72–73

Kolars J C, Allen M O, Ansel H et al 1989 Pancreatic pseudocysts: clinical and endoscopic experience. American Journal of Gastroenterology 84: 259–264

Kozarek R A, Brayleo C M, Harlan J et al 1985 Endoscopic drainage of pancreatic pseudocysts. Gastrointestinal Endoscopy 31: 322–328

Kozarek R A, Ball T J, Patterson D J et al 1991 Endoscopic transpapillary therapy for disrupted pancreatic duct and peripancreatic collections. Gastroenterology 100: 1362–1370

Kreel L, Sandin S 1973 Changes in pancreatic morphology associated with aging. Gut 14: 962–970

Lack E E 1989 Primary tumors of the exocrine pancreas. American Journal of Surgical Pathology 13 (Suppl 1): 66–88

Lambert R, Ponchon A, Chauaillon F et al 1988 Laser treatment of tumors of the papilla of Vater. Endoscopy 20: 227–231

Lang C, Gyr K, Stalder G A et al 1981 Assessment of exocrine pancreatic function by oral administration of N-benzoyl-L-tyrosyl-P-aminobenzoic acid (Bentiromide) 5 years' clinical experience. British Journal of Surgery 68: 771–775

Lang C, Gyr R, Tonko I et al 1984 The value of serum PABA as a pancreatic function test. Gut 25: 508–512

Langergren C 1962 Calcium carbonate precipitation in the pancreas, gallstones and urinary calculi. Acta Chirurgica Scandinavica 124: 320–325

Lankisch P G, 1982 Exocrine pancreatic function test. Gut 23: 777–798

Lankisch P G, Chreiber A, Otto J 1983 Pancreolauryl test. Digestive Diseases and Sciences 28: 490–493

Lankisch P G, Brauneis J, Otto J et al 1986 Pancreolauryl and PABA tests. Are serum tests more practical alternatives to urine tests in the diagnosis of exocrine pancreatic insufficiency? Gastroenterology 90: 350–354

Lans J I, Geenen J E, Johanson A F et al 1991 Endoscopic therapy in patients with pancreatitis divisum and acute pancreatitis: a prospective randomized controlled clinical trial. Gastroenterology 100: 831A (abstract)

Laxson L C, Fromkes J J, Cooperman M 1985 ERCP in the management of pancreatic pseudocysts. American Journal of Surgery 150: 683–686

Leese T, Shaw D 1988 Comparison of three Glasgow multifactor prognostic scoring systems in acute pancreatitis. British Journal of Surgery 75: 460–462

Leese T, Neoptolemos J P, West K P et al 1986 Tumours and pseudotumours of the ampulla of Vater: an endoscopic, clinical and pathological study. Gut 27: 1186–1192

Ligoury C, Lefebvre J F, Canard L N 1986 Pancreas division: therapeutic results in 12 patients. Digestive Diseases and Sciences 31: 53

Lindstrom E, Ihse I 1989 Computed tomography findings in pancreas divisum. Acta Radiologica 30: 609–613

Lindstrom E, Ihse I 1990 Dynamic CT scanning of pancreatic duct after secretin provocation in pancreas divisum. Digestive Diseases and Sciences 35: 1371–1376

Lindstrom E, Von Schenk H, Ihse I 1990 Pancreatic exocrine and endocrine function in patients with pancreas divisum and abdominal pain. International Journal of Pancreatology 6: 17–24

Lowes J R, Lees W R, Cotton P B 1989 Pancreatic duct dilatation after secretin stimulation in pancreas divisum. Pancreas 21: 111–126

Lumsden A, Bradley E L 1989 Pseudocyst or cystic neoplasm? Differential diagnosis and initial management of cystic pancreatic lesions. Hepato-gastroenterology 36: 462–466

McCarthy J, Fumo D, Geenen J E 1987 Pancreas divisum: a new method for cannulating the accessory papilla. Gastrointestinal Endoscopy 33: 440–442

McCarthy J H, Geenen J E, Hogan W J 1988 Preliminary experience with endoscopic stent placement in pancreatic disease. Gastrointestinal Endoscopy 34: 16–18

Macarty R L, Stephens D H, Brown J A L 1975 Retrograde pancreatography in autopsy specimens. American Journal of Roentgenology 123: 359–366

McCune W S, Short P E, Moscovitz H 1968 Endoscopic cannulation of the ampulla of Vater: a preliminary report. Annals of Surgery 167: 752–756

Madura J A 1986 Pancreas divisum: stenosis of the dorsally dominant pancreatic duct. A surgically correctable lesion. American Journal of Surgery 151: 742–745

Madura J A, Fiore A C, O'Connor K W et al 1985 Pancreas divisum: correction and management. American Journal of Surgery 51: 353–357

Malfertheiner P, Büchler M 1989 Correlation of imaging and function in chronic pancreatitis. Radiologic Clinics of North America 27: 51–64

Marshall J B, Eckhauser M L 1985 Pancreas divisum. A cause of chronic relapsing pancreatitis. Digestive Diseases and Sciences 30: 582–587

Mayer A D, McMahon M J, Benson E A et al 1984 Operations upon the biliary tract in patients with acute pancreatitis: aims, indications and timing. Annals of the Royal College of Surgeons of England 66: 179–183

Mayo J H 1936 Pancreatic calculi. Mayo Clinic Proceedings 11: 456–457

Minami M, Itai Y, Ohtomo K et al 1989 Cystic neoplasms of the pancreas: comparison of MR imaging with CT. Radiology 171: 53–56

Moreira V F, Merono E, Ledo L et al 1991 Incomplete pancreas divisum. Gastrointestinal Endoscopy 37: 104–105

MRC Multicentre Trial 1977 Death from acute pancreatitis. Lancet 2: 632–635

Mullens J E, Barr J R, Barron P T 1983 Cystadenoma and cystadenocarcinoma of the pancreas. Canadian Journal of Surgery 26(6): 529–531

Nakao M, Siegel J, Stenger R et al 1982 Tumors of the ampulla of Vater: early diagnosis by intra-ampullary biopsy during endoscopic cannulation. Gastroenterology 83: 459–464

Neoptolemos J P 1988 The urgent diagnosis and treatment of biliary (gallstone asociated) acute pancreatitis. Hunterian Lecture, presented at the Royal College of Surgeons of England, London

Neoptolemos J P, Fossard D P, Berry J M 1983 A prospective study of radionuclide biliary scanning in acute pancreatitis. Annals of the Royal College of Surgeons of England 65: 180–182

Neoptolemos J P, Hall A W, Finlay D F et al 1984 The urgent diagnosis of gallstones in acute pancreatitis: a prospective study of three methods. British Journal of Surgery 71: 230–233

Neoptolemos J P, London N, Slater N D et al 1986 A prospective study of ERCP and endoscopic sphincerotomy in the diagnosis and treatment of gallstone acute pancreatitis. Archives of Surgery 121: 696–702

Neoptolemos J P, London N, Bailey I et al 1987a The role of clinical and biochemical criteria and endoscopic retrograde cholangiopancreatography in the urgent diagnosis of common bile duct stones in acute pancreatitis. Surgery 100: 732–742

Neoptolemos J P, Talbot I C, Carr–Locke D L et al 1987b Treatment and outcome in 52 consecutive cases of ampullary carcinoma. British Journal of Surgery 74: 957–961

Neoptolemos J P, Carr–Locke D L, London N J 1988a Controlled trial of urgent endoscopic retrograde cholangiopancreatography and endoscopic sphincterotomy versus conservative treatment for acute pancreatitis due to gallstones. Lancet 2: 979–983

Neoptolemos J P, Davidson B R, Vallance D et al 1988b The role of duodenal bile crystal analysis in the investigation of 'idiopathic' pancreatitis. British Journal of Surgery 75: 450–453

Nickl N J, Lawson J M, Cotton P B 1991 Mucinous pancreatic tumors. ERCP findings. Gastrointestinal Endoscopy 37: 133–138

O'Connor K W, Lehman G A 1985 An improved technique for accessory papilla cannulation. Gastrointestinal Endoscopy 31: 13–17

O'Connor M, Kolars J, Ansel H et al 1986 Preoperative ERCP in the surgical management of pancreatic pseudocysts. American Journal of Surgery 151: 18–24

Oi I, Takemoto T, Kondo T 1969 Fibreduodenoscope. Direct observations of the papilla of Vater. Endoscopy 1: 101–103

Opie E L 1901 The etiology of acute hemorrhagic pancreatitis. Johns Hopkins Hospital Bulletin 121: 182–188

Osborne D H, Imrie C W, Carter D C 1981 Biliary surgery in the same admission for gallstone associated acute pancreatitis. British Journal of Surgery 68: 758–761

Paloyan D, Simonowitz D, Skinner D B 1975 The timing of biliary tract operations in patients with pancreatitis associated with gallstones. Surgery, Gynecology, and Obstetrics 141: 737–739

Parker H W 1987 Congenital anomalies of the pancreas. In: Sivak M V Jr (ed) Gastrointestinal Endoscopy. W B Saunders, Philadelphia, p 770–779

Pereyra-Lima L, Kalil A N, Wilson T J 1989 Surgical treatment of chronic pancreatic cholangiopathy. British Journal of Surgery 76: 1129–1131

Pitt H A 1984 Is endoscopic sphincterotomy a safe and effective method for the management of stones in the distal common bile duct? In Gitnick G (ed) Churchill Livingstone, London, p 89–116

Ponchon T, Berger F, Chavaillon A et al 1989 Contribution of endoscopy to diagnosis and treatment of tumors of the ampulla of Vater. Cancer 64: 161–167

Prinz R A, Badrinath K, Cheijfec G et al 1983 Nonfunctioning islet cell carcinoma of the pancreas. American Surgeon 49: 345–349

Prinz R A, Pickelman J, Hoffman J P 1988 Treatment of pancreatic cutaneous fistulas with a somatostatin analog. American Journal of Surgery 155: 36–42

Ranson J H C 1979 The timing of biliary surgery in acute pancreatitis. Annals of Surgery 189: 654–662

Ranson J H C 1982 Etiologic and prognostic factors in human acute pancreatitis: a review. American Journal of Gastroenterology 77: 633–638

Ranson J H C 1990 The role of surgery in the management of acute pancreatitis. Annals of Surgery 211(4): 382–393

Reshef R, Stamler B, Novis B G 1987 Recurrent acute pancreatitis associated with pancreas divisum. American Journal of Gastroenterology 83: 86–88

Richter J M, Schapiro R H, Mulley A G et al 1981 Association of pancreas divisum and pancreatitis, and its treatment by sphincteroplasty of the accessory ampulla. Gastroenterology 81: 1101–1110

Rickaert F, Cremer M, Deviere J et al 1991 Intraductal mucin-hypersecreting neoplasms of the pancreas. Gastroenterology 101: 512–519

Robertson J F R, Imrie C W, Hole D J et al 1987 Management of periampullary carcinoma. British Journal of Surgery 74: 816–819

Roberts-Thomson I C 1987 Therapeutic endoscopy in the biliary tract. Australia and New Zealand Journal of Surgery 57: 345–348

Roesch W, Demling L 1982 Endoscopic management of pancreatitis. Surgical Clinics of North America 62: 845–852

Rosseland A R, Osnes M 1989 Biliary concrements: the endoscopic approach. World Journal of Surgery 13: 178–185

Rosseland A R, Solhaug J H 1984 Early or delayed endoscopic papillotomy (EPT) in gallstone pancreatitis. Annals of Surgery 199: 165–167

Rusnak C H, Hosie R T, Kuechler P M et al 1988 Pancreatitis assóciated with pancreas divisum: results of surgical intervention. American Journal of Surgery 155: 641–643

Russell R C G, Wong N W, Cotton P B 1984 Accessory sphincterotomy (endoscopic and surgical) in patients with pancreas divisum. British Journal of Surgery 71: 954–957

Rustgi A, Kelsey P, Guelrud M et al 1989 Malignant tumors of the bile ducts: diagnosis by biopsy during endoscopic cannulation. gastrointestinal Endoscopy 35(3): 248–251

Rustin R E, Broughan T A, Hermann R E et al 1986 Papillary cystic epithelial neoplasms of the pancreas. A clinical study of four cases. Archives of Surgery 121: 1073–1076

Ryan M E 1991 Cytologic brushings of ductal lesions during ERCP. Gastrointestinal Endoscopy 37(2): 139–142

Sachs J R, Deren J J, Sohn M et al 1989 Mucinous cystadenoma: pitfalls of differential diagnosis. American Journal of Gastroenterology 84: 811–816

Safrany L 1978 Endoscopic treatment of biliary tract diseases. Lancet 2: 983–985

Safrany L 1982 Controversies in acute pancreatitis. In: Hollender L F (ed) Controversies in acute pancreatitis. Springer-Verlag, New York, p 214–218

Sahel J, Cros R C, Bourry J et al 1982 Clinico-pathological conditions associated with pancreas divisum. Digestion 23: 1–8

Sahel J, Bastid C, Pellat B et al 1987 Endoscopic cystoduodenostomy of cysts of chronic calcifying pancreatitis: a report of 20 cases. Pancreas 2: 447–453

Saltzberg D M, Schreiber J B, Smith K et al 1990 Isolated ventral pancreatitis in a patient with pancreas divisum. American Journal of Gastroenterology 85: 1407–1410

Sanfey H, Mendelsohn G, Cameron J L 1983 Solid and papillary neoplasm of the pancreas. A potentially curable lesion. Annals of Surgery 197: 272–275

Sarles S, Sahel J 1976 Pathology of chronic calcifying pancreatitis. American Journal of Gastroenterology 66: 117–136

Sarner M, Cotton P B 1984 Classification of pancreatitis. Gut 25: 756–759

Satterfield S T, McCarthy J H, Geenen J E et al 1988 Clinical experience in 82 patients with pancreas divisum: preliminary results of manometry and endoscopic therapy. Pancreas 3: 248–253

Sauerbruch T, Holl J, Sackmann M et al 1987 Disintegration of pancreatic duct stones with shock waves in a patient with chronic pancreatitis. Endoscopy 19: 207–208

Schleintz P F, Katon R M 1984 Blunt tipped needle catheter for cannulation of the minor papilla. Gastrointestinal Endoscopy 30: 263–266

Schlippert W, Kucke D, Anuras S et al 1978 Carcinoma of the papilla of Vater. A review of fifty-seven cases. American Journal of Surgery 135: 754–770

Schott B, Neuhaus B, Portocarrero G et al 1982 Endoskopische Papillotomie bei akuter bilaren Pankreatitis. Klinikarzt 11: 52–54

Schwartz M S, Brandt L J 1989 The spectrum of pancreatic disorders in patients with the acquired immune deficiency syndrome. American Journal of Gastroenterology 84: 459–462

Scudera P, Koizumi J, Jacobson I 1990 Brush cytology evaluation of lesions encountered during ERCP. Gastrointestinal Endoscopy 36(3): 281–284

Seifert E 1978 Endoscopic papillotomy and removal of gallstone. American Journal of Gastroenterology 69: 154–159

Semba D, Wada Y, Ishihara Y et al 1990 Massive pancreatic pleural effusion: pathogenesis of pancreatic duct disruption. Gastroenterology 99: 528–532

Seto H, Kamei T, Bandba Y et al 1990 Pancreas divisum: CT and ERCP findings. Radiation Medicine 8: 20–21

Shemesh E, Nass S, Czerniak A 1989 Endoscopic sphincterotomy and endoscopic fulguration in the management of adenoma of the papilla of Vater. Surgery, Gynecology and Obstetrics 169: 445–448

Sherman S, Lehman G, Nisi R et al 1990 Results for endoscopic sphincterotomy for pancreas divisum. Gastrointestinal Endoscopy 36: 198A (abstract)

Siegel J H, Ben-Zvi J S, Pullano W et al 1990 Effectiveness of endoscopic drainage for pancreas divisum: endoscopic and surgical results in 31 patients. Endoscopy 22: 129–133

Siegelman S S, 1980 CT of fluid collections associated with pancreatitis. American Journal of Radiology 134: 1121–1125

Sigfusson B F, Wehlin L, Lindstrom C G 1983 Variants of pancreatic duct system of importance in endoscopic retrograde cholangiopancreatography. Observations on autopsy specimens. Acta Radiol Diag 24: 113–128

Silverman P M, McVay L, Zeman R K et al 1989 Pancreatic pseudotumor in pancreas divisum: CT characteristics. Journal of Computer Assisted Tomography 13: 140–141

Singer M V, Gyr K, Sarles H 1985 Revised classification of pancreatitis. Report of the Second International Symposium on the Classification of Pancreatitis, Marseille, France, March 28–30, 1984. Gastroenterology 89: 683–685

Sivak M V 1988 Clinical and endoscopic aspects of tumor of the ampulla of Vater. Endoscopy 20: 211–217

Soehendra N, Kempeneers I, Nam V C et al 1986 Endoscopic dilatation and papillotomy of the accessory papilla and internal drainage in pancreas divisum. Endoscopy 18: 129–132

Soehendra N, Grimm H, Berger B et al 1989 Malignant jaundice: Results of diagnostic and therapeutic endoscopy. World Journal of Surgery 13: 171–177

Soulen M C, Serhouni E A, Fishman E K et al 1989 Enlargement of the pancreatic head in patients with pancreas divisum. Clinical Imaging 13: 51–57

Spinetti P, Meroni E, Prada A 1988 Endoscopic treatment of a pancreatic pseudocyst by nasocystic tube. Endoscopy 20: 27–29

Staritz M, Meyer zum Buschenfelde K H 1988 Elevated pressure in dorsal part of pancreas divisum: the cause of chronic pancreatitis? Pancreas 3: 108–110

Steiner E, Stark D D, Hahn P F et al 1989 Imaging of pancreatic neoplasms: comparison of MR and CT. American Journal of Radiology 152: 487–491

Stern C D 1986 A historical perspective on the discovery of the accessory duct of the pancreas, the ampulla 'of Vater' and the pancreas divisum. Gut 27: 203–212

Stobbé C K, ReMine W H, Baggenstoss A H 1970 Pancreatic lithiasis. Surgery, Gynecology and Obstetrics 131: 1090–1099

Stone H H, Fabian T C, Dunlop W E 1981 Gallstone pancreatitis: biliary tract pathology in relation to time of operation. Annals of Surgery 194: 305–310

Sugawa C, Lucas C E 1988 The case for preoperative and intraoperative ERCP in pancreatic trauma. Gastrointestinal Endoscopy 34: 145–147

Taft D A, Freeny P C 1981 Cystic neoplasms of the pancreas. American Journal of Surgery 142: 30–35

Taxier M, Sivak M V, Cooperman A M et al 1980 Endoscopic retrograde pancreatography in the evaluation of trauma to the pancreas. Surgery, Gynecology and Obstetrics 150: 65–68

Tio T L, Tytgat N K 1986 Endoscopic ultrasonography in staging local resectability of pancreatic and periampullary malignancy. Scandinavian Journal of Gastroenterology 21 (Suppl 123): 135–142

Tondelli P, Stutz K, Harder F et al 1982 Acute gallstone pancreatitis: best timing for biliary surgery. British Journal of Surgery 69: 709–710

Tulassay A, Papp J 1980 New clinical aspects of pancreas divisum. Gastrointestinal Endoscopy 26: 143–146

Tulassay A, Papp J, Farkas I E 1986 Diagnostic aspects of incomplete pancreas divisum. Gastrointestinal Endoscopy 32: 428

Uflacker R, Amaral N M, Lima S et al 1980 Angiography in cystadenoma and cystadenocarcinoma of the pancreas. Acta Radiologica 21: 189–195

Van Spuy D S 1981 Endoscopic sphincterotomy in the management of gallstone pancreatitis. Endoscopy 13: 25–26

Venu R, Geenen J, Kini M et al 1990 Endoscopic retrograde brush cytology: a new technique. Gastroenterology 99: 1475–1479

Von Riemann J F, Lux G 1984 Therapeutische Strategie bei der akuten Pankreatitis (1). Fortschritte der Medizin 102: 179–182

Wagner C W, Golladay E S 1988 Pancreas divisum and pancreatitis in children. American Surgeon 54: 22–26

Warshaw A L 1988 Pancreas divisum: a case for surgical treatment. Advances in Surgery 21: 93–109

Warshaw A L 1991 Mucinous cystic tumours and mucinous ductal ectasia of the pancreas. Gastrointestinal Endoscopy 37: 199–201

Warshaw A L, Rattner D W 1985 Timing of surgical drainage for pancreatic pseudocyst: clinical and chemical criteria. Annals of Surgery 202: 720–724

Warshaw A L, Rutledge P L 1987 Cystic tumors mistaken for pancreatic pseudocysts. Annals of Surgery 205(4): 393–398

Warshaw A L, Richter J M, Schapiro R H 1983 The cause and treatment of pancreatitis associated with pancreas divisum. Annals of Surgery 198: 443–452

Warshaw A L, Compton C C, Lewandrowsk K et al 1990a Cystic tumors of the pancreas. Annals of Surgery 212(4): 432–445

Warshaw A L, Simeone J F, Schapiro R H et al 1990b Evaluation and treatment of the dominant dorsal duct syndrome (pancreas divisum redefined). American Journal of Surgery 159: 56–64

Whittwell A E, Gomez G A, Byers P et al 1989 Blunt pancreatic trauma: prospective evaluation of early endoscopic retrograde pancreatography. Southern Medical Journal 82: 586–591

Williamson R C N 1984 Early assessment of severity in acute pancreatitis. Gut 25: 1331–1339

Wilson C, Auld C D, Schlinkert R et al 1989 Hepatobiliary complications in chronic pancreatitis. Gut 30: 520–527

Wittenberg J, Ferrucci J, Warshaw A 1984 Contribution of computed tomography to patients with pancreatic adenocarcinoma. World Journal of Surgery 8: 831–838

Yamaguchi K, Enjoji M 1987a Carcinoma of the ampulla of Vater. A clinicopathologic study and pathologic staging of 109 cases of carcinoma and 5 cases of adenoma. Cancer 59: 506–515

Yamaguchi K, Enjoji M 1987b Cystic neoplasms of the pancreas. Gastroenterology 92: 1934–1943

Yamaguchi K, Munetomo E, Kitamura K 1990 Endoscopic biopsy has limited accuracy in diagnosis of ampullary tumors. Gastrointestinal Endoscopy 36: 588–592

Yasuda K, Mukai H, Cho E et al 1988a The use of endoscopic ultrasonography in the diagnosis and staging of carcinoma of the papilla of Vater. Endoscopy 20: 218–222

Yasuda K, Mukai H, Fujimoto S et al 1988b The diagnosis of pancreatic cancer by endoscopic ultrasonography. Gastrointestinal Endoscopy 34(1): 1–8

Yedlin S T, Dubois R S, Philippart A I 1984 Pancreas divisum: a cause of pancreatitis in childhood. Journal of Pediatric Surgery 19: 793–794

Yvergeneaux J P, Van der Boer H, De Keyser R et al 1985 Pancreas divisum: a teenager with calculi in the duct of Santorini. Report of a case treated by double drainage procedure. Acta Chirurgica Belgica 85: 67–70

Zeman R K, McVay L V, Silverman P M et al 1988 Pancreas divisum: thin section CT. Radiology 169: 395–398

11. Endoscopic ultrasonography

T. L. Tio

INTRODUCTION

Pancreatic cancer is a highly malignant disease, the prognosis of which has remained unchanged despite advances in diagnostic imaging. The disease has usually reached an advanced stage by the time of diagnosis. Transcutaneous abdominal ultrasonography is widely used to detect and stage pancreatic carcinoma. However, the technique is frequently hindered by bowel gas, adipose tissue or postsurgical scarring. In Western countries, ideal sonogenic patients are rare because obesity is common. Moreover, small pancreatic cancers and periampullary carcinomas may not be imaged with abdominal ultrasonography. Endoscopic ultrasonography, generally known as endosonography (ES), was developed to overcome these limitations by approaching the target of interest via the gastrointestinal lumen. Approximately 10 years ago, the pioneer work was done by cardiologists and gastroenterologists (Hisanaga & Hisanaga 1978, et al 1980, Di Magno et al 1980, Strohm et al 1980, Lux et al 1982). Through close contact with the target, a high frequency real-time ultrasonic beam can be used to improve image quality and diagnostic accuracy. ES has been reported to be an accurate means of staging pancreatic and periampullary carcinomas due to its ability to image ductular and parenchymal abnormalities (Tio & Tytgat 1984, 1986a, Yasuda et al 1988a, b).

In the TNM system tumours are staged by defining the anatomical extent of the primary tumour (T), detecting involved regional lymph nodes (N) and detecting distant metastases (M). Recently, pancreatic and periampullary carcinoma have been included in a new 1987 International Union Against Cancer (Union Internationale Contre le Cancer, UICC) TNM classification (Hermanek & Sobin 1987, Sobin et al 1988). The depth of carcinoma has been used as the main criterion to categorize the tumour and predict resectability of the carcinoma. Clinical TNM staging (c-TNM) requires a high resolution imaging modality, and should show a close correlation with pathological TNM classification (p-TNM) (Sobin & Ros 1990,

Tio et al 1990). TNM classification with ES is defined as C2, with surgery as C3, with the histology of a resected specimen as C4 and with the histology of an autopsy specimen as C5. The aim of this chapter is to review the usefulness of ES in preoperative TNM staging (c-TNM). Selected case reports are described to illustrate the role of ES in planning treatment.

INSTRUMENTS

Since 1983 we have been using a prototype Olympus echoendoscope (EU-M2) and a commercially available Olympus echoendoscope (EU-M3). The latter emits ultrasound at an adjustable frequency of 7.5 MHz or 12 MHz and has an instrumental channel for ES-guided cytological puncture or endoscopic biopsy (Fig. 11.1). Recently, a prototype echoendoscope with a smaller echoprobe has become available and incorporates an elevator for manoeuvring the puncture needle (Fig. 11.2). Finally, a small catheter echoprobe has also been devel-

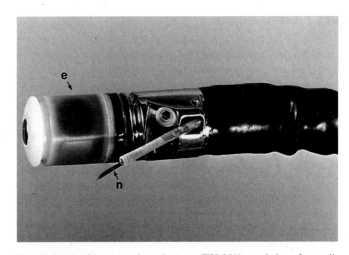

Fig. 11.1 An Olympus echoendoscope (EU-M3) consisting of a small echoprobe (e) attached at the tip of a side-viewing gastroscope. A Sclerning needle (n) passing through the biopsy channel is used for endosonographically guided puncture.

111

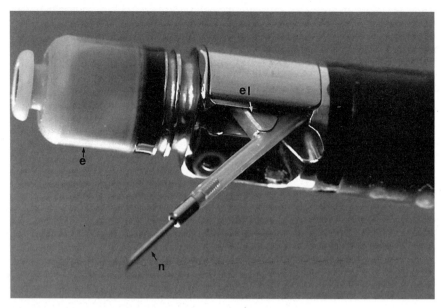

Fig. 11.2 An Olympus echoduodenoscope consisting of a smaller echoprobe (e). An elevator (el) is available for better endoscopic manoeuvring of the puncture needle (n).

oped which can be introduced through the biopsy channel of conventional forward-viewing endoscopes (Fig. 11.3). Table 11.1 summarizes the specifications of these instruments.

TECHNIQUE OF ENDOSONOGRAPHY

The echoendoscope is introduced into the oesophagus after oropharyngeal anaesthesia and intravenous sedation with diazepam or midazolam. Intravenous sedation is necessary to reduce discomfort during insertion of the instrument into the oesophagus, and during intubation of the pylorus and duodenal bulb. The echoprobe is passed blindly down

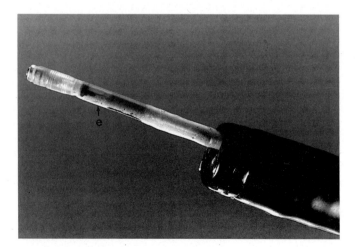

Fig. 11.3 A catheter echoprobe (e) of 2 mm outer diameter for endoscopic guided endosonography through the biopsy channel of a large calibre gastroscope.

the oesophagus because the side-viewing optics do not allow visualization. The echoprobe is then passed through the distal part of the stomach and into the duodenum. The papilla of Vater is first identified endoscopically. Thereafter, the echoprobe should be positioned beyond the papilla. After inflating the balloon with water the instrument is drawn back gradually under endosonographic control until the target lesion is imaged. The adjacent lymph nodes should also be imaged in their known anatomical locations, usually adjacent to the primary tumour and major blood vessels.

Then the instrument is gradually withdrawn into the stomach for complete imaging of the pancreas. The configuration of the stomach plays an important role in endosonography of the pancreas because of the close anatomical relationship of the two organs. The body and tail of the pancreas can be imaged from the posterior wall of the mid-body of the stomach.

In patients who have undergone partial gastrectomy, particularly Billroth II resection, complete pancreas imaging may be difficult or impossible. Lymph nodes along the splenic artery and splenic vein should be identified for complete staging. In the case of periampullary carcinoma, lymph nodes at the splenic hilum must be imaged because malignant involvement in this region is classified as distant metastasis, presumably due to the relatively large distance from the primary lesion. Thus, widespread disease can readily be staged. For complete staging of regional lymph nodes the extrahepatic portal vein must also be examined.

Knowledge of topographic anatomy is essential in endosonographic examination. In the duodenum, cross-sections similar to those obtained with computed tomography (CT) scans should be obtained for standardization

Table 11.1   Technical data for various Olympus echoendoscopes

Echoendoscope	GIF-EUM2	GIF-EUM3	VU-M2 (video)	XIF-UM3	Endoscopic-catheter echoprobe
Endoscope	Side-viewing gastroscope	Side-viewing duodenoscope	Side-viewing gastroscope	Side-viewing gastroscope	Forward-viewing (GIF-IT10/GIF20)
Echoprobe	Mechanical sector or radial scanning (180°)	Mechanical sector or radial scanning (180° or 360°)	Mechanical sector or radial scanning (180° or 360°)	Mechanical sector or radial scanning (180° or 360°)	Catheter echoprobe (radial scanning 180° or 360°)
Specifications					
Length	42 mm	42 mm	44 mm	42 mm	In total 14 mm with the catheter
Diameter	13 mm	13 mm	10.4 mm	10 mm	3 mm
Frequency	7.5 MHz	7.5 MHz/12 MHz*	7.5 MHz	7.5 MHz	7 MHz
Depth of penetration	10 cm	10 cm/3 cm	10 cm	10 cm	3 cm
Axial resolution	0.2 mm	0.2 mm/0.12 mm	0.2 mm	0.2 mm	Not known presently (prototype)
ES-guided puncture/biopsy	No	Yes	No	A bridge (elevator) for sonographically guided puncture or biopsy	No

* Switchable frequency

of the ES investigation. Ductular abnormalities seen on endoscopic retrograde cholangiopancreatography (ERCP) should be compared with those visualized endosonographically; the cause of ductular abnormality can usually be imaged clearly with ES. In this manner, both the parenchymal and ductular aspects of the target lesion can be visualized. In the stomach, cross-sections similar to those seen on CT can also be obtained with ES. Longitudinal and oblique sections can be integrated as in the case of conventional transcutaneous ultrasonography to allow accurate assessment of tumour extent. The most important aspects of vascular imaging with ES are visualization of the portal vein, superior mesenteric vein and splenic vein, and in particular, the splenoportal junction. Segmental portal hypertension is diagnosed by the presence of segmental splenic vein obstruction with the development of gastric fundal varices. The lymph node distribution in and around the pancreatic head, along the common bile duct, and adjacent to the mesenteric vessels, splenic vein, splenic hilum and coeliac axis should be carefully examined to detect regional and distant metastases.

INTERPRETATION OF ES IMAGES

The endosonographic diagnosis of pancreatic and peri-ampullary carcinoma is based on the results of previous studies (Tio & Tytgat 1984, 1986b). Pancreatic carcinoma is imaged as a hypoechoic lesion, usually located at a distance from the ampulla, and which causes prestenotic dilatation of the pancreatic duct often in association with a dilated common bile duct, the so-called 'double duct sign'. Periampullary carcinoma is imaged as a hypoechoic (echo-poor) pattern with destruction of the normal architecture of the ampulla of Vater, often in association with dilatation of the common bile duct and/or pancreatic duct.

Lymph nodes with hypoechoic patterns and clearly defined boundaries lead to suspicions of malignancy. Direct tumour penetration into adjacent lymph nodes is defined as regional lymph node metastasis. Lymph nodes with a hyperechoic (echogenic) pattern and poorly demarcated boundaries are usually benign. The ES classifications used in the TNM system for pancreatic and periampullary carcinomas are summarized in Tables 11.2 and 11.3.

In our own prospective study, ES has proved to be reliable in the staging of pancreatic and periampullary tumours. The depth and size of tumour can be assessed and carcinomas at an early stage can be distinguished from advanced cancers.

A T1 pancreatic carcinoma is usually imaged as a sharply demarcated hypoechoic tumour without evidence of penetration into the adjacent structures (Fig. 11.4). A T2 pancreatic carcinoma is usually imaged as a hypoechoic tumour with penetration into the duodenal wall, peripancreatic tissue and/or adjacent common bile duct (Fig. 11.5). A T3 pancreatic carcinoma is usually imaged as a hypoechoic tumour with penetration into the splenoportal venous confluence, stomach or superior mesenteric artery (Fig. 11.6). In our experience the accuracy of ES in assessing T1 carcinoma was 100%, in T2 carcinoma 88%, and in T3 carcinoma 93%. The overall accuracy was 92%.

In the assessment of regional lymph node metastasis the accuracy of ES was relatively high in our experience at 91%. However, in the assessment of non-metastatic lymph nodes its accuracy was low (42%). The overall accuracy of ES was 74%, the sensitivity 91% and the specificity 42%. The positive predictive value was 75% and the negative predictive value was 71%. The incidence of lymph node involvement relative to the depth of tumour infiltration was as follows: in T1 carcinomas it was 40%, in T2 carcinomas 59% and in T3 carcinomas 85%. Even

Table 11.2   ES classification of the depth of tumour infiltration, regional lymph node metastasis, distant metastasis and stage grouping of pancreatic carcinoma

T:	Primary tumour	T1	Hypoechoic tumour limited to the pancreas
		T1a	Tumour with a maximal diameter of 2 cm or less
		T1b	Tumour with a maximal diameter of more than 2 cm
		T2	Tumour extends directly to any of the following: duodenum, bile duct, peripancreatic tissue
		T3	Tumour extends directly to any of the following: stomach, spleen, colon, adjacent blood vessels
		Tx	Primary tumour cannot be assessed
N:	Regional lymph node metastasis	N0	No regional lymph node metastasis
		N1	Regional lymph node metastasis as follows: pancreatic head, along the common bile duct and adjacent major blood vessels
		NX	Regional lymph nodes cannot be assessed
M:	Distant metastasis	M0	No evidence of distant metastasis
		M1	Liver metastasis or peritoneal dissemination
Stage grouping		Stage I	T1 N0 M0 or T2 N0 M0
		Stage II	T3 N0 M0
		Stage III	any T N1 M0
		Stage IV	any T any N M1

Table 11.3   ES criteria for assessing the depth of tumour infiltration, regional lymph node metastasis distant metastasis and stage grouping of periampullary carcinoma

T:	Primary tumour	T1	Hypoechoic tumour limited to the ampulla of Vater
		T2	Hypoechoic tumour invading duodenal wall
		T3	Hypoechoic tumour invading 2 cm or less into pancreas
		T4	Hypoechoic tumour invading more than 2 cm into pancreas and/or other adjacent structures
N:	Regional lymph nodes	N0	No regional lymph node metastasis
		N1	Regional lymph node metastasis in the pancreatic head, along the common bile duct, liver hilum and adjacent major blood vessels except for splenic hilum lymph nodes
M:	Distant metastasis	M0	No distant metastasis
		M1	Lymph node metastasis at the splenic hilum, liver metastases or peritoneal dissemination
Stage grouping		Stage I	T1 N0 M0
		Stage II	T2 N0 M0 or T3 N0 M0
		Stage III	T1 N1 M0 or T2 N1 M0 or T3 N1 M0
		Stage IV	T4 any N M0 or any T any N M1

'early' pancreatic carcinoma can be associated with lymph node metastasis.

In the case of periampullary carcinoma a T1 carcinoma is usually imaged as a hypoechoic tumour limited to the papilla of Vater without penetration into the muscularis propria of the duodenum; such lesions were correctly diagnosed in 2 of our 3 patients. A T2 carcinoma is usually imaged as a hypoechoic tumour with penetration into the adjacent duodenal wall; such lesions were correctly diagnosed in 11 of our 12 patients (Fig. 11.7). A T3 carcinoma is usually imaged as a hypoechoic tumour penetrating the adjacent pancreatic parenchyma (with pancreatic invasion measuring less than 2 cm in its greatest diameter) and was correctly diagnosed in 7 of our 8 patients (accuracy, 87%; Fig. 11.8). A T4 carcinoma is usually imaged as a hypoechoic tumour with deep penetration into the pancreatic parenchyma, with a diameter of more than 2 cm; such a lesion was correctly diagnosed in one patient in our series. The overall accuracy of ES in staging periampullary carcinoma was 87%.

In the assessment of regional lymph node involvement periampullary carcinoma, the accuracy of ES in our hands was 54%, with a sensitivity of 91% and a specificity of 36%. The positive predictive value and negative predictive value were 47% and 71% respectively. The incidence of lymph node metastases, relative to the depth of tumour infiltration, was as follows: in T1 carcinomas, zero; in T2 carcinomas, 42%; in T3 carcinomas, 50%, and in T4 carcinomas, 100%. In contrast to our experience with pancreatic cancer, 'early' periampullary carcinoma was not associated with lymph node metastases. In the assessment of distant metastasis, ES has proved disappointing due to

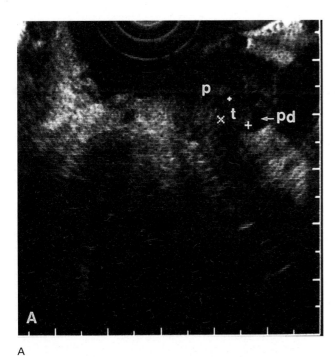

A

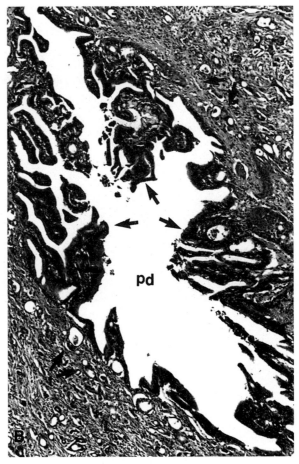

B

Fig. 11.4 A Endosonogram reveals a small hypoechoic pancreatic carcinoma (t) with circumscribed transductal spread of diameter 2 cm. Note the prestenotic dilated pancreatic duct (pd) with epithelial dysplasia; p, pancreas. **B** Corresponding histology of resected specimen shows a small pancreatic carcinoma (arrows) surrounding the dilated pancreatic duct (pd).

the limited penetration of ultrasound. Thus, accuracy its in diagnosing distant metastasis was zero in our cases of pancreatic carcinoma, while distant metastases were not found in our patients with periampullary carcinomas.

Illustrative case reports

Case 1

A 76-year-old man was referred for gastroscopy because of abdominal discomfort, pain in the upper left quadrant and weight loss. Endoscopy revealed a bulging lesion in the fundus of the stomach, the appearance of which was thought to be suspicious of a submucosal lesion. Histological examination of the biopsy specimen revealed no abnormality. For further evaluation endosonography was performed. A hypoechoic tumour was revealed in the tail of the pancreas with direct tumour penetration of the fundic wall. The tumour was obstructing the splenic vein with segmental portal hypertension and development of fundal varices. Multiple regional lymph nodes with suspicion of metastases were seen. Surgery was not recommended due to the advanced stage of carcinoma.

Case 2

A 65-year-old woman presented with painless obstructive jaundice. Abdominal ultrasonography and a CT scan revealed a mass in the body of the pancreas without evidence of liver metastases. ERCP showed obstruction of the duct of Wirsung as it crossed the vertebral column. ES performed for cancer staging revealed an extensive hypoechoic mass in the pancreatic body with obstruction of the duct of Wirsung. Segmental splenic vein obstruction with fundal varices directly adjacent to the tumour mass was also revealed (Fig. 11.9). Hypoechoic, sharply demarcated lymph nodes were found adjacent to the tumour and in the splenic hilum and were interpreted as suspicious of metastasis. After consultation with the surgeon, surgery was not recommended due to the advanced stage of disease and in view of the presence of portal hypertension. Six weeks after the diagnosis the patient died suddenly at home. Autopsy revealed diffuse peritoneal metastases with an extensive tumour mass in the body of the pancreas, with obstruction of the inferior vena cava and multiple thrombi in the pulmonary vein and left atrium.

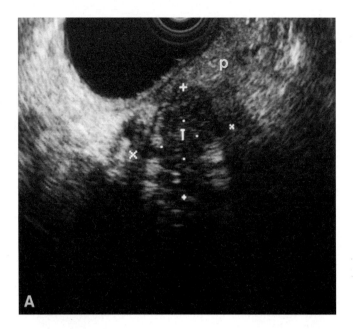

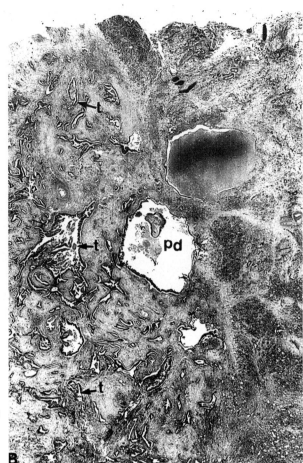

Fig. 11.5   **A** Endosonogram shows a hypoechoic tumour (T) in the pancreatic head with penetration into the adjacent pancreatic tissue; p, adjacent normal pancreatic parenchyma. **B** Corresponding histology shows a pancreatic carcinoma (t) adjacent to the dilated pancreatic duct (pd) and penetrating into the surrounding peripancreatic fat tissue.

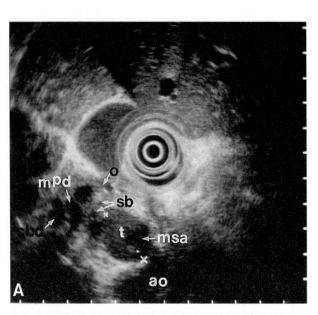

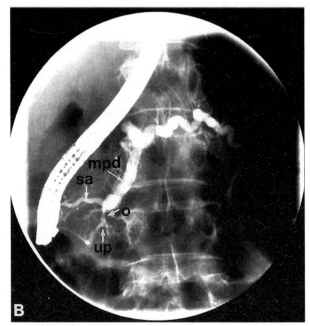

Fig. 11.6   **A** Endosonogram reveals a round hypoechoic tumour (t) obstructing (o) the main pancreatic duct (mpd) and side branches (sb), without involvement of the common bile duct. Note the location of tumour in the uncinate process with close proximity to the aorta (ao) and involvement of the superior mesenteric artery (msa). **B** Endoscopic retrograde cholangiopancreatogram reveals a narrowing (arrow;) of the main pancreatic duct (mpd) and abnormal side branches in the uncinate process (up), without filling of the common bile duct; sa, duct of Santorini.

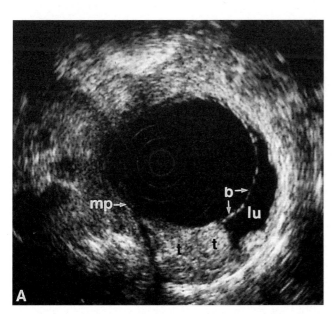

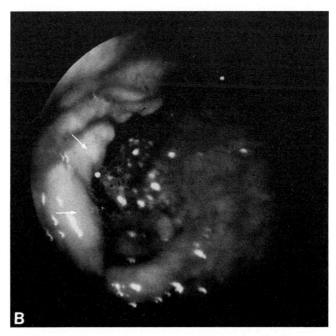

Fig. 11.7 **A** Endosonogram of a hypoechoic periampullary carcinoma (t) penetrating into the muscularis propria (mp) of the duodenum. Note the clear image of polypoid tumour after filling the duodenal lumen (lu) with water; b, waterfilled balloon. **B** Endoscopic picture shows a polypoid periampullary carcinoma (arrows). Figure 11.7B is reproduced in colour in the plate section at the front of the volume.

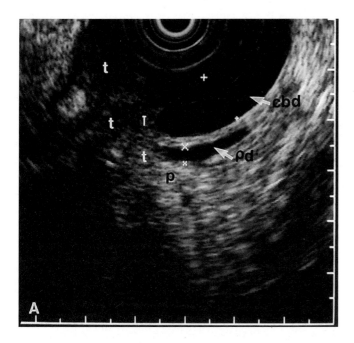

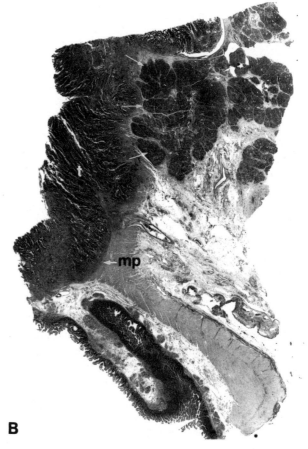

Fig. 11.8 **A** Endosonogram shows a hypoechoic periampullary carcinoma (t) involving the common bile duct (cbd) and pancreatic duct (pd) and adjacent pancreatic parenchyma (p). **B** Corresponding histology of resected specimen shows a polypoid periampullary carcinoma (t) penetrating through the muscularis propria (mp) with tiny penetration into the adjacent pancreas (arrows).

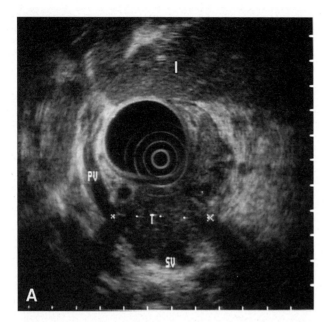
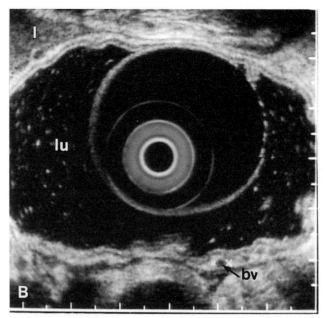

Fig. 11.9 **A** Endosonogram shows an extensive hypoechoic tumour (T) in the body of the pancreas, involving the splenic vein (sv) with multiple hypoechoic clearly defined lymph nodes with suspicion of metastasis; pv, portal vein; l, left liver lobe. **B** Another cross-section shows some small hypoechoic blood vessels (bv) in the submucosa of the stomach compatible with fundal varices; lu, water in the gastric lumen; l, left liver lobe.

DISCUSSION

It is now clear that pancreatic carcinoma obstructing the pancreatic duct and common bile duct can be accurately imaged with ES. The extent and size of tumour according to the new TNM classification can be assessed, and the ES findings show a close correlation with the histology of the resected specimen. This is important in that tumour size can now be assessed before surgery, and depth of tumour infiltration can be used as the main criterion for staging. An interesting observation in our series was the detection of segmental portal hypertension with fundal varices due to carcinoma in the pancreatic body and tail. Moreover, if submucosal gastric infiltration is present it can usually be diagnosed by ES-guided cytological puncture. Patients with such advanced carcinomas are not candidates for surgical resection.

The TNM classification is more suitable for use with pancreatic head carcinoma than for cancers of the pancreatic body and tail (P. Hermanek 1986, personal communication). Periampullary carcinomas can usually be distinguished from pancreatic cancers by their anatomical location and the extent of the primary tumour. However, extensive periampullary carcinomas may be difficult, or even impossible, to distinguish from pancreatic cancer. Early stage cancers can be distinguished from advanced carcinomas by the depth and extent of tumour infiltration at ES. However it must be stressed that in pancreatic carcinomas, even early cancer can be associated with regional lymph node metastasis. In our series, regional lymph node metastasis was not found in early stage periampullary carcinomas (Tio et al 1990, 1992).

In a Japanese study of periampullary carcinoma which employed the p-TNM pathological classification, the 5-year survival of periampullary carcinoma patients in stage I was 100%, in stage II, 64.8%, in stage III, 15%, and stage IV zero (Mori et al 1990). Therefore it is imperative to diagnose this disease in its early stages if appropriate patients are to be selected for surgery. The 5-year survival rate is 53% for patients with periampullary carcinoma without lymph node metastasis, whereas it decreases to 27% for patients with lymph node metastasis (Hayes et al 1987).

In the assessment of regional lymph nodes ES is an accurate means of detecting metastatic involvement when present, but it is not an accurate means of assessing non-metastatic lymph nodes. In the near future, ES-guided cytological puncture may be introduced to enhance diagnostic accuracy. In assessing distant metastasis, ES is not accurate due to the limited penetration of ultrasound used. Thus additional abdominal ultrasonography or CT is still needed to detect liver metastases and/or peritoneal dissemination.

In the assessment of stage grouping the overall accuracy of ES was 66% and 54% for pancreatic and peri-ampullary carcinomas respectively (Tio et al 1990). In this approach, each stage is a combination of T, N and M, and so incorrect diagnosis of any category on ES may result in incorrect staging. Clinically, lymph node metastasis is a negative parameter in predicting prognosis. In our 7-year experience we have also found that invasion of the splenic or portal vein by tumour in association with segmental portal hypertension and fundal varices is an absolute contraindication to surgery. Direct tumour infiltration into the adjacent fundus of the stomach may result in mucosal thickening at endoscopy which cannot be distinguished from fundal varices by gross appearance alone. This, however, can readily be resolved by ES; the presence of a hypoechoic submucosal pattern communicating with the hypoechoic pancreatic mass leaves no doubt as to the true diagnosis. ES-guided cytology can be performed to achieve a tissue diagnosis. In the case of carcinomas located in the uncinate process, even small cancers may nevertheless be irresectable due to the close proximity of major blood vessels such as the superior mesenteric artery and aorta, and involvement of the mesocolon.

In conclusion, ES offers promise in the clinical TNM staging of pancreatic and periampullary carcinoma. It is an accurate method of staging T categories and valuable in the detection of regional lymph node metastasis; it is not accurate in the detection of distant metastases and conventional ultrasonography and/or CT is still necessary for complete staging.

REFERENCES

Di Magno E P, Boxton J L, Regan P T et al 1980 The ultrasonic endoscope. Lancet 1: 629–631

Di Magno E P, Regan P T, Clain J E, James E M, Buxton J L 1982 Human endoscopic ultrasonography. Gastroenterology 83: 824–829

Hayes D H, Bolton J S, Willis G W, Bower J C 1987 Carcinoma of the ampulla of Vater. Annals of Surgery 206: 572–577

Hermanek P, Sobin L H 1987 TNM Classification of malignant tumors, 4th edn. Springer-Verlag, Heidelberg

Hisanaga K, Hisanaga A 1978 A new real-time sector scanning system of ultra-wide angle and real-time recording of entire cardiac images: transesophagus and transchest methods. Ultrasound Medicine 4: 391–402

Hisanaga K, Hisanaga A, Hibi N 1980 High speed rotating scanner for transesophageal cross-sectional echocardiography. American Journal of Cardiology 41: 832

Lux G, Heyder N, Demling L 1982 Endoscopic ultrasonography – technique, orientation and diagnostic possibilities. Endoscopy 4: 220–225

Mori K, Ikei T, Yamaguchi T, Katsumori Y, Shibata Y, Arai T 1990 Pathological factors influencing survival of carcinoma of the ampulla of Vater. European Journal of Surgical Oncology 16:183–188

Sobin L H, Ros P R 1990 Radiology and the new TNM classification of tumors: the future. Radiology 176:1–4

Sobin L H, Hermanek P, Hutter R V P 1988 TNM classification of malignant tumors: a comparison between the new (1987) and old editions. Cancer 6: 2310–2314

Strohm W D, Phillip E, Hagenmüller F, Classen M 1980 Ultrasonic tomography by means of an ultrasonic fiber endoscope. Endoscopy 12: 241–244

Tio T L, Tytgat G N J 1984 Endoscopic ultrasonography in the assessment of intra-and transmural infiltration of tumors of the esophagus, stomach and papilla of Vater and extraesophageal lesions. Endoscopy 16: 220–225

Tio T L, Tytgat G N J 1986a Endoscopic ultrasonography in staging local resectability of pancreatic and periampullary malignancy. Scandinavian Journal of Gastroenterology 21 (Suppl 123):135–142

Tio T L, Tytgat G N J 1986b Endoscopic ultrasonography in analysing periintestinal lymph node abnormality. Scandinavian Journal of Gastroenterology 21 (Suppl 123):158–163

Tio T L, Tytgat G N J 1986c Atlas of transintestinal ultrasonography. Mur Kostverloren, Aalsmeer, The Netherlands

Tio T L, Tytgat G N J, Cikot R J L M, Houthoff H J, Sars R A 1990 Ampullopancreatic carcinoma: Preoperative TNM Classification with Endosonography. Radiology 175: 455–461

Tio T L, Mulder C J J, Eggink W F 1992 Endosonography in staging early carcinoma of the ampulla of Vater. Gastroenterology 102:1392–1395

Yasuda K, Mukai H, Cho E, Nakayima M, Kawai K 1988a The use of endoscopic ultrasonography in the detecting and staging of carcinoma of the papilla of Vater. Endoscopy 20: 218–222

Yasuda K, Mukai H, Fujimoto S, Nakayima M, Kawai K 1988b The diagnosis of pancreatic cancer by endoscopic ultrasonography. Gastrointestinal Endoscopy 34:1–8

12. Percutaneous fine-needle aspiration cytology

I. Ihse   Å. Andrén-Sandberg

INTRODUCTION

During the last two decades the introduction of an increasing number of non-operative imaging techniques has added new dimensions to the clinical management of patients with suspicion of pancreatic disease. Ultrasonography, computerized tomography (CT), endoscopic retrograde cholangiopancreatography (ERCP) and percutaneous transhepatic cholangiography (PTC) all have a high diagnostic accuracy. The role of magnetic resonance (MR) imaging has still to be proven. However, a serious drawback with all these new methods is their uncertainty in discriminating between malignant and inflammatory disease, making further characterization desirable. In 1972 Oscarson et al described a small series of patients who underwent percutaneous fine-needle aspiration for cytological diagnosis of pancreatic lesions. Since then this technique has been used widely throughout the world. The puncture is most often done under ultrasonographic guidance (Hancke et al 1975, Kocjan et al 1989) but CT (Dickey et al 1986), ERCP (Ihre et al 1978) and PTC (Evander et al 1978) have also been used. The rationale of fine-needle aspiration cytology in a patient with suspicion of a pancreatic lesion is to establish a definite diagnosis with a minimum of time, investigation, cost and suffering. In the following pages we will discuss the extent to which the method has fulfilled expectations.

INDICATIONS

The accepted indications for percutaneous fine-needle cytology of pancreatic lesions have varied between different countries and hospitals, and have also changed with time within the same hospital. In many places in Scandinavia the technique was used initially in almost all patients with radiologically suspected tumours, whereas today it is practised much more selectively. This swing in policy is the result of experience gained during the years, and which will be discussed below.

At present percutaneous fine-needle aspiration is performed to verify the diagnosis of cancer in patients who are too old and/or frail for surgery, and to verify metastases to the liver, lungs or lymph nodes in those patients with pancreatic cancer for whom non-operative palliation is the best option. Percutaneous punctures should be avoided in patients who will undergo laparotomy for attempted curative surgery or palliation (e.g. gastroenterostomy). Instead biopsies should be taken intraoperatively, especially if a non-resective operation is undertaken. In our opinion biopsy is not mandatory before resection if there is a strong clinical suspicion of cancer and if the operating team is experienced. As the main value of fine-needle cytology is to prove the *presence* of malignant cells without detailed classification, it provides only scanty information regarding the type of the tumour. To obtain this information, histological specimens are generally required.

TECHNIQUE

After localization of the lesion by the chosen imaging technique, the aspirates are taken using a needle 0.6–0.9 mm in external diameter. The needle is attached to a 20 ml disposable plastic syringe in an adaptor permitting single-handed manipulation. The puncture is done from the abdominal wall with the patient in the supine position. Local anaesthesia is only occasionally necessary. After reaching the desired site with the tip of the needle, aspiration is performed by moving the needle back and forth under maximal suction which, however, is released before the needle is withdrawn from the lesion. This prevents the negative pressure from forcing the aspirates into the syringe. The aspirated material is then ejected from the needle and carefully smeared out on to one or more glass slides and either air-dried or fixed in alcohol. Staining is done by the May–Grünwald–Giemsa or the Papanicolau method. It is possible to evaluate the alcohol-fixed slides in the microscope within a few minutes.

Slides may also be kept at –20°C for immuno-cytochemical studies to detect the presence of markers such as carcinoembryonic antigen (CEA), neuron specific enolase (NSE) and chromogranin (Kocjan et al 1989) or for DNA analysis. However, experience with such studies is still limited, and their role therefore uncertain. Finally, in this discussion on technique, it must be stressed that the experience of the examiner greatly influences the results (Evander et al 1978), and that at several centres shortage of trained cytologists is a major drawback to the use of the method.

RESULTS

Since the introduction of the technique, the reported sensitivity of fine-needle aspiration cytology in diagnosing malignant disease of the pancreas has varied between 49 and 86% (Tylén et al 1976, Evander et al 1978, Mitchell et al 1988, Kocjan et al 1989, Parsons & Palmer 1989, Soudah et al 1989). Although advances in imaging technique have improved localization of pancreatic tumours, there does not seem to have been any further increase in diagnostic yield. However, as the specificity of examination for cancer is usually reported to be 100% (Evander et al 1978, Kocjan et al 1989, Glenthöj et al 1990), the cytological results may provide a sound basis for the decision on further treatment and obviate an unnecessary exploratory laparotomy.

It must however be remembered that a few false positive results have been reported (Holm et al 1985, Waldner et al 1987, Mitchell et al 1988) and we have ourselves seen one false positive in some 400 patients (unpublished). Whereas positive results are of clinical value, negative results do not exclude malignancy. The rate of false negatives among verified cancers is often as high as one in four (Soudah et al 1989). This is related both to sampling error and to problems with technical preparation and interpretation. Poor sampling can be due to fibrosis of the tumour but is probably most often explained by the needle missing the tumour.

Problems of interpretation, again, underline the need for a trained cytologist. However, experienced examiners possess similar diagnostic abilities as reflected by small differences between intraobserver and interobserver kappa values in the study of Glenthöj et al (1990).

From what has been noted above it is obvious that the value of percutaneous pancreatic cytodiagnosis is related to its ability to prove the presence of tumours, whereas their classification generally requires further investigation involving histological techniques. However, it is generally possible to decide whether the tumour is of exocrine (Fig. 12.1) or endocrine (Fig. 12.2) origin. Sometimes the cytologist may have a problem of interpretation when distinguishing epithelial atypia due to chronic pancreatitis (Fig. 12.3) or duct obstruction from well-differentiated neoplasms (Fig. 12.4). This dilemma may constitute a risk of false negative as well as false positive results.

To overcome the drawbacks of fine-needle cytology, i.e. too many false negative results and unprecise information regarding tumour type and origin, ultrasound-guided pancreatic core biopsy was introduced (Jennings et al 1989). However, initial results show that cytological

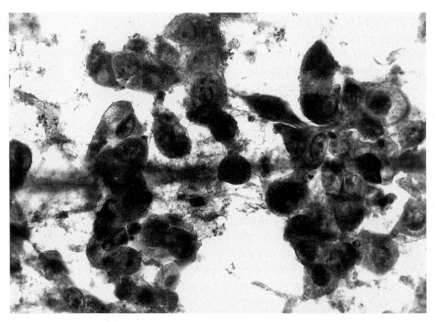

Fig. 12.1   Poorly differentiated carcinoma. A group of loosely cohesive cells exhibiting marked nuclear atypia. Haematoxylin and eosin; × 392. (Courtesy or Dr Måns Åkerman, Lund, Sweden.)

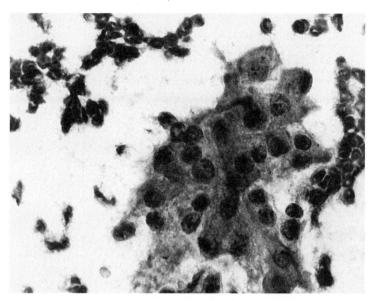

Fig. 12.2   Endocrine tumour (insulinoma). A group of moderately cytoplasm-rich cells with finely granular cytoplasma and rounded nuclei with evenly distributed chromatin. Haematoxylin & eosin: × 392. (Courtesy of Dr Måns Åkerman, Lund, Sweden.)

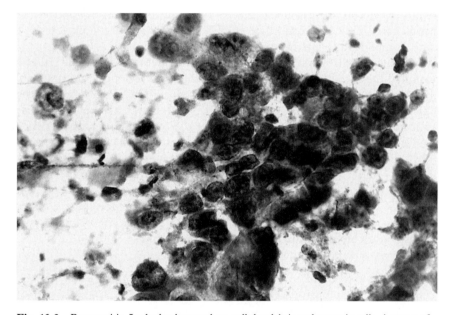

Fig. 12.3   Pancreatitis. In the background are cellular debris and necrotic cells. A group of ductal cells are loosely attached to each other. The nuclei vary in size and the nucleoli are enlarged. Haematoxylin and eosin; × 392. (Courtesy of Dr Måns Åkerman, Lund, Sweden.)

fine-needle biopsy is more sensitive in making a consistent diagnosis of malignancy than histological fine-needle biopsy, and the predictive values of both malignant and benign diagnosis were similar with the two techniques (Glenthöj et al 1990). Further studies are needed to determine whether core biopsy has any advantages over cytological investigation.

COMPLICATIONS

Livraghi et al (1983) reported a mortality rate of 0.008%

and an incidence of major complications of 0.005% in 11 700 patients undergoing fine-needle abdominal biopsy. The corresponding figures found by Smith (1984) were 0.006% and 0.16% respectively, in 15 777 patients. Fornari et al (1989) reported a similar collective study involving 10 766 patients and found a mortality rate of 0.018% and a major complication rate of 0.18%. Of 12 fatalities reported in the literature after abdominal fine-needle aspiration cytology, three followed pancreatic punctures (Fornari et al 1989, Howard & Campbell 1990). Papers dealing exclusively with pancreatic biopsies

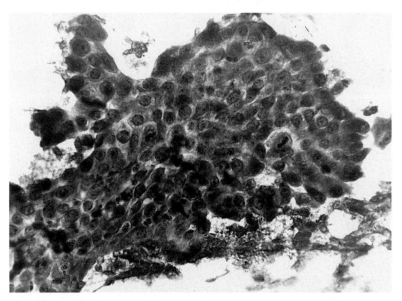

Fig. 12.4 Well-differentiated carcinoma. A cluster of closely packed cells with slight nuclear atypia and scattered mitotic figures is seen. Haematoxylin and eosin; × 315. (Courtesy of Dr Måns Åkerman, Lund, Sweden.)

have also reported without exception, an extremely low mortality and complication rate. Thus, the technique is safe regarding immediate complications but the risk of needle-tract seeding of tumour cells should not be ignored. Following abdominal fine-needle biopsy Fornari et al (1989) collected eight such cases from the literature, five of which occurred after pancreatic puncture. Another two cases with pancreatic cancer seeding were reported by Bergenfeldt et al (1988) and one case by us (Ihse & Isaksson 1984).

CURRENT ROLE OF PANCREATIC FINE-NEEDLE CYTOLOGY

Percutaneous fine-needle aspiration biopsy of the pancreas is a safe procedure with a very low early complication rate, but the risk of needle-tract seeding of tumour cells is a reality that has contributed to a narrowing of the initially wide indications.

The method is reliable in proving the presence of a malignant lesion, but unreliable in excluding such disorder. Therefore, its present role is restricted to verification of the malignant diagnosis in patients, who for various reasons are not candidates for surgery, be it exploratory, palliative or attempted radical. Patients in whom an operation is planned should be investigated intraoperatively and not percutaneously.

In the group of patients where percutaneous fine-needle cytology does have a place, it is definitely valuable in both proving the diagnosis and providing information on prognosis.

REFERENCES

Bergenfeldt M, Genell S, Lindholm K, Ekberg O, Aspelin P 1988. Needle-tract seeding after percutaneous fine-needle biopsy of pancreatic carcinoma. Acta Chirurgica Scandinavica 154: 77–79

Dickey J E, Haaga J R, Stellato T A, Schultz C L, Hau T 1986 Evaluation of computed tomography guided percutaneous biopsy of the pancreas. Surgery, Gynecology and Obstetrics 163: 497–50

Evander A, Ihse I, Lunderquist A, Tylén U, Åkerman M 1978 Percutaneous cytodiagnosis of carcinoma of the pancreas and the bile duct. Annals of Surgery 188: 90–92

Fornari F, Civardi G, Cavanna M, Distasi S, Rossi G, Sbolli L, Buscarini L and The Cooperative Italian Study Group 1989 Complication of ultrasonically guided fine-needle abdominal biopsy . Scandinavian Journal of Gastroenterology 24: 949–955

Glenthöj A, Sehested M, Torp-Pedersen S 1990 Ultrasonically guided histological and cytological fine needle biopsies of the pancreas. Reliability and reproducibility of diagnoses. Gut 31: 930–933

Hancke S, Holm H H, Kock F 1975 Ultrasonically guided fine needle biopsy of the pancreas. Surgery, Gynecology and Obstetrics 140: 361–363

Holm H H, Torp-Pedersen S, Larsen T, Juul N 1985 Percutaneous fine needle biopsy. Clinics in Gastroenterology 14: 423–449

Howard J M, Campbell E W 1989 Fatal clostridial pancreatitis following ERCP and percutaneous needle biopsy. International Journal of Pancreatology 5: 305–310

Ihre T H, Pyk E, Raaschou-Nielsen T, Seligson U 1978 Percutaneous fine needle aspiration biopsy during endoscopic retrograde cholangiopancreatography. Scandinavian Journal of Gastroenterology 13: 657–662

Ihse I, Isaksson G 1984 Preoperative and operative diagnosis of pancreatic cancer. World Journal of Surgery 8: 846–853

Jennings P E, Coral A, Donald J J, Rode J, Lees W R 1989 Ultrasound-guided core biopsy. Lancet 1369–1371

Kocjan G, Rode J, Lees W R 1989 Percutaneous fine needle aspiration cytology of the pancreas: advantages and pitfalls. Journal of Clinical Pathology 42: 341–347

Livraghi T, Damascelli B, Lombardi C, Spagnoli J 1983 Risk in fine-

needle abdominal biopsy. Journal of Clinical Ultrasound
11: 77–81

Mitchell M L, Bittner C A, Wills J S, Parker E P 1988 Fine needle
aspiration cytology of the pancreas. A retrospective study of 73 cases.
Acta Cytologica 32: 447–451

Oscarson J, Stormby N, Sundgren R 1972 Selective angiography and
fine needle aspiration cytodiagnosis of gastric and pancreatic tumors.
Acta Radiologica 12: 737–741

Parsons L Jr, Palmer C H 1989 How accurate is fine-needle biopsy in
malignant neoplasia of the pancreas? Archives of Surgery 124:
681–683

Smith E H 1984 The hazards of fine-needle aspiration biopsy.
Ultrasound in Medicine and Biology 10: 629–634

Soudah B, Fritsch R S, Witrekind C, Hilka B, Spindler B 1989 Value of
the cytologic analysis of fine needle aspiration biopsy specimens in the
diagnosis of pancreatic carcinomas. Acta Cytologica 33: 875–880

Tylén U, Arnesjö B, Lindberg L G, Lunderquist A 1976 Percutaneous
biopsy of carcinoma of the pancreas guided by angiography. Surgery,
Gynecology and Obstetrics 142: 737–739

Waldner B, Dorral E D, Anthonioz P 1987 Cytoponction pancréatique
à l'aiguille fine. A propos de 45 observations. Gastroenterologie
Clinique et Biologique 11: 12–16

13. Laboratory evaluation of pancreatic function and disease

R. Klapdor

The relative inaccessibility of the pancreas to direct examination, and the non-specific nature of abdominal pain and symptoms of maldigestion, explain the efforts undertaken during the past decades to evaluate function and develop laboratory tests to diagnose and monitor exocrine pancreatic insufficiency and pancreatic disease. Function tests and laboratory investigations may be divided into three main groups;

1. direct and indirect assessment of exocrine activity
2. assessment of endocrine function
3. measurement of tumour-associated substances secreted or shed by exocrine and endocrine tumours of the pancreas.

EXOCRINE PANCREATIC FUNCTION TESTS

The exocrine pancreas, the organ with the highest protein turnover in the body (25–50 g/day), involves about 98–99% of the gland. The exocrine tissue consists of the acini and the duct system. Clusters of acini are arranged in lobules which are separated by loose connective tissue and which secrete proteolytic enzymes, lipolytic enzymes, glycosidases and nucleases (Table 13.1). Amylases, esterases and nucleases are produced in activated form, whereas proteases, peptidases and phospholipases are secreted as inactive proenzymes which are later activated within the duodenum, following the activation of trypsinogen to trypsin by duodenal enterokinase.

The duct system draining the acini begins with the so-called centroacinar cells, and is the part of the pancreas responsible for the secretion of water and electrolytes. Pancreatic proteases, lipase and amylase are essential for the normal digestion of nutrients, while pancreatic bicarbonate secretion neutralizes gastric acid and maintains the duodenum at the alkaline pH required for pancreatic enzyme activity.

Exocrine function is controlled and stimulated by various neural and humoral factors via cephalic, gastric and intes-

Table 13.1 Components of pancreatic juice

Acinar secretion	Ductal secretion
Proteolytic enzymes	Water
Trypsin	
Chymotrypsin	Electrolytes
Elastase	Bicarbonate
Collagenase	Chloride
Kallikrein	Phosphate
Carboxypeptidases	Sodium
	Potassium
Lipolytic enzymes	Calcium
Lipase	Magnesiun
Phospholipase	
Cholinesterase	
Glycosidases	
α-amylase	
Nucleases	
Desoxyribonuclease	
Ribonuclease	

tinal phases and by direct substrate stimulation (see Ch. 3).

Both anatomical and physiological changes occur with ageing. The paramount change is dilatation of the main pancreatic duct associated histologically with ductal epithelial hyperplasia and intralobular fibrosis. This fibrosis may lead to pancreatic atrophy. Such alterations do not always result in altered pancreatic function although enzyme output diminishes progressively with advancing age after the fourth decade. Malabsorption in the elderly may also be caused by bacterial overgrowth in the small intestine, a change found in about 55% of elderly patients (McEvoy et al 1983), or by impaired absorption of fat and carbohydrates, as has been reported in patients over 65 years of age, although the mechanism is unclear (Webster et al 1977).

Maldigestion and subsequent malabsorption and diarrhoea or steatorrhoea do not appear until more than 90% of exocrine pancreatic function is lost (Di Magno et al 1973). As protein digestion is aided by gastric pepsin and carbohydrate digestion is aided by salivary and intestinal amylase, pancreatic insufficiency affects fat absorption more than absorption of protein and carbohydrate. Steatorrhoea is mild to moderate if 2–10% of normal function is preserved and severe if less than 2% of normal function remains.

Though vitamin B_{12} malabsorption is reported in 20–40% of cases, malabsorption of vitamins is rarely a significant clinical problem. Fat soluble vitamins, although dependent on micellar formation of bile salts, do not require pancreatic enzymes for their uptake. Water-soluble vitamins are absorbed throughout the small intestine.

Exocrine pancreatic function tests are based on direct measurement of secreted substances (direct tests) or on measurement of the products of enzymatic activity (indirect tests) in pancreatic/duodenal juice, intestinal content, or faeces and urine (Table 13.2).

Direct exocrine function tests

Secretin–Cholecystokinin (caerulein) test

Direct function tests, involving intubation of the duodenum and collection of the pancreatic or duodenal juice after a specific stimulus, remain the gold standard (Lankisch 1982). The most widely employed test uses a maximal or near-maximal dose of secretin and cholecystokinin (CCK) or caerulein. After peroral intubation, secretion is measured under basal conditions for 15 minutes and thereafter 1 clinical unit per kg body weight of secretin is injected intravenously. After 30 minutes one Ivy dog unit of CCK per kg body weight is injected intravenously and duodenal content collected for a further 30 minutes. Parameters to be determined are volume, bicarbonate concentration, and output of the enzymes amylase, lipase and trypsin. Some clinicians try to correct for incomplete collection of secreted juice by using a dilution indicator, such as polyethylene-glycol or ^{58}Co-vitamin B_{12}, by using a double balloon tube technique, or by combining balloon tubes and dilution indicators (Klapdor et al 1982). In general, loss of

Table 13.2 Exocrine pancreatic function tests

Direct tests
  With duodenal/intestinal intubation
    Secretin–CCK test
    Lundh test
  Without duodenal/intestinal intubation
    Faecal chymotrypsin determination

Indirect tests (all without duodenal/intestinal intubation)
  Stool
    Stool fat determination
  Urine
    Pancreolauryl test
    Para-amino benzoic acid (PABA) test
    Dual-labelled Schilling test
  Breath
    ^{14}C-labelled triolein test

duodenal juice amounts to no more than 5% of the total secreted volume and does not play a significant role in evaluation (Lankisch 1982).

The secretin–CCK test allows the differentiation between mild, moderate and severe pancreatic insufficiency (mild, volume and bicarbonate secretion normal, enzyme secretion diminished; moderate volume and bicarbonate secretion unchanged, all enzymes decreased; severe volume, bicarbonate and enzyme secretion diminished). In a series involving more than 2000 patients, an 8% rate of false positive tests and a 6% false normal result rate reflects the high specificity and sensitivity of the secretion–CCK test (Otte 1979).

However, the test is cumbersome, uncomfortable for the patient, and time-consuming. Consequently it is now rarely used clinically. Furthermore, this test cannot be performed in patients after Billroth II gastrectomy or Whipple resection because of the impossibility of positioning the duodenal tube correctly. Nevertheless, it remains the standard test and can detect pancreatic insufficiency even when there has been loss of less than 70% of the exocrine tissue, that is, even in the case of clinically latent exocrine insufficiency.

Lundh test

Another commonly used direct test is the Lundh test (Lundh 1962). In this test the patient also undergoes duodenal intubation but the gland is stimulated with a liquid test meal containing fat, protein and sugar. Trypsin concentration is measured in the duodenal aspirates over the 2 hours following ingestion of the test meal. This test measures secretion capacity by physiological (neural and humoral) stimulation of the gland.

The Lundh test is easier to perform and is less expensive than the secretin–CCK test but it does not allow measurement of volume or bicarbonate secretion or quantitative measurement of enzyme output. In the healthy patient, trypsin output doubles or triples relative to basal rates of secretion, while in patients with severe pancreatic malabsorption there is virtually no rise in trypsin secretion after the meal.

The Lundh test also needs an intact upper gastro-intestinal tract and additionally requires intact innervation of the pancreas. Consequently, this test cannot be used after resectional gastric surgery or the Whipple operation. This test is also less reliable in patients with severe inflammatory disease of the intestine.

Chymotrypsin in the faeces

The enzymatic activity which remains in the faeces amounts to less than 5% of the enzyme activity secreted by the pancreas. Nevertheless, the stool excretion of chymotrypsin does allow conclusions to be reached concerning pancreatic secretion (Banwell et al 1965).

The chymotrypsin test is a non-invasive test which allows detection of insufficiency without duodenal intubation, an advantage when compared to the secretion–CCK test and the Lundh test. Moreover, new developments replacing the titrimetric methods allow rapid determinations to be made. However, sensitivity and specificity are lower than those of the secretin–CCK and the Lundh test. False normal and false pathological results can be found, as in cases of mild and moderate insufficiency, and in patients with decreased endogenous stimulation of the pancreas such as those with diseases of the intestine, protein malnutrition, and after gastric resection (Dürr et al 1978, Lankisch et al 1983).

Indirect exocrine function tests

Qualitative and quantitative faecal fat determination

Qualitative tests are useful for screening individuals with suspected fat malabsorption. Excretion of more than 10% of a daily intake of 60 g of fat is found in more than 90% of patients with moderate and severe fat malabsorption, while excretion of 6–10% of the dietary fat intake is found in mild to moderate malabsorption (Bin et al 1983). The test is less sensitive than direct function testing.

The measurement of quantitative fat excretion over 3 days in a patient on a daily diet containing 80–100 g of fat is the best method for evaluating fat malabsorption. Faecal fat levels greater than 6 g per day are abnormal and suggest underlying small intestinal, pancreatic or hepatobiliary diseases. The stool fat is analysed by the van de Kamer method, based on extraction and titration of long-chain fatty acids by NaOH (van de Kamer et al 1949).

Faecal fat excretion represents the most reliable global test of malabsorption. It allows reliable control of efficacy of enzyme treatment of exocrine pancreatic insufficiency. However, because of its low specificity this test cannot be used as a specific pancreatic function test.

[^{14}C] triolein breath test

In order to avoid the known disadvantages of the quantitative faecal fat determination, attempts have been made to produce other tests of fat absorption. The most widely used is the [^{14}C] triolein breath test following oral administration of glyceryltri(1, ^{14}C)oleate that normally is hydrolysed by pancreatic lipase in the small intestine. Exhaled ^{14}C-labelled in carbon dioxide is trapped by hyamine and then quantitated by scintillation counting. In cases of impaired fat absorption, the amount of ^{14}C-labelled carbon dioxide exhaled in 6 hours after an oral dose of ^{14}C-labelled triolein is reduced. This test is easier to perform than faecal fat determination but again it provides little information about the cause of malabsorption in any particular patient.

Pancreolauryl test

A number of oral tolerance tests have been developed for the diagnosis of pancreatogenous malabsorption all of which depend on the detection of metabolites in the breath, blood or urine. The best current non-invasive test of exocrine function is the pancreolauryl test (Lankisch et al 1986). The test is based on the fact that fluorescein-dilaurate is hydrolysed by pancreatic arylesterase to water-soluble fluorescein. This is absorbed by the small intestine, conjugated by the liver and excreted into the urine. Release and absorption of fluorescein thus depend on the action of the pancreatic arylesterases and therefore reflects exocrine pancreatic secretory activity (Newcomer et al 1979, Butler et al 1984).

These tests are non-invasive, relatively inexpensive and have a sensitivity of about 80% for the diagnosis of severe exocrine insufficiency when compared with the direct secretin–CCK test. However, in early or mild pancreatitis the sensitivity is less than 50%. In order to avoid falsely abnormal results in renal insufficiency, intestinal disease and liver disease, the test is performed over 3 days. On the first day fluorescein-dilaurate is given, and on the third day fluorescein alone. On the basis of the test and the control study, a quotient is calculated which reflects pancreatic exocrine function. There have been some attempts to replace the urine analyses by serum determinations. The available data indicate that the serum determinations are as accurate as the urine analyses (Lankisch et al 1986).

NBT-PABA test

The underlying principle of the NBT-PABA test is that an adequate duodenal concentration of chymotrypsin is necessary to cleave free para-aminobenzoic acid (PABA) from the synthetic peptide N-benzoyl-L-trysoyl-para-amino-benzoic acid (NBT-PABA). PABA excretion in the urine is reduced when enzyme output is less than 5% of normal. If performed during only one day, then renal, liver and intestinal diseases may influence the test results.

In a comparative study in patients with steatorrhoea due to exocrine pancreatic insufficiency, comparable sensitivity (range 92–100%) was found for the pancreolauryl test, NBT-PABA test and faecal chymotrypsin determination. In cases of mild and moderate insufficiency, the tubeless pancreolauryl test appears to be superior when compared to measurement of chymotrypsin in the faeces (Lankisch et al 1983).

These indirect tests may also be affected by drugs such as vitamin B_{12} and salazosulphapyridine, so that the oral intake of such drugs must be stopped for 5 days before performing the test.

Dual-labelled Schilling test

Approximately 20–40% of patients with exocrine pancreatic insufficiency have impaired absorption of vitamin B_{12} as measured by the standard Schilling test, and which can be corrected by administration of oral pancreatic enzymes. The dual-labelled Schilling test was developed to provide information about pancreatic exocrine function in relation to reduced vitamin B_{12} absorption (Brugge et al 1980). Pancreatic insufficiency may induce abnormal B_{12} absorption because proteases are required for release of vitamin B_{12} from the so called R-proteins of gastric juice, which preferentially bind the vitamin.

The test compares the absorption of ^{58}Co-labelled vitamin B_{12} given orally, bound to R-proteins, and ^{57}Co-labelled vitamin B_{12} given orally bound to intrinsic factor. In pancreatic insufficiency the ratio ^{58}Co/^{57}Co in urine specimens is significantly decreased compared to normal. The test allows differentiation between different forms of vitamin B_{12} malabsorption including bacterial overgrowth of the small intestine and distal ileal disease. Although theoretically attractive, this test is no longer in clinical use because attempts at standardization have not been successful. Moreover, normalization of vitamin B_{12} absorption after pancreatic enzyme replacement, as measured by the standard Schilling test, in itself suggests pancreatogeneous malabsorption.

Other tests

A variety of other laboratory tests have been proposed for use in the diagnosis of exocrine insufficiency and chronic pancreatitis. These tests are of uncertain worth, and include synthesis of pancreatic digestive enzymes using a radiolabelled amino acid, the measurement of human pancreatic polypeptide after stimulation of the exocrine pancreas, and nuclear magnetic resonance spectrometry of lyophylized samples of reconstituted stools.

Serum enzyme determinations

Determination of α-amylase and isoamylase levels in the serum is useful in the evaluation of acute pancreatitis or of acute relapses of chronic pancreatitis. Isoamylase represents about 35–45% of the amylase in normal serum and does not return to normal as rapidly as total serum amylase in patients with acute pancreatitis. However, serum amylase and isoamylase do not have a significant role in the detection of exocrine insufficiency in chronic pancreatitis (Goebell 1976, Otte et al 1976).

Some authors have reported decreased circulating levels of trypsin and lipase in patients suffering from chronic pancreatitis and exocrine insufficiency. Conversely, elevated serum concentrations of elastase, DNase and RNase have also been reported. However, these relatively simple blood tests have only been proposed for use in severe pancreatitis, and so far they have not demonstrated a sufficient degree of sensitivity and specificity to be useful in early or mild pancreatitis.

EXOCRINE PANCREATIC FUNCTION AND PANCREATIC SURGERY

Chronic pancreatitis is the commonest cause of exocrine pancreatic insufficiency. About 50–70% of pancreatic cancer patients show maldigestion before surgery and in about 90% of cases there is decreased enzyme secretion after stimulation by secretin–CCK (Perez et al 1983).

Total pancreatectomy results in about 75% of fat malabsorption. After partial resection symptoms of exocrine pancreatic insufficiency may develop or become more severe. According to Frey et al (1976), the Whipple operation may lead to clinically significant steatorrhoea in 55% of cases. The severity of steatorrhoea depends on the extent of resection and on whether the pancreatic remnant is abnormal. Distal resection of 40–80% of the gland induced postoperative steatorrhoea in 19% of Frey's patients, whereas resection of 80–95% caused steatorrhoea in 38%. In cases where the pancreatic remnant is normal, subtotal resection has little effect on fat absorption.

In contrast, in patients suffering from chronic pancreatitis, abstinence from alcohol and surgical intervention in the form of pancreaticojejunostomy is thought by some to improve secretory activity of the pancreas (Lankisch et al, 1975, Nealon et al, 1988).

The differential diagnosis of malabsorption after pancreatic surgery, with or without concomitant gastric resection, also has to involve motility studies and absorption tests, such as the D-xylose test, lactose tolerance test, H_2-breath test, and cholyl-^{14}C-glycine breath test. It is well known that factors other than absolute exocrine pancreatic insufficiency may also cause malabsorption after such forms of surgery. These factors include postcibal asynchronization; the various forms of dumping syndrome; the afferent loop, blind loop and efferent loop syndromes, and syndromes due to technical mistakes such as construction of a gastroenterostomy using ileum rather than jejunum.

ENDOCRINE PANCREATIC FUNCTION TESTS

The endocrine tissue amounts to about 1–2% of the pancreas. The endocrine cells are principally aggregated in the islets of Langerhans which lie interspersed in the loose connective tissue between the lobules of the exocrine pancreas. These endocrine cells normally secrete the gastrointestinal peptides insulin, glucagon, somatostatin and pancreatic polypeptide. The main function of the endocrine pancreas is to facilitate storage of foodstuffs by release of insulin during a meal and to provide a mechanism for the metabolism of these foodstuffs by release of glucagon during periods of fasting.

The major diagnostic procedures involving the endocrine pancreas are the various oral and intravenous glucose tolerance tests; calculation of glucose assimilation coefficients or insulin/glucose ratios; determination of fasting glucose levels and glucose profile over the day; determination of serum insulin and C-peptide levels, and the determination of haemoglobin A_1 and/or haemoglobin A_{1C} (Table 13.3).

As part of the study of changes in gastrointestinal peptide secretion in patients with pancreatic disease and after pancreatic surgery (Vinik & Jackson 1980, Bestermann et al 1982, Domschke et al 1988), attention has focused on glucagon and pancreatic polypeptide (PP) as specific indicators of endocrine failure in chronic pancreatitis, and as a possible sensitive index of pancreatic exocrine impairment. In spite of some correlation to urinary PABA excretion, the glucagon response after arginine infusion has not proved to have clinical relevance. Plasma PP response, however, is significantly reduced in patients with chronic pancreatitis of varied severity, following the i.v. infusion of CCK-8, even in those without steatorrhoea. Furthermore, the integrated PP response to maximal stimulation with i.m. caeruletide clearly separates normal control subjects from patients with mild to moderate impairment of exocrine pancreatic function, as well as those with pancreatic steatorrhoea. There is some evidence that near-maximal PP stimulation may be required to detect patients with chronic pancreatitis of mild to moderate severity. Further studies are necessary to evaluate whether PP has a definitive role in the diagnosis of chronic pancreatitis or exocrine insufficiency.

Other studies also indicate a correlation between exocrine insufficiency and alterations of insulin/glucose metabolism or ratios (Domschke et al 1975, Klapdor et al 1982)

ENDOCRINE FUNCTION AND PANCREATIC SURGERY

Benign and malignant disease as well as pancreatic surgery can effect endocrine pancreatic function. Clinically, diabetes does not become manifest until more than 90% of endocrine pancreatic function is lost.

About 75% of patients with calcific chronic pancreatitis and 30% of those with non-calcific pancreatitis have insulin-dependent diabetes (Vinik & Jackson 1980). Most of the rest have either abnormal glucose tolerance curves or abnormally low serum insulin levels after a test meal. In patients with cystic fibrosis, diabetes mellitus occurs

Table 13.3 Endocrine pancreatic function tests

Fasting serum glucose
Serum glucose profile

Oral glucose tolerance test
Intravenous glucose tolerance test
Glucose assimilation coefficient
Insulin/glucose ratio

Integrated insulin/glucose response to test meals
Arginine-stimulated glucagon response
CCK-stimulated pancreatic polypeptide (PP) response

significantly more often in the second decade of life compared to healthy controls. About 20–30% of pancreatic cancer patients have clinical manifestations of diabetes mellitus at the time of diagnosis (Klöppel et al 1976).

After total pancreatectomy all patients exhibit insulin-dependent diabetes. Partial pancreatectomy often converts a patient who does not require insulin into one who does require it postoperatively. Altogether, the incidence of diabetes after Whipple resection is about 20–40% (Stone et al 1988). Decisive factors for development of diabetes after pancreatic surgery are the extent of resection, involvement of the pancreatic remnant in the primary disease, effects of decompression of the main pancreatic duct, and maintenance or non-maintenance of the enteroinsular axis. For example Christiansen et al (1971) did not find clinical diabetes in four patients after pancreaticoduodenectomy or pancreaticogastrectomy for cancer of the duodenum or the papilla of Vater. In a study published by Bittner et al (1992) duodenum-preserving pancreatic head resection led to improvement of the glucose tolerance in the majority of patients. Only one patient (7%) developed diabetes postoperatively, and it is speculated that maintenance of the enteroinsular axis by duodenum-preserving resection, together with efficient decompression of the main duct, explains why the results appear to be better than those of the Whipple resection. Development of abnormal glucose tolerance in experimental animals depends on the relationship between atrophy and sclerosis after pancreatic duct ligation and/or occlusion (Klapdor et al 1984, Grossner et al 1989). Thus, atrophy of the exocrine pancreas affected glucose-stimulated insulin release and arginine-induced glucagon release to a nonsignificant extent for up to 2 years after duct ligation (Reis 1980). Postoperative improvement in metabolic state and retardation of development of diabetes is also reported by Nealon et al (1988) in patients with chronic pancreatitis after longitudinal pancreaticojejunostomy where duct dilatation preoperatively exceeded 7–9 mm.

LABORATORY DIAGNOSIS OF ENDOCRINE TUMOURS OF THE PANCREAS

The most common endocrine tumours of the pancreas are listed in Table 13.4 (Modlin 1979, Kreijs 1987). With

Table 13.4 Pancreatic endocrine tumours

Syndrome	Tumour-associated peptides.
Gastrinoma (Zollinger Ellison Syndrome)	Gastrin
Insulinoma	Insulin
Glucagonoma	Glucagon
Somatostatinoma	Somatostatin
PP-oma	Pancreatic peptide
VIP-oma	Vasoactive intestinal peptide
	Gastric inhibitory polypeptide (GIP)? pancreatic polypeptide (PP)?
GRF-oma	Growth releasing factor (GRF)
CRF-oma	Corticotropin releasing factor (CRF)
Carcinoid	Serotonin, prostaglandins, bradykinin
Multiple endocrine neoplasia (MEN-I)	Associated with neoplastic lesions of the pancreas, parathyroid, pituitary, adrenal cortex and thyroid

respect to tumorigenesis, the bulk of evidence now points to a non-islet ductular origin of these endocrine tumours, although endocrine tumours associated with excessive hormone production are frequently called islet cell tumours. The tumours are thought to arise from pluripotent stem cells in the duct epithelium. Under normal conditions in the fetus these stem cells called nesidioblasts give rise to islets by budding, but under pathological conditions they may differentiate into neoplasms producing ectopic hormones.

Unlike other gastrointestinal neoplasms these frequently are slow-growing tumours, causing symptoms from excess hormone secretion rather than from growth, invasion or local anatomical effects. The diagnosis is suggested by the history, physical examination, and by finding elevated blood levels of the relevant peptides, or elevated urinary levels of major metabolites. Further confirmation of the presence of hormone-producing tumours may be provided by provocative tests that reveal abnormalities in the regulation of hormone secretion.

Examples of abnormal regulation of endocrine tumour cells include enhancement by secretin of gastrin secretion in gastrinoma; pentagastrin stimulation of calcitonin secretion in medullary thyroid (C-cell) tumour, and tolbutamide-induced enhancement of somatostatin secretion from somatostatinoma cells.

Other function tests include the calcium infusion test for diagnosing gastrinomas, and the demonstration of fasting hypoglycaemia in the presence of inappropriately high levels of serum insulin as the most reliable test for diagnosis of organic hyperinsulinism. A ratio of plasma insulin to glucose of greater than 30 is diagnostic. (Editor's comment: The ratios of immunoreactive insulin (IRI) to glucose in the blood stream, after fasting for 12–15 hours, show overlap between control subjects and insulinoma patients. Some recommend the use of an 'amended IRI/ glucose ratio', i.e. $(100 \times IRI)/(glucose -1.7 \text{ mmol/l})$. The subtraction of 1.7 mmol/l from the value of the fasting blood glucose concentration is based on the assumption that at glucose concentrations below this value, insulin

secretions from normal β cells should be undetectable. An amended IRI/glucose ratio of >30 is usually taken as strong evidence of an insulinoma. D.C.) Ratios should be calculated before and after fasting for 12–15 hours. Proinsulin levels greater than 40% suggest a malignant islet cell tumour.

Provocative tests employing drugs that release insulin (tolbutamide, glucagon, leucin and others) are now obsolete. In contrast to first impressions, euglycaemic clamp experiments are less reliable for detecting or excluding a functioning insulinoma than the relationship between glucose and insulin values during starvation (Nauck et al 1990). Trials to distinguish insulin-secreting adenomas from carcinomas by their response to somatostatin have failed so far.

Recently, clinicians have focused their interest on two other markers, namely chromogranin-A and neuron-specific enolase (NSE). Chromogranin-A is useful for detection of endocrine tumours and in patient follow-up. It is a 48 kd acidic monomeric protein which is co-stored and co-released with resident peptides by a wide variety of normal neuroendocrine tissues and by benign and malignant neuroendocrine tumours (Stabile et al 1990). NSE is a glycolytic enzyme found in the neurones of the brain and peripheral nervous tissue. It is also present in cells belonging to the neuroendocrine system (Tapia et al 1981). There is some evidence that chromogranin-A and NSE can serve as useful endocrine markers even in the absence of secretion of the usual resident peptides by the tumour. Their definitive value in the clinical diagnosis and management of patients with these tumours has yet to be established by prospective studies.

In the case of endocrine tumours of the pancreas the secreted endocrine products not only allow diagnosis. They may also help to localize islet tumours of less than 1–2 cm in diameter (by transhepatic portal vein catheterization and venous sampling) in cases where imaging methods, including superselective angiography and endoscopic ultrasound, fail to provide localization (Doppman et al 1991, Vinik et al 1991).

LABORATORY DIAGNOSIS OF EXOCRINE TUMOURS OF THE PANCREAS

Carcinoma of the pancreas stems in over 90% of cases from the cuboidal epithelium of the pancreatic duct. For the vast majority of patients there are few early suggestive signs and symptoms. In general, clinical symptoms such as weight loss, upper abdominal pain and jaundice indicate advanced disease. In the earlier stages, imaging studies such as CT and ultrasonography are often indeterminate, leading to repetition of studies where symptoms continue or progress. Consequently, diagnosis is achieved in most cases several months after onset of the complaints, usually too late for resection and especially for curative resection. Less than 20–30% of diagnosed cancer patients have resectable cancer, and more than 95% will die from the disease. A palpable mass, which is found in about 10% of cases, virtually always signifies surgical incurability.

This gloomy stituation explains the search during the past decades for laboratory tests which might allow easier non-invasive diagnosis and monitoring of patients with this tumour. Prior to 1983 tumour markers could not be considered helpful in the detection or follow-up of patients with pancreatic cancer. Serum amylase, alkaline phosphatase, 4-nucleotidase, aspartate aminotransferase (SGOT), lactic dehydrogenase (LDH), serum albumin, pancreatic RNase, α-fetoprotein, oncofetal protein (POA), galactosyltransferase isoenzyme II, trypsin-creatinine clearance, as well as secondary phenomena such as decreased serum testosterone levels, were neither useful for early detection nor for follow-up because of their low sensitivity and specificity. Initially promising methods of overcoming these problems by measuring pancreatic enzyme profiles in pancreatic or duodenal juice (Filippini & Amman 1967, Reber et al 1981, Rinderknecht et al 1983), or α_1-fetoprotein and lactoferrin in pancreatic juice proved disappointing and of no clinical relevance. However, there was some evidence that lactoferrin in pancreatic and duodenal juice may be a sensitive and specific marker of early or mild chronic pancreatitis (Nicolai et al 1984).

The development of hybridoma technology followed by the detection and clinical introduction of new associated antigens such as CA 19-9 (Del Villano et al 1983, Klapdor et al 1983), CA 50 (Haglund et al 1987), CA 195 (Guptka et al 1987), Du-Pan-2 (Metzgar et al 1984, Suzuki et al 1988) and SPan 1 (Takeda et al 1991), changed this situation, at least to some extent. For example, CA 19-9 has a sensitivity of about 80% and a specificity of 95% at the time of primary diagnosis of pancreatic cancer. Simultaneous determination of CA 19-9 and CA 125, CA 72-4 or CEA increases the sensitivity to more than 90% (Klapdor et al 1984, 1990). CA 19-9 also differentiates between exocrine pancreatic ductal carcinoma and endocrine pancreatic cancer as well as chronic inactive pancreatitis (Fig. 13.1).

In spite of this high sensitivity at the time of primary diagnosis these new tumour-associated substances do not represent ideal tumour markers; they do not show tumour specificity or organ specificity (Del Villano et al 1983, Klapdor et al 1984) and do not allow early diagnosis, in other words, the detection of stage T1a and T1b pancreatic cancer on screening (Manabe et al 1988, Satake et al 1991). For example, acute pancreatitis and acute cholangitis may induce significant transient increases of CA 19-9 levels to up to more than 1000 u/ml. Elevated CA 19-9 serum levels may be detected not only in pancreatic cancer patients, but also in the course of other malignant diseases (Fig. 13.2), and the sensitivity is significantly lower in the case of early (30%) or resectable stages (60%) compared to advanced stages (80–90%).

Animal experiments clearly demonstrate the correlation between tumour mass and elevation of the levels of these tumour markers in the serum (Klapdor et al 1984, 1989), and suggest that the relatively high sensitivity of about 80% at the time of primary diagnosis simply reflects the fact that even today, pancreatic exocrine cancer is diagnosed at a more advanced stage than say, colorectal cancer.

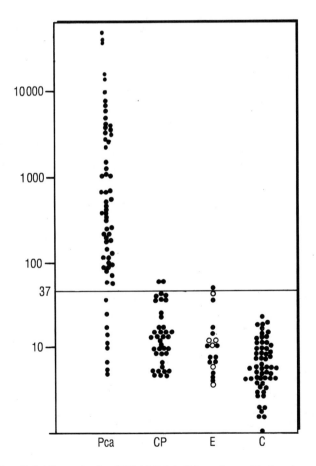

Fig. 13.1 Serum levels of CA 19-9 (u/ml) in patients with ductal pancreatic cancer (PCa), inactive chronic pancreatitis (CP), endocrine tumours of the pancreas or gastrointestinal tract (E) and healthy controls (C). The cut-off value of 37 u/ml corresponds to a 95% specificity; ○ = benign, ● = malignant endocrine tumour.

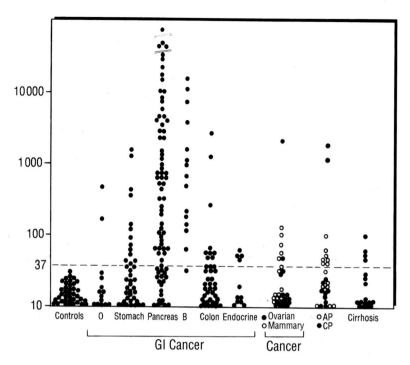

Fig. 13.2 Serum levels of CA 19-9 (u/ml) in healthy controls, patients with gastrointestinal cancer (O, oesophageal; B, biliary), ovarian or breast cancer, pancreatitis (AP, acute pancreatitis; CP, chronic pancreatitis) and hepatic cirrhosis.

A review of the experience of the past decade allows us to summarize the actual clinical relevance of CA 19-9 or related tumour-associated antigens in the detection and follow-up of exocrine pancreatic cancer (Table 13.5) as follows:

1. Tumour markers have no role in screening for early cancer in the asymptomatic population. However, there is some evidence (CA 19-9 sensitivity in resectable cancer about 60%, tumour marker doubling time in the serum about 0.5–3.5 months) that earlier determination of CA 19-9 would allow earlier diagnosis that might offer a higher rate of resectional surgery. This factor might be of interest when discussing adjuvant therapeutic trials in patients with pancreatic cancer (Klapdor 1990). From the available data it might be concluded that earlier determination of serum CA 19-9 might allow the diagnosis of pancreatic cancer to be brought forward by 3–12 months. Therefore we suggest that CA 19-9 serum determination could be valuable in patients over 45–50 years of age with upper abdominal complaints of unknown origin which have persisted for more than 2–3 weeks (Klapdor et al 1989).

2. CA 19-9, CA 50 and CA 195 also have no role in preoperative staging. There is no doubt that there is some correlation between stage of disease and serum CA 19-9 (Klapdor et al 1984, see Fig. 13.3) and between serum CA 19-9 and prognosis (Glenn et al 1988). However, animal studies clearly show that CA 19-9 secretion may vary to a significant extent from one tumour to another (Klapdor et al 1989), preventing definitive conclusions concerning tumour staging in individual patients on the basis of one marker determination. It is recommended that the surgeon should base his decisions concerning resectability on the results of the imaging methods and the intraoperative findings. However, in patients with extremely elevated CA 19-9 levels (that means levels above 10 000 u/ml), non-resectability is the rule.

3. Despite these comments on staging, the serum concentration of CA 19-9 should still be determined preoperatively to serve as a basis for monitoring progress postoperatively (Dallek et al 1986).

In the majority of resected patients, postoperative CA 19-9 determinations allow earlier differentiation between those who will suffer from recurrence in the near future

Table 13.5 Clinical relevance of CA 19-9 in the diagnosis and follow-up of exocrine pancreatic carcinoma

Screening	
For early cancer (T1a) in asymptomatic population	–
For cancer in symptomatic patients	(+)
Preoperative determination	
Confirmation of cancer diagnosis	(+)
Staging	(+)
Prognosis	(+)
Basis for follow-up	+++
Follow-up	
Postoperative determination after 2–4 weeks	+++
Detection of recurrence	+++
Follow-up during palliative therapy	+++

–, No relevance; (+), limited value; +++ clinical relevance.

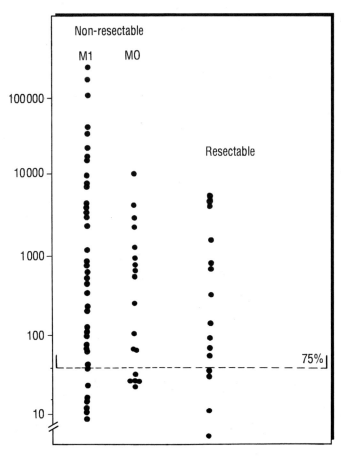

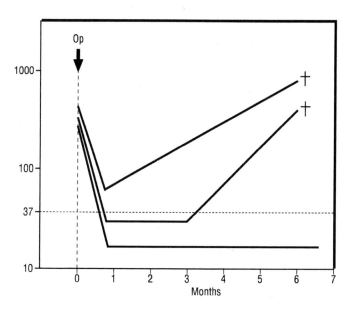

Fig. 13.4 Typical patterns of serum CA 19-9 levels (u/ml) in three patients following potentially curative resection of pancreatic cancer. The one patient who continues to survive showed a sustained fall in CA 19-9 levels to within the normal range.

Fig. 13.3 Serum levels of CA 19-9 (u/ml) in patients with non-resectable (M1, metastatic disease present; MO, metastatic disease absent) and resectable pancreatic cancer. The dotted horizontal line represents a cut-off level of 37 u/ml; 75% of the patients had higher CA 19-9 levels including a large proportion of those with resectable disease.

achieved by imaging methods, it might be possible in the near future to perform immunoscintigraphy with radiolabelled monoclonal antibodies directed against the antigen expressed by the tumour (Klapdor et al 1986, 1989, Montz et al 1985). However, this method cannot be recommended for routine use as yet because of the sensitivity and specificity of the presently available antibodies are too low. Similarly, while intraoperative immunoscintigraphy might allow early tumour detection

and those with a real chance of cure. In our experience all patients who do not show decrease of CA 19-9 into the normal range within 2–4 weeks of resection will suffer from recurrence within the next months, even in the case of Ro resection (Klapdor et al 1987, Glenn et al 1988). All patients with a fall in CA 19-9 levels below the cut-off retain a chance of cure. This knowledge is of importance not only for the patient, but for the clinicians planning adjuvant therapeutic trials (Fig. 13.4).

With respect to the early diagnosis of tumour recurrence we now have a similar situation as with colorectal cancer. In tumours with expression and secretion of CA 19-9, a new increase in the levels of this marker indicates tumour recurrence, often some months earlier than clinical signs or modern imaging methods (Glenn et al 1988). The lead time amounts to about 3–6 months. As a consequence we recommend measurement of the relevant tumour-associated antigen, in most cases CA 19-9, at 1–3 month intervals in the postoperative period.

If serial determinations of a tumour-associated antigen indicate recurrence when localization has not been

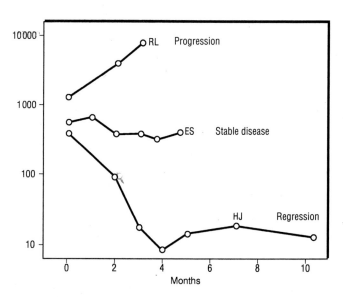

Fig. 13.5 Typical patterns of serum CA 19-9 levels (u/ml) in patients with progressive, stable or regressing disease following treatment of pancreatic cancer.

or earlier diagnosis of recurrence, this method does not yet have a role in pancreatic cancer (Reuter et al 1992).

4. Tumour markers such as CA 19-9 also provide useful follow-up in patients treated palliatively. CA 19-9 levels under these circumstances may show the three different courses known from imaging studies (Klapdor 1985) namely, a stable course, a decrease even to normality (Fig. 13.5), and a further increase. A sensitive tumour marker often indicates antitumoral effects of the treatment more rapidly than imaging. Furthermore, a sensitive tumour-associated substance often allows a more precise differentiation between progressive and stable disease (Klapdor 1991). On the basis of available clinical data and experimental studies in nude mice bearing xenografts of human pancreatic carcinomas, two statements are of clinical importance. First, in the case of progressive increase of a tumour marker in the serum we have to assume a progressive disease even if imaging methods suggests a stable course for 2 or 3 months, and secondly, stable disease as indicated by imaging methods should be accepted as stable disease only if the relevant tumour marker remains stable or decreases with normalization of the serum levels.

Thus, imaging methods should always be combined with determinations of CA 19-9 or other sensitive markers in order to monitor the course of palliative treatment in individual patients. This combination is particularly important in the evaluation of response rates to new therapies in controlled trials.

REFERENCES

Banwell J G, Leonhard P J, Lobo R M 1965 Measurement of trypsin and chymotrypsin in stools to detect chronic pancreatitis. Gut 6: 143–145

Bestermann H S, Adrian T E, Bloom S R, Christofides N D, Mallison D N, Ponti V, Lombardo L, Modigliani R, Guerin S, South M 1982 Pancreatic and gastrointestinal hormones in chronic pancreatitis. Digestion 24: 195–208

Bin T L, Stopard M, Anderson S, Grant A, Quantrill D, Wilkinson R H, Jewell D P 1983 Assessment of fat malabsorption. Journal of Clinical Pathology 36: 1362–1366

Bittner R, Büchler M, Butters M, Leibl B, Nägele S, Roscher R, Beger H G 1992 Der Einfluss der duodenumerhaltenden Pankreaskopfresektion (DPKR) auf die endokrine Pankreasfunktion bei Patienten mit chronisch Pankreatitis. Zeitschrift für Gastroenterologie 30: 12–16

Brugge W R, Godd J S, Allen N C, Podell E R, Allen R H 1980 Development of a dual labelled Schilling test of pancreatic exocrine function based on the differential absorption of cobalamin bound to intrinsic factor and R protein. Gastroenterology 78: 937–949

Butler R N, Gehling N J, Lawson M J, Grant A K 1984 Clinical evaluation of the ^{14}C-triolein breath test: A critical analysis. Australian and New Zealand Journal of Medicine

Christiansen J, Olsen J H, Worning H 1971 The pancreatic function following subtotal pancreatectomy for cancer. Scandinavian Journal of Gastroenterology Suppl 9: 189–193

Dallek M, Klapdor R, Helling K, van Ackeren H, Kranz H W 1986 Diagnosis of recurrence and follow-up of cancers in the large intestine using CEA and the new tumor markers CA 19-9 and CA 125. In: Greten H, Kladpor R (eds) Clinical relevance of new monoclonal antibodies, 3rd Symposium on Tumor Markers, Hamburg 1985. Thieme, Stuttgart, p 38–44

Del Villano B C, Brennan S, Brock P 1983 Radioimmunometric assay for monoclonal antibody-defined tumor marker CA19–9. Clinical Chemistry 29: 549–552

Di Magno E P, Go V L W, Summerskill W H J 1973 Relations between pancreatic enzyme outputs and malabsorption in severe pancreatic insufficiency. New England Journal of Medicine 288: 813–815

Domschke W, Tympner F, Domschke S, Demling L 1975. Exocrine pancreatic function in juvenile diabetes. American Journal of Digestive Diseases 20: 309–321

Domschke S, Bloom S R, Adrian T E, Lux G, Domschke W 1988 Chronic pancreatitis and diabetes mellitus: Plasma and gastroduodenal mucosal profiles of regulatory peptides (gastrin, motilin, secretin, cholecystokinin, gastric inhibitory polypeptide, somatostatin, VIP, substance P, pancreatic polypeptide, glucagon, enteroglucagon, neurotensin). Hepato-Gastroenterology 35: 229–237

Domschke S, Adrian T E, Bloom R, Lux G, Domschke W 1982 Pancreatic and gut hormones in chronic pancreatitis and diabetes mellitus. Digestion 25: 24

Doppman J L, Miller D L, Chang R, Shawker T H, Gordon P, Norton J A 1991 Insulinomas: Localization with selective intraarterial injection of calcium. Radiology 178: 237–241

Dürr H K, Otte M, Forell M M, Bode J C 1978 Fecal chymotrypsin: A study on its diagnostic value by comparison with the secretin-cholecystokinin test. Digestion 17: 404–409

Filippini L, Amman R 1967 Klinisch-funktionelle Diagnostik des Pankreaskarzinoms. Schweizerische medizinische Wochenschrift 97: 803–810

Frey C F, Child C G, Fry W 1976 Pancreatectomy for chronic pancreatitis. Annals of Surgery 184: 403–414

Glenn J, Steinberg W M, Kurtzmann S H, Steinberg S M, Sindelar W F 1988 Evaluation of the utility of a radioimmunoassay for serum CA 19-9 levels in patients before and after treatment of carcinoma of the pancreas. Journal of Clinical Oncology 6: 462–468

Goebell H 1976 Enzymevokationstest. In: Forell M (ed) Pankreas. Springer Berlin, Issue 3, ch 6 p 473–477

Grossner D, Kroge H, Berkhoff M, Klapdor R, Klöppel G 1989 Insulinreserve und Morphologie des Pankreasschwanzes nach Pankreaskopfresektion bei unterschiedlicher Methoden der Versorgung. Langenbecks Archiv für Chirurgie 374: 4–11

Guptka M K, Arciaga R, Bukowsky R, Gaur P K 1987 CA 195: A new sensitive monoclonal antibody defined tumor marker for pancreatic cancer. Journal of Tumor Marker Oncology 2: 201–205

Haglund C, Kuusela P, Jalanko H, Roberts P J 1987 Serum Ca 50 as a tumor marker in pancreatic cancer: a comparison with CA19-9. International Journal of Cancer 39: 477–481

Klapdor R 1985 Clinical course and follow-up of patients suffering from pancreatic carcinoma. In: Greten H, Klapdor R (eds) New tumor associated antigens, Proceedings of the 2nd Symposium on tumor markers, Hamburg 1984. Thieme, Stuttgart, p 2–10

Klapdor R 1989 Zum Stand der Früherkennung des Pankreaskarzinoms. Internist 30: 752–758

Klapdor R 1990 Ist eine neo- oder adjuvante Chemotherapie beim Pankreaskarzinom sinnvoll? Langenbecks Archiv für Chirurgie 375 (Suppl II): 135–147

Klapdor R 1991 Perspectives in chemotherapy of pancreatic cancer. European Journal of Surgical Oncology 17: 153–166

Klapdor R, Greten H 1984 Das tumor-assoziierte Antigen CA 19-9 in der Differentialdiagnostik und Verlaufkontrolle von Malignomen des Pankreas und Magen-Darm-Traktes. Deutsche Medizinische Wochenschrift 109: 1935–1937

Klapdor R, Humke R 1976 About the efficiency of the duodenal balloon tube technique using polyethylene glycol as duodenal marker. Acta Hepatogastroenterologica 23: 250–254

Klapdor R, Montz R 1989 Immunoscintigraphy of pancreatic cancer: relevance for diagnosis and therapy. In: Chatal J F (ed) Monoclonal antibodies in immunoscintigraphy. CRC Press, Boca Raton, Florida, p 154–163

Klapdor R, Lehmann U, Grossner D, Bahlo, M, Heling C, Schmidt-Thiedemannn K, Strüven D 1982 Postprandiale Sekretion von pankreatischem Polypeptid, Insulin und Gastric inhibitory Polypeptid nach Pankreasoperationen. Zeitschrift für Gastroenterologie 20: 59

Klapdor R, Lehmann U, Bahlo M, Greten H, van Ackeren H, Dallek M, Schreiber H W 1983 CA 19-9 in der Diagnostik und Differentialdiagnostik des exkretorischen Pankreaskarzinoms. Tumordiagnostik und Therapie 4: 197–201

Klapdor, R, Otremba H, Grossner D, Klöppel G, v. Kroge H 1984 B-cell function after pancreatic duct ligation–comparative studies in pigs after ligation and after pancreas resection. European Journal of Clinical Investigations 14: 23

Klapdor R, Bahlo M, Montz R, Dietel M, Kremer B, Dimigen J, Chatal J F, Douillard J Y, Saccavini, J C 1986 Immunoscintigraphy of gastrointestinal carcinomas especially pancreatic cancer with 131-I-anti-CA 19-9, 131-I-anti-CEA and 131-I-anti-CA 125. Experimental studies on xenografts in nude mice. In: Greten H, Klapdor R (eds) Clinical relevance of new monoclonal antibodies, Proceedings of the 3rd Symposium on tumor markers, Hamburg 1985. Thieme, Stuttgart, p 362–375

Klapdor R, Klapdor U, Montz R, Dietel M, Arps H, Schreiber H W, Greten H 1987 New tumor associated antigens and their monoclonal antibodies in the follow-up of exocrine pancreatic carcinoma. In: Klapdor R (ed) New tumor markers and their monoclonal antibodies – Actual relevance for diagnosis and therapy of solid tumors. Proceedings of the 4th Symposium on Tumor markers, Hamburg, 1948 Thieme, Stuttgart, p 154–166

Klapdor R, Harms F, Bahlo M, Arps H, Dietel M 1989 Tumor marker secretion (CA 19-9, CEA, CA 125) by xenografts of eight different human pancreatic carcinomas compared to the human tumors. Strahlentherapie und Onkologie 165: 496–497

Klapdor R, Bahlo M, Strüven D 1990 Role of tumor markers in the diagnosis of pancreatic carcinoma. In: Klapdor R (ed) Recent results in tumor diagnosis and therapy. Proceedings of the 5th Symposium on Tumor Markers, Hamburg 1989. W Zuckschwerdt, Munich, p 46–50

Klöppel G, Sosnowski J, Eichfuss H-P, Rückert K, Klapdor R 1976 Aktuelle Aspekte des Pankreaskarzinomas. Deutsche medizinische Wochenschrift 104: 1801–1813

Kreijs G J (ed) 1987 Gastrointestinal endocrine tumors: Diagnosis and management. American Journal of Medicine 82 (Suppl 5B)

Lamers C B H, van Tongeren J H M 1977 Comparative study of the value of calcium, secretin and the meal stimulated increase in serum gastrin in the diagnosis of the Zollinger-Ellison syndrome. Gut 18: 128–134

Lankisch P G 1982 Progress report: Exocrine pancreatic function tests. Gut 23: 777–798

Lankisch P G, Fuchs K, Schmidt H, Peiper H-J, Creutzfeld W 1975 Ergebnisse der operativen Behandlung der chronischen Pankreatitis mit besonderer Berücksichtigung der exokrinen und endokrinen Funktion. Deutsche Medizinische Wochenschrift 105: 1418–1423

Lankisch P G, Schreiber A, Otto J 1983 Pancreolauryl test. Evaluation of a tubeless pancreatic function test in comparison with other indirect and direct tests for exocrine pancreatic function. Digestive Diseases and Sciences 28: 490–493

Lankisch P G, Brauneis J, Otto J, Göke B 1986 Pancreolauryl and NBT-PABA test. Are serum tests more practicable alternatives to urine tests in the diagnosis of exocrine pancreatic insufficiency? Gastroenterology 90: 350–354

Lundh G 1962 Pancreatic exocrine function in neoplastic and inflammatory disease; a simple and reliable new test. Gastroenterology 42: 275–280

Manabe T, Miyashita T, Ohshio G, Monaka A, Suzuki T, Endo K, Takahashi M, Tobe T 1988 Small carcinoma of the pancreas. Cancer 62: 135–141

McEvoy A, Dutton J, James O F 1983 Bacterial contamination of the small intestine is an important cause of occult malabsorption in the elderly. British Medical Journal 287: 789–793

Metzgar R, Rodriguez N, Finn O 1984 Detection of a pancreatic cancer associated antigen (Du-Pan-2 antigen) in serum and ascites of patients with adenocarcinoma. Proceedings of the National Academy of Sciences of the USA 81: 5242–5246

Modlin I M 1979 Endocrine tumors of the pankreas. Surgery, Gynecology and Obstetrics 149: 751–769

Montz R, Klapdor R, Rothe B, Heller M 1985 Immunoscintigraphy and radioimmunotherapy in patients with pancreatic carcinoma. Nuclear Medicine 25: 239–244

Nauck M, Stöckmann F, Creutzfeld W 1990 Evaluation of a euglycaemic clamp procedure as a diagnostic test in insulinoma patients. European Journal of Clinical Investigations 20: 15–28

Nealon W H, Townsend C M, Thompson J C 1988 Operative drainage of the pancreatic duct delays functional impairment in patients with chronic pancreatitis. Annals of Surgery 208: 321–329

Newcomer A D, Hofmann A F, Di Magno E P, Thomas P J, Carlson G L 1979 Triolein breath test: A sensitive and specific test for fat malabsorption. Gastroenterology 76: 6–13

Nicolai J J, Teunen A, Zuyderhoudt F, Hoek F, Tytgat G N J 1984 Lactoferrin in pure pancreatic juice. Scandinavian Journal of Gastroenterology 19: 765–769

Nishida K, Tasaki N, Miyagawa H, Yoshikawa T, Kondo M 1988 Estimation of carbohydrate antigen (CA) 19-9 levels in pure pancreatic juice of patients with pancreatic cancer. American Journal of Gastroenterology 83: 126–129

Otte M, Thurmayr R, Thurmayr G R, Forell M M 1976 Diagnostic value of the provocative test with secretin and cholecystokinin/pancreozymin. Scandinavian Journal of Gastroenterology (Suppl) 41:11:75

Otte M 1979 Pankreasfunktionsdiagnostik. Internist 20: 560–566

Perez M M, Newcomer A D, Moertel C G, Go V L, Di Magno E P 1983 Assessment of weight loss, food intake, fat metabolism, malabsorption and treatment of pancreatic insufficiency in pancreatic cancer. Cancer 52: 346–352

Reber H A, Tweedie H, Austin J L 1981 Pancreatic secretions as a clue to the presence of pancreatic cancer. Cancer 47: 1646–1651

Reis H E, Hoffmann E, Drost H, Usmiani J, Gebhardt C, Jahnke K, Gries F A 1980 Insulin und Glucagonsekretion nach Pankreasgangokklusion bei chronischer Pankreatitis. Zeitschrift für Gastroenterologie 18: 407–417

Reuter M, Montz R, de Heer K, Schäfer H, Klapdor R, Desler K, Schreiber H W 1992 Detection of colorectal carcinomas by intraoperative RIS in addition to preoperative RIS: surgical and immunohistological findings. European Journal of Nuclear Medicine 18: 102–109

Rinderknecht H, Renner I G, Stace N H 1983 Abnormalities in pancreatic secretory profiles of patients with cancer of the pancreas. Digestive Diseases and Sciences 28: 103–110

Satake K, Chung Y-S, Umeyama K, Takeuchi T, Kim Y S 1991 The possibility of diagnosing small pancreatic cancer (less than 4.0 cm) by measuring various serum tumor markers. Cancer 68: 149–152

Schilling R F 1953 A new test for intrinsic factor activity. Journal of Laboratory and Clinical Medicine 42: 946

Stabile B E, Howard T J, Passaro E, O'Connor D T 1990 Source of plasma chromogranin A elevation in gastrinoma patients. Archives of Surgery 125: 451–454

Stone W M, Sarr M G, Nagorney D M, McIllrath D C 1988 Chronic pancreatitis. Results of Whipple's resection and total pancreatectomy. Archives of Surgery 123: 815–919

Suzuki Y, Ichihara T, Nakao A, Sakamoto J, Takagi H, Nagura H 1988 High levels of Dupan-2 antigen and CA 19-9 in pancreatic cancer: Correlation with immunohistochemical localization of antigens in cancer cells. Hepato-Gastroenterology 35: 128–135

Takeda S, Nakao A, Ichihara T, Suzuki Y, Nonami Z T, Harada A, Koshikawa T, Takagi H 1991 Serum concentration and immunhistochemical localization of SPan-1 antigen in pancreatic cancer. A comparison with CA 19-9 antigen. Hepato-Gastroenterology 38: 143–148

Tapia F J, Barbrosa A J A, Marangos P J, Polak J M, Bloom S R, Dermody C 1981 Neuron-specific enolase in produced by neuroendocrine tumors. Lancet 1: 808–811 van de Kamer J H, Bokkel Huinink H ten, Weijers H A 1949 Rapid method for the determination of fat in feces Journal of Biological Chemistry 117: 347–355

Vinik A I, Jackson W P U 1980 Endocrine secretions in chronic pancreatitis. In: Podolsky S, Viswanathan M (eds) Secondary diabetes. Raven Press, New York, p 165–183

Vinik A I, Delbridge L, Moattari R, Kyung C, Thompson N 1991 Transhepatic portal vein catheterization for localization of insulinomas: A ten-year experience. Surgery 109: 1–11

Webster S G P, Wilkinson E M, Gowland E A 1977 A comparison of fat absorption in young and old subjects. Age and Ageing 6: 113–116

Intraoperative diagnostic procedures

14. Approaches to the pancreas and abdominal exploration

M. Trede

THE INCISION

With the patient lying supine on a table that will permit radiographic examination, if required, the incision chosen depends on the patient's build, presence of scars from previous operations and on the expected pathology. The various possibilities are shown in Figure 14.1. In practice only two of these are of any importance, namely the curved transverse upper abdominal incision and the vertical midline laparotomy incision.

The author prefers the former for most situations. If the patient has a narrow subcostal angle, if there is a median scar already or if he is being explored for blunt abdominal (and possibly pancreatic) trauma, a vertical incision is

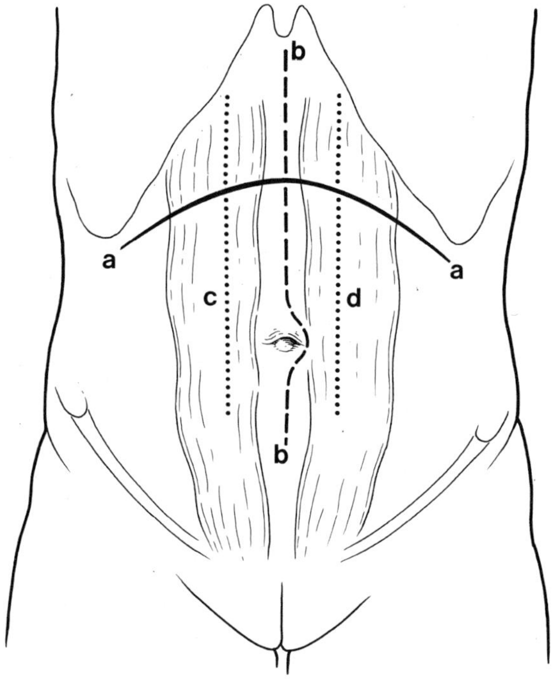

Fig. 14.1 Incisions for pancreatic operations.
a, bilateral transverse subcostal incision;
b, median laparotomy; c, d, right and left paramedian incision.

equally adequate for all pancreatic procedures. In my hands, laparotomy begins with a right subcostal incision that is not extended over the midline and to the left until gross signs of inoperability have been excluded. With the abdomen open the ligamentum teres is divided between clamps. With this wide exposure through a curved incision, retractors fixed to a frame in all four directions are cumbersome and superfluous. If necessary, a large Rochard retractor, as modified by Stuhler, can be used to retract the costal margin cranially so as to improve access to the hepatic hilus on the right and the pancreatic tail and spleen on the left.

THE EXPLORATION

The next step depends very much on the pathology encountered: e.g. whether one is dealing with necrotizing pancreatitis, a malignant tumour or an insulinoma. As specific situations are dealt with in the appropriate chapters, for the purpose of this section let us assume that the presumptive diagnosis is pancreatic carcinoma but–as happens not infrequently–chronic pancreatitis has not been excluded.

Preliminary exploration, by a rapid but systematic palpation of the entire abdominal cavity aims at detecting ascites, peritoneal nodules or hepatic metastases. If any one of these is found, time can be saved by sending a sample for frozen section examination before the operation progresses very much further. While sizeable metastases are surprisingly rare in patients who come to operation with pancreatic carcinoma, careful bimanual palpation of both lobes of the liver may uncover barely visible grey subcapsular nodules of about 1–2 mm in size. The majority of these will turn out to be benign hamartomas but some are identified histologically as metastatic nodules. If so, nothing beyond a palliative bypass should be performed, if indeed this is required.

Warshaw correctly points out that each of these eventualities can and should be excluded by laparoscopy *before* the patient is submitted to an unnecessary laparotomy

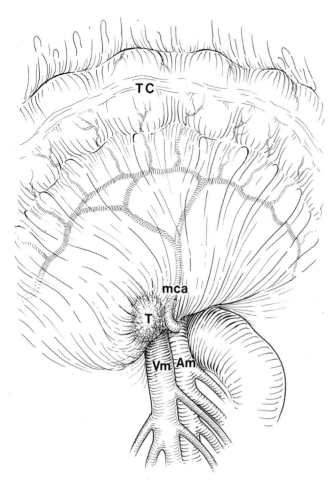

Fig. 14.2 Tumour infiltration (T) at the base of the mesocolon and close to the mesenteric vessels (Vm, Am).
TC, transverse colon; mca, middle colic artery.

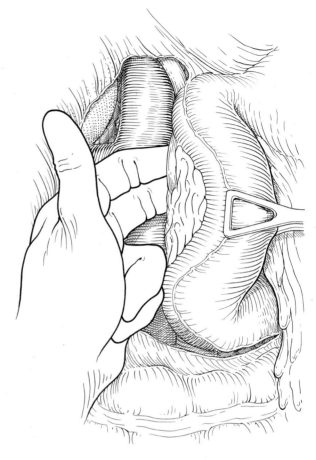

Fig. 14.3 The Kocher manoeuvre for mobilizing the head of the pancreas.

(Warshaw et al 1990). However, in the author's experience, laparoscopy has only rarely been utilized, because peritoneal carcinomatosis and visible hepatic metastases are rarely found even in patients whose condition finally turns out to be inoperable on thorough exploration. This may be due to prior selection of patients before they are referred for surgical treatment.

Courvoisier's law still holds good for most cases. Although obstructive jaundice is by no means rare in chronic pancreatitis, a thin-walled distended gallbladder and a grossly dilated common duct, shimmering with a blue-green hue within the hepatoduodenal ligament are pathognomonic signs of cancer.

Exploration of the pancreas itself begins with superficial palpation to assess the localization, size and mobility of any tumour. Although tumour size does not of itself relate to inoperability, any carcinoma of more than 5 cm in diameter is very unlikely to be resectable. The same applies, of course, to a fixed immobile mass particularly if it is located in the midline close to the coeliac and mesenteric vessels.

Next, the root of the mesentery and base of the mesocolon are exposed by lifting the transverse colon upwards, thus putting the mesocolon under tension. Puckering of the peritoneum in the vicinity of a hard nodule, usually involving the uncinate process, points at incurability, even though the tumour may still be resectable if part of the mesocolon and the stem of the middle colic artery are included in the specimen. Another sinister sign is marked dilatation of mesenteric and gastroepiploic veins (Fig. 14.2).

Any suspicious nodes at the root of the mesentery must be removed for histological examination at this stage. Random biopsy of normal looking lymph nodes is, however, not advisable. Even if foci of malignant cells are found in lymph nodes close to the pancreas, this would not preclude resection in an otherwise operable case.

If the tumour is located in the head of the pancreas, a liberal mobilization from the right by means of a Kocher manoeuvre is performed next. This involves incision of the peritoneal reflection close to the lateral curve of the duodenum from the hepatoduodenal ligament above to the mesocolon below. After cauterizing the small vessels coursing under this part of the peritoneum, blunt dissection between the pancreas in front and the vena cava behind is rapidly possible in an avascular plane (Fig. 14.3). If this manoeuvre is prevented by tumour infiltration, again the situation is inoperable.

For complete mobilization, the right colonic flexure is freed and reflected downwards. The avascular peritoneal reflection tethering the third part of the duodenum is divided right up to the large vessels at the mesenteric root. This dissection is carried along the avascular outer curve of the duodenum, until the peritoneal cavity is entered below the mesocolon.

Dissection between the inner curve of the duodenum and the uncinate process leads next to the large superior mesenteric vein (Fig. 14.4). If tumour clearly infiltrates this vein caudal to the lower border of the pancreas, the situation is inoperable because of numerous tributaries (jejunal and middle colic veins) entering it at this point. Resection of the vein at this level would leave insufficient length of the main venous trunk for anastomosis.

If, however, the vein is infiltrated in its retropancreatic course, the tumour (including vein) may still be resectable even though the disease is unlikely to be curable.

Next the pancreatic head and duodenum are lifted up and reflected to the left, thus, exposing the inferior vena cava (with left renal and right spermatic or ovarian veins) and aorta (Fig. 14.5) in the retropancreatic space.

The origin of the superior mesenteric artery can now be checked for signs of tumour encasement (Fig. 14.6).

In addition, the lymphoid tissue occupying the space between vena cava and aorta is carefully examined and excised, if at all suspicious. Tumour involvement of these nodes is classified as distant metastatic spread and spells

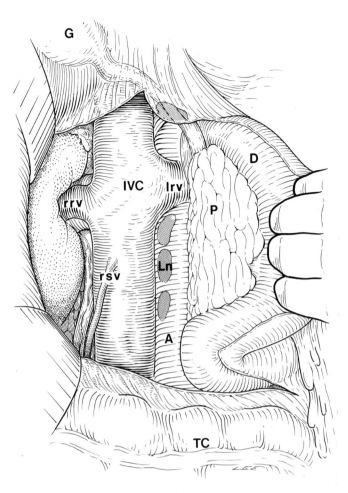

Fig. 14.5 The Kocher manoeuvre exposes the inferior vena cava (IVC), the aorta (A), the left renal vein (lrv), the right renal vein (rrv), the right spermatic vein (rsv) as well as the retropancreatic lymph nodes (Ln); G, gall bladder; P pancreas; D, duodenum; TC, transverse colon.

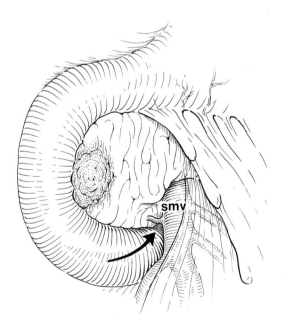

Fig. 14.4 Dissection between the third part of the duodenum and the uncinate process leads to the superior mesenteric vein (smv).

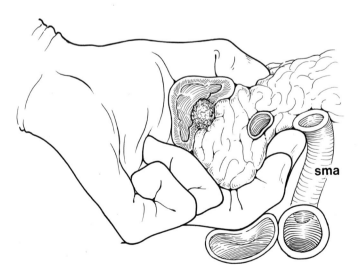

Fig. 14.6 Bidigital palpation of the pancreatic head and mesenteric root (sma).

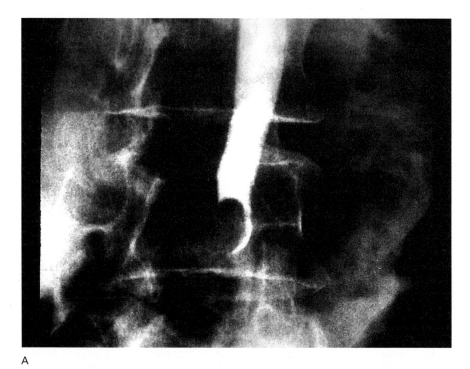

A

B

Fig. 14.7 **A** Endoscopic retrograde cholangiopancreatogram (ECRP) in a 61-year-old patient. In spite of the curiously rectangular configuration of the lesion (mimicking a stone) a prepapillary tumour was correctly predicted. **B** Operative specimen.

incurability. Under favourable circumstances, however, with a locally resectable tumour, we have gone ahead with pancreatic resection nonetheless since this does provide the best palliation.

With the pancreatic head mobilized it is possible to palpate it and the hepatoduodenal ligament between finger and thumb (Fig. 14.6). Here particular attention is paid to the distal retropancreatic portion of the common bile duct.

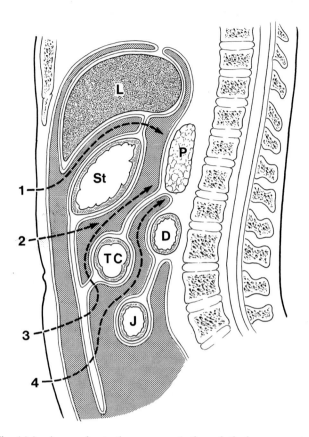

Fig. 14.8 Approaches to the pancreas: 1, through the lesser omentum; 2, through the greater omentum; 3, behind the greater omentum; 4, below the root of the transverse mesocolon. L, liver; St, stomach; P, pancreas; TC, transverse colon; D, duodenum; J, jejunum.

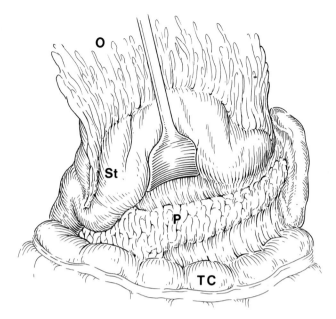

Fig. 14.9 The lesser sac is opened widely after detaching the greater omentum (O) from the transverse colon (TC). Retraction of the stomach (St) reveals the body of the pancreas (P)

If a hard discrete nodule is palpable here, this may be a papillary carcinoma – but it is well to remember that Whipple resections have been inadvertently performed for duodenal ulcer and impacted prepapillary stones (Jordan 1987).

However, with an expert endoscopic department at our disposal such mishaps can be avoided (Fig. 14.7). Intra-operative exploration, either via the common duct or the duodenum, so as to clarify doubtful lesions is hardly ever required.

Access to the anterior aspect of the pancreas is next gained by opening the lesser sac (Fig. 14.8). If the case is clearly inoperable, then standard skeletonization of the gastrocolic ligament in its central portion is adequate. If, however, pancreatic resection is anticipated, it is better to detach the greater omentum from its avascular attachments to the transverse colon, beginning at the right flexure. Following a standard Whipple resection this right half of the omentum invariably becomes ischaemic (and then has to be resected anyway), so that it is better to keep it en bloc with the specimen from the start. Should total pancrea-tectomy be planned, the whole of the omentum has to be detached from the transverse colon in this way.

On retracting the stomach and greater omentum up-wards, and the transverse colon caudally, the whole of the pancreas from head to tail lies exposed to inspection and palpation (Fig. 14.9). In doubtful cases suspicious lesions can now be sampled either directly by a fine needle (for cytology) or by means of a Trucut needle (for histological examination). For the latter, we feel that the transduo-denal route is safer.

Intraoperative evaluation by modern imaging and biopsy methods will be dealt with in the following sections. Valuable as these modalities are in practised hands, in the vast majority of cases one can rely on the preoperative findings. With the abdomen open, and faced with a symptomatic lesion of the pancreas (causing duodenal, biliary or pancreatic duct obstruction and/or pain), it is best to achieve histological diagnosis and treatment by one and the same procedure: an appropriate resection. If this can be done with reasonably low risk for the patient, then it is indeed justifiable to say that 'the best biopsy is resection' (Grieco et al 1980, Porter 1985).

REFERENCES

Grieco M B, Braasch J W, Rossi R L 1980 Mass in the head of the pancreas. Surgical Clinics of North America 60: 33
Jordan G L Jr 1987 Operative decisions. In: Howard J M, Jordan G L Jr, Reber H A (eds) Surgical diseases of the pancreas. Lea and Febiger, Philadelphia, p 657–665
Porter M R 1958 Carcinoma of the pancreatico-duodenal area. Operability and choice of procedure. Annals of Surgery 148: 711–724
Warshaw A L, Gu Z, Wittenberg J, Waltman A C 1990 Preoperative staging and assessment of resectability of pancreatic cancer. Archives of Surgery 125: 230–233

15. Intraoperative ultrasonography

J. Machi   B. Sigel

INTRODUCTION

Recent advances in various imaging methods have improved the accuracy of preoperative diagnostic evaluation of pancreatic diseases. Intraoperative imaging can provide further diagnostic information. During pancreatic operations, operative pancreatography and ultrasonography may prove useful methods of assessment. Operative pancreatography is discussed in Chapter 28, and the remainder of this chapter will be devoted to consideration of ultrasonography. High-resolution ultrasonography appears to be a useful imaging technique that is easily applicable (Sigel et al 1984, 1985, 1987, Norton et al 1985, Smith et al 1985, Klotter et al 1987, Machi 1987, Plainfosse et al 1987, Sigel 1988, Angelini et al 1989). We have used ultrasonography during pancreatic surgery for more than 10 years (Sigel 1988, Machi & Sigel 1989, Zaren et al 1989a, b, Machi et al 1990). In this chapter we report our experience of the techniques, indications and benefits of intraoperative ultrasonography, and report on our clinical results obtained during surgery of the pancreas. A new imaging method, intraoperative colour Doppler imaging, is also described (Zaren et al 1989a, b).

INSTRUMENTATION AND TECHNIQUES

A high-frequency real-time B-mode ultrasound system is the instrument of choice for intraoperative ultrasonography. Ultrasound transducers of 5–10 MHz (most frequently 7.5 MHz) are employed during pancreatic surgery and provide high-resolution images (Fig. 15.1). Small intraoperative probes with different shapes are available (e.g. flat, side-viewing, and pencil-like front-viewing probes). Recently, a colour Doppler imaging system that demonstrates blood flow in colour on real-time images has been introduced for intraoperative use (Fig. 15.2).

The pancreas can be scanned through the stomach, the gastrocolic ligament, or the transverse mesocolon, immedi-

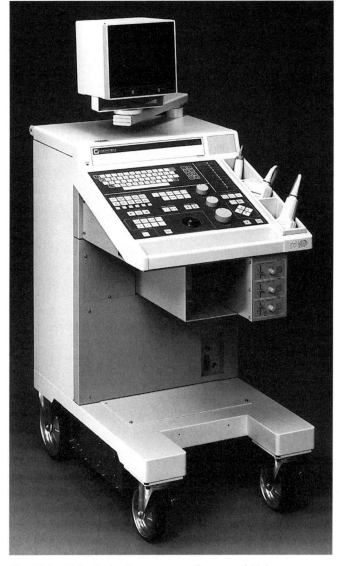

Fig. 15.1 Aloka duplex B-scan system. Courtesy of Aloka.

ately after laparotomy. However, the best imaging of the pancreas is obtained by direct scanning after exposure of

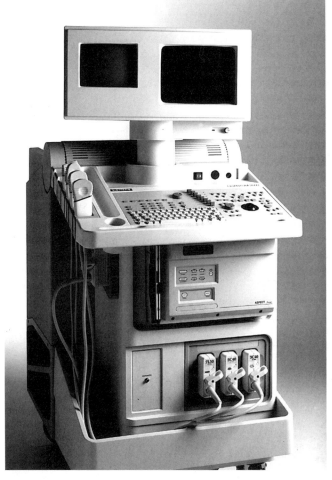

Fig. 15.2 Quantum colour Doppler imaging system. Courtesy of Quantum Medical Systems, Inc.

the organ. The pancreas should be examined thoroughly from head to tail by both transverse and longitudinal scanning. The pancreatic head may also be imaged from the right side after performance of a Kocher manoeuvre. In addition to contact scanning, probe-standoff scanning should be performed (after pouring saline solution into the abdominal cavity) in order to clearly visualize the superficial surface of the pancreas. The normal main pancreatic duct is almost always demonstrated by intraoperative scanning. With the use of colour Doppler imaging, blood vessels around the pancreas can be readily delineated and evaluated.

INDICATIONS AND BENEFITS

Intraoperative ultrasonography is indicated during pancreatic surgery for the complications of pancreatitis, pancreatic cancer, and islet cell tumour. It can provide accurate imaging information with which to detect, localize, or exclude complications of pancreatitis, such as pseudocyst, abscess, pancreatic duct dilatation, biliary duct calculi

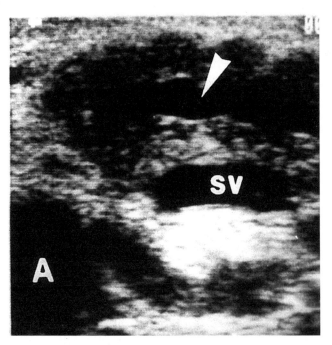

Fig. 15.3 Pancreatic duct dilatation in chronic pancreatitis (Machi 1987). The main pancreatic duct (arrowhead) of the body of the pancreas was moderately dilated; however, it was not palpated from the pancreatic surface. SV, splenic vein behind the pancreas; A, aorta.

and stenosis, or portal vein thrombosis. Operative imaging may detect associated problems, such as a second pseudocyst that was not recognized preoperatively. Intraoperative ultrasonography localizes precisely dilated ducts or cystic lesions that cannot be palpated during an operation because of dense inflammation (Fig. 15.3). An exploratory needle can be guided into these structures

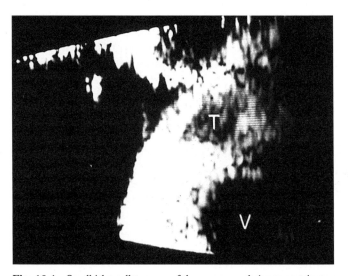

Fig. 15.4 Small islet cell tumour of the pancreas. A 4 mm gastrinoma (T) was detected in the tail of the pancreas by intraoperative ultrasonography. The tumour exhibited a characteristic hypoechoic appearance compared to surrounding pancreatic tissue. This tumour was not localized with preoperative imaging studies. V, splenic vein. (Reprinted, with permission of Annals of Surgery, from Sigel et al 1984 The role of imaging ultrasound during pancreatic surgery, 200:486.)

under ultrasound imaging, thereby facilitating aspiration or internal drainage of these abnormalities. In the presence of pancreatic tissue swelling, intraoperative ultrasonography is also helpful in excluding the presence of a pseudocyst or duct dilatation.

During operations for pancreatic cancer, intraoperative ultrasonography demonstrates the extent of tumour spread to involve the portal system, lymph nodes, and liver more accurately than preoperative studies. This ultrasound information helps to stage the tumour and to select the type of operation to perform, prior to extensive tissue dissection. Intraoperative biopsy of primary or metastatic tumours such as liver metastases can be carried out safely under operative ultrasound guidance, thus avoiding a blind biopsy which may be associated with complications such as bleeding or pancreatic fistula.

Surgical management of islet cell tumours (including insulinomas and gastrinomas) is also improved by the use of intraoperative ultrasonography. Islet cell tumours as small as 4 mm are identifiable by high-resolution ultrasonography (Fig. 15.4). Even non-palpable tumours can be precisely localized, thus facilitating less invasive operations such as tumour enucleation, and so avoiding extensive procedures such as blind pancreatic resection. Multiple tumours can be diagnosed or excluded by thorough scanning of the entire pancreas.

Intraoperative ultrasonography is further enhanced by the use of colour Doppler imaging, which provides precise information regarding vascular structures within and around the pancreas. For example, small blood vessels, such as

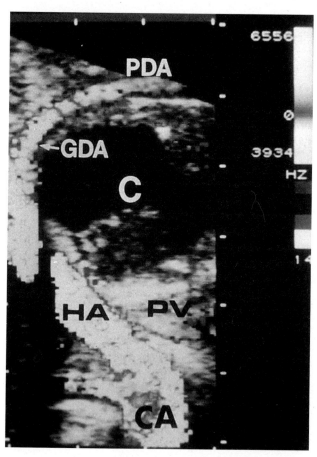

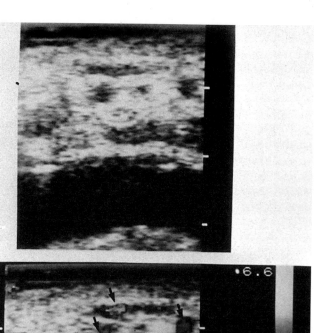

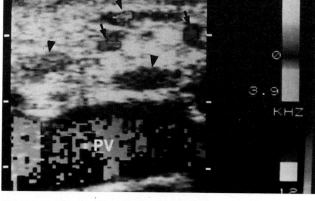

Fig. 15.5 Intraoperative colour Doppler imaging of the vascular structures around the pancreatic head during an operation for a pancreatic pseudocyst. The pseudocyst (C) contained debris. The course of the coeliac artery (CA) was clearly demonstrated; the common hepatic artery (HA), gastroduodenal artery (GDA) and pancreaticoduodenal artery (PDA) and their relationship to the pseudocyst were delineated. Usually, small blood vessels such as the pancreaticoduodenal artery cannot be visualized well with B-mode imaging. PV, portal vein. (Reprinted, with permission of Dynamic Cardiovascular Imaging, from Zaren et al 1989a Operative color Doppler imaging of pancreatic pseudocysts, 2:49–51.) This figure is reproduced in colour in the plate section at the front of the volume.

Fig. 15.6 The use of colour Doppler imaging to distinguish blood vessels from tissue spaces during operation. Pancreatitis causes tissue swelling associated with multiple spaces between tissues due to inflammation. It is often difficult to identify small blood vessels in these tissues with B-mode ultrasonography as seen in the upper print. However, intraoperative colour Doppler imaging which demonstrates blood flow in vessels enables distinction between blood vessels (arrows) and tissue spaces (arrowheads) as seen in the lower print. PV, portal vein. (Reprinted, with permission of Dynamic Cardiovascular Imaging, from Zaren et al 1989a Operative color Doppler imaging of pancreatic pseudocysts, 2:49–51.) This figure is reproduced in colour in the plate section at the front of the volume.

the pancreaticoduodenal artery can be delineated (Fig. 15.5). Tissue spaces associated with pancreatic inflammation (pancreatitis) are readily distinguished from blood vessels (Fig. 15.6). Pancreatic cancer invasion or tumour encasement is more clearly demonstrated with intraoperative colour Doppler imaging (Fig. 15.7). Tiny, intratumoural vessels are also depicted (Fig. 15.8), and this information is helpful for avoiding bleeding complications during needle biopsy.

RESULTS OF INTRAOPERATIVE ULTRASONOGRAPHY

Over a period of 10 years, we have performed intraoperative ultrasonography during a total of 232 pancreatic operations: 139 operations for chronic pancreatitis; 19 operations for acute pancreatitis; 61 operations for pancreatic cancer; 10 operations for islet cell tumours, and 3 operations for pancreatic trauma. Intraoperative ultrasonography was deemed useful in 72.4% of pancreatic operations (Table 15.1). The benefits provided by intraoperative ultrasonography for pancreatic surgery included acquisition of new information (146 operations), guidance of surgical manipulation (80 operations), confirmation of completion of operation (12 operations), and complementing or replacing operative contrast radiography (6 operations) (Sigel et al 1984, 1985, 1987, Machi & Sigel 1989).

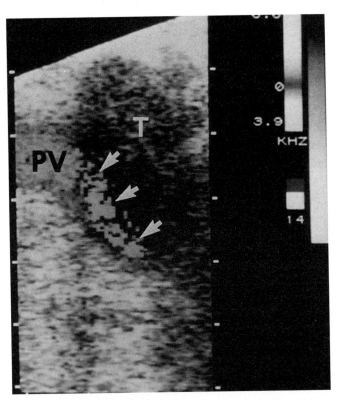

Fig. 15.7 Pancreatic head cancer with invasion of the portal vein. Preoperative studies failed to diagnose tumour involvement of the vein. Intraoperative colour Doppler imaging immediately after laparotomy demonstrated tumour (T) encasement of the portal vein (PV) causing vessel stenosis (arrows), indicative of tumour invasion (Reprinted, with permission of Dynamic Cardiovascular Imaging, from Zaren et al 1989b Operative color Doppler imaging of carcinoma of the pancreas, 2:100–103.) This figure is reproduced in colour in the plate section at the front of the volume.

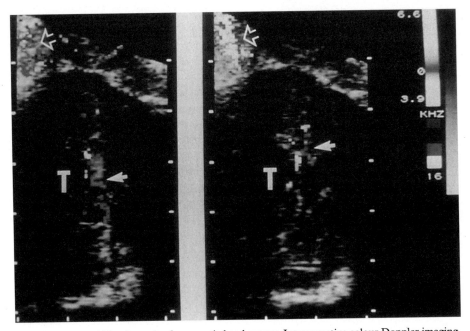

Fig. 15.8 Intratumural blood vessels of pancreatic head cancer. Intraoperative colour Doppler imaging delineated many tiny vessels (arrows) in the tumour (T). Usually, such small intratumoral vessels cannot be depicted with B-mode ultrasonography. This tumour caused complete obstruction of the portal system, and multiple collateral portal tributaries (open arrows) were seen around the pancreas. (Reprinted, with permission of Dynamic Cardiovascular Imaging, from Zaren et al 1989b Operative color Doppler imaging of carcinoma of the pancreas, 2:100–103.) This figure is reproduced in colour in the plate section at the front of the volume.

Table 15.1 Results of intraoperative ultrasonography during pancreatic surgery

Disease	Number of operations	Useful applications of intraoperative ultrasound (%)
Pancreatitis	158	116 (73.4)
Pancreatic cancer	61	43 (70.5)
Islet cell tumour	10	7 (70.0)
Pancreatic trauma	3	2 (60.7)
Total	232	168 (72.4)

CONCLUSION

Intraoperative ultrasonography with high-resolution instruments provides useful information in more than 70% of pancreatic operations. The precise anatomical information obtained by intraoperative ultrasonography facilitates safe and definitive surgical treatment of the complications of pancreatitis. Unsuspected associated conditions, such as a second pseudocyst, may be discovered by intraoperative ultrasound. Evaluating the extent of tumour spread can be aided by intraoperative ultrasonography thereby facilitating decision-making for selection of the best procedure during pancreatic cancer operations. Ultrasonography is currently the most sensitive method for the intraoperative detection and localization of islet cell tumours of the pancreas. Various pancreatic procedures can be guided by intraoperative ultrasonography (Machi et al 1990). Colour Doppler imaging is a new intraoperative ultrasound technique that is particularly useful for demonstrating the vasculature in and around the pancreas. Intraoperative ultrasonography is, therefore, a valuable means for improving the outcome of pancreatic surgery.

REFERENCES

Angelini L, Bezzi M, Tucci G et al 1989 The ultrasonic detection of insulinomas during surgical exploration of the pancreas. World Journal of Surgery 11: 642–647

Klotter H J, Ruckert K, Kummerle F, Rothmund M 1987 The use of intraoperative sonography in endocrine tumors of the pancreas. World Journal of Surgery 11: 635–641

Machi J 1987 Operative ultrasonography – fundamentals and clinical applications. (In Japanese.) Life Science Co Ltd, Tokyo

Machi J, Sigel B 1989 Overview of benefits of operative ultrasonography during a ten-year period. Journal of Ultrasound in Medicine 8:647–652

Machi J, Sigel B, Kurohiji T, Zaren H A, Sariego J 1990 Operative ultrasound guidance for various surgical procedures. Ultrasound in Medicine and Biology 16:33–42

Norton J A. Sigel B. Baker A R. et al 1985 Localization of an occult insulinoma by intraoperative ultrasound. Surgery 97:381–384

Plainfosse M C, Bouillot J L, Rivaton F, Vaucamps P, Hernigou A,. Alexandre J H 1987 The use of operative sonography in carcinoma of the pancreas. World Journal of Surgery 11:654–658

Sigel B, Machi J, Ramos J R, Duarte B, Donahue P E 1984 The role of imaging ultrasound during pancreatic surgery. Annals of Surgery 200:486–493

Sigel B, Machi J, Anderson K W et al 1985 Operative sonography of the biliary tree and pancreas. Seminars in Ultrasound, CT and MR 6:2–14

Sigel B, Machi J, Kikuchi T, Anderson K W, Horrow M, Zaren H A 1987 The use of ultrasound during surgery for complications of pancreatitis. World Journal of Surgery 11:659–663

Sigel B 1988 Operative ultrasonography, 2nd edn. Raven Press, New York

Smith S J, Vogelzang R L, Donavan J, Atlas S W, Gore R M, Heiman H L 1985 Intraoperative sonography of the pancreas. American Journal of Radiology 144:557–562

Zaren H A, Sariego J, Clarke L E et al 1989a Operative color Doppler imaging of pancreatic pseudocysts. Dynamic Cardiovascular Imaging 2:49–51

Zaren H A, Sariego J, Machi J et al 1989b Operative color Doppler imaging of carcinoma of the pancreas. Dynamic Cardiovascular Imaging 2:100–103

16. Intraoperative needle aspiration and biopsy

E. Bodner   K. Glaser

THE NEED FOR BIOPSY IN PANCREATIC SURGERY

A clear indication is the most important precondition for high quality surgery, especially in elective interventions; this becomes more important if surgery is associated with a high risk of postoperative morbidity and mortality. Therefore decision-making in curative tumour surgery has to be based on an exact, microscopically confirmed diagnosis of the lesion. This dictum is especially true for masses of the pancreas, since not only the preoperative findings, but also the intraoperative exploration may not enable one to distinguish chronic inflammation from a neoplastic process.

The smaller the tumour, the more important is the microscopic diagnosis. An early cancer submitted to radical surgery has a potential chance, although small, for cure whereas a Whipple resection may be contraindicated if the lesion proves to be benign. On the other hand, it can be argued that the indications for surgical exploration in most neoplastic pancreatic lesions should be somewhat broader and that a definite preoperative diagnosis is not essential. Laboratory tests and the findings obtained by modern diagnostic imaging methods may be sufficient to indicate that at least a bilioenteric anastomosis is advisable and feasible. However, before the final intraoperative decision for pancreatic resection is made, the diagnosis of pancreatic cancer should be confirmed microscopically.

Additionally, the case for pancreatic biopsy as the basis for intraoperative decision-making is supported by the following considerations:

1. In the case of pancreatic cancer, resection should be carried out according to oncosurgical criteria with systematic regional lymphadenectomy.

2. Multimodal therapy (for example, adjuvant external radiotherapy, chemotherapy or intraoperative irradiation) can only be undertaken on the basis of a proven diagnosis.

3. Chronic inflammatory diseases should be managed by non-resectional measures if possible.

4. If resection is not undertaken, a scientific evaluation of patient outcome is impossible without microscopical diagnosis.

Despite these arguments, many surgeons do not obtain a pancreatic biopsy as a routine (Gudjonsson et al 1978). This may reflect the pitfalls connected with the method.

PROBLEMS WITH PANCREATIC BIOPSY

The main criteria which determine the value of different methods of pancreatic biopsy are:

a. the likelihood of obtaining representative tissue samples
b. the degree of diagnostic accuracy in the microscopic assessment of the biopsy material
c. the time needed for the whole diagnostic procedure (intraoperative frozen section or cytology)
d. the danger of complications connected with the biopsy of pancreatic tissue.

The circumstances are especially difficult in pancreatic cancer since, due to chronic duct congestion and induration of the surrounding tissue, the macroscopic appearances can closely resemble those of chronic pancreatitis. Furthermore, in the presence of chronic inflammation, the tumour itself may be difficult to localize by mere palpation. Accordingly, the original method of wedge biopsy did not prove to be successful in that the results were unreliable and biopsy was associated with a significant risk of bleeding, fistula formation and pancreatitis (Schultz & Sanders 1963, Lightwood et al 1976).

The surgeon's fear of such complications remained unchanged with the advent of core needle biopsy using the Vim-Silverman or Trucut needle, and this prevented their general acceptance and application. A transduodenal or transcholedochal approach to the pancreatic mass is generally recommended. A cylinder-shaped tissue specimen of 1.6 mm in diameter can be extracted for frozen section examination. Publications in the literature on microscopic assessment show considerable variation in diagnostic accuracy and risk of complications following core needle

153

biopsies (Isaacson et al 1974, Beazley 1981, Weiss et al 1982, Hermanek 1983).

In the early seventies, the method of fine-needle aspiration cytology (FNAC), which at that time had already been in use for tumours of the thyroid, breast and prostate, was put to the test in pancreatic cancer (Arnesjö et al 1972, Bodner 1973). On account of the much-reduced tissue trauma associated with use of a fine needle, a minimal complication rate was expected. That in itself would have meant a major advantage over conventional core biopsy procedures, especially if the diagnostic accuracy was as good. A modification of Papanicolaou staining allowed adaptation of FNAC for rapid intraoperative fine-needle cytological investigations (Lederer & Bodner 1976). Furthermore, microscopic tumour diagnosis in FNAC proved to be at least equal to that of conventional biopsy and major complications concerning the method were not observed for a long time (Bodner & Lederer 1976, Ihse et al 1979, Beazley 1981, Sellner & Jelinek 1984, Soreide et al 1985).

FINE-NEEDLE ASPIRATION CYTOLOGY

Equipment

A standard 20 ml syringe topped with a fine needle (outer diameter 0.7 mm) is sufficient. A special device for fixation of the syringe is recommended in that it enables one to perform the FNAC with one hand, while the other is free to fix the tumour.

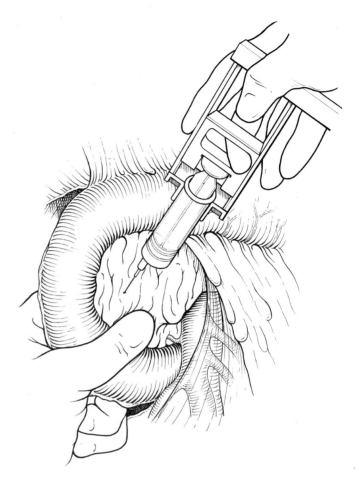

Fig. 16.1   Technique of fine-needle aspiration cytology.

Operative technique

At first the pancreas has to be explored surgically to localize and expose the most suspicious part of the gland. For carcinomas of the head of the pancreas, this includes a Kocher manoeuvre to give the probing hand access to the dorsal aspect of the head of the gland. The most appropriate position for the needle puncture can be selected and the needle is advanced into the tumour (Fig. 16.1) from any suitable direction or through the duodenal wall. During maximum aspiration the needle is quickly moved back and forth for a few seconds. Care is taken that the aspiration is discontinued before withdrawal of the needle from the tissue, otherwise the aspirate will be spread on to the syringe walls, making it difficult to expel.

The aspirate is immediately expelled on to a slide and carefully smeared out using a second slide. Squashing of the aspirate during smearing should be strictly avoided because the morphology of the cell complexes will be destroyed, possibly simulating pleomorphism. The smears are then fixed with ether-alcohol or cyto-spray. In our own experience, air-drying of the specimens is much less satisfactory. In general, more than one puncture is carried

out (2–5) and all slides are forwarded to the pathologist for staining and cytological evaluation.

Staining procedure

Different staining methods can be used, e.g. the modified Papanicolaou procedure (Lederer & Bodner 1976), as well as staining with haematoxylin and eosin. The staining process using the special modifications takes about 5–8 minutes. A different technique has been recommended by Ihse et al (1979).

Cytological judgement

Microscopic diagnosis in specimens obtained by fine-needle aspiration is based on cytological criteria. Most of the time, pancreatic cancer smears will contain malignant cells together with ductal epithelia and cell clusters, allowing some evaluation according to histological criteria. Infiltrative tumour growth, however, cannot be assessed in cytodiagnosis. An admixture of blood makes specimens unsuitable for evaluation.

Assessment of form and diameter of nuclei is of major importance and a strong nuclear polymorphism is the most reliable indicator of malignancy (Fig. 16.2). Experienced pathologists can even grade the micromorphological tumour type. As in histological frozen sections, highly differentiated tumours may cause difficulties in assessment. On the other hand, atypical and rare pancreatic neoplasms can be identified very reliably (Ihse et al 1979, Bodner et al 1982, Foote et al 1986, Gupta et al 1989). In the case of chronic pancreatitis the specimens contain only inflammatory cells, blood and cellular detritus.

RESULTS OF FNAC

Diagnostic accuracy of cytodiagnosis

From 1972 to 1989, intraoperative FNAC was carried out in 414 of our patients with pancreatic tumours. In 359 out of 414 cases, a reliable diagnosis was achieved in addition to cytological diagnosis, i.e. resection specimens in 199 patients; conventional biopsy (wedge excision) from the tumour or metastases in 118 patients; in 13 patients through autopsy findings; in 8 cases by the intraoperative finding of liver metastases, and in 21 patients who were followed up for more than 3 years, thus excluding malignant disease.

Table 16.1 shows the final diagnosis in those 359 patients. The frequency of the different tumour subtypes is consistent with the distribution found in collective studies published in the literature (Ihse et al 1979, Eggert et al 1984, Soreide et al 1985). According to the report provided by the pathologist, in 11 out of 359 patients, the fine-needle specimens were not suitable for cytological

Table 16.1 Experience of intraoperative fine-needle aspiration cytology in pancreatic tumours (II Universitätsklinik für Chirurgie, Innsbruck)

Total number of cases (until 1989)	414
Number with proven diagnosis	359
Pancreatic carcinoma	207
Periampullary carcinoma	63
Carcinoma of the papilla	13
Pancreatic metastasis	7
Retropancreatic tumour	8
Lymphoma	1
Insulinoma	1
Chronic pancreatitis	59

evaluation because there was too much blood or too many mucinous epithelial cells; however, no specific tumour or pancreatic cells were present. This probably reflects technical problems in tissue sampling during the initial learning period, but since intraoperative repetition of FNAC is always possible, this should not constitute a major problem.

To assess the accuracy of intraoperative FNAC in the differentiation of malignant and non-malignant masses of the pancreas, 348 patients are available for analysis. The cytodiagnostic findings are listed in Table 16.2

In our patient population the sensitivity of FNAC for a positive test of malignancy is 0.95 and its specificity is 0.92, underlining the impressive quality of the method. Comparable accuracy is also reported in the literature even though a relatively wide range is observed (Table 16.3). One has to bear in mind that almost all published papers report early experiences with FNAC, and that both surgeon and pathologist were still in the learning

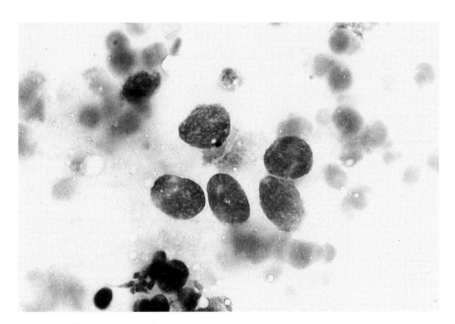

Fig. 16.2 Haematoxylin and eosin stained smears of a ductal pancreatic cancer showing the typical enlarged and irregular nuclei with a high chromatin content.

Table 16.2   Results of fine-needle aspiration cytology (FNAC) in pancreatic masses (II Universitätsklinik für Chirurgie, Innsbruck)

	FNAC positive	FNAC negative	Total
Definitive diagnosis			
Malignant	283	14	297
Not malignant	4	47	51
Total	287	61	348

phase of their part of the procedure. This fact may explain the published reports which have results that are less encouraging than our own experience. In our institution, most of the patients were operated upon by the same surgeon, especially skilled in the field of pancreatic cancer, and cytological assessments have been evaluated and further developed since the beginning of the 1970s.

It is accepted that histological diagnosis gives excellent results in the hands of skilled pathologists. The results published by Hermanek (1983), obtained from Trucut biopsy material of the pancreas indicate tremendous expertise. Nevertheless, false negative frozen section judgements were made in 1.6% of patients when compared with assessment based on the final resection specimens. Furthermore, in 2 out of 438 patients with disease classified as non-malignant, the clinical course surprisingly revealed the presence of carcinoma. Due to the absence of full follow-up data, it is possible that there were further false negative results.

Incorrect negative findings in cytodiagnosis are mostly due to aspiration of unrepresentative material when small carcinomas are not sampled by the needle tip.

False positive diagnosis is caused by atypia of the ductal epithelium occurring in the framework of regeneration in chronic pancreatitis.

In about 80% of all patients with pancreatic masses, the diagnosis is already certain from clinical features (medical history, diagnostic imaging methods, intra-operative findings). In many cases, resection of the tumour appears technically impossible, and the question of resection does not arise. However, intraoperative FNAC should not only be performed in diagnostically uncertain cases; it should be carried out in all pancreatic tumours so as to increase the experience of the surgeon and pathologist and so ensure accurate diagnosis on every occasion (Sellner & Jelinek 1984). During the first 15 years after the introduction of FNAC, we have made an effort to puncture every pancreatic cancer or suspected malignancy, without exception.

We should emphasize that our patient population is preselected and that the incidence of malignant tumours is high, as shown by a prevalence of 0.85. This also influences the positive predictive value which is 0.986, close to 100%.

A diagnostic method has to be reliable if it is to serve the surgeon as a basis for therapeutic decisions with considerable consequences for the patient. Therefore, the accuracy of FNAC must be compared to the histology of the resected tumours. We were able to do this in 199 patients (Table 16.4). For these cases a sensitivity of 0.94, a specificity of 0.86, a positive predictive value of 0.98 and a negative predictive value of 0.69 was calculated. The prevalence amounts to 0.86, but patients with the clinical appearance of chronic pancreatitis without suspicion of malignancy were only submitted to FNAC exceptionally.

In 11 patients with false negative cytology, intra-operative FNAC was not repeated due to the unequivocal intraoperative macroscopic appearance of malignancy. On the other hand, resection was clinically indicated in the 4 patients with non-malignant masses of the pancreas who had a false positive cytological assessment, so that the cytological findings were not relevant in reaching the decision to resect the pancreatic mass.

The accuracy of FNAC of the pancreas for resected cases is quite similar to that of the overall patient population. As yet this has not been confirmed for all other conventional methods of biopsy and diagnosis.

Risk of complications

Each method of tissue sampling has a certain complication rate. Following conventional biopsy, bleeding, pancreatitis,

Table 16.3   Proportion of correct results reported for intraoperative fine-needle aspiration cytology (FNAC) in pancreatic malignancies

Authors	FNAC positive (%)
Arnesjö et al (1972)	16/18 (88.9)
Koivuniemi et al (1972)	68/75 (90.7)
Forsgren & Orell (1973)	28/29 (96.6)
Akashi et al (1974)	44/46 (95.7)
Shorey (1975)	18/18 (100.0)
Hastrup et al (1978)	17/19 (89.5)
Kline & Neal (1978)	39/41 (95.1)
Decker & Lloyd (1979)	15/17 (88.2)
Ihse et al (1979)	65/75 (86.7)
Schick et al (1980)	10/11 (90.7)
Willems & Löwenhagen (1980)	18/22 (81.8)
Eggert et al (1984)	52/65 (80.0)
Keighley et al (1984)	42/46 (91.3)
Soreide et al (1985)	54/76 (71.1)

Table 16.4   Results of intraoperative fine-needle aspiration cytology (FNAC) in resectable pancreatic tumours (II Universitätsklinik für Chirurgie, Innsbruck)

	FNAC positive	FNAC negative	Total
Definitive diagnosis			
Malignant	160	11	171
Not malignant	4	24	28
Total	164	35	199

fistulae, abscesses and pancreatic ascites have all been observed.

Most reports on FNAC (Ihse et al 1979, Beazley 1981, Sellner & Jelinek 1984, Soreide et al 1985), including our own publications (Bodner 1986), emphasize the absence of complications as a major advantage of the method. Recently, we have observed abscess formation in the right upper abdomen in one of our patients subsequent to intraoperative FNAC from the pancreatic head. The abscess required drainage by incision and must almost certainly be ascribed to FNAC. In the 215 patients who underwent FNAC (with an average of 2–3 punctures per patient) and in whom the site of puncture was left in situ, this has been the only clinically relevant complication that has occurred.

Meanwhile, complications following FNAC have been reported in the literature (Table 16.5). The first two reports in Table 16.5 were from the same institution and described cases of pancreatitis after percutaneous FNAC with a lethal outcome in one patient. Of three other complications following intraoperative FNAC, two patients needed surgical reintervention, while in one patient (Rosenbaum & Frost 1990) a pancreatic fistula subsided spontaneously. In one further case, haemorrhage from the puncture site had to be oversewn, thus preventing a postoperative complication (Eggert et al 1984). Eggert et al (1984) observed an elevation of urine amylase levels in 25% of patients undergoing FNAC of the pancreas, but this is of uncertain clinical significance.

The risk of tumour cell spread by intraoperative FNAC seems to be of no clinical relevance according to the collective experience (Ihse et al 1979). Needle-tract seeding of tumour cells with implantation metastases in the outer subcutaneous puncture site has been observed after percutaneous FNAC (Ferrucci et al 1979, see Ch. 12). We have seen such a late complication in one patient, in the epigastric region 2 months after percutaneous FNAC of an inoperable carcinoma of the body of the gland. The implantation metastasis presented as a subcutaneous indolent lump 5 mm in diameter. Two

further implantation metastases with a similar macroscopic appearance were seen in the right lower chest wall at the exact location where previous FNAC of liver metastases had been carried out.

CONCLUSION

The rationale for tissue sampling in patients with pancreatic masses is to avoid overtreatment of benign diseases and in particular to help to diagnose small tumours which are clinically difficult to assess, but potentially curable by radical resection.

The publications on FNAC, as well as our own experience which is the largest of any single institution, allow us to claim that this method is suitable for the differentiation of pancreatic masses, and that it is almost never necessary to resect without a confirmed diagnosis. The high diagnostic accuracy, simple and quick application, unhindered access to almost all locations within the gland and low complication rate confirm that FNAC is superior to other forms of conventional biopsy. For the future, it is expected that a combination of FNAC and DNA ploidy assessment of tumour cells will become a valuable measure for prognosis (Weger et al 1991).

When compared to conventional biopsy, FNAC is a relatively new method, the value of which can only be judged after some experience has been acquired by the surgeon in tissue sampling and by the pathologist in cytological assessment. Simultaneous use of intraoperative ultrasonography with exact location of the tumour will undoubtedly reduce the incidence of false negative findings. Furthermore, complications such as accidental puncture of a distended pancreatic duct and subsequent fistula formation can be avoided completely (Klotter et al 1985).

It remains to be clarified whether or not intraoperative FNAC can be replaced by percutaneous fine-needle aspiration biopsy. If the diagnostic accuracy turns out to be comparable to that of open FNAC it must be appreciated that only very favourable cases will be submitted to percutaneous FNAC. The complication risk, at least as far as needle-tract seeding is concerned, is likely to be higher in percutaneous FNAC.

In patients where a preoperative diagnosis will avoid operation (i.e. cases where unresectable lesions do not require palliative surgery or where bile duct drainage can be accomplished with non-surgical methods), percutaneous FNAC is a most valuable means of obtaining a final diagnosis and will lead to a shorter hospital stay and reduce medical costs (Mitty et al 1981). Percutaneous and intraoperative FNAC should be considered as complementary rather than competitive methods.

Table 16.5 Reported complications after fine-needle aspiration cytology (FNAC) of pancreatic tumours

Authors	Complication	Cases
McLoughlin et al (1978)	Pancreatitis*	1
Evans et al (1981)	Necrotizing pancreatitis*	1**
Simms et al (1982)	Pancreatic ascites/fistula	1
Rosenbaum & Frost (1990)	Pancreatic ascites	1
Bodner & Glaser	Parapancreatic abscess	1

* following percutaneous FNAC; ** fatal

REFERENCES

Akashi M, Hemmi T, Kondo N 1974 Pancreatic biopsy. Stomach and Intestine 9:1563–1570

Arnesjö B, Stormby N, Akerman M 1972, Cytodiagnosis of pancreatic lesions by means of fine-needle biopsy during operation. Acta Chirurgica Scandinavica 138:363–369

Beazley R M 1981 Needle biopsy diagnosis of pancreatic cancer. Cancer 47:1685–1687

Bodner E 1973 Das Problem der intraoperativen Abklärung von Pankreaskopftumoren. Langenbecks Archiv für Chirurgie 333:165–190

Bodner E, Lederer B 1976 La biopsie pancréatique peropératoire à l'aiguille fine. Lyon Chirurgical 72:64–67

Bodner E, Schwamberger K, Mikuz G 1982 Cytological diagnosis of pancreatic tumors. World Journal of Surgery 6:103–106

Bodner E 1986 Intraoperative Punktionsdiagnostik. In: Beger H G, Bittner R (eds) Das Pankreaskarzinom, Springer-Verlag, Berlin

Decker A, Lloyd J D 1979 Fine-needle aspiration biopsy in ampullary and pancreatic carcinoma. Archives of Surgery 114:592–595

Eggert A, Lattmann E, Kopf R, Pfeiffer M, Klöppel G 1984 Intraoperative Pankreaspunktionszytologie. Zentralblatt für Chirurgie 109:540–544

Evans W, Ho C, McLoughlin M, Tao L 1981 Fatal necrotizing Pancreatitis following fine-needle aspiration biopsy of the pancreas. Radiology 141:61–62

Ferrucci J T, Wittenberg J, Margolies M N, Carey R W 1979 Malignant seeding of the tract after thin-needle aspiration biopsy. Radiology 130:345–346

Foote A, Simpson J S, Steward R J, Wakefield J St, Buchmann A, Gupta R K. 1986 Diagnosis of the rare solid and papillary epithelial neoplasm of the pancreas by fine needle aspiration cytology. Acta Cytologica 30:519–522

Forsgren L, Orell S 1973 Aspiration cytology in carcinoma of the pancreas. Surgery 73:38–42

Gudjonsson B, Livstone E M, Spiro H M 1978 Cancer of the pancreas. Diagnostic accuracy and survival statistics. Cancer 42:2494–2506

Gupta R K, Wakefield S J, Fauck R, Stewart R J 1989 Immunocytochemical and ultrastructural findings in a case of rare carcinoma of the pancreas with predominance of malignant squamous cells in an intraoperative needle aspirate. Acta Cytologica, 33:153–156

Hastrup J, Thommesen P, Frederiksen P 1978 Pancreatitis and pancreatic carcinoma, diagnosed by peroperative fine-needle aspiration biopsy. Acta Cytologica 21:731–734

Hermanek P 1983 Intraoperative Diagnostik des Pankreascarcinoms. Langenbecks Archiv für Chirurgie 359:289–299

Ihse I, Toregard B M, Akerman M 1979 Intraoperative fine needle aspiration cytology in pancreatic lesions. Annals of Surgery 190:732–734

Isaacson R, Weiland L H, McIlrath D C 1974 Biopsy of the pancreas. Archives of Surgery 109:227–230

Keighley M B, Moore J, Thompson H 1984 The place of fine needle aspiration cytology for the intraoperative diagnosis of pancreatic malignancy. Annals of the Royal College of Surgeons of England 66:405–408

Kline T S, Neal H S 1978 Needle aspiration biopsy: A critical appraisal. Journal of the American Medical Association 239:36–39

Klotter H J, Rückert K, Dzieniszewski G P, Brückner R, Kuhn F P 1985 Sonographiegesteuerte intraoperative Feinnadelaspirationszytologie bei Pankreaserkrankungen. Ultraschall 6:139–143

Koivuniemi A, Lempinen M, Pantzar P 1972 Fine needle aspiration biopsy of the pancreas. Annales Chirurgiae et Gynaecologiae Fenniae 61:273–280

Lederer B, Bodner E 1976 Fine needle cytopathology of the periampullary region. Journal of Abdominal Surgery 18:163–166

Lightwood R, Reber H A, Way L W 1976 The risk and accuracy of pancreatic biopsy. American Journal of Surgery 132:189–194

McLoughlin M J, Ho C J, Langer B, McHattie J, Tao L C 1978 Fine needle aspiration biopsy of malignant lesions in and around the pancreas. Cancer 41:2413–2419

Mitty H A, Efremidis S C, Yeh H C 1981 Impact of fine-needle biopsy on management of patients with carcinoma of the pancreas. American Journal of Radiology 137:1119–1121

Rosenbaum D A, Frost D B 1990 Fine-needle aspiration biopsy of the pancreas complicated by pancreatic ascites. Cancer 65:2537–2538

Schick P, Goldberg I, Nieberg R, State D 1980 Peroperative pancreatic aspiration for evaluating pancreatic disease. American Journal of Surgery 139:851–854

Schultz N J, Sanders R J 1963 Evaluation of pancreatic biopsy. Annals of Surgery 158:1053–1057

Sellner F, Jelinek R 1984 Erfahrungen mit der intraoperativen Feinnadelpunktionszytologie bei Pankreastumoren. Acta Chirurgia Austrica 16:35–38

Shorey B A 1975 Aspiration biopsy of carcinoma of the pancreas. Gut 16:645–647

Simms M H, Tindall N, Allan R N 1982 Pancreatic fistula following operative fine-needle aspiration. British Journal of Surgery 69:548

Soreide O, Skaarland E, Pedersen O M, Larssen T B, Arnesjö B 1985 Fine-needle biopsy of the pancreas: results of 204 routinely performed biopsies in 190 patients. World Journal of Surgery 9:960–965

Weger A R, Glaser K S, Schwab G, Oefner D, Bodner E, Auer G U, Mikuz G 1991 Quantitative nuclear DNA content in fine needle aspirates of pancreatic cancer. Gut 32:325–328

Weiss S M, Skibber J, Dobelbower R R, Whittington R, Rosato F E 1982 Operative pancreatic biopsy. American Surgeon 48:214–216

Willems J S, Löwenhagen T 1980 Aspiration biopsy cytology of the pancreas. Schweizerische Medizinische Wochenschrift 110:845–848

Acute pancreatitis

17. Definition and classification of pancreatitis

D. C. Carter

In 1963 the participants at a symposium held in Marseilles (Sarles 1965) agreed upon a classification of pancreatic inflammatory disease. Four forms of pancreatitis were recognized namely, acute, acute relapsing, chronic relapsing (i.e. chronic pancreatitis with acute exacerbations) and chronic pancreatitis. Diagnostic criteria were not elaborated and formal clinical definitions were not developed. By definition, acute pancreatitis and acute relapsing pancreatitis were followed by a return to clinical and biochemical normality once the precipitating cause for pancreatitis was removed. In the two chronic forms of the disease, pancreatic anatomy and function did not return to normal even if the precipitating causes were eliminated. While the possibility of progression from acute forms to chronic forms of pancreatitis was recognized, this was regarded as rare.

In the years that followed it became apparent that this classification had major limitations, particularly with regard to the difficulty of distinguishing between acute relapsing and chronic relapsing pancreatitis in clinical practice.

CAMBRIDGE–MARSEILLES CLASSIFICATION 1983–1984

Given the limitations of the original Marseilles classification, further symposia were held in 1983 in Cambridge (Sarner & Cotton 1984) and in 1984 in Marseilles (Sarles 1985). These symposia built on the clinical experience acquired with the earlier system and on the increasing body of morphological and functional data obtained following the advent of investigations such as ultrasonography, computed tomography (CT) scanning and endoscopic retrograde pancreatography (ERP). In Cambridge acute pancreatitis was defined as

. . . an acute condition typically presenting with abdominal pain, and usually associated with raised pancreatic enzymes in blood or urine, due to inflammatory disease of the pancreas.

This clinical definition was expanded at the Marseilles meeting to include description of the spectrum of accompanying morphological changes:

In the mild form peripancreatic fat necrosis and interstitial edema can be recognised but, as a rule, pancreatic necrosis is absent. The mild form may develop into severe form with extensive peri- and intrapancreatic fat necrosis, parenchymal necrosis, and hemorrhage. The lesions may be either localised or diffuse. Occasionally, there may be little correlation between the severity of the clinical features and the morphological findings.

It was accepted that after an attack of acute pancreatitis, exocrine and endocrine function might be impaired for a variable time and to a variable extent. While acute pancreatitis may recur, it seldom progresses to chronic pancreatitis and a return to clinical, morphological and functional normality is usual if the primary cause is eliminated and complications do not supervene.

The Cambridge–Marseilles symposia in 1983—1984 abolished the categories of acute relapsing and chronic relapsing pancreatitis. Chronic pancreatitis was defined as

. . . a continuing inflammatory disease of the pancreas, characterised by irreversible morphological change, and typically causing pain and/or permanent loss of function.

It was accepted that not all patients have pain despite morphological evidence of chronic inflammation, and that pain can be recurrent or persistent.

The Marseilles meeting developed descriptions of the morphological changes involved, stressing the irregular sclerosis with accompanying destruction and permanent loss of exocrine parenchyma. The changes may be focal, segmental or diffuse, and calculi may be present. The large and/or small ducts may be dilated and such dilatation is frequently, but not invariably, associated with strictures or intraductal protein plugs which may calcify to produce calculi. Cysts and pseudocysts are common and may or may not communicate with the duct system. The islets of Langerhans are less affected than the acini, at least until the late stages of the disease. According to the predominant structural changes, the Marseilles symposium suggested that three descriptive terms might be employed: chronic pancreatitis with focal necrosis; chronic pancreatitis with segmental or diffuse fibrosis, and chronic pancreatitis with or without calculi. In practice, it is difficult to know whether this categorization has proved useful.

The Marseilles symposium also highlighted a distinct morphological variant of chronic pancreatitis, namely obstructive chronic pancreatitis. This variant is characterized by dilatation of the duct system following obstruction of a major duct by agencies such as scarring or neoplasia. Calculi are uncommon and the affected portion of the gland undergoes diffuse atrophy of the acinar parenchyma with diffuse fibrosis. In contrast to the other forms of chronic pancreatitis, structural and functional changes may show some improvement when the obstruction is relieved. In an important addendum, the revised Marseilles classification (Sarles 1985) indicated that

... the first manifestation of alcoholic chronic pancreatitis may be an episode of clinically acute pancreatitis. In the early phases of alcoholic chronic pancreatitis, exacerbations closely resemble attacks of acute pancreatitis.

The Cambridge meeting also attempted to classify the morphological changes seen with various imaging techniques in chronic pancreatitis (Table 17.1), and agreed international definitions of changes seen on pancreatography have been published in detail (Axon et al 1984).

LIMITATIONS OF THE CAMBRIDGE–MARSEILLES CLASSIFICATION

Although it represented a significant advance, classification of pancreatitis by the Cambridge–Marseilles system still suffers from difficulties in the following areas.

Histopathological data. Histological material with which to underpin the diagnosis is not available in the majority of patients with acute pancreatitis, and in many diagnosed as having chronic pancreatitis.

Unreliability of functional assessment. It is generally accepted that tests of exocrine pancreatic function are insensitive and will fail to detect anything less than moderately severe or marked functional impairment. Many centres no longer use pancreatic exocrine function tests, relying on clinical assessment to determine whether steatorrhoea is present or absent.

Serum amylase determination. The well-recognized problem of the shortcomings of serum amylase determination in the diagnosis of acute pancreatitis is dealt with in detail elsewhere (p. 196).

Variability of function. As indicated earlier, exocrine and endocrine function may be impaired to a variable degree and for a variable period after an attack of acute pancreatitis. It follows that sequential assessment over a period of many months may be needed before it can be accepted that function has been impaired irreversibly.

Morphological data. This may be lacking, as although the three key imaging techniques (endoscopic retrograde pancreatography (ERP), ultrasonography and CT scanning) are now readily available in most hospitals, they are not yet available universally. Furthermore, even in specialist centres, ERP is not always successful in outlining the duct system in patients thought to have chronic pancreatitis.

Lack of correlation between assessments. The lack of correlation between clinical, morphological, functional

Table 17.1 Grading of chronic pancreatitis by imaging methods*

	Endoscopic retrograde pancreatography	Ultrasound (US) or computed tomography (CT)
Normal	Good quality study visualizing the whole gland without abnormal features	Good quality study visualizing the whole gland without abnormal features
Equivocal	<3 abnormal side branches	One or more abnormal feature (see below)
Mild	>3 abnormal side branches	Two or more abnormal features, such as: Main duct enlarged (<4 mm) Gland enlarged (up to twice normal) Cavities <10 mm Duct irregularity Focal acute pancreatitis Parenchymal heterogeneity Increased echogenicity of duct wall Irregularity of head/body contour
Moderate	>3 abnormal side branches and abnormal main duct	As above
Marked	All of above plus one or more of: Large cavity (>10 mm) Gross gland enlargement (> twice normal) Cavities <10 mm Intraduct filling defects Calculi/pancreatic calcification Duct obstruction Severe duct dilatation or irregularity Contiguous organ invasion on US or CT	

*Based on reports by Sarner & Cotton (1984) and Axon et al (1984)

and histopathological assessments remains one of the major obstacles to development of a simple classification system. In acute pancreatitis clinically severe disease is not always associated with major morphological change, while in chronic pancreatitis major functional upset may be present in the face of minor morphological abnormality on pancreatography. It is also well recognized that marked morphological change including calcification may be present without pain, and that many of the changes regarded as typical of chronic pancreatitis can affect the elderly without producing symptoms or overt functional insufficiency.

Inadequate understanding of the aetiology of pancreatitis. Any attempts to refine existing classifications of pancreatitis are restricted by our imperfect understanding of the aetiology and pathophysiological mechanisms involved. In a substantial number of patients with acute pancreatitis, an aetiological factor cannot be identified while the exact role of alcohol in both the acute and chronic forms of the disease remains uncertain. It is becoming apparent that nutritional and dietary factors may be much more important than had been appreciated, and that many patients labelled as having pancreatitis due to alcohol abuse may have underlying metabolic derangements which render the gland more susceptible to damage.

THE PRESENT POSITION

An ideal classification of pancreatitis remains an elusive goal, given the difficulties outlined above. However, there is widespread agreement that it is useful to retain the two main categories of acute pancreatitis and chronic pancreatitis as defined by the Cambridge and Marseilles meetings in 1983 and 1984.

Thus *acute pancreatitis* is defined as an acute condition typically presenting with abdominal pain, usually associated with raised levels of pancreatic enzymes in blood (or urine), and due to an inflammatory disease of the pancreas. Serum amylase elevation (p. 196) seems destined to remain the key diagnostic criterion but as suggested by Frey (1991) the following elements should be included in the classification system:

1. The clinical definition of acute pancreatitis and its complications should be underpinned by radiological investigations (ultrasonography, CT scan and angiography as appropriate). In patients coming to surgery or autopsy,

histological findings can also be included.

2. The aetiology of the acute pancreatitis should be documented, recognizing that in some cases, no cause will be found.

3. An assessment of the severity of the attack should be made using prognostic criteria such as those described by Ranson (Ranson et al 1975) or Imrie (Osborne et al 1981), supplemented by means of the APACHE II scoring system (Larvin & McMahon 1989).

Frey (1991) has summarized a useful clinicopathological subdivision of acute pancreatitis as follows:

- *Acute interstitial pancreatitis* consists of sterile inflammation and oedema of pancreas. Fat necrosis may be present. Peripancreatic tissues may become involved in a persistent inflammatory process or fluid collection. On dynamic CT scanning, uniform enhancement of pancreatic tissue is seen. If needle aspiration is employed no bacteria or necrotic material will be recovered.

- *Acute necrotising pancreatitis* consists of inflammation with devitalized pancreas and/or peripancreatic tissue. Necrosis may be local or diffuse, may result in loss of integrity of the major pancreatic duct, and may be complicated by splenic vein thrombosis. Peripancreatic fluid collections may occur. Dynamic CT scanning will reveal local or diffuse areas of non-enhancement. If needle aspiration reveals bacteria on Gram stain or culture, *infected necrosis* is present.

Some authors also use two additional categories, namely pancreatic pseudocyst and abscess. In my view, these are complications of acute pancreatitis rather than distinct forms of the disease, as discussed in Chapter 23.

Chronic pancreatitis is defined as continuing inflammatory disease of the pancreas characterized by irreversible morphological change and typically causing pain and/or permanent impairment of function. This clinical definition should be underpinned by documentation of morphological changes on imaging as defined in Table 17.1. It is arguable whether tests of pancreatic exocrine function are worthwhile but overt steatorrhoea and the presence of diabetes mellitus should be recorded. As discussed in acute pancreatitis, the aetiological factors should be documented where possible; the pattern, localization and severity of pain should be recorded, and the presence of complications (e.g. pseudocyst, portal hypertension) noted.

REFERENCES

Axon A T R, Classen M, Cotton P B, Cremer M et al 1984 Pancreatography in chronic pancreatitis: international definitions. Gut 25: 1107–1112

Frey C F 1991 Classification of acute pancreatitis. International Journal of Pancreatology 9:39–49

Larvin M and McMahon M J 1989 APACHE II score for assessment and monitoring of acute pancreatitis. Lancet 2: 201–204

Osborne D H, Imrie C W, Carter D C 1981 Biliary surgery in the same admission for gallstone-associated acute pancreatitis. British Journal of Surgery 68: 758–761

Ranson J H, Rifkind K M, Roses D G et al 1975 Prognostic signs and the role of operative management in acute pancreatitis. Surgery, Gynecology and Obstetrics 139: 69–80

Sarles H 1965 Pancreatitis symposium of Marseilles 1963. Karger, Basle

Sarles H 1985 Revised classification of pancreatitis – Marseille. Digestive Diseases and Sciences 30: 573–574

Sarner M, Cotton P B 1984 Classification of pancreatitis. Gut 25: 756–759

18. Aetiology and pathogenesis of acute pancreatitis

J. L. Cameron   J. A. Clemens

INTRODUCTION

The clinical syndrome of acute pancreatitis has been recognized since antiquity and its manifestations well documented since 1856, but its pathogenesis is still not well understood. Although much has been learned of the predisposing risk factors, pathology, and biochemical events within the pancreas through a large number of clinical and experimental studies, the earliest changes in the gland, the so-called initiator or trigger mechanisms, await discovery. Until a better understanding of the pathogenesis is achieved, it is unlikely that specific effective treatment will alter the course of the disease, and management will remain primarily supportive.

Gallstone disease and ethanol are the most important of the clinical scenarios in which acute pancreatitis occurs, accounting for 90% of the cases (Ranson 1979). A number of infrequent clinical presentations are also thought to be associated with the condition, accounting for the remaining 10% of cases. Table 18.1 lists the additional predisposing factors. The clinical disease varies in severity, but the basic response of the pancreas to the injurious stimulus appears to be limited to one or two sequences of events, giving credence to the idea of a 'final common pathway' for the initiation of pancreatitis, despite the disparate predisposing factors. The latter must lead to similar cellular alterations, which are manifest as clinically similar forms of pancreatitis. Any encompassing theory of the pathogenesis of pancreatitis must explain the diversity of the initiating stimuli, the varying clinical and pathological pictures, and the systemic manifestations of the disease. While chronic pancreatitis will not be discussed in this chapter, it may result from repeated attacks of acute pancreatitis. The pathophysiology of this disease appears to be different and a separate discussion is required.

This chapter contains a discussion of the clinical situations which precede or coexist with acute pancreatitis, theories of the cellular and biochemical events which may trigger the local disease and its systemic complications, and a description of the animal models of acute pancreatitis, including their strengths and limitations.

Table 18.1 Clinical associations and acute pancreatitis

Clinical setting	Proposed aetiologies
Alcoholism	Hypersecretion
	Diet
	Hyperlipidaemia
	Direct toxicity
	Hereditary factors
	Free radical production
	Protein plugs
Gallstone disease	Bile reflux
	Duodenal fluid reflux
	Pancreatic duct obstruction
	Free radical production
Familial hyperlipidaemia	Direct toxicity of free fatty acids
Hypercalcaemia	Increased calcium
	Increased parathormone
Familial	Defect of membranes/metabolism
Malnutrition	Unknown
Trauma (external, operative)	Direct injury, duct obstruction
Post endoscopic retrograde cholangio pancreatography	Interstitial extravasation
Haemodynamic	Ischaemia, free radical production
Mechanical duct obstruction	Increased pressure, extravasation
Drug-induced	Direct toxicity, altered secretions
Viral infection	Direct cellular injury
Miscellaneous	Unknown
Idiopathic	Unknown

CLINICAL SCENARIOS

Alcohol-associated pancreatitis

Alcohol has been known to be associated with acute pancreatitis since the 1930s. The incidence varies in different populations, and appears to correlate with the amount of ethanol consumed; it is greater in men, probably related to a greater ethanol intake. There is no evidence that an occasional drinker can develop clinical pancreatitis (Strum & Spiro 1971), and indeed most patients have a history of several years of heavy drinking, either on a daily basis or as 'binge' drinking (Durbec & Sarles 1978).

Many authors have attempted to relate the drinking pattern, type, and amount of alcohol consumed to the eventual risk of developing pancreatitis. Stigendal & Olsson (1984) compared 27 men with alcoholic liver disease and

24 men with alcoholic pancreatitis, and found a more intermittent 'binge' drinking pattern in the individuals with pancreatitis.

Patients with pancreatitis tended to be younger and consume less alcohol than cirrhotics, while the cirrhotics had a longer drinking history, suggesting that the pancreas is more susceptible to the toxic effects of ethanol. However, others have found a greater degree of similarity in the drinking patterns of patients with pancreatitis and cirrhosis (Angelini et al 1985). Although pancreatitis and cirrhosis have been found to correlate in autopsy series (Sobel & Waye 1963, Shader & Paxton 1966), clinically evident pancreatitis and alcoholic cirrhosis rarely occur simultaneously, regardless of the alcohol intake (Dutta et al 1978). The type of alcoholic beverage consumed was not noted to be a factor in the incidence of pancreatitis in a study by Wilson et al (1985). Patients consuming beer, wine, and hard liquor were equally at risk.

A troublesome observation is that the majority of patients who drink excessive ethanol do not, in fact, develop pancreatitis (Wilson et al 1985). Others who consume equivalent amounts of ethanol appear susceptible to the disease, perhaps due to dietary factors or an inherited predisposition.

Malnutrition is a known predisposing factor for pancreatitis independent of alcohol abuse, particularly in third world countries (Wilson et al 1985). While malnourished alcoholics may be at a significantly increased risk, experimental and epidemiological studies in affluent countries suggest more an association with poor dietary composition. Durbec & Sarles (1978) found that alcoholics consume more fat and protein and less carbohydrate than age-matched controls. A dietary predisposition to acute pancreatitis is not universally accepted however.

Several studies have identified genotypes which are associated with alcoholic pancreatitis. An increased frequency of HLA types B40, Aw23, Aw24, and B13 has been found in patients with alcoholic pancreatitis, as well as blood groups O and Le (a-b) (Wilson et al 1984). However, the majority of these studies have compared alcoholic pancreatitis patients to normal non-alcoholic controls, and thus may have been confounded by the known genetic tendency towards alcoholism itself. In a more appropriately controlled study, Wilson found an increased frequency of HLA Bw39 in alcoholics with pancreatitis while alcoholics without pancreatitis did not differ from the general population in HLA frequency.

The mechanism linking particular genotypes with pancreatitis is obscure. Since there is no evidence that cell-mediated or humoral immunity plays a role in the initiation of acute alcoholic pancreatitis, a likely explanation for the association is the close linking of structural genes coding for abnormal enzymes or membrane components with the HLA complex. The enzymatic or membrane alterations presumably would predispose some alcoholics to the development of pancreatitis, and because of the close linking to HLA genes, these patients would show a preponderance of certain HLA types.

Mechanisms of alcohol injury to the pancreas: toxicity

A number of theories have been advanced concerning the mechanism by which ethanol injures the pancreas. Perhaps the simplest is that ethanol or its metabolites are directly toxic to the pancreatic cells. Ethanol is metabolized in the body to acetaldehyde by the enzyme alcohol dehydrogenase. This occurs primarily in the liver, although there may be limited breakdown in the pancreas as well. It is unclear whether the pancreas contains sufficient alcohol dehydrogenase to account for any direct toxicity (Balart & Ferrante 1982), although other toxic metabolic products could be produced. Most experimental studies have failed to demonstrate any direct ethanol toxicity to the pancreas.

By contrast, ethanol does appear to have direct toxicity in the liver where there is an abundance of alcohol dehydrogenase and acetaldehyde production. Acetaldehyde has recently been shown to induce pancreatitis in the isolated perfused canine pancreas, when given directly into the arterial circulation (Nordback et al 1989). Clinically, Bordalo et al (1976) have shown acinar cell damage in alcoholics without clinical pancreatitis, which resembles acetaldehyde-induced hepatic toxicity, including hypertrophy of the smooth endoplasmic reticulum, mitochondrial swelling, and intracellular fat accumulation.

The mechanism of acetaldehyde toxicity may involve oxygen free radical generation by the enzyme xanthine oxidase. Acetaldehyde can serve as a substrate for this ubiquitous enzyme which is thought to be central in several forms of experimental pancreatitis (see below). The pancreas and the liver have high concentrations of xanthine oxidase, and this could perhaps account for preferential ethanol injury to these organs.

Perhaps the oldest theory of the initiation of acute alcohol-induced pancreatitis was advanced by Paxton & Payne (1948) who stressed the secretory state of the gland as a predisposing factor in the development of pancreatic inflammation and oedema. Alcohol stimulates gastric secretion by a direct effect on the mucosa, and the hydrochloric acid produced is itself a potent stimulus for secretin release. Secretin directly stimulates pancreatic secretion and could result in an increase in pancreatic ductal pressure. In addition ethanol may cause chemical duodenitis and ampullitis which could partially obstruct the ampulla of Vater, and further increase intraductal pressure in the pancreas, already stimulated to secrete greater volumes. The resultant high pressures could then result in ductal disruption with extravasation of activated intraluminal enzymes into the interstitium where autodigestion of the gland would occur. This theory has lead to the concept of interruption of secretory stimulation as the standard treatment of acute pancreatitis, but a large number of experimental and clinical studies have failed to confirm this mechanism.

Atempts to inhibit pancreatic secretion. The pressure required to disrupt pancreatic ductules appears to be far above physiological values (Harvey et al 1988), and intragastric ethanol may simply increase pancreatic ductal permeability and allow back-diffusion of activated enzymes into the interstitium without physical disruption of the ducts. A number of treatments aimed at decreasing pancreatic secretion have failed to be of clinical benefit. Nasogastric suction and cimetidine decrease gastric acid output and theoretically should diminish secretin stimulation of the pancreas. Nasogastric suction (Levant et al 1974, Naeije et al 1978, Sarr et al 1986) and H_2 blockers (Meshkinpour et al 1979, Regan et al 1981, Broe et al 1982b) have both failed to improve the clinical course of acute pancreatitis or reduce the mortality rate.

The hormones glucagon and somatostatin directly antagonize the stimulatory effect of secretin, but neither has been effective in patient studies (Kronberg et al 1976, Durr et al 1978, Usadel et al 1980, Lankisch 1984). A long-acting somatostatin analogue, SM201-995, has been efficacious in interrupting bile salt-induced pancreatitis in a dog model when given prophylactically (Augelli et al 1989), but human trials have not yet been conducted.

Atropine is a theoretically appealing treatment for acute pancreatitis, since it blocks cholinergic-induced pancreatic secretion, relaxes the sphincter of Oddi, and inhibits gastric acid secretion. A clinical study of atropine has failed to confirm a beneficial effect however (Cameron et al 1979).

Two other stimulants of pancreatic secretion have slightly different mechanisms of action. While secretin and cholinergic stimulation tend to increase the volume and bicarbonate content of secretions, cholecystokinin (CCK) disproportionately increases the enzyme content of the juice while increasing the volume. There is ample experimental evidence that CCK is detrimental in some models of acute pancreatitis. The hormone caerulein (a CCK analogue) increases pancreatic secretory enzyme content when administered to animals at low doses. At higher, so-called supramaximal doses, pancreatitis develops (Lampel & Kern 1977). It is of note that alcohol itself appears to increase enzyme release and total enzyme content of the gland (Wilson & Pirola 1983), and this could favour activation of zymogens by altering the protease/antiprotease ratio.

Recently a number of synthetic CCK inhibitors have become available, although none has yet been evaluated in a human trial. CCK receptor blockade with the asperlicin analogue L 364,718 (Clemens 1988) and the less specific agent CR1392 (Tani 1988) effectively ameliorate secretagogue-induced experimental pancreatitis.

The effect may be specific for secretagogue-induced pancreatitis however, since these agents were ineffective in a bile salt injection model of pancreatitis (Sjovall et al 1988).

Intraduodenal trypsin exerts an inhibitory effect on pancreatic enzyme secretion via a feedback loop, and oral trypsin supplementation has been proposed as a strategy to decrease pancreatic secretion. There is no evidence to support such an approach in the treatment of pancreatitis, however.

The general failure of therapies aiming to decrease pancreatic secretion has led to abandonment of Paxton & Payne's sequence of hypersecretion, partial obstruction, and ductal disruption as the major pathophysiological events leading to acute alcoholic pancreatitis.

Other proposed mechanisms

A second theory of the generation of alcoholic pancreatitis proposes ethanol-induced spasm of the sphincter of Oddi. This could conceivably simultaneously block the common bile duct and main pancreatic duct creating a 'common channel' similar to the situation that many believe is responsible for gallstone pancreatitis (Wilson & Pirola 1983). Bile reflux into the pancreatic duct might then injure the ductal mucosa and lead to activation of pancreatic zymogens. The most significant argument against this theory is that alcoholic pancreatitis occurs with equal frequency in patients with separate orifices of the pancreatic and biliary ducts, clearly a situation in which biliary reflux does not occur.

A related theory holds that alcohol in fact causes incompetence of the sphincter and this allows duodenal contents to reflux into the pancreatic duct. In fact, a well-established animal model relies on this very mechanism to induce pancreatitis. The duodenum is ligated above and below the ampulla, and as intraduodenal pressure increases, reflux occurs into the pancreatic duct and pancreatitis results. The intraluminal duodenal enzymes are activated by the brush border enzyme enterokinase and would prove much more toxic to the ductal mucosa than bile alone. The relevance of this mechanism to human disease has not been demonstrated however.

Sarles (1974) and Nakamura et al (1972) have postulated a popular theory of the initiation of alcoholic pancreatitis in which protein deposition occurs in the small ductules of the pancreas and obstruction results. Histological examination of diseased human glands has demonstrated protein plugs in the small ductules of the gland and these may be precursors of the calcified stones seen with chronic pancreatitis. The plugs consist of albumin and a low molecular weight protein with a high affinity for calcium (stone protein) (Wilson & Pirola 1983). There is some controversy as to whether the protein plugs precede acute pancreatitis or result secondarily, since they are more prominent in advanced disease. Alcohol has been shown to interfere with solubilization of intraductal proteins by decreasing pancreatic bicarbonate secretion in chronically alcoholic dogs (Noel-Jorand et al 1981, Lohse et al 1981) and citrate is also important in maintaining the solubility of pancreatic secretions. A citrate deficiency in alcoholic patients may predispose to pancreatic stone formation (Wilson & Pirola 1983) although this has not been demonstrated clinically. There is no accepted animal model in which protein deposition in the ductules plays an important role in pancreatitis.

Many alcoholics demonstrate abnormalities of lipid metabolism which may have aetiological significance (Isselbacher & Greenberger 1964). Estimates of the frequency of lipid abnormalities in acute alcoholic pancreatitis have ranged from 4–53% (Cameron et al 1973). Some of these patients in fact, have a recognized hyperlipoproteinaemia syndrome (Table 18.2). Cameron et al (1973) showed that 10 of 48 patients admitted with acute alcoholic and gallstone pancreatitis had lactescent serum with markedly elevated triglycerides with a range of 493–7520 mg/100 ml. An additional eight patients without lactescent serum had triglyceride elevations, although not as severe. A total of 38% of these patients had some degree of triglyceride elevation. Of the 10 patients with lipaemic serum, nine had type V hyperlipidaemia, and the tenth had a type I pattern which reverted to a type V pattern during convalescence. Seven of the eight patients with elevated triglycerides but no lactescence had lipoprotein electrophoresis and four of these had a type IV pattern and two a type I pattern. The remaining patient had a normal electrophoresis. None of 34 control patients admitted for abdominal disease other than pancreatitis had lactescent serum and only three had triglyceride levels exceeding 175 mg/100 ml. Of the 34 control patients, 33 underwent lipoprotein electrophoresis, and only two had hyperlipidaemia patterns, one a type II and one a type IV.

While studies such as these suggest an association of hyperlipidaemia and pancreatitis, the aetiological significance remains controversial. It is possible that pancreatitis causes the hyperlipidaemia or that some third factor is responsible for both. In a second study, Cameron et al (1974) readmitted 22 patients with pancreatitis and hyperlipidaemia 2–24 months after the acute attack. Of the 22, 21 admitted to heavy alcohol consumption and the remaining one had familial hyperlipidaemia. A control group of 23 patients was composed of six normal adults, 12 patients with a history of pancreatitis but without hyperlipidaemia, two diabetics, and three patients with acute non-pancreatic illnesses.

In the study group, 17 of 22 had abnormal lipoprotein electrophoresis (Type I, 2 patients, Type III, 1 patient, Type IV, 8 patients, and Type V, 6 patients). Twenty of these patients had lipoprotein electrophoresis during the earlier admission for acute pancreatitis, and at that time, 18 had a type V pattern and two had a type I pattern. In the control group, 21 of the 23 had normal lipoprotein electrophoresis and two had a type IV pattern. Fasting triglyceride levels were normal in 17 of the 23 control patients but in only six of the study patients.

After a 250 g lipid meal, serum triglycerides exceeded 500 mg/100 ml in one control patient, but a similar elevation was present in 20 of the study group. Two of the study patients developed acute abdominal pain similar to acute pancreatitis after ingestion of the lipid meal. No control patient developed abdominal pain.

This study demonstrates that pre-existent primary lipid disorders are common in patients with pancreatitis, and do not resolve with resolution of pancreatitis. In two patients an acute elevation of serum lipids was associated with abdominal complaints resembling pancreatitis, suggesting that hyperlipidaemia was the primary event.

Pancreatitis occurs in other situations in which serum lipids are elevated. Hazzard et al (1969) demonstrated an increased frequency of pancreatitis in hyperlipidaemic women taking oral birth control medication. Patients with chronic renal failure and hyperlipidaemia may develop acute pancreatitis as well (Brunzell & Schrott 1973). Familial hyperlipidaemias types I and V are strongly associated with attacks of pancreatitis.

Havel (1969) has proposed an explanation of the toxic effects of serum lipids on the pancreas. The pancreas contains a high concentration of the digestive enzyme lipase which hydrolyses triglycerides to glycerol and free fatty acids. Normally serum free fatty acids are bound to albumin and are non-toxic. High local concentrations of free fatty acids may develop locally in the pancreas if elevated serum triglycerides are hydrolysed in the gland by the endogenous lipase. Saturation of albumin binding could then occur with the release of cytotoxic free fatty acids into the gland.

Experimental studies in the isolated perfused canine pancreas confirm that a direct triglyceride or free fatty

Table 18.2   Frederickson's familial hyperlipoproteinaemias

Type	Serum lipid	Electrophoretic pattern	Clinical pattern
I	Triglycerides	Chylomicrons	Childhood onset, hepatosplenomegely pancreatitis
II	Cholesterol	β lipoproteins	Tendinous xanthomas, atherosclerosis
III	Cholesterol, triglycerides	Abnormal β-lipoproteins	Palmar xanthomas, atherosclerosis
IV	Triglycerides	Pre-β lipoproteins	Tuberous xanthomas, atherosclerosis
V	Triglycerides	Pre-β lipoproteins, chylomicrons	Adult onset, pancreatitis.

acid infusion into the arterial supply of the gland is toxic (Saharia et al 1977). Mineral oil, which has similar physical properties but is not hydrolysed to free acids, has no ill effects. Free fatty acid toxicity may occur secondary to a vascular injury with relative ischaemia of the pancreatic tissue (Janes et al 1986, Clemens et al 1989). Recent experimental work in this model has also implicated oxygen derived free radicals as a mechanism of injury (see below). Whether this will prove to have clinical implications remains to be demonstrated.

Gallstone-associated pancreatitis

Gallstone disease is the second major clinical precursor of acute pancreatitis. Its frequency varies with the population under consideration, accounting for 5–57% of all cases of pancreatitis (Durr 1979). Alcoholic disease appears to predominate in the United States as a cause of acute pancreatitis, while gallstones are more frequently responsible in Europe (Trapnell 1968, Ranson 1979). Together, alcohol and gallstones account for about 90% of all cases of acute pancreatitis.

The natural history of patients with gallstone pancreatitis is different from those with alcohol-induced disease. The age and sex distribution of patients with this aetiology parallels the age and sex distribution of gallstones. There is a preponderance of females and older patients when compared with patients with alcoholic pancreatitis (Durr 1979). There is a spectrum of severity, similar to alcoholic pancreatitis, but if the patient recovers, endocrine or exocrine deficiencies are much less likely than in alcoholics. Patients with gallstone pancreatitis seldom have pathological evidence of chronic fibrosis and inflammation, unlike alcoholic disease, and in most cases the gland is normal histologically after clinical recovery (Frey 1981). Gallstone pancreatitis is very likely to recur if the biliary disease is not corrected.

Fluid reflux theories

The association between gallstones and acute pancreatitis was first noted in 1882 by Prince. In an autopsy case he noted impaction of a gallstone in the common bile duct distal to the point of entry of the pancreatic duct creating a 'common channel'. The theory of a common biliary and pancreatic channel was further popularized by Opie (1901), who reported a case of stone impaction in the ampulla distal to the opening of the pancreatic duct on autopsy of a patient of Dr Halsted, who had died of pancreatitis Halsted had discovered a dilated common bile duct at laparotomy and suspected choledocholithiasis but could not palpate a stone in the duct. The patient died 24 hours later and on autopsy Opie demonstrated an impacted stone acting as a ball valve in the distal common bile duct, with a common channel proximal to the obstruction.

Opie proposed that the impacted stone created forcible bile reflux into the pancreatic duct through the common channel, and that this reflux had initiated the pancreatitis. He later supported this theory with experimental injections of bile into the pancreatic duct of dogs which reproducibly initiated pancreatitis.

This theory has now fallen into disfavour since other autopsy studies have failed to demonstrate the expected frequency of impacted ampullary stones in patients dying of pancreatitis. Trapnell (1968) found a common channel in only 50% of patients with gallstone pancreatitis, and in a recent study, Kelly (1974) found that less than 10% of patients dying of gallstone pancreatitis had a stone impacted in the common duct. In an elegant study in 1974, Acosta and Ledesma demonstrated that impaction of a stone in the common bile duct is probably not the crucial event, but rather the passage of a gallstone of a suitable size through the ampulla of Vater. These authors found small gallstones in the stools of 94% of patients with gallstone pancreatitis, whereas only 8% of control patients with cholelithiasis without pancreatitis had stones recovered from the stool. Kelly (1976) repeated this study and found 84% of patients with gallstone pancreatitis had small stones in the stool compared with only 11% of controls with cholelithiasis alone.

In a further study Kelly (1984) examined operative cholangiography in 75 patients undergoing cholecystectomy for gallstone pancreatitis compared with 75 undergoing cholecystectomy for cholelithiasis alone. Reflux of dye from the common bile duct into the pancreatic duct occurred in 67% of those with pancreatitis, compared with only 18% of controls with cholelithiasis alone. Various anatomical features were identified which seemed to predispose to biliary reflux into the pancreatic duct. Stones in the gallbladder or impacted in the common duct (when present) were smaller in the group with pancreatitis. Intraoperative cholangiography demonstrated a large cystic duct in the pancreatitis patients and significantly more of these patients had reflux of contrast into the pancreatic duct than control patients (67 vs. 18%).

Armstrong et al (1985) confirmed these findings in a prospective study of 769 patients undergoing biliary operation for stones; 7.7% of these patient had a history of pancreatitis. Operative cholangiography was performed in every case. Patients with pancreatitis had smaller and more numerous gallbladder stones and a larger cystic duct. Common bile duct stones were found in greater numbers, and the common bile duct tended to be more dilated in the pancreatitis group. Reflux of dye into the pancreatic duct occurred much more frequently in those with pancreatitis (62.3% vs. 14.6% of controls). A common channel (if present) was longer in patients with pancreatitis. Armstrong concluded that these anatomical conditions facilitate migration of small gallstones through an enlarged cystic and common duct into the ampulla, where relative obstruction and reflux of bile into the pancreatic duct could occur through a common channel.

While these anatomical features suggest that reflux of bile into the pancreatic duct may occur in patients with gallstone pancreatitis, the mechanism of toxicity to the pancreas is still unclear. Cholangiography produces supra-physiological biliary pressures which probably have little relevance to clinical pancreatitis. Csendes et al (1979) has reported that maximal pancreatic duct pressures exceed maximal biliary pressures in many patients, and clearly reflux could not occur in this situation even with the common bile duct transiently obstructed, but others believe that straining or coughing can disproportionally raise the common bile duct pressure and promote bile reflux. Experimental studies have shown that bile in the pancreatic duct is relatively innocuous at physiological pressures, and that pancreatitis occurs only when the bile is under supraphysiological pressure (Robinson & Dunphy 1963). The intrapancreatic pressure may be the injurious mechanism, rather than the presence of bile, since even normal saline induces pancreatitis when injected under sufficient pressure.

A second problem with the theory of bile reflux is that activation of pancreatic zymogens is unlikely to occur. Bile alone activates pancreatic proteases but only after prolonged incubation periods of 8–12 hours, too long a period to be produced by transient reflux (Frey 1981). Infected bile can hasten enzyme activation and it is known that 25–50% of patients with chronic cholelithiasis and 75–100% of patients with acute cholelithiasis have bacterial colonization of the bile (Frey 1981). In this situation it is possible that transient reflux of infected bile under near physiological pressures could be deleterious (Keynes 1988).

Duodenal fluid reflux. There remains, however, the most serious objection to the bile reflux theory of gallstone pancreatitis. Apparent gallstone-induced pancreatitis has been reported in patients without an anatomical common pathway, a situation in which bile reflux is clearly impossible. A related theory has been proposed (Tuzhilin et al 1981) to resolve this paradox, namely that repeated passage of small stones through the ampulla leads to fibrosis and incompetence of the sphincter of Oddi, allowing chronic reflux of duodenal fluid into the pancreatic duct. Duodenal juice contains digestive enzymes activated by the brush border enzyme enterokinase and has a high bacterial count, and is probably much more toxic to the pancreas than the sterile non-protease-containing bile. An experimental model of pancreatitis relies on exactly this mechanism to induce pancreatitis. In this model, the duodenum is ligated above and below the pancreatic duct, producing a 'closed loop' which allows reflux of duodenal fluid into the pancreatic duct under high pressure producing severe pancreatitis.

There are several serious objections to this theory, as well. The ampulla is usually normal in patients with gall-stone pancreatitis, not incompetent, and reflux into the pancreatic duct has not been observed. In fact sphincterotomy is often used to treat patients with gallstone pancreatitis or a stenotic ampulla as in pancreas divisum, a situation in which duodenal reflux is facilitated. Patients with chronically incompetent sphincters and gallstones rarely continue to have bouts of acute pancreatitis after cholecystectomy, implicating the gallstones, not reflux, in the disease. Transient sphincter incompetence with reflux from the duodenum after stone passage seems to be less likely than simple transient obstruction.

Obstruction theory

Transient obstruction of the pancreatic duct without bile or duodenal fluid reflux into the duct is an attractive alternative to both theories of gallstone pancreatitis.

Obstruction of Wirsung's duct is associated with acalculous pancreatitis in pancreas divisum and ampullary stenosis. Obstruction of the pancreatic duct can occur without a common channel or even without a common orifice for the two ducts. Even if the pancreatic and common bile ducts open separately into the duodenum, a stone of the proper size passing through the bile duct could compress the adjacent pancreatic duct sufficiently to cause relative obstruction. Presumably, transient pressure increases in Wirsung's duct could lead to extravasation of pancreatic juice into the interstitium of the gland and subsequent injury to the gland. Many cases of clinical gallstone pancreatitis seem to occur after a meal, a situation in which the gallbladder contracts and the pancreas is stimulated to secrete. Such hypersecretion would then enhance pressure increases in a duct partially or completely obstructed by a migrating gallstone and intensify the injury (Broe & Cameron 1982). If the pancreatitis was self-sustaining, later therapeutic manoeuvres to decease pancreatic secretion would be expected to be ineffective. In the isolated perfused canine pancreas model of gallstone pancreatitis, partial obstruction of the secretory duct with secretin stimulation produces pancreatitis comparable to that seen in the clinical setting. Again, the cellular mechanism by which injury might occur is unclear, but free radical generation is involved in several forms of experimental secretory pancreatitis (see discussion below).

Ischaemic pancreatitis

Pancreatic inflammation and necrosis have long been associated with ischaemia, both clinically and in experimental models.

Clinical experience

Langerhans (1890) noted pancreatic necrosis in association with vessel thrombosis in a small autopsy series. In the last decade, reviews of patients incurring periods of shock or low flow have reported an increased incidence of pancreatitis.

Feiner (1976) recorded 34 cases of autopsy-proven pancreatitis amongst 182 patients who died following cardiopulmonary bypass. He suggested that either intraoperative hypotension while on cardiopulmonary bypass or postoperative shock was the initiating stimulus. In a retrospective study, Warshaw & O'Hara (1978) examined the autopsy records of 63 patients dying of a ruptured aortic aneurysm, and noted a 50% incidence of acute pancreatitis in those patients who had concurrent acute tubular necrosis (ATN) compared with a 9% incidence of pancreatitis in cases in which ATN was absent. ATN serves as a pathological marker for a period of sustained antemorbid hypotension, and this study suggests that ischaemia of some duration is necessary before pancreatitis develops.

In a retrospective study, Haas et al (1985) examined the records of 5400 patients undergoing cardiopulmonary bypass. Of these patients 12 (0.2%) had a diagnosis of postoperative pancreatitis made antemortem, although six of the 12 had other risk factors besides cardiopulmonary bypass. Severe pancreatitis was present in nine of the 12, and all nine required pharmacological and mechanical circulatory support postoperatively. The clinical presentation in these patients was unclear, with only persistent fever, ileus, mild abdominal pain, transient hyperamylasaemia, and progressive systemic deterioration, in spite of the severity of the pancreatitis. Laparotomy was usually necessary to make the diagnosis.

The study further examined the autopsy records of 138 patients who died after cardiac surgery and a control group of 93 nonsurgical patients who died with acute cardiac disease. A total of 35 (25%) of the 138 study patients had evidence of acute interstitial or necrotizing pancreatitis, and most (31 of 35) of these patients had survived longer than 24 hours postoperatively; and 28 had experienced prolonged hypotension. Of the 93 control patients, 38 died in a low flow state, and nine of these had evidence of pancreatitis. None of the 55 control patients who died without a period of hypotension had pancreatitis on autopsy, again suggesting that a sustained period of hypotension is necessary before pancreatitis develops. A total of 30 unselected patients undergoing cardiopulmonary bypass were selected prospectively, and a 27% incidence of asymptomatic hyperamylasaemia was noted postoperatively, perhaps representing unsuspected subclinical pancreatitis.

In addition to intraoperative or postoperative hypotension, cardiac surgery has been suggested to predispose to pancreatitis by embolization of cholesterol from plaques during cannulation, or by non-pulsatile perfusion, hypothermia, and venous sludging on cardiopulmonary bypass. While clinical studies such as these support an association between cardiopulmonary bypass and prolonged postoperative shock with pancreatic injury, the incidence of clinical pancreatitis is low. There may be many subclinical cases which are manifest only as transient amylase elevation, mild abdominal pain, and prolonged ileus. Autopsy series of patients dying after cardiopulmonary bypass demonstrate a much higher incidence of pancreatitis, especially when a greater than 24-hour-period of hypotension has preceded death.

The disparity between the incidence of pancreatitis in those dying after cardiopulmonary bypass and the low incidence in survivors may be explained by the difficulty of making the diagnosis in the minimally symptomatic patients who go on to survive. Those with more severe disease would be subject to more extensive diagnostic studies, including laparotomy and autopsy, leading to a more accurate estimate of the incidence of pancreatitis in this group.

Experimental studies

In experimental studies, Smyth (1940) induced necrosis of pancreatic parenchyma by injection of mercury droplets into the arterial circulation, and this work was later expanded by Pfeffer et al (1962) who injected polyethylene microspheres of varying sizes into the pancreatic circulation. He observed that the smaller microspheres produced more severe pancreatitis than larger microspheres. Presumably the larger spheres did not block end vessels and the collateral circulation was left intact to maintain viability of the gland.

The isolated perfused canine pancreas is ideally suited to studies of ischaemic pancreatitis. Two hours of complete cold ischaemia is sufficient to produce pancreatitis in this model (Broe et al 1982a), but hypoxia alone, or shorter periods of ischaemia do not lead to pancreatitis. Kvietys et al (1982) found that the totally isolated canine pancreas could compensate for relative (but not total) ischaemia by autoregulation with vasodilation and increased oxygen extraction.

In addition, dopaminergic stimulation of pancreatic blood flow appears to improve survival in some forms of experimental pancreatitis in which ischaemia is not the initiating factor (Donahue et al 1984), suggesting that ischaemia may play a global role in promoting gland injury in several types of acute pancreatitis (Berry et al 1982). There is evidence that blood flow is normally increased *early* in the course of experimental acute pancreatitis (Berry et al 1982), and Goodhead (1969) has postulated that relative ischaemia in this situation could lead to thrombosis, increased permeability of the capillary endothelium leading to increased oedema, and haemorrhage.

These findings may account for the conversion of oedematous pancreatitis to haemorrhagic pancreatitis

(Popper et al 1948). Pancreatic oedema may compress the capillary beds and further worsen ischaemia, leading to intraparenchymal thrombosis and haemorrhage and eventually disruption of the ductal system and enzyme extravasation.

Electron microscopic histological studies in the isolated perfused canine pancreas (Clemens et al 1989) have demonstrated a primary endothelial cell injury with ischaemic pancreatitis, with damage to the acinar cells only occurring later in the course of the disease. The vascular injury consisted of thrombosis and platelet plugging of small vessels, similar to that seen with free fatty acid infusion into the pancreatic arterial circulation.

In the small bowel, liver, and heart, production of oxygen derived free radicals is responsible for much of the injury produced by ischaemia-reperfusion (Parks et al 1983c). Similar studies in the isolated perfused canine pancreas have implicated oxygen free radical production in ischaemia-induced pancreatitis (see below).

Miscellaneous causes of pancreatitis

Drugs

Acute pancreatitis has been associated with at least 25 different drugs (Table 18.3) (Mallory & Kern 1980). There is little or no information regarding the pathogenesis of drug-associated pancreatitis, although direct parenchymal toxicity and alteration of the pancreatic secretions with the production of ductal stones and obstruction have been suggested. The delay of several weeks between drug ingestion and the development of pancreatitis has suggested an allergic aetiology in some patients (Sturdevant et al 1979). The incidence of drug-related disease and dose relationships are unclear since the number of patients taking any given drug (the number at risk) is difficult to estimate.

Excluding ethanol, the drugs most definitely associated with pancreatitis are azathioprine and oestrogens. Nogueria & Freedman (1972) reported a series of patients who

developed pancreatitis after receiving azathioprine, and had recurrent disease after the drug was restarted. The frequency of this complication in 113 Crohn's disease patients receiving azathioprine alone was 5.3% (Sturdevant et al 1979), and was significantly increased compared to groups taking placebo, sulphasalazine, and prednisone. The incidence of pancreatitis in patients without Crohn's disease who take azathioprine is unclear, and indeed the aetiological relationship has been questioned since Crohn's disease itself has been reported as a rare cause of pancreatitis (Matsumoto et al 1989). A study of renal transplant patients receiving azathioprine (Corrodi et al 1975) was complicated by the simultaneous ingestion of multiple drugs, including steroids, in addition to azathioprine. A study in the isolated perfused canine model (Broe & Cameron 1983) failed to confirm azathioprine toxicity but did demonstrate alterations in the composition of the pancreatic secretions. Whether these changes might have pathogenetic significance over a longer period in humans is unknown.

Exogenous oestrogens are also frequently cited as causes of acute pancreatitis. Pancreatitis has been noted in women taking oral contraceptives and in men receiving oestrogens for cancer of the prostate. Bank & Marks (1960) and Davidoff et al (1973) have each reported a series of patients who developed clinical pancreatitis within several weeks of starting oral contraceptives and later became asymptomatic once the drug was stopped. Rechallenge with oestrogens resulted in recurrence of the pancreatitis, and there were no further episodes once oestrogens were permanently discontinued (Bank & Marks 1960).

Marked hypertriglyceridaemia was noted in all of these patients during the attack of pancreatitis, and in many some form of lipid abnormality (Frederickson's types IV and V most commonly) persisted after remission of the pancreatitis. These patients may have had pre-existent lipid abnormalities which were exacerbated by oestrogen.

Glueck et al (1972) studied four patients with covert type V hyperlipidaemia who became severely hypertriglyceridaemic after starting estrogens and later developed pancreatitis. He noted that all these patients had poor glucose tolerance and decreased postheparin lipolytic activity (PHLA, a measure of lipoprotein lipase activity). Triglyceride levels fell, carbohydrate tolerance improved, and PHLA levels increased after the oestrogens were stopped.

In a study of normal females without lipid abnormalities, Hazzard et al (1969) found that triglyceride levels increased over baseline in 9 of 10 patients within 2 weeks of starting oestrogens, but only one of the 10 had triglyceride levels exceeding the upper limits of normal. None developed pancreatitis. Hazzard also noted decreased PHLA levels and increased immunoreactive insulin in these patients suggesting that increased triglyceride syn-

Table 18.3   Drug associations and acute pancreatitis

Definite	Ethanol	Oestrogens
	Azathioprine	
Probable	Chlorothiazide	Iatrogenic hypercalcaemia
	Hydrochlorothiazide	Chlorthalidone
	Tetracycline	Corticosteroids
	Furosemide	Ethacrynic acid
	Sulphonamides	Phenformin
	L-Asparaginase	Procainamide
Possible	Amphetamines	Isoniazid
	Cholestyramine	Mercaptopurine
	Cyproheptadine	Opiates
	Propoxyphene	Rifampicin
	Diazoxide	Salicylates
	Histamine	Cimetidine
	Indomethacin	Acetaminophen

thesis by the oestrogen-stimulated liver with decreased peripheral metabolism by lipoprotein lipase caused the biochemical abnormalities.

In summary, oestrogens appear to cause a slight increase in serum triglycerides in nearly all patients (but not exceeding the limits of normal in most). In patients with pre-existing lipid abnormalities, severe hypertriglyceridaemia and pancreatitis can result. Only a small percentage of patients receiving oestrogens develop pancreatitis and there have been no reported cases which developed with normal triglyceride levels. Abstinence from oestrogens in patients who have pancreatitis results in prompt resolution of symptoms and an indefinite remission, while rechallenge often leads to further attacks. Poor glucose tolerance, increased insulin levels, and decreased PHLA levels occur during the attack. The aetiology of the hypertriglyceridaemia appears to be increased hepatic triglyceride synthesis and decreased peripheral utilization by lipoprotein lipase.

Several clinical studies (Johnston & Cornish 1959, Cornish et al 1961, Ances & McClean 1971, Diamond 1972), and an experimental study in mice (Cornish 1961) have implicated thiazide diuretics in the production of pancreatits, but the number of reported cases is small, and rechallenge with the drug has not been reported, questioning the aetiological association.

The other drugs listed in Table 18.3 have been reported in small series or case reports and their potential for initiating pancreatitis is not well documented. They will not be discussed in detail.

Hyperparathyroidism and hypercalcaemia

Hyperparathyroidism has also been proposed as a predisposing factor for acute pancreatitis. Early series documented a 7–12% incidence of pancreatitis in hyperparathyroid patients (Cope et al 1957, Mixter et al 1962), with resolution of symptoms after resection of parathyroid adenomas. Reeve & Delbridge (1982) have reported postoperative hyperamylasaemia in 35% of patients undergoing parathyroid resection, and clinical pancreatitis in 9%. They attributed these findings to transient hypercalcaemia occurring during surgery. Hypercalcaemia from total parenteral nutrition (TPN) infusion (Izsak et al 1980), and malignancy (Gafter et al 1976) have also been associated with pancreatitis.

Others (Romanus et al 1973, Werner et al 1974, Rosin 1976) have questioned this relationship however. In a study of 1153 patients with hyperparathyroidism, Bess et al (1980) found only a 1.5% incidence of pancreatitis, and 11 of these 17 patients had other risk factors which may have accounted for the pancreatitis. The discrepancy between the incidence of pancreatitis in early reports from the 1960s when the association was first noted and more recent reports might be explained by the different patient base in the more recent reports. The advent of multichannel electrolyte screening has led to a marked increase in the number of patients with asymptomatic biochemical hypercalcaemia, compared with the symptomatic patients included in earlier reviews. The symptomatic patients of early studies may well have presented late in the course of the disease when secondary manifestations (such as pancreatitis) had become manifest, whereas today's patients are diagnosed before such manifestations have developed.

Several theories have been proposed to explain the proposed association of hypercalcaemia and hyperparathyroidism with pancreatitis (Rosin 1976). Calcium is known to accelerate the conversion of trypsinogen to trypsin, and may thereby promote autodigestion of the pancreas. Increased calcium levels within the pancreatic juice may also promote calculus formation and obstruction of the ductules. Parathormone (PTH) itself may have direct toxic effects on the gland as well.

Abdominal trauma

Some cases of blunt abdominal trauma are complicated by the development of pancreatitis, presumably because of direct ductal disruption or obstruction (Durr 1979). Intraoperative injury to the gland after pancreatic, biliary, or gastric procedures can result in postoperative pancreatitis, and even non-abdominal surgery has been reported as a rare cause of pancreatitis. Presumably these cases are later related to the anaesthetic rather than the operation itself. A penetrating peptic ulcer eroding into the pancreas is another example of direct injury which can result in pancreatitis.

Endoscopic retrograde cholangiopancreatography

The development of endoscopic retrograde cholangiopancreatography (ERCP) has resulted in an increased frequency of patients with iatrogenic disease, and in some series this is the third most frequent cause of pancreatitis, following alcohol and gallstones. Pancreatitis is one of the most frequent complications of ERCP, occurring after 0.7–12% of all procedures (Roszler & Campbell 1985). Asymptomatic hyperamylasaemia is even more frequent and occurs in up to one-half of all patients.

Several studies have identified specific risk factors for the development of post-ERCP pancreatitis. These include a prior history of pancreatitis, multiple injections into the pancreatic duct, high injection pressures, acinarization (entry of contrast into the acini with appearance of a 'pancreatogram' on fluoroscopy), and inexperience of the operator.

Pancreatitis, if it develops, is usually manifest within 24 hours of the procedure and is almost always mild and self-limited. Fatal post-ERCP pancreatitis is very rare

(Ruppin et al 1974). Pancreatitis following ERCP probably results from a direct ductal injury when the contrast material is injected under high pressure. Ductal disruption and enzyme extravasation may then occur.

Obstructing lesions

Mechanical obstruction of Wirsung's duct by various space-occupying lesions has also been associated with pancreatitis. Pancreatic cancer, periampullary tumours, duodenal diverticula, and choledochal cysts are examples of anatomically obstructing lesions which may result in pancreatitis.

Guelrud & Siegal (1984) have recently reported four patients with isolated hypertensive (and presumably obstructing) ampullary sphincters and episodes of pancreatitis, who were successfully treated by balloon dilatation of the pancreatic duct. Congenital papillary stenosis has been implicated in some cases of otherwise idiopathic pancreatitis. Helminthic colonization of Wirsung's duct can lead to obstruction of the pancreatic duct and has been reported in association with pancreatitis as well (Choi & Wong 1984). Acute pancreatitis may sometimes be the initial presentation of cystic fibrosis (Masaryk & Achkar 1983), and pathological studies in these young patients have shown progressive obstruction of the pancreatic ductal system due to mucus plugging.

In all of these clinical situations with some degree of obstruction, the initiating stimulus is probably the development of elevated pressures in the ductal system with ductal disruption, extravasation of juice into the parenchyma, and resultant pancreatic injury.

Duodenal obstruction, usually from stricture, has also been reported as a cause of acute pancreatitis (Durr 1979). In this situation high intraduodenal pressure may force reflux of duodenal fluid into the pancreatic duct where injury occurs.

Pancreas divisum

Pancreas divisum is a congenital anomaly in which the two main ducts draining the gland fail to fuse normally. The anomaly has been noted in 4–11% of unselected autopsy cases (Richter et al 1981), but it may be difficult to identify on ERCP. Radiographic studies have demonstrated pancreas divisum in only about 4% of cases (Richter et al 1981, Warshaw et al 1983). The appearance of a foreshortened Wirsung's duct on ERCP is virtually diagnostic, although Warshaw & Cambria (1984) have pointed out that acquired ductal stenoses can sometimes simulate this picture.

During embryonic development, the pancreas exists as a dorsal and ventral bud, with the dorsal portion draining through Santorini's duct into the accessory papilla, and the ventral portion through Wirsung's duct into the ampulla of Vater. Normally the dorsal bud rotates around the duodenum and fuses with the ventral bud and Santorini's duct fuses with Wirsung's duct proximal to the ampulla. Santorini's duct then loses its separate connection with the duodenum through the accessory papilla. The entire pancreas thus comes to drain through Wirsung's duct and the ampulla, and the accessory papilla becomes a vestigial structure. In pancreas divisum, there is no ductal fusion, and the superior portion of the head, and the body and tail drain through Santorini's duct and the accessory papilla. Only the ventral pancreas (forming the inferior portion of the head) drains through the ampulla.

While about 12% of patients with pancreatitis have pancreas divisum demonstrated on ERCP, only 3% of patients who have pancreatography for other reasons have the anomaly, suggesting that pancreas divisum predisposes to attacks of acute pancreatitis (Cotton 1980, Richter et al 1981, Gregg et al, 1983). Although the pathogenetic mechanism is unclear, it is likely that the inadequate drainage of the dorsal pancreas through the small accessory papilla results in relative obstruction of the most of the pancreatic parenchyma.

Warshaw et al (1983) have published a report of 32 patients with pancreas divisum, who had recurrent acute pancreatitis (22) or persistent pain (10), presumably of pancreatic origin but without hyperamylasaemia or pancreatic oedema on CT scan. A total of 29 of the 32 patients were treated by operative sphincterotomy of the accessory papilla. Out of the accessory ducts, 22 were judged to be stenotic at laparotomy with a diameter of 0.75 mm or less. In the 25 patients in whom follow-up exceeded 6 months, 17 had good relief of symptoms, while eight had only fair or poor results. Patients with stenotic ducts, demonstrated at operation, and a history of discrete attacks rather than chronic pain, tended to fare better. Two patients had reoperation at 5 and 15 months postoperatively to relieve recurrent stenosis and were again rendered asymptomatic. The remaining group of eight patients had chronic pancreatitis as defined by changes of chronic pancreatitis on ERCP or fibrosis of the gland at laparotomy, and received no benefit from surgical sphincterotomy. Of these eight patients, seven eventually required a formal drainage or ablative procedure.

This study suggests that pancreas divisum may be a cause of acute pancreatitis in some patients, and that those with discrete attacks, and evidence of papillary stenosis at laparotomy, may benefit from surgical sphincterotomy. Patients with changes of chronic pancreatitis in association with pancreas divisum are unlikely to benefit from sphincterotomy. The recent technique of secretin stimulation during ultrasound examination of the pancreas may be helpful in identifying preoperatively the subset of patients who may benefit from sphincterotomy.

Other factors

Autoimmune disease. Autoimmune disease, usually systemic lupus erythematosus (SLE), and rarely rheumatoid arthritis or polyarteritis nodosa, have been associated with acute pancreatitis in some patients (Goebell & Hotz 1979). This aetiology is uncommon, and the association is complicated by the frequent ingestion of drugs such as azathioprine or steroids which have the potential to lead to pancreatitis in their own right. Autoantibodies directed against cell fractions from the pancreas have been described, although the aetiological significance is unclear (Durr 1979). Vasculitis of pancreatic vessels has been reported in resection and autopsy specimens, implicating ischaemia as the more proximate cause of the disease in these cases (Phat et al 1984).

Familial factors. About 250 case reports exist in the literature of a familial form of pancreatitis. There does not appear to be sex-linked expression but it is is unclear whether the condition is inherited as an autosomal dominant or recessive trait. Pancreatitis may also occur in inherited connective tissue disorders (Sarra-Carbonell & Jimenez 1989).

Infection. Infectious causes of acute pancreatitis have been implicated in some patients. Mumps virus antigens have been localized in the acinar and islet cells of pancreatitis patients by fluorescent antibody techniques suggesting this virus as an aetiological factor (Durr 1979). Serum antibody titres have also implicated infection with mycoplasma, hepatitis, echo, and coxsackie viruses in patients with otherwise unexplained pancreatitis (Durr 1979), and a single case of cytomegalovirus infection associated with pancreatitis has been reported (Iwasaki et al 1987). The potential for treatment with antiviral therapy in patients with infectious pancreatitis has not been evaluated.

Malnutrition. Malnutrition is associated with pancreatitis in third world countries and while the aetiology is not known with certainty a vitamin or trace mineral deficiency may be the causative factor. In developed countries, malnutrition is rarely associated with pancreatitis except in alcoholics.

Scorpion bites. Scorpion bites have also been implicated in some cases of human pancreatitis (Poon-King 1963), and injection of the venom into the arterial supply of the gland in experimental models reproduces the disease (Pantoja et al 1983). The biochemical mechanisms have not been elucidated.

Absence of predisposing factors

After the above aetiological factors have been eliminated, there remain a number of patients on which no predisposing factor can be identified. Such patients and their families should be carefully questioned for a history of ethanol abuse, as this is sometimes not readily apparent. A thorough search should be made for gallstones, hypercalcaemia, pancreas divisum, hypertriglyceridaemia, and obstructing lesions of the pancreatobiliary tree. An appropriate drug history should be taken and symptoms suggestive of viral infection or autoimmune disease should be sought. A small number of patients, after thorough investigation, never have a recognized aetiological factor identified and are best termed idiopathic.

MODELS OF ACUTE PANCREATITIS

A number of animal models of acute pancreatitis have been developed to facilitate study of the condition. The pancreas is anatomically inaccessible in the retroperitoneum and until the development of sonography, CT scanning, MR imaging, and ERCP, it was beyond the reach of even radiological examination. Physiological studies of the gland are difficult to perform in humans and sometimes give contradictory results, and biopsies of the pancreas are seldom performed in cases of acute pancreatitis, even if a laparotomy is required. Most studies of the pathological changes in acute pancreatitis are accordingly from autopsy material, seriously limiting the type of data which may be collected, since only severe cases of the disease in the late stages come to autopsy. Little is known about the early pathological changes of acute human pancreatitis.

All of these factors have led to widespread use of animal models in study of the disease, but the question of how closely models approach human disease remains open to discussion. Steinberg & Schlesselman (1987) have reviewed this issue in a comparison of 25 drug studies in acute experimental pancreatitis and 13 drug studies in clinical pancreatitis. They found that most of the agents which were effective in the animal models were later proven ineffective in human trials. A number of less than ideal conditions in the human studies may explain the contradictory results, including inadequate sample size, too short a duration of therapy, and an unavoidable delay in the initiation of therapy for several hours after the initiating event.

Duodenal ligation model

One of the oldest methods of inducing pancreatitis in animals is simple ligation of the duodenum, proximal and distal to the pancreatic duct so as to produce a closed loop. Duodenal and pancreatic secretion in the presence of the closed loop leads to increased intraduodenal pressure and eventually the resistance of the sphincter of Oddi is overcome and reflux of duodenal contents occurs into the pancreatic duct. The duodenal fluid contains digestive proteases activated by the brush border enzyme enterokinase, and severe injury occurs to the pancreatic ductal mucosa. With a continued increase in pressure, disruption of the ducts occurs, and the enzymes gain entry into the parenchyma of the gland where autodigestion of the acinar cells and recognizable pancreatitis occurs.

While the model is easily reproducible and has the advantage of being technically simple, its relevance to human pancreatitis is minimal, since duodenal obstruction is only a rare cause of clinical pancreatitis in humans. Duodenal discontinuity and necrosis occur as well, which add additional pathogenetic factors to the pancreatitis in any assessment of treatment efficacy or mortality rates. Because of these problems the model is of limited utility and is rarely used.

Bile injection model

A second time-honoured mechanism of inducing pancreatitis in experimental animals is through bile injection under pressure into the pancreatic duct. Bile salts appear to be the most injurious component of the bile, but the pressure of injection is of key significance. Even normal saline induces acute pancreatitis if injected under sufficient pressure. Bile requires a high injection pressure before injury is apparent, and some investigators have added bacteria, trypsin, or even blood to the bile to increase the toxicity and pancreatic injury. A major problem with the reproducibility of the model is standardization of the injection rate and pressure, key factors in determining the degree of injury.

The clinical significance of bile reflux under high pressure into the pancreatic duct is uncertain, and thus the relevance of the model to most forms of human disease is doubtful. Injection of bile under supraphysiological pressures or the addition of exogenous activated proteases to the injectate are necessary before experimental pancreatitis occurs. Bile reflux in humans, if it occurs at all, is likely to be at physiological pressure, and activated proteases are unlikely to be present. These factors limit the clinical relevance of this model as well.

In a related model, bile salts are directly injected into the parenchyma of the gland but this obviously has almost no clinical relevance.

Feline duct perfusion

Studies of ductal factors in acute pancreatitis have been performed in the feline duct perfusion model described by Reber et al (1979). In this model, the main pancreatic duct is cannulated in the tail of the gland, and the duct perfused progradely with a perfusate which empties into the duodenum through the unobstructed ampulla. If a bile salt solution is perfused through the duct at physiological pressures and concentrations, permeability changes in the mucosa and histological alterations in the ductal cells are noted (Farmer et al 1984), but no pan-

creatitis results. If activated proteases are perfused through the duct at physiological pressures, no pancreatitis results, but when ductal permeability is altered with either aspirin or ethanol, protease infusion does result in pancreatitis (Steer 1985). Intravenous isoproterenol decreases pancreatic inflammation in this model, perhaps by altering microvascular permeability (Harvey et al 1987). The earliest histological changes which are seen in this model are to the ductal cells, and the changes in both the ductal and acinar cells resemble those seen with human acute pancreatitis.

These factors make this model an excellent choice for the study of early histological and ductal factors in acute pancreatitis. The model does have the drawback of being technically difficult, and like the bile injection model, assumes that reflux of activated proteases into the pancreatic duct occurs in clinical pancreatitis.

Austin (see Steer 1985) has described a similar model which focuses more on duct hypertension than protease injury to the pancreas. In this model, a perfusion catheter is placed in the major pancreatic duct in the tail, as with Reber's model. In addition, the common pancreatic duct, formed by the confluence of the major and minor ducts is ligated at the duodenum. A second cannula is placed in the minor duct to monitor pressure changes. Perfusion of the duct through the cannula or stimulation of the gland to secrete produces hypertension in the range of 20 mmHg. Ductal permeability is assessed by the addition of radiolabelled dextrans to the perfusate, and measuring the amount of sequestration into the parenchyma, or concentration of the tracer in the portal venous blood. This model shares the advantages and disadvantages of Reber's preparation.

Non-invasive induction of experimental pancreatitis

Choline-deficient ethionine-supplemented diet model

There are several non-invasive methods of inducing experimental pancreatitis. Perhaps the most unique is the choline-deficient ethionine-supplemented diet model (CDE diet model) developed by Lombardi et al (1975). Farber & Popper (1950) and Goldberg et al (1950) were the first to report the induction of pancreatitis in mice by an ethionine-supplemented diet, and this has subsequently been observed in a number of species. Ethionine supplementation alone produces focal necrosis and atrophy of the gland, but not necrotizing lethal pancreatitis. Lombardi & Rao (1975) found that young female mice fed diets supplemented with DL-ethionine and deficient in choline and marginally deficient in methionine, develop haemorrhagic pancreatitis which is almost uniformly fatal in 4–5 days. The age, sex, and species of the animal are crucial in determining the outcome: male mice develop only pancreatic necrosis and atrophy similar to ethionine supplementation alone, and adult female mice develop less severe forms of pancreatitis. Only immature female mice develop the lethal form of pancreatitis which Lombardi believes is due to the hormonal milieu and a greater susceptibility of young animals to choline deficiency. Female mice have also been shown to have lower levels of endogenous pancreatic antiproteases, which may increase the likelihood of injury in these animals.

An ethionine-supplemented diet which is not deficient in choline or methionine produces a less severe form of pancreatitis, suggesting that the toxic effects of ethionine are potentiated by choline or methionine deficiency. Ethionine has several deleterious effects in mammalian cells (Lombardi et al 1975) including interference with ATP generation. Ethionine traps adenine as S-adenosyl ethionine, a compound with a very low turnover rate, which blocks synthesis of S-adenosyl methionine, a cofactor necessary for methylation in a number of pathways, including choline synthesis from dietary precursors. Ethionine also inhibits incorporation of labelled phosphorus into pancreatic phospholipids, and may be directly capable of activating pancreatic proteases. Supplementation of the CDE diet with methionine (Lombardi 1976) ameliorates the deficiency of S-adenosyl methionine to a degree, and can reduce the mortality rate of the diet-induced pancreatitis. This addition of choline to the ethionine-supplemented diet also lessens the severity of the disease, but adenine supplementation has no effect. These findings indicate that while a choline or methionine deficiency potentiate toxicity, depletion of adenosine by incorporation into S-adenosyl ethionine is probably not the key factor, since exogenous adenine does not alter the severity of pancreatitis. Whatever the biochemical basis of injury, the normal secretory mechanism of the acinar cell is interrupted (see below).

The CDE diet model is a non-invasive, reproducible, and slowly evolving model of lethal pancreatitis, which is species-, sex- and age-specific. It lends itself to study of the early morphological changes and biochemical events in acute pancreatitis. The CDE diet probably produces pancreatitis by a combination of the direct toxic effects of ethionine with potentiation by methionine and choline deficiency. Alteration of membrane phospholipid synthesis and metabolism probably occur as well. The pathological changes in this model resemble those seen on autopsy of patients dying with severe pancreatitis. The model has the disadvantage of having no clear correlation with human disease, as nutritional factors are rarely implicated in clinical pancreatitis.

Caerulein model

Non-invasive induction of pancreatitis can also be ac-complished in several species by infusion of the secretagogue caerulein in a model first developed by Lampel & Kern (1977). Caerulein is a synthetic decapeptide analogue of cholecystokinin (CCK) and was originally isolated from the skin of an Australian frog. At low doses, it has a stimulatory effect similar to that of CCK, i.e. an increased enzyme content in the pancreatic juice out of proportion to the volume increase. When caerulein is given as a continuous intravenous infusion for several hours, severe haemorrhagic pancreatitis results. This is a supramaximal dose in that it exceeds the dose which produces a maximal secretory rate. Even when given at submaximal doses, caerulein is capable of potentiating pancreatitis initiated by another agent (Evander et al 1981).

Mechanisms of action of caerulein and the CDE diet. Both caerulein and the CDE diet appear to alter the normal secretory pathway of the acinar cell in such a way as to allow intracellular activation of digestive proteases. The pancreatic cell has several defence mechanisms against such premature activation of digestive enzymes. Trypsin and other enzymes are normally secreted as inactive proenzymes, or zymogens, which undergo proteolytic cleavage in the duodenum with release of the active form. The pancreas also contains a number of endogenous antiproteases which migrate along with the zymogens through the secretory pathway and further inhibit activation. Finally, zymogens are physically segregated from other enzymes which can initiate activation, such as the lysosomal hydrolase cathepsin B, which activates trypsin and other proteases in vitro (Greenbaum & Hirshkowitz 1961). Both zymogens and lysosomal enzymes are synthesized on the rough endoplasmic reticulum, and each class of enzyme undergoes a post-translational modification (addition of sugar moieties) which determines whether the enzyme will be packaged in a lysosome or zymogen granule by the Golgi apparatus.

Normal segregation appears to fail for unknown reasons in caerulein pancreatitis (Fig. 18.1) (Watanabe et al 1984), theoretically exposing trypsinogen and other inactive proteases to lysosomal enzymes (such as cathepsin B) which are capable of activating these enzymes. Caerulein blunts the response of the gland to exogenous secretagogues (Watanabe et al 1984), suggesting a block in the secretory pathway. Steer et al (1984) have confirmed these findings by demonstrating, on electron microscopy, a failure of normal secretion in the acinar cell, with the accumulation of large immature condensing vacuoles and a depletion of mature zymogen granules. The normal segregation of lysosomal and digestive enzymes appears to be defective in caerulein-treated glands and both enzyme types are present within the condensing vacuoles. Co-localization of these enzymes favours intracellular protease activation. Unlike the CDE diet model, secretory granule accumulation and crinophagy (the fusion

ACINAR LUMEN

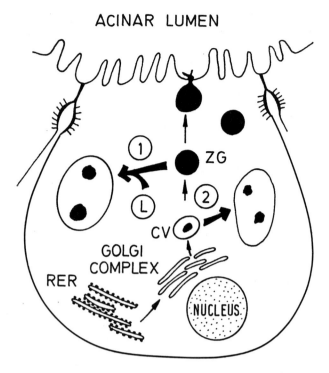

Fig. 18.1 Proposed normal and abnormal secretory pathways in the pancreatic acinar cell. The thin arrows illustrate the physiological pathway, beginning with synthesis of zymogens in the rough endoplasmic reticulum (RER). The enzymes are next transported to the Golgi complex. Lysosomal hydrolases are segregated into the lysosomes (L), and digestive enzymes into the condensing vacuoles (CV) which mature into zymogen granules (ZG). Zymogen granules are discharged into the acinar lumen by fusion with the cell membrane. The heavy arrows show abnormal secretory pathways. In pathway 1 the zymogen granules fuse with lysosomes (crinophagy) as is seen in diet-induced (CDE) pancreatitis. Hypersecretory (caerulein) pancreatitis is outlined by pathway 2 in which condensing vacuoles fail to mature. Large vacuoles form which contain both digestive and lysosomal enzymes (solid black areas represent digestive enzymes and stippled areas represent lysosomal hydrolases). (Reprinted from Steer M, Meldolesi J, Figarella C, Pancreatitis: the role of lysosomes. Digestive Diseases and Sciences (1984) 29: 934.)

of mature secretory granules and lysosomes) does not occur in caerulein preparations. Protease inhibitors which are active against trypsin lower amylase levels and limit histological evidence of injury in the caerulein model (Otsuki et al 1990, Tani 1988). Ohshio et al (1989) found that the antiproteases FOY and FOY 305 significantly improved both CDE and caerulein-induced pancreatitis, and demonstrated diminished redistribution (mixing) of the lysosomal and zymogen cellular compartments when these agents were employed. These results suggest that admixture of the two enzyme classes and intracellular activation of trypsin is the central mechanism in both the caerulein and CDE models.

A second morphological change, seen on electron microscopy in acinar cells treated with caerulein, is misdirected exocytosis (Alder et al 1985). Ordinarily the contents of the secretory granules are discharged into the

pancreatic ductules by exocytosis from the apical surface of the acinar cells. In caerulein-treated glands the process is disrupted and the zymogen granules are discharged into the intercellular space from the basolateral cell surface. The release of activated zymogens into the intercellular spaces in such a fashion obviously has the potential to cause great injury to the pancreas and may initiate pancreatitis.

The CDE diet also disrupts the orderly secretion of zymogen granules but in a different manner (Fig. 18.1) (Lombardi et al 1975). In CDE pancreatitis the earliest morphological change seen is the accumulation of *mature* secretory granules within the acinar cell, suggesting a block in the secretory pathway, perhaps mediated by an ethionine-induced membrane alteration. Crinophagy has been observed. While the segregation of the lysosomal and digestive enzymes is initially normal with the CDE diet model, crinophagy could place digestive proteases in an environment favouring intracellular activation. Secretory granule antiproteases are inactive at lysosomal pH values. Experimental evidence for this mechanism includes the demonstration of activated proteases in pancreatic homogenates of CDE-fed animals (Rao et al 1976), increased cathepsin B levels in the homogenates (Rao et al 1980), and a modulation of the severity of CDE pancreatitis by antiproteases active against cathepsin B (Lombardi & Rao 1982).

Although ultrastructural changes in secretory granules in both CDE diet and caerulein models may be responsible for the initiation of pancreatitis, it is unclear how these changes are initiated. Furthermore, the pertinence of either of these models to human pancreatitis is purely speculative. Secretory granule changes have not been demonstrated in human tissue, and treatment with antiproteases is not beneficial in clinical studies. Therefore, the applicability of these models to human pancreatitis is questionable.

Ex vivo isolated perfused canine model

The final model of acute pancreatitis to be considered is the ex vivo isolated perfused canine pancreas preparation. This model was first described by Babkin & Starling (1926) and later refined by Nardi et al (1963) and Hermon-Taylor (1969). The pancreas is isolated surgically with its major vasculature intact. Perfusion catheters are placed in the superior mesenteric artery and a branch of the splenic artery, and the gland perfused with oxygenated autologous blood. Venous drainage is collected via a portal venous cannula, which carries the blood to a small oxygenator, after which it is pumped back to the preparation. The pancreatic duct is cannulated and secretions are collected. The preparation is monitored by hourly measurements of weight, secretory output, perfusion pressure, blood gases, haemoglobin, haematocrit, glucose, and amylase levels. Control glands harvested in this fashion remain physiological for periods of several hours.

A variety of stimuli are capable of initiating pancreatitis in this model. The infusion of small amounts of free fatty acid (oleic acid) into the arterial perfusion line quickly produces pancreatitis with marked weight gain and hyperamylasaemia (Saharia 1977), but if a similar amount of mineral oil is infused, pancreatitis does not develop, suggesting that free fatty acids have a toxic effect but that esterified fatty acids do not. Free fatty acid infusion mimics the initiation of acute alcoholic pancreatitis associated with lipaemia. If the pancreatic duct is partially obstructed with a small gauge cannula, and the gland is maximally stimulated to secrete, weight gain and marked hyperamylasaemia develop (Partial Obstruction plus Secretin Stimulation or POSS, Broe & Cameron 1982). Partial obstruction of the pancreatic duct in a stimulated gland simulates acute gallstone pancreatitis. A third method of inducing pancreatitis in this model is to allow a period of complete ischaemia prior to initiating perfusion. As in the other two models, hyperamylasaemia and weight gain develop (Broe et al 1982a). Supramaximal caerulein infusion also induces acute pancreatitis in this model, similar to that seen in intact animals (Clemens et al 1989).

A major advantage of the ex vivo isolated perfused canine preparation is the ease of duplicating conditions proposed as initiators in clinical pancreatitis. In addition the preparation is versatile in that a number of initiating stimuli can be studied. Since the gland is isolated, complicating systemic factors such as hypotension or hypovolemia are eliminated. A disadvantage is that since the preparation is stable for only several hours, only the early events in the development of acute pancreatitis can be studied. Further drawbacks include technical complexity and expense.

SPECIFIC ISSUES OF PATHOGENESIS

Proteases, antiproteases and protease-activated cascades

The pancreas is a unique organ in that it contains enzymes which are capable of autodigestion. Chiari (1896) first suggested that tryptic autodigestion of the pancreas might play an aetiological role in pancreatitis, and since then numerous clinical and experimental studies have examined the role of activated proteases and protease inhibitors in the initiation and treatment of pancreatitis, although some doubt the role of this mechanism (Keynes, 1988). Activated proteolytic enzymes have been detected in the gland itself, the serum, and ascitic fluid of patients and animals with pancreatitis (Masoero et al 1980, Artigas et al 1981, Geokas et al 1981, Wellborn et al 1983, Lasson & Ohlsson 1984b).

There are a number of safeguards which ordinarily prevent protease activation except in the bowel lumen. Proteolytic enzymes are physically segregated during secretion from lysosomal enzymes which have the potential for activating trypsin, as discussed above. Several protease inhibitors are secreted with the digestive enzymes, preventing intracellular activation. Most importantly, several serum and tissue antiproteases quickly inactivate enzymes before injury occurs. However, if a sufficient amount of the activated enzyme is present, all of these defences can be overwhelmed with resultant tissue injury.

Proteases

Trypsin is the most important of the pancreatic proteases, because, once activated, it can activate the other proteases in a self-sustaining process. Trypsin is a 24 000 Da endopeptidase (meaning that it can cleave peptide bonds at any point along a chain) which is found in the pancreas of most vertebrates (Keil 1971). Trypsin cleaves peptide bonds in which the carbonyl group is contributed by a lysine or arginine residue, and is termed a serine protease since a serine residue is essential in the active site. The pancreas secretes an inactive form of the enzyme, trypsinogen, which is then activated by irreversible proteolytic cleavage of a hexapeptide from the N-terminal end of the molecule. Trypsinogen can be activated by the duodenal brush border enzyme enterokinase or by other activated trypsin molecules or thrombin. Trypsin activates chymotrypsin, elastase, phospholipase A_2, plasmin, thrombin, and the complement cascade. Although trypsin is assumed to play a pivotal role in severe pancreatitis, it is unknown how the initial intraparenchymal activation occurs. The initial activation of trypsin in some models of acute pancreatitis may be due to the lysosomal enzyme cathepsin B.

Chymotrypsin may also have some importance in the initiation of pancreatitis. It is secreted by the pancreas as two inactive isoenzyme precursors, chymotrypsinogen A and chymotrypsinogen B, both of which can be activated by trypsin. There are a number of active forms of the enzyme as well, including alpha, beta, gamma, delta and pi (α, β, γ, δ and π) which appear to result form varying degrees of proteolysis. The alpha form is the most studied and has a molecular weight of about 25 000. Chymotrypsin catalyses the hydrolysis of peptide bonds adjacent to the carboxyl groups of tryptophan, tyrosine and phenylalanine. Chymotrypsin, like trypsin, has a serine residue as a crucial constituent of the active site, and is therefore a serine protease (Keil 1971).

Pancreatic elastase is another enzyme which has special properties which may contribute to necrotizing pancreatitis. Elastase hydrolyses the elastin fibres of connective tissue, and may promote spread of proteolysis through tissue planes. It has a molecular weight of about 25 000 and is secreted in an inactive form, pro-elastase, by the pancreas. Elastase is activated by the trypsin mediated proteolytic cleavage of a single peptide bond. An N-terminal peptide is released which allows the molecule to assume its active conformation. Elastase is less specific than other pancreatic proteases and preferentially hydrolyses peptide bonds involving an alanine residue. Elastase is also a serine protease.

The pancreas secretes a number of other proteases, including carboxypeptidase A and B, ribonuclease, and deoxyribonuclease but these will not be discussed in detail. The saccharogenic enzyme amylase probably has no role in the pathophysiology of the disease except as a diagnostic marker, but the lipolytic enzymes lipase and, in particular, phospholipase A_2 have greater potential for causing injury. These enzymes are discussed in more detail below.

Antiproteases

There are several major antiproteases in the plasma which limit the potential for injury from activated proteases released from the pancreas. For instance, α_2-macroglobulin is a high molecular weight (725 000 Da) inhibitor of endoproteases, including trypsin, elastase, plasmin, thrombin and kallikrein (Lasson 1984). It is synthesized by the liver, alveolar macrophages and fibroblasts, and is distributed mainly in the intravascular space because of its large size. Protease inhibition occurs by covalent bonding to the target enzyme, sterically hindering the active site. However, the complex retains some proteolytic activity until it is eliminated from the circulation by the reticuloendothelial system. The half life for elimination is about 10 minutes. Serum levels of α_2-macroglobulin are low in septic shock, after major surgery, and with streptokinase infusion.

A second serum protease inhibitor synthesized by the liver is α_1-protease inhibitor (molecular weight 54 000) and it inhibits several serine proteases, including thrombin, plasmin, and kallikrein (Lasson 1984). It is mainly distributed in the extravascular space and may serve as a carrier of activated proteases from the extravascular space to the serum where α_2-macroglobulin is located.

The pancreas also secretes its own protease inhibitor, pancreatic secretory trypsin inhibitor (Lasson 1984). This protein accompanies the zymogens as they are secreted into the ductal system, and constitutes about 1% of the protein content of the pancreatic juice. Proteases bound to this inhibitor are cleaved in the presence of serum, binding α_2-macroglobulin preferentially.

Changes in protease and inhibitor levels

Alterations of the serum levels of proteases and their inhibitors have been noted in experimental and clinical acute pancreatitis. Geokas et al (1981) studied the time course of the appearance of activated trypsin in the blood, using a bile injection canine model. Trypsin was found bound to α_2-macroglobulin and α_1-protease inhibitor in the serum early in the course of the disease, and in animals that died the antiprotease–protease complex retained proteolytic activity, suggesting that the antiprotease system had been overwhelmed by a massive protease release. In a series of 34 patients with acute pancreatitis, Artigas et al (1981) found a significant increase in serum trypsin levels in every patient compared with 26 healthy controls. Trypsin elevation was not specific however, and was present in 11 of 12 patients with chronic renal failure, and in four of 23 with acute non-pancreatic abdominal disease. Masoero et al (1980) have reported a 100% incidence of elevated serum trypsin levels in 28 patients with pancreatitis. Several other studies have documented elevated serum trypsin levels in acute pancreatitis (Brodrick et al 1979, Elias et al 1977).

Rinderknecht et al (1984) reported a novel form of trypsin (mesotrypsin) which is not inhibited by the usual trypsin inhibitors, but is capable of degrading trypsinogen to inactive products without the release of activated trypsin. While mesotrypsin itself may have some deleterious proteolytic effects, it is more likely to serve a protective role by reducing extrapancreatic trypsinogen to inactive products. Reduced levels of mesotrypsin were found in patients with acute pancreatitis, and this may have pathogenetic significance.

Increased serum elastase activity has also been noted. In a study of 14 unselected patients with acute pancreatitis, Wellborn et al (1983) found increased elastase levels and decreased elastase inhibitory activity compared with 21 healthy controls and seven patients with chronic pancreatitis. Elastase levels tended to fall with resolution of the disease, and inhibitory activity increased.

Lasson & Ohlsson (1984b) have extensively studied the levels of serum antiproteases in patients with acute pancreatitis. In a study of 25 patients suffering 27 attacks, they found a marked reduction in α_2-macroglobulin in nine severe attacks of pancreatitis, as classified by Ranson's criteria (Ranson et al 1976), compared with 18 mild or moderately severe attacks, although these later patients also had subnormal levels when compared with healthy controls. The nadir was reached 3 days after admission and the levels did not normalize for 14 days.

The levels of α_1-protease inhibitor were increased above normal regardless of the severity of the disease, but severe attacks gave higher values. This inhibitor is an acute phase reactant, and unlike α_2-macroglobulin, is rapidly synthesized by the liver if consumed in protease complexes. The increased levels are presumably protective against injury caused by activated proteases which accumulate when α_2-macroglobulin is depleted. Trypsin–α_1-protease inhibitor complexes were found in severe cases and persisted for about a week. Pancreatic secretory trypsin inhibitor levels varied considerably within the groups, and while the levels did not follow a consistent pattern, increased levels were common. Lasson believes this to be due to leakage of the inhibitor from an injured gland.

Protease and inhibitor levels were measured in the peritoneal fluid in patients who underwent therapeutic or diagnostic peritoneal lavage; trypsin was found complexed to both α_2-macroglobulin and α_1-protease inhibitor. Normal levels of protease inhibitors and proteases in the peritoneal fluid have not been established, but α_2-macroglobulin levels were decreased in severe attacks compared with mild attacks. Peritoneal lavage has been effective in lowering levels of proteases in the peritoneal exudate of patients with severe pancreatitis, although the therapeutic importance of these findings is unknown (Aasen et al 1989). Levels of trypsin–α_1-protease inhibitor complexes were higher in the peritoneal fluid than the blood, suggesting that the initial protease activation had occurred in the peritoneal cavity.

Importance of protease activation

The importance of protease activation in acute pancreatitis is twofold. In addition to probable systemic effects, activated proteolytic enzymes in the peripancreatic tissues have profound local effects such as sequestration of fluid in the retroperitoneum and peritoneal cavity, necrosis of the pancreas, erosion into surrounding structures, and disruption of the ductal system. Fat necrosis with calcium precipitation also occurs in the peripancreatic tissues, but this is primarily the result of lipase-mediated triglyceride hydrolysis and saponification. The lipolytic enzymes are considered separately below.

Antiprotease therapy

Because of clear evidence of protease activation in some patients with pancreatitis, exogenous antiprotease therapy has received considerable attention as a specific form of treatment. Aprotinin (Trasylol) is the best known of these agents. This drug is an excellent inhibitor of trypsin, chymotrypsin, kallikrein, plasmin and thrombin in vitro. Aprotinin has beneficial effects in experimental pancreatitis (Fujii 1979, Imrie & Mackenzie 1981) if given early enough, but most clinical studies (Imrie et al 1978, Medical Research Council Multicentre Trial 1980, Balldin et al 1983) have shown no benefit in morbidity or mortality, and the drug is seldom if ever used clinically. Fritz & Wunderer (1983) suggested that the failure of aprotinin in clinical studies was due to inadequate dosing and a very short half-life (7 minutes). In addition, a key protease cascade may escape inhibition completely, since Sipila & Louhija (1982) found that aprotinin does not prevent kallikrein-mediated kininogen activation in vivo.

Newer antiprotease agents such as leupeptin have shown promise in experimental pancreatitis (Lombardi & Rao 1982, Jones et al 1982), but have not been subjected to human trials. The antimetabolite 5-fluorouracil has been evaluated as an experimental inhibitor of enzyme synthesis (Saario 1983), but its clinical efficacy has not been demonstrated.

Systemic manifestations.

In addition to the local effects of activated proteases in pancreatitis, systemic manifestations of the disease may result from the systemic release of proteases and depletion of the protease inhibitor defences. Serum or ascitic fluid trypsin activates the complement, kininogen and clotting cascades, and a number of inflammatory mediators may thus be released. These three cascade systems appear to be important in the pathophysiology of pancreatitis and contribute to its evolution and systemic toxicity. Each will be considered separately.

The complement cascade. This is shown for reference in Figure 18.2. There are two mechanisms of activation, the classical and alternative pathways. Classical activation can be initiated by a number of agents, including immunoglobulins, endotoxin, and serine proteases (trypsin, plasmin and kallikrein). Once activated, the q and r subunits of C1 interact with the s subunit to form activated C1s. C1s interact with the C2–C4 complex to

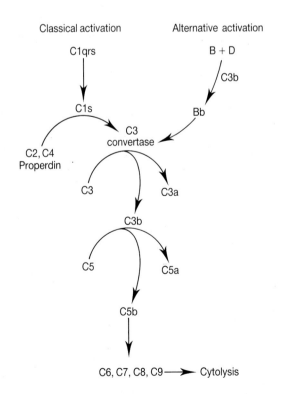

Fig. 18.2 The complement cascade.

cleave both C2 and C4 into large and small fragments. The large subunits of cleaved C2 and C4 associate to form C3 convertase (activated C4C2). C3 convertase produces two active fragments C3a and C3b. C3b continues the activation process by cleaving C5 into two active subunits, C5a and C5b. C5b then activates the later components of the system. Activated C3a and C5a have chemotactic properties for leucocytes and may play a role in some forms of respiratory insufficiency.

Description of the alternative pathway is beyond the scope of this discussion, but this pathway also results in the formation of C3 convertase.

Trypsin is capable of direct activation of several complement proteins. A number of complement cascade inhibitors have been described including C1INH which inhibits C1s, Factor I (which inactivates C3b) and Factor H (a regulator of C3b inactivation).

Seelig & Seelig (1975) have advanced the complement system as the initiator of acute pancreatitis, but this view is not widely shared. Most authors agree there is evidence of classical and alternative complement activation in pancreatitis, although its significance is unclear. Whicher et al (1982) studied complement changes in 26 patients with acute pancreatitis. Of the 26, 19 had reduced C3 levels with C3 breakdown products present, but the presence of breakdown products did not predict the clinical course. C4 and Factor B breakdown products were not present, suggesting that early activation of classical pathway and the alternative pathway did not occur. The inhibitors C1INH and Factor H were elevated, but this may represent only an acute phase response. Whicher attributed the complement changes seen in acute pancreatitis to tryptic activation of C3.

Balldin et al (1981) examined the relationship of serum and peritoneal serine protease inhibitors to complement activation. C3 levels were decreased in 32 patients with severe acute pancreatitis, and C3 breakdown products were present. Proteases in the serum did not complex with α_2-macroglobulin and α_1-antitrypsin, but extensive complex formation was present in peritoneal fluid. The authors demonstrated depletion of serum complement factors in acute pancreatitis, presumably due to consumption of the factors by activated proteases in the peritoneal cavity. Complement activation in vitro occurs only if protease inhibitors are saturated by a sufficient amount of activated trypsin.

In a study of 15 patients with pancreatitis, Lasson et al (1985) found decreased C1q, C3, C4, properdin, and Factors I and H in the serum and the peritoneal fluid, supporting both classical and alternative pathway activation. Trypsin–antiprotease complexes were present in the serum and peritoneal fluid. The authors concluded that complement activation occurs in severe cases of acute pancreatitis and is probably initiated by tryptic digestion of the early complement components in the peritoneal cavity.

The kininogen cascade. The second major cascade susceptible to proteolytic activation is the kininogen system, which is outlined in Figure 18.3. The final product of this pathway is bradykinin, a compound which relaxes vascular smooth muscle, stimulates catecholamine release by the adrenal gland, and increases vascular permeability. The precursor molecule kininogen is present in the serum in both a high molecular weight (20% of total) and low molecular weight form (80%). Activation of the kininogen cascade classically begins with the conversion of inactive prekallikrein to kallikrein by the Hagemann Factor, but trypsin also catalyses this conversion. Kallikrein cleaves high molecular weight kininogen to bradykinin. Bradykinin is metabolized to inactive fragments in the lung by the enzyme kinase II. Kallikrein activation is inhibited by C1INH and α_2-macroglobulin.

Lasson & Ohlsson (1984a) examined changes in the kininogen system in 19 attacks of pancreatitis and found that severe attacks were associated with lowered prekallikrein and kininogen levels, and deficient kallikrein inhibition, changes which were more marked in the peritoneal fluid than in the serum. In a series of 14 patients, Aasen et al (1982) found reduced prekallikrein levels in both survivors and those dying of acute pancreatitis, although the levels were lower in those who died. Decreased prekallikrein and increased kallikrein activity has been noted in experimental pancreatitis in the peritoneal cavity (Ruud et al 1982).

The clotting cascade. Alterations in the clotting cascade have been reported in acute pancreatitis as well. Trypsin can simultaneously initiate thrombosis and fibrinolysis by activation of both prothrombin and

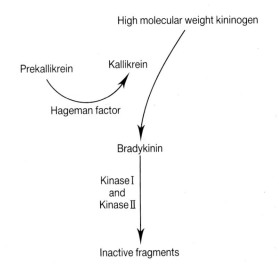

Fig. 18.3 The kallikrein kinin system.

plasminogen, in a situation similar to that occurring in disseminated intravascular coagulopathy.

Clinically, an increased tendency toward thrombosis has been noted in some patients with acute pancreatitis and pancreatic carcinoma (Kwaan et al 1971). In a study of the clotting profiles of 35 patients with acute pancreatitis, Ranson et al (1977) reported elevated fibrinogen, platelet, and fibrinogen–fibrin related antigen levels, with the changes being more marked in severe cases. A total of 9% of the patients had impaired euglobulin clot lysis on presentation, but this figure increased to 25% by the eleventh hospital day. There were no consistent changes in the prothrombin time (PT) and the partial thromboplastin time (PTT). An initial fall in fibrinogen and platelet counts has been observed in burn and trauma patients due to a consumptive coagulopathy, followed within 24 hours by a rebound hyperfibrinogenaemia and thrombocytosis. Ranson states that a similar situation probably occurs in acute pancreatitis due to tryptic activation of the clotting cascade.

In an experimental study, Satake et al (1981) studied coagulation changes in dogs after pancreatitis was induced by intraductal trypsin injection. He found significantly reduced fibrinogen levels and platelet counts, prolongation of partial thromboplastin and prothrombin times, and elevated fibrin degradation products. Microthrombi were present in the lungs and kidneys of the animals. Intravenous injection of pancreatic juice in another set of experiments was associated with hypofibrinogenaemia, thrombocytopenia, and slight prolongation of the PT and PTT. The pancreatic juice did not contain activated proteases, however. Other animals developed marked consumptive coagulopathy after the intravenous injection of activated trypsin in the absence of pancreatitis. Ascitic fluid from animals with pancreatitis produced similar changes when given intravenously to control animals. Agarwal et al (1982) noted a mild consumptive coagulopathy in the canine bile injection model of pancreatitis. No evidence of systemic thrombosis was found however.

Interactions between cascades. These can occur between the three cascade systems (Lasson & Ohlsson 1984a), since some activated factors (e.g. the Hageman factor, Factor XII) can activate components of other cascades. Likewise, while some inhibitors are specific for specific pathways (antithrombin III for example), others are less selective (alpha$_2$-macroglobulin). A few proteases such as trypsin and plasmin activate a number of factors in all the cascades.

Peritoneal lavage

Pullos et al (1982) and Frey et al (1982) have demonstrated the accumulation of toxic substances in the ascitic fluid in experimental models of severe acute pancreatitis. These substances included activated proteases, bradykinin, histamine, complement components, prostaglandins, phospholipase A$_2$, and others. Therapeutic peritoneal lavage has been proposed as a means of diluting the toxic substances in the abdominal cavity and reducing their systemic absorption.

Several studies have found an improvement in the mortality rate when animals with experimental pancreatitis were treated with peritoneal lavage (Rasmussen 1967, Rodgers & Carey 1966, Rosato et al 1973). Van Hee et al (1981) produced a temporary improvement in biochemical parameters in dogs with experimental pancreatitis by a single peritoneal lavage, but there was no improvement in survival.

Ranson et al (1976) found marked biochemical improvement and improved morbidity and mortality rates in five patients with severe pancreatitis who received peritoneal lavage, compared with a group of five controls with similar prognostic signs. Stone & Fabian (1980) reported an 85% response rate to peritoneal lavage in 34 patients with severe acute alcoholic pancreatitis compared with a 36% response rate in 36 patients treated conservatively. A total of 17 of these latter patients crossed over to the peritoneal lavage arm of the study after 24 hours, and 14 of these improved. The overall mortality rates were 15% in the 51 patients who received peritoneal lavage at some point in their illness, compared with 31% in the 19 patients who never received lavage.

In a larger series, Ranson & Spencer (1978) examined biochemical parameters, and morbidity and mortality in 24 patients with severe pancreatitis who were lavaged compared with a group of 79 patients, with equally severe disease, managed without lavage. Patients receiving lavage had a striking clinical improvement, and there were no deaths within the first 10 days of the illness in this group. By comparison, 45% of the deaths in the non-lavaged patients occurred in the first 10 days. Late deaths from intra-abdominal sepsis occurred more often in the lavaged group, and the overall mortality rate for the non-lavaged and lavaged patients were similar. Ranson advocates peritoneal lavage in patients with severe pancreatitis to reduce the early complication and mortality rate, but notes that the late sequelae of pancreatic necrosis are not prevented.

There is still considerable controversy concerning the optimal dosing schedule and timing for therapeutic peritoneal lavage and some investigators (Mayer et al 1985) question whether the technique is of any value.

Oxygen derived free radicals

Recent experimental work in the isolated perfused canine pancreas and other models has implicated the involvement of toxic oxygen-derived free radicals in the initiation of some forms of pancreatitis. Free radicals are molecular species which contain an unpaired electron in the outer shell of at least one atom, and are unstable, short-lived, and very reactive. Free radicals have been implicated in the pathogenesis of necrotizing enterocolitis, inflammatory conditions of the gastrointestinal tract, radiation injury, gastric ulceration, ischaemic hepatic injury and cirrhosis, deterioration of transplant organs during transport, necrosis of skin flaps, myocardial infarction, and other conditions (Bulkley 1983, Parks et al 1983b). Many enzyme systems produce free radicals (initiation), including neutrophil myeloperoxidase, cytochrome oxidases, aldehyde oxidase and xanthine oxidase. Once formed, free radicals can lead to formation of other free radicals (propagation) before they are metabolized (termination).

Although a number of free radicals have been described in biological systems, this discussion will be limited to two oxygen-derived free radicals, superoxide (O_2^-) and the hydroxyl radical, and a non-free-radical intermediate, hydrogen peroxide. Oxygen-derived free radicals are unstable and potent oxidizing agents, and produce tissue injury by peroxidation of the lipid components of mitochrondrial and cellular membranes, and degradation of hyaluronic acid and collagen. Superoxide released into the blood may also sitmulate production of a neutrophil chemotactic factor (McCord & Roy 1982, McCord 1983) which may lead to a non-specific inflammatory response. Oxygen-derived free radicals cause endothelial injury and increased capillary permeability in a number of experimental models (Parks & Granger 1983).

Cytochrome oxidase system. The major endogenous source of biological free radicals is the reduction of molecular oxygen to water in the mitochondria by oxidative phosphorylation. Approximately 98% of molecular oxygen undergoes tetravalent reduction (the addition of four electrons) to water by the cytochrome oxidase system (McCord 1983) (Fig. 18.4). The remaining 1–2% of oxygen undergoes univalent (single electron) reduction with the formation of superoxide free radical. While superoxide radical has some inherent toxicity, the trivalent reduction product of oxidative phosphorylation, hydroxyl radical, has even more potential toxicity.

Aerobic cells have evolved efficient scavenging systems (Fig. 18.5) to metabolize these toxic molecules to inert substances. Superoxide dismutase (SOD), first described by McCord & Fridovich in 1969, is an intracellular enzyme (actually several enzymes) which catalyses the conversion of O_2^- to hydrogen peroxide and molecular oxygen. It is a specific scavenger of the superoxide radical. The hydrogen peroxide which is formed is converted to water and oxygen by the enzyme catalase. At normal low levels of free radical production by oxidative phosphorylation, the two free radical scavengers SOD and catalase prevent the accumulation of significant amounts of superoxide and hydrogen peroxide. Injury to the cell only occurs if free radical production exceeds the scavenging capacity of these enzymes. Significant accumulation of hydrogen peroxide and superoxide favours formation of the highly toxic hydroxyl radical by the iron catalysed Haber Weiss reaction. No biological scavenger system has been identified for the hydroxyl radical, although dimethylsulphoxide (DMSO) scavenges the radical in vitro.

Xanthine oxidase. Other enzymes besides cytochrome oxidase produce free radicals as well. McCord & Fridovich (1968) demonstrated that the ubiquitous gastrointestinal enzyme xanthine oxidase produces superoxide radical. Xanthine oxidase has since been implicated as the source of superoxide radical production and reperfusion injury in a variety of ischaemia–reperfusion models. The evidence implicating xanthine oxidase is based on the amelioration of the ischaemia–reperfusion injury in these models by the specific xanthine oxidase inhibitor allopurinol (Hille & Massey 1981). An active metabolite of allopurinol, oxypurinol, binds tightly but reversibly at the active site of xanthine oxidase, sterically inhibiting the binding of substrate molecules.

Xanthine oxidase is widely distributed within the gastrointestinal tract but is most concentrated in the small bowel mucosa and the liver, where it is localized in the cell cytoplasm (Ibrahim & Stoward 1978, Auscher & Amory 1976). In small bowel mucosal cells, it is localized to the tips of the microvilli (Auscher & Amory 1976). The pancreas contains less xanthine oxidase than the small bowel, but a considerable amount is still present. The substrates which are oxidized by xanthine oxidase include hypoxanthine, acetaldehyde (a metabolite of ethanol), and unsubstituted purines and pyrimidines. Xanthine oxidase has two physiological functions: the oxidation of hypoxanthine to xanthine and xanthine to uric acid (the rate-limiting steps in purine degradation), and the facilitation of iron absorption across small bowel

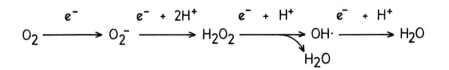

Fig. 18.4 The tetravalent reduction of O_2 to H_2O. Mitochondrial cytochrome oxidase catalyses the reduction of 98% of molecular oxygen to water with release of only minor amounts of free radicals.

$$O_2^- + O_2^- + 2H^+ \longrightarrow H_2O_2 + O_2 \qquad \text{Superoxide dismutase}$$

$$H_2O_2 + H_2O_2 \longrightarrow 2H_2O + O_2 \qquad \text{Catalase}$$

$$O_2^- + H_2O_2 \xrightarrow{Fe^{2+}} OH^- + OH\cdot + O_2 \qquad \text{Haber Weiss reaction}$$

Fig. 18.5 Oxygen-derived free radicals and scavengers.

mucosa by oxidation of ferrous ion to ferric ion, which is then incorporated into transferrin.

Xanthine oxidase exists in two interconvertible forms. The 'D' form, or xanthine dehydrogenase, utilizes NAD^+ (nicotinamide–adenine dinucleotide) as the electron receptor during oxidation of hypoxanthine to xanthine. NADH is released as a reaction byproduct. The 'O' form of the enzyme (xanthine oxidase proper) utilizes molecular oxygen as the electron receptor and superoxide free radical is a reaction product (Roy & McCord 1983). In healthy cells, the majority of the enzyme exists as the D form (Parks & Granger 1983), but certain conditions promote conversion to the O form, including proteolysis, low oxygen tension, heating at 37°C, and incubation with subcellular fractions (Parks & Granger 1986). Conversion to the O form occurs within seconds.

'D to O' conversion occurs via at least two biochemical pathways, including the proteolytic cleavage of a 20 000 Da peptide fragment from the 'D' form and oxidation of sulphydryl to disulphide bonds (Parks & Granger 1986) within the molecule. Ischaemia is thought to contribute to D to O conversion by increasing intracellular calcium and stimulating a calmodulin regulated protease to cleave a fragment from the xanthine dehydrogenase molecule (McCord & Roy 1982). Ischaemia also increases hypoxanthine levels by a factor of five by degradation of ATP to adenine and inosine (Jones et al 1968, DeWall et

al 1971, Schoenberg et al 1983), increasing the substrate for xanthine oxidase. Most of the injury in ischaemia–reperfusion appears to occur with reperfusion (McCord & Roy 1982) when molecular oxygen is available in excess. A burst of free radical production occurs with reperfusion when both molecular oxygen and hypoxanthine are present in excess and the majority of xanthine oxidase is present in the 'O' form. Figure 18.6 shows the sequence of events which occur with ischaemia–reperfusion which stimulate production of O_2^-.

Experimental evidence regarding oxygen-derived free radicals

Isolated perfused canine model. Studies in the isolated perfused ex vivo canine pancreas model have implicated oxygen-derived free radicals in the initiation of ischaemic pancreatitis. Addition of the scavengers SOD and catalase together, but not alone, prior to reperfusion decreased the severity of ischaemic pancreatitis in this model (Sanfey et al 1984). Surprisingly, the SOD and catalase combination was as effective in reducing injury in the oleic acid injection (FFA) and partial duct obstruction and secretin stimulation (POSS) models. Since these models mimic alcoholic and gallstone pancreatitis respectively, it is possible that the production of free radicals is a basic final common pathway by which several injurious stimuli initiate pancreatitis.

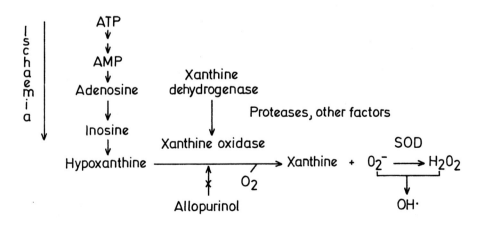

Fig. 18.6 Initiation of free radical production by D to O conversion.

In other experiments with these three models, allopurinol was equally efficacious in preventing injury (Sanfey et al 1985), but was ineffective if given after the injury occurred (Sarr et al 1987a), suggesting that xanthine oxidase is the source of the free radical production. Sarr et al (1987b) also eliminated leucocytes as the source of free radicals in these models by perfusing the isolated canine pancreas with leucocyte-depleted blood. No reduction in the degree of injury was observed in any model, evidence against the involvement of such enzymes as leucocyte myeloperoxidase in the initiation of pancreatitis.

How free radical production is stimulated in these three models (ischaemia, FFA, and POSS) is unknown, but promotion of D to O conversion by chymotrypsin-mediated proteolytic cleavage has been proposed (Fig. 18.7). Crist et al (1986) lowered the calcium permeability of pancreatic cells with the calcium channel blocker verapamil and reduced the severity of FFA-induced pancreatitis, confirming a role for this ion in the initiation of some forms of experimental pancreatitis.

The evidence linking free radical generation and caerulein-induced pancreatitis in intact animals is suggestive as well. In 1986 Guice et al demonstrated that free radical scavengers effectively ameliorate the ultrastructural and biochemical sequelae of caerulein pancreatitis even if given 12 hours after injury. Polyethylene glycol (PEG) conjugated catalase was ineffective as a one-time dose (Guice et al 1989), but was effective as a high dose continuous infusion (Wisner et al, 1988). Yamagishi et al (1987) and Saluja et al (1986) have confirmed a partially protective effect of free radical scavengers in the caerulein model and Wisner & Renner (1988) demonstrated a similar beneficial effect for a continuous allopurinol infusion. Dabrowski et al (1988) reported elevated xanthine oxidase and malondialdeylde levels (a product of free radical generation) in the pancreata of rats treated with caerulein. Tissue SOD activity was reduced as well, creating a milieu favourable for free radical production.

However, Clemens et al (1988) were unable to show a beneficial effect for unconjugated superoxide dismutase and catalase given as a single dose in a caerulein model in the isolated perfused canine pancreas preparation.

CDE diet model. In studies with the CDE diet model of pancreatitis, Degertekin et al (1985) demonstrated a detrimental effect of hyperbaric oxygen and a protective effect of allopurinol pretreatment. Pancreatic xanthine oxidase and lipoperoxide levels have been shown to be increased in the CDE diet model, while SOD levels are decreased (Nonaka et al 1989), an environment favourable for free radical generation.

Bile salt injection. In yet another model (bile salt injection in rats), MacGowen et al (1987) discounted the importance of free radical generation in acute pancreatitis.

Summary

Most experimental evidence supports the involvement of oxygen-derived free radicals in the initiation of acute experimental pancreatitis, although a beneficial effect from allopurinol or free radical scavengers has yet to be demonstrated in a clinical population. In a single clinical study, allopurinol was ineffective in reducing post-ERCP hyperamylasaemia or pancreatitis when given in a prospective fashion (Clemens et al 1991).

Prostaglandins

The role of prostaglandins in the pathogenesis of acute pancreatitis is unclear. A number of experimental studies (usually the CDE diet model or a variation thereof) have demonstrated conflicting results concerning the influence of prostaglandins. A single clinical study of a prostaglandin synthesis inhibitor (indomethacin) (Ebbehøj et al 1985) failed to improve the course of acute pancreatitis. No human trials of prostaglandin infusion have been reported.

Prostaglandins have a number of effects in the gastrointestinal tract, most notably a protective influence on the

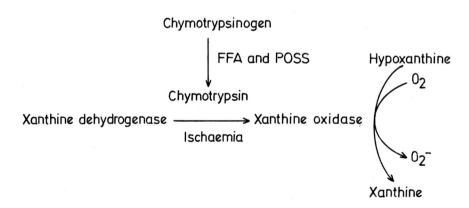

Fig. 18.7 Possible role of chymotrypsinogen activation in D to O conversion.

gastric mucosa (Miller & Jacobson 1979). The effects on the pancreas appear to involve the secretory state of the gland and the maintenance of normal perfusion and vascular permeability. In the perfused feline pancreatic duct model, 16,16-dimethyl prostaglandin E_2 (PGE_2) converts oedematous to haemorrhagic pancreatitis, perhaps by increasing microvascular permeability (Wedgwood et al 1986). Increased levels of PGE_2 (Glazer & Bennett 1976), the leukotrienes LTC4 and LTD4, prostacyclin, and thromboxane (Vollmar et al 1989) have all been reported in the portal venous effluent in experimental pancreatitis. These arachadonic acid metabolites seem likely to have some role in the systemic toxicity seen with acute pancreatitis. PGE_2 is a known stimulant of small bowel and pancreatic secretion (Matuchansky & Coutrot 1978, Coelle et al 1983) and may have deleterious effects in some cases of obstructive pancreatitis. Indomethacin, a prostaglandin synthesis inhibitor, reduces pancreatic blood flow both in the basal state and with pancreatitis (Studley et al 1983), supporting a role for prostaglandins in the maintenance of normal splanchnic blood flow. Prostaglandins also appear to stabilize organelle and cellular membranes (Robert 1979).

Prostaglandin infusion has been beneficial in several models of pancreatitis (Reber et al 1980, Tweedie et al 1981, Manabe & Steer 1980), but ineffective in others (Martin et al 1981, Lankisch et al 1983). Phenylbutazone (a prostaglandin synthesis inhibitor) did not alter mortality rates in a rat model in which intraductal trypsin injection initiated pancreatitis (Louagie et al 1984). The histological changes in the pancreas in treated animals were less severe than in untreated animals, however, and Louagie attributed this to a non-specific anti-inflammatory effect of the drug independent of prostaglandins.

In a study of PGE_2 infusion in the CDE diet-induced pancreatitis model, Coelle et al (1983) demonstrated a significant dose-related reduction in the degree of histological injury and mortality rate in treated animals. The mortality rate in animals treated with indomethacin (another prostaglandin synthesis inhibitor) was increased. Coelle attributes some of the contradictory results obtained with PGE_2 infusion to the varying potency of different PGE_2 derivatives used in the studies. The reduction in mortality rate in animals treated with prostaglandin infusion was attributed to a membrane-stabilizing effect which could theoretically prevent secretory vacuole and lysosomal fusion (recall that fusion of these two organelles is thought to lead to intracellular protease activation in the CDE model). Prostaglandins may also stimulate pancreatic secretion and reduce crinophagy by clearing cells of secretory vacuoles.

Phospholipase A_2

In addition to the proteolytic enzymes implicated in the pathogenesis of acute pancreatitis, the lipolytic pancreatic enzymes phospholipase A_2, lecithinase, and lipase may each have a role to play. Phospholipase is synthesized by the pancreas as the trypsin activated proenzyme prophospholipase A_2. Phospholipase A_2 is synthesized primarily in the pancreas, although there may be other sources (Eskola et al 1988). The active enzyme hydrolyses various lipids, triglycerides, and phospholipids including cephalin and lecithin. Serum phospholipase A_2 attacks pulmonary surfactant, and this may partially explain the pulmonary injury seen with severe pancreatitis. In addition, the product of the lecithin hydrolysis (lysolecithin) is a potent detergent which is toxic to cell membranes and capillaries. The pancreatic content of lecithin has been shown to drop during experimental pancreatitis while the level of lysolecithin increases (Aho et al 1980). High levels of phospholipase A_2 have been found in the ascitic exudate in clinical and experimental pancreatitis (Schmidt & Creutzfeldt 1969, Zeive & Vogel 1961), and in the serum in acute pancreatitis, while pancreatic levels are decreased (Nordback et al 1989).

Serum phospholipase A_2 levels also correlate with the severity of experimental and clinical pancreatitis. In the CDE diet model in mice, Mizuma et al (1984) found a better correlation between the mortality rate and phospholipase A_2 levels than with amylase levels. Nevalainen et al (1985) found elevated mean immunoreactive phospholipase A_2 levels in 103 patients with acute pancreatitis and in eight patients with pancreatic cancer. In this study phospholipase A_2 levels distinguished between mild and severe alcoholic pancreatitis but did not predict the severity in gallstone pancreatitis. In a series of 66 patients with alcoholic, biliary, and idiopathic pancreatitis, Schroder et al (1980) distinguished severe pancreatitis form mild disease by following phospholipase A_2 levels over a 5-day-period. The levels correlated well with Ranson's criteria.

Local anaesthetic agents inhibit the action of phospholipase A_2, probably by stabilizing membranes (Schroder et al 1981). These drugs have been studied as possible therapeutic agents in both animal and clinical studies. In a study of bile salt injection pancreatitis in rats, Aho et al (1980) increased survival in animals treated with procaine. Human studies also suggest a beneficial effect, although not conclusively (Nevalainen 1988). Tykka et al (1985) administered $CaNa_2EDTA$, a calcium chelator and inhibitor of phospholipase A_2, to 33 patients with alcoholic, gallstone, and idiopathic pancreatitis. A control group of 31 patients received a placebo and supportive therapy. Patients in the study group had more severe disease as ranked by Ranson's criteria. A total of 20 of the patients in the study group and 13 in the placebo group had elevated phospholipase A_2 levels on admission. Phospholipase A_2 activity levels decreased significantly and standard laboratory tests normalized more quickly in the treatment group compared with controls, despite the more severe initial disease in this group. However, the clinical condition at the time of discharge (assessed by laboratory determinations), complication rate, and mortality rate of the two groups were similar.

There is direct experimental evidence that lipase may play a central role in cell membrane injury in pancreatitis (Nagai et al 1989). In this study, activated trypsin, lipase, and phospholipase failed to injure suspended rat pancreatic acini, but a triglyceride and lipase-containing mixture injured the acinar cells and allowed leakage of newly synthesized proteins into the medium, suggesting a lack of cell membrane integrity. The authors speculate that the resultant free fatty acids and diglycerides are directly toxic to the acinar cells.

CONCLUSIONS

In spite of over 100 years of study, the pathogenesis of acute pancreatitis remains largely unknown. A number of markedly disparate clinical situations are associated with pancreatitis, including alcohol abuse, gallstone disease hypotension, certain drugs and anatomical anomalies. In none of these clinical scenarios is there sufficient data to offer a single unifying concept which ties together the known information into a pathogenetic sequence. Because of the lack of information concerning pathogenetic mechanisms, the current treatment of pancreatitis is purely supportive, i.e. there is no accepted effective treatment which interrupts the disease process once it is initiated. Hopefully, with increased understanding of the pathophysiology, gained in large part through animal studies, the development of an effective therapy will be possible during the next decade.

REFERENCES

Aasen A, Kierulf P, Rund T, Godal J, Aune S 1982 Studies on pathological plasma proteolysis in patients with acute pancreatitis: a preliminary report. Acta Chirurgica Scandanavica (Suppl) 509: 83

Aasen A, Ruud T, Roeise O, Bouma B, Stadaas J 1989 Peritoneal lavage efficiently eliminates protease-α_2-macroglobulin complexes and components of the contact system from the peritoneal cavity in patients with severe acute pancreatitis. European Surgical Research 21: 1

Acosta J, Ledesma C 1974 Gallstone migration as a cause for acute pancreatitis. New England Journal of Medicine 290: 484

Adler G, Hahn C, Kern H, Rao K 1985 Cerulein-induced pancreatitis in rats: increased lysosomal enzyme activity and autophagocytosis. Digestion 32: 10

Agarwal M, Kamdar M, Bapat R, Mehta B, Suryaprabha R, Rao P 1982 Consumptive coagulopathy and fibrinolysis in experimental acute pancreatitis. Journal of Postgraduate Medicine 28: 214

Aho H, Nevalainen T, Lindberg R, Aho A 1980 Experimental pancreatitis in the rat. The role of phospholipase A in sodium taurocholate-induced acute haemorrhagic pancreatitis. Scandinavian Journal of Gastroenterology 15: 1027

Ances I, McClean C 1971 Acute pancreatitis following the use of thiazide in pregnancy. Southern Medical Journal 64: 267

Angelini G, Merigo F, Degani G et al 1985 Association of chronic alcoholic liver and pancreatic disease: a prospective study. American Journal of Gastroenterology 80: 998

Armstrong C, Taylor T, Jeacock J, Lucas S 1985 The biliary tract in patients with acute gallstone pancreatitis. British Journal of Surgery 72: 551

Artigas J, Garcia M, Faure M, Gimeno A 1981 Serum trypsin levels in acute pancreatic and non-pancreatic abdominal conditions. Postgraduate Medical Journal 57: 219

Augelli N, Hussain S, McKain M et al 1989 Effect of SMS201-995 (a long-acting somatostatin analog) on bile-induced acute hemorrhagic pancreatitis in the dog. American Surgeon 55: 389–391

Auscher C, Amory W 1976 The histochemical localization of xanthine oxidase in the rat liver. Biomedicine 25: 37

Babkin B, Starling E 1926 A method for the study of the perfused pancreas. Journal of Physiology (London) 61: 245

Balart L, Ferrante W 1982 Pathophysiology of acute and chronic pancreatitis. Archives of Internal Medicine 142: 113

Balldin G, Eddeland A, Ohlasson K 1981 Studies on the role of the plasma protease inhibitors on in vitro C3 activation and in acute pancreatitis. Scandinavian Journal of Gastroenterology 16: 603

Balldin G, Borgstrom A, Genell S, Ohlsson K 1983 The effect of peritoneal lavage and aprotinin in the treatment of severe acute pancreatitis. Research and Experimental Medicine 183: 203

Bank S, Marks I 1960 Hyperlipemic pancreatitis and the Pill. Postgraduate Medical Journal 46: 576

Berry A, Millar A, Taylor T 1982 Pancreatic blood flow in experimental acute pancreatitis. Digestive Diseases and Sciences 27: 444

Bess M, Edis A, van Heerden J 1980 Hyperparathyroidism and pancreatitis. Journal of the American Medical Association 243: 246

Bordalo O, Noronha M, Dreiling D 1976 Morphologic evidence of cytologic damage to the pancreatic parenchyma in alcoholics. Scandinavian Journal of Gastroenterology 11: 78

Brodrick J, Geokas M, Largman C, Johnson J 1979 Molecular forms of immunoreactive pancreatic cationic trypsin in pancreatitis patient sera. American Journal of Physiology 237: E474

Broe P, Cameron J 1982 Experimental gallstone pancreatitis: pathogenesis and response to different treatment modalities. Annals of Surgery 195: 566

Broe P, Cameron J 1983 Azathioprine and acute pancreatitis: studies with an isolated perfused canine pancreas. Journal of Surgical Research 34: 159

Broe P, Zuidema G, Cameron J 1982a The role of ischemia in acute pancreatitis: studies with an isolated perfused canine pancreas. Surgery 91: 377

Broe P, Zinner M, Cameron J 1982b A clinical trial of cimetidine in acute pancreatitis. Surgery, Gynecology and Obstetrics 154: 13

Brunzell J, Schrott H 1973 Interaction of familial and secondary causes of hypertriglyceridemia: role in pancreatitis. Clinical Research 21: 723

Bulkley G 1983 The role of oxygen free radicals in human disease processes. Surgery 94: 407

Cameron J, Capuzzi D, Zuidema G, Margolis S 1973 Acute pancreatitis with hyperlipemia: the incidence of lipid abnormalities in acute pancreatitis. Annals of Surgery 177: 483

Cameron J, Capuzzi D, Zuidema G, Margolis S 1974 Acute pancreatitis with hyperlipemia: evidence for a persistent defect in lipid metabolism. American Journal of Medicine 56: 482

Cameron J, Mehigan D, Zuidema G 1979 Evaluation of atropine in acute pancreatitis: a prospective randomized clinical trial. Surgery, Gynecology and Obstetrics 148: 206

Chiari H 1896 Uber die Selbstverdauung des menschlichen Pankreas. Zeitschrift für Heilkunde 17: 69

Choi T, Wong J 1984 Severe acute pancreatitis caused by parasites in the common bile duct. Journal of Tropical Medicine and Hygiene 87: 211

Clemens J 1988 Cerulein and SOD/catalae study

Clemens J, Olsen, J, Cameron J 1989 Histology of the pancreas study

Clemens J et al 1991 ERCP and allopurinol study

Coelle E, Adham N, Elashoff J, Lewin K, Taylor I 1983 Effects of prostaglandin and indomethacin on diet-induced acute pancreatitis in mice. Gastroenterology 85: 1307

Cope O, Gulliver P, Mixter G, Nardi C 1957 Pancreatitis, a diagnostic clue to hyperparathyroidism. Annals of Surgery 145: 857

Cornish A, McClellan J, Johnston D 1961 Effects of Chlorothiazide on the pancreas. New England Journal of Medicine 265: 673

Corrodi P, Knoblanch M, Binswanger U, Scholzel E, Largiader F 1975 Pancreatitis after renal transplantation. Gut 16: 285

Cotton P 1980 Congenital anomaly of pancreas divisum as cause of obstructive pain and pancreatitis. Gut 21: 105

Crist D, Bulkley G, Cameron J 1986 The role of calcium influx in the pathogenesis of experimental acute pancreatitis, Surgical Forum 37: 151

Csendes A, Kruse A, Funch-Jensen P, Oster M, Ornsholt J, Amdrup E 1979 Pressure measurements in the biliary and pancreatic duct systems in controls, and in patients with gallstones, previous cholecystectomy, or common bile duct stones. Gastroenterology 77: 1203

Dabrowski A , Gabryelewicz A, Wereszczynske-Siemiatkowska U, Chyczewski L 1988 Oxygen-derived free radicals in cerulein-induced acute pancreatitis. Scandanavian Journal of Gastroenterology 23: 1245

Davidoff F, Tishler S, Rosoff C 1973 Marked hyperlipidemia and pancreatitis associated with oral contraceptive therapy. New England Journal of Medicine 289: 552

Degertekin H, Ertan A, Yates R, Van Meter K, Akdamar K 1985 Hyperbaric oxygen, allopurinol, and diet-induced acute pancreatitis. (Letter to the editor) Annals of Internal Medicine 103: 474

De Wall R, Vasko K, Stanley E, Kezdi P 1971 Responses of the ischemic myocardium to allopurinol. American Heart Journal 82: 362

Diamond M 1972 Hyperglycemic hyperosmolar coma associated with hydrochlorothiazide and pancreatitis. New York State Journal of Medicine 72: 1741

Donahue P, Akimoto H, Ferguson J, Nyhus L 1984 Vasoactive drugs in acute pancreatitis. Archives of Surgery 119: 477

Durbec J, Sarles H 1978 Multicenter survey of the etiology of pancreatic diseases: relationship between the relative risk of developing chronic pancreatitis and alcohol, protein and lipid consumption. Digestion 18: 337

Durr G 1979 Acute pancreatitis. In: Howat HT, Sarles H (eds) The exocrine pancreas, W B Saunders, London p 352

Durr H, Maroske D, Zelder O, Bode J 1978 Glucagon therapy of acute pancreatitis: report of a double blind trial. Gut 19: 175

Dutta S, Mobrahan S, Iber F 1978 Associated liver disease in alcoholic pancreatitis. American Journal of Digestive Diseases 23: 618

Ebbehøj N, Friis J, Svendsen L, Bulow S, Donahue P, Madsen P 1985 Indomethacin treatment of acute pancreatitis. Scandinavian Journal of Gastroenterology 20: 798

Elias E, Redshaw M, Wood T 1977 Diagnostic importance of changes in circulating concentrations of immunoreactive trypsin. Lancet 2: 66

Eskola J, Nevalainen T, Kortesuo P 1988 Immunoreactive pancreatic phospholipase A_2 and catalytically active phospholipase A_2 in serum from patients with acute pancreatitis. Clinical Chemistry 34(6): 1052

Evander A, Ihse I, Lundquist I 1981 Influence of hormonal stimulation by caerulein on acute experimental pancreatitis in the rat. European Surgery Research 13: 257

Farber E, Popper H 1950 Production of acute pancreatitis with ethionine and its prevention by methionine. Proceedings of the Society of Experimental Biology and Medicine 74: 838

Farmer R, Tweedie J, Maslin S, Reber H, Adler G, Kern H 1984 Effects of bile salts on permeability and morphology of main pancreatic duct in cats. Digestive Diseases and Sciences 29: 740

Feiner H 1976 Pancreatitis after cardiac surgery: a morphological study. American Journal of Surgery 131: 684

Frey C 1981 Gallstone pancreatitis. Surgical Clinics of North America 61: 923

Frey C, Wong H, Hickman D, Pullos T 1982 Toxicity of hemorrhagic ascitic fluid associated with hemorrhagic pancreatitis. Archives of Surgery 117: 401

Fritz H, Wunderer G 1983 Biochemistry and applications of aprotinin, the kallikrein inhibitor from bovine organs. Arzneimittel Forsch 33: 479

Fujii S 1979 Inhibitors of kinin-forming enzymes. Advances in Experimental Medicine and Biology 120A: 75

Gafter U, Mandel E, Har-Zahav L, Weiss S 1976 Acute pancreatitis secondary to hypercalcemia: occurrence in a patient with breast carcinoma. Journal of the American Medical Association 235: 2004

Geokas M, Largman C, Durie P, Brodrick J, Ray S, O'Rourke M, Vollmer J 1981 Immunoreactive forms of cationic trypsin in plasma and ascitic fluid of dogs in experimental pancreatitis. American Journal of Pathology 105: 31

Glazer G, Bennett A 1976 Prostaglandin release in canine acute haemorrhagic pancreatitis. Gut 17: 22

Glueck C, Scheel D, Fishback J, Steiner P 1972 Estrogen-induced pancreatitis in patients with previously covert familial type V hyperlipoproteinemia. Metabolism 21: 657

Goebell H, Hotz J 1979 Die Aetiologie der Akuten Pankreatitis. In : Forell M M (ed) Handbuch der Inneren Medizin, Band 3, Teil 6: Pankreas 5 Auflage. Springer-Verlag, Berlin.

Goldberg R, Chaikoff I, Dodge A 1950 Destruction of pancreatic acinar tissue by DL-ethionine. Proceedings of the Society of Experimental Biology and Medicine 74: 869

Goodhead B 1969 Vascular factors in the pathogenesis of acute haemorrhagic pancreatitis. Annals of the Royal College of Surgeons of England 45: 80

Greenbaum L, Hirshkowitz A 1961 Endogenous cathepsin activates trypsinogen in extracts of dog pancreas. Proceedings of the Society of Experimental Biology and Medicine 107: 74

Gregg J, Monaco A, McDermott W 1983 Pancreas divisum: results of surgical intervention. American Journal of Surgery 145: 488

Guelrud M, Siegal J 1984 Hypertensive pancreatic duct sphincter as a cause of pancreatitis: successful treatment with hydrostatic balloon dilatation. Digestive Diseases and Sciences 29: 225

Guice K, Miller D, Oldham K, Townsend C, Thompson J 1986 Superoxide dismutase and catalase: a possible role in established pancreatitis. American Journal of Surgery 151: 163

Guice K, Oldham K, Johnson K 1989 Failure of antioxidant therapy (polyethylene glycol-conjugated catalase) in acute pancreatitis. American Journal of Surgery 157: 145–149

Haas G, Warshaw A, Daggett W, Aretz H 1985 Acute pancreatitis after cardiopulmonary bypass. American Journal of Surgery 149: 508

Harvey M, Wedgwood K, Reber H 1987 Isoproterenol treatment of acute pancreatitis. Abstract Book of the Society of University Surgeons, 48th Annual Meeting, Columbus, Ohio, p 29

Harvey M, Cates M, Reber H 1988 Possible mechanisms of acute pancreatitis induced by ethanol. American Journal of Surgery 155: 49

Havel R 1969 Pathogenesis, differentiation and management of hypertriglyceridaemia. Advances in Internal Medicine 15: 117

Hazzard W, Spiger M, Bagdale J, Bierman E 1969 Studies on the mechanism of increased plasma triglyceride levels induced by oral contraceptives. New England Journal of Medicine 280: 471

Hermon-Taylor J 1969 A technique for perfusion of the isolated canine pancreas. Gastroenterology 55 (4): 488

Hille R, Massey V 1981 Tight binding inhibitors of xanthine oxidase. Pharmacologic Therapy 14: 249

Ibrahim B, Stoward P 1978 The histochemical localization of xanthine oxidase. Histochemistry Journal 10: 617

Imrie C, Mackenzie M 1981 Effective aprotinin therapy in canine experimental bile-trypsin pancreatitis. Digestion 22: 32

Imrie C, Benjamin I, Ferguson J, McKay A, Mackenzie I, O'Neill J, Blumgart L 1978 A single-centre double-blind trial of trasylol therapy in primary acute pancreatitis. British Journal of Surgery 65: 337

Isselbacher K, Greenberger N 1964 Metabolic effects of alcohol on the liver. New England Journal of Medicine 270: 351

Iwasaki T, Tashiro A, Satodate R, Sata T, Kurata T 1987 Acute pancreatitis with cytomegalovirus infection. Acta Pathologica Japan 37 (10): 1661

Izsak E, Shike M, Roulet M, Jeejeebhoy K 1980 Pancreatitis in association with hypercalcemia in patients receiving total parenteral Nutrition. Gastroenterology 79: 555

Janes N, Clemens J, Chacko V, Cameron J 1986 NMR study demonstrating ischemia.

Johnston D, Cornish A 1959 Acute pancreatitis in patients receiving chlorothiazide. Journal of the American Medical Association 170: 2054

Jones C, Crowell J, Smith E 1968 Significance of increased blood uric acid following extensive hemorrhage. American Journal of Physiology 214: 1374

Jones P, Hermon-Taylor J, Grant D 1982 Antiprotease chemotherapy of acute experimental pancreatitis using the low molecular weight oligopeptide aldehyde leupeptin. Gut 23: 939

Keil B 1971 Trypsin. In: Boyer P (ed) The Enzymes, 3rd ed. Academic Press, New York, vol 3

Kelly T 1974 Gallstone pancreatitis. Archives of Surgery 109: 294

Kelly T 1976 Gallstone pancreatitis: pathophysiology. Surgery 80: 488

Kelly T 1984 Gallstone pancreatitis: local predisposing factors. Annals of Surgery 200: 479

Keynes M 1988 Heretical thoughts on the pathogenesis of acute pancreatitis. Gut 29: 1413

Kronberg O, Jorgensen P, Bulow S 1976 A controlled randomized trial of glucagon in the treatment of first attack of severe acute pancreatitis with associated biliary disease: Interim report. Scandinavian Journal of Gastroenterology, 38 (Suppl): 13

Kvietys P, McLendon J, Bulkley G, Perry M, Granger D 1982 Pancreatic circulation: Intrinsic regulation. American Journal of Physiology 242: G596

Kwaan H, Anderson M, Gramatica L 1971 A study of pancreatic enzymes as a factor in the pathogenesis of disseminated intravascular coagulation during acute pancreatitis. Surgery 69: 663

Lampel M, Kern H 1977 Acute pancreatitis in the rat induced by excessive doses of pancreatic secretagogue. Virchows 373: 97

Langerhans P 1890 Veber Multiple Fettgewebsnekrose. Virchows Archiv für Pathologie und Anatomie 122: 252

Lankisch P 1984 Acute and chronic pancreatitis: An update on management. Drugs 28: 554

Lankisch P, Goke B, Kunze H, Otto J, Winckler K 1983 Does PGE_2 have a beneficial effect on acute experimental pancreatitis in the rat? Hepato-Gastroenterology 30: 148

Lasson A 1984 Acute pancreatitis in man: a clinical and biochemical study of pathophysiology and treatment. Scandinavian Journal of Gastroenterology 99 (Suppl): 1

Lasson A, Ohlsson K 1984a Changes in the kallikrein kinin system during acute pancreatitis in man. Thrombosis Research 35: 27

Lasson A, Ohlsson K 1984b Protease inhibitors in acute human pancreatitis: correlation between biochemical changes and clinical course. Scandinavian Journal of Gastroenterology 19: 779

Lasson A, Laurell A, Ohlsson K 1985 Correlation among complement activation, protease inhibitors, and clinical course in acute pancreatitis in man. Scandinavian Journal of Gastroenterology 20: 335

Levant J, Secrist D, Resin H, Sturdevant R, Guth P 1974 Nasogastric suction in the treatment of alcoholic pancreatitis: a controlled study. Journal of the American Medical Association 229: 51

Lohse J, Verine H, Sarles H 1981 Studies on pancreatic stones. 1. In vitro dissolution. Digestion 21: 125

Lombardi B 1976 Influence of dietary factors on the pancreatotoxicity of ethionine. American Journal of Pathology 84: 633

Lombardi B, Rao N. 1975 Acute hemorrhagic pancreatic necrosis in mice: influence of the age and sex of the animals and of dietary ethionine, choline, methionine, and adenine sulfate. American Journal of Pathology 81: 87

Lombardi B, Rao K 1982 Acute hemorrhagic pancreatic necrosis in mice: effects of protease inhibitors on its induction. Digestion 23: 57

Lombardi B, Estes L, Longnecker D 1975 Acute hemorrhagic pancreatitis (massive necrosis) with fat necrosis induced in mice by DL ethionine fed with a choline-deficient diet. American Journal of Pathology 79: 465

Louagie Y, Hancotte-Lahaye C, Delloye Ch, Mairy Y, DeMuylder C 1984 The effect of phenylbutazone on acute hemorrhagic pancreatitis in the rat. International Surgery 69: 265

MacGowan S, Bouchier-Hayes D, Broe P 1987 Experimental pancreatitis: the effect of allopurinol. Gut 28: A368 (abstract)

Mallory A, Kern F 1980 Drug-induced pancreatitis: a critical review. Gastroenterology 78: 813

Manabe T, Steer M 1980 Protective effect of PGE_2 on diet induced acute pancreatitis in mice. Gastroenterology 78: 777

Martin D, Someren A, Nasrallah S 1981 The effect of prostaglandin E_2 on ethionine-induced pancreatitis in the rat. Gastroenterology 81: 736

Masaryk T, Achkar E 1983 Pancreatitis as initial presentation of cystic fibrosis in young adults: A report of two cases. Digestive Diseases and Sciences 28: 874

Masoero G, Andruilli S, Recchia S, Marchetto M, Benitti V, Verme G 1980 Trypsin-like immunoreactivity in the diagnosis of acute pancreatitis. Scandinavian Journal of Gastroenterology 62 (Suppl): 21

Matsumoto T, Matsui T, Iida M, Nunoi K, Fujishima M 1989 Acute pancreatitis as a complication of Crohn's disease. American Journal of Gastroenterology 84 (7): 804

Matuchansky C, Coutrot S 1978 The role of prostaglandins in the study of intestinal water and electrolyte transport in man. Biomedicine 28: 143

Mayer A, McMahon M, Corfield A et al 1985 Controlled clinical trial of peritoneal lavage for the treatment of severe acute pancreatitis. New England Journal of Medicine 312: 399

McCord J, Fridovich I 1969 Superoxide dismutase: an enzymic function for erythrocuprein (Hemocuprein). Journal of Biologic Chemistry 244: 6049

McCord J, Fridovich I 1968 The reduction of cytochrome c by milk xanthine oxidase. Journal of Biologic Chemistry 243: 5753

McCord J, Roy R 1982 The pathophysiology of superoxide: roles in inflammation and ischemia. Canadian Journal of Physiology and Pharmacology 60: 1346

McCord J 1983 The superoxide free radical: its biochemistry and pathophysiology. Surgery 94: 412

Medical Research Council Multicentre Trial 1980 Morbidity of acute pancreatitis: the effect of aprotinin and glucagon. Gut 21: 334

Meshkinpour H, Molinari M, Gardner L, Berk J, Hoehler F 1979 Cimetidine in the therapy of acute alcoholic pancreatitis: a randomized double-blind study. Gastroenterology 77: 687

Miller T, Jacobson E 1979 Progress report. Gastrointestinal cytoprotection by prostaglandins. Gut 20: 75

Mixter C, Keynes W, Cope O 1962 Further experience with pancreatitis as a diagnostic clue to hyperparathyroidism. New England Jounal of Medicine 266: 265

Mizuma K, Schrodeer T, Kaarne M, Korpela H, Lempinen M 1984 Serum phospholipase A_2 in diet-induced pancreatitis. European Surgical Research 16: 156

MRC Multicentre Trial of Glucagon and Aprotinin 1977 Death from acute pancreatitis, Lancet, p 632

Naeije R, Salingret E, Clumeck N, De Troyer A, Devis G 1978 Is nasogastric suction necessary in acute pancreatitis? British Medical Journal 2: 659

Nagai H, Henrich H, Hans Wunsch P, Fischbach W, Mossner J 1989 Role of pancreatic enzymes and their substrates in autodigestion of the pancreas. In vitro studies with isolated rat pancreatic acini. Gastroenterology 96: 838

Nakamura K, Sarles H, Payan H 1972 Three dimensional reconstruction of the pancreatic ducts in chronic pancreatitis. Gastroenterology 62: 942

Nardi G, Greep J, Chambers D, McCrae C, Skinner D 1963 Physiologic peregrinations in pancreatic perfusion. Annals of Surgery 158: 830

Nevalainen T 1988 Phospholipase A_2 in acute pancreatitis. Scandinavian Journal of Gastroenterology 23: 897

Nevalainen T, Eskola J, Aho A, Havia V, Lovgren T, Nanto V 1985 Immunoreactive phospholipase A_2 in serum in acute pancreatitis and pancreatic cancer. Clinical Chemistry 31: 1116

Noel-Jorand M, Colomb E, Astier J, Sarles H 1981 Pancreatic basal secretion in alcohol fed and normal dogs. Digestive Diseases and Sciences 26: 783

Nogueira J, Freedman M 1972 Acute pancreatitis as a complication of imuran therapy in regional enteritis. Gastroenterology 62: 1040

Nonaka A, Manabe T, Tamura K, Asano N, Imanishi K, Tobe T 1989 Changes of xanthine oxidase, lipid peroxide and superoxide dismutase in mouse acute pancreatitis. Digestion 43: 41

Nordback I, Teerenhovi O, Auvinen O et al 1989 Human pancreatic phospholipase A_2 in acute necrotizing pancreatitis. Digestion 42: 128

Opie E 1901 The etiology of acute haemorrhagic pancreatitis. Bulletin of the Johns Hopkins Hospital 12: 182

Ohshio G, Saluja A, Leli U, Sengupta A, Steer M 1989 Esterase inhibitors prevent lysosomal enzyme redistribution in two noninvasive models of experimental pancreatitis. Gastroenterology 96: 853

Otsuki M, Tani S, Okabayashi Y et al 1990 Beneficial effects of the synthetic trypsin inhibitor camostate in cerulein-induced acute pancreatitis in rats. Digestive Diseases and Sciences 35 (2): 242

Pantoja J, Renner I, Abramson S, Edmondson H 1983 Production of acute hemorrhagic pancreatitis in the dog using venom of the scorpion, *Buthus quinquestriatus*. Digestive Diseases and Sciences 28: 429

Parks D, Granger N 1983 Ischemia-induced vascular changes: role of xanthine oxidase and hydroxyl radicals. American Journal of Physiology 8: G285

Parks D, Granger N 1986 Xanthine oxidase: biochemistry, distribution, and physiology. Acta Physiologica Scandanavica 548 (Suppl): 87

Parks D, Bulkley G, Granger D 1983a Role of oxygen derived free radicals in digestive tract diseases. Surgery 94: 415

Parks D, Bulkley G, Granger D 1983b Role of oxygen free radicals in shock, ischemia, and organ preservation. Surgery 94: 428

Paxton J, Payne J 1948 Acute pancreatitis: a statistical review of 307 established cases of acute pancreatitis. Surgery, Gynecology and Obstetrics 86: 69

Pfeffer R, Lazzarini-Robertson A, Safadi D, Mixter G, Secoy C, Hinton J 1962 Gradations of pancreatitis, edematous through hemorrhagic, experimentally produced by controlled injection of microspheres in blood vessels in dogs. Surgery 51: 764

Phat V, Guerrieri M, Alexandre J, Camilleri J 1984 Early histological changes in acute necrotizing hemorrhagic pancreatitis. Pathology Research and Practice 178: 273

Poon-King T 1963 Myocarditis from scorpion stings. British Medical Journal 1: 374

Popper H, Necheles H, Russell K 1948 Transition of pancreatic edema into pancreatic necrosis. Surgery, Gynecology and Obstetrics 87: 79

Prince M 1882 Pancreatic apoplexy with a report of two cases. Boston Medical and Surgical Journal 7: 28, 55

Pullos T, Frey C, Zaiss C 1982 Toxicity of ascitic fluid from pigs with hemorrhagic pancreatitis. Journal of Surgical Research 33: 136

Ranson J 1979 Acute pancreatitis. In: Current problems in surgery, Year Book Medical Publishers, Chicago, Vol 16 (2)

Ranson J, Spencer F 1978 The role of peritoneal lavage in severe acute pancreatitis. Annals of Surgery 187: 565

Ranson J, Rifkind K, Turner J 1976 Prognostic signs and nonoperative peritoneal lavage in acute pancreatitis. Surgery, Gynecology and Obstetrics 143: 209

Ranson J, Lackner H, Berman I, Schinella R 1977 The relationship of coagulation factors to clinical complications of acute pancreatitis. Surgery 81: 502

Rao K, Tuma J, Lombardi B. 1976 Acute hemorrhagic pancreatic necrosis in mice: intraparenchymal activation of zymogens and other enzyme changes in pancreas and serum. Gastroenterology 70: 720

Rao K, Zuretti M, Baccino F, Lombardi B 1980 Acute hemorrhagic pancreatic necrosis in mice: the activity of lysosomal enzymes in the pancreas and the liver. American Journal of Pathology 98: 45

Rasmussen B 1967 Hypothermic peritoneal dialysis in the treatment of acute experimental hemorrhagic pancreatitis. American Journal of Surgery 114: 716

Reber H, Roberts C, Way L 1979 The pancreatic duct mucosal barrier. American Journal of Surgery 147: 128

Reber H, Tweedie J, Mosley J 1980 The cytoprotective effect of 16,16-dimethyl prostaglandin E_2 (PG) on bile salt induced damage to the pancreas. Gastroenterology 78: 1241 (abstract)

Reeve T, Delbridge L 1982 Pancreatitis following parathyroid surgery. Annals of Surgery 195: 158

Regan P, Malagelada J, Go W, Wolf A, Di Magno E 1981 A prospective study of the antisecretory and therapeutic effects of cimetidine and glucagon in human acute pancreatitis. Mayo Clinic Proceedings 56: 499

Richter J, Schapiro R, Mulley A, Warshaw A 1981 Association of pancreas divisum and pancreatitis, and its treatment by sphincteroplasty of the accessory ampulla. Gastroenterology 81: 1104

Rinderknecht H, Renner I, Abramson S, Carmack C 1984 Mesotrypsin: a new inhibitor-resistant protease in human pancreatic tissue and fluid. Gastroenterology 86: 681

Robert A 1979 Cytoprotection by prostaglandins. Gastroenterology 77: 761

Robinson T, Dunphy J 1963 Continuous perfusion of bile protease activators through the pancreas. Journal of the American Medical Association 183: 530

Rodgers R, Carey L 1966 Peritoneal lavage in experimental pancreatitis in dogs. American Journal of Surgery 111: 792

Romanus R, Helmann P, Nilsson O, Hansson G 1973 Surgical treatment of hyperparathyroidism. Progress in Surgery 12: 22

Rosato E, Mullis W, Rosato F 1973 Peritoneal lavage therapy in hemorrhagic pancreatitis. Surgery 74: 106

Rosin R 1976 Pancreatitis and hyperparathyroidism. Postgraduate Medical Journal 52: 95

Roszler M, Campbell W 1985 Post-ERCP pancreatitis: association with urographic visualization during ERCP. Radiology 157: 595

Roy R, McCord J 1983 Superoxide and ischemia: conversion of xanthine dehydrogenase to xanthine oxidase. In : Greenwald R, Cohen G (eds) Oxy radicals and their scavenger systems, vol 2: Cellular and medical aspects. Elsevier Science, p 145

Ruppin H, Amon R, Ettl W, Classen M, Demling L 1974 Acute pancreatitis after endoscopic/radiological pancreaticography (ERCP). Endoscopy 6: 94

Ruud T, Aasen A, Kierulf P, Stadaas J, Aune S 1982 Studies on components of the plasma kallikrein–kinin system in peritoneal fluid and plasma before and during experimental acute pancreatitis in pigs. A preliminary report. Acta Chirurgica Scandanavica 509 (Suppl): 89

Saario I 1983 5-fluorouracil in the treatment of acute pancreatitis. American Journal of Surgery 145: 349

Saharia P, Margolis S, Zuidema G, Cameron J 1977 Acute pancreatitis with hyperlipemia: studies with an isolated perfused canine pancreas. Surgery 82: 60

Saluja A, Powers R, Saluja M, Rutledge P, Steer M 1986 The role of oxygen derived free radicals in caerulin induced pancreatitis. Abstract Book of the Pancreas Club, Inc., 20th Annual Meeting, San Francisco, p 14

Sanfey H, Bulkley G, Cameron J 1984 The role of oxygen derived free radicals in the pathogenesis of acute pancreatitis. Annals of Surgery 200: 405

Sanfey H, Bulkley G, Cameron J 1985 The pathogenesis of acute pancreatitis: the source and role of oxygen derived free radicals in three different experimental models. Annals of Surgery 201: 633

Sarles H 1974 Chronic calcifying pancreatitis – chronic alcoholic pancreatitis. Gastroenterology 66: 604

Sarr M, Sanfey H, Cameron J 1986 Prospective randomized trial of nasogastric suction in patients with acute pancreatitis. Surgery 100: 500

Sarr M, Bulkley G, Cameron J 1987a Temporal efficacy of allopurinol during the induction of pancreatitis in the ex vivo perfused canine pancreas. Surgery 101: 342

Sarr M, Bulkley G, Cameron J 1987b The role of leukocytes in the production of oxygen derived free radicals in acute experimental pancreatitis. Surgery 101: 292

Sarra-Carbonell S, Jimenez S 1989 Ehlers–Danlos syndrome associated with acute pancreatitis. Journal of Rheumatology 16 (10): 1390

Satake K, Uchima K, Umeyama K, Appert H, Howard J 1981 The effects upon blood coagulation in dogs of experimentally induced pancreatitis and the infusion of pancreatic juice. Surgery, Gynecology and Obstetrics 153: 341

Schmidt H, Creutzfeldt W 1969 The possible role of phospholipase A in the pathogenesis of acute pancreatitis. Scandinavian Journal of Gastroenterology 4: 39

Schoenberg M, Younes M, Muhl E, Hagland U, Sellin D, Schildberg F 1983 Free radical involvement in ischemic damage of the small intestine. In: Greenwald R, Cohen G (eds) Proceedings of the Third International Conference on Superoxides and Superoxide Dismutase. Biomedical Press, New York, p 154

Schroder T, Kivilaakso E, Kinnunen P, Lempinen M 1980 Serum phospholipase A_2 in human acute pancreatitis. Scandinavian Journal of Gastroenterology 15: 633

Schroder T, Lempinen M, Nordling S, Kinnunen P 1981 Chlorpromazine treatment of experimental acute fulminant pancreatitis in pigs. European Surgical Research 13: 143

Seelig R, Seelig H 1975 The possible role of serum complement system in the formal pathogenesis of acute pancreatitis. Acta Hepato-Gastroenterologica 22: 263

Shader A, Paxton J 1966 Fatal pancreatitis. American Journal of Surgery 111: 369

Sipila R, Louhija A 1982 Aprotinin in acute pancreatitis: effect on the plasma kallikrein–kinin system. Acta Medica Scandanavica 668 (Suppl): 118

Sjovall S, Ahren B, Stenram U 1988 Effects of the specific cholecystokinin antagonist L364, 718 in experimental acute pancreatitis in the rat. European Surgical Research 20: 325

Smyth C 1940 Etiology of acute pancreatitis with special reference to vascular factors. Archives of Pathology 30: 651

Sobel H, Waye J 1963 Pancreatic changes in various types of cirrhosis in alcoholics. Gastroenterology 45: 341

Steer M, Meldolesi J, Figarella C 1984 Pancreatitis: the role of lysosomes. Digestive Diseases and Sciences 29: 934

Steer M 1985 Workshop on experimental pancreatitis. Digestive Diseases and Sciences 30: 575

Steinberg W, Schlesselman S 1987 Treatment of acute pancreatitis, a comparison of animal and human studies. Gastroenterology 93: 1420

Stigendal L, Olsson R 1984 Alcohol consumption pattern and serum lipids in alcoholic cirrhosis and pancreatitis: a comparative study. Scandinavian Journal of Gastroenterology 19: 582

Stone H, Fabian T 1980 Peritoneal dialysis in the treatment of acute alcoholic pancreatitis. Surgery, Gynecology and Obstetrics 150: 878

Strum W, Spiro H 1971 Chronic pancreatitis. Annals of Internal Medicine 74: 264

Studley J, Lee J, Schenk W 1982 Pathophysiology of acute pancreatitis: evaluation of the effects and mode of action of indomethacin in experimental pancreatitis in dogs. Journal of Surgical Research 32: 563

Sturdevant R, Singleton J, Deren J, Law D, McCleery J 1979 Azathioprine-related pancreatitis in patients with Crohn's disease. Gastroenterology 77: 883

Tani S 1988 Experimental acute pancreatitis induced by excessive doses of caerulein in rats; protective and therapeutic effects of trypsin inhibitor urinastatin and CCK receptor antagonist CR1392. Kobe Journal of Medical Science 34: 93

Trapnell J 1968 The pathogenesis of gallstone pancreatitis. Postgraduate Medical Journal 44: 497

Tuzhilin S, Podolsky A, Dreiling D 1981 The role of insufficiency of the sphincter of Oddi in the pathogenesis of pancreatitis. Mount Sinai Journal of Medicine 48: 133

Tweedie J, Mosley J, Austin J, Reber H 1981 Effect of 16,16 dimethyl prostaglandin E_2 on aspirin-induced permeability changes in the pancreatic duct. American Journal of Surgery 141: 22

Tykka H, Vaittinen E, Mahlberg K, Railo J, Pantzar P, Sarna S, Tallberg T 1985 A randomized double-blind study using $CaNa_2$ EDTA, a phospholipase A_2 inhibitor, in the management of human acute pancreatitis. Scandinavian Journal of Gastroenterology 20: 5

Usadel K, Leuschner U, Uberla K 1980 Treatment of acute pancreatitis with somatostatin: a multicenter double-blind trial. New England Journal of Medicine 303: 999 (letter)

Van Hee R, Van Elst F, Van Rooy F, Van Haasen R, Hubens A 1981 Peritoneal lavage in acute pancreatitis: an experimental and clinical study. Acta Chirurgica Belgica 6: 397

Vollmar B, Waldner H, Schman J et al 1989 Release of arachidonic acid metabolites during acute pancreatitis in pigs. Scandinavian Journal of Gastroenterology 24: 1253

Warshaw A, Cambria R 1984 False pancreas divisum: acquired pancreatic duct obstruction simulating the congenital anomaly. Annals of Surgery 200: 595

Warshaw A, O'Hara P 1978 Susceptibility of the pancreas to ischemic injury in shock. Annals of Surgery 188: 197

Warshaw A, Richter J, Schapiro R 1983 The cause and treatment of pancreatitis associated with pancreas divisum. Annals of Surgery 198: 443

Watanabe O, Baccino F, Steer M, Meldolesi J 1984 Supramaximal caerulein stimulation and ultrastructure of rat pancreatic acinar cell: early morphological changes during development of experimental pancreatitis. American Journal of Physiology 246: G457

Wedgwood K, Farmer R, Reber H 1986 A model of hemorrhagic pancreatitis in cats – role of 16,16-dimethyl prostaglandin E_2. Gastroenterology 90: 32

Wellborn J, Alston J, Cannon D, Read R 1983 Serum proteolytic and antiproteolytic activity in acute pancreatitis. American Journal of Surgery 146: 834

Werner S, Hjern B, Sjoberg H 1974 Primary hyperparathyroidism: analysis of findings in a series of 129 patients. Acta Chirurgica Scandinavica 140: 618

Whicher J, Barnes M, Brown A 1982 Complement activation and complement control proteins in acute pancreatitis. Gut 23: 944

Wilson J, Pirola R 1983 Pathogenesis of alcoholic pancreatitis. Australian and New Zealand Journal of Medicine 13: 307

Wilson J, Gossat D, Tait A, Rouse S, Jeng Juan X, Pirola R 1984 Evidence for an inherited predisposition to alcoholic pancreatitis: a controlled HLA typing study. Digestive Diseases and Sciences 9: 727

Wilson J, Bernstein L, McDonald C, Tait A, McNeil D, Pirola R 1985 Diet and drinking habits in relation to the development of alcoholic pancreatitis. Gut 26: 882

Wisner J Renner I 1988 Allopurinol attenuates caerulein induced acute pancreatitis in the rat. Gut 29: 926

Wisner J, Green D, Ferrell L, Renner I 1988 Evidence for a role of oxygen derived free radicals in the pathogenesis of caerulein induced acute pancreatitis in rats. Gut 29: 1516–1523

Yamagishi T, Haggit R, Garcia R, Goto Y, Debas H 1987 Comparison of drugs with therapeutic potential in cerulein induced acute pancreatitis in the rat. Gastroenterology 92 (5) part 2: 1702

Zieve L, Vogel W 1961 Measurement of lecithinase A in serum and other body fluids. Journal of Laboratory and Clinical Medicine 57: 586

19. Diagnostic assessment and prognostication in acute pancreatitis

D. C. Carter

INTRODUCTION

Acute pancreatitis remains a common and potentially lethal condition that is not always easy to diagnose and the severity of which may be notoriously difficult to assess when the patient is first seen. A number of studies have suggested that the disease may be increasing in incidence although it seems likely that much of this apparent increase reflects increasing awareness and improvements in diagnosis (O'Sullivan et al 1972, Trapnell & Duncan 1975). For example, the Scottish Hospitals' Statistics show that the number of patients with a primary discharge diagnosis of acute pancreatitis rose 11-fold in males (from 69 to 750 patients/year) and four-fold in females (from 112 to 484 patients/year), when the years 1961 and 1985 are compared (Fig. 19.1) (Wilson & Imrie 1990). The trend in males affected all age groups and the incidence apparently continues to increase, whereas in females the increase was most marked in those over 60 years of age and now appears to have reached a plateau. In Bristol, the mean annual incidence of acute pancreatitis rose from 55.1 per million population in the period 1968–1973 to 90.5 per million for the years 1974–1979 (Corfield et al 1985a). Similarly in Nottingham the mean annual incidence rose from 75.1 per million between 1969 and 1976 to 116.9 per million between 1977 and 1983 (Katschinski et al 1990). These three studies were all conducted in the United Kingdom, a country where the proportion of cases of acute pancreatitis due to gallstones is particularly high. In Japan where alcohol is the predominant cause, recent studies suggest an annual incidence of 120 per million population (Saitoh & Yamamoto 1991), a figure not greatly different from the UK experience.

It is of interest that a recent Swedish study showed that the incidence of non-gallstone pancreatitis in Stockholm county fell in the period 1969–1986, a fall which took place at the same time as a drop in the consumption of distilled spirits (Schmidt 1991).

Most studies of the incidence of acute pancreatitis rely on clinical diagnosis which in turn is based on a compatible

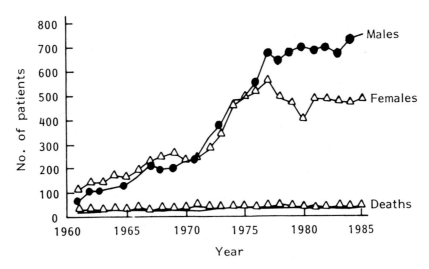

Fig. 19.1 Annual incidence and mortality from acute pancreatitis in Scotland by recorded discharge diagnoses in the period 1961–1985. (From Wilson C, Imrie C W, British Journal of Surgery 1990, 77: 731–734. Reproduced by permission of the publishers, Butterworth–Heinemann Ltd.)

193

clinical picture and 'diagnostic' elevation of serum amylase levels. As will be discussed, hyperamylasaemia may not be the reliable basis for diagnosis that was once believed (see below). It has become apparent that a number of patients with acute pancreatitis escape the diagnostic net, a problem which is particularly apparent in children, patients dealt with in wards other than general surgical wards, and those with atypical presentation. This has important implications when attempting to define the mortality of acute pancreatitis and the statement that mortality continues to diminish must be treated with some caution. Thus the fall in mortality from 17.8% in 1961 to 5.8% in 1985 in the Scottish study (Wilson & Imrie 1990) has to be taken in conjunction with the observation that no less than 42% of the 126 patients dying from acute pancreatitis in Glasgow Royal Infirmary in the period 1974–1984 were diagnosed as suffering from pancreatitis for the first time at autopsy (Wilson et al 1988, see Table 19.1). Similarly, in the Bristol study 35% of the fatal cases were diagnosed for the first time at necropsy, while case mortality remained at around 20% throughout the study (Corfield et al 1985a). Lankisch et al (1991) also found that the diagnosis was not made in life in 30% of their 43 fatal cases of acute pancreatitis collected between 1980 and 1985. Important findings to emerge from this study were that only one of these patients complained of abdominal pain while 12 had been given analgesics immediately on admission which may have masked their pain. Serum amylase levels were often normal, not obtained or obtained too late.

It is clear that we have no grounds for complacency regarding our ability to diagnose and treat acute pancreatitis. The elderly are at particular risk and mortality rates for those over 60 years of age in Bristol were 28% compared with 9% for younger patients (Corfield et al 1985a). In Hong Kong, mortality rates rose from 6% in those under 50 years to 21% in those over 75 years, the increase in mortality being attributed primarily to a greater incidence of concomitant medical or surgical disease in the elderly (Fan et al 1988).

DIAGNOSIS OF ACUTE PANCREATITIS

There are no symptoms and signs which are pathognomonic of acute pancreatitis and as already indicated, the standard diagnostic test, namely determination of the serum amylase concentration, is far from infallible. Acute pancreatitis may affect all age groups but is rare in children. Recent series indicate that the mean age at presentation ranges from 52–60 years (Blamey et al 1984, Corfield et al 1985a, Fan et al 1988). Most series show a male:female ratio that is close to unity (Corfield et al 1985) or has a slight female preponderance (Blamey et al 1984, Fan et al 1988). In general, the peak age incidence of the disease is higher in females, reflecting the high proportion of females with gallstone pancreatitis, whereas the lower peak age incidence in men reflects their propensity to alcohol-associated disease. These demographic patterns may change with time as evidenced by the recent Scottish data showing a move from an almost equal sex incidence to a recent male preponderance of 1.5:1 (Wilson & Imrie 1990).

Clinical presentation

Pain is usually the cardinal symptom in acute pancreatitis. It characteristically develops relatively quickly, taking minutes rather than hours to attain maximum intensity and persisting thereafter for many hours or several days. The pain is usually experienced first in the epigastrium but may be localized to either upper quadrant or felt diffusely throughout the abdomen. There is radiation to the back in about 50% of cases and some patients obtain some relief by sitting or leaning forwards. Alternatively, the patient may find that lying on one or other side curled up in bed eases, although rarely, if ever, banishes, the pain. Radiation to the chest may simulate myocardial infarction, pneumonia or pleuritic irritation. The pain varies in severity from patient to patient but frequently it is severe or agonizing, refractory to relief by usual doses of analgesics, and constant in nature and intensity.

Dramatic and sudden onset of epigastric pain may simulate perforated peptic ulcer, while pain in the right upper quadrant can suggest biliary colic or acute cholecystitis. It should be stressed that acute pancreatitis can mimic virtually every cause of the acute abdomen and should always be considered in differential diagnosis.

It is also now well recognized that acute pancreatitis may be painless and failure to make the diagnosis early in such cases is particularly liable to a fatal outcome (Read et al 1976, Lankisch et al 1991). As Amman (1976) has

Table 19.1 Aetiology of fatal acute pancreatitis in relation to patient age and sex, and proportion of patients diagnosed at autopsy (Wilson et al 1988)

Aetiology	n(%)	Male:female	Mean age (years)	Percentage undiagnosed before autopsy
Gallstones	39(30%)	19:20	68	33
Alcohol	20(15%)	16:4	48	40
Other causes	23(17%)	12:11	62	74
Unknown causes	50(38%)	21:29	66	42
Total	132(100%)	68:64	63	42

stressed, the diagnosis must also be considered in any patient who:

1. Suddenly develops shock and/or anuria regardless of whether they have abdominal pain
2. has fever, marked abdominal pain or unexplained shock following abdominal surgery, particularly when this has involved the biliary tree or stomach
3. presents with apparent diabetic coma and shock, or
4. shows clinical features suggestive of myocardial infarction.

To this list should now be added patients who are unwell following ERCP and associated procedures, and those who develop abdominal signs and symptoms after cardiopulmonary bypass procedures.

Nausea, *vomiting* and *retching* are marked accompaniments of acute pancreatitis in the majority of cases. The vomiting is often frequent and persistent, and retching may persist despite keeping the stomach empty by means of a nasogastric tube. A combination of factors is probably responsible, including severe pain, side-effects of opiate analgesics, irritation of the stomach by the inflamed pancreas, and development of ileus. *Hiccoughs* can also prove troublesome and may reflect irritation of the diaphragm by retroperitoneal inflammation tracking upwards from the inflamed pancreas and lesser sac.

Examination

Patients exhibit a wide spectrum of appearances, ranging from those who appear completely well to those who from the time of admission are gravely ill with profound shock, toxicity and confusion. *Tachypnoea* is common and can be associated with pleuritic pain, *tachycardia* is usual and *hypotension* may be present. The *temperature* may be normal or even subnormal on admission but frequently becomes elevated as pancreatic and peripancreatic inflammation extends and complications develop. Mild *icterus* may reflect the fact that the pancreatitis is due to gallstones and an associated swinging pyrexia suggests acute cholangitis. *Facial flushing* is found in some patients, while in severe acute pancreatitis there may be areas of cyanotic marbling of the abdominal wall or brawny pitting oedema of the flanks. *Bruising* from entry of blood into fascial planes may produce bluish discoloration of the flanks (Grey-Turner's sign) or umbilicus (Cullen's sign). The prognostic significance of these signs will be considered below but it should be emphasized that neither is pathognomonic of acute pancreatitis; in fact Cullen's sign was first described following rupture of an ectopic pregnancy (Cullen 1918). Subcutaneous fat necrosis may produce small red tender nodules which affect the limbs more often than the torso. These lesions may be misdiagnosed as erythema nodosum and have been described in association with pancreatic cancer as well as acute pancreatitis (Higgins & Ive 1990).

If biopsy is undertaken it reveals panniculitis with basophilic 'ghost' cells which are remnants of fat cells, the contents of which have been replaced by calcium soap formation. Occasionally such necrosis involves joint spaces and synovitis can occur.

Apart from skin changes, abdominal examination may reveal distension due to ileus, or more rarely, due to ascites. A *mass* is rarely present on admission but can develop in patients with severe and continuing pancreatic and peripancreatic inflammation. *Tenderness* in the epigastrium is usually present on palpation but may seem surprisingly mild when compared to the severity of pain and prostration. There may be some muscle *guarding* over the areas of tenderness but marked rigidity is seldom seen in acute pancreatitis in contrast to perforated peptic ulcer. The presence of *ileus* may result in a tympanitic abdomen on percussion as well as resulting in diminished or absent bowel sounds on auscultation. When there is a considerable amount of free fluid in the peritoneal cavity, shifting dullness may be elicited. Hepatomegaly and splenomegaly are not features of acute pancreatitis but may reflect underlying liver disease in those with alcohol-associated disease.

Examination of the *chest* reveals the presence of a pleural effusion in 10–20% of patients with acute pancreatitis. The effusion is usually left-sided, but can be bilateral, and probably reflects inflammation tracking upwards behind the peritoneum from the body and tail of the pancreas and lesser sac. In rare cases the effusion results from an internal pancreaticopleural fistula following rupture of a major pancreatic duct. Air entry at the bases is usually diminished and pulmonary oedema and/or pneumonitis may be present. It is now appreciated that arterial hypoxia and the full adult respiratory distress syndrome may develop in patients who initially have little obvious clinical or radiological chest abnormality at the time of admission.

Other features occasionally seen in acute pancreatitis include a combination of disorientation, confusion, delirium and hallucination, sometimes referred to as 'pancreatic encephalopathy'. The mechanism responsible is uncertain but metabolic upset, circulating pancreatic enzymes, toxins and vasoactive substances, and hypoxaemia may be involved. The derangements may be more common in patients with alcoholic pancreatitis in whom alcohol withdrawal can contribute. Although hypocalcaemia is a recognized feature of severe acute pancreatitis (see below), tetany is exceptional and it is unusual to be able to elicit positive tests of neuromuscular irritability such as Trousseau's test or Chvostek's test.

Past medical history

The importance of detailed documentation of the patient's past medical history cannot be over-emphasized. Some patients are already known to have gallstones or have suffered from previous attacks of biliary colic, acute cholecystitis, obstructive jaundice or episodes or gallstone pancreatitis. Alcohol consumption must be defined, drug ingestion noted, and the nature of any previous abdominal surgery clarified. Postoperative pancreatitis has a particularly bad reputation, given that it is often difficult to evaluate the abdomen and assess the significance of pain in someone who has recently undergone laparotomy. Operations involving surgery to the stomach, duodenum and bile duct are particularly liable to cause postoperative pancreatitis and its association with cardiopulmonary bypass surgery is now well-recognized. Recent ERCP and associated procedures such as endoscopic papillotomy, stenting and gallstone extraction are all potential causes of acute pancreatitis. A history of recent abdominal trauma may well be relevant, as is a family history of pancreatitis in children with abdominal pain.

Laboratory aids to diagnosis

Routine blood tests

The haemoglobin concentration and haematocrit are frequently elevated early in the course of acute pancreatitis reflecting the loss of protein-rich fluid into the inflamed pancreas and retroperitoneal tissues: the so-called 'retroperitoneal burn' effect. Serum electrolyte levels are not usually deranged at the time of admission, but elevation of the blood urea may reflect dehydration and impending renal failure in severe disease. Derangement of liver function is not a result of acute pancreatitis per se but elevation of serum aminotransferases, alkaline phosphatase and bilirubin is often seen in gallstone pancreatitis.

Transient hyperglycaemia is common in severe pancreatitis and the combination of abdominal pain and a raised blood glucose in a patient not known to have diabetes mellitus should be taken as extremely suggestive of acute pancreatitis. The fact that hyperamylasaemia and abdominal pain may be present in diabetic ketacidosis can cause confusion. However, ketoacidosis is most unusual in acute pancreatitis and when hyperamylasaemia accompanies ketoacidosis it is due to raised levels of salivary amylase rather than pancreatic amylase (Warshaw et al 1977).

Serum calcium levels fall slightly in about one-quarter of patients with acute pancreatitis and a fall to beneath 2 mmol/l signifies the presence of severe disease (see below). As mentioned above, neuromuscular irritability and tetany are exceptional. It is now appreciated that much of the hypocalcaemia is apparent rather than real, and that most patients are in fact normocalcaemic when allowances are made for the degree of hypoalbuminaemia (Allam & Imrie 1977). Nevertheless, true hypocalcaemia does occur in severe disease; it cannot be explained simply on the basis of calcium deposition in the calcium soaps of fat necrosis and factors implicated include hyperglucagonaemia

(Paloyan et al 1976), promotion of calcitonin secretion (Pickleman et al 1969) and reduced levels of circulating parathormone (McMahon et al 1978).

Serum amylase

Serum amylase concentrations increase rapidly during the first 24 hours of an attack of acute pancreatitis. Enzymes leaking from the acinar cells or pancreatic duct system are initially absorbed directly into the venous drainage of the pancreas and peripancreatic tissues, whereas later in the attack, enzyme-rich fluid is absorbed transperitoneally into the peritoneal lymphatics and passes from there into thoracic duct lymph (Egdahl 1958, Mayer et al 1985). Serum amylase levels usually return to normal within a few days; a more rapid fall may reflect rapid resolution of mild inflammation or more rarely, destruction of the gland in fulminant pancreatitis with loss of enzyme production.

The lack of a standardized international method for amylase measurement is reflected in the varied range of normal values, and chosen thresholds range from one to nine times the upper value of normal for the laboratories concerned (Clavien et al 1989a). In Britain where gallstones are the predominant cause of acute pancreatitis, diagnostic levels for serum amylase are usually set at a higher level (i.e. at some point between 1000 and 2000 iu/l) than in the United States (200–1000 Somogyi units/dl) where alcoholic pancreatitis predominates. In our own practice a serum amylase level of greater than 1000 iu/l is regarded as strongly suggestive of acute pancreatitis.

Specificity of serum amylase. Many abdominal and non-abdominal conditions other than acute pancreatitis can be associated with hyperamylasaemia (Table 19.2). In general the serum amylase elevation is less marked than that found in acute pancreatitis but while specificity can be improved by raising the level required for diagnosis, this is only achieved at the price of reduced sensitivity. When isoenzyme determinations (see below) are performed, as many as one-third of patients diagnosed as having acute pancreatitis on the basis of hyperamylasaemia and abdominal pain are found not to be suffering from acute pancreatitis (Weaver et al 1982, Koehler et al 1982).

Macroamylasaemia. This is another potential diagnostic pitfall. In this condition normal serum amylase is bound to an abnormal serum protein, which may be an IgG, IgM or IgA or non-immunoglycoprotein. The resulting high molecular weight complex is too large to be excreted by the kidney and produces hyperamylasaemia with normal or low levels of urinary amylase excretion. While macroamylasaemia is found in up to 3% of cases of acute pancreatitis (Durr et al 1977) this does not pose problems; the real problems are that 1–2% of the normal population may have persistent or transient macroamylasaemia in the absence of any particular disease

Table 19.2   Conditions associated with hyperamylasaemia

Abdominal causes	Non-abdominal causes
Pancreatitis	Thoracic
Pancreatic cancer	Myocardial infarct
Biliary tract disease	Pulmonary embolism
Perforated peptic ulcer	Pneumonia
Acute perforated appendicitis	Metastatic lung cancer
Intestinal obstruction	Cardio-pulmonary bypass
Mesenteric infarction	Salivary gland
Liver disease	Salivary trauma
Dissecting aortic aneurysm	Infection (mumps)
Ruptured ectopic pregnancy	Salivary duct obstruction
Prostatic disease	Irradiation
Ovarian neoplasm	Metabolic
	Diabetic ketoacidosis
Recent abdominal operation	Drugs
Afferent loop syndrome	Opiates
	Phenylbutazone
	Trauma
	Cerebral trauma
	Burns
	Renal disease
	Renal insufficiency
	Renal transplantation

process and that macroamylasaemia is responsible for between 10 and 20% of all cases of unexplained hyperamylasaemia (Levitt et al 1980, Forsman 1986, Kleinmann & O'Brien 1986). When macroamylasaemia is suspected as the cause hyperamylasaemia in a patient who may or may not have acute pancreatitis the situation can be clarified by direct demonstration of the macromolecule (which is technically complex); measurement of the amylase:creatinine clearance ratio (usually less than 1% in macroamylasaemia but greater than 6% in acute pancreatitis), or more simply, by measurement of serum lipase levels (elevated in acute pancreatitis but normal in non-pancreatic disease).

Sensitivity of serum amylase. The sensitivity of serum amylase as a diagnostic test for acute pancreatitis is difficult to determine given that most authors use hyperamylasaemia as the very basis of their definition of the disease. It was frequently taught that only about 5% of patients with acute pancreatitis have normal amylase levels when first seen but it is now clear that acute pancreatitis and normoamylasaemia is a far from uncommon combination. Spechler et al (1983) disregarded serum amylase values in a series of 68 patients thought clinically to have acute alcoholic pancreatitis. In one-third of cases, serum amylase levels were normal, but the ultrasonographic and CT findings supported the diagnosis of acute pancreatitis as frequently in patients with normoamylasaemia as in those with hyperamylasaemia. It is possible that amylase levels may have been elevated at an earlier stage in some of these patients with normoamylasaemic pancreatitis; alternatively they may have been suffering from an acute exacerbation of underlying chronic alcoholic pancreatitis with a pancreas incapable

of producing hyperamylasaemia. Clavien et al (1989b) used CT scanning to evaluate 318 patients with 352 attacks of acute pancreatitis; no less than 67 (19%) of these patients had normoamylasaemia on admission. Such normoamylasaemic pancreatitis was commoner in patients with an alcoholic aetiology but was seen in gallstone pancreatitis, postoperative pancreatitis and idiopathic pancreatitis. Patients with normoamylasaemic and hyperamylasaemic pancreatitis did not differ significantly in terms of severity, CT findings or clinical course but normoamylasaemic patients had a longer duration of symptoms before admission (2.4 vs. 1.5 days).

Under normal circumstances only about 40% of total serum amylase is of pancreatic origin. Electrophoresis now allows differentiation between three forms of this pancreatic amylase, the p-3 fraction being the most specific for acute pancreatitis. It also allows pancreatic amylase to be distinguished from the so-called salivary amylase which is found in all tissues that contain amylase. Although pancreatic isoamylase levels may be elevated for longer than total amylase levels in acute pancreatitis (Kolars et al 1984), isoamylase determinations have proved to have little clinical value in increasing the diagnostic sensitivity of amylase measurement. Unfortunately, a number of important abdominal causes of hyperamylasaemia other than acute pancreatitis, notably mesenteric infarction and perforated peptic ulcer, are associated with raised levels of pancreatic isoamylase. However, as mentioned earlier, isoamylase determinations can increase specificity by identifying patients in whom hyperamylasaemia is due to non specific salivary isoamylase (Koehler et al 1982, Weaver et al 1982).

Hyperlipidaemia. This can cause difficulty in diagnosis

in that high levels of plasma triglyceride suppress or inhibit amylase activity and may produce false negative assay results in patients with acute pancreatitis and hyperamylasaemia. The problem is found particularly in patients with alcoholic pancreatitis, of whom some 20% have lipaemic serum. Serial dilution of the serum will usually allow the true level of serum amylase activity to be revealed. Alternatively, urinary amylase levels can be used for diagnosis (Dickson et al 1984).

Urinary amylase

Urinary amylase levels in acute pancreatitis generally parallel serum amylase levels and are subject to the same limitations in diagnosis. A rapid colorimetric test for urinary amylase, the Rapignost-Amylase test (Hoescht UK) has been advocated as a screening test for acute pancreatitis (Thompson et al 1987). Although simple to perform, on one drop of urine, and taking only 3 minutes to read, the need to distinguish between positive (+) and strongly positive (+ +) results has given rise to controversy and in some hands, sensitivities and specificities of around only 70% (Holdsworth et al 1984, Burkitt 1987). The test is not widely used.

Amylase : creatinine clearance ratio (ACCR). This measure was described by Levitt et al (1969) as a means of detecting the increased amylase clearance which takes place in acute pancreatitis. The test requires a simultaneous sample of blood and urine but avoids the need for prolonged urine collection with all its inherent difficulties. Normally, the ACCR is less than 1–2% and a rise above 6% was at first thought to be specific for acute pancreatitis. Unfortunately, it is now apparent that a number of circumstances including burns, perforated peptic ulcer, renal failure, and the performance of an operation can all elevate the ACCR (see Clavien et al 1989a), and the test is seldom used.

Serum lipase

It has been recognized since 1932 that pancreatic injury produces high serum lipase levels (Cherry & Crandall 1932) but methodological problems led to the more easily measurable serum amylase being adopted as the standard marker of acute pancreatitis. Although lipase is also produced by non-pancreatic sources such as the stomach, it is probably one of the most reliable tests for acute pancreatitis with a specificity of almost 90% (Ventrucci et al 1989). Serum lipase levels remain elevated for longer than amylase levels, do not rise in conditions where hyperamylasaemia is due to salivary isoamylase, and remain normal in patients with macroamylasaemia not due to pancreatitis (Kolars et al 1984). The fact that the earlier cumbersome turbidimetric and nephelometric lipase assays have been replaced by rapid reliable methods, such as the lipase latex agglutination test, with encouraging results (Moller-Petersen et al 1985), means that lipase measurements may come to be used more widely in clinical practice.

Other pancreatic enzymes

A number of other enzymes normally produced by the pancreas such as trypsin, phospholipase A_2, carboxylic ester hydrolase and RNase also show changes in their serum levels in acute pancreatitis. The potential role of these markers has been reviewed recently (Clavien et al 1989a) but at present none seem to offer significant advantages relative to the use of amylase and lipase measurements.

Diagnostic peritoneal lavage

Peritoneal lavage has been advocated as a means of diagnosing acute pancreatitis and assessing its severity (Pickford et al 1977). In this technique a peritoneal catheter is introduced through a small midline stab incision sited 2.5 cm below the umbilicus, using local anaesthesia (20 ml 1% lignocaine with adrenaline), first having ensured that the stomach and bladder are empty. The cannula is passed into the pelvis and an attempt made to aspirate any free peritoneal fluid. One litre of warmed normal saline is then run in as quickly as possible. The patient is moved from side to side and the foot of the bed is elevated momentarily to distribute the fluid widely, and it is then allowed to siphon back into its bag with the aid of gravity. Any free fluid and the lavage return fluid is sniffed for odour and inspected for colour before samples are sent for bacteriological culture, microscopy and amylase determinations. In the early stages of acute pancreatitis the ascitic fluid which accumulates is odourless and sterile and the presence of odour, uncharacteristic colour, or organisms or fibres on microscopy suggests that the diagnosis is incorrect.

McMahon (1987) has instanced several patients, who were thought clinically and biochemically to have acute pancreatitis, in whom lavage suggested the true diagnosis, namely perforation of the gallbladder or bile duct (4 cases), mesenteric infarction (2 cases) or perforated duodenal ulcer (1 case). In McMahon's view the potential to save life in such patients more than compensates for the invasive nature of the technique and its 0.5–1% misadventure rate. He argues that lavage is still indicated in all patients who appear clinically to have severe pancreatitis except where contraindicated by multiple laparotomy scars, grossly distended bowel or pregnancy.

Although this is not routine practice in most centres, diagnostic peritoneal lavage should still be regarded as a viable alternative to laparotomy when a surgically remediable cause of the acute abdomen cannot be excluded from the differential diagnosis of acute pancreatitis.

Radiological diagnosis (Freeny & Lawson 1982)

Abdominal plain films

Plain films of the abdomen taken in erect and supine positions may be of more value in excluding other causes of the acute abdomen as there are no radiological signs which are specific to acute pancreatitis. However, abnormal gastrointestinal gas patterns are common in acute pancreatitis and there may be evidence of a generalized adynamic ileus or in some instances, a gasless abdomen. Focal ileus can involve the duodenum and the gas-filled first and second part may show effacement of its medial wall from oedema of the head of the pancreas; these appearances of focal ileus may in fact be due to compression of the third part of the duodenum by an inflamed oedematous root of mesentery. An isolated 'sentinel' gas-filled loop of jejunum is often seen in the left upper abdomen, although like duodenal ileus, this sign is far from specific. Inflammation tracking into the transverse mesocolon may produce irritation, paresis and even necrosis of the transverse colon. The 'colon cut-off' sign as originally described by Price (1956) was characterized by gaseous distension of the hepatic and splenic flexures, separated by a gasless transverse colon. In some patients, no gas is seen beyond the hepatic flexure while in others there is distension of the ascending and transverse colon with an abrupt cut-off at the splenic flexure.

Necrosis within the pancreas and peripancreatic tissues in patients with severe acute pancreatitis may produce areas of mottling, although this is seldom manifest when patients are first seen. Retroperitoneal inflammation occasionally causes blurring of the psoas and renal outlines, and a large amount of free fluid can produce the 'ground-glass' appearance of ascites on the erect film. Extensive pancreatic swelling and accumulation of fluid in the lesser sac can displace the transverse colon downwards, and on lateral films may give rise to anterior displacement of the stomach.

Pancreatic calcification may be visible in patients experiencing an acute exacerbation of chronic pancreatitis while calcified gallstones may be seen in the gallbladder (and occasionally at the lower end of the common bile duct) in patients with gallstone pancreatitis.

Chest radiographs

Splinting and elevation of the left hemidiaphragm is seen in many patients with acute pancreatitis and associated pleural and lung changes are apparent radiologically in some 20% of cases (Jacobs et al 1977). Pleural effusion, focal atelectasis, and lower lobe consolidation are more often restricted to the left side but are occasionally bilateral. When there is diagnostic doubt, aspiration of the effusion reveals an amylase content that is higher than that of serum in acute pancreatitis. Large pleural effusions may be the result of the rare complication of pancreatico-pleural fistula, although this is a most unusual finding at the time of first presentation with acute pancreatitis. In patients with severe pancreatitis, extensive perihilar alveolar oedema may reflect development of the adult respiratory distress syndrome; it must be stressed that significant arterial hypoxia can be present in severe acute pancreatitis in the absence of marked radiological change. On rare occasions, acute pancreatitis produces pericardial effusions.

Barium studies

These are not required for the diagnosis of acute pancreatitis but barium or the water-soluble contrast medium, gastrografin, is sometimes instilled in an attempt to exclude other causes of the acute abdomen. In the presence of acute pancreatitis there may be forward displacement of the stomach, widening of the duodenum with engorgement of its folds from contiguous pancreatic inflammation, and a prominent oedematous papilla of Vater. Gastric outlet obstruction and/or duodenal ileus is found in some cases.

Ultrasonography

Ultrasonography is being used more extensively as a means of diagnosing acute pancreatitis now that the shortcomings of serum amylase measurements are more widely appreciated. The technique is relatively inexpensive, non-invasive and can be repeated as often as necessary. The equipment is portable and can be taken to the bedside of ill patients. The drawbacks of ultrasonography are that its value depends greatly on the skill of the operator, that comprehensive permanent records are not easy to obtain, and that in some 20% of cases of acute pancreatitis the quality of the ultrasonograms is compromised by gaseous distension of the gastrointestinal tract.

Inflammation of the pancreas with its attendant oedema results in diminished echogenicity; under normal circumstances the echogenicity is equal to or greater than that of the liver whereas the acutely inflamed pancreas becomes less echogenic. In the later stages of severe acute pancreatitis, echogenicity may increase as a consequence of bleeding, saponification of fat and necrosis. The pancreas usually enlarges as a result of inflammation although this is not invariable in acute pancreatitis. Complications of acute pancreatitis such as pseudocysts and abscess are readily detectable on ultrasonography. Gallstones within the gallbladder are normally seen well on ultrasonography as echogenic foci with posterior acoustic shadowing, but in the early stages of acute pancreatitis the accuracy of ultrasonography falls to around 70% due to problems of interpretation in the presence of ileus (McKay et al 1982). Biliary tract dilatation may be apparent, particularly in patients with gall stone pancreatitis, and pancreatic duct dilatation is also seen in some cases.

Computerized tomography (CT) scanning

CT scanning is being used more widely in the assessment of severe acute pancreatitis, and has helped to highlight some of the limitations of serum amylase measurement in diagnosis. In acute pancreatitis the gland may show focal or diffuse enlargement, with blurring of its boundaries due to inflammation involving the peripancreatic tissues. The pancreas frequently has a heterogenous appearance with decreased enhancement (see below) but may retain a homogenous texture. Collections of fluid are usually apparent in the pararenal spaces and lesser sac, and a halo of oedema is sometimes seen surrounding the pancreas. Inflammation may also be seen to extend into the mesentery and mesocolon giving the so-called 'smoke and fire' appearance on CT scanning.

CT scanning is particularly valuable in defining the presence and extent of pancreatic necrosis and the complications of severe pancreatitis (see Ch. 22). It may also reveal the presence of gallstones, calcification in chronic pancreatitis, and the presence of biliary and pancreatic duct dilatation. Magnetic resonance imaging may complement CT scanning in the diagnosis and assessment of acute pancreatitis; as yet it remains available in only a few centres and its definitive role is uncertain.

In most centres, CT scanning is not used routinely to diagnose acute pancreatitis but is reserved for cases where there is diagnostic doubt or where the development of necrosis and other complications is suspected.

ASSESSMENT OF SEVERITY OF ACUTE PANCREATITIS

A large proportion of attacks of acute pancreatitis are mild and settle promptly on conservative treatment. However, in approximately one in four patients the disease proves to be severe with a significant risk of progression to potentially lethal complications. Separation of patients into 'good' and 'bad' prognostic groups as soon as possible after admission to hospital has three major advantages (Williamson 1984):

1. Those patients with severe pancreatitis can be resuscitated vigorously and monitored intensively.

2. Detection of severe pancreatitis and its complications may signal the need to consider urgent intervention, such as the need for endoscopic papillotomy in patients with severe gallstone pancreatitis (see Ch. 21).

3. Use of internationally agreed criteria for severity would facilitate comparisons between centres and prove useful as a basis for prospective studies.

The following section will be devoted to consideration of various methods of assessing the severity of an attack of acute pancreatitis.

Clinical evaluation

At one end of the spectrum it is easy for the experienced clinician to diagnose the presence of severe acute pancreatitis in a patient admitted with profound circulatory collapse, fever, cyanosis and dyspnoea, abdominal distension, and staining of the body wall. However, it is well-recognized that many patients who go on to develop major complications from which they may die, do not exhibit such grave signs at the time of admission. Conversely, many patients with the ominous clinical signs mentioned above may now be expected to survive their attack with modern management. There has been debate about whether obese patients are at greater risk when they develop acute pancreatitis; in one recent report obesity was not a predictor of pancreatic necrosis or need for surgery but was associated with an increased risk of respiratory failure (Porter & Banks 1991).

The presence of flank staining (Grey-Turner 1919) and periumbilical staining (Cullen 1918) used to be regarded as particularly ominous. The reported incidence of such body wall ecchymoses in acute pancreatitis ranges from 1 to 3% (Dickson & Imrie 1984) but it is now apparent that death is far from inevitable. In the 23 patients reported by Dickson & Imrie (1984), 63% survived although no less than 96% developed serious complications. In the elderly these signs may remain a poor prognostic sign but in younger patients Dickson & Imrie argue that they signify no greater risk of dying than that experienced by patients identified as having severe disease on multifactor grading (see below).

The difficulty of early detection of severe pancreatitis is highlighted by reports that severe attacks are identified by experienced clinicians in only 34–39% of cases at the time of admission (McMahon et al 1980, Corfield et al 1985b). Conversely, of 365 attacks initially classified as mild in one multicentre study, only 292 had an uncomplicated outcome (Corfield et al 1985b).

Single prognostic factors

Given the fallibility of clinical evaluation, a number of authors have attempted to use single biochemical or haemodynamic parameters as a means of identifying patients liable to develop complications or die. Although serum amylase values are useful in diagnosis, it is generally accepted that the height of the amylase level bears little relationship to prognosis; if anything, amylase levels may have an inverse relationship with severity in that some patients with severe disease have normal or modestly elevated amylase values when first seen (Clavien et al 1989a). On the other hand hyperamylasaemia which persists for more than 5–7 days may have prognostic significance in that it may signal the development of complications such as pseudocyst or abscess.

Haemolysis and coagulopathy

Methaemalbuminaemia reflects intravascular haemolysis with subsequent combination of the haemoglobin breakdown product haematin (methaem) with albumin. Once canvassed as a predictor of severity in acute pancreatitis (Lankisch et al 1978), the search for methaemalbuminaemia never established a role in clinical practice. Similarly, despite early promise (Berry et al 1982) serum *fibrinogen* levels have not been used widely as a means of identifying severe disease.

Proteases and protease inhibitor

Plasma concentrations of the pancreatic proteases trypsin, chymotrypsin and elastase rise during an attack of acute pancreatitis, but these enzymes remain largely in zymogen form (trypsinogen, chymotrypsinogen and proelastase). Although protease activity is not detectable in the plasma, the fact that active proteases have been present can be inferred by falling concentrations of the protease inhibitor α_2-macroglobulin. In patients with mild acute pancreatitis, α_2-macroglobulin concentrations remain in the lower limits of the normal range whereas patients with severe disease show a gradual decrease to a nadir on day 6 (Banks et al 1991). Although measurement of α_2-macroglobulin concentration is not likely to be used to predict outcome, interest surrounds the observation that levels of α_2-macroglobulin–protease complexes are maintained at abnormally high levels in the majority of patients with severe disease. As such complexes are normally removed rapidly from the circulation by cells of the reticuloendothelial system, their persistence may reflect impaired reticuloendothelial function, a factor currently attracting considerable interest in pathogenesis. Of further interest, Banks et al (1991) found little or no evidence that uncomplexed α_2-macroglobulin levels were exhausted in acute pancreatitis, a finding in keeping with the failure of fresh frozen plasma (which contains α_2-macroglobulin) to influence the course of the disease (Leese et al 1987).

Wilson et al (1989) have also evaluated the relationship between the circulating antiproteases, α_2-macroglobulin and α_1-antiprotease, and the severity of acute pancreatitis. The levels of α_2-macroglobulin were significantly lower in patients with complicated attacks during days 3–8, while α_1-antiprotease levels were significantly higher during days 4–8. It is doubtful whether either agent will prove useful in clinical practice as a means of assessing severity, and neither provided the discrimination achieved with C-reactive protein (see below).

Gudgeon et al (1990) have shown recently that urinary levels of *trypsinogen activation peptides* (TAP) are increased in patients with severe acute pancreatitis. These peptides are normally produced when trypsinogen is activated by duodenal enterokinase. In severe acute pancreatitis, there may be extensive activation of trypsinogens and other zymogens (and thus TAP liberation) within the pancreas and this may have adverse effects on the nature and severity of subsequent local and distant complications. In the study referred to above, urinary TAP assay was performed on admission in 55 patients with acute pancreatitis. None of the 30% of patients who were TAP-negative on admission and remained so throughout 5 days of sampling developed complications. TAP concentrations on admission correlated correctly with subsequent disease severity in 87% of cases, whereas the correlation for C-reactive protein (CRP) levels and multifactor grading at 48 hours were 55% and 84% respectively. The urinary TAP assay has yet to become widely available so that its definitive role in diagnosis and management can be assessed; in time it is hoped that a rapid serum assay might also become available.

Phospholipase A_2

This enzyme converts lecithin and cephalin in cell membranes and bile into cytotoxic lysocompounds and may make a major contribution to necrosis and systemic complications in severe acute pancreatitis. Phospholipase A_2 concentrations are significantly higher in patients with severe pancreatitis than in those with mild disease, the difference being apparent even by the first day (Puolakkainen et al 1987). Patients with fatal attacks have particularly high levels of serum phospholipase A_2 activity. However, it is unlikely that phospholipase A_2 measurements will become a routine method of evaluation in clinical practice as CRP levels are easier to measure and provide equal discrimination (Puolakkainen et al 1987).

Serum ribonuclease

Despite claims that raised serum levels of an acid low molecular weight ribonuclease (presumably resulting from cell breakdown in anoxic pancreas) are a reliable indication of pancreatic necrosis (Warshaw & Lee 1979), the sensitivity of this marker has been questioned (Kemmer et al 1991) and the approach has not found a place in clinical practice.

Complement levels

Complement activation in acute pancreatitis may reflect direct attack on C3 complement factors by trypsin or activation of the alternative complement pathway. While a fall in C1q levels has been described in severe pancreatitis and a rise in C3d levels (reflecting activation) has been observed, the wide scatter of results rules out the use of complement levels as a useful index of severity (Wilson et al 1989).

C-reactive protein (CRP) and inflammatory mediators

CRP is a non-specific acute phase protein which is synthesized by hepatocytes in a number of conditions including major trauma, sepsis and acute pancreatitis. Elevated serum levels are detected within hours of injury but 24–48 hours usually elapse before peak levels are attained (Wilson et al 1989). The precise role of CRP is uncertain but it may recognize, bind and help to detoxify toxic materials released by damaged tissues. While CRP is of no value in the diagnosis of acute pancreatitis, there is general agreement that monitoring serum levels is an excellent method of detecting pancreatic necrosis and that this makes it a useful early marker of severity (Fig. 19.2) (Mayer et al 1984, Büchler et al 1986, Puolakkainen et al 1987, Wilson et al 1989).

Differing methods of measurement have given rise to differing criteria for use in assessing severity. For example, Wilson et al (1989) found that a peak level of ≥ 210 mg/l on days 2–4 after admission offered the best discrimination between mild and complicated attacks,

and that either the peak or day 7 levels had a similar accuracy to that of multiple factor grading systems. Puolakkainen et al (1987) suggest that a cut-off value of 110 mg/l is optimal; in this study the mean CRP level on admission was 45 mg/l in patients with mild disease and 289 mg/l in those with verified haemorrhagic pancreatitis.

The cytokine, interleukin-6 (IL-6) may be responsible for the induction of hepatic synthesis of CRP and other acute phase proteins. Recent studies (Leser et al 1991) indicate that patients with mild acute pancreatitis have only slightly elevated IL-6 levels at the time of admission and that these fall rapidly. On the other hand, patients with severe disease have greater and persisting rises in IL-6 levels, while those who go on to die have marked elevations at the time of admission. CRP levels followed the course of IL-6 concentrations after an interval of 1 day. Thus IL-6 levels, probably reflecting activation of the monocyte–macrophage system in severe acute pancreatitis, may prove a useful early, prognostic parameter. Activation of granulocytes is also implicated in severe acute pancreatitis and granulocyte elastase levels also appear to be a promising early marker of severity (Gross et al 1990, Uhl et al 1991).

Individual factors from multifactor scoring systems

Blamey et al (1984) conducted a detailed evaluation of 405 attacks of acute pancreatitis to assess the power of individual factors to discriminate between mild and severe attacks, the definition of 'severe' being an attack which led to the development of complications, need for

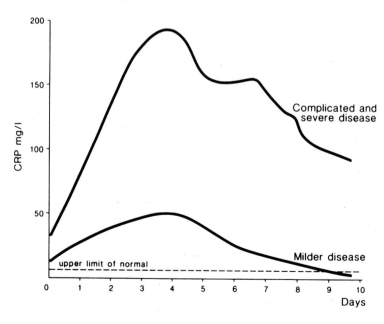

Fig. 19.2 Schematic diagrams of the C-reactive protein (CRP) levels found in patients with severe pancreatitis compared with milder disease (From Imrie C W and Wilson C, 1989, in Carter D C & Warshaw A L (eds) Pancreatitis, Churchill Livingstone; reproduced with permission.)

operation, or death. Factors showing a significant difference between the two groups were calcium, urea, lactic dehydrogenase (LDH), arterial oxygen saturation, white cell count, albumin, glucose and age; aminotransferase, alkaline phosphatase, bilirubin, and amylase levels did not differ significantly between the groups. Ranking of the importance of individual factors (Table 19.3) showed that serum calcium levels provided the most powerful discrimination, in that while levels of less than 2.00 mmol/l were found in 58 episodes, 38% of which proved to be severe, levels greater than 2.00 mmol/l were found in 305 episodes, with 91% of these being mild attacks and 9% being severe attacks. Use of the Glasgow multifactor system (see below) in the same group of patients resulted in correct prediction of severity in 72% of cases; 31% of the 131 episodes with three or more factors were severe while 8% of the 274 with less than three factors were severe. It is clear that individual factors do have prognostic significance but none has emerged, with the recent exception of CRP, as a prognostic indicator for use in isolation in clinical practice.

Peritoneal lavage in assessment of severity

Abdominal paracentesis using the technique described above has been used to predict severity in acute pancreatitis (McMahon et al 1980). Pancreatitis is classified as severe if there is more than 10 ml of free fluid and its colour is dark, or assessment may be made on the basis of a colour chart used to grade the colour of the return fluid. The accuracy of prediction (72%) is comparable to that of multifactor grading systems, with the advantage that the assessment is made at the time of admission rather than over 48 hours, and that other causes of the acute abdomen such as perforation of a viscus can be excluded. Visceral puncture is a potential hazard but its incidence is less than 1%. Despite this, peritoneal lavage is not used widely as a means of assessing severity at the time of admission, although McMahon (1987) has argued cogently for its use in the setting of investigative research.

Multiple factor grading systems

Ranson system

Ranson and his group in New York developed an objective grading system in the 1970s in an attempt to separate patients with mild and severe pancreatitis. After analysis of 43 parameters, 11 of them, which correlated with severity and which could be determined with 48 hours of admission, were combined into a prognostic system, (Table 19.4) (Ranson et al 1974). In a prospective evaluation of 200 patients, severity was predicted correctly in 93% of cases; of the 162 patients classified as having mild disease only one died whereas 24 of the 38 patients deemed to have severe disease died or developed complications (Ranson & Pasternak 1977).

Glasgow systems. Imrie et al (1978) in Glasgow originally used a nine factor system (Table 19.4) in the hope that it might prove more valuable in areas where gallstones are a more important cause of acute pancreatitis than in the urban North American setting in which Ranson's system was developed. The system differed from Ranson's original in that haematocrit, base deficit and fluid sequestration were eliminated but serum albumin was added. In fact the system proved unsatisfactory in the assessment of severity in gallstone pancreatitis, given that so many patients were over 55 years of age. In an attempt to overcome this problem in gallstone patients, age was deleted and the threshold for serum aminotransferase was doubled (Osborne et al 1981). In their more recent analysis of 405 episodes of acute pancreatitis from all causes, the Glasgow group have attempted to return to a uniform system by retaining eight of the original nine factors (Table 19.4) and dispensing totally with aminotransferase as it proved to have no discriminatory value (Blamey et al 1984). Using this modified eight factor Glasgow system, 39% of 92 episodes classified as severe were associated with death, development of complications or need for operation, as opposed to 9% of the 313 episodes assessed as mild on prognostic grading. Overall, 79% of the episodes had the outcome predicted correctly.

Table 19.3 Significant factors in predicting severity of acute pancreatitis (Blamey et al 1984)

Factors	Episodes		
	n	Mild %	Severe %
Calcium (mmol/l)			
<2.00	58	62	38
>2.00	305	91	9
Urea (mmol/l)			
>16	13	31	69
<16	385	86	14
Lactic dehydrogenase (LDH) (u/l)			
>600	70	67	33
<600	165	94	6
Glucose (mmol/l)			
>10	29	48	52
<10	181	74	26
Arterial oxygen saturation (PaO_2) (mmHg)			
<60	114	75	25
>60	262	89	11
White blood cell count ($\times 10^9$/l)			
>15	130	73	27
<15	237	90	10
Albumin (g/l)			
<32	28	64	36
>32	344	87	13
Age (years)			
>55	198	80	20
<55	207	88	12

Table 19.4 Basis of factor scoring systems to predict the severity of acute pancreatitis. In both systems disease is classified as severe when three or more factors are present

Ranson et al (1974)	Imrie et al (1978)
On admission	Age >55 years
Age >55 years	White blood cell count >15 x 10^9/l
White blood cell count 16×10^9/l	Blood glucose >10 mmol/l (no diabetic history)
Blood glucose >10 mmol/l	Serum urea >16 mmol/l (no response to i.v. fluids)
Lactic dehydrogenase >700 u/l	Arterial oxygen saturation (PaO_2) <60 mmHg
Aspartate aminotransferase >250 Sigma Frankel units%	
Within 48 hours	Serum calcium <2.0 mmol/l
Blood urea nitrogen rise >5 mg%	Serum albumin <32 g/l
Arterial oxygen saturation (PaO_2) < 60 mmHg	Lactic dehydrogenase >600 u/l
Serum calcium < 2.0 mmol/l	Aspartate aminotransferase/alanine aminotransferase >100u/l
Haematocrit fall >10%	
Base deficit >4 mmol/l	
Fluid sequestration >6 l	

Leese & Shaw (1988) from Leicester have published an independent appraisal of the Glasgow systems, endorsing the suggestion that aminotransferase levels should no longer be considered. Using the modified Glasgow system proposed by Blamey et al (1984), they reported that it had a sensitivity of 79%, specificity of 80% and correct prediction rate of 80%.

In a three-centre study involving Glasgow, Leeds and Bristol, multiple factor grading has been compared with the predicitive capacity of clinical assessment and peritoneal lavage (Corfield et al 1985). Clinical assessment on admission identified only 34% of the patients whose attack proved to be fatal or complicated. Multiple factor grading and peritoneal lavage were more sensitive (61% and 53% respectively) while retaining reasonable diagnostic accuracy (79% and 74%). When used together the three indices correctly identified the 82% of attacks which proved fatal or complicated and identified all patients destined to die within 10 days of admission.

Hong Kong system

Fan et al (1989) in Hong Kong have suggested that a simple system based on measurement of only serum urea and glucose provides sensitivity (75%), specificity (80%) and accuracy (79%) comparable with the Glasgow multi-factor system. Discriminant analysis was the technique used to identify the independent significance of these two factors and it should be noted this technique may not prove to be particularly robust when used in other patients in other centres. The use of discriminant analysis in Glasgow (Blamey et al 1984) and Leicester (Leese & Shaw 1988) resulted in the emergence of lactic dehydrogenase and serum calcium (Glasgow) or a combination of white cell count, urea, arterial oxygen saturation (PaO_2) and lactic dehydrogenase (Leicester). Further evaluation in other groups of patients will be needed to confirm the value of the Hong Kong system.

Japanese system

A recent national survey of acute pancreatitis in Japan has attempted to develop criteria for the definition of severe acute pancreatitis (Saitoh & Yamanoto 1991). This system combines clinical and laboratory parameters (Table 19.5), appears to be even more cumbersome than the Ranson or Glasgow systems, and will require unequivocal prospective demonstration of its worth before gaining clinical acceptance.

Table 19.5 Criteria for severe acute pancreatitis developed by Japanese Research Committee for Intractable Diseases of the Pancreas (Saitoh & Yamamoto 1991). Cases were classified as severe if one or more asterisked criteria were fulfilled or if two or more non-asterisked criteria were fulfilled

Parameters	Definition
Clinical	
*Shock	Blood pressure <80 mmHg
*Dyspnoea	Respirator employed
*Neurological symptoms	Disturbance of central nervous system with loss of consciousness
*Severe infection	Fever >38°C, with leucocytosis, endoxaemia and/or intra-abdominal abscess
*Haemorrhagic tendency	Gastrointestinal bleeding Intra-abdominal haemorrhage (including Cullen or Grey-Turner's sign) Disseminated intravascular coagulation
Laboratory	
*Base excess	≤3 mmol/l
*Haematocrit	≤30% (after fluid sequestration)
*Blood urea nitrogen	≥40 mg/dl (or creatinine ≥ 2 mg/dl)
Calcium	≤7.5 mg/dl
Fasting blood sugar	≥200 mg/dl
Arterial oxygen saturation (PaO_2)	≤60 mmHg (on room air)
Lactic dehydrogenase	≥700 u/l
Total protein	≤6 g/dl
Prothrombin time	≥15 s
Platelet count	≥10 × 10^4/mm^3

APACHE II Score

The modified APACHE II score was introduced in 1985 in an attempt to overcome some of the difficulties associated with its more complex forerunner (Knaus et al 1985). The system is already used widely in intensive care units and it would be useful to have one internationally accepted scoring system for use in all critical illness, including acute pancreatitis. Larvin and McMahon (1989) studied 290 attacks of acute pancreatitis, 231 of which were uncomplicated (mild) while 59 were associated with major organ failure or development of a pancreatic collection (severe). APACHE II scores on admission correctly predicted outcome in 77% of attacks and identified 6% of the severe attacks, compared with a 44% identification rate on clinical assessment. After 48 hours, APACHE II scoring was more accurate than Ranson and Glasgow scoring, correctly predicting outcome in 88% of attacks (Table 19.6). Comparable studies from Glasgow (Wilson et al 1990) have confirmed the value of the APACHE II score in this context, not only as an initial means of assessment but as a means of monitoring progress. In Glasgow no deaths occurred in patients with a peak APACHE II score of less than 10 whereas rising scores were associated with clinical deterioration in those dying early.

Radiological assessment of severity

While some studies have shown a correlation between outcome and early CT scan changes in acute pancreatitis (Ranson et al 1985, Nordestegaard et al 1986), others have suggested that early CT scanning may be no more valuable than conventional means of assessment such as the Glasgow multifactor system (Rotmann et al 1986, London et al 1989). A number of scoring systems have been developed for objective assessment of CT scans (Kivisaari et al 1983, Schröder et al 1985). In such assessments the abdomen is first scanned without giving

intravenous contrast so as to assess pancreatic and extrapancreatic changes; one point each is given for oedema around part of the pancreas, oedema around the entire pancreas, mesenteric fat oedema, perirenal fat oedema, bowel distension, peritoneal exudate and pleural effusions. It was claimed that a score of 4 or more was associated with a high incidence of haemorrhagic pancreatitis and risk of developing pancreatic pseudocyst or abscess (Schröder et al 1985). Although others have found that such extrapancreatic changes are always found in patients who prove to have severe pancreatitis, they may also be present in patients with mild disease (Puolakkainen 1989).

London et al (1989) developed a 'pancreatic size index' in which the maximum anteroposterior measurement of the pancreatic head and body are multiplied; although a result of 10 cm^3 or greater has a sensitivity of 71% and specificity of 77% in predicting clinically severe attacks, it proved inferior to the use of the modified Glasgow criteria in this regard.

Regardless of the debate surrounding the predictive value of an admission CT scan, there is now general agreement that rapid-bolus contrast-enhanced dynamic CT scanning offers a reliable means of defining the presence and extent of pancreatic necrosis (Kivisaari et al 1984, Bradley et al 1989, Larvin et al 1990, London et al 1991). The pancreas has an abundant blood supply and its density on CT scans is normally enhanced after giving an intravenous contrast medium. Necrosis and the associated reduced or absent perfusion leads to reduced enhancement on dynamic CT scanning and enhancement of less than 30 Hounsefield units is normally taken as the threshold level for the diagnosis of necrosis (Kivisaari et al 1984). While necrosis of the pancreas and extrapancreatic tissues undoubtedly reflects the presence of severe pancreatitis and an increased risk of developing complications, its presence is not in itself an indication for surgical intervention (London et al 1991). The subject of operative intervention in necrotizing pancreatitis is dealt with in detail elsewhere (see Ch. 22).

Table 19.6 Prediction of severity of acute pancreatitis by various prognostic systems on admission and after 24 or 48 hours (Larvin & McMahon 1989). All figures are percentages

	Sensitivity	Specificity	Positive predictive value	Negative predictive value	Overall accuracy
Admission					
Clinical	44	95	68	87	84
APACHE II	63	81	46	89	77
24 hours					
Clinical	59	96	78	90	88
APACHE II	71	91	67	93	87
48 hours					
Clinical	66	95	76	92	89
Ranson*	75	68	37	91	69
Glasgow**	61	89	59	90	83
APACHE II	75	92	71	93	88

*Ranson et al 1974; **Blamey et al 1984

CONCLUSIONS

While serum amylase determinations seem destined to remain the mainstay in the diagnosis of acute pancreatitis for some time, this marker is far from foolproof. False positive and false negative amylase results will continue to pose problems and consideration must be given to more widespread use of serum lipase assays and the diagnostic use of ultrasonography (and perhaps CT scanning in selected cases). Early assessment of severity remains worthwhile as a means of identifying patients who require more intensive monitoring, and who may benefit from surgical or endoscopic intervention. Clinical assessment on admission is an unreliable means of identifying those patients who will run a complicated course and who may die. Multiple factor prognostic scoring systems have proved valuable in this context but are cumbersome and it may take 24–48 hours before all the results become available. Peritoneal lavage is invasive (but not as invasive as laparotomy), as reliable as multiple factor systems and can be carried out at the time of admission; however its potential benefits do not justify its routine use outside the setting of investigative clinical research protocols. C-reactive protein levels have emerged as a reliable marker for the development of necrosis while the APACHE II scoring system has also proved useful as a means of monitoring progress. These two means of assessment seem likely to replace other means of assessing severity, and will be used widely as an indication for the need for dynamic rapid-bolus contrast-enhanced CT scanning and identification of patients who may require surgical intervention.

REFERENCES

Allam B F, Imrie C W 1977 Serum ionized calcium in acute pancreatitis. British Journal of Surgery 64: 665–668

Amman R 1976 Acute pancreatitis In: Bockus H L (ed) Gastroenterology, 3rd edn, W B Saunders, Philadelphia, ch 137, p 1020

Banks R E, Evans S W, Alexander D, Leuven V F, Whicher J T, McMahon M J 1991 Alpha$_2$ macroglobulin state in acute pancreatitis. Raised values of α_2-macroglobulin-protease complexes in severe and mild attacks. Gut 32: 430–434

Berry A R, Taylor T V, Davies G C 1982 Diagnostic tests and prognostic indicators in acute pancreatitis. Journal of the Royal College of Surgeons, Edinburgh 27: 345–352.

Blamey S L, Imrie C W, O'Neill J, Gilmour W H, Carter D C 1984 Prognostic factors in acute pancreatitis. Gut 25: 1340–1346

Bradley E L, Murphy F, Ferguson C 1989 Prediction of pancreatic necrosis by dynamic pancreatography. Annals of surgery 210: 495–504

Büchler M, Malfertheiner P, Beger H G 1986 Correlation of imaging procedures, biochemical parameters and clinical stage in acute pancreatitis. In: Malfertheiner P, Ditschuneit H (eds) Diagnostic procedures in pancreatic disease. Springer-Verlag, Berlin p 123–129

Burkitt D S 1987 The Rapignost–amylase test in acute pancreatitis. British Journal of Surgery 74: 1063

Cherry I S, Crandall A L 1932 Specificity of pancreatic lipase: its appearance in blood after pancreatic injury. American Journal of Physiology 100: 266–273

Clavien P-A, Burgan S, Moossa A R 1989a Serum enzymes and other laboratory tests in acute pancreatitis. British Journal of Surgery 76:1234–1243

Clavien P-A, Robert J, Meyer P 1989b. Acute pancreatitis and normoamylasemia. Annals or Surgery 210: 614–620

Corfield A P, Cooper M J Williamson R C N 1985a Acute pancreatitis: a lethal disease of increasing incidence. Gut, 26: 724–729

Corfield A P, Williamson R C N, McMahon M J et al 1985b Prediction of severity in acute pancreatitis: prospective comparison of three prognostic indices. Lancet 2: 403–407

Cullen T S 1918 A new sign in ruptured extrauterise pregnancy. American Journal of Obstetrics and Gynecology 78: 457–460

Dickson A P, Imrie C W 1984. The incidence and prognosis of body wall ecchymosis in acute pancreatitis. Surgery, Gynecology and Obstetrics 159: 343–347

Dickson A P, O'Neill J, Imrie C W 1984 Hyperlipidaemia, alcohol abuse and acute pancreatitis. British Journal of Surgery 71: 685–688

Durr H K, Bindrich D, Bode J C 1977 The frequency of macroamylasaemia and the diagnostic value of the amylase to creatinine clearance ratio in patients with elevated serum amylase activity. Scandinavian Journal of Gastroenterology 12: 701–705

Egdahl R H 1958 Mechanism of blood enzyme changes following production of experimental pancreatitis. Annals of Surgery 148: 389–400

Fan S T, Choi T K, Lai C S, Wong J 1988 Influence of age on the mortality from acute pancreatitis. British Journal of Surgery 75: 463–466

Fan S T, Choi T K, Lai E C S, Wong J 1989 Prediction of severity of acute pancreatitis: an alternative approach. Gut 30: 1591–1599

Forsman R W 1986 Macroamylase: prevalence, distribution of age, sex, amylase activity and electrophoretic mobility. Clinical Biochemistry 19: 250–253

Freeny P C, Lawson T L 1982 Radiology of the pancreas. Springer-Verlag, Berlin

Grey-Turner G 1919 Local discolouration of the abdominal wall as a sign of acute pancreatitis. British Journal of Surgery 7: 394–395

Gross V, Schölmerch J, Leser H-G et al 1990 Granulocyte elastase in assessment of severity of acute pancreatitis. Comparison with acute-phase proteins C-reactive protein, α-antitrypsin and protease inhibitor α_2-macroglobulin. Digestive Diseases and Sciences 35:97–105

Gudgeon A M, Health D I, Hurlcy P, Jchanli A 1990 Trypsinogen activation peptides assay in the early prediction of severity of acute pancreatitis. Lancet 335: 4–8

Higgins E, Ive F A 1990 Subcutaneous fat necrosis in pancreatic disease. British Journal of Surgery 77: 532–533

Holdsworth P J, Mayer A D, Wilson D H, Flowers M W, McMahon M J 1984 A simple test for acute pancreatitis. British Journal of Surgery 71: 958–959.

Imrie C W, Benjamin I S, Ferguson J C et al 1978 A single centre double blind trial of Trasylol therapy in primary acute pancreatitis. British Journal of Surgery 65: 337–341

Imrie C W, Wilson C 1989 In: Carter D C, Warshaw A L (eds) Pancreatitis. Churchill Livingstone

Jacobs M L, Daggett W M, Civetta J M et al 1977 Acute pancreatitis: Analysis of factors influencing survival. American Surgeon 185: 43–51

Katschinski B D, Giggs J A, Bourke J B 1990, Inzidenz und geographische verteilung der akuten pankreatitis in Nottingham von 1969 bis 1983. Zeitschrift für Gastroenterologie 28: 183–187

Kemmer T P, Malfertheiner P, Büchler M, Kemmer M L, Ditschumeit H 1991. Serum ribonuclease activity in the diagnosis of pancreatic disease. International Journal of Pancreatology 8: 23–33

Kivisaari L, Somer K, Standertskjold-Nordenstam C G, Schroder T, Kivilaakso E, Lempinen M 1983 Early detection of acute fulminant pancreatitis by contrast enhanced computed tomography. Scandinavian Journal of Gastroenterology 18: 39–41

Kivisaari L, Somer K, Standertskjold-Nordenstam C G, Kivilaakso E, Lempinen M 1984. A new method for the diagnosis of acute haemorrhagic necrotising pancreatitis using contrast-enhanced CT scanning. Gastrointestinal Radiology 9: 27–30

Kleinmann D S, O'Brien J F 1986 Macroamylase. Mayo Clin Proceedings 61: 669–670

Knaus W A, Draper E A, Wagner D P, Zimmerman J E 1985 APACHE-II: a severity of disease classification. Critical Care Medicine 13: 818–829

Koehler D F, Eckfeld J H, Levitt M D 1982 Diagnostic value of routine isoamylase assay of hyperamylasaemia serum. Gastroenterology 82: 887–890

Kolars J C, Ellis C J, Levitt M D 1984 Comparison of serum amylase pancreatic isoamylase and lipase in patients with hyperamylasemia. Digestive Diseases and Sciences: 29: 289–293

Lankisch P G, Koop H, Otto J, Oberdeck U 1978 Evaluation of methaemalbumin in acute pancreatitis. Scandinavian Journal of Gastroenterology 13: 975–978

Lankisch P G, Schirren C A, Kunze E 1991 Undetected fatal acute pancreatitis: why is the disease so frequently overlooked? American Journal of Gastroenterology 86: 322–326

Larvin M, McMahon M J 1989 APACHE-II score for assessment and monitoring of acute pancreatitis. Lancet 2: 201–204

Larvin M, Chalmers A G, McMahon M J 1990 Dynamic contrast enhanced computed tomography: a precise technique for identifying and localising pancreatic necrosis. British Medical Journal 300: 1425–1428

Leese T, Shaw D 1988 Comparison of three Glasgow multifactor prognostic scoring systems in acute pancreatitis. British Journal of Surgery 75: 460–462

Leese T, Holliday T, Heath D, Hall A W, Bell P R F 1987 Multicentre trial of low volume fresh frozen plasma therapy in acute pancreatitis. British Journal of Surgery 74: 907–911

Leser H-G, Gross V, Scheibenbogen C, Heinisch A et al 1991 Elevation of serum interleukin-6 concentration precedes acute-phase response and reflects severity in acute pancreatitis. Gastroenterology 101: 782–785

Levitt M D, Rapaport M, Cooperland S R 1969 The role of amylase in renal insufficiency, acute pancreatitis and macroamylasaemia. Annals of Internal Medicine 71: 919–926

Levitt M D, Ellis C, Meier P B 1980 Extrapancreatic origin of chronic unexplained hyperamylasaemia. New England Journal of Medicine 302: 670–671

London N J M, Neoptolemos J P, Lavelle J, Bailey I, James D 1989 Contrast-enhanced abdominal computed tomography scanning and prediction of severity of acute pancreatitis: a prospective study. British Journal of Surgery 76: 268–272

London N J M, Leese T, Lavelle J M, Miles K, West K P, Watkin D F L, Fossard D P 1991 Rapid-bolus contrast-enhanced dynamic computed tomography in acute pancreatitis: a prospective study. British Journal of Surgery 78: 1452–1456

McKay A J, Imrie C W, O'Neill J, Duncan J G 1982. Is an early ultrasound scan of value in acute pancreatitis? British Journal of Surgery 69: 369–372

McMahon M 1987. Peritoneal fluid and the diagnosis and prognosis of acute pancreatitis. In: Beger H G, Büchler M (eds) Acute Pancreatitis, Springer-Verlag, Berlin, ch 4, p 159–163

McMahon M J, Woodhead J S, Hayward R D 1978 The nature of hypocalcaemia in acute pancreatitis. British Journal of Surgery 65: 216–218

McMahon M J, Playforth M J, Pickford I R 1980. A comparative study of methods for the prediction of severity of attacks of acute pancreatitis. British Journal of Surgery 67: 22–25

Mayer A D, McMahon M J, Bowen M, Cooper E H 1984 C-reactive protein: an aid to assessment and monitoring of acute pancreatitis. Journal of Clinical Pathology 37: 207–211

Mayer A D, Airey M, Hodgson J, McMahon M J 1985 Enzyme transfer from pancreas to plasma during acute pancreatitis. The contribution of ascitic fluid and lymphatic drainage of the pancreas. Gut 26: 876–881

Moller-Petersen J K, Klaerbe M, Dali T, Toth T 1985 Immunochemical qualitative latex agglutination test for pancreatic lipase in serum evaluated for use in diagnosis of acute pancreatitis. Clinical Chemistry 31: 1207–1210

Nordestgaard A G, Wilson S E, Williams R A 1986 Early computerised tomography as a predictor of outcome in acute pancreatitis. American Journal of Surgery 152: 127–132

Osborne D H, Imrie C W, Carter D C 1981 Biliary surgery in the same admission for acute pancreatitis. British Journal of Surgery 68: 758–761

O'Sullivan J N, Nobrega F T, Morlock C G, Brown A L, Bartholomew L G 1972 Acute and chronic pancreatitis in Rochester, Minnesota 1940–1969. Gastroenterology 62: 373–379

Paloyan D, Paloyan E, Harper P V 1967 Glucagon-induced hypocalcaemia. Metabolism 16: 35–39

Pickford I R, Blackett R L, McMahon M J 1977 Early assessment of severity of acute pancreatitis using peritoneal lavage. British Medical Journal 2: 1377–1379

Pickleman J R, Ernst K, Brown S 1969 Glucagon-induced hypocalcaemia: effect of the thyroid gland. Surgical Forum 20: 85–87

Price C W R 1956 The 'colon cut-off' sign of acute pancreatitis. Medical Journal of Australia 1: 313–314

Porter K A, Banks P A 1991 Obesity as predictor of severity in acute pancreatitis. International Journal of Pancreatology 10: 247–252

Puolakkainen P A 1989. Early assessment of acute pancreatitis. Acta Chirurgica Scandinavica 155: 25–30

Puolakkainen P, Valtonen V, Paananen A, Schroder T 1987 C-reactive protein (CRP) and serum phospholipase A_2 in the assessment of the severity of acute pancreatitis. Gut 28: 754–761

Ranson J H, Pasternak B S 1977 Statistical methods for quantifying the severity of clinical acute pancreatitis. Journal of Surgical Research 22: 77–79

Ranson J H, Rifkind K M, Roses D F, Fink S D, Eng K, Spencer J 1974 Prognostic signs and the role of operative management in acute pancreatitis. Surgery Gynecology and Obstetrics 139: 69–81

Ranson J H C, Balthazar E, Caccavale R, Cooper M 1985 Computed tomography and the prediction of pancreatic abscess in acute pancreatitis. Annals of Surgery 201: 656–665

Read G, Bragamza J M, Howat H T 1976 Pancreatitis – a retrospective study. Gut 17: 945–952

Rotmann N, Bonnet F, Larde D, Fagniez P L 1986 Computerised tomography in the evaluation of late complications of acute pancreatitis. American Journal of Surgery 152: 286–289

Saitoh Y, Yamamoto, M 1991 Evaluation of severity of acute pancreatitis. 9: 51–58

Schmidt D N 1991. Apparent risk factors for chronic and acute pancreatitis in Stockholm county. International Journal of Pancreatology 8: 45–50

Schröder T, Kivisaari L, Somer K, Standertskjold-Nordenstam C G Kivilaakso E, Lempinen M, 1985 Significance of extrapancreatic findings in computed tomography of acute pancreatitis. European Journal of Radiology 5: 273–275

Spechler S J, Dalton J W, Robbins A H et al 1983 Prevalence of normal serum amylase levels in patients with acute alcoholic pancreatitis. Digestive Diseases and Sciences 28: 865–869

Thomson H J, Brydon W G, Obekpa P O, Smith A N 1987 Screening for acute pancreatitis. Journal of the Royal College of Surgeons (Edinburgh) 32: 348–351

Trapnell J E, Duncan E H L 1975 Patterns of incidence in acute pancreatitis. British Medical Journal 2: 179–183

Uhl W, Buchler M, Malfertheiner P, Martini M, Beger H G 1991 PMN-elastase in comparison with CRP, antiproteases, and LDH as indicators of necrosis in human acute pancreatitis. Pancreas 6: 253–259

Ventrucci M, Pezilli R, Gullo L et al 1989 Role of serum pancreatic enzyme assays in diagnosis of pancreatic disease. Digestive Diseases and Sciences 34: 39–45

Warshaw A L, Lee K H 1979. Serum ribonuclease elevations and pancreatic necrosis in acute pancreatitis. Surgery 86: 227–234

Warshaw A L, Feller E R, Lee K H 1977 On the cause of raised serum amylase in diabetic ketoacidosis. Lancet 1: 929

Weaver D W, Bouwman D L, Walt A J et al 1982 A correlation between clinical pancreatitis and isoenzyme pattern of amylase. Surgery 9: 576–580

Williamson R C N 1984. Early assessment of severity in acute pancreatitis. Gut 25: 1331–1339

Wilson C, Imrie C W 1990 Changing patterns of incidence and mortality from acute pancreatitis in Scotland, 1961–1985. British Journal of Surgery 77: 731–734

Wilson C, Imrie C W, Carter D C 1988 Fatal acute pancreatitis. Gut 29: 782–788

Wilson C, Heads A, Shenkin A, Imrie C W 1989 C-reactive protein, antiproteases and complement factors as objective markers of severity in acute pancreatitis. British Journal of Surgery 76: 177–181

Wilson C, Heath D I, Imrie C W 1990 Prediction of outcome in acute pancreatitis: a comparative study of APACHE II, clinical assessment and multiple factor scoring systems. British Journal of Surgery 77: 1260–1264

20. Non-operative management of acute pancreatitis

J. H. C. Ranson

INTRODUCTION

The term acute pancreatitis includes pancreatic inflammation associated with a wide range of aetiological, pathological and clinical findings. The discussion of acute pancreatitis as a single entity is analogous to the consideration of all forms of acute pulmonary inflammation under one category whether initiated by bacterial or viral agents, by smoke inhalation or aspiration. Until a more precise classification of patients with acute pancreatitis is developed, it is clear that no overall course of management will be appropriate for all patients and treatment must be individualized. Furthermore, the heterogeneity of patients with acute pancreatitis has severely hampered the rational evaluation of proposed treatments (Steinberg & Schlessman 1987).

There are three primary objectives of treatment in patients with acute pancreatitis. The first is to support the patient and treat the specific complications which may occur. The second is to limit the severity of pancreatic inflammation, and the third is to ameliorate complications by interrupting their pathogenesis. Distinctions between these categories are often blurred. However, some of the non-operative measures which have been proposed are listed in Table 20.1.

SUPPORTIVE AND SYMPTOMATIC TREATMENT

The basic management of all patients with acute pancreatitis is supportive and symptomatic. It includes monitoring, restoration and maintenance of intravascular volume, electrolyte balance and respiratory and cardiovascular function, together with nutritional support and pain relief.

Intravascular volume management

Evaluation and monitoring of intravascular volume and cardiovascular function require regular measurements of

Table 20.1 Medical measures proposed for the treatment of acute pancreatitis

To support the patient and treat complications
    Restoration and maintenance of intravascular volume
    Electrolyte replacement
    Respiratory support
    Nutritional support
    Pain relief
    Heparin

To limit pancreatic inflammation
    Inhibition of pancreatic exocrine secretion
        Nasogastric suction, cimetidine
        Pharmacological: anticholingerics, propylthiouracil, glucagon, somatostatin, 5-fluorouracil, acetazolamide, calcitonin
        Hypothermia
        Pancreatic irradiation
    Inhibition of pancreatic enzymes
        Aprotinin, epsilon-amino caproic acid, fresh frozen plasma, soybean trypsin inhibitor, insulin, snake antivenom, chlorophyll, xylocaine, gabexelate mesilate, camostate,
    Prostaglandin
    Corticosteroids
    Endoscopic sphincterotomy

To interrupt the pathogenesis of complications
    Antibiotics
    Antacids, cimetidine
    Heparin, fibrinolysin
    Low molecular weight dextran
    Peritoneal lavage
    Plasmapheresis
    Haemofiltration

pulse rate and blood pressure. In most patients, a central venous catheter should be inserted and an indwelling urethral catheter introduced for regular measurement of central venous pressure, venous blood gases and hourly urine output. In patients with associated cardiovascular disease, large fluid requirements or severe respiratory complications, monitoring of pulmonary arterial pressures and cardiac output using a Swan Ganz catheter may be essential for appropriate management. Haemodynamic evaluation of patients with severe pancreatitis has demonstrated a high cardiac output and low peripheral vascular resistance (Di Carlo et al 1981, Bradley et al 1983, Beger et al 1986). These findings are similar to those observed in sepsis or hepatic cirrhosis and have been attributed to circulating vasoactive substances which are released in severe pancreatitis. Since ischaemia may convert mild pancreatitis to more severe disease, it is especially important that pharmacological cardiovascular support should be directed toward maintaining tissue perfusion and avoiding vasoconstricton.

Electrolyte replacement

Hypokalaemia is frequent and potassium replacement is usually required (Edmondson et al 1952). Intravenous replacement of calcium and magnesium has also been recommended (Wills 1966, Zimberg 1968). Symptoms and complications referable to hypocalcaemia, however, are uncommon and since hypercalcaemia has been implicated in the genesis of pancreatitis, calcium should be administered cautiously (Imrie et al 1976, Manson 1974).

Respiratory monitoring and support

Clinically occult respiratory failure is a frequent feature of acute pancreatitis (Imrie et al 1977, Ranson et al 1973, 1974) and may occur in patients who do not have severe disease by the usual clinical criteria. Changes in oxyhaemoglobin affinity during acute pancreatitis may increase the physiological consequences of respiratory failure (Greenburg et al 1977) and early hypoxaemia may certainly be lethal if undiagnosed or untreated (Ranson et al 1973). Therefore, it is essential that arterial blood gas values are determined at the time of diagnosis and at intervals of not less than 12 hours for the initial 48–72 hours of treatment. Subsequent measurements depend on the patient's course.

Progressive respiratory insufficiency, pulmonary infiltration and pleural effusions occur in approximately 30% of patients. These complications are related to the patient's age, initial serum amylase level, early hypocalcaemia and early fluid sequestration (Ranson et al 1974). These intrathoracic complications are more common in patients undergoing early intra-abdominal surgery for pancreatitis and occur in approximately 60% of this group.

Early hypoxaemia usually resolves as the underlying pancreatitis subsides and the only treatment which is required is administration of oxygen, chest physiotherapy, and close monitoring of arterial blood gas measurements. Patients with progressive pulmonary insufficiency require early endotracheal intubation and mechanical ventilatory assistance. Early institution of positive end-expiratory pressure ventilation may be beneficial (Nath & Warshaw 1982).

Nutritional support

The occurrence of marked nutritional depletion in patients with acute pancreatitis is well known (Feller et al 1974, Blackburn et al 1976). In those with mild pancreatitis, oral feeding can usually be resumed within a few days. In patients with severe pancreatitis, oral feeding is usually not tolerated for prolonged periods and alternative nutritional support must be instituted as early as possible. Initially, the only possible route is intravenous alimentation. After intestinal peristalsis returns, enteral feeding is a possible alternative route.

For most patients, standard total parenteral nutrition, initiated as soon as early cardiovascular instability has subsided, is the most practical form of nutritional support (Goodgame & Fischer 1977). Glucose levels must be carefully monitored and insulin given as needed. The safety of intravenous lipid as a caloric source has been controversial. Konturek et al (1979) found that intravenous administration of amino acids and of fat emulsion caused an increase in pancreatic secretion in dogs. Further studies in dogs (Fried et al 1982) and man (Silberman et al 1982, Edelman & Valenzuela 1983, Van Gossum 1988) have not confirmed this finding.

It should be emphasized that total parenteral nutrition is only appropriate for patients in whom oral feeding is not possible for a substantial period. A recent randomized controlled clinical study compared total parenteral nutrition with standard supportive care in 54 unselected patients with acute pancreatitis. In this study most patients had mild pancrcatitis and the morbidity related to central intravenous catheters far outweighed any benefits of nutritional support (Sax et al 1987).

In patients in whom gastrointestinal function has returned, enteral feeding of a low-fat chemically defined diet is usually well tolerated. Food may be introduced directly into the jejunum by a fine weighted feeding tube positioned fluoroscopically or by a feeding jejunostomy in patients undergoing abdominal surgery.

Pain relief

The pain associated with acute pancreatitis may be very severe. It is traditional to recommend demerol (pethidine) for its relief rather than morphine because of the spasm of the ampulla of Vater associated with the latter drug (Anderson 1969, Elmslie 1967). Splanchic block or continuous epidural anaesthesia have been recommended because they avoid ampullary spasm and may increase pancreatic blood flow (Howard & Jordan 1960). They are not, however, widely used.

Heparin

Serial studies of coagulation factors show that elevated platelet counts in the range of 1 000 000/mm³ and fibrinogen levels as high as 10 g/l occurred during the second and third weeks of treatment in some patients with severe pancreatitis (Ranson et al 1977). Furthermore, pulmonary embolism has been a major problem in the late course of some patients, particularly those who require surgical drainage of infected pancreatic abscesses. It is, therefore, our practice to monitor fibrinogen levels and platelet counts in patients with severe pancreatitis. In those with marked thrombocytosis or hyperfibrinogenaemia, and those who require surgical drainage of pancreatic abscesses, heparin is administered by constant infusion. A dose of 750–1000 units/h is used, depending on the partial thromboplastin time. Bleeding from drain tracts has been a problem in some patients and has led to permanent suspension of heparin in two cases. Pulmonary embolism has not, however, been recognized in patients who were able to continue heparin.

MEASURES TO LIMIT PANCREATIC INFLAMMATION

Inhibition of pancreatic secretion

Nasogastric suction, cimetidine and the timing of oral feeding

Nasogastric suction has traditionally been instituted in patients with acute pancreatitis to reduce vomiting and abdominal distension. It has also been suggested that aspiration of gastric acid may decrease pancreatic exocrine secretion by reducing secretin release (Anderson 1969, Elmslie 1967, White 1966).

The therapeutic efficacy of nasogastric suction has been evaluated recently in controlled clinical trials. These studies are summarized in Table 20.2. In most studies, nasogastric suction is compared to simple withholding of oral feeding. In Lange and Pedersen's study (1983), the control group received a clear liquid diet and in that of Goff et al (1982), the control group received cimetidine.

None of these studies demonstrated any significant benefit from the nasogastric suction. It should be noted, however, that the great majority of patients studied had alcoholic pancreatitis. Furthermore, in some studies many patients were experiencing their third or subsequent episode of pancreatitis and might more accurately be classified as suffering from relapses of chronic pancreatitis. The overwhelming majority of patients in these studies had mild pancreatitis; the average duration of pain and other symptoms was low and although 408 patients are included, there were only five deaths. In addition, the average duration of pain was reduced by nasogastric suction in five of the eight studies in which pain duration was reported. Finally, the number of patients included in individual studies remains small, averaging 45 patients per study. In a disease as heterogeneous as acute pancreatitis, this number is far too small to evaluate therapeutic measures unless patients are carefully stratified. Hence, present data indicate that nasogastric suction is not essential for recovery from mild pancreatitis, especially when associated with alcohol abuse. Further studies are needed to evaluate the role of this measure in more severe pancreatitis and in other aetiological subgroups. We continue to recommend nasogastric suction for most patients with acute pancreatitis because of the symptomatic relief which is usually afforded, and because it occasionally appears to be associated with decreased evidence of pancreatic inflammation.

Inhibition of gastric acid production by the administration of H_2 receptor antagonist, cimetidine, has also been evaluated in acute pancreatitis (Evander & Ihse 1979, Meshkinpour et al 1979, Broe et al 1982, Goff et al 1982, Loiudice et al 1984). The clinical studies again predominantly include patients with mild alcoholic pancreatitis and the numbers of patients studied have been small. In the studies of Meshkinpour et al (1979) and Loiudice et al (1984), cimetidine appeared to delay somewhat the

Table 20.2 Studies evaluating the effect of nasogastric (NG) suction in patients with acute pancreatitis. The average number of patients/study was 45.

Study	Number of patients		Days of pain		Death	
	NG suction	No NG suction	NG	No NG	NG	No NG
Levant et al (1974)	15	14	2.9	3.7	0	0
Naeije et al (1978)	27	31	3.0	2.5	0	0
Field et al (1979)	20	17	3.3	4.0*	0	0
Loiudice et al (1984)	16	11	3.1	3.3	0	0
Fuller et al (1981)	10	11†	1.6	1.8	0	0
Sarr et al (1986)	29	28‡	4.7	4.2	0	0
Lange & Pedersen (1983)	25	25**	3.0	3.0	2	3
Switz et al (1975)	16††	16	No details but reports no benefit			
Goff et al (1982)	46	57‡‡	5.0	5.3	0	0
Total number of patients	198	210				

*Six patients with 'severe' pancreatitis were excluded; †1 patient in no NG suction group withdrawn because of clinical deterioration; ‡3 patients required NG suction; **control group received clear liquid oral diet; ††one-half of each group received anticholinergics; ‡‡control group received cimetidine clinical or biochemical recovery. In experimental studies, (Evander & Ihse 1979, Hadas et al 1979) cimetidine was associated with an increased mortality from acute pancreatitis. Thus, cimetidine has, at present, no demonstrated value in decreasing the overall morbidity of acute pancreatitis and may even have some hazards. It may, however, be helpful in decreasing the incidence of acute gastroduodenal ulceration.

Whatever the role of nasogastric suction or cimetidine, it has been shown experimentally that gastric feeding during acute pancreatitis results in increased pancreatic inflammation (Lium & Maddock 1948, Wangensteen et al 1931). Furthermore it has been our repeated clinical experience that oral feeding prior to resolution of pancreatitis may often be followed by reactivation of pancreatic inflammation and further complications (Ranson & Spencer 1977). In a study by Lange and Pederson (1983), early administration of clear liquids by mouth did not appear to be harmful in mild pancreatitis. Nonetheless, this has clearly not been our experience in moderate or severe disease. It remains our practice to withhold feeding until abdominal pain and tenderness, fever and leucocytosis have subsided. When oral feeding is resumed, it is important that the intake should be low in fat.

Anticholinergics

Anticholinergic drugs have been widely recommended in the treatment of acute pancreatitis in order to decrease vagally mediated exocrine pancreatic secretion and reduce ampullary spasm (Howard & Jordan 1960, Elliott & Williams 1961, White 1966, Anderson 1969). It is uncertain whether these drugs add significantly to pancreatic suppression in patients receiving nasogastric suction. Furthermore, in patients with severe pancreatitis, high fever and tachycardia frequently contraindicate their use. Finally, a controlled clinical study (Cameron et al 1979) compared the outcome in 19 patients given atropine with that in 32 control patients with mild, predominantly alcoholic pancreatitis. Although nasogastric suction was not controlled in this study, no benefit was apparent in the atropine treated group.

Glucagon

The administration of glucagon has been recommended in the treatment of acute pancreatitis because of its inhibitory effect on exocrine pancreatic secretion (Knight et al 1971, 1972, Condon et al 1973, Rossi et al 1974). Experimental studies were encouraging in pigs (Waterworth et al 1976) but not in rats (Lankisch et al 1974) or dogs (Eckhauser et al 1985, Condon et al 1974). Controlled clinical studies have shown no amelioration of any aspect of this disease (Ohlsson 1971, Gauthier 1978, Cox et al 1980).

Calcitonin

Administration of calcitonin has been evaluated in the treatment of acute pancreatitis because of the inhibition of pancreatic secretion effected by this substance (Nakashima et al 1977). Three controlled clinical trials of calcitonin have been reported and include a total of 228 patients (Paul et al 1979). Two studies suggest that pain and hyperamylasaemia resolve more rapidly with calcitonin treatment (Paul et al 1979, Goebell et al 1979) but no reduction in complications or mortality has been demonstrated.

Somatostatin

Like calcitonin, somatostatin inhibits pancreatic exocrine secretion (Boden et al 1975, Raptis et al 1978, Susini et al 1980) and has been recommended for the treatment of acute pancreatitis. Experimental studies have yielded conflicting results concerning the efficacy of this measure (Lankisch et al 1977, Schwedes et al 1979, Mann et al 1980, Baxter et al 1985). Initial controlled clinical studies did not show any clear benefit (Moreau et al 1976, Usadel et al 1980). A more recent interinstitutional study from Italy (D'Amico et al 1990) compared 82 patients treated with somatostatin to 82 patients who were not. Somatostatin was given at a dose of 3.5 µg/kg body weight per hour by continuous intravenous infusion for periods of 72–100 hours. Although there appeared to be a trend to more rapid pain relief and lower morbidity in the somatostatin-treated patients, the differences did not achieve statistical significance.

Other proposed methods for the inhibition of pancreatic secretion include acetazolamide (Anderson & Copass 1966, Banks & Sum 1971), external irradiation of the pancreas (Wachtfeidl & Vitez 1968), hypothermia (Eichelter et al 1966, Eichelter 1967, Eichelter & Schenk 1968), administration of 5-fluorouracil (Johnson et al 1973, Saario 1983, Mann & Mann 1979), fotorafur (Hudvagner et al 1984), propylthiouracil (Reid et al 1958) or cycloheximide (Mann et al 1980). Most of these measures have been recommended on the basis of experimental or uncontrolled clinical studies and their clinical effectiveness is not known.

Inhibition of pancreatic enzymes

The concept that the severity of acute pancreatitis and of its complications may be reduced by inhibitors of pancreatic enzymes has received much attention over the past 30 years. The most extensively investigated agent has been aprotinin, a polypeptide that is extracted from bovine parotid glands and which inhibits trypsin and kallikrein. Experimental studies have produced conflicting results (Kelly et al 1953, Mallet-Guy et al 1961, Beck et al 1965,

Schutt et al 1965, Tountas et al 1966), but a controlled clinical trial in 1965 showed no benefit in patients (Skyring et al 1965). Interest in aprotinin was rekindled by a further controlled clinical trial in 1974 that indicated that aprotinin reduced mortality from 25 to 7.5% (Trapnell et al 1974). However, subsequent randomized double-blind clinical studies have shown no benefit from this agent (Gauthier et al 1978, Imrie et al 1978, Cox et al 1980).

Preliminary controlled clinical studies of the synthetic protease inhibitors gabexelate mesilate (FOY) and camostate (Freise et al 1985, Yang et al 1987) have been reported. The numbers of patients included are small. However, serum α-amylase levels appeared to fall more rapidly in the treatment group and there was some trend toward lower morbidity in patients receiving gabexelate mesilate. A preliminary trial by Konttinen (1971) and a further randomized double-blind evaluation of the influence of $CaNa_2$ EDTA, a phospholipase A_2 inhibitor have been completed. The controlled clinical trial included 64 patients. In the 33 treated patients, 3 g of $CaNa_2$ EDTA was infused intravenously in 100 ml of 5% glucose for 12 hours on the first and second day, to a total dose of 6 g. Serum phospholipase activity fell significantly more rapidly in the treatment group and early clinical improvement seemed more marked. An improvement in overall morbidity and mortality was not demonstrated (Tykka et al 1985).

Other enzyme inhibitors which have been studied experimentally include soybean trypsin inhibitor (Rush & Clifton 1952, Hoffman et al 1953, Cannon & Turner 1961), snake antivenom (Rittenbury & Hanback 1969), xylocaine (Schroeder et al 1978), chlorophyll-a (Mann & Mann 1979) and leupeptin (Jones et al 1982). There is no evidence that any of these agents would be effective clinically. Hallberg & Theve (1974) proposed the infusion of insulin and glucose in order to inactivate adipose tissue lipase, but a controlled clinical trial of this regimen has demonstrated no significant therapeutic effect.

Anti-inflammatory agents

Adrenocorticosteroids have been administered to patients with acute pancreatitis because of their anti-inflammatory effects (Anderson et al 1964, Stefanini et al 1965). Experimental studies in whole animals suggested that steroid administration may be beneficial (Anderson et al 1964, Studley & Schenk 1982) especially if administered early after the induction of pancreatitis. On the other hand, studies using an isolated perfused pancreas model suggested that steroids led to worsening of pancreatitis (Kimura et al 1980). No adequate clinical studies have been reported.

Recent experimental studies have begun to evaluate the influence of prostaglandins, and drugs which influence their metabolism, on the course of pancreatitis. Reported results at present are conflicting (Lankisch et al 1978,

Manabe & Steer 1980, Olazabal & Nasciemento 1980, Coelle et al 1983, Farias et al 1985). A randomized double-blind controlled clinical trial of indomethacin has been reported in which 50 mg was administered twice daily for 7 days. Only 30 patients were included in the study and most had mild pancreatitis. However, the duration and intensity of pain were significantly reduced in indomethacin treated patients (Ebbehøj et al 1985). This observation requires further study.

Endoscopic retrograde cholangiopancreatography sphincterotomy

The hypothesis that persistent calculous obstruction of the ampulla of Vater is responsible for progression of acute gallstone pancreatitis, has led to the suggestion that urgent endoscopic sphincterotomy may benefit such patients (Safrany & Cotton 1981). This therapeutic intervention has been evaluated by a controlled clinical trial. A total of 59 patients underwent endoscopic retrograde cholangiopancreatography (ERCP), within 72 h of hospital admission, and endoscopic sphincterotomy and stone extraction if common duct stones were demonstrated. Another 62 patients were treated by standard measures for the first 5 days. In patients who were predicted to have mild pancreatitis, no benefit was demonstrated. However, in patients predicted to have severe pancreatitis, both morbidity and mortality were significantly reduced (Neoptolemos et al 1988). It may be exceedingly difficult to distinguish between cholangitis associated with hyperamylasaemia and true pancreatitis associated with gallstones. Because of the potential for ERCP and endoscopic sphincterotomy to initiate acute pancreatitis, the findings in this study require confirmation.

MEASURES TO INTERRUPT THE PATHOGENESIS OF COMPLICATIONS

Antibiotics

Antibiotics have traditionally been recommended in the treatment of acute pancreatitis and experimental evidence suggests that they may, in some instances, decrease the severity of pancreatitis (Byrne & Joison 1964, Williams & Byrne 1968). Recent prospective controlled clinical trials evaluated the role of ampicillin in pancreatitis (Craig et al 1975, Howes et al 1975, Finch et al 1976) and found no benefit from this antibiotic. The studies were small and the great majority of patients included had alcoholic pancreatitis. The three studies together include a total of 199 patients. There were only three patients who developed pancreatic abscesses and only one who died. Death was due to aspiration pneumonia. Thus, while it seems clear that ampicillin probably confers no benefit on patients with mild, alcoholic pancreatitis, it may be unwise to extrapolate this finding to other aetiological groups or those with severe disease. I continue to recommend broad spectrum antibiotic treatment for patients with gallstone-associated pancreatitis, because of the frequency of positive biliary cultures in this group, and also for patients with severe pancreatitis. In this last group, positive cultures may be obtained from blood during the first few days of illness even in the absence of an identifiable source.

Antacids

In patients with pancreatitis, acute gastroduodenal ulceration and bleeding may occur. The risk of this complication can be substantially reduced by monitoring of gastric pH and maintenance above pH4. This can usually be accomplished with antacids although H_2-blocking drugs such as cimetidine may sometimes be helpful.

Anticoagulants

Pathological studies of human and experimental pancreatitis by Rich and Duff in 1936 documented the occurrence of intravascular thrombosis in the pancreas and led to the hypothesis that trypsin-mediated vascular injury might be responsible. Further experimental studies by Popper et al (1948) and Goodhead (1969) suggested that ischaemic injury may play a critical role in the evolution of necrotizing pancreatitis. Subsequent clinical and experimental studies (Ranson & Lackner 1982) have clearly established that the intravascular deposition of coagulation factors occurs during the early phase of acute pancreatitis. The degree to which this deposition contributes to the genesis of local systemic complications remains uncertain. If intravascular clotting is secondary to enzyme-mediated changes in coagulation, inhibition of clotting may ameliorate the sequelae of pancreatitis. It is possible, however, that observed coagulation changes are secondary to vascular or other tissue injury and play little or no causative role.

Experimental studies of the influence of heparin administration on the course of acute pancreatitis, by Gabryelewicz & Niewiarowski (1968) and Wright & Goodhead (1970), found that mortality was dramatically reduced compared with untreated controls. In these experiments, the coagulation changes, serum amylase elevations, and degree of pancreatic inflammation were all reported to be reduced by heparin. Wright & Goodhead (1970) also found that administration of fibrinolysin immediately after the induction of pancreatitis improved survival and reduced the histological evidence of pancreatic inflammation (Simmons et al 1969). By contrast, Hureau and co-workers (1968) reported that the administration of heparin to animals with pancreatitis resulted uniformly in death owing to internal haemorrhage. Furthermore, Byrne and associates found that the administration of aspirin, sodium salicylate, or dipyridamole neither prevented the early fall in circulating platelet counts after induction of acute pancreatitis nor reduced the degree of pancreatic inflammation (Byrne et al 1971).

Our own experimental studies evaluated the influence of heparin on a model of acute pancreatitis in dogs. Changes in coagulation factor levels following induction of pancreatitis were reduced by heparin administration but mortality was not improved. In a further study, circulating fibrinogen levels were reduced almost to zero by the administration of Ancrod, which is the purified coagulation fraction of Malaysian pit viper venom, before induction of pancreatitis. Although virtually no fibrinogen was present for intravascular deposition, mortality was not improved (Ranson & Lackner 1982). It seems probable, therefore, that observed changes in coagulation factors and intravascular thrombosis represent a response to tissue or vascular injury rather than a cause.

Whatever the theoretical value of anticoagulant therapy in acute pancreatitis may be, a review of 10 patients who had received heparin (5000 units subcutaneously at 6-hourly intervals during the initial 48 hours after diagnosis) did not demonstrate any apparent benefit in any aspect of the disease (Ranson & Lackner 1982). One of these patients who appeared to have mild pancreatitis had a major retroperitoneal haemorrhage, requiring transfusions before eventual recovery. This experience suggests that anticoagulants should, if possible, be avoided during the early phase of acute pancreatitis.

Low molecular weight dextran and vasopressin

Modification of pancreatic blood flow by administration of vasopressin, low molecular weight dextran and other vasoactive drugs or by surgical sympathectomy ameliorates the severity of experimental acute pancreatitis (Andreadis et al 1967, Williams & Byrne 1968, Goodhead & Wright 1969, Carey 1970, Pissiotis et al 1972, Mann & Mann 1979, Donaldson & Schenk 1980, Donahue et al 1984). The clinical applicability of these observations is, however, unknown.

Peritoneal lavage

Interest in the possibility that peritoneal lavage might benefit patients with acute pancreatitis was initiated by an observation by Wall in 1965. He undertook peritoneal dialysis in three patients judged to have severe acute pancreatitis, two of whom had frank renal failure. Marked clinical improvement was noted following the institution of peritoneal dialysis and two patients survived. Following this, a number of reports appeared, all of which suggested that peritoneal lavage was of benefit to patients with severe acute pancreatitis (Gjessing 1967, Bolooki & Gliedman 1968, Geokas et al 1978, Lasson & Ohlsson 1984). Reynaert et al, in 1985, reviewed 203 reported patients treated by peritoneal lavage for severe pancreatitis with an overall mortality of 22.6%. Unfortunately, the criteria used to identify patients with severe acute pancreatitis varied considerably. Furthermore, the timing and duration of peritoneal lavage were not standardized, and in some patients, placement of lavage catheters was combined with formal intra-abdominal surgical procedures.

In 1976, we reported a small controlled clinical trial of peritoneal lavage which suggested that morbidity was reduced by this measure (Ranson et al 1976). In 1980, Stone & Fabian reported a larger controlled trial in which 29 of 34 patients treated with lavage showed 'a decided improvement in the overall condition' compared to only 13 of 36 patients treated without lavage. In this study 11 patients underwent formal early laparotomy. Further interpretation of this group is also clouded by the fact that 17 non-lavage group patients were later transferred to lavage therapy. However, mortality in the final group of 51 patients treated with lavage was 15.7% compared to 31.6% in those treated without lavage.

Two other small controlled clinical trials (Cooper et al 1982, Ihse et al 1986) and a large cooperative study (Mayer et al 1985) found no benefit from peritoneal lavage in severe acute pancreatitis. The large cooperative trial included 91 patients, 45 of whom received peritoneal lavage for 3 days. No difference was found between the lavage and non-lavage groups in overall mortality nor in the cause or timing of death. These findings may have been influenced by the fact that 34 of the 46 non-lavage patients underwent diagnostic lavage of the peritoneal cavity for prognostic assessment. Furthermore, patients in the study were cared for in different hospitals which may have had differing patterns of treatment.

Our own initial experience with peritoneal lavage for the management of severe acute pancreatitis was summarized in 1978 (Ranson & Spencer 1978). At that time, the course of 103 patients with three or more positive prognostic signs was reviewed. This included 24 patients whose early management included laparotomy. Of the 103 patients 24 had received lavage of the peritoneal cavity for periods of 2–4 days. A number of observations were made at that time. First, overall mortality was not affected by lavage but was influenced by early laparotomy. It was 67% in six patients who underwent laparotomy and placement of lavage catheters alone and 67% in 18 patients who underwent other early operative procedures. Mortality was 17% in 18 patients who underwent lavage using catheters introduced under local anaesthesia and 16% in 61 patients who received standard non-operative treatment without peritoneal lavage. Peritoneal lavage did, however, appear to influence the cause and timing of death. No lavaged patient died during the first 10 days of treatment while 10 of 22 deaths (45%) in non-lavaged patients occurred during this early period, primarily as a result of cardiovascular or respiratory failure. Almost all

deaths in lavaged patients were due to late pancreatic sepsis. It was our conclusion that peritoneal lavage for periods of 2–4 days was a valuable adjunct to the management of early cardiovascular and respiratory complications of severe acute pancreatitis, but did not influence the occurrence of the sequelae of pancreatic and peripancreatic necrosis, specifically sepsis.

It was also noted at that time that in clinical reports of acute pancreatitis, published during the period 1962–1974, death had been attributed to 'shock' or pulmonary complications in 66–80% of patients (Foster & Ziffren 1962, Trapnell 1966, Kune 1968, Gliedman et al 1970, Olsen 1974), and most such deaths had occurred during the first 14 days of treatment (Thal et al 1957, Enquist & Gliedman 1958, Trapnell 1966). Death was due to pancreatic sepsis in 14–35% of cases (Trapnell 1966, Kune 1968, Gliedman et al 1970) and these deaths usually occurred after the first 2 weeks of treatment (Enquist & Gliedman 1958, Trapnell 1966, Ranson & Spencer 1977). In our series of 450 patients reported in 1978, death was due to cardiovascular, respiratory or cerebrovascular insufficiency in 10 patients (32%). These deaths occurred on days 1–16 (median, day 5). A total of 22 deaths (68%) were associated with intra-abdominal sepsis and occurred on days 8–131 (median, day 23). It was clear that, with improvements in early supportive care of patients and possibly the use of peritoneal lavage, the major cause of morbidity and death in acute pancreatitis had become infection of devitalized pancreatic and peripancreatic tissue (Buggy & Nostrant 1983).

A recent controlled clinical trial has suggested that a period of 7 days of peritoneal lavage may dramatically reduce the incidence and mortality of late pancreatic infection (Ranson & Berman 1990). This study included 29 patients judged to have severe pancreatitis and the differences did not achieve statistical significance.

The possible mode of action of peritoneal lavage is obscure, but its efficacy has usually been attributed to the removal of toxic materials in the peritoneal exudate in acute pancreatitis (Baslov et al 1962, Wall 1965, Ancarani et al 1972, Rosato et al 1973). This is, in part, due to an observation in 1962 that haemodialysis did not improve survival in severe acute pancreatitis (Baslov et al 1962). The conclusion that peritoneal lavage acts by removing substances in the peritoneal exudate rather than dialysable material from the blood may not be appropriate. Studies of the peritoneal exudate found during acute pancreatitis have shown that this exudate contains numerous substances including amylase, lipase, phospholipase A, protease–antiprotease complexes, trypsinogen, proteolytic pro-enzymes, prostaglandin-like activity and kinin-forming enzymes. Furthermore, the exudate has been shown to produce systemic hypotension, histamine release, increased vascular permeability and inhibition of hepatic mitochondrial function. While removal of such material might explain the dramatic immediate clinical improvement which is sometimes observed following the initiation of peritoneal lavage, it is not clear why prolonged lavage should influence pancreatic or peripancreatic necrosis or the risk of infection of such devitalized tissue (Ranson & Berman 1990).

Studies of peritoneal lavage in the treatment of pancreatitis in dogs (Rogers & Carey 1966, Rasmussen 1967, Ancarani et al 1972, Rosato et al 1973, Bassi et al 1989), guinea pigs (Rosato et al 1972) and rats (Lankisch et al 1979) have shown immediate improvement and reduced mortality. Furthermore, lavage is reported to have reduced necrosis of the pancreas and peripancreatic fat in some of these experimental studies. Experimental studies suggest that the addition of protease inhibitors to lavage fluid may increase the therapeutic efficacy of this measure (Lankisch et al 1979, Satake et al 1985, Bassi et al 1989). However, in a controlled clinical trial including 55 patients treated by peritoneal lavage (Balldin et al 1983), no benefit was observed in those patients randomized to receive aprotinin in their lavage fluid.

Evidence that periods of lavage that are longer than 2–4 days may be beneficial in human acute pancreatitis has also been provided by studies from Germany. Gebhardt & Gall in 1981 advocated operative debridement of necrotic tissue combined with postoperative irrigation and sump drainage of the peritoneal cavity. Mortality, in their report, was 54% in 84 patients treated for necrotizing pancreatitis without postoperative peritoneal irrigation compared to 37% when irrigation was added. Beger has also advocated operative debridement of necrotic tissue and combines this with postoperative lavage of the lesser omental sac (Beger et al 1988, see Chapter 22). Lavage was continued for an average of 25 days (range 5–90 days) and it was found that markedly elevated levels of pancreatic trypsin, amylase and phospholipase A were present in the lavage effluent for periods of 10–15 days post-operatively. If active pancreatic enzymes are released for similarly prolonged periods in unoperated patients, this may provide an explanation for the benefits of long lavage observed in the recent controlled clinical study (Ranson & Berman 1990). In Beger's report, the overall mortality was 8.1% in 74 patients, who had an average of 4.5 positive prognostic signs, treated in this way. It is possible that these excellent results may, in large part, be due to prolonged peritoneal lavage.

By contrast, a controlled clinical trial in Finland (Teerenhovi et al 1989) compared laparotomy with postoperative pancreatic drainage to laparotomy and postoperative lavage of the lesser omental sac for a mean of 6.8 days (range 4–12 days). A total of 24 patients were included in this study and had an average of 4.7–4.5 positive prognostic signs. No reduction in the frequency of pancreatic infection was observed and overall mortality was higher in the lavage group (36%) than in the drainage group (17%). It must be emphasized that all patients in this last study underwent laparotomy and that lavage was begun on day 4.1 ± 3.6 of symptoms.

Clearly further studies are needed.

Attempts to remove toxic substances by plasmapheresis (Larvin et al 1988) and haemofiltration (Bodecker et al 1990) have also appeared promising in preliminary reports.

CONCLUSIONS

While many therapeutic measures have been proposed for patients with acute pancreatitis, no single measure has been convincingly shown to limit the severity of pancreatic inflammation or prevent the development of complications. This is in part due to the wide spectrum of illnesses grouped under this one diagnosis. However, until more specific treatments are developed, the most important steps in management are supportive and symptomatic.

REFERENCES

Ancarani E, Tersigni R, Vincenti R 1972 Peritoneal dialysis in the treatment of experimental acute pancreatitis. Bulletin de la Société Internationale de Chirurgie 31:142–145

Anderson M C 1968 Review of pancreatic disease. Surgery 66:434–439

Anderson M C, Booher D L, Lim T B 1964 Treatment of acute pancreatitis with adrenocorticosteroids. Surgery 55:551–558

Anderson M C, Copass M K 1966 Use of carbonic anhydrase inhibitor in the treatment of pancreatitis. American Journal of Digestive Diseases 11:367–376

Andreadis P, Kirakou K, Tountas C 1967 Vasopressin in the treatment of acute experimental pancreatitis. Annals of Surgery 166:913–918

Balldin G, Borgstrom A, Genell S, Ohlsson K 1983 The effect of peritoneal lavage and aprotinin in the treatment of severe acute pancreatitis. Research and Experimental Medicine 183:203–13

Banks P A, Sum P T 1971 Mode of action of acetazolamide on pancreatic exocrine secretion. Archives of Surgery 102:505–508

Baslov J T, Jorgensen H E, Nielsen R 1962 Acute renal failure complicating severe acute pancreatitis. Acta Chirurgica Scandinavica 124:348–354

Bassi C, Gianfranco B, Vesentini S et al 1989 Continuous peritoneal dialysis in acute experimental pancreatitis in dogs. International Journal of Pancreatolology 5:69–75

Baxter J N, Jenkins S A, Day D W et al 1985 Effects of somatostatin and a long-acting somatostatin analogue on the prevention and treatment of experimentally induced acute pancreatitis in the rat. British Journal of Surgery 72:382–385

Beck I T, McKenna R D, Zylberszac B et al 1965 The effect of trypsin inhibitor, Trasylol, on the course of bile- and trypsin-induced pancreatitis in dogs. Gastroenterology 48:478–483

Beger H G, Bittner R, Büchler M et al 1986 Hemodynamic data pattern in patients with acute pancreatitis. Gastroenterology 90:74–79

Beger H G, Büchler M, Bittner R, Oettinger W, Block S, Nevalainen T 1988 Necrosectomy and postoperative local lavage in patients with necrotizing pancreatitis: results of a prospective clinical trial. World Journal of Surgery 12:255–62

Blackburn G L, Williams L F, Bristrian B R et al 1976 New approaches to the management of severe acute pancreatitis. American Journal of Surgery 131:114–124

Bodecker H, Blinzer L, Krauss D et al 1990 Conservative treatment of severe necrotic pancreatitis using continuous hemofiltration.

(Summary of Pancreas Club Meeting). American Journal of Surgery 160:464

Boden G, Sivitz M C, Owen O E, Essa-Koumar N, Landor J H 1975 Somatostatin suppresses secretin and pancreatic exocrine secretion. Science 190:163–164

Bolooki H, Gliedman M L 1968 Peritoneal dialysis in treatment of acute pancreatitis. Surgery 64:466–471

Bradley E L, Hall J R, Lutz J, Hamner L, Lattouf O 1983 Hemodynamic consequences of severe pancreatitis. Annals of Surgery 198:130–133

Broe P J, Zinner M J, Cameron J L 1982 A clinical trial of cimetidine in acute pancreatitis. Surgery, Gynecology and Obstetrics 154:13–16

Buggy B P, Nostrant T T 1983 Lethal pancreatitis. American Journal of Gastroenterology 78:810–814

Byrne J J, Joison J 1964 Bacterial regurgitation in experimental pancreatitis. American Journal of Surgery 107:317–320

Byrne J J, Migliore J J, Beekley W et al 1971 Platelet response to induction of hemorrhagic pancreatitis. Proceedings of the Society of Experimental Biology and Medicine 136:994–996

Cameron J L, Mejigan D, Zuidema G D 1979 Evaluation of atropine in acute pancreatitis. Surgery, Gynecology and Obstetrics 148:206–208

Cannon R H, Turner M D 1961 Retardation of the progress of experimental pancreatitis with trypsin inhibitors. Surgical Forum 13:367–369

Carey L B C 1970 Low molecular weight dextran in experimental pancreatitis. American Journal of Surgery 119:197–199

Cavuoti O P, Moody F G, Martinez G 1988 Role of pancreatic duct occlusion with prolamine (Ethibloc) in necrotizing pancreatitis. Surgery 103:361–366

Coelle E F, Adham N, Elashoff J, Lewin K, Taylor I L 1983 Effects of prostaglandin and indomethacin on diet-induced acute pancreatitis in mice. Gastroenterology 85:1307–1312

Condon J R, Knight M, Day J L 1973 Glucagon therapy in acute pancreatitis. British Journal of Surgery 60:509–511

Condon R E, Woods J H, Poulin T L, Wagner W G, Pissiotis O A 1974 Experimental pancreatitis associated with glucagon or lacted ringer solution. Archives of Surgery 109:154–158

Cooper M J, Williamson R C N, Pollock A V 1982 The role of peritoneal lavage in the prediction and treatment of severe acute pancreatitis. Annals of the Royal College of Surgeons of England 64:422–427

Cox A G, Armitage P, Hogg R 1980 Morbidity of acute pancreatitis: the effect of aprotinin and glucagon. Gut 21:334–339

Craig R, Dordal E, Myles L 1975 The use of ampicillin in acute pancreatitis. Annals of Internal Medicine 83:831–832

D'Amico D, Favia G, Biasiato R et al 1990 Hepato-gastroenterology 37:92–98

Di Carlo V, Nespoli A, Chiesa R et al 1981 Hemodynamic and metabolic impairment in acute pancreatitis. World Journal of Surgery 5:329–339

Donahue P E, Akimoto H, Ferguson J L, Nyhus L M 1984 Vasoactive drugs in acute pancreatitis. Archives of Surgery 119:477–480

Donaldson L A, Schenk W G 1980 The effect of Trasylol and vasopressin on experimental pancreatitis. Surgery, Gynecology and Obstetrics 150:657–660

Ebbehøj N, Friis J, Svendsen L B, Bulow S, Madsen P 1985 Indomethacin treatment of acute pancreatitis. Scandinavian Journal of Gastroenterology 20:798–800

Eckhauser F E, Knol J A, Inman M G, Strodel W E 1985 Efficacy of pharmacologic glucagon in acute experimental pancreatitis. Archives of Surgery 120:355–360

Edelman K, Valenzuela J E 1983 Effect of intravenous lipid on pancreatic secretion. Gastroenterology 85:1063–1066

Edmondson H A, Berne C J, Homann R E, Wertman M 1952 Calcium, potassium, magnesium and amylase disturbances in acute pancreatitis. American Journal of Medicine 12:34–42

Eichelter P 1967 Influence of hypothermia on the course of experimental pancreatitis. Archives of Surgery 94:280–285

Eichelter P, Schenk W G 1968 The influence of hypothermia on pancreatic secretion and blood flow. Archives of Surgery 96:883–886

Eichelter P, Schenk W G, Schueller E F 1966 Histopathology of experimental pancreatitis in the dog. Archives of Surgery 93:606–613

Elliott D W, Williams R D 1961 A reevaluation of serum amylase determinations. Archives of Surgery 83:130–153

Elmslie R G 1967 Aspects of the management of acute pancreatitis. Medical Journal of Australia 1:211–213

Enquist I F, Gliedman M L 1958 Gross autopsy findings in cases of fatal acute pancreatitis. Archives of Surgery 77:985–991

Evander A, Ihse I 1979 Influence of cimetidine on acute experimental pancreatitis. Danish Medical Bulletin 26:13

Farias L R, Frey C F, Holcroft J W, Gunther R 1985 Effect of prostaglandin blockers on ascites fluid in pancreatitis. Surgery 98:571–578

Feller J H, Brown R A, Toussaint G P M, Thompson A G 1974 Changing methods in the treatment of severe pancreatitis. American Journal of Surgery 127:196–201

Field B E, Hepner G W, Shabot M M et al 1979 Nasogastric suction in alcoholic pancreatitis. Digestive Diseases and Sciences 24:339–344

Finch W T, Sawyer J L, Schenker S 1976 A prospective study to determine the efficacy of antibiotics in acute pancreatitis. Annals of Surgery 183:667–670

Foster P D, Ziffren S E 1962 Severe acute pancreatitis. Archives of Surgery 85:252–259

Freise J, Schmidt F W, Magerstedt P, Schmid K 1985 Gabexelate mesilate and camostate: new inhibitors of phospholipase A_2 and their influence on the α-amylase activity in serum of patients with acute pancreatitis. Clinical Biochemistry 18:224–229

Fried G M, Ogden W D, Rhea A, Greely G, Thompson J C 1982 Pancreatic protein secretion and gastrointestinal hormone release in response to parenteral amino acids and lipids in dogs. Surgery 92:905–905

Fuller R K, Loveland J P, Frankel M H 1981 An evaluation of the efficacy of nasogastric suction treatment in alcoholic pancreatitis. American Journal of Gastroenterology 75:349–353

Gabryelewicz A, Niewiarowski S 1968 Activation of blood clotting and inhibition of fibrinolysis in acute pancreatitis. Thrombosis et Diathesis Haemorrhagica 20:409–411

Gauthier A, Gillet M, Di Costanzo J, Camelot G, Maurin P, Sarles H 1978 Étude controlée multicentrique de l'aprotinine et du glucagon dans le traitement des pancréatitis aigues. Gastroenterologie Clinique et Biologique 2:777–784

Gebhardt C, Gall F P 1981 Importance of peritoneal irrigation after surgical treatment of hemorrhagic, necrotizing pancreatitis. World Journal of Surgery 5:379–385

Geokas M C, Rinderknecht H, Brodrick J W, Largman C 1978 Studies on the ascites fluid of acute pancreatitis in man. American Journal of Digestive Diseases 23:182–188

Gjessing J 1967 Peritoneal dialysis in severe acute hemorrhagic pancreatitis. Acta Chirurgica Scandinavica 133:645–647

Gjone E, Ofstad E, Marton P F, Amundsen E 1967 Experimental acute pancreatitis. Scandinavian Journal of Gastroenterology 2:181

Gliedman M L, Bolooki H, Rosenn R G 1970 Acute pancreatitis. Current Problems In Surgery. Year Book Medical Publishers, Chicago, p 1–52

Goebell H, Ammann R, Herfarth C et al 1979 A double-blind trial of synthetic salmon calcitonin in the treatment of acute pancreatitis. Scandinavian Journal of Gastroenterology 14:881–889

Goff J S, Feinberg L E, Brugge W R 1982 A randomized trial comparing cimetidine to nasogastric suction in acute pancreatitis. Digestive Diseases and Sciences 27:1085–1088

Goodgame J T, Fischer J E 1977 Parenteral nutrition in the treatment of acute pancreatitis: effect on complications and mortality. Annals of Surgery 186:651–658

Goodhead B 1969 Vascular factors in the pathogenesis of acute hemorrhagic pancreatitis. Annals of the Royal College of Surgeons of England 45:80–97

Goodhead B, Wright P W 1969 The effect of postganglionic sympathectomy on the development of hemorrhagic pancreatitis in the dog. Annals of Surgery 170:951–960

Greenburg A G, Terlizzi L, Peskin G W 1977 Oxyhemoglobin affinity in acute pancreatitis. Journal of Surgical Research 22:561

Hadas N, Wapnick S, Grosberg S J, Sugaar S 1979 Cimetidine induced mortality in experimental pancreatitis. Gastroenterology 76:1148

Hallberg D, Theve N O 1974 Observations during treatment of acute pancreatitis with insulin and glucose infusion. Acta Chirurgica Scandinavica 140:138–142

Hoffman H L, Jacobs J, Freedlander S O 1953 Use of crystalline soybean trypsin inhibitor in acute hemorrhagic pancreatitis in dogs. Archives of Surgery 66:617–623

Howard J M, Jordan G L 1960 Surgical Diseases of the Pancreas. J B Lippincott, Philadelphia, p 92–202

Howes R, Zuidema G D, Cameron J L 1975 Evaluation of prophylactic antibiotics in acute pancreatitis. Journal of Surgical Research 18:197–200

Hudvagner S, Gecser G, Tekeres M, Illenyi L 1984 Fotorafur therapy in acute pancreatitis. Acta Physiologica Hungarica 64:485–488

Hureau J, Forlot P, Raby C, Vairel E 1968 Évidence de la présence de trypsine dans le sang périphérique au cours des pancréatites aigues hemorragiques. Revue Français des Études Cliniques et Biologiques 13:80–82

Ihse I, Evander A, Holmberg J T, Gustafson I 1986 Influence of peritoneal lavage on objective prognostic signs in acute pancreatitis. Annals of Surgery 204:122–127

Imrie O W, Allam B F, Ferguson J C 1976 Hypocalcemia of acute pancreatitis: the effect of hypoalbuminemia. Current Medical Research and Opinion 4:101–115

Imrie O W, Ferguson J C, Murphy D, Blumgart L H 1977 Arterial hypoxia in acute pancreatitis. British Journal of Surgery 64:185–188

Imrie O W, Benjamin I S, Ferguson J C et al 1978 A single-centre double-blind trial of Trasylol therapy in primary acute pancreatitis. British Journal of Surgery 65:335–341

Johnson R M, Barone R M, Newson B L, Das Dupta T K, Nyhus L M 1973 Treatment of experimental acute pancreatitis with 5-fluorouracil (5-FU). American Journal of Surgery 125:211–222

Jones P A, Hermon-Taylor J, Grant D A W 1982 Antiproteinase chemotherapy of acute experimental pancreatitis using the low molecular weight oligopeptide aldehyde leupeptin. Gut 23:939–943

Kelly T R, Bratcher E P, Falor W H 1953 Trypsin inhibitor in acute hemorrhagic pancreatitis in dogs. Archives of Surgery 66:317–321

Kimura T, Zuidema G D, Cameron J L 1980 Acute pancreatitis. Experimental evaluation of steroid, albumin and trasylol therapy. American Journal of Surgery 140:403–408

Knight M J, Condon J R, Smith R 1971 Possible use of glucagon in the treatment of acute pancreatitis. British Medical Journal 2: 440

Knight M J, Condon J R, Day J L 1972 Possible role of glucagon in pathogenesis of acute pancreatitis. Lancet i:1097–1099

Konttinen Y P 1971 Epsilon-aminocaproic acid in treatment of acute pancreatitis. Scandinavian Journal of Gastroenterology 6:715–718

Konturek S J, Tasler J, Cieszkowski M, Jaworek J, Konturek J 1979 Intravenous amino acids and fat stimulate pancreatic secretion. American Journal of Physiology 236:E678–E684

Kune G A 1968 The challenge of severe acute pancreatitis. Medical Journal of Australia 2:8–12

Lange P, Pedersen T 1983 Initial treatment of acute pancreatitis. Surgery, Gynecology and Obstetrics 157:332–334

Lankisch P G, Winkler K, Bokermann M, Schmidt H, Creutzfeldt W 1974 The influence of glucagon on acute experimental pancreatitis in the rat. Scandinavian Journal of Gastroenterology 9:725–729

Lankisch P G, Koop H, Winckler K, Folsch U R, Creutzfeldt W 1977 Somatostatin therapy of acute experimental pancreatitis. Gut 18:713–716

Lankisch P G, Koop H, Winckler K, Kunze H, Vogt W 1978 Indomethacin treatment of acute experimental pancreatitis in the rat. Scandinavian Journal of Gastroenterology 13:629–633

Lankisch P G, Koop H, Winckler K, Schmidt H 1979 Continuous peritoneal dialysis as treatment of acute experimental pancreatitis in the rat. I. Effect on length and rate of survival. Digestive Diseases and Sciences 24:111–115

Larvin M, Lansdown M R J, McMahon M J, Chalmers A G, Turney J H, Brownjohn A M 1988 Plasmapheresis: a rational treatment for fulminant acute pancreatitis? British Medical Journal 297:593–594

Lasson A, Ohlsson K 1984 Peritoneal lavage in severe acute pancreatitis. Scandinavian Journal of Gastroenterology 19 (Suppl 99):6

Levant J A, Secrisr D M, Resin H, Studevant R A L, Guth P H 1974

Nasogastric suction in the treatment of alcoholic pancreatitis. Journal of the American Medical Association 229:51–52

Lium R, Maddock S 1948 Etiology of acute pancreatitis. Surgery 24:593–604

Loiudice T A, Lang J, Mehta H, Banta L 1984 Treatment of acute alcoholic pancreatitis: the roles of cimetidine and nasogastric suction. American Journal of Gastroenterology 89:553–558

Mallet-Guy P, Bosser C, Michoulier J, Topis D 1961 Antienzymes en pancréatite aigue. Lyon Chirurgical 57:801–824

Manabe T, Steer M L 1980 Protective effects of PGE$_2$ on diet induced-acute pancreatitis in mice. Gastroenterology Mann N S 1980 Experimental acute pancreatitis in rats: protective effect of cycloheximide. Gastroenterology 78:1215

Mann S K, Mann N S 1979 Effect of chlorophyll-A, fluorouracil, and pituitrin on experimental acute pancreatitis. Archives of Pathology and Laboratory Medicine 103:79–81

Mann N S, Mauch M J, Barnett R 1980 Intraductal somatostatin protects against experimentally induced pancreatitis. Gastroenterology 78:1216

Masson R R 1974 Acute pancreatitis secondary to iatrogenic hypercalcemia. Annals of Surgery 108: 213–219

Mayer D A, McMahon M J, Corfield A P et al 1985 Controlled clinical trial of peritoneal lavage for the treatment of severe acute pancreatitis. New England Journal of Medicine 312:399–404

Meshkinpour H, Molinari M-D, Gardner L, Berk J E, Hoehler F K 1979 Cimetidine in the treatment of acute alcoholic pancreatitis. Gastroenterology 77:687–690

Moreau L, Bommelaer L, Buscail A et al 1976 Preliminary results of a multicentric double blind trial of somatostatin (S) vs placebo (P) in acute pancreatitis (AP). Digestive Diseases and Sciences 31:24S

Naeije R, Salingret E, Clumeck N, De Troyer A, Devis G 1978 Is nasogastric suction necessary in acute pancreatitis? British Medical Journal 2:659–660

Nakashima Y, Appert H E, Howard J M 1977 The effects of calcitonin on pancreatic exocrine secretion in dogs. Surgery, Gynecology and Obstetrics 144:71–76

Nath B J, Warshaw A L 1982 Pulmonary insufficiency. In: Bradley E L (ed). Complications of pancreatitis. W B Suanders, Philadelphia, p 51–71

Neoptolemos J P, London N J, James D, Carr-Locke D L, Bailey I A, Fossard D P 1988 Controlled trial of urgent endoscopic retrograde cholangiopancreatography and endoscopic sphincterotomy versus conservative treatment for acute pancreatitis due to gallstones. Lancet 2: 979–983

Olazabal A, Nasciemento L 1980 Effect of prostoglandin (PG) inhibition on dexycolic acid (DOC) induced pancreatitis (P) in the rat. Gastroenterology 78:1230

Olsen H 1974 Pancreatitis. American Journal of Digestive Diseases 19:1077–1090

Ohlsson K 1971 Experimental pancreatitis in the dog. Appearance of complexes between proteases and trypsin inhibitors in ascitic fluid, lymph, and plasma. Experimental Pancreatitis 645–652

Paul F, Ohnhaus E E, Hesch R D et al 1979 Einfluss von Salm-Calcitonin auf den Verlauf der akuten pancreatitis. Deutsche medizinische Wochenschrift 104:615–622

Pissiotis C A, Condon R E, Nyhus L M 1972 Effect of vasopressin on pancreatic blood flow in acute hemorrhagic pancreatitis. American Journal of Surgery 123:203–207

Popper H L, Necheles H, Russell K C 1948 Transition of pancreatic edema into pancreatic necrosis. Surgery, Gynecology and Obstetrics 87:79

Ranson J H C, Roses D F, Fink S D 1973 Early respiratory insufficiency in acute pancreatitis. Annals of Surgery 178:75–79

Ranson J H C, Berman I R 1990 Long peritoneal lavage decreases pancreatic sepsis in acute pancreatitis. Annals of Surgery 211:708–716

Ranson J H C, Lackner H 1982 Coagulopathies. In: Bradley E L (ed) Complications of pancreatitis. W B Saunders, Philadelphia, p 154–175

Ranson J H C, Spencer F C 1977 Prevention, diagnosis and treatment of pancreatic abscess. Surgery 82:99–106

Ranson J H C, Spencer F C 1978 The role of peritoneal lavage in severe acute pancreatitis. Annals of Surgery 187:565–576

Ranson J H C, Turner J W, Roses D F, Rifkind K M, Spencer F C 1974 Respiratory complications in acute pancreatitis. Annals of Surgery 179:557–565

Ranson J H C, Rifkind K M, Turner J W 1976 Prognostic signs and non-operative peritoneal lavage in acute pancreatitis. Surgery Gynecology and Obstetrics 143:209–219

Ranson J H C, Lackner H, Berman I R, Schinella R 1977 The relationship of coagulation factors to clinical complications of acute pancreatitis. Surgery 81:502–511

Raptis S, Schlegel W, Lehmann E, Dollinger H C, Zoupas C 1978 Effects of somatostatin on the exocrine pancreas and the release of duodenal hormones. Metabolism 27 (Suppl 1):1321–1328

Rasmussen B L 1967 Hypothermic peritoneal dialysis in the treatment of acute experimental hemorrhagic pancreatitis. American Journal of Surgery 114:716–720

Reid L C, Paulette R E, Challis T W, Hinton J W 1958 The mechanism of the pathogenesis of pancreatic necrosis and the therapeutic effect of propylthiouracil. Surgery 43:538–549

Reynaert M S, Bshouty Z H, Otte J B, Kestens P J, Tremouroux J 1985 Percutaneous peritoneal dialysis as an early treatment of acute necrotic hemorrhagic pancreatitis. Intensive Care Medicine 11: 123–128

Rich A R, Duff G L 1936 Experimental and pathological studies on the pathogenesis of acute haemorrhagic pancreatitis. Johns Hopkins Bulletin 58:212–258

Rittenbury M S, Hanback L D 1969 Snake antivenom. Archives of Surgery 99:179–184

Rogers R E, Carey L C 1966 Peritoneal lavage in experimental pancreatitis in dogs. American Journal of Surgery 111:792–794

Rosato E F, Chu W H, Mullen J L, Rosato F 1972 Peritoneal lavage treatment of experimental pancreatitis. Journal of Surgical Research 12:138–140

Rosato E F, Mullis W F, Rosato F E 1973 Peritoneal lavage therapy in hemorrhagic pancreatitis. Surgery 74:106–115

Rossi T C, Pissiotis C A, Taube R R, Condon R E 1974 Hemodynamic and metabolic effects of glucagon in acute hemorrhagic pancreatitis. European Surgical Research 6:209–218

Rush B, Clifton E E 1952 The role of trypsin in the pathogenesis of acute hemorrhagic pancreatitis and the effect of antitryptic agent in treatment. Surgery 31:349–360

Saario I A 1983 5-Fluorouracil in the treatment of acute pancreatitis. American Journal of Surgery 145:349–352

Safrany L, Cotton P B 1981 A preliminary report: urgent duodenoscopic sphincterotomy for acute gallstone pancreatitis. Surgery 89:424–428

Sarr M G, Sanfey H, Cameron J L 1986 Prospective, randomized trial of nasogastric suction in patients with acute pancreatitis. Surgery 100:500–504

Satake K, Koh I, Nishiwaki H, Umeyama K, 1985 Toxic products in hemorrhagic ascitic fluid generated during experimental acute hemorrhagic pancreatitis in dogs and a treatment which reduces their effect. Digestion 32:99–105

Sax H C, Warner B W, Talamini M A et al 1987 Early total parenteral nutrition in acute pancreatitis: lack of beneficial effects. American Journal of Surgery 153:117–124

Schroeder T, Kinnunen P K J, Lempinen M 1978 Xylocaine treatment in experimental pancreatitis in pigs. Scandinavian Journal of Gastroenterology 13:863–865

Schutt A J, Wakim K G, Bartholomew L G et al 1965 Acute experimental pancreatitis – role of proteolytic enzyme inhibitor in treatment. Journal of the American Medical Association 191:905–913

Schwedes U, Althoff P H, Klempa I et al 1979 Effect of somatostatin on bile-induced acute hemorrhagic pancreatitis in the dog. Hormone and Metabolic Research 11:655–661

Silberman H, Dixon N P, Eisenberg D 1982 The safety and efficacy of a lipid-based system of parenteral nutrition in acute pancreatitis. American Journal of Gastroenterology 77:494–497

Simmons R L, Collins J A, Heisterkamp C A et al 1969 Coagulation disorders in combat casualties: I. Acute changes after wounding.

II. Effects of massive transfusion. III. Post-resuscitative changes. Annals of Surgery 169:455–482

Skyring A, Singer A, Tornya P 1965 Treatment of acute pancreatitis with Trasylol: report of a controlled therapeutic trial. British Medical Journal 2:627–629

Stefanini P, Erminii M, Carboni M 1965 Diagnosis and management of acute pancreatitis. American Journal of Surgery 110:866–874

Steinberg W M, Schlessman S E 1987 Treatment of acute pancreatitis. Gastroenterology 93:1420–1427

Stone H H, Fabian T C 1980 Peritoneal dialysis in the treatment of acute alcoholic pancreatitis. Surgery, Gynecology and Obstetrics 150:878–882

Studley J G N, Schenk W G 1982 Pathophysiology of acute pancreatitis. Evaluation of the effect and mode of action of steroids in experimental pancreatitis in dogs. American Journal of Surgery 143:761–864

Susini C, Esteve J P, Vaysse N, Pradayrol L, Ribert A 1980 Somatostatin 28: effects on exocrine pancreatic secretion in conscious dogs. Gastroenterology 79:720–724

Switz D M, Vlahcevic Z R, Farrar J T 1975 The effect of anticholinergic and/or nasogastric suction on the outcome of acute alcoholic pancreatitis. Gastroenterology 68:974

Teerenhovi O, Nordback I, Eskola J 1989 High volume lesser sac lavage in acute necrotizing pancreatitis. British Journal of Surgery 76:370–373

Thal A P, Perry J F, Egner W 1957 A clinical and morphologic study of 42 cases of fatal acute pancreatitis. Surgery, Gynecology and Obstetrics 105:191–202

Tountas C, Kiriakou K, Marselos A, Carapistolis E 1966 Local intra-arterial infusion of antienzymes in the treatment of acute pancreatitis. Surgery 60:1235–1241

Trapnell J E 1966 The natural history and prognosis of acute pancreatitis. Annals of the Royal College of Surgeons 38:265–287

Trapnell J E, Rigby C C, Talbot C H, Duncan E H L 1974 A controlled trial of Trasylol in the treatment of acute pancreatitis. British Journal of Surgery 61:177–182

Tykka H T, Vaittinen E J, Mahlberg K L et al 1985 A randomized double-blind study using CaNa$_2$ EDTA, a phospholipase A$_2$ inhibitor, in the management of human acute pancreatitis. Scandinavian Journal of Gastroenterology 20:5–12

Usadell K-H, Leuschner U, Uberla K K 1980 Treatment of acute pancreatitis with somatostatin; a multicentre double-blind trial. New England Journal of Medicine 303:999

Van Gossum A, Lemoyne M, Greig P D, Jeejeebhoy K 1988 Lipid-associated total parenteral nutrition in patients with severe acute pancreatitis. Journal of Parenteral and Enteral nutrition 12:250–255

Wachtfeidl V, Vitez M 1968 X-ray therapy for acute pancreatitis. American Journal of Surgery 116:853–867

Wall A J 1965 Peritoneal dialysis in the treatment of severe acute pancreatitis. Medical Journal of Australia 2:281–283

Wangensteen O H, Leven N L, Manson M H 1931 Acute pancreatitis (pancreatic necrosis). An experimental and clinical study with special reference to the significance of the biliary tract factor. Archives of Surgery 23:47–73

Waterworth M W, Barbezat G O, Hickman R, Terblanche J 1976 A controlled trial of glucagon in experimental pancreatitis. British Journal of Surgery 63:617–620

White T T 1966 Pancreatitis. Williams and Wilkins, Baltimore, p 1–19

Williams L F, Byrne J J 1968 The role of bacteria in hemorrhagic pancreatitis. Surgery 64:967–972

Wills M R 1966 Hypocalcaemia and hypomagnesaemia in acute pancreatitis. British Journal of Surgery 53:174–176

Wright P W, Goodhead B 1970 Prevention of hemorrhagic pancreatitis with fibrinolysin or heparin. Archives of Surgery 100:42–46

Yang C H, Chang-Chien C-S, Liaw Y-F 1987 Controlled trial of protease inhibitor gabexelate mesilate (FOY) in the treatment of acute pancreatitis. Pancreas 2:698–700

Zimberg Y H 1968 Pancreatitis: principles of management. Surgical Clinics of North America 48:889–905

21. Special aspects of gallstone pancreatitis

D. C. Carter

INTRODUCTION

The first description of the association between gallstones and acute pancreatitis is variously attributed to Bernard (1856, quoted by Kirchner et al 1990) or Prince (1882) who reported impaction of a gallstone in a common channel just distal to the point of entry of the pancreatic duct. In 1901, Opie also described impaction of a stone in a common channel in a patient with acute pancreatitis who died after surgery (Opie 1901a, b). Since then the role of gallstones as an aetiological factor in acute pancreatitis has been recognized increasingly, although the nature of the mechanism responsible remains controversial. Acute pancreatitis occurs in only some 3–7% of patients with gallstones (Ranson 1979, Moreau et al 1988) but gallstones accounted for between 3 and 63% of cases of acute pancreatitis in series reported in the decade up to 1980 (Ranson 1983). In Ranson's review (Ranson 1983) gallstones were implicated in 27% of the total of 5019 patients with acute pancreatitis. In a study involving residents of Rochester, Minnesota who were known to have gallstones in the period 1950–1970, the relative risk of developing acute pancreatitis was increased by 14– 35-fold in men and by 12– 25-fold in women (Moreau et al 1988). Cholecystectomy in patients who had not had pancreatitis reduced relative risk to 1.9 and 2.0 in men and women respectively.

The relative importance of gallstones in acute pancreatitis varies from country to country and within a given country it is influenced by socioeconomic, ethnic and cultural factors in the patient population under review. In general there is an inverse relationship between alcohol and gallstones as aetiological factors (Fig. 21.1). In some reports based on inner city North American hospitals, alcohol accounts for some 70–92% of cases of pancreatitis whereas gallstones account for only 3–16% (Howes et al 1975, Ranson & Spencer 1978, Satiani & Stone 1979). In the United Kingdom, alcohol has been a less common cause of acute pancreatitis, accounting for 8–33% of cases (Blamey et al 1983a, b, Corfield et al 1985, Mayer & McMahon 1985),

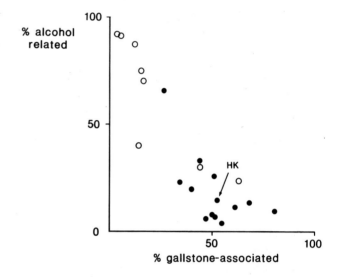

Fig. 21.1 Proportion of cases of acute pancreatitis associated with alcohol and gallstones in series reported from American (○) or European (●) centres. A series reported from Hong Kong (HK) is marked with an arrow.

with gallstones accounting for some 40–50% of cases (Blamey et al 1983a, b, Corfield et al 1985). In Scandinavia, gallstones used to account for some two-thirds of all cases of acute pancreatitis, but some 58–68% of cases are now attributed to alcohol (Svensson et al 1979, Mero 1982). As will be discussed, it is probable that all of these figures underestimate the importance of gallstones in that some patients labelled as having idiopathic pancreatitis, may well have passed small calculi which escape detection on routine evaluation. It should also be borne in mind that in the vast majority of cases, gallstones are responsible for the so-called pancreatitis of pregnancy (McKay et al 1980).

The age and sex distribution of patients with gallstone pancreatitis parallels that of patients with gallstones, and in contrast to alcoholic pancreatitis there is a preponderance of females and older patients (Durr 1979). In a large review from Bristol, the female:male ratio was 60:40 with mortality rates of 10% and 17% respectively (Corfield et al 1985). Patients with stones impacted at the ampulla of Vater had a much higher mortality rate (71%) than those with mobile stones (11%), and the mortality of recurrent attacks was not significantly lower than that of the first attack (Corfield et al 1985). Overall mortality rates for acute gallstone pancreatitis still ranged recently from 8–13% (Imrie & Whyte, 1975, Corfield et al 1985, Fielding et al 1989, Windsor 1990). In our own study of fatal acute pancreatitis, gallstones were implicated in no less than 39 (30%) of 132 deaths and in one-third of these patients the diagnosis of pancreatitis was made for the first time at autopsy (see Table 19.1, p. 194). Similarly, Corfield et al (1985) found that just over one-third of patients dying with acute pancreatitis did not have the diagnosis made in life. In the review of 667 fatal cases of acute pancreatitis reported by Ivy and Gibbs (1952) gallstones were present in 55%, while Bell (1958) found that gallstones were the aetiological factor leading to lethal acute pancreatitis in one-third of men over 40 and in one-half of women, irrespective of age.

It is clear that we cannot be complacent about our ability to diagnose and manage acute gallstone pancreatitis and a high index of suspicion must be exercised, particularly when assessing elderly patients, many of whom present atypically and in wards other than general surgical wards. It is important to emphasize that overlooked or neglected gallstones accounted for no less than 51% of the recurrent attacks of acute pancreatitis in Bristol (Corfield et al 1985), and every effort must be made to avoid unnecessary suffering and mortality by eradicating gallstones when the patient first presents with acute pancreatitis. The success of this policy is attested by studies such as that reported from Rochester, Minnesota where 58 patients who had undergone cholecystectomy after an attack of pancreatitis were followed for a median of 15 years; only two developed a further attack of pancreatitis and in both cases this was unrelated to gallstones (Moreau et al 1988).

PATHOGENESIS OF GALLSTONE PANCREATITIS

Opie's description of gallstone pancreatitis in a patient with a stone acting as a ball-valve obstruction in a common channel (Opie 1901a) led to the proposal that reflux of bile into the pancreatic duct might be the initiating event in acute pancreatitis. Before this theory of pathogenesis can be accepted, three critical issues must be addressed:

1. Is there a common channel for the termination of the common duct and main pancreatic duct in patients who develop gallstone pancreatitis?
2. Is impaction of a gallstone in the ampullary region a feature of gallstone pancreatitis?

3. Does impaction promote reflux of bile into the pancreatic duct and, equally important, does such reflux trigger the development of acute pancreatitis?

Each of these issues will be addressed separately.

Incidence of a common channel

Opie (1901b) using formalin-fixed autopsy material found a common channel ranging in length from 1–11 mm in 89 of 100 individuals, an incidence which was confirmed by subsequent studies employing beeswax injection or contrast radiology (Newman et al 1958, Hand 1963). Osborne (1982) using contrast radiology and an operating microscope found a common channel in 64% of unselected autopsies; interestingly less than 10% of individuals showed any dilatation of the channel, calling into question the validity of the term 'ampulla of Vater'. In studies based on findings at operative cholangiography, Armstrong et al (1985) compared 59 patients with acute gallstone pancreatitis with 710 patients undergoing cholecystectomy who had no history of pancreatic disease. Reflux into the pancreatic duct was seen more frequently in pancreatitis patients (see below) and such individuals had a wider pancreatic duct and a common channel which was on average twice as long as in non-pancreatitis patients. A common channel of 5 mm or longer was identified in 73% of pancreatitis patients as opposed to 20% of 'control' patients. The length of the common channel also exceeded the diameter of the smallest stone (so allowing the possibility of bile reflux into the pancreatic duct), in 30% of patients with gallstone pancreatitis as opposed to 14% of those without pancreatitis. The fact that a common channel was not present in all gallstone pancreatitis patients indicates that additional factors may be involved, or that operative cholangiography may be an insensitive method of detection, or that the common channel may be present transiently only during gallstone impaction. Kelly (1984) also found a common channel with bile reflux on cholangiography in 67% of patients with acute gallstone pancreatitis as opposed to 18% of patients with gallstones but no pancreatitis.

Thus, there is good evidence that the majority of individuals do have a common channel, and that this is longer and more frequently associated with bile reflux into the pancreatic duct in those with gallstones who have had an attack of acute pancreatitis.

Impaction of gallstones (See Fig. 21.2)

The theory that impaction of a gallstone in the distal common bile duct might cause acute pancreatitis was initially called into question when autopsy in patients dying from gallstone pancreatitis frequently failed to reveal an impacted stone. However, it is now apparent that *transient* impaction may be sufficient to trigger pancreatitis and that the offending stone may then migrate into the gastro-

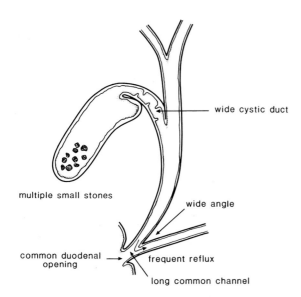

Fig. 21.2 Summary of anatomical and other abnormalities predisposing to the development of acute gallstone pancreatitis.

intestinal tract. In support of this contention, Acosta and Ledesma (1974) recovered stones from the faeces in 34 of 36 (94%) of patients with gallstone pancreatitis in the 5 days following the attack whereas stones were retrieved in only 3 of 36 (8%) of control patients with no attacks of pancreatitis. Furthermore, the finding of stones in pancreatitis patients was usually preceded by relief of symptoms and a rapid fall in serum amylase levels. The stones recovered ranged in diameter from 1–12 mm and were ultimately shown to have the same chemical composition as stones recovered from the gallbladder at cholecystectomy. In a subsequent study, Acosta et al (1980) showed that the frequency with which stones are found impacted in the distal bile duct in acute pancreatitis depends on the timing of biliary surgery; if operation is undertaken within 48 hours of the onset of pancreatitis stones will be found impacted in 75% of cases whereas if surgery is delayed beyond 4 days the figure falls to 25%. Gallstone migration in acute gallstone pancreatitis has also been confirmed by Kelly (1976) who recovered stones from the faeces in 84% of 45 pancreatitis patients as opposed to 11% of patients with gallstones but no pancreatitis.

The transient nature of the impaction in the majority of patients with gallstone pancreatitis must be emphasized. As indicated above, the offending stone has usually passed on by the time the patients come to biliary surgery. In a review of some 1450 collected cases, Goebell & Hotz (1979) found stones in the gallbladder alone in 72%, in the common bile duct in 20%, and impacted in the distal bile duct in only 2%. In our own experience, operative cholangiography revealed that the diameter of the common bile duct was often increased in patients who have had gallstone pancreatitis, regardless of whether stones

were still present in the duct at the time of cholecystectomy (Osborne et al 1983). Conversely, gallstone patients who had never had pancreatitis tended to show significant ductal enlargement only when stones were still present.

As might be expected, patients who have had gallstone pancreatitis often have *small* stones in the biliary system at the time of surgery. Taylor & Armstrong (1987) showed that gallbladder stones in pancreatitis patients could be passed through the cystic duct in 67% of cases whereas passage was possible in only 3% of patients who had not experienced pancreatitis. Furthermore, the diameter of the cystic duct was greater in patients with pancreatitis than in those without. Even very small stones i.e. less than 2–3 mm in diameter have been implicated in the pathogenesis of gallstone pancreatitis and there is some evidence that they may frequently give rise to severe necrotizing forms of the disease (Farinon et al 1987, Negro et al 1984). Such small stones and crystal microaggregates may escape detection on ultrasonography or cholecystography but can be identified by microscopic analysis of bile recovered at operation, endoscopy or duodenal intubation (Freund et al 1976). The importance of 'biliary sludge' as a cause of acute pancreatitis has been highlighted recently in a study of 31 patients thought to have idiopathic acute pancreatitis and in whom gallstones or biliary duct dilatation were not present on ultrasonography (Lee et al 1992). Samples of bile recovered from the duodenum at endoscopic retrograde cholangiopancreatography (ERCP) or on duodenal intubation showed microscopic evidence of sludge, in the form of suspension of precipitates of cholesterol monohydrate crystals or calcium bilirubinate granules, in 23 of the 31 patients, but this was detected ultrasonographically in the gallbladder in only 11 of the 23 (48%). In the 21 of the 23 patients in whom biliary sludge was the only finding (two also had dilated bile ducts), the six treated by cholecystectomy and the four treated by papillotomy had fewer recurrent attacks of pancreatitis than the 11 untreated patients (Tables 21.1, 21.2). It appears that

Table 21.1 Detection of biliary sludge in patients with idiopathic acute pancreatitis (Lee et al 1992)

Cases	Proportion of total (%)
Idiopathic acute pancreatitis	31/86 (36%)
Microscopic biliary sludge	23/31 (74%)
Sludge detected on ultrasonography	11/23 (48%)

Table 21.2 Recurrent acute pancreatitis after treatment of biliary sludge (Lee et al 1992)

Treatment of sludge	n	Patients with recurrent attacks of acute pancreatitis
Cholecystectomy	6	0
Endoscopic papillotomy	4	1
No treatment	11	8

biliary sludge is an underestimated cause of acute idiopathic pancreatitis and that it may have important therapeutic implications.

Thus there is good evidence that impaction of gallstones in the distal common bile duct is implicated in the pathogenesis of gallstone pancreatitis. Such stones are frequently small and in the majority of cases they impact transiently before migrating into the intestine. Even the microscopic particles found in biliary sludge may be capable of causing acute pancreatitis.

Reflux of bile

As indicated earlier, reflux of bile into the pancreatic duct systems is frequently observed at operative cholangiography in patients who have had gallstone pancreatitis. Armstrong & Taylor (1986) found reflux in 63% of such patients but in only 15% of those with no history of pancreatic disease, findings remarkably similar to those of other authors (Cuschieri & Hughes 1973, Kelly 1980, Mayer & McMahon 1983, Osborne et al 1983). However, it can be argued that reflux demonstrated on operative cholangiography may have little pathophysiological relevance given the injection pressures involved. A further problem relates to the fact that not all patients with gallstone pancreatitis appear to have a common channel on operative cholangiography (see above). Furthermore, even if bile does reflux it has but a weak capacity to activative pancreatic zymogens, although infected bile may cause more rapid enzymic activation.

The effect of bile and its constituents on the integrity of the pancreatic duct has been studied extensively in animal models. Robinson & Dunphy (1963), using goats, and Elmslie et al (1966), using dogs, found that the contents of the common bile duct could reflux into the pancreatic duct under physiological pressures without producing ill effects. Konok & Thompson (1969) used a cat model for such studies, emphasizing that this animal normally has a terminal common pancreaticobiliary channel, a sterile biliary tree and pancreatic ducts, and parenchyma histologically similar to those of man. At low infusion pressures, the cat pancreatic duct proved remarkably resistant to bile, activated pancreatic enzymes and bacteria; on the other hand, bile infected with *Escherichia coli* showed marked mucolytic and cytotoxic effects, damaged mucosal permeability and initiated in vivo activation of trypsinogen (as evidenced by the presence of free trypsin in the gland parenchyma).

Reber & Mosley (1980) working with the same model also found that sterile cat bile did not damage the permeability of the pancreatic duct whereas infected bile did. In subsequent studies, exposure of the pancreatic duct to individual bile salts at physiological pressures was found to render the duct permeable to molecules as large as 20 000 Da, the effect being more marked after perfusion with higher but still physiological concentrations of bile salt (Farmer et al 1984). The changes in permeability were accompanied by marked morphological changes in the duct including disruption of tight junctions, swelling of intercellular spaces and epithelial cell loss. In our own studies in this model (Simpson et al 1983), increasing luminal pressure to 30 cmH_2O markedly potentiated the ability of physiological concentrations of bile salt to increase mucosal permeability and cause epithelial damage.

Armstrong et al (1985) have performed comparable studies in a rat model. Perfusion of the pancreatic duct with a bacterial solution of *Esch. coli* had little effect on mucosal permeability or ultrastructure. Sterile human bile increased ionic permeability and caused reversible ultrastructural changes, particularly when infused at higher pressure (35 cmH_2O). However, infected human bile under high or low infusion pressure was by far the most toxic substance tested, leading to irreversible duct damage and complete loss of integrity. It is estimated that some 25–50% patients with chronic cholelithiasis and 75–100% with acute cholelithiasis have bacterial colonization of the bile (Frey 1981) and so reflux of infected bile could well be implicated in the pathogenesis of gallstone pancreatitis.

The exact agent(s) responsible for pancreatic ductal damage remains uncertain. Deconjugation of bile acids by bacteria may increase their cytotoxic potential in that deconjugated bile acids have a higher pK_a than their conjugated counterparts; this could result in an increase in the fraction of the bile acid that is unionized and so capable of absorption into the duct epithelial cells. Bile salts could also promote activation of phospholipase A_2, an enzyme capable of converting lecithin to the highly cytotoxic lysolecithin. It is also conceivable that it is reflux of duodenal juice (rather than bile) which is the initiating factor in gallstone pancreatitis. Duodenal contents certainly contain high concentrations of the brush border enzyme, enterokinase, and could readily cause activation of pancreatic zymogens. The contents of the upper small intestine normally contain some 1000 organisms/ml opening the possibility of further damage to the pancreatic duct lining.

Thus there is evidence that some constituents of bile, particularly in the presence of infection, may be injurious to the pancreatic duct system. Bile reflux during transient impaction of a gallstone at the lower end of the bile duct is almost certainly implicated in the pathogenesis of pancreatitis in patients with a common channel. Whether duodenal reflux is also implicated is more controversial. While reflux of bacteria and enterokinase offers a seductive explanation for zymogen activation and duct injury, the fact remains that destruction of the sphincter mechanism by endoscopic sphincterotomy is now regarded as beneficial in some patients with gallstone pancreatitis (see below). Sphincterotomy has also been used widely to treat patients with choledocholithiasis who have never had pancreatitis, and has not been incriminated as a cause of pancreatitis in the long term. Furthermore, it seems likely that migration of a gallstone into the duodenum might be followed by transient incompetence of the sphincter of Oddi and duodenal reflux, yet such migration is thought to lead to resolution rather than aggravation of the pancreatic inflammation.

Occlusion of the pancreatic duct. In addition to reflux of bile or duodenal juice, one more factor deserves consideration, namely that a stone impacted in the lower common bile duct might occlude the pancreatic duct regardless of the presence of a common channel. Obstruction of the pancreatic duct by agencies such as neoplasia, parasites and strictures is a recognized cause of 'obstructive' pancreatitis (Warshaw 1989), and in the isolated perfused canine pancreas, partial obstruction of the duct system in conjuction with stimulation of secretion by secretin has been shown to cause acute pancreatitis (Broe & Cameron 1982).

DIAGNOSIS OF GALLSTONE PANCREATITIS

Clinical and biochemical prediction of gallstone disease

It is frequently difficult to determine whether gallstones are responsible for an attack of acute pancreatitis. In patients known to have gallstones, acute pancreatitis should be assumed to be gallstone-associated until proved otherwise, but many patients present with pancreatitis as the first manifestation of their gallstone disease and have no preceding history of biliary colic, acute cholecystitis or obstructive jaundice. It should also be remembered that gallstones and alcohol abuse are both common and that acute pancreatitis attributed initially to alcohol may turn out to be due to gallstone disease. The problem is complicated further by the possibility that some patients with gallstones and hyperamylasaemia may prove at laparotomy to have acute cholecystitis with little or no evidence of pancreatic inflammation (Ranson 1979, Mackie et al 1985).

Clinical and biochemical parameters can be used to identify patients in whom there is a strong probability that their attack of acute pancreatitis is gallstone-related. In our own retrospective analysis of 177 episodes of gallstone pancreatitis and 135 attacks of alcohol-associated disease, seven variables showed a significant association with gallstones (Blamey et al 1983, see Table 21.3). For example 82% of attacks in females were attributed to gallstones as opposed to only 31% in males; similarly 82% of attacks of pancreatitis in patients over 50 were gallstone-associated as opposed to only 28% of attacks in younger patients. As might be predicted serum bilirubin, alkaline phosphatase and aminotransferase levels were higher in gallstone pancreatitis (Table 21.3), but perhaps surprisingly, serum amylase level was also a significant discriminant. Amylase

Table 21.3 Factors of significance in distinguishing between episodes of acute pancreatitis due to gallstones and those associated with alcohol (Blamey et al 1983)

Factor	Value	Percentage with gallstone
Alkaline phosphate (i.u./l)	< 300	28*
	> 300	86
Age (years)	< 50	28*
	> 50	82
Alanine aminotransferase (i.u./l)	< 100	34*
	> 100	89
Sex	M	31*
	F	82
Asparate aminotransferase (i.u./l)	< 100	38*
	> 100	37
Amylase (u/l)	< 4000	41*
	> 4000	73
Bilirubin (μmol/l)	< 25	45*
	> 25	73

Chi-squared analysis: *$p < 0.001$

levels greater than 4000 units/1 were associated with gallstone pancreatitis in 73% of our patients whereas only 41% of attacks in patients with lower amylase levels proved to be gallstone-related.

Further analysis by stepwise logistic regression showed that only five of these seven factors had independent significance in predicting the presence of gallstones. As shown in Table 21.4, use of these five factors in a simple numerical scoring system allows immediate identification of groups of patients with differing probabilities of gallstone pancreatitis. For example, patients with four of five positive criteria had a probability of gallstone pancreatitis ranging from 95–100% whereas their probability of alcohol-related disease ranged from 0–5%. Conversely, the probability of gallstone pancreatitis was less than 5% in patients with a score of zero or one.

Although we have confirmed the validity of this system in a prospective analysis of a further group of patients (Blamey et al 1984), its value must not be overestimated. The analysis was performed to discriminate only between gallstone pancreatitis and alcohol pancreatitis and the discriminatory value of the system has yet to be defined in patients with acute pancreatitis due to other causes.

Table 21.4 Simple scoring system to distinguish gallstone pancreatitis from alcohol-associated disease (Blamey et al 1983). The five factors are drawn from those listed in Table 21.3, with the exception of asparate aminotransferase and bilirubin

Positive factors	Number of Episodes	Percentage with gallstones	Percentage alcohol-related
0	43	5	95
1	50	4	96
2	47	55	45
3	53	86	14
4	62	95	5
5	35	100	0

Furthermore, the system provides at best an estimate of the probability that gallstones are responsible for the attack, and in a substantial group of patients such as those with two positive factors, there is an almost even chance that their pancreatitis is due to causes other than gallstones.

Nevertheless, such approaches may be useful in that they allow early definition of the likelihood that gallstones are responsible for an attack of acute pancreatitis, particularly when the attack is judged to be severe and non-invasive diagnostic tests such as ultrasonography (see below) have proved equivocal. Other workers have come to a similar conclusion. For example, Neoptolemos et al (1984) found that a combination of ultrasonography and biochemical testing (serum bilirubin, gamma glutamyl-transpeptidase, alanine amino transferase) allowed the correct diagnosis of 81% of their gallstone pancreatitis patients without any false positive diagnoses. The biochemical tests alone had a sensitivity of 73% and specificity of 94% in diagnosing gallstone pancreatitis, and in nine gallstone patients with negative ultrasonography and oral cholecystography, a positive biochemical test correctly suggested the presence of stones in six cases (Goodman et al 1985). In their most recent report, this group have now compared three systems for their ability to predict the presence of gallstones in 391 attacks of acute pancreatitis (Davidson et al 1988). The simplest system, namely an aminotransferase (aspartate or alanine, AST or ALT) level in excess of 60 i.u./l detected gallstones with a sensitivity of 75% and specificity of 74%. Of interest, addition of other variables such as alkaline phosphatase and bilirubin had little effect, whereas addition of age and sex lowered the sensitivity to 62% while increasing specificity to 80%.

McMahon & Pickford (1979) have also highlighted the association between elevation of plasma aspartate aminotransferase (AST, previously known as glutamate oxalo-acetic transaminase, or GOT) levels on admission and biliary pancreatitis, provided there was no history of excessive alcohol consumption. In a more recent report, Mayer & McMahon (1985) showed that AST levels were elevated above 60 i.u./l in 84% of attacks of gallstone pancreatitis as opposed to 15% of attacks not associated with gallstones. Although some have doubted the discriminatory ability of aminotransferase levels (Damman et al 1980), it has been postulated that early transient AST rises reflect hepatocyte disruption following obstruction to the biliary tree in gallstone pancreatitis.

Although all of the positive studies referred to above were carried out in the United Kingdom, there is evidence that the approach remains valuable in other parts of the world. For example, Wang et al (1988) in Taiwan found that biochemical tests (ALT–AST ratio, bilirubin, γ-glutamyl transferase, alkaline phosphatase) performed in the first 2 days of admission gave a sensitivity of 85% in identifying gallstones as the cause of acute pancreatitis; ultrasonography had a similar sensitivity (86%) and a combination of the two increased sensitivity to 95%. In Germany, Scholmerich et al (1989) found that alanine aminotransferase (ALT, previously known as glutamyl pyrurate transaminase, or GPT) was the best biochemical predictor of the presence of gallstones in 50 patients with acute pancreatitis in that it had a positive predictive value of 53% and a negative predictive value of 94% at a cut-off value of 40 i.u./l.

Radiological diagnosis

There is general agreement that the radiological tests originally used to detect gallstones (i.e. oral cholecystography and intravenous cholangiography) are of little value in the early period following an attack of acute pancreatitis (Kaden et al 1955, Freund et al 1976). Percutaneous transhepatic cholangiography was once used to detect gallstones in patients with severe acute pancreatitis where surgery was contemplated (Coppa et al 1981) but did not become popular in this context. Early reports of scanning with radionuclides, such as ^{99m}Tc-labelled HIDA, suggested that non-visualization of the gallbladder was linked to gallstone pancreatitis (Glazer et al 1981). However, subsequent studies failed to confirm the ability of radionuclide scanning to discriminate between gallstone pancreatitis and pancreatitis due to alcohol (Neoptolemos et al 1984).

Ultrasonography has emerged as a useful investigation in patients thought to have acute pancreatitis due to gallstones. It is non-invasive, readily repeatable, and does not depend on the excretion of contrast or radionuclides by the liver. It offers a means of detecting gallstones in the gallbladder and bile ducts, allows measurement of bile duct diameter, detects inflammation of the gallbladder, and frequently provides useful information regarding pancreatic inflammation. Unfortunately, ultrasonography may be less reliable than usual in the early period following an attack of gallstone pancreatitis. Ileus and gaseous distension may prevent visualization of the biliary tree while the gallstones responsible for the attack are frequently small and easily missed, particularly as they may be located at the lower end of the common bile duct, an area not well visualized by ultrasonography. McKay et al (1982) scanned 114 patients with grey-scale ultrasonography in the first week of admission with acute pancreatitis. The gallbladder was visualized in only 70% of cases but when it was seen, ultrasonography had a 96% accuracy in gallstone detection. Similarly, Neoptolemos et al (1984) using real-time ultrasonography within 72 hours of admission in 83 patients, reported that the investigation was accurate in 92% of the 80% patients in whom the gallbladder was visualized. There were no false positive results but only 67% of the patients with gallstone pancreatitis had their gallstones detected at this stage. Schlömerich et al (1989) also reported that the investigation failed to detect stones in 10 of their 50 patients, stones which incidentally also escaped detection on CT scanning. As mentioned earlier, ultrasonography had a sensitivity of 86% in gallstone detection when used in Taiwan, a sensitivity far better than the value of 53% reported for CT scanning (Wang et al 1988).

Thus it is well recognized that ultrasonography may fail to reveal gallstones in the critical early period after admission to hospital with acute pancreatitis. With clinical improvement the rate of diagnosis of gallstones rose from 67% to 78% in Leicester (Neoptolemos et al 1984) and in a review of 99 pancreatitis patients discharged without a defined aetiological factor, ultrasonography at 6 weeks had a sensitivity of 87% and specificity of 93% in gallstone detection (Goodman et al 1985). However, even at this stage stones can escape detection in that ultrasonography and oral cholecystography failed to detect stones in no less than 13% of patients in whom gallstones were finally recovered at surgery or visualized at ERCP.

Practical guidelines in diagnosis

The following guidelines are suggested as a basis for evaluation of patients in the first 24 hours after admission to hospital with an attack of acute pancreatitis which may be gallstone-associated:

1. Gallstones should always be entertained as a possible cause of acute pancreatitis when a patient is first seen, regardless of whether other factors such as alcohol may appear to be the responsible cause.

2. The probability that an attack of acute pancreatitis is due to gallstones increases if the plasma aminotransferase (ALT or AST) levels are increased on admission. Other factors which increase the probability of gallstone pancreatitis are abnormalities in other liver function tests (bilirubin, alkaline phosphatase, γ-glutamyl transpeptidase), female sex, increasing age and marked hyperamylasaemia (>4000 i.u./l).

3. The most useful screening test to detect gallstones is ultrasonography. Unequivocal demonstration of gallstones whether in the gallbladder, bile ducts or both means that gallstones should be regarded as the responsible agent. An equivocal ultrasonogram is usually the result of technical difficulties posed by gastrointestinal gas and means that gallstones cannot be excluded. The ultrasonogram should be repeated some days later if the patient is not judged to have severe acute pancreatitis on prognostic scoring systems (e.g. Ranson or Glasgow system) or settles promptly on admission. In patients deemed to have severe acute pancreatitis, consideration should be given at this stage to urgent endoscopic retrograde cholangiography (ERC), particularly if clinical and biochemical factors point to gallstones as the likely cause. The use of ERC for thera-

peutic as well as diagnostic purposes will be considered below. A negative ultrasonogram where gallstones are not revealed but the technical quality of the investigation is considered satisfactory by an experienced radiologist, makes it unlikely but not impossible that the attack of pancreatitis was gallstone-associated. The offending stone(s) may have escaped detection in the lower common bile duct or may already have migrated into the gut. As discussed earlier it is now appreciated that very small stones or crystal micro-aggregates can cause pancreatitis. Assuming, that the patient settles on conservative management, ERC should be considered subsequently to exclude biliary pathology if other causes for pancreatitis are not apparent.

4. While CT scanning is invaluable as a means of detecting pancreatic necrosis and defining its extent (see Chs 22, 23), it is inferior to ultrasonography in the detection of gallstones and is not recommended in this context.

TREATMENT OF GALLSTONE PANCREATITIS

General measures to treat acute pancreatitis

The supportive measures described in Chapter 20 should be instituted as part of the general management of acute pancreatitis, regardless of cause. The severity of the attack should be assessed as soon as possible using one of the prognostic scoring systems (eg. Ranson et al 1974, Blamey et al 1984) and the course of the attack should be monitored using conventional clinical assessment or the APACHE II system (Knaus et al 1981, Wilson et al 1990). In patients with mild disease or those in whom severe disease settles promptly on conservative treatment, subsequent investigation to detect gallstones can proceed without urgency. When severe pancreatitis is present, ultrasonography should be ordered as a matter of urgency and consideration given to urgent diagnostic, and if appropriate, therapeutic ERC. In some patients delayed presentation may preclude any attempts to abort the attack by removal of bile duct stones. Monitoring of clinical progress, APACHE II score, C-reactive protein (see p. 202) and CT scan appearances will signal the need to intervene surgically in such cases to deal with complications such as infected pancreatic and peripancreatic necrosis.

Role of endoscopic retrograde cholangiography (ERC)

There are three situations in which ERC may be of value in gallstone pancreatitis:

1. Urgent ERC and sphincterotomy
2. ERC and sphincterotomy as an alternative to surgery
3. Delayed diagnostic ERC.

Urgent ERC and sphincterotomy

It may be indicated urgently when the presence of gallstones is suspected in patients with severe acute pancreatitis who fail to settle promptly on conservative treatment. Given that acute pancreatitis is one of the recognized complications of ERC there was originally some understandable reluctance to recommend the investigation in patients already suffering from pancreatic inflammation. However, there is growing confidence that when used carefully the technique need not exacerbate the pancreatitis. In a review of seven studies in which ERC and endoscopic sphincterotomy were performed, complications developed in only nine (5%) of 152 patients with gallstone pancreatitis, four of whom died (Neoptolemos et al 1988). It should be emphasized that cholangiography rather than pancreatography is the prime objective; indeed filling the pancreatic duct system must be scrupulously avoided. The early experience of urgent ERC and endoscopic papillotomy in gallstone pancreatitis proved sufficiently encouraging (Safrany & Cotton, 1981, Rosseland & Solhaug 1984) for Carr-Locke and his colleagues in Leicester to undertake a prospective controlled trial of its use. In this important study (Neoptolemos et al 1988), patients with acute pancreatitis thought to be due to gallstones were first stratified into those with mild or severe disease using Glasgow criteria. They were then randomized to receive conventional treatment or undergo ERC within a 72-hour period. There were fewer complications in the 59 patients randomly allocated to undergo ERC (with endoscopic sphincterotomy if appropriate) than among the 62 conventionally treated controls. In patients with mild disease there was little morbidity and no mortality, regardless of the form of treatment, whereas patients with severe disease receiving conventional treatment had significantly more morbidity and a higher mortality than those undergoing ERC (see Table 21.5). The only complication attributable to ERC–endoscopic sphincterotomy was a late presentation of lumbar osteitis in a patient with acute cholangitis; postsphincterotomy bleeding was not encountered.

A number of aspects of this important study deserve comment. It remains to be demonstrated whether the excellent results can be reproduced in other centres, where the same endoscopic skills may not be available. Even in Leicester, the success rate of ERC was only 80% in severe cases as opposed to 94% in mild cases, and particular care was taken to avoid injudicious injury to the papilla of Vater. Finally, this study only involved patients in whom the presence of gallstones was confirmed; it remains unclear whether ERC with or without sphincterotomy has a role in patients who have passed all their stones or who have acute pancreatitis as a consequence of microlithiasis.

ERC and sphincterotomy as an alternative to surgery

As will be discussed, cholecystectomy is still regarded as the definitive treatment of gallstone pancreatitis. When the pancreatitis is mild or settles promptly on conservative management and gallstones are known to be present, most surgeons would proceed to surgical eradication of biliary tract disease. However, in the elderly, the unfit and those unwilling to have surgery, a case can be made for endoscopic sphincterotomy. Even though this may not eradicate gallstones and will leave the gallbladder in situ as a potential source of problems, it will at least minimize the chance of developing another attack of gallstone pancreatitis. From time to time, patients who have already undergone cholecystectomy will develop acute pancreatitis because of retained (or on rare occasions, recurrent) ductal stones; endoscopic sphincterotomy and gallstone removal is indicated to avoid subsequent attacks of pancreatitis (Kelly & Swaney 1982).

Delayed diagnostic ERC

ERC/ERCP may also have a valuable role when the cause of acute pancreatitis remains obscure. Goodman et al (1985) reported a series of 99 patients who were discharged following an attack of acute pancreatitis without a defined aetiological cause. Of 35 patients with normal ultrasonography and oral cholecystectography, 33 agreed to undergo ERCP; gallstones were revealed in seven cases, two of whom had been labelled as having had alcohol-associated pancreatitis. However, ERCP was not universally successful in that two further patients with negative findings were found to have gallstones at subsequent laparotomy. In Hong Kong, Lee et al (1986) have also strongly recommended ERCP within 2 weeks of recovery from acute pancreatitis as a means of detecting biliary tract pathology.

Surgical treatment

Consideration will be given here to the question of biliary surgery in gallstone pancreatitis. The treatment of complications, such as pancreatic, necrosis are considered elsewhere (Ch. 22) but it is worth emphasizing that when

Table 21.5 Controlled trial of urgent ERCP (with or without endoscopic sphincterotomy, ±ES) and conventional treatment in patients with acute gallstone pancreatitis (Neoptolemos et al 1988)

	Group A (ERCP ± ES within 72 hours	Group B (conventional treatment)
Mild acute pancreatitis*(n)	34	34
With complications (%)	4 (12%)	4 (12%)
Deaths	0	0
Severe acute pancreatitis(n)	25	28
With complications (%)	6 (24%)	17 (61%)
Deaths	1	5

*Severity assessed by Glasgow criteria (Blamey et al 1984)

gallstones are detected in the course of surgery for complications, the gallbladder should be removed whenever this is deemed to be acceptably safe. In our experience, biliary drainage by cholecystostomy or choledochotomy are less satisfactory alternatives. At the same time, exploration and manipulation of the bile duct is usually unacceptably hazardous when undertaken in the course of emergency surgery for complicated acute pancreatitis.

Returning to the question of biliary surgery in patients who have not developed complications such as necrosis, there has been considerable debate as to the timing of cholecystectomy. The traditional approach was to allow the acute attack to settle, discharge the patient and arrange readmission for surgery 6–8 weeks later. This policy of 'deferred' surgery came under attack with the realization that as many as 50% of patients experienced a further attack of pancreatitis while awaiting readmission (Paloyan et al 1975, Kelly 1980, Osborne et al 1981). In many cases the problem lay in the fact that readmission was unduly delayed but it is worth emphasizing that in our own recent report of fatal acute pancreatitis, three patients dying from gallstone pancreatitis had been discharged only 6, 7 and 12 days respectively before the onset of their final fatal attack (Wilson et al 1988).

Recognition of the potential dangers of deferred biliary surgery led some to adopt a more aggressive approach involving urgent surgical intervention. Acosta et al (1978, 1980) advocated that surgery should be undertaken immediately after admission, and hopefully, within 48 hours of the start of the attack. Much of their argument rested on the need to prevent prolonged ampullary obstruction, and in apparent support for their policy, stones were found impacted at the ampulla in 75% of patients operated on within 48 hours of the onset of symptoms. Delaying surgery for 2–4 days reduced this figure to 45% and when surgery was delayed for more than 4 days it fell to 25%. Restoration of ampullary patency following surgery within 48 hours resulted in immediate and complete remission of symptoms and rapid normalization of serum amylase and bilirubin values in all but one of their 41 patients. In contrast, when operation was carried out within 48–96 hours, four of their five patients died from necrotizing pancreatitis, despite restoration of biliary and pancreatic duct patency. Three patients in whom an impacted stone could not be removed also died from necrotizing pancreatitis (Acosta et al 1980). Neither of the group's publications deals in detail with the problem of early diagnosis of gallstones in patients with acute pancreatitis, and it should be noted that in the later paper no less than 40 of the 78 patients with gallstone pancreatitis had 'clinical jaundice' (Acosta et al 1980). It may be that this experience was based on a selected group of patients. A further difficulty relates to the dwindling number of patients found to have impacted stones as the interval between surgery and the onset of symptoms

lengthened. It can be argued that deferral of surgery would have allowed many of these stones to migrate spontaneously into the duodenum and so obviate the need for choledochotomy and/or transduodenal sphincterotomy.

Stone et al (1981) have conducted a prospective controlled trial in which patients with gallstone pancreatitis were assigned randomly to undergo biliary surgery (i.e. cholecystectomy plus transduodenal sphincteroplasty and pancreatic duct septotomy) within 73 hours of admission or after an interval of 3 months. As expected, patients coming to early surgery had a higher incidence of common bile duct stones (75% versus 28%). Morbidity was very similar in the two groups, and the one death in the early surgery group was balanced by two deaths after deferred operation. The relatively small sample size (65 patients) prevented firm conclusions but the authors commented on the sudden gush of pancreatic juice following sphincteroplasty in the early surgery group, and clearly believed that early intervention offered the greater certainty of relieving obstruction and allowing pancreatitis to settle. As with the work of Acosta's group, reservations must be expressed about the reliability of diagnostic tests in this critical early period, although Stone et al (1981) reported that ultrasonography detected gallstones in 93% of the 35 patients coming to early surgery. It can also be contended that the amount of surgery performed was excessive in that avoidance of early surgery may have obviated the need for transduodenal sphincteroplasty; the need for pancreatic duct septotomy also remains extremely debatable.

A number of uncontrolled studies have highlighted the dangers which can be associated with early biliary surgery in gallstone pancreatitis. For example, Ranson (1979) reported a mortality rate of 23% in 22 patients having surgery within the first week of admission; conversely surgery carried out at a later stage in the same admission resulted in no deaths in the 37 patients so treated. Similarly, Tondelli et al (1982) reported a mortality rate of 31% (five of 16 patients) in patients having immediate operation as opposed to 2% in those having later surgical treatment. Mayer et al (1984) undertook urgent surgery in five of 159 patients with gallstone pancreatitis; three of these five patients died whereas there were only two deaths in the 84 patients having non-urgent surgery during the index hospital admission.

In our own review of the timing of operation we examined the outcome of biliary surgery in a consecutive series of 147 patients with gallstone pancreatitis, 47 of whom had biliary surgery during their first hospital admission (Osborne et al 1981). Of these 47 patients, 37 had early biliary surgery after prompt resolution of signs and symptoms while in 10 cases surgery was undertaken because of failure of resolution of pancreatitis or because of the development of complications. The 37 patients coming to surgery after clinical resolution progressed well in that none died and morbidity was minimal. On the other hand, the 10 patients failing to resolve experienced major morbidity and five died. Our interpretation of this study was that the majority of patients admitted with gallstone pancreatitis will settle on conservative treatment and that biliary surgery can be carried out safely but without urgency in the course of the same hospital admission. It is now well recognized that failure to eradicate gallstone during the first admission with acute pancreatitis leaves the patient with an unacceptably high risk of developing further potential lethal attacks (Fielding et al 1989, Windsor 1990).

It is also recognized that as in our experience a significant proportion of patients admitted with severe acute pancreatitis will not settle on conservative management and undue deferment of intervention may allow them to drift into difficulty and danger. It is this important group of patients with severe disease who may now benefit from endoscopic intervention to relieve ampullary obstruction and allow resolution of inflammation. However, by analogy with the work of Acosta et al (1978, 1980) it seems likely that there is a critical window for intervention of some 48 hours and that delay beyond this critical period may create a vicious circle of pancreatic inflammation that will no longer resolve promptly once the obstructing gallstone is removed. In this context, Neoptolemos (1989) has suggested that small migrating gallstones may initiate an attack of acute pancreatitis, whereas it is larger 'persisting' ductal stones that are responsible for the development of severe pancreatic inflammation.

CONCLUSIONS REGARDING THE TREATMENT OF GALLSTONE PANCREATITIS

Recommendations for the management of patients with gallstone pancreatitis can now be summarized as follows:

1. Gallstone pancreatitis remains a potentially lethal condition which must always be regarded seriously.

2. Investigation to detect gallstones should be undertaken as a matter of urgency in patients admitted with acute pancreatitis.

3. In patients admitted with mild acute pancreatitis and in those with severe disease who settle promptly, invasive investigation such as ERC may not be needed.

4. In those with severe disease who fail to settle promptly, ERC is advocated to confirm that gallstones are present and relieve ampullary obstruction by endoscopic sphincterotomy.

5. If ERC is indicated it should be performed within 48 hours of the onset of the attack whenever possible and over-filling of the pancreatic duct system should be avoided.

6. With resolution of the acute attack of pancreatitis, cholecystectomy should be carried out on a non-urgent basis during the same hospital admission.

7. Operative cholangiography should be performed at the time of cholecystectomy, recognizing that the bile duct may remain dilated after stones have passed on into the duodenum.

8. No patient who has suffered from gallstone pancreatitis should be allowed to leave hospital with gallstones. In the majority of cases this means that biliary surgery should be undertaken; an exception may be justified in the elderly and high-risk patient where the dangers of laparoscopic or open cholecystectomy may be regarded as unacceptably high. In such cases, endoscopic eradication of duct stones with sphincterotomy to prevent any further episodes of impaction may be an acceptable compromise.

9. Finally, it must be emphasized that some patients with gallstone pancreatitis will develop necrosis and other life-threatening complications despite attempts to abort the attack by endoscopic sphincterotomy. If surgery is indicated to deal with these complications, cholecystectomy should be performed whenever feasible as part of the operative intervention.

REFERENCES

Acosta J L, Ledesma C L 1974 Gallstone migration as a cause of acute pancreatitis. New England Journal of Medicine 270:484–487
Acosta J M, Rossi R, Gallio M R 1978 Early surgery for acute gallstone pancreatitis: evaluation of a systemic approach. Surgery 83:367–370
Acosta J M, Pellegrini C A, Skinner D B 1980 Etiology and pathogenesis of acute biliary pancreatitis. Surgery 88:118–125
Armstrong C P, Taylor T V 1986 Pancreatic duct reflux and acute gallstone pancreatitis. Annals of Surgery 204:59–64
Armstrong C P, Taylor T V, Torrance H B 1985 Effects of bile, infection and pressure on pancreatic duct integrity. British Journal of Surgery 72:792–795
Bell E T 1958 Pancreatitis. Surgery 43:527–537
Blamey S L, Osborne D H, Gilmour W H et al 1983a The early identification of patients with gallstone associated pancreatitis using clinical and biochemical factors only. Annals of Surgery 198:574–578
Blamey S L, Osborne D H, O'Neill J et al 1983b Identification of patients with gallstone-associated pancreatitis using clinical and biochemical parameters only. British Journal of Surgery 70:301

Blamey S L, Imrie C W, O'Neill J, Gilmour W H, Carter D C 1984 Prognostic factors in acute pancreatitis. Gut 25:1340–1346
Broe P, Cameron J 1982 Experimental gallstone pancreatitis:pathogenesis and response to different treatment modalities. Annals of Surgery 195:566–571
Coppa G F, Le Fleur R, Ranson J H C 1981 The role of Chiba-needle cholangiography in the diagnosis of possible acute pancreatitis with cholelithiasis. Annals of Surgery 193:393–398
Corfield A P, Cooper M J, Williamson R G N 1985 Acute pancreatitis: A lethal disease of increasing incidence. Gut 26:724–729
Cuschieri A, Hughes J H 1973 Pancreatic reflux during operative choledochography. British Journal of Surgery 60:933–936
Damman H, Dopner M, Wichert P, Harders H, Hornborstel H 1980 Gallstones and acute pancreatitis. Lancet 1:308
Davidson B R, Neoptolemos J P, Leese T, Carr-Locke D L 1988 Biochemical prediction of gallstones in acute pancreatitis: a prospective study of three systems. British Journal of Surgery 75:213–215
Durr G H K (1979) In: Howat H T, Sarles H (eds) the exocrine pancreas W B Saunders, London, Ch 15, p 373
Elmslie R, White T, McGee D 1966 The significance of reflux of

tryspin and bile in the pathogenesis of acute pancreatitis. British Journal of Surgery 53:809–816

Farinon A M, Ricci G L, Sianesi M, Percudani M, Zanella E 1987 Physiopathologic role of microlithiasis in gallstone pancreatitis. Surgery, Gynecology and Obstetrics 164:252–256

Farmer C R, Tweedie J, Maslin S, Reber H, Adler G, Kern H 1984 Effects of bile salts on permeability and morphology of main pancreatic duct in cats. Digestive Diseases and Sciences 29:740–746

Fielding G A, Mok F, Wilson C, Imrie C W, Carter D C 1989 Management of gallstone pancreatitis. Australian and New Zealand Journal of Surgery 59:775

Freund H, Pfeffermann R, Durst A L, Rabinovici N 1976 Gallstone pancreatitis: exploration of the biliary system in acute and recurrent pancreatitis. Archives of Surgery 111:1106–1107

Frey C F 1981 Gallstone pancreatitis. Surgical Clinics of North America 61:923–938

Glazer G, Murphy F, Clayden G S (1981) Radionuclide biliary scanning in acute pancreatitis. British Journal of Surgery 68:766–770

Goebell H, Hotz J 1979 In: Howat H T, Sarles H (eds) The exocrine pancreas. W B Saunders, London Ch 15 p 37

Goodman A J, Neoptolemos J P, Carr-Locke D L, Finlay D B, Fossard D P 1985 Detection of gallstones after acute pancreatitis. Gut 26:125–132

Hand B H 1963 Anatomical study of the choledochoduodenal area. British Journal of Surgery 50:486–489

Howes R, Zuidema G D, Cameron J L 1975 Evaluation of prophylatic antibiotics in acute pancreatitis. Journal of Surgical Research 18:197–200

Imrie C W, Whyte A S 1975 A prospective study of acute pancreatitis. British Journal of Surgery 62:490–494

Ivy A C, Gibbs G E 1952 Pancreatitis: A review. Surgery 31:614–642

Kaden V G, Howard J M, Doubleday L C 1955 Cholecystographic studies during and immediately following acute pancreatitis. Surgery 38:1082–1086

Kelly T R 1976 Gallstone pancreatitis; pathophysiology. Surgery 80:488–492

Kelly T R 1980 Gallstone pancreatitis: the timing of surgery. Surgery 88:654–663

Kelly T R 1984 Gallstone pancreatitis: local predisposing factors. Annals of Surgery 200:479–484

Kelly T R, Swaney P E 1982 Gallstone pancreatitis: the second time around. Surgery 92:571–575

Kirchner R, Lausen M, Salm R, Scholmerich J 1990 Acute gallstone pancreatitis. Digestive Surgery 7:1–7

Knaus W A, Zimmerman J E, Wagner D P, Draper E A, Lawrence D E (1981) APACHE – acute physiology and chronic health evaluation: a physiologically based classification system. Critical Care Medicine 9:591–597

Konok G P, Thompson A G 1969 Pancreatic ductal mucosa as a protective barrier in the pathogenesis of pancreatitis. American Journal of Surgery 117:18–23

Lee M J R, Choi T K, Lai E C S, Wong K P, Ngan H, Wong J 1986 Endoscopic retrograde cholangiopancreatography after acute pancreatitis. Surgery, Gynecology and Obstetrics 163:354–358

Lee S P, Nicholls J F, Park H Z 1992 Biliary sludge as a cause of acute pancreatitis. New England Journal of Medicine 326:589–593

McKay A J, O'Neill J, Imrie C W 1980 Pancreatitis, pregnancy and gallstones. British Journal of Obstetrics and Gynaecology 87:47–50

McKay A J, Imrie C W, O'Neill J, Duncan J G 1982 Is an early ultrasound scan of value in acute pancreatitis? British Journal of Surgery 69:369–372

Mackie C R, Wood R A B, Preece P E, Cuschieri A 1985 Surgical pathology at early elective operation for suspected acute gallstone pancreatitis: preliminary report of a prospective clinical trial. British Journal of Surgery 72:179–181

McMahon M, Pickford I 1979 Biochemical prediction of gallstones early in attack of acute pancreatitis. Lancet 2:541–543

Mayer A D, McMahon M J 1983 Gallstone migration and early diagnosis of cholelithiasis in acute pancreatitis. Gut 24:A988 (abstract)

Mayer A D, McMahon M J 1985 Biochemical identification of patients with gallstones associated with acute pancreatitis on the day of admission to hospital. Annals of Surgery 201:68–75

Mayer A D, McMahon M J, Benson E A, Axon A T R 1984 Operations upon the biliary tract in patients with acute pancreatitis: aims, indications and timing. Annals of the Royal College of Surgeons of England 66:179–183

Mero M 1982 Changing aetiology of acute pancreatitis. Annales de Chirurgie et Gynaecologie 71:126–129

Moreau J A, Zinsmeister A R, Melton I J, Di Magno E P 1988 Gallstone pancreatitis and the effect of cholecystectomy: a population based cohort study. Mayo Clinic Proceedings 63:466–473

Negro P, Falti G, Porowska B, Tuscano D, Carboni M 1984 Occult gallbladder microlithiasis causing acute recurrent pancreatitis. Acta Chirurgica Scandinavica 150:503–506

Neoptolemos J P 1989 The theory of 'persisting' common bile duct stones in severe gallstone pancreatitis. Annals of the Royal College of Surgeons of England 71:326–331

Neoptolemos J P, Hall A W, Finlay D F, Berry J M, Carr-Locke D L, Fossard D P 1984 The urgent diagnosis of gallstones in acute pancreatitis: a prospective study of three methods. British Journal of Surgery 71:230–233

Neoptolemos J P, Carr-Locke D L, Leese T, James D 1988 ERCP findings and the role of endoscopic sphincterotomy in acute gallstone pancreatitis. British Journal of Surgery 75:915–917

Newman H F, Weinberg S B, Newman E B, Northup J D 1958 The papilla of Vater and distal portion of the common bile duct and duct of Wirsung. Surgery, Gynecology and Obstetrics 106:687–694

Opie E L 1901a The relation of cholelithiasis to disease of the pancreas and to fat necrosis. Bulletin of the Johns Hopkins Hospital 12:19–22

Opie E L 1901b The etiology of acute haemorrhagic pancreatitis. Bulletin of the Johns Hopkins Hospital 12:182–188

Osborne D H 1982 Surgical implications in gallstone associated acute pancreatitis. MD Thesis, Trinity College, Dublin

Osborne D H, Imrie C W, Carter D C 1981 Biliary surgery in the same admission for gallstone associated acute pancreatitis. British Journal of Surgery 68:758–761

Osborne D H, Harris N W S, Gilmour H, Carter D C 1983 Operative cholangiography in gallstone associated acute pancreatitis. Journal of the Royal College of Surgeons (Edinburgh) 28:96–100

Paloyan D, Simonowitz D, Skinner D B 1975 The timing of biliary tract operations in patients with pancreatitis associated with gallstones. Surgery, Gynecology and Obstetrics 141:737–739

Prince M 1882 Pancreatic apoplexy with a report of two cases. Boston Medical Surgery Journal 107:28–32, 55–57

Ranson J H C 1979 The timing of biliary surgery in acute pancreatitis. Annals of Surgery 189:654–663

Ranson J H C 1983 Acute pancreatitis. In: Brooks J R (ed) Surgery of the pancreas. W B Saunders, Philadelphia, p 146–181

Ranson J H C, Rifkind K M, Roses D F 1974 Prognostic signs and the role of operative management in acute pancreatitis. Surgery, Gynecology and Obstetrics 139:69–81

Ranson J H C, Spencer F C 1978 The role of peritoneal lavage in severe acute pancreatitis. Annals of Surgery 187:565–575

Reber H A, Mosley J G 1980 The effect of bile salts on the pancreatic duct mucosal barrier. British Journal of Surgery 67:59–62

Robinson T M, Dunphy J E 1963 Continuous perfusion of bile protease activators through the pancreas. Journal of the American Medical Association 183:530–533

Rosseland A R, Solhaug J M 1984 Early or delayed endoscopic papillotomy (EPT) in gallstone pancreatitis. Annals of Surgery 199:165–168

Safrany L, Cotton P B 1981 Urgent duodenoscopic sphincterotomy for acute gallstone pancreatitis. Surgery 89:424–428

Satiani B, Stone H H 1979 Predictability of present outcome and future recurrence in acute pancreatitis. Archives of Surgery 114:711

Scholmerich J, Gross V, Johannesson T, Brobmann G, Ruckauer K, Wimmer B, Gerok W, Farthmann, E H 1989 Detection of biliary origin of acute pancreatitis. Digestive Diseases and Sciences 34:830–833

Simpson C J, Toner P G, Carr K E, Anderson J D, Carter D C 1983 Effect of bile salt perfusion and intraduct pressure on ionic flux and mucosal ultrastructure in the pancreatic duct of the cat. Virchows Arch (Cell Pathology) 42:327–342

Stone H H, Fabian T C, Dunlop W E 1981 Gallstone pancreatitis:

biliary tract pathology in relation to time of operation. Annals of Surgery 194:305–312

Svensson J-O, Nordback B, Bokey E L, Edlund Y 1979 Changing patterns in aetiology of pancreatitis in an urban Swedish area. British Journal of Surgery 66:159–162

Taylor T, Armstrong C P 1987 Migration of gall stones. British Medical Journal 294:1320–1322

Tondelli P, Stutz K, Harder F et al 1982 Acute gallstone pancreatitis: best timing for biliary surgery. British Journal of Surgery 69:709–710

Wang S D, Lin X-Z, Tsai Y-E et al 1988 Clinical significance of ultrasonography, computed tomography and biochemical tests in the rapid diagnosis of gallstone-related pancreatitis: a prospective study. Pancreas 3:153–158

Warshaw A L 1989 Obstructive pancreatitis: acute and chronic pancreatitis due to ductal obstruction by causes other than gallstone. In: Carter D C, Warshaw A L (eds) Pancreatitis. Churchill Livingstone, Edinburgh. Clinical Surgery International, vol 16 p 71–89

Wilson C, Imrie C W, Carter D C 1988 Fatal acute pancreatitis. Gut 29:782–788

Wilson C, Heath D I, Imrie C W 1990 Prediction of outcome in acute pancreatitis: a comparative study of APACHE II, clinical assessment and multiple factor scoring systems. British Journal of Surgery 77:1260–1264

Windsor J A 1990 Gallstone pancreatitis: a proposed management strategy. Australian and New Zealand Journal of Surgery 60:589–594

22. Operative management of acute pancreatitis

H. G. Beger   W. Uhl

INTRODUCTION

Acute pancreatitis is a disease with varied signs and symptoms which produces a clinical picture lacking homogeneity. The condition may range from a mild, self-limiting disease to a most severe illness with a fatal outcome. In up to 90% of cases acute pancreatitis takes a mild course, being accompanied by abdominal pain and raised levels of pancreatic enzymes in the blood and urine. Severe acute pancreatitis is characterized morphologically by pancreatic parenchymal necrosis and extrapancreatic fat necrosis. This necrosis is the critical feature which is responsible for the high morbidity and mortality rates in severe acute pancreatitis (Gerzof et al 1981, Allardyce 1987) and the frequency and degree of severity of local and systemic complications are directly related to its extent (Table 22.1). Recognition of this association is not new in that it was described 100 years ago by the Boston surgeon, Ronald Fitz (1889).

Early prediction of the severity of acute pancreatitis is mandatory in order to define the optimal therapeutic approach (Büchler et al 1987a). In the past, various efforts have been made to stage acute pancreatitis with the aid of clinical and/or laboratory findings (Ch. 19 and also Ranson et al 1974, Warshaw & Lee 1979, Bank et al 1983, McMahon et al 1984, Corfield et al 1985, Puolakkainen et al 1987). However, it is now apparent that the morpho-

logical changes produced by the inflammatory process in and around the pancreas provide a better predictor of severity than any other factor. Contrast-enhanced CT scanning, which can be used by radiologists throughout the world, is the best method available with which to stage acute pancreatitis (Kivisaari et al 1984, Block et al 1986, Balthazar 1989). Serum indicators can also be used to predict the presence of necrosis with a high degree of accuracy; such indicators include C-reactive protein (CRP), PMN-elastase, and lactic dehydrogenase (LDH) (Mayer et al 1984, Büchler et al 1986, 1987a, Uhl et al 1991). The use of contrast-enhanced CT-scanning can then be restricted to patients with increased levels of these serum indicators to determine the extent of pancreatic and extrapancreatic necrosis.

ACUTE PANCREATITIS: THE ULM CLASSIfiCATION

The classification of acute pancreatitis into mild or severe forms as suggested by the Marseilles classification consensus of 1984 (Singer et al 1985; Ch. 17) must now be regarded as inadequate for clinical decision-making in individual patients who may go on to develop a complicated course (Beger & Büchler 1986). On the basis of morphological, pathophysiological, clinical and bacteriological observations, four different entities can be distinguished in acute pancreatitis, each requiring a different therapeutic approach (Table 22.2). These entities are interstitial-oedematous pancreatitis, necrotizing pancreatitis (with sterile or infected necrosis), pancreatic abscess and pancreatic pseudocyst (Beger & Uhl 1990).

Interstitial oedematous pancreatitis. In the majority of cases, acute pancreatitis is characterized by a periacinar, interstitial oedema associated with accumulation of inflammatory cells. This may lead to the release of biologically active compounds into the inflammatory exudate with generation of spots of fatty tissue calcification. This oedematous form of the disease generally has a low morbidity and mortality (Beger et al 1986). Conservative

Table 22.1 Necrotizing pancreatitis: correlation between complications and the extent of the necrotizing process. Wet weight of dissected necrosis: focal, <50 g; extensive, 51–120 g; subtotal, 121–190 g; total, >190 g.

Complication	Extent of necrosis		
	Focal (n = 62)	Extensive (n = 57)	Subtotal/total (n = 42)
Pulmonary insufficiency	26%	40%	59%
Renal failure	19%	23%	55%
Shock	5%	12%	21%
Sepsis	11%	28%	45%

Table 22.2   Classification of acute pancreatitis in 987 patients treated in the University of Ulm; May 1982–March 1990

Classification	No. of patients (%)	Treatment	
		Surgical	Medical
Interstitial-oedematous pancreatitis	737 (75%)	0.4%	99%
Necrotizing pancreatitis	178 (18%)	83%*	17%
Pancreatic abscess	23 (2%)	100%	0
Pseudocyst (post-acute)	49 (5%)	65%	34%
Total	987 (100%)	21%	79%

*Biliary tract surgery not included

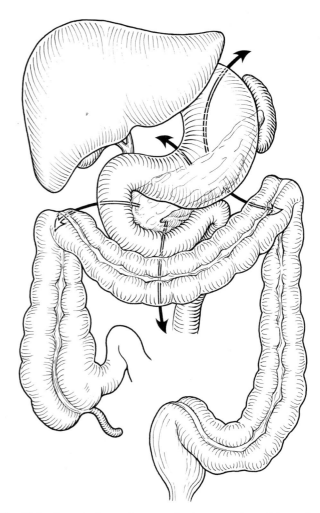

Fig. 22.1   Spread of necrotic process in the retroperitoneal tissues in acute necrotizing pancreatitis.

treatment usually results in a rapid improvement of symptoms, even in the rare patients with cardiovascular, respiratory, or renal dysfunction, and the retroperitoneal inflammation usually recedes completely in a matter of weeks. Hospital mortality rates in this form of acute pancreatitis are below 2% in most published clinical series (Allardyce 1987, Beger et al 1988).

Necrotizing pancreatitis. In 8–15% of patients with acute pancreatitis, necrotizing disease develops (Warshaw 1980, Allardyce 1987, Beger et al 1988). This form, even if it appears at first to be of moderate severity, may still proceed to local or systemic complications that can be life-threatening. Morphologically, necrotizing pancreatitis is characterized by interstitial oedematous inflammation combined with necrosis of the pancreatic exocrine and endocrine parenchyma, and invariably there is fatty tissue necrosis which extends beyond the pancreas (Fig. 22.1). The necrotic areas in the parenchyma are mostly focal and multicentric; total necrosis of the pancreas is exceptional. The necrotizing process tends to spread diffusely into the retroperitoneal tissue, liberating a variety of vasoactive and toxic substances, and peripancreatic fluid collections are common.

The critical development in necrotizing pancreatitis is bacterial contamination of the necrotic areas, contamination which is responsible for the late mortality from septic complications. Today, patients rarely die in the early phase of acute pancreatitis from cardiocirculatory complications produced by the liberation of vasoactive and toxic substances (Bradley 1982). Bacterial infection of the necrotic pancreatic and retroperitoneal tissue occurs in 40–60% of patients with necrotizing pancreatitis and Gram-negative organisms are usually responsible (Gerzof et al 1984, Beger et al 1988).

Not every patient with necrotizing pancreatitis has to undergo operation (Table 22.2). Patients with minor pancreatic necrosis which responds to intensive care frequently recover from severe acute pancreatitis without surgical intervention. However, infection of necrotic areas should be carefully excluded by fine-needle aspiration

(Warshaw 1974, Gerzof et al 1984, Beger et al 1986, Büchler et al 1988).

Pancreatic abscess This is a late complication of acute pancreatitis which may develop between the third and fifth week of the disease as a result of bacterial colonization of the necrotic tissue (Bittner et al 1987). In morphological terms a pancreatic abscess is a cavity containing purulent fluid and surrounded by an inflammatory pseudocapsule. In a clinical context, necrotizing pancreatitis with infected necrosis should be regarded as a severe form of acute pancreatitis with generalized sepsis, whereas pancreatic abscess occurs after the actual attack of acute pancreatitis has subsided. The course taken by a pancreatic abscess is similar to that seen during the development of any intra-abdominal abscess and the signs of acute pancreatitis are no longer present. Drained early, pancreatic abscess does not necessarily progress to generalized sepsis.

Pseudocysts. Similarly, weeks after the onset of acute pancreatitis, one of more pseudocysts may form. Such pseudocysts represent peripancreatic collections of exudate which may or may not be connected with the pancreatic duct system; alternatively they may be sequestra of liquefied necrotic tissue, in which case they originate within the pancreas. Such collections are also surrounded by a pseudocapsule of fibrous tissue.

Based on this morphological and pathological classification and our clinical experience, we were able to divide 987 patients admitted to our hospital with acute pancreatitis over the last 8 years, into a group of 75% with interstitial-oedematous pancreatitis and 18% with necrotizing pancreatitis. Pancreatic abscess and postacute pseudocysts, occurring in the more advanced stages of the disease were rare entities, affecting 2% and 5% respectively of our patient population (Table 22.2).

TREATMENT OF ACUTE PANCREATITIS

The initial clinical management of acute pancreatitis is based on the knowledge that most patients suffer from a mild self-limiting disease. However, there are considerable uncertainties with regard to medical management (see Ch. 20) since specific and effective pharmacological treatment is not available, while the effectiveness of surgical treatment of necrotizing pancreatitis has not yet been substantiated by controlled clinical data.

The treatment of interstitial-oedematous and necrotizing pancreatitis is in the first instance conservative (Goebell & Singer 1987, Ranson 1981). As necrotizing pancreatitis has come to be regarded as a severe and most unpredictable disease, so different approaches to surgical management have been proposed. These proposals include pancreatic resection (Edelmann & Boutelier 1974, Alexandre & Guerreri 1981, Hollender et al 1981, Kivilaakso et al 1984, Aldridge et al 1985); peritoneal dialysis (Wall 1965, Bolooki & Gliedman 1978, Ihse et al 1982, Lasson et al 1984, Mayer et al 1985); multiple tube drainage (McCarthy & Dickermann 1982); surgical debridement and suction drainage (Watermann et al 1968, Warshaw & Jin 1985); necrosectomy with postoperative continuous local lavage of necrotic cavities (Beger et al 1985); various forms of open packing (Knol et al 1984, Stone et al 1984, Wayand & Waclawiczek 1985, Teichmann et al 1986, Wertheimer & Norris 1986, Bradley 1987, Wittmann et al 1990), and non-operative drainage using percutaneous techniques (Gerzof et al 1981, van Sonnenberg et al 1984, Freeny et al 1988, Larvin et al 1989, Pederzoli et al 1990). All of the proposals for surgical management of necrotizing pancreatitis have stressed the removal of toxic fluid collections and/or the debridement of devitalized tissue from the pancreas and surrounding retroperitoneal fatty tissue.

Indication for surgical treatment

In patients classified as having acute interstitial-oedematous

pancreatitis there is usually no indication for pancreatic surgery even if complications develop (Ranson 1986, Goebell & Singer 1987). In patients with gallstone pancreatitis there is a need to eradicate cholelithiasis but this specific problem is considered elsewhere (Ch. 21).

Confusion has arisen about the role of surgery in necrotizing pancreatitis for four reasons. First, the condition runs a variable clinical course; secondly, there is no universally accepted classification of its stages; thirdly, the early diagnosis of complications may be difficult; and fourthly, there is lack of agreement regarding the timing of surgical intervention (Kümmerle & Neher 1981, Mercadier 1981, Aldridge et al 1985, Trapnell & Anderson 1986, Poston & Williamson 1990). However nobody denies that patients with severe necrotizing pancreatitis should be treated in an intensive care unit, because even the early phase of the disease is characterized by organ complications such as cardiorespiratory and renal failure caused by the release of vasoactive and toxic substances. A significant proportion of patients with necrotizing pancreatitis and organ complications can be successfully treated by intensive care measures without recourse to surgery. Intensive care treatment includes specific treatment of pulmonary, renal and cardiocirculatory dysfunction, recognition and treatment of metabolic and haematological disorders, and appropriate antibiotic treatment (Table 22.3).

Surgical treatment of necrotizing pancreatitis is based on the observation that patients who develop local septic complications have a chance of survival only following operation. From a clinical viewpoint surgical management is indicated in patients with necrotizing pancreatitis who develop signs of an acute 'surgical' abdomen or sepsis, or who have persisting organ failure, such as pulmonary and/or renal insufficiency. Severe gastrointestinal bleeding and metabolic derangement are also indications for surgical treatment if these complications worsen over a period of 3–5 days despite full intensive care treatment. Patients with proven necrotizing pancreatitis who develop an upper abdominal mass with abdominal pain (despite analgesic therapy) after the second week of their illness, who have increasing leucocytosis despite absence of pyrexia, and who develop increasing ileus, are also potential candidates for surgical intervention (Table 22.4).

In a prospective clinical study in Ulm involving 110 of our patients with necrotizing pancreatitis, a surgical acute abdomen developed in 9%, sepsis in about 24%, and a shock syndrome in 8% (9 cases). Over one-third of the patients had to be operated upon because of organ complications or systemic upset resulting from failure of intensive therapy (Table 22.5). Since there are no clinically substantiated data which allow assessment of the response to conservative therapy and the effectiveness of intensive care treatment, a minimum period of intensive care therapy should be observed. In Ulm, surgery was carried out on average on the 9th day of the disease (range,

Table 22.3   Intensive care and acute pancreatitis. (Pao_2, arterial oxygen saturation)

Organ/system	Parameter	Treatment
Pulmonary insufficiency	Pao_2 <70 mmHg	Oxygen
	Pao_2 <60 mmHg, on oxygen	Mechanical ventilation
Renal insufficiency	Serum creatinine >120μmol/l, urine output <30 ml/h	Dopamine (low dose + diuretics)
	Serum creatinine >400 μmol/l or blood urea >30 mmol/l	Haemofiltration Haemodialysis
Cardiocirculatory dysfunction shock	Falling central venous pressure	Volume replacement
	Mean arterial blood pressure <70 mmHg	Dopamine (high dose)
	Systolic blood pressure <90 mmHg for more than 10 minutes	Swan Ganz catheter, noradrenaline
Metabolic upset	Hyperglycaemia >11.1 mmol/l	Insulin
	Disseminated intravascular coagulation	Fresh frozen plasma
Sepsis	Rectal temperature >38.5°C	Antibiotics
	White cell count <4.0 × 10⁹/l >12.0 × 10⁹/l	Surgical intervention
	Platelet count <150 × 10⁹/l	
	Metabolic acidosis (base excess > −4 mmol/l)	

1–64 days) and after an average of 5 days' treatment in the intensive care unit (range, 0–56 days).

Further, studies are needed to determine the extent to which recently introduced methods of haemodialysis or haemofiltration can influence the early phase of the disease and thus avoid surgery (Gebhardt et al 1991, unpublished data). This would also be particularly interesting with regard to the second or late phase of acute pancreatitis, in which septic complications predominate, particularly as multi-organ failure in association with sepsis is now the most frequent cause of death in necrotizing pancreatitis. Patients who develop a septic clinical picture in the course of severe acute pancreatitis should receive antibiotics, followed by an ultrasound- or CT-guided aspiration of the necrotic tissue to determine the presence, type and antibiotic sensitivity of infecting bacteria. If bacteria contamination is detected, surgical intervention is of course indicated.

From a morphological point of view, contrast-enhanced CT and guided fine-needle aspiration can also indicate the need for surgery. Patients with infected necrosis, extended pancreatic necrosis (involving more than 50% of the gland) with or without extrapancreatic fatty tissue necrosis, and those with local complications (such as stenosis of the common bile duct, duodenum or colon) are also candidates for surgical intervention.

Timing and goals of surgical intervention

The timing of surgical intervention in severe acute pancreatitis is still controversial (Lawson et al 1970, Kivilaakso et al 1981, Kümmerle & Neher 1981, Ranson 1986, Freeny et al 1988). It is, of course, very difficult to establish generally applicable rules for the ideal timing of surgical intervention. Each case has to be judged individually and the indications for surgical treatment must be carefully evaluated. Figure 22.2 provides an algorithm

Table 22.4   Necrotizing pancreatitis: indications for surgical management

Clinical criteria	Surgical acute abdomen
	Sepsis syndrome
	Non-response to intensive care unit treatment (>3 days),
	Persisting or increasing local/systemic complications:
	Pulmonary insufficiency
	Renal failure
	Cardiocirculatory insufficiency
Bacteriological criterion	Infected necrosis
Morphological criteria	Extensive pancreatic necroses (>50%)
	Extensive pancreatic and/or retroperitoneal necroses
	Stenosis of common bile duct, duodenum, large bowel

Table 22.5   Indication for surgical management in 110 prospectively studied patients with proven necrotizing pancreatitis at the University of Ulm, May 1982–June 1987 (ICU, intensive care unit)

Indication	No. patients (%)
Acute surgical abdomen	10 (9%)
Sepsis	28 (24%)
Cardiocirculatory failure/shock	9 (8%)
Multiple organ failure (despite ICU treatment ≥3 days)	40 (36%)
Pulmonary (n = 29)	
Renal failure (n = 15)	
Metabolic insufficiency (n = 31)	
Gastrointestinal tract	
Bleeding (n = 10)	
Severe ileus (n = 12)	
Persisting acute upper abdominal mass (despite ICU treatment ≥8 days)	23 (21%)

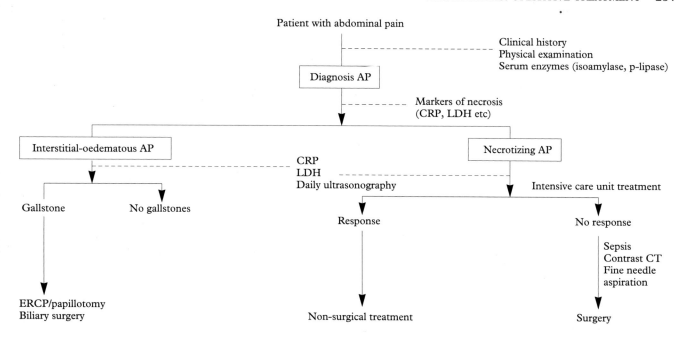

Fig. 22.2 Algorithm for decision-making in interstitial-oedematous and necrotizing acute pancreatitis (AP, acute pancreatitis; CRP, C-reactive protein; LDH, lactic dehydrogenase.)

which outlines one model of assessment and management. Intervention can be undertaken 'early', that is in the acute phase, if complications arise which make early operation absolutely necessary (Kivilaakso et al 1981, Poston & Williamson 1990) or on rare occasions if the diagnosis is still uncertain (Ranson 1986). Intervention can also be 'delayed' (Larvin et al 1989), the rationale being to wait until the necrosis has become demarcated. However, the problem remains that the demarcation process cannot yet be evaluated objectively. Surgical treatment of patients with necrotizing pancreatitis focuses on the debridement of devitalized tissue from the pancreas and retroperitoneal fatty tissue spaces (Table 22.6). It is generally accepted that in most cases of necrotizing pancreatitis there is still viable pancreatic tissue between the necrotic areas and that this tissue may survive. Careful surgical treatment of pancreatic necrosis should preserve functional pancreatic tissue between or deep to areas of devitalized pancreas so as to minimize or avoid subsequent exocrine and endocrine insufficiency. The combination of necrosectomy with intraoperative and postoperative local lavage of the lesser sac

provides atraumatic and continuous evacuation of devitalized and infected tissues as well as removing biologically active substances (in order to interrupt the process of inflammation and necrosis).

Pancreatic resection using the classical surgical techniques of partial or total pancreaticoduodenectomy, was proposed as a means of radical removal of the diseased tissue in necrotizing acute pancreatitis. However, standard forms of resectional surgery cannot be applied in this context in view of the presence of retroperitoneal and intraperitoneal necrosis and inflammation which frequently involves the mesentery of the small and large intestine. Even in patients with 'total' pancreatic necrosis, pancreatectomy is difficult to justify, because an intraoperative distinction between fatty tissue necrosis and necrosis of the pancreatic parenchyma cannot be made visually. In quite a number of cases only the superficial parts of the pancreas are necrotic, while the parenchyma around the pancreatic duct remains intact. Such superficial necrotizing pancreatitis (Leger et al 1978, Becker 1981, Mercadier 1981) can easily be mistaken for total necrosis by the surgeon, and lead to inappropriate removal of viable pancreas unless the surgeon is aware of the pancreatic morphology as seen on a contrast-enhanced CT scan.

Partial or total pancreaticoduodenectomy (Alexandre & Guerreri 1981, Kivilaakso et al 1984) also requires the removal of otherwise healthy organs (duodenum, distal stomach, extrapancreatic bile ducts) and this imposes additional stress on the severely ill patient. Surgical treatment of necrotizing pancreatitis using such classical

Table 22.6 Goals of surgical management of necrotizing pancreatitis

Removal of necrotic tissue
Drainage of bacterially infected areas
Removal of pancreatic ascites
Arrest of pancreatic inflammatory/necrotizing process
Arrest of release and systemic spread of vasoactive/toxic substances
Preservation of functioning pancreatic tissue

resection techniques resulted in high complication rates and a mortality rate above 30% (Alexandre & Guerreri 1981, Kümmerle & Neher 1981). Except for the exceptionally rare cases of near-total pancreatic necrosis where resection may be seen as a heroic last-ditch manoeuvre, pancreatic resection involves the risk of overtreatment and an increase in late morbidity.

Peritoneal lavage and triple-tube drainage

Modern surgical treatment of necrotizing pancreatitis centres on the removal of necrosis followed by continuous evacuation of pancreatic fluids and exudates, which may contain bacterial and biologically active compounds. Thus, peritoneal dialysis alone (Wall 1965, Ihse et al 1982, Lasson et al 1984, Mayer et al 1985, Beger et al 1986) cannot be regarded as adequate therapy for acute pancreatitis. In the controlled study conducted by Mayer et al (1985), hospital mortality was the same in the control group as in the group randomized to have peritoneal dialysis (27% and 28% respectively). According to current clinical studies, significant reduction in the incidence of organ complications and in mortality rate is not achieved, nor is it to be expected, as the effects of peritoneal lavage are restricted to the peritoneal cavity and do not influence the persisting necrotizing process in the retroperitoneum. Evacuation of all necrotic and infected tissue is therefore impossible. For the same reason, therapeutic improvement cannot be expected from the addition of protease inhibitors such as aprotinin to the lavage fluid.

Operative placement of several large-bore drainage tubes into the lesser sac, combined with T-tube drainage of the common bile duct (after cholecystectomy), gastrostomy and jejunostomy became known as 'triple-tube drainage'. The method was used mostly in North American clinics from 1970 onwards, and aimed to drain ascitic fluid from the lesser sac and inhibit exocrine pancreatic secretion (McCarthy & Dickermann 1982). However, the approach failed to reduce morbidity and mortality substantially. As necrotic and infected pancreatic and retropancreatic tissue is not removed, it is not surprising that pancreatic abscesses develop with a frequency of up to 40% after the use of 'triple-tube drainage' (Warshaw 1974).

Necrosectomy and lesser sac lavage

As lavage or drainage of the peritoneal cavity is in itself not able to bring down the high morbidity and mortality rates associated with necrotizing pancreatitis, our group have developed a therapeutic approach in which necrosectomy is combined with intraoperative and postoperative closed continuous lavage of the lesser sac. This procedure proved so successful that it has now been adopted as our clinical routine. The method provides continuous atraumatic evacuation of devitalized necrotic tissue and removes

bacterially contaminated dead tissue and biologically active potentially hazardous substances.

Our technique is as follows. After opening the abdominal cavity, usually by an upper abdominal midline incision, the gastrocolic and duodenocolic ligaments are divided, and the pancreas is fully exposed. The extent of necrosis in the head, body and tail of the gland can easily be assessed and its extent assessed. Debridement or necrosectomy, either by digital means or by the careful use of instruments, permits the removal of demarcated and devitalized tissue while preserving vital pancreatic parenchyma. After surgical debridement, meticulous haemostasis is obtained using transfixion stitches of monofilament suture material. It has become increasingly clear that it is not necessary to remove every gram of devitalized tissue, as any remaining tissue which is necrotic or which will become necrotic may be rinsed out later by the lavage fluid.

After haemostasis has been obtained, an extensive intraoperative lavage is performed using 3–6 litres of normal saline, so as to cleanse the surface of the pancreas and peripancreatic tissues.

For the postoperative closed continuous local lavage (the necrotizing process is of course still progressing), two large (28–34 Fr) double-lumen silicone rubber tubes are inserted to allow regional lavage of the lesser sac. On the left side, the drain passes behind the large bowel, below the spleen and in front of the kidney. On the right, the tube is usually placed so that it passes through the infrahepatic space passing behind the hepatoduodenal ligament and hepatogastric ligament; the tip of the tube lies in the lesser sac behind the stomach. The drains emerge in the midaxillary line on each side (Fig. 22.3). If there are large

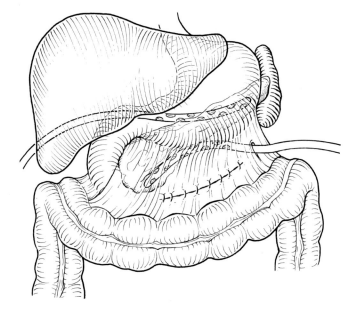

Fig. 22.3 Lavage of the lesser sac following necrosectomy. Note the repair of the gastrocolic omentum aimed at reconstituting the lesser sac.

retroperitoneal cavities lined by fatty tissue necroses, additional tubes are inserted as required to allow complete evacuation of all devitalized tissue and exudates. The opening made in the gastrocolic and duodenocolic ligaments to gain access to the lesser sac is then closed by sutures to recreate the lesser sac compartment for closed postoperative continuous lavage. In patients with severe haemorrhagic ascites, a Tenckhoff catheter is also placed in the lower abdomen for short-term peritoneal lavage. The operation ends with layered closure of the abdominal wall and lavage commences immediately after closure of the peritoneum.

In the first few postoperative days we use 24 litres of lavage fluid daily per tube. The amount is reduced quickly over the following few days, the rate of reduction depending on the clinical course and the appearance of the outflow fluid. For lavage purposes we employ a slightly hyperosmotic fluid, usually the solution used for chronic ambulatory peritoneal dialysis.

Postoperative flow of lavage fluid through the lesser sac and associated cavities mechanically cleans the inflamed areas. As demonstrated in Figure 22.4, the inflammatory process may continue to be active after necrosectomy for as long as 2–3 weeks, the returning lavage fluid still containing enzyme activity and other toxins. Lavage can be discontinued when there are no longer any signs of acute pancreatitis and once the necrosis cavities have been completely cleansed. This is confirmed by measurement of pancreatic enzyme levels in the lavage fluid, assessing its sterility, and taking note of the amount of returned

devitalized tissue. As a rule of thumb, lavage should continue if the amount of devitalized tissue exceeds 7 g in 24 hours. Once lavage has ceased, the drainage tubes are removed successively.

A total of 95 patients with necrotizing pancreatitis have been treated by our group according to this protocol (Beger et al 1988) and the results are shown in Table 22.7. These patients had severe acute pancreatitis, the mean value of their Ranson score amounting to 4.5 points, and the infection rate was 42%. Postoperative lavage was kept going for a median of 25 days, the median quantity of lavage fluid amounting to 8 litres per day.

Postoperative organ complications were rare and occurred mainly in patients who developed local complications or who needed re-operation. In total, 26 patients had to undergo re-operation and 23 of them had developed a secondary abscess in the area of the original necrosis cavity. Other causes of re-operation were massive diffuse local bleeding (one patient), progressive necrosis (one patient), and development of a colonic fistula leading to intra-abdominal sepsis (one patient). Pancreatic fistulas developed in 10 patients but in all cases closed spontaneously. An interesting finding was that the local complication rate was proportional to the extent of intrapancreatic necrosis; thus the re-operation rate was 18% in patients with focal necrosis, 28% in those with extended necrosis and 42% in those with subtotal or total pancreatic necrosis. The median hospital stay of surviving patients was 65 days (range 16–150 days).

In this group of 95 patients with severe necrotizing pancreatitis, the hospital mortality rate was 8% (eight patients). Death was related to both the extent of necrosis and the presence of bacterial infection of the necrosis. The mortality rate of patients with infected necrosis was twice as high as that of patients with sterile pancreatic necrosis (Table 22.8). Death was caused by sepsis in five patients, massive diffuse local haemorrhage in two, and cardiogenic shock in one patient. When one compares the results of necrosectomy plus continuous closed local lavage of the lesser sac with results from other centres, the hospital mortality of less than 10% in this group of patients is

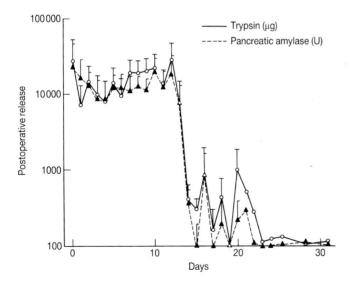

Fig. 22.4 Postoperative release of pancreatic trypsin and isoamylase into the lavage fluid per day ($\bar{x} \pm$ S E M; n = 18) in necrotizing pancreatitis. Local lavage with 7.5 l for 24 hours (median). The release of trypsin and isoamylase into the lavage fluid hints at contamination by acute pancreatitis up to postoperative day 12–14 in these patients, day 0 = day of operation. Note the logarithmic scale of the ordinate. Normal calculated ranges: trypsin < 1000 μg per 24 hours; isoamylase < 700 U per 24 hours.

Table 22.7 Results of necrosectomy and continuous local lavage in necrotizing pancreatitis in 95 patients studied prospectively at the University of Ulm, May 1982–June 1987

Preoperative status	Severity of pancreatitis (median)	4.5 Ranson points
	Infected necrosis	42%
Postoperative data	Duration of hospitalization (median)	65 days (in surviving patients)
	Duration of lavage (median)	25 days
	Amount of lavage fluid per 24 hours (median)	8 litres
	Need for re-operation	27%
	Hospital mortality	8% (8/95 patients)

Table 22.8 Hospital mortality in patients with infected and non-infected necrotizing pancreatitis after necrosectomy and local lavage

	Bacterial culture +ve			Bacterial culture –ve		
	n	No. of deaths	(%)	n	No. of deaths	(%)
Focal necrosis (n = 38)	12	1	(8%)	26	1	(4%)
Extended necrosis (n = 29)	17	2	(12%)	12	0	–
Subtotal/total necrosis (n = 22)	8	2	(25%)	14	2	(14%)
Total number of patients (n = 89)	37	5*	(14%)	52	3**	(6%)

* Five patients dying of sepsis; ** two patients dying from massive diffuse local bleeding and one from cardiogenic shock

remarkably low. Further controlled clinical trials will be necessary to confirm the favourable results obtained by this approach when compared to other non-operative and/or surgical methods of treatment.

Necrosectomy and methods of management other than closed lesser sac lavage

Other methods of management following debridement of necroses have been assessed over the years. In the Mayo series, published by Becker et al (1984), the hospital mortality of patients with pancreatic abscess was found to be 40%, and their re-operation rate was 31% (Table 22.9). Dissatisfied with these results and feeling that surgical necrosectomy with drainage alone was not enough to reduce mortality, these authors developed additional treatment protocols following surgical debridement. These methods of management included open packing with multiple redressing, multiple sump drainage with lavage, and planned frequent re-operations with or without placement of a zipper to facilitate multiple re-entry to the abdomen (Hollender et al 1981, Knol et al 1984, Stone et al 1984, Wayand & Waclawiczek 1985, Teichmann et al 1986, Wertheimer & Norris 1986, Bradley 1987, Wittmann et al 1990). Multiple re-dressings and frequent re-operations were used to remove the necroses and intra-operative lavage was employed at the time of surgery.

The Boston series reported by Warshaw & Jin (1985), showed a significant decrease in hospital mortality in patients with necrotizing pancreatitis or pancreatic abscess.

The overall hospital mortality in the Boston series was 24% and in the later part of the study only one of 19 patients died. In Atlanta, an open packing technique was employed by Bradley (1987). Multiple re-dressings, however, entail many re-operations, prolonged intensive care, and great additional stress for the patients. Multiple re-operations are also responsible for the increased occurrence of intestinal fistulas, gastric outlet stenosis, ileus, incisional hernia, and other complications such as local severe bleeding.

Percutaneous drainage

Thanks to the availability of CT scanning and ultrasonography, interventional techniques have attained increasing importance over the last few years, particularly with regard to achieving a more defined diagnosis of infection in areas of necrosis and fluid collections, and in the treatment of acute necrotizing pancreatitis. Using ultrasonography or CT scanning fine-needle aspiration of necrotic areas can be guided accurately and Gram-staining of the aspirate can be used to differentiate promptly between infected and sterile necrosis (Watermann et al 1968, Gerzof et al 1984, 1987, van Sonnenberg et al 1985, Steiner et al 1988). The bacteria can then be identified on culture and antibiotic sensitivity determined. Specific antibiotics can then be administered to cover surgical intervention, which by then has become absolutely necessary.

Recently, good results have also been reported following percutaneous insertion of large drainage tubes into necrotic areas using imaging procedures and without any surgical

Table 22.9 Results of surgical debridement/necrosectomy in necrotizing pancreatitis and pancreatic abscess. (Postoperative complications included pancreatic fistula, enteric fistula, gastric obstruction, incisional hernia and retroperitoneal haemorrhage)

	Additional treatment	No. of patients	No. of deaths (%)	Hospitalization (days)	Postoperative complications	Re-operation
Becker et al (1984)	Drainage	62	25 (40%)		80%	31%
Warshaw & Jin (1985)	Multiple suction drainage	45	11 (24%)*	49	84%	27%
Bradley (1987)	Open packing	28	3 (11%)	46	4–36%	100%

* In a later part of the study only one of 19 (5%) patients died

intervention (Gerzof et al 1981, van Sonnenberg et al 1984, 1985, Freeny et al 1988, Pederzoli et al 1990). However, this method cannot guarantee complete removal of necrotic areas and every second patient in the series reported by van Sonnenberg et al (1984, 1985) had to be operated upon subsequently as the removal of necrotic tissue and bacterially contaminated necroses proved to be inadequate.

Late complications after necrosectomy

The evolution of pancreatic damage during acute pancreatitis has not been adequately investigated to date although a few studies have examined functional recovery of the exocrine pancreas after acute pancreatitis. In man, exocrine function appears to be impaired in the initial phase following onset of the attack (Mitchell et al 1983), although some authors have reported increased pancreatic secretion in two-thirds of patients during acute pancreatitis (Regan et al 1981). Other reports on exocrine and endocrine function and its relationship to morphological changes after severe acute pancreatitis have been conflicting (Angelini et al 1984, Büchler et al 1987b).

There are two major problems in objective assessment of the pancreatic functional state after acute pancreatitis. Firstly, there is no possibility of investigating a patient before the acute attack so that the pre-existing functional state of the organ is unknown; this is particularly important in alcoholic patients. Secondly, it is difficult to distinguish between changes due to acute pancreatitis, those due to chronic pancreatitis, and those that may be due to ageing.

With regard to later exocrine pancreatic function, 80% (16 out of 20) of our patients showed abnormal results within 4 months of an attack of necrotizing pancreatitis. There was no change in the proportion with abnormal function in the period between 5 and 12 months, but after that time exocrine function recovered in a number of patients (Table 22.10). Half of the patients with necrotizing pancreatitis developed subclinical or overt diabetes mellitus within 4 months, a rate which did not change significantly thereafter. There was a significantly greater number of patients with abnormal exocrine and endocrine function after alcohol-induced pancreatitis than

after gallstone-induced pancreatitis (Büchler et al 1987b). Diabetes mellitus developed twice as often in patients with extensive necrosis (subtotal or total pancreatic necrosis) as in patients with focal necrosis, less than 30% of whom developed diabetes.

In contrast to the general opinion that full recovery is routine after acute pancreatitis, about two-thirds of the patients have impairment of endocrine and exocrine function, as well as morphological changes in the gland, after necrotizing pancreatitis.

SUMMARY

The most important diagnostic step in the management of patients with acute pancreatitis is the discrimination between interstitial-oedematous and necrotizing forms of the disease. Indicators of necrosis, such as C-reactive protein, PMN-elastase and LDH, are easy to monitor, and may be helpful in detecting patients who have or who are developing necrotizing acute pancreatitis. Contrast-enhanced CT scanning can then define the exact extent of pancreatic and extrapancreatic necrosis and fine-needle aspiration of necrotic fluid and tissue should be undertaken to obtain material for bacteriological examination.

Surgical decision-making in necrotizing pancreatitis should be based on clinical, bacteriological (fine-needle aspiration), and contrast-enhanced CT scan data. Generally, patients with focal pancreatic necrosis respond well to medical and intensive care treatment and do not need surgical intervention. Extended pancreatic necrosis (subtotal or total pancreatic necrosis) and/or extrapancreatic fatty tissue necrosis, especially when infected, needs surgical management. In patients with proven necrotizing pancreatitis, the decision regarding the need for surgery and its timing must also be based on clinical criteria and has to be individualized. Systemic or local organ complications which present or worsen despite a minimum of 3–5 days of intensive care treatment, are also indications for surgical management.

Major pancreatic resection in the management of necrotizing pancreatitis represents overtreatment, and is accompanied by high morbidity and mortality rates. Resectional treatment may however become necessary in the rare event of total pancreatic necrosis but is unlikely to be successful in this extreme circumstance. The surgeon should always keep in mind that at operation it is easy to misjudge necrosis as total, especially if he is not aware of the morphology of the entire pancreas as defined by preoperative contrast-enhanced CT scanning. Drainage procedures alone, drainage combined with necrosectomy, and peritoneal lavage alone are now, in our view, obsolete methods of management. Carefully performed necrosectomy or debridement with continuous or repeated elimination of necrotic tissue, bacteria and biologically

Table 22.10 Incidence of abnormal findings in pancreatic function studies performed at varying intervals after an attack of necrotizing acute pancreatitis

Interval (months)	Proportion of patients with abnormal result	
	Exocrine function	Endocrine function
2–4	16/20 (80%)	11/22 (50%)
5–12	22/28 (79%)	9/21 (43%)
13–40	21/36 (58%)	14/30 (45%)

active compounds have proved very effective in experienced treatment centres. Necrosectomy with postoperative closed continuous lavage now represents a well-characterized, safe and atraumatic procedure resulting in hospital mortality rates of less than 10% in necrotizing pancreatitis.

REFERENCES

Aldridge M C, Ornstein M, Glazer G 1985 Pancreatic resection for severe acute pancreatitis. British Journal of Surgery 72: 796–800

Alexandre J H, Guerreri M T 1981 Role of total pancreatectomy in the treatment of necrotizing pancreatitis. World Journal of Surgery 5: 376–377

Allardyce D B 1987 Incidence of necrotizing pancreatitis and factors related to mortality. American Journal of Surgery 154: 259–299

Angelini G, Pederzoli P, Caliari S 1984 Long-term outcome of acute necrohemorrhagic pancreatitis. Digestion 30: 131–137

Balthazar E J 1989 CT diagnosis and staging of acute pancreatitis. Radiologic Clinics of North America 27: 19–37

Bank S, Wise L, Gerstein M 1983 Risk factors in acute pancreatitis. American Journal of Gastroenterology 78: 637–640

Becker V, 1981 Pathological anatomy and pathogenesis of acute pancreatitis. World Journal of Surgery. 5: 303–313

Becker J M, Pamberton J H, Di Magno E P 1984 Prognostic factors in pancreatic abscess. Surgery 96: 455–460

Beger H G, Büchler M 1986 Decision-making in surgical treatment of acute pancreatitis: operative or conservative management of necrotizing pancreatitis. Theoretical Surgery 1: 61–68

Beger H G, Uhl W 1990 Severe acute pancreatitis: II: The surgical approach. Clinical Intensive Care 1: 223–227

Beger H G, Krautzberger W, Bittner R 1985 Results of surgical treatment of necrotizing pancreatitis. World Journal of Surgery 90: 972–979

Beger H G, Bittner R, Büchler M 1986 Hemodynamic data pattern in patients with acute pancreatitis. Gastroenterology 90: 74–79

Beger H G, Krautzberger W, Bittner R 1986 Bacterial contamination of pancreatic necrosis. A prospective clinical study. Gastroenterology 91: 433–438

Beger H G, Büchler M, Bittner R 1988 Necrosectomy and postoperative local lavage in necrotizing pancreatitis. British Journal of Surgery. 75: 207–221

Bittner R, Block S, Büchler M 1987 Pancreatic abscess and infected pancreatic necrosis different local septic complications in acute pancreatitis. Digestive Diseases and Sciences 32: 1082–1087

Block S, Maier W, Clausen C 1986. Identification of pancreas necrosis in severe acute pancreatitis. Gut 27: 1035–1087

Bolooki H, Gliedman M L 1978 Peritoneal dialysis in the treatment of acute pancreatitis. Surgery 64: 466–471

Bradley E L III (ed) 1982 Complications of pancreatitis. Medical and surgical management. W B Saunders, Philadelphia

Bradley E L III 1987 Management of infected pancreatic necrosis by open drainage. Annals of Surgery 206: 542–550

Büchler M 1991 Severity staging of acute pancreatitis. Hepatogastroenterology 38: 101–108

Büchler M, Malfertheiner P, Schoetensack C 1986 Sensitivity of antiproteases, complement factors and C-reactive protein in detecting pancreatic necrosis. Results of a prospective clinical study. International Journal of Pancreatology 1: 227–235

Büchler M, Uhl W, Malfertheiner P, 1987a. Biochemical staging of acute pancreatitis. In: Beger H G, Büchler M (eds) Acute pancreatitis: research and clinical management. Springer-Verlag, Heidelberg p 144–153

Büchler M, Haucke A, Malfertheiner P, 1987b Follow up after acute pancreatitis: morphology and function. In: Beger H G, Büchler M (eds) Acute pancreatitis: research and clinical management. Springer-Verlag, Heidelberg p 367–374

Büchler M, Malfertheiner P, Uhl W, Beger H G 1988 Conservative treatment of necrotizing pancreatitis in patients with minor pancreatic necrosis. Pancreas 3: 592

Corfield A P, Copper M J, Williamson R C N 1985 Prediction of severity in acute pancreatitis: prospective comparison of three prognostic indices. Lancet 2: 403–407

Edelmann G, Boutelier P 1974 Le traitement des pancréatites aigues nécrosantes par l'ablation chirurgicale précoce des portions nécrosées. Chirurgie 100: 155–167

Fitz R H 1889 Acute pancreatitis: a consideration of pancreatic hemorrhage, hemorrhagic suppurative and gangrenous pancreatitis and of disseminated fat necrosis. Boston Medical and Surgical Journal 120: 181–187

Freeny P C, Lewis G P, Traverso L W, Ryan J A 1988 Infected pancreatic fluid collections: percutaneous catheter drainage. Radiology 167: 435–441

Gebhardt C 1981 Chirurgische Therapie der akuten Pankreatitis. In: Gebhardt C (ed) Chirurgie des exokrinen Pankreas. Georg Thieme Verlag, Stuttgart, 48–68

Gerzof S G, Robbins A J, Johnson W C 1981 Percutaneous catheter drainage of abdominal abscess: a five-year experience. New England Journal of Medicine. 29: 950

Gerzof S G, Banks P A, Robbins A H 1984 Role of guided percutaneous aspiration in early diagnosis of pancreatic sepsis. Digestive Diseases and Sciences 29: 950

Gerzof S G, Banks P A, Robbins A H 1987 Early diagnosis of pancreatic infection by computed tomography-guided aspiration. Gastroenterology 93: 1315–1320

Goebell H, Singer M V 1987 Acute pancreatitis: standards of conservative treatment. In: Beger H G, Büchler M (eds) Acute pancreatitis. Research and clinical management. Springer-Verlag, p 259–265

Hollender L F, Meyer C, Marrie A 1981 Role of surgery in the management of acute pancreatitis. World Journal Surgery 5: 361–368

Ihse I, Evander A, Gustafson I 1982 A controlled randomized study on the value of peritoneal lavage in acute pancreatitis. In: Hollender L F (ed) Controversies in acute pancreatitis. Springer-Verlag, Berlin, p 200–222

Kivilaakso E, Fräki O, Nikki P, Lempinen M 1981 Resection of the pancreas for acute fulminant pancreatitis. Surgery, Gynecology and Obstetrics 152: 493–498

Kivilaakso E, Lempinen M, Mäkeläinen A 1984 Pancreatic resection versus peritoneal lavation for acute fulminant pancreatitis. Annals of Surgery 199: 426–431

Kivisaari L, Somer K, Standertskjöld-Nordenstam C G 1984 A new method for the diagnosis of acute hemorrhagic necrotising pancreatitis using contrast-enhanced CT. Gastrointestinal Radiology 9: 27–30

Knol J A, Eckhauser F E, Strodel W E 1984 Surgical treatment of necrotizing pancreatitis by marsupialization. American Surgeon 50: 324–328

Kümmerle F, Neher M 1981 Management of complications after operations for acute pancreatitis. World Journal of Surgery 5: 387–392

Larvin M, Chalmers A G, Robinson P J, McMahon M J 1989 Debridement and closed cavity irrigation for the treatment of pancreatic necrosis. British Journal of Surgery 76: 465–471

Lasson A, Balldin G, Genell S, Ohlsson K 1984 Peritoneal lavage in severe acute pancreatitis. Acta Chirurgica Scandinavica 150: 479–484

Lawson D W, Daggett W M, Civetta J M 1970 Surgical treatment of acute necrotizing pancreatitis. Annals of Surgery 172: 605–616

Leger L, Chiche B, Ghouti A, Lovel A 1978 Pancréatites aigués nécrose capsulaire superficielle et atteinte parenchymateuse. Journal de Chirurgie (Paris) 115: 65–70

Mayer A D, McMahon M J, Corfield A P 1984 C-reactive protein: an aid to assessment and monitoring of acute pancreatitis: Journal of Clinical Pathology 37: 207–211

Mayer A D, McMahon M J, Corfield A P 1985 Controlled clinical trial of peritoneal lavage for the treatment of severe acute pancreatitis. New England Journal of Medicine 312: 399–404

McCarthy M C, Dickermann R M 1982 Surgical management of severe acute pancreatitis. Archives of Surgery 117: 476–480

McMahon M J, Bowen M, Mayer A D, Cooper E H 1984 Relationship of α_2-macroglobulin and other antiproteases to the clinical features of acute pancreatitis. American Journal of Surgery 147: 164–169

Mercadier M 1981 Surgical treatment of acute pancreatitis: tactics, techniques, and results. World Journal of Surgery 5: 393–400

Mitchell C J, Playforth M J, Kelleher J, McMahon M J 1983 Functional recovery of the exocrine pancreas after acute pancreatitis. Scandinavian Journal of Gastroenterology 18: 5–8

Pederzoli P, Bassi C, Vesentini S, Girelli R 1990 Retroperitoneal and peritoneal drainage and lavage in the treatment of severe necrotizing pancreatitis. Surgery, Gynecology and Obstetrics 170: 197–203

Poston G J, Williamson R C N 1990 Surgical management of acute pancreatitis. British Journal of Surgery 77: 5–12

Puolakkainen P, Valtanen V, Paananen A, Schröder T 1987 C-reactive protein and serum phospholipase A_2 in the assessment of severity of acute pancreatitis. Gut 28: 764–771

Ranson J H C 1981 Conservative surgical treatment of acute pancreatitis. World Journal of Surgery 5: 351–359

Ranson J H C 1986 Acute pancreatitis: surgical management. In Go V L W et al (eds) The exocrine pancreas: biology, pathology, and diseases. Raven Press, New York, p 503–511

Ranson J H C, Rifkind K M, Roses D F 1974 Prognostic signs and the role of operative management in acute pancreatitis. Surgery, Gynecology and Obstetrics 139: 69–81

Regan P T, Malagelada J R, Go V L W 1981 A prospective study of the antisecretory and therapeutic effects of cimetidine and glucagon in human acute pancreatitis. Mayo Clinic Proceedings 56: 499–503

Singer M V, Gyr K, Sarles H 1985 Revised classification of pancreatitis. Gastroenterology 89: 683–685

Steiner E, Mueller P R, Hahn P F 1988 Complicated pancreatic abscesses: problems in interventional management. Radiology 167: 443–446

Stone H H, Strom P R, Mullins R J 1984 Pancreatic abscess management by subtotal resection and packing. World Journal of Surgery 8: 340–345

Teichmann W, Wittmann D H, Andeone P A 1986 Scheduled reoperations (Etappenlavage) for diffuse peritonitis. Archives of Surgery 121: 147–152

Trapnell J E, Anderson M C 1986 Role of early laparotomy in acute pancreatitis. Annals of Surgery 165: 49–55

Uhl W, Büchler M, Nevalainen T J 1991 PMN-elastase in comparison with CRP, antiproteases and LDH as indicators of necrosis in human acute pancreatitis. Pancreas 6: 253–259

Van Sonnenberg E, Wing V W, Casola G 1984 Temporizing effect of percutaneous drainage of complicated abscesses in critically ill patients. American Journal of Radiology 142: 821–826

Van Sonnenberg E, Wittich G R, Casola G 1985 Complicated pancreatic inflammatory disease: diagnostic and therapeutic role of interventional radiology. Radiology 155: 335–340

Wall A J 1965 Peritoneal dialysis in the treatment of severe acute pancreatitis. Medical Journal of Australia 2: 281–287

Warshaw A L 1974 Inflammatory masses following acute pancreatitis. Surgical Clinics of North America 54: 620–637

Warshaw A L 1980 A guide to pancreatitis. Comprehensive Therapy 6: 49–55

Warshaw A L, Jin G 1985 Improved survival in 45 patients with pancreatic abscess. Annals of Surgery 202: 408–417

Warshaw A, Lee K 1979 Serum ribonuclease elevations and pancreatic necrosis in acute pancreatitis. Surgery 86: 227–232

Watermann N G, Walsky R S, Kasdan M L 1968 The treatment of acute hemorrhagic pancreatitis by sump drainage. Surgery, Gynecology and Obstetrics 126: 963–974

Wayand W, Waclawiczek H W 1985 The treatment of acute necrotizing pancreatitis, using a mediastinoscope postoperatively and antiseptic rinses. Journal of Hospital Infection 6: 93–95

Wertheimer M D, Norris C S 1986 Surgical management of necrotizing pancreatitis. Archives of Surgery 121: 484–487

Wittmann D H, Aprahamian C H, Bergstein J M 1990 Etappenlavage: advanced diffuse peritonitis managed by planned multiple laparotomies utilizing zippers, slide fastener, and velcro analogue for temporary abdominal closure. World Journal of Surgery 14: 218–226

23. Complications of acute pancreatitis and their management

E. L. Bradley   K. A. Allen

INTRODUCTION

As a result of widespread improvements in supportive and intensive care, recovery from acute pancreatitis has become the rule rather than the exception. In fact, three out of every four patients with acute pancreatitis will recover with supportive therapy alone. Unfortunately, however, the fourth will suffer a complication of acute pancreatitis, and will stand a one-in-three chance of dying from the complication. In effect, this observation serves to focus our therapeutic attention on the recognition and management of the complications of acute pancreatitis.

Systemic complications of acute pancreatitis, such as acute respiratory distress syndrome, renal insufficiency, encephalopathy, and various coagulopathies have been well covered elsewhere (Allen & Bradley 1990; see also Ch. 20), and will not be considered further in this discussion. In contrast to such remote developments, local or regional complications of pancreatitis account for the majority of instances of surgical interest.

PANCREATIC NECROSIS

Primarily as a result of systematic pancreatic resection for acute pancreatitis in several European centres (Hollender et al 1981, Beger et al 1985), a wealth of histological information regarding severe acute pancreatitis has been obtained. We now know that the clinical course of a patient with acute pancreatitis principally reflects the presence and extent of pancreatic necrosis (Beger et al 1985). As a result, clinicopathological correlation has now become established as a cornerstone for successful management of patients with acute pancreatitis.

In a prospective study from our institution using dynamic pancreatography as the standard for detection of necrotizing pancreatitis, we found that pancreatic necrosis developed in 38 of 194 patients (19.5%) admitted with acute pancreatitis (Bradley & Allen 1991). In an earlier retrospective study, Büchler and his co-workers (1988)

estimated that pancreatic necrosis was present in 20% of their patients admitted with acute pancreatitis. As a consequence of these combined observations, it seems reasonable to propose that pancreatic necrosis develops in approximately one patient in five requiring admission for acute pancreatitis.

Sterile necrosis

Little attention has been paid to the natural history of pancreatic necrosis, perhaps because a positive tissue diagnosis of necrosis could previously be obtained only by surgical intervention. Today, given that the overall accuracy rate for dynamic pancreatography in detecting pancreatic necrosis has been shown to exceed 90% (Maier 1987, Bradley et al 1989, Larvin et al 1990), information regarding the natural history of pancreatic necrosis has become available (Fig. 23.1). While the mere presence of pancreatic necrosis has previously been considered to be a sufficient indication for surgical resection in some centres (Alexandre & Guerrieri 1981, Aldridge et al 1985, Beger et al 1985), others have begun to question the wisdom of this ablative approach (Smadja & Bismuth 1986). Teerenhovi and his associates (1988) were unable to demonstrate any retrospective benefit from resection of sterile pancreatic necrosis in 84 patients with acute pancreatitis and associated organ failure. In 11 consecutive patients with sterile pancreatic necrosis documented by dynamic pancreatography and transcutaneous aspiration cultures, a prospective policy of supportive management was successful in each case, including six patients with pulmonary or renal insufficiency (Bradley & Allen 1991). Accordingly, it would seem clear that sterile pancreatic necrosis, even when associated with co-existing organ failure, can no longer be considered a pressing indication for surgical intervention. While these observations seem to contradict the 'commonsense' surgical dictum that necrotic tissue should be removed whenever and wherever recognized, necrotic tissues in other organ systems are not always resected. Consider for a moment that infarcted

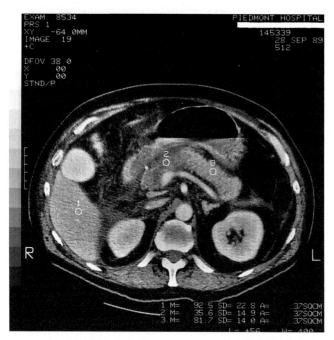

Fig. 23.1 Dynamic pancreatogram in a patient with necrotizing pancreatitis following endoscopic retrograde cholangiopancreatography. Following an intravenous contrast load, liver (1 m = 92.5 Hounsfield units) and tail of pancreas (3 m = 81.7 Hounsfield units) are approximately equal in density. Head of pancreas (2 m = 35.6 Hounsfield units) does not enhance. Pancreatic necrosis involving the cephalic portion of the pancreas was found at surgery.

tissue in the heart, brain, and lung are most often left to heal by secondary fibrosis.

In our experience with the conservative management of sterile pancreatic necrosis, the clinical course has varied from uncomplicated healing by fibrosis, to pseudocyst formation, and even to secondary infection, resulting in infected pancreatic necrosis. It would appear that the frequency with which secondary infection develops in patients with pancreatic necrosis is of the order of 40–70% (Beger et al 1986, Bradley & Allen 1991).

Infected pancreatic necrosis

The development of infection in pre-existing pancreatic necrosis represents a quantum leap in mortality risk. Mortality rates for patients with infected pancreatic necrosis are at least three times the risk for patients with sterile necrosis (Machado et al 1986, Allardyce 1987, Bittner et al 1987, Pederzoli et al 1989). Moreover, fully 80% of patients dying from acute pancreatitis today will die as a result of secondary infection (Buggy & Nostrant 1983, Renner et al 1985). Accordingly, any efforts directed at reducing the mortality rate in acute pancreatitis must directly address the issue of secondary infection.

Primary pancreatic infections, those arising in a previously normal gland, are rare indeed. Primary infections usually consist of viral infections (Joe et al 1989), and other exotic uncommon infections, such as tuberculosis (Stambler et al 1982). Even less common are primary bacterial infections of the pancreas. Several anatomical and physiological features of the pancreas may contribute to the rarity of primary bacterial infections; these include the pancreatic duct sphincter, the higher pressure in the pancreatic ductal system, the epithelial barrier of the pancreatic duct, and the relative paucity of bacteria in the upper gastrointestinal tract due to gastric acidity. Furthermore, pancreatic juice itself appears to demonstrate intrinsic antibacterial activity (Rubinstein et al 1985). It is becoming increasingly apparent that bacterial infections can only occur following pre-existing injury to pancreatic tissues, and that such injuries occur most commonly after necrotizing pancreatitis.

The exact mechanism by which bacteria colonize the tissues injured by pancreatitis is unknown. However, recent work by a number of investigators suggests that host endogenous bacteria may be translocated to the necrotic tissues by a number of mechanisms such as transmural migration from the colon, the result of bacteraemia from distant sites, and defective phagocytosis (Wells et al 1987, Dietch 1990, Widdison et al 1990a).

Since the majority of bacteria resulting in secondary pancreatic infections are endogenous Gram negative organisms (Lumsden & Bradley 1990), there exists the intriguing possibility that secondary pancreatic infections could be prevented by the judicious administration of antibiotics. However, the precise role of prophylactic antibiotics in the prevention of secondary infections is currently unknown. Earlier prospective studies in patients with acute pancreatitis purporting to show no difference between placebo and antibiotic in secondary infection rates (Howes et al 1975, Finch et al 1976) used ampicillin, a drug which we now know does not cross the lipophilic 'blood–pancreas barrier' (Bradley 1989). Furthermore, these studies were conducted in patients with mild acute pancreatitis, suggesting that the degree of necrotizing pancreatitis required to permit the development of secondary pancreatic infection was not present. Although recent experimental studies suggest that prophylactic antibiotics may be useful in necrotizing pancreatitis (Widdison et al 1990b), randomized prospective studies of antibiotics known to cross the blood–pancreas barrier in patients with demonstrated pancreatic necrosis are urgently needed. Until such studies have clarified these issues and specific drugs have been identified, we have found the parenteral combination of ceftazidime and metronidazole useful. It remains to be seen whether the alternative concept of selective decontamination of the gut (administration of non-absorbable antibiotics to reduce endogenous gut flora) will prove to be a valuable adjunct to parenteral antibiotics, or will be shown to be of as much prophylactic use in sterile pancreatic necrosis as it appears to have been in preventing nosocomial pneumonia in intensive care unit patients.

From a clinical standpoint, the distinction in an individual case between the systemic inflammatory response to the presence of sterile pancreatic necrosis, and the systemic response to secondary bacterial infection of pancreatic necrosis can be exceedingly difficult to make, if not impossible (Sostre et al 1985, Block et al 1987). Since each condition may result in the clinical signs of 'toxaemia' (fever, leukocytosis, abdominal tenderness), and since sterile necrosis can often be successfully managed by conservative means, accurate clinical differentiation is mandatory for appropriate therapy. Fine-needle CT-guided transcutaneous aspiration (FNA) of non-enhancing pancreatic tissue for bacterial and fungal smears and culture has proved to be both safe and remarkably accurate in distinguishing between sterile and infected pancreatic necrosis (Gerzof et al 1987, Banks et al 1990) (Fig. 23.2). Currently, in order to recognize that secondary infection has developed, we recommend that FNA should be undertaken in all patients with demonstrated pancreatic necrosis and signs of clinical sepsis which persist after 1 week of maximal supportive treatment.

Once the diagnosis of infected pancreatic necrosis is made, operative debridement and drainage is mandatory. Infected pancreatic necrosis is virtually 100% fatal without drainage (Frey et al 1979), and attempts at transcutaneous radiological drainage of infected pancreatic necrosis have proved to be remarkably unsuccessful (Bittner et al 1987, Gerzof et al 1987, Steiner et al 1988, Adams et al 1990). The tenacious, particulate nature of infected pancreatic necrosis defies percutaneous drainage through

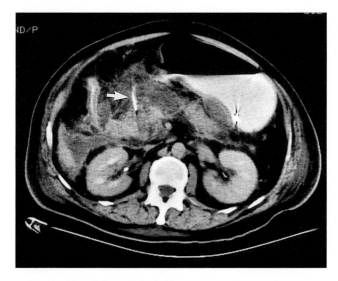

Fig. 23.2 Fine-needle aspiration (arrow) for bacterial smear and culture in a patient with pancreatic necrosis demonstrated by dynamic pancreatogram, who continued to exhibit signs of 'toxaemia' 2 weeks after admission.

even relatively large bore transcutaneous catheters (Banks et al 1990).

While almost all workers agree that operative debridement of infected pancreatic necrosis is necessary, the actual form of drainage has become controversial. Given the observation that infected pancreatic necrosis often results in loss of integrity of the pancreatic ductal system (Bradley 1987) (Fig. 23.3), and that the digestion of the retroperitoneum by activated pancreatic proteases and lipases continues for as long as 2–3 weeks after initial surgical debridement (Beger et al 1988, Bradley 1991), the fact that necrotic material re-accumulates in the retroperitoneum following surgical debridement in patients with extensive infected necrosis should not be surprising. It is precisely this feature of progressive re-accumulation of necrotic tissue which separates infected pancreatic necrosis from all other forms of infections that the surgeon is called upon to treat. No doubt the persistent nature of pancreatic infections occurring in necrotizing pancreatitis accounts for the comparatively high operative mortality rates when conventional drainage systems are used. In fact, in an extensive review of the literature involving more than 1200 cases of secondary pancreatic infection, operative debridement of infected pancreatic necrosis combined with conventional drainage led to death in 30–60% of cases, and more than three-quarters of postoperative deaths were due to persistent or recurrent infection (Lumsden & Bradley 1990).

Although even today conventional closed drainage continues to have its advocates (Warshaw 1987), two forms of continuous active drainage have emerged as preferable surgical techniques. The first involves initial surgical debridement and packing, with re-laparotomy and re-debridement every 2–3 days until granulation tissue develops in the retroperitoneal tissues (Pemberton et al 1986, Waclawiczeck et al 1986, Wertheimer & Norris 1986, Bradley 1987, Stanten & Frey 1990). While the actual technical details vary somewhat between the investigators, the underlying principle is similar; periodic re-debridement is continued until the progressive necrotic process is controlled, and no further evidence of infection is present. Beginning with this approach in 1976, we have to date treated 73 patients with proven infected pancreatic necrosis by this technique, with a current overall mortality rate of 14%.

The second approach to continuous removal of re-accumulated infected necrotic tissue has been that of surgical debridement followed by continuous high volume lesser sac lavage through large bore catheters placed at the time of surgery (see Ch. 22). Mortality rates attributed to this approach range from 14–28% (Beger et al 1988, Nicholson et al 1988, Larvin et al 1989, Pederzoli et al 1990). Whether this approach will achieve mortality rates comparable to relaparotomy remains to be demonstrated. In a prospective study of 24 patients under-

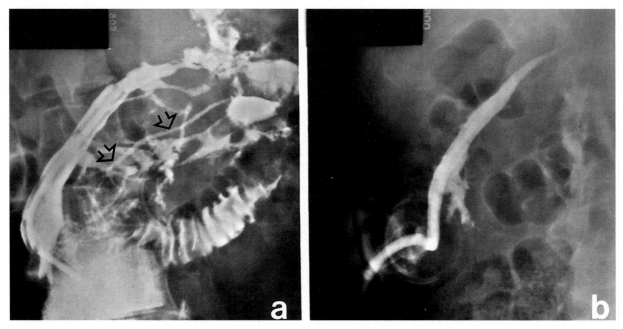

Fig. 23.3   Fistulogram through a drainage tube 3 weeks after initial surgical debridement and open drainage of infected pancreatic necrosis limited to the head of the pancreas. **A** Note the scattered pockets of contrast still remaining, the connection with the duodenum (present on transfer), and the loss of integrity of the proximal pancreatic duct (arrows). **B** One month later, duodenal and pancreatic duct fistulas have closed spontaneously.

going surgical debridement, with subsequent randomization to conventional drainage or prolonged lesser sac lavage, Teerenhovi and his associates (1989) found no demonstrable clinical benefits associated with lavage. Perhaps even more importantly, they noted a 36% mortality rate in patients managed by lesser sac lavage, as compared to 17% in the conventional drainage group. Clearly, many of these surgical issues will require prospective study before the optimal approach to continuous drainage of infected pancreatic necrosis can be determined.

ACUTE PSEUDOCYSTS

By definition, an acute pseudocyst is an effusion of pancreatic juice which arises in conjunction with an episode of acute pancreatitis, and which is less than 6 weeks old (Bradley et al 1976). Acute pseudocysts must be differentiated from non-specific peripancreatic fluid collections which can be imaged in over 50% of patients with acute pancreatitis (Gonzalez et al 1976). Acute pseudocysts presumably arise in patients with acute pancreatitis from loss of pancreatic duct integrity as a result of necrosis of ductular tissues. Unlike chronic pseudocysts (pseudocysts older than 6 weeks), acute pseudocysts will resolve spontaneously in approximately one-half of cases (Bradley et al 1979) (Fig. 23.4). Furthermore, complications common to chronic pseudocysts occur infrequently with acute pseudocysts (Bradley & Clements 1974, Crass & Way 1981).

Historically, the diagnosis of an acute pseudocyst in a patient with pancreatitis is suspected when signs and symptoms of pancreatic inflammation (notably pain, nausea, vomiting and fever) continue beyond 7 days, when an abdominal mass develops, or when there is persistent hyperamylasaemia. Clinical suspicion that an individual episode of acute pancreatitis has become complicated by a pseudocyst is best confirmed by CT (Foley et al 1980). Once an uncomplicated acute pseudocyst is initially identified by CT, the subsequent course is best followed by serial ultrasonography (Silverstein et al 1981). The collection is found most often in the lesser sac or left anterior pararenal space, but any area of the retroperitoneum may be involved and fluid tracking upwards can, on occasion, cause pseudocyst formation in the mediastinum.

Considering their demonstrated propensity for spontaneous resolution, and in view of their low complication rate, acute pseudocysts can be managed expectantly in the first instance. Surgical intervention is usually restricted to the infrequent case of development of a complication, such as infection, obstruction, rupture, or haemorrhage.

The diagnosis of secondary infection complicating an acute pseudocyst can be difficult. As we have noted, clinical parameters suggestive of sepsis, such as tachycardia, fever, leukocytosis, and abdominal tenderness, often occur in severe acute pancreatitis without infection (Sostre et al 1985, Block et al 1987). When, however, the clinical picture is correlated with CT findings which suggest that a cystic structure is present, diagnosis of secondary in-

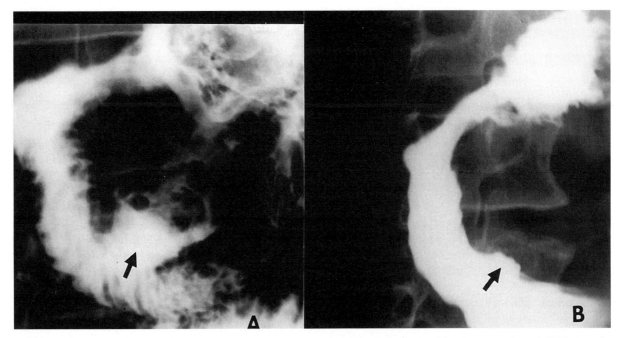

Fig. 23.4   **A** Spontaneous rupture of an acute pancreatic pseudocyst into the third portion of the duodenum (arrow). **B** Two weeks later the fistula (arrow) has been obliterated.

fection can be confirmed by transcutaneous CT-directed fine-needle aspiration for smear and culture (Gerzof et al 1987). If percutaneous aspiration bacteriological testing of the cystic lesion is positive, and dynamic pancreatography fails to demonstrate any associated pancreatic necrosis, then the lesion is likely to be an infected acute pseudocyst.

As opposed to infected necrosis, infected acute pseudocysts can frequently be managed successfully by CT-guided percutaneous drainage (van Sonnenberg et al 1989). In general, infected acute pseudocysts are more effectively managed by percutaneous drainage than their non-infected counterparts, as there is anxiety regarding the risk of introducing infection into previously uninfected collections (Gerzof et al 1984, van Sonnenberg et al 1985, Torres et al 1986).

The space-occupying nature of acute pseudocysts may occasionally result in gastrointestinal (Bradley 1982a) or biliary obstruction (Bradley 1982b) (Fig. 23.5). In the absence of other complicating factors, observation is prudent, in anticipation of spontaneous resolution of the obstruction associated with spontaneous resolution of the acute pseudocyst. Persistent biliary or gastrointestinal obstruction caused by an acute pseudocyst may be effectively relieved by percutaneous CT-directed catheter drainage of the pseudocyst (van Sonnenberg et al 1985).

Regardless of whether external drainage is performed radiologically or surgically, persistent communication between the acute pseudocyst and the pancreatic duct will result in an external pancreatic fistula. Premature

removal of the drainage catheter in the face of a pancreatic fistula may result in re-accumulation of the pseudocyst. The drainage catheter can be safely removed when serial fistulograms through the catheter no longer

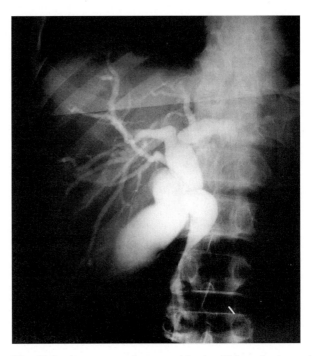

Fig. 23.5   An acute pseudocyst resulting in a high grade obstruction of the common duct. (Reproduced with permission from Bradley E L III (ed) Complications of pancreatitis, 1982, W B Saunders, Philadelphia.)

demonstrate ductal communication, and when the pseudocyst cavity has been obliterated. Somatostatin analogues may prove to have value in hastening the obliteration of pseudocysts and external pancreatic fistulas.

In general, acute pseudocysts which are secondarily infected, and complicated pseudocysts in poor surgical candidates, can be treated initially by percutaneous catheter drainage. Patients with non-infected pseudocysts who are good surgical candidates should still be treated by traditional methods until such time as prospective randomized trials demonstrate the efficacy and safety of percutaneous catheter drainage techniques. However, it does seem likely that percutaneous drainage may be used as the intial approach to all complicated pseudocysts in the future. It remains to be seen whether endoscopic drainage techniques (endoscopic cystgastrostomy and endoscopic cystduodenostomy, see Ch. 10) will find a place in the therapy of acute pseudocysts, but the early results in patients with chronic pancreatitis suggest that this approach may allow safe internal drainage provided that the pseudocyst is actually indenting the gut lumen (Kozarek et al 1985, Sahel et al 1987). Kozarek et al (1991) have recently described the transpapillary placement of stents to bridge disrupted pancreatic ducts in patients with peripancreatic fluid collections, but the place of this technique is as yet uncertain.

The traditional surgical approach to pancreatic pseudocysts has been internal drainage into the stomach, jejunum or duodenum. Resection of the affected part of the pancreas including the pseudocyst represents another option but although it has a low cyst recurrence rate, it is a more major undertaking and is less frequently performed. Internal drainage requires a mature cyst wall that will hold sutures and it is generally held that 4–6 weeks are needed for the wall of the pseudocyst to mature to this degree. This means that external drainage may be needed if at surgery the cyst wall is found not to be mature or if there is gross infection of the contents, bleeding or free rupture into the peritoneal cavity. External drainage is associated with a complication rate and mortality rate that are about twice as great as those attending internal drainage (see below). When internal drainage is performed, the choice of procedure depends on the circumstances. Mature collections adherent to the stomach are best dealt with by cystgastrostomy, creating a stoma between the posterior gastric wall and the anterior aspect of the pseudocyst. An ellipse of the pseudocyst wall is routinely sent for frozen section analysis as it is always necessary to exclude the presence of a cystic neoplasm when dealing with what is believed to be a pancreatic cyst or pseudocyst. Bleeding from the stoma must be avoided by inserting closely spaced, interrupted sutures of non-absorbable material around the stoma margin.

Large lesser sac collections may be unsuitable for drainage into the stomach if a large dependent sump will be left below the level of the stoma. Such giant collections and pseudocysts arising in association with the distal pancreas are usually best dealt with by drainage into a Roux loop of jejunum. Occasionally, pseudocysts in the region of the head of the pancreas will be suitable for drainage into the duodenum, taking care to avoid injury to the common bile duct or the large vessels associated with the pancreatic head.

In series reporting the results of operative treatment of pancreatic pseudocysts, mortality rates have varied from 5–12%, while morbidity rates have varied from 21–53% with recurrence rates of 5–20% (Yeo et al 1990). In general, internal drainage has had a lower complication rate (around 33%) and mortality rate (5% or less) than external drainage, although this almost certainly reflects the fact that patients undergoing external drainage have been a group of higher risk patients with more complicated disease.

HAEMORRHAGE

Life-threatening haemorrhage into the gastrointestinal tract, retroperitoneum, or peritoneal cavity complicates acute pancreatitis in only 1–3% of patients (Marks et al 1967, Trapnell 1971). Unfortunately, this uncommon complication often results in a considerable escalation in risk, with an associated mortality rate of 50–80% (Stroud et al 1981, Frey et al 1982, Stabile et al 1983).

Stress ulceration

Haemorrhage from superficial mucosal erosions is common in patients with severe acute pancreatitis (Siler & Wulsin 1951, Thal et al 1951). As a result of improved techniques for resuscitation, when stress ulceration develops today in the course of severe acute pancreatitis, it most commonly coincides with the onset of sepsis (Frey et al 1982). Prophylactic use of H_2 blockers, antacids, or enteric mucosal protectants such as sucralfate, have been equally effective in reducing the incidence of stress-induced ulcer bleeding (Borrero et al 1985, Tryba et al 1985). Recent data, however, suggests that the risk of ventilator-associated pneumonia can be reduced by maintaining prophylaxis against stress ulceration with sucralfate rather than antacids or H_2 blockers (Dricks et al 1987). Surgical intervention for massive haemorrhage from stress ulceration is often fatal in these critically ill patients, and therefore, stress ulceration is a condition better prevented than treated.

Left-sided portal hypertension and variceal haemorrhage

Splenic vein thrombosis is an underdiagnosed complication of acute pancreatitis. While the exact incidence is unknown, data from two large autopsy series documented splenic vein thrombosis in approximately 15% of patients in whom death was attributed to acute pancreatitis (Renner et al 1985, Rogers & Klatt 1989). Left-sided segmental portal hypertension, a sequela of splenic vein thrombosis, may lead to the development of gastric (Little & Moossa 1981), oesophageal (Moossa & Gadd 1985), and even colonic (Burbidge et al 1978) varices. Although variceal haemorrhage associated with chronic, long-standing splenic vein thrombosis has been reported to occur in 30–70% of cases (Longstreth et al 1971, Salam et al 1973, Little & Moossa 1981), variceal haemorrhage during an episode of acute pancreatitis is rare.

At laparotomy, the absence of cirrhosis and the presence of a dilated gastroepiploic vein is pathognomonic of splenic vein occlusion. Recognition of splenic vein thrombosis is critical, since portosystemic shunts are contraindicated, and splenectomy is curative. Although prospective studies have not followed patients with asymptomatic splenic vein thrombosis, it may be prudent to consider prophylactic elective splenectomy in good risk patients with demonstrable gastroesophageal varices.

Vascular necrosis

Vascular necrosis resulting in haemorrhage is a rare but catastrophic complication of acute necrotizing pancreatitis. This dramatic complication is almost always associated with the development of a secondary pancreatic infection (Stroud et al 1981, Frey et al 1982, Waltman et al 1986). Peripancreatic and splanchnic arteries in contact with activated proteolytic enzymes and products of pancreatic suppuration frequently demonstrate arteritis and splitting of the internal elastic membrane (Rich & Duff 1936). These pathological changes may be manifested as either segmental vascular thrombosis or pseudoaneurysm formation, and presumably occur as a result of necrotic changes in the arterial wall. Unlike atherosclerotic splanchnic aneurysms, pancreatitis-related pseudoaneurysms appear to result from loss of nutritive flow to the arterial wall due to inflammatory thrombosis of the vasa vasorum.

The frequency of pseudoaneurysm formation in patients with pancreatitis has been estimated to be as high as 10% (White et al 1976). Arterial proximity to a septic or inflammatory focus appears to be the only prerequisite to the formation of pseudoaneurysms. In descending order of frequency, false aneurysms most commonly affect the splenic, gastroduodenal, pancreaticoduodenal, gastric and hepatic arteries (Stanley et al 1976, Eckhauser et al 1980).

Early utilization of contrast-enhanced computed tomography (Burke et al 1986) and duplex ultrasonography (Lim et al 1989) in severe acute pancreatitis may detect unsuspected pseudoaneurysms. Selective arteriography, however, remains the diagnostic gold standard for localizing

active bleeding secondary to vascular necrosis (Stabile et al 1983, Vugic 1989).

Haemorrhage resulting from erosive arteritis may follow several courses. While fatal haemorrhage from direct intraperitoneal rupture has been reported, indirect rupture into the gastrointestinal tract is the most common presentation (Frey et al 1982). Often patients will experience a series of intermittent, self-limiting, bleeding episodes ('herald bleeding'), which precede a final exsanguinating haemorrhage (Gadacz et al 1978, Steckman et al 1984). Haemorrhage can also occur into a pre-existing acute pseudocyst, with conversion of the acute pseudocyst to a pseudoaneurysm (Wolstenholme 1974, Wu et al 1977) (Fig. 23.6). The sudden development of a pulsatile abdominal mass, often associated with a bruit, and increased abdominal pain is a triad almost pathognomonic of intracystic haemorrhage (Bradley 1988). Rarely, a pseudoaneurysm may erode directly into the pancreatic duct with subsequent gastrointestinal haemorrhage by way of the ampulla (Bivens et al 1978, Cahow et al 1983). This syndrome has been called 'hemosuccus pancreaticus' (Sandblom 1970).

Traditionally, vascular complications of acute pancreatitis have been managed by surgical means. In the light of mortality rates of 25–53% with surgical management alone (Stanley et al 1976, Eckhauser et al 1980), some investigators have advocated angiographic embolization as primary therapy (Steckman et al 1984, Mandel et al 1987, Vugic 1989). While some enthusiasm for the angiographic approach to complicated pseudoaneurysms is justified, proper patient selection is mandatory. Failure to correct the frequently associated infected pancreatic necrosis will lead to a high rate of recurrent haemorrhage, since the erosive process will continue and infected arteritis may result (Waltman et al 1986).

If permitted by time and the patient's clinical condition, our initial approach to patients with acute pancreatitis and massive haemorrhage is to perform diagnostic angiography along with concomitant embolization of the offending artery, all as part of a preoperative evaluation. Angiographic embolization is considered to be definitive therapy only in selected patients in whom infected necrosis can be ruled out (Fig. 23.7). Even if initial arterial embolization is unsuccessful, intravascular balloon occlusion or vasopressin infusion may serve to control brisk bleeding until surgical therapy can be initiated (Vugic 1989).

When emergency surgical intervention for haemorrhage is required in patients without prior angiographic location and control, several paramount principles must be observed. Blood noted to be within the stomach is approached through a prepyloric longitudinal gastrotomy in search of duodenal, gastric, or variceal haemorrhage. If this manoeuvre is unhelpful, then 'hemosuccus pancreaticus' must be ruled out by visualization of the papilla

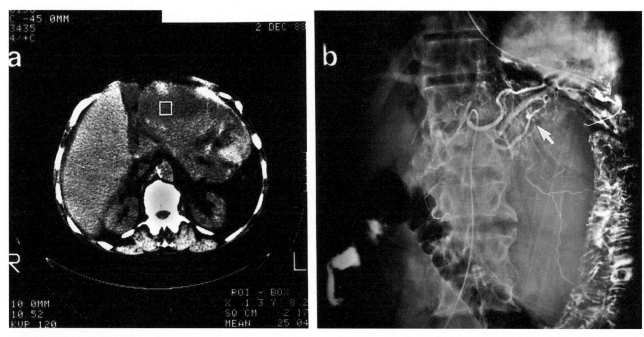

Fig. 23.6 Spontaneous haemorrhage into a pancreatic pseudocyst. **A** Large mass with relatively high density material (25 Hounsfield units). **B** Splenic arteriogram demonstrating pseudoaneurysm of the pancreatic magna (arrow) and large left upper quadrant intracystic haematoma.

of Vater. If the haemorrhage is coming from a pseudocyst or a pseudoaneurysm which has eroded into the gastro-intestinal tract, the offending vessel can often be identified by the location of the inflammatory mass. Masses within

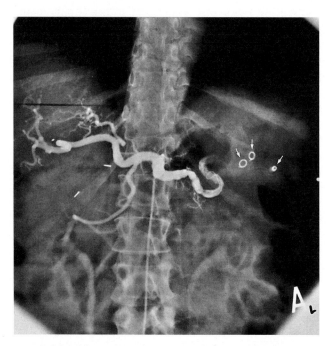

Fig. 23.7 Splenic artery embolization using coils for occlusion (arrows) in a poor risk patient with massive haemorrhage from a splenic pseudoaneurysm.

the head of the pancreas usually involve the gastro-duodenal or pancreaticoduodenal arteries, while the splenic artery is associated with masses in the body or tail of the pancreas. Initial treatment should consist of compression of the suspected vessel followed by ligation at its origin if local conditions permit. While definitive management of distal vascular lesions may be provided by distal pancreatectomy and splenectomy, proximal pancreatic resection is a formidable procedure in these precarious patients and is best avoided if at all possible.

Massive haemorrhage complicating acute pancreatitis is a diagnostic and therapeutic challenge with ominous prognostic implications. Initiation of early and definitive therapy is the cornerstone for successful management.

INTESTINAL COMPLICATIONS

Intestinal obstruction

The spectrum of enteric involvement in the process of acute pancreatitis is often unappreciated. At the simplest level, a self-limiting, regional paralytic ileus involving the contiguous duodenum, jejunum, and transverse colon is a common radiographic finding. Sentinel loop, a regional jejunal ileus frequently observed radiographically, is neither sensitive nor specific for acute pancreatitis (Stanely et al 1983). Colonic ileus confined to the transverse colon, and manifested by proximal dilatation and distal collapse (the 'colon cutoff' sign), is also an often-cited but non-specific finding in acute pancreatitis (Pierce 1956).

At the next level of involvement, reversible duodenal atony and mucosal oedema have been identified in 25% of patients with pancreatitis undergoing upper gastrointestinal studies. However, frank duodenal obstruction is rare (Bradley & Clements 1981). Unlike chronic pancreatitis, where fibrotic duodenal obstruction may require surgical intervention, idiopathic duodenal obstruction associated with acute pancreatitis can be expected to resolve with conservative management (Bradley & Clements 1981, Aranha et al 1984).

Mechanical small bowel obstruction rarely complicates acute pancreatitis. When present, however, mechanical small bowel obstruction is usually the result of adhesions secondary to peritoneal inflammation (Bradley 1982a).

Mechanical colonic obstruction occurring during acute pancreatitis, is also extremely uncommon. First described in 1927 (Forlini 1927), in an extensive 1982 review, only 34 reported cases of colonic obstruction due to inflammatory stenosis could be found (Bradley 1982a). The observed predilection for the transverse colon in 94% of reported cases is best explained by the spread of inflammatory pancreatic exudate between mesenteric leaves to the contiguous colon, which results in an inflammatory pericolitis (Bradley 1982a) (Fig. 23.8). Histologically, these inflammatory strictures demonstrate an inflammatory infiltrate, muscle destruction, and fibrosis similar to changes found in the analogous group of patients with idiopathic duodenal obstruction (Hancock et al 1973).

Surgical intervention is rarely required in patients with inflammatory stenosis and colonic pseudo-obstruction. Reports of spontaneous resolution of the pericolitis (and with it the resultant obstruction) speak in support of

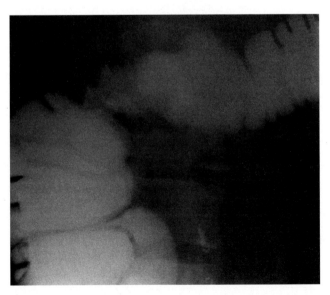

Fig. 23.8 Barium enema in a patient with acute pancreatitis and partial colonic obstruction. Note the inflammatory appearance of the stricture at the hepatic flexure. This inflammatory stricture resolved spontaneously.

conservative management (Bradley 1982a, Hudson & De Beer 1988). If conservative therapy must be abandoned because of persistent obstruction, proximal colostomy without any attempt at resection is the procedure of choice. Resection is indicated only when a colonic stricture persists following resolution of the acute inflammatory episode. Prior to any resection of a colonic obstruction in a patient with pancreatitis, endoscopic evaluation is essential since the mucosa is normal in these patients when an inflammatory stricture is present. Reliance upon barium studies alone may result in misdiagnosis of the lesion as a carcinoma (Hunt & Mildenhall 1975). Using these guidelines, it should be possible to reduce the 20% surgical mortality rate currently seen in patients with acute pancreatitis complicated by colonic obstruction (Hudson & De Beer 1988).

Intestinal necrosis

Intestinal necrosis is considered to be a rare complication of acute pancreatitis. In a 1982 review, only 33 reported cases could be found in the English literature (Bradley 1982a). Subsequently, perhaps an additional 60 cases have been reported (Kukora 1985, Schein et al 1985, Bouillot et al 1989). It is likely, however, that the actual frequency of intestinal necrosis in acute pancreatitis may be underestimated, since single cases of a recognized complication are seldom reported. The authors have personal knowledge of 11 unreported cases in the Southeastern United States alone.

The pathogenesis of intestinal necrosis in acute pancreatitis is unknown. Focal intestinal necrosis, often with an associated fistula, usually involves intestinal segments which are in close anatomical proximity to a localized septic complication, such as a pancreatic abscess or infected pancreatic necrosis (Bradley 1982a, Schein et al 1985) (Fig. 23.9). In cases with focal necrosis, enteric digestion by contiguous activated proteolytic and lipolytic enzymes is a possible mechanism for pathogenesis (Schroeder et al 1980, Dubnick et al 1985). Vascular thrombosis may be responsible for cases with more extensive segmental intestinal necrosis. Both arterial (Kukora 1985, Bouillot et al 1989, Nordback & Sisto 1989) and venous (Gatch & Brickley 1951, Collins et al 1968, Jensen & Bradley 1989) mesenteric thrombosis have been histologically documented in segments of necrotic intestine removed at surgery in patients with acute pancreatitis. Arterial thrombosis in patients with acute pancreatitis is a common arteriographic finding (Reuter et al 1969). A vasculitis induced by adjacent perivascular vasoactive substances, cytotoxic enzymes, and pancreatic suppuration is a likely candidate mechanism responsible for segmental mesenteric vascular occlusion.

The site of visceral infarction appears to be primarily determined by anatomical peritoneal reflections (Meyer &

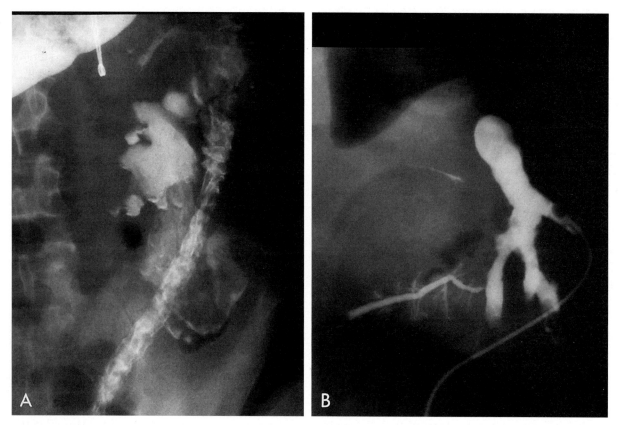

Fig. 23.9 **A** Segmental necrosis of the splenic flexure of the colon with a large retrocolic abscess in a patient with acute pancreatitis. **B** A fistulogram 2 weeks after proximal colostomy and surgical drainage demonstrating connection of the cavity to the main pancreatic duct. (Reproduced with permission from Bradley E L III (ed) Complications of pancreatitis, 1982, W B Saunders, Philadelphia.)

Evans 1976) (Fig. 23.10). Inflammatory pancreatic exudate can diffuse between mesenteric leaves with direct access to the transverse colon, duodenum, and the small bowel. Furthermore, it is likely that anatomical continuity of the pancreas with the base of the mesocolon and the root of the small bowel mesentery may potentiate segmental vascular occlusion.

Enteric necrosis, which is anatomically remote from sites of pancreatic inflammation, is less easily explained. Segmental intestinal infarction of the small bowel has been reported in four cases associated with acute pancreatitis, in which the afflicted segment of bowel was anatomically remote from the pancreatic inflammatory process (Collins et al 1968, Griffith & Brown 1970, Jensen & Bradley 1989). Pancreatitis-induced hypercoagulability, resulting in secondary mesenteric arterial or venous thrombosis may offer one explanation (Jensen & Bradley 1989).

The diagnosis of intestinal necrosis in acute pancreatitis requires a high index of suspicion by an alert clinician. The triad of an abdominal mass, sepsis, and gastrointestinal haemorrhage in a patient with acute pancreatitis has been associated with intestinal necrosis in approximately 50% of reported cases (Bradley 1982a). Findings suggestive of intestinal ischaemia on a plain abdominal

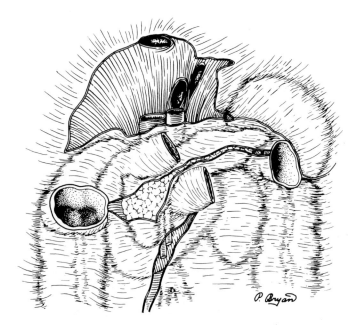

Fig. 23.10 Relationship of peritoneal reflections to the pancreas. Note the anatomical pathways enabling inflammatory exudate from acute pancreatitis to reach the transverse colon, the duodenum, and the enteric vessels. (Reproduced with permission from Bradley E L III (ed) Complications of pancreatitis, 1982, W B Saunders, Philadelphia.)

radiograph, computed tomography, or a careful water-soluble contrast study include: oedematous mucosal folds ('thumbprinting'), pneumatosis, 'toxic megacolon', or perforation (Miller et al 1970) (Fig. 23.11).

If diagnostic manoeuvres confirm or strongly suggest intestinal necrosis, surgical intervention is mandatory, since untreated intestinal necrosis is uniformly fatal. Surgical management should include resection of the involved segment with proximal enterostomy. Even with early diagnosis and aggressive surgical management, a mortality rate greater than 50% is typical when intestinal necrosis complicates acute pancreatitis (Bradley 1982a, Schein et al 1985, Bouillot et al 1989).

COMMON DUCT OBSTRUCTION

Biochemical and clinical jaundice occur in approximately 20% of patients with acute pancreatitis at some time during their hospital course (Bradley & Salam 1978). Extrahepatic ductal obstruction from biliary lithiasis (see Ch. 21), or compression by a pancreatic abscess (Holden et al 1976) or pseudocyst (Bradley et al 1979, Skellinger et al 1983) are recognized causes of hyperbilirubinaemia.

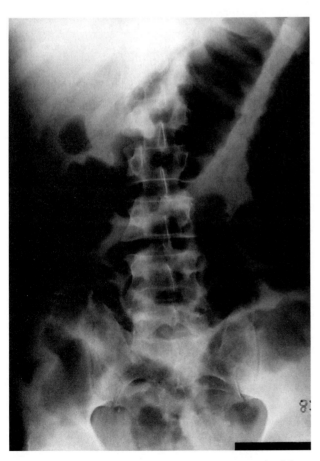

Fig. 23.11 Flat plate in a patient with extensive necrosis of the transverse and descending colon associated with necrotizing pancreatitis. Note the similarity in appearance to 'toxic megacolon'.

In almost half of these cases associated with acute pancreatitis, however, cholestasis has been unassociated with any known cause. This idiopathic hyperbilirubinaemia, so called acute pancreatic cholangiopathy, has been attributed to periductular oedema and cholangitis (Bradley & Salam 1978).

From a clinical standpoint, hyperbilirubinaemia due to acute cholangiopathy is mild (<6 mg%, 100 μmol/l) and transient (<10 days) (Bradley & Salam 1978). An important clinical corollary is that if the serum bilirubin exceeds 6 mg% (100 μmol/l), or if hyperbilirubinaemia lasts longer than 10 days, other causes should be sought. In the absence of other demonstrable causes, spontaneous resolution of inflammatory duct compression is the usual course, and surgical intervention is unnecessary. Unlike the transient hyperbilirubinaemia due to acute cholangiopathy, chronic cholangiopathy with hyperbilirubinaemia is the result of periductal fibrosis from long-standing chronic inflammation caused by chronic pancreatitis, and requires surgical bypass (Bradley 1982b).

INTERNAL PANCREATIC FISTULA

Pancreatic ascites and massive pancreatic pleural effusions, collectively termed internal pancreatic fistulas, result from pancreatic duct disruption or a leaking pancreatic pseudocyst. Over the past 20 years, internal pancreatic fistulas have become increasingly recognized as complications of inflammatory pancreatic disease rather than clinical curiosities (Cameron et al 1967, Donowitz et al 1974). In 1976, Sankaran & Walt noted a 14.5% incidence of pancreatic ascites in 131 pseudocysts treated over a 17-year period (Sankaran & Walt 1976). Iacono et al reported a 1.3% incidence of massive pancreatic pleural effusion in 670 patients with inflammatory pancreatic disease (Iacono et al 1989). Although the exact incidence of internal pancreatic fistulas is unknown, the frequency of recognition of these complications appears to be directly related to heightened clinical awareness.

Even though the precise initiating events in the development of internal pancreatic fistulas are unknown, the mechanics of their formation is understood. Disruption of a pseudocyst or the pancreatic duct in an anterior direction produces intraperitoneal ascites (Smith et al 1973). Posterior leaks may track through the oesophageal or aortic hiatus, thereby creating a mediastinal pseudocyst (Jaffe et al 1972). A massive pancreatic pleural effusion results from rupture of the mediastinal pseudocyst into one or both pleural cavities.

Internal pancreatic fistulas are rarely diagnosed during the initial stages of acute pancreatitis. When seen in patients with acute pancreatitis, they are usually a reflection of underlying chronic pancreatitis with an acute exacerbation.

Parenthetically, it is of interest to note that internal pancreatic fistulas have not been reported in association with acute biliary pancreatitis. A history of alcohol ingestion is a common feature in the majority of patients who develop internal pancreatic fistulas. Trauma is the aetiology in approximately 10% of patients who develop internal pancreatic fistulas, and is the cause in virtually all cases involving children (Broe & Cameron 1982). In an extensive review of 185 cases, Broe and Cameron identified the typical patient as a male alcoholic, age 20–50 years who presents with tense ascites, mild abdominal discomfort, and malnutrition, often without a clear history of pancreatitis (Broe & Cameron 1982).

Internal pancreatic fistulas can be differentiated accurately and rapidly from other forms of ascites and pleural effusions by biochemical examination of the aspirated fluid. Aspiration of straw coloured or serosanguinous fluid with a markedly elevated amylase level, and a protein concentration greater than 25 g/l is diagnostic in most cases (Cameron et al 1967, Sankaran & Walt 1976).

Initial management of patients with internal pancreatic fistulas is conservative. Non-operative management should include total parenteral nutrition, pharmacological inhibition of pancreatic secretion, and nasogastric suction. Frequent paracentesis, thoracentesis, or even occasional chest tube placement, will minimize peritoneal or pleural fluid accumulation, and will help to promote fistula closure through serosal or pleural apposition. Utilizing this approach, approximately 50% of the patients with internal pancreatic fistulas will experience spontaneous remission (Weaver et al 1982). Medical management is not recommended beyond 2 weeks, however, since sudden unexplained deaths have been frequent among patients treated with prolonged supportive care (Broe & Cameron 1982). In fact, mortality in several series with prolonged conservative management approaches 20% (Donowitz et al 1974, Sankaran & Walt 1976). Low-dose irradiation to the pancreas to diminish pancreatic secretion may prove useful in patients who are a prohibitive operative risk (Morton et al 1976). Somatostatin and its long-acting analogues have recently been reported to be successful in the treatment of pancreatic ascites (Ellison et al 1988).

Persistence of pancreatic ascites or pleural effusion after 2–3 weeks of maximal conservative therapy is an indication for surgery. Endoscopic retrograde pancreatography is mandatory to assist in surgical planning. Operative mortality in the 130 surgical patients collected by Broe & Cameron was 14%. This excessive mortality can be reduced to between zero and 7% when pancreatography is used to plan a rational surgical approach (Sankaran et al 1979, Sanfey & Cameron 1984). Leaks in the body or tail of the pancreas are best managed by pancreatic resection. However, if proximal duct obstruction is present, the pancreatic remnant should be drained into a Roux-en-Y loop. Leaks in the head of the pancreas can be treated satisfactorily with a Roux-en-Y drainage procedure, the jejunal loop being applied directly to the site of ductal rupture.

REFERENCES

Adams D B, Harvey T S, Anderson M C 1990 Percutaneous catheter drainage of infected pancreatic and peripancreatic fluid collections. Archives of Surgery 125:1554–1557

Aldridge M C, Ornstein M, Glazer G et al 1985 Pancreatic resection for severe acute pancreatitis. British Journal of Surgery 72:796–800

Alexandre J H, Guerrieri M T 1981 Role of total pancreatectomy in the treatment of necrotizing pancreatitis. World Journal of Surgery 5:369–377

Allardyce D B 1987 Incidence of necrotizing pancreatitis and factors related to mortality. American Journal of Surgery 154:295–299

Allen K A, Bradley E L III 1990 Modern management of acute pancreatitis. Surgery Report 1:220–249

Aranha G V, Prinz R A, Greenlee H B, Freeark R J 1984 Gastric outlet and duodenal obstruction from inflammatory pancreatic disease. Archives of Surgery 119:833–835

Banks P A, Gerzof S G, Chong F K et al 1990 Bacteriologic status of necrotic tissue in necrotizing pancreatitis. Pancreas 5:330–333

Beger H G, Krautzberger W, Bittner R, Block S, Büchler M 1985 Results of surgical treatment of necrotizing pancreatitis. World Journal of Surgery 9:972–979

Beger H G, Bittner R, Block S, Büchler M 1986 Bacterial contamination of pancreatic necrosis. A prospective clinical study. Gastroenterology 91:433–438

Beger H G, Büchler M, Bittner R, Oettinger W, Block S, Nevalainen T 1988 Necrosectomy and postoperative local lavage in patients with necrotizing pancreatitis: Results of a prospective clinical trial. World Journal of Surgery 12:255–262

Bittner R, Block S, Büchler M, Beger H G 1987 Pancreatic abscess and infected pancreatic necrosis. Different local septic complications in acute pancreatitis. Digestive Diseases and Sciences 32:1082–1087

Bivens B A, Sachatello C R, Chuang V P, Brady P 1978 Hemosuccus pancreaticus (hemoductal pancreatitis). Archives of Surgery 113:751–753

Block S, Büchler M, Bittner R, Beger H G 1987 Sepsis indicators in acute pancreatitis. Pancreas 2:499–505

Borrero S, Bank S, Margolis I, Schulman N D, Chardavoyne R 1985 Comparison of antacid and sucralfate in the prevention of gastrointestinal bleeding in patients who are critically ill. American Journal of Medicine 79 (Suppl 2C):62–64

Bouillot J L, Alexandre J H, Vuong N P 1989 Colonic involvement in acute necrotizing pancreatitis: Results of surgical treatment. World Journal of Surgery 13:84–87

Bradley E L III 1982a Enteropathies. In: Bradley E L III (ed) Complications of pancreatitis. W B Saunders, Philadelphia, p 265–292

Bradley E L III 1982b Jaundice. In: Bradley E L III (ed) Complications of pancreatitis. W B Saunders, Philadelphia, p 223–244

Bradley E L III 1987 Management of infected pancreatic necrosis by open drainage. Annals of Surgery 206:542–550

Bradley E L III 1988 Later complications of acute pancreatitis. In Glazer G, Ranson J H C (eds) Acute pancreatitis: experimental and clinical aspects of pathogenesis and management. W B Saunders, Philadelphia, p 390–431

Bradley E L III 1989 Antibiotics in acute pancreatitis. Current status and future directions. American Journal of Surgery 158:472–477

Bradley E L III 1991 The role of open packing in the management of infected pancreatic necrosis. In: Boeckl O, Waclawiczek H W (eds) Proceedings of the International Symposium on Open Packing (Laparostomy), Springer-Verlag, Berlin, p 105–192

Bradley E L III, Allen K B 1991 Observation vs. surgical intervention in acute necrotizing pancreatitis: Results of a prospective longitudinal trial. American Journal of Surgery 161:19–25

Bradley E L III, Clements L J 1974 Implications of diagnostic ultrasound in the surgical management of pancreatic pseudocysts. American Journal of Surgery 127:163–173

Bradley E L III, Clements L J 1975 Spontaneous resolution of pancreatic pseudocysts: Implications for timing of operative intervention. American Journal of Surgery 129:23–28

Bradley E L III, Clements L J 1981 Idiopathic duodenal obstruction: an unappreciated complication of pancreatitis. Annals of Surgery 193:638–648

Bradley E L III, Salam A A 1978 Hyperbilirubinemia in inflammatory pancreatic disease: Natural history and management. Annals of Surgery 188:626–629

Bradley E L III, Gonzalez A C, Clements L J 1976 Acute pancreatic pseudocysts: Incidence and implications. Annals of Surgery 184:734–737

Bradley E L III, Clements L J, Gonzales A C 1979 The natural history of pancreatic pseudocysts: a unified concept of management. American Journal of Surgery 137:135–141

Bradley E L III, Murphy F, Ferguson C 1989 Prediction of pancreatic necrosis by dynamic pancreatography. Annals of Surgery 210:495–504

Broe P J, Cameron J L 1982 Pancreatic ascites and pancreatic pleural effusion. In: Bradley E L III (ed) Complications of pancreatitis. W B Saunders, Philadelphia, p 245–264

Büchler M, Malfertheiner P, Uhl W, Beger H G 1988 Conservative treatment of necrotizing pancreatitis in patients with minor pancreatic necrosis. Pancreas 3 (No 5) Abstract 592

Buggy B P, Nostrant T T 1983 Lethal pancreatitis. American Journal of Gastroenterology 78:810–814

Burbidge E R, Tarder G, Carson S, Eugene J, Frey C F 1978 Colonic varices: A complication of pancreatitis with splenic vein thrombosis. American Journal of Digestive Diseases 23:752–755

Burke J W, Erickson S J, Kellum C D, Tegtmeyer C J, Williamson B R J, Hansen M F 1986 Pseudoaneurysms complicating pancreatitis: Detection by CT. Radiology 161:447–450

Cahow C E, Gusberg R J, Gottlieb L J 1983 Gastrointestinal hemorrhage from pseudoaneurysms in pancreatic pseudocysts. American Journal of Surgery 145:534–541

Cameron J L, Anderson R P, Zuidema G D 1967 Pancreatic ascites. Surgery, Gynecology and Obstetrics 125:328–332

Collins J J, Peterson L M, Wilson R E 1968 Small intestinal infarction as a complication of pancreatitis. Annals of Surgery 167:433–436

Crass R A, Way L W 1981 Acute and chronic pseudocysts are different. American Journal of Surgery 142:660–664

Dietch E A 1990 The role of intestinal barrier failure and bacterial translocation in the development of systemic infection and multiple organ failure. Archives of Surgery 125:403–404

Donowitz M, Kerstein M D, Spiro H M 1974 Pancreatic ascites. Medicine 53:183–195

Dricks M R, Craven D E, Celli B R 1987 Nosocomial pneumonia in intubated patients given sucralfate as compared with antacids or histamine type 2 blockers. New England Journal of Medicine 317:1376–1382

Dubnick M A, Geokas M C, Mar G, McMahon M J, Mayer A D, Majmudar A P N 1985 Digestive enzymes and protease inhibitors in ascites fluid from patients with acute pancreatitis. Gastroenterology 88:1370

Eckhauser F E, Stanley J C, Zelenock G B, Borlaza G S, Ferier D T, Lindenauer S M 1980 Gastroduodenal and pancreaticoduodenal artery aneurysms: a complication of pancreatitis causing spontaneous gastrointestinal hemorrhage. Surgery 88:335–344

Ellison E C, Garner W L, Mekhjian H S 1988 Successful treatment of pancreatic ascites with somatostatin analog. Gastroenterology 90, Abstract 1405

Finch W T, Sawyers J L, Schenker S 1976 A prospective study to determine the efficacy of antibiotics in acute pancreatitis. Annals of Surgery 183:667–671

Foley W D, Stewart E T, Lawson T L et al 1980 Computerized tomography, ultrasonography and ERCP in the diagnosis of pancreatic disease: A comparative study. Gastrointestinal Radiology 5:29–35

Forlini E 1927 Stenosis del colon bar pancreatite. Giornale di Clinica Medica 8:609–620

Frey C F, Lindenauer S M, Miller T A 1979 Pancreatic abscess. Surgery, Gynecology and Obstetrics 149:722–726

Frey C F, Stanley J C, Eckhauser F 1982 Hemorrhage. In: Bradley E L III (ed) Complications of pancreatitis. W B Saunders, Philadelphia, p 96–119

Gadacz T R, Trunkey D, Kieffer R F 1978 Visceral vessel erosion associated with pancreatitis. Archives of Surgery 113:1438–1440

Gatch W D, Brickley R A 1951 Perforation of colon following acute necrosis of pancreas. Archives of Surgery 63:698–704

Gerzof S G, Johnson W C, Robbins A H, Spechler S J, Nabseth D C 1984 Percutaneous drainage of infected pancreatic pseudocysts. Archives of Surgery 119:888–893

Gerzof S G, Banks P A, Robbins A H et al 1987 Early diagnosis of pancreatic infection by CT-guided aspiration. Gastroenterology 93:1315–1320

Gonzalez A C, Bradley E L III, Clements J L 1976 Pseudocyst formation in acute pancreatitis: Ultrasonic evaluation of 99 cases. American Journal of Radiology 127:315–317

Griffith R W, Brown P W W 1970 Jejunal infarction as a complication of pancreatitis. Gastroenterology 58:709–712

Hancock R J, Christensen R M, Osler T R, Cassim M M 1973 Stenosis of the colon due to pancreatitis and mimicking carcinoma. Canadian Journal of Surgery 16:393–396

Holden J L, Berne T V, Rosoff L 1976 Pancreatic abscess following acute pancreatitis. Archives of Surgery 111:858–867

Hollender L F, Meyer C, Marrie A et al 1981 Role of surgery in the management of acute pancreatitis. World Journal of Surgery 5:364–365

Howes R, Zuidema G D, Cameron J L 1975 Evaluation of prophylactic antibiotics in acute pancreatitis. Journal of Surgical Research 18:197–200

Hudson D A, De Beer J V 1988 Acute large bowel obstruction complicating acute pancreatitis. Southern Medical Journal 81:804–805

Hunt D R, Mildenhall P 1975 Etiology of strictures of the colon associated with pancreatitis. American Journal of Digestive Diseases 20:941–946

Iacono C, Procacci C, Frigo F et al 1989 Thoracic complications of pancreatitis. Pancreas 4:228–236

Jaffe B M, Ferguson T B, Holtz S, Shields J B 1972 Mediastinal pancreatic pseudocysts. American Journal of Surgery 124:600–606

Jensen K, Bradley E L III 1989 Mesenteric venous infarction in acute pancreatitis. International Journal of Pancreatology 5:213–219

Joe L, Ansher A F, Gordin F M 1989 Severe pancreatitis in an AIDS patient in association with cytomegalovirus infection. Southern Medical Journal 82:1444–1445

Kivilaakso E, Fräki O, Nikki P, Lempinen M 1981 Resection of the pancreas for acute fulminant pancreatitis. Surgery, Gynecology and Obstetrics 152:493–498

Kozarek R A, Brayleo C M, Harlan J et al 1985 Endoscopic drainage of pancreatic pseudocysts. Gastrointestinal Endoscopy 31:322–328

Kozarek R A, Ball T J, Patterson D J et al 1991 Endoscopic transpapillary therapy for disrupted pancreatic duct and peripancreatic collections. Gastroenterology 100:1362–1370

Kukora J S 1985 Extensive colonic necrosis complicating acute pancreatitis. Surgery 97:290–293

Larvin M, Chalmers A G, Robinson P J, McMahon M J 1989 Debridement and closed cavity irrigation for the treatment of pancreatic necrosis. British Journal of Surgery 76:465–471

Larvin M, Chalmers A G, McMahon M J 1990 Dynamic contrast enhanced computed tomography: a precise technque for identifying and localising pancreatic necrosis. British Medical Journal 300:1425–1428

Lim G M, Jeffrey R B, Tolentino C S 1989 Pancreatic pseudoaneurysm: Monitoring the success of transcatheter embolization with duplex sonography. Journal of Ultrasound Medicine 8:643–646

Little A G, Moossa A R 1981 Gastrointestinal hemorrhage from left-sided portal hypertension: An unappreciated complication of pancreatitis. American Journal of Surgery 141:153–158

Longstreth G F, Newcomer A D, Green P A 1971 Extrahepatic portal hypertension caused by chronic pancreatitis. Annals of Internal Medicine 75:903–908

Lumsden A, Bradley E L III 1990 Secondary pancreatic infections. Surgery, Gynecology and Obstetrics 170:459–467

Machado M C C, Bacchella T, Monteiro da Cunha J E et al 1986 Surgical treatment of pancreatic necrosis. Digestive Diseases and Sciences 31 (Suppl):25S

Maier W 1987 Early objective diagnosis and staging of acute pancreatitis by contrast-enhanced computed tomography. In: Beger H G, Büchler M (eds) Acute pancreatitis. Springer-Verlag, Berlin, p 132–140

Mandel S R, Jacques P J, Mauro M A, Sonofsky S 1987 Nonoperative management of peripancreatic arterial aneurysms: A 10 year experience. Annals of Surgery 205:126–128

Marks I N, Bank S, Louw J H et al 1967 Peptic ulceration and gastrointestinal bleeding in pancreatitis. Gut 8:253–259

Meyer M A, Evans J A 1976 Effects of pancreatitis on the small bowel and colon spread along mesenteric planes. Radiology 149:151–160

Miller W T, Scott J, Rosato E F, Rosato F E, Crow H 1970 Ischemic colitis with gangrene. Radiology 94:291–297

Moossa A R, Gadd M A 1985 Isolated splenic vein thrombosis. World Journal of Surgery 9:384–390

Morton R E, Deluca R, Reisman T N 1976 Pancreatic ascites: Successful treatment with pancreatic radiation. American Journal of Digestive Diseases 21:333–336

Nicholson M L, Mortensen N J McC, Espiner H J 1988 Pancreatic abscess: results of prolonged irrigation of the pancreatic bed after surgery. British Journal of Surgery 75:88–91

Nordback I, Sisto T 1989 Peripancreatic vascular occlusions as a complication of pancreatitis. International Surgery 74:36–39

Pederzoli P, Bassi C, Elio A, Corrà S, Nifosì F, Benetti G 1989 The infected necrosis is a prognostic factor in necrotizing pancreatitis. Gastroenterology 96 (5): Abstract 1389

Pederzoli P, Bassi C, Vesentini S et al 1990 Retroperitoneal and peritoneal drainage and lavage in the treatment of severe necrotizing pancreatitis. Surgery, Gynecology and Obstetrics 170:197–203

Pemberton J H, Becker J M, Dozois R R, Nagorney D M, Ilstrup D, ReMine W H 1986 Controlled open lesser sac drainage for pancreatic abscess. Annals of Surgery 203:600–604

Pierce C W 1956 The 'colon cutoff' sign in acute pancreatitis. Medical Journal of Austria 1:313–317

Renner I G, Savage W T III, Pantoja J L, Renner V J 1985 Death due to acute pancreatitis. A retrospective analysis of 405 autopsy cases. Digestive Diseases and Sciences 30:1005–1017

Reuter S R, Redman H C, Joseph R R 1969 Angiographic findings in pancreatitis. American Journal of Radiology 107:56–67

Rich A R, Duff G L 1936 Experimental and pathologic studies on pathogenesis of acute hemorrhagic pancreatitis. Johns Hopkins Medical Journal 58:212–228

Rogers C, Klatt E C 1989 Splenic vein thrombosis in patients with acute pancreatitis. International Journal of Pancreatology 5:117–121

Rubinstein E, Mark Z, Haspel J et al 1985 Antibacterial activity of the pancreatic fluid. Gastroenterology 88:927–932

Sahel J, Bastid C, Pellat B et al 1987 Endoscopic cystoduodenostomy of cysts of chronic calcifying pancreatitis: a report of 20 cases. Pancreas 2:447–453

Salam A A, Warren W D, Tyras D H 1973 Splenic vein thrombosis: a diagnosable and curable form of portal hypertension. Surgery 74:961–972

Sandblom P 1970 Gastrointestinal hemorrhage through the pancreatic duct. Annals of Surgery 171:61–66

Sanfey H, Cameron J L 1984 The management of internal pancreatic fistulas. Surgical Rounds 8:26–37

Sankaran S, Walt A J 1976 Pancreatic ascites: Recognition and management. Archives of Surgery 111:430–434

Sankaran S, Sugawa C, Walt A J 1979 Value of endoscopic retrograde pancreatography in pancreatic ascites. Surgery, Gynecology and Obstetrics 148:185–192

Schein M, Saadia R, Decker G 1985 Colonic necrosis in acute pancreatitis: A complication of massive retroperitoneal suppuration. Diseases of the Colon and Rectum 28:948–950

Schroeder T, Kivilakso E, Kianunen D K J, Lempinen M 1980 Serum phospholipase A$_2$ in human acute pancreatitis. Scandinavian Journal of Gastroenterology 15:633–635

Siler V E, Wulsin J H 1951 Consideration of the lethal factors in acute pancreatitis. Archives of Surgery 63:496–502

Silverstein W, Isikoff M B, Hill M C, Barkin J 1981 Diagnostic imaging of acute pancreatitis: Prospective study using CT and sonography. American Journal of Radiology 137:497–502

Skellinger M E, Patterson D, Foley M T, Jordan P H 1983 Cholestasis due to compression of the common bile duct by pancreatic pseudocysts. American Journal of Surgery 145:343–348

Smadja C, Bismuth H 1986 Pancreatic debridement in acute necrotizing pancreatitis: an obsolete procedure? British Journal of Surgery 73:408–410

Smith R B III, Warren W D, Rivard A A, Amerson R J 1973 Pancreatic ascites: Diagnosis and management with particular reference to surgical technique. Annals of Surgery 177:538–546

Sostre C F, Flournoy J G, Bova J G, Goldstein H M, Schenker S 1985 Pancreatic phlegmon: clinical features and course. Digestive Diseases and Sciences 30:918–927

Stabile B E, Wilson S E, Debas H T 1983 Reduced mortality from bleeding pseudocysts and pseudoaneurysms caused by pancreatitis. Archives of Surgery 118:45–51

Stambler J B, Klibaner M I, Bliss C M, La Mont J T 1982 Tuberculous abscess of the pancreas. Gastroenterology 83:922–925

Stanely J H, Schabel S I, Seymour E Q 1983 Pancreatic imaging. Southern Medical Journal 76:625–631

Stanley J C, Frey C F, Miller T A, Lindenauer S M, Child C G 1976 Major arterial hemorrhage: a complication of pancreatic pseudocysts and chronic pancreatitis. Archives of Surgery 111:435–440

Stanten R, Frey C F 1990 Comprehensive management of acute necrotizing pancreatitis and pancreatic abscess. Archives of Surgery 125:1269–1275

Steckman M L, Dooley M C, Jaques P F, Powell D W 1984 Major gastrointestinal hemorrhage from peripancreatic blood vessels in pancreatitis: Treatment by embolotherapy. Digestive Diseases and Sciences 29:486–497

Steiner E, Mueller P R, Hahn P F et al 1988 Complicated pancreatic abscesses: problems in interventional management. Radiology 167:443–446

Stroud W H, Cullom J W, Anderson M C 1981 Hemorrhagic complications of severe pancreatitis. Surgery 90:658–665

Teerenhovi O, Nordback I, Isolauri J 1988 Influence of pancreatic resection of systemic complications in acute necrotizing pancreatitis. British Journal of Surgery 75:793–795

Teerenhovi O, Nordback I, Eskola J 1989 High volume lesser sac lavage in acute necrotizing pancreatitis. British Journal of Surgery 76:370–373

Thal A P, Perry J F, Egner W 1951 A clinical and morphologic study of 42 cases of fatal acute pancreatitis. Surgery, Gynecology and Obstetrics 105:191–198

Torres W E, Evert M B, Baumgartner B R, Bernadino M E 1986 Percutaneous aspiration and drainage of pancreatic pseudocysts. American Journal of Radiology 147:1007–1009

Trapnell J T 1971 Management of the complications of acute pancreatitis. Journal of the Royal College of Surgeons of England 49:361–372

Tryba M, Zevounou F, Torok M, Zeuz M 1985 Prevention of acute stress bleeding with sucralfate, antacids or cimetidine: a controlled study with pirenzepine as a basic medication. American Journal of Medicine 79 (Suppl 2C): 55–61

Van Sonnenberg E, Wittich G R, Casola G et al 1985 Complicated pancreatic inflammatory disease: diagnostic and therapeutic role of interventional radiology. Radiology 155:335–341

Van Sonnenberg E, Wittich G R, Casola G et al 1989 Percutaneous drainage of infected and noninfected pancreatic pseudocysts: experience in 101 cases. Radiology 170:757–761

Vugic I 1989 Vascular complications of pancreatitis. Radiologic Clinics of North America 27:81–91

Waclawiczek H W, Pimpl W, Chmelizek F 1986 Perioperative interdisciplinary management in acute necrotizing pancreatitis. Digestive Diseases and Sciences 31 (10) (Suppl) Abstract 1426:359S

Waltman A C, Luers P R, Athanasoulis C A, Warshaw A L 1986 Massive arterial hemorrhage in patients with pancreatitis: Complementary roles of surgery and transcatheter occlusive techniques. Archives of Surgery 121:439–443

Warshaw A L 1987 Management of pancreatic abscesses. In: Beger H G, Büchler M (eds). Acute pancreatitis. Springer-Verlag, Berlin, p 354–363

Weaver D W, Walt A J, Sugawa, Bouwman D L 1982 A continuing appraisal of pancreatic ascites. Surgery, Gynecology and Obstetrics 154:845–848

Wells C L, Maddaus M A, Simmons R L 1987 Role of the macrophage in the translocation of intestinal bacteria. Archives of Surgery 122:48–53

Wertheimer M D, Norris C S 1986 Surgical management of necrotizing pancreatitis. Archives of Surgery 121:484–487

White A F, Baum S, Buranasiri S 1976 Aneurysms secondary to pancreatitis. American Journal of Radiology 127:393–396

Widdison A L, Karanjia N D, Reber H A 1990a Route(s) of spread of bacteria to the pancreas in acute necrotizing pancreatitis (ANP). Pancreas 5 (6) (Abstract):736

Widdison A L, Karanjia N D, Reber H A 1990b The outcome of pancreatic colonization in acute necrotizing pancreatitis (ANP) and the efficacy of cefotaxime (CEF) treatment. Pancreas 5 (6) (Abstract):736

Wolstenholme J T 1974 Major gastrointestinal hemorrhage associated with pancreatic pseudocyst. American Journal of Surgery 127:377–381

Wu T K, Zaman S N, Gullick H D, Powers S R 1977 Spontaneous hemorrhage due to pseudocysts of the pancreas. American Journal of Surgery 134:408–410

Yeo C J, Bastidas J A, Lynch-Nyhan A et al 1990 The natural history of pancreatic pseudocysts documented by computed tomography. Surgery, Gynecology and Obstetrics 170:411–417

Chronic pancreatitis

24. Aetiology and pathogenesis of chronic pancreatitis

M. K. Müller   M. V. Singer

Chronic pancreatitis is a chronic inflammatory disease with irreversible destruction of pancreatic tissue. The clinical course is characterized by a dynamic but progressive process leading to 'cirrhosis' of the pancreas. In the early stages of its evolution, it is frequently complicated by attacks of acute pancreatitis that are responsible for the recurrent pain which may be the only clinical symptom. An interval of several years (on average just over 5 years) between the onset of symptoms and the manifestation of permanent pancreatic dysfunction and/or calcification is typical. Exocrine tissue is destroyed first and, at least in the later stages, endocrine tissue is also damaged.

AETIOLOGY AND EPIDEMIOLOGY OF CHRONIC PANCREATITIS

The aetiology of the pancreatic inflammation plays an important role in the long-term progression of the disease and epidemiological data reveal distinct differences between different forms of pancreatitis. Acute biliary pancreatitis virtually never progresses to chronic pancreatitis (see below), in contrast to acute alcoholic pancreatitis, which proceeds to chronic pancreatitis in the majority of patients. Chronic pancreatitis caused by alcohol has a much higher rate of progression of pancreatic dysfunction, causes more pain, and is more often calcific than non-alcoholic chronic pancreatitis (Ammann 1989). The parallel development of calcification and exocrine (and/or endocrine) insufficiency is also more evident in alcoholic pancreatitis, whereas in non-alcoholic pancreatitis calcification precedes exocrine insufficiency in nearly half the patients.

It is not clear whether acute (reversible) pancreatitis can progress to chronic pancreatitis once the cause of the disease (in most cases gallstones) has been removed. Strictures of pancreatic ducts which may remain after episodes of acute necrotizing pancreatitis or pseudocyst formation can cause obstruction and consequently give rise to chronic pancreatitis (Sarles 1986a). This form of pancreatitis, however, is usually non-progressive and by definition is generally regarded as a separate subtype of chronic pancreatitis (Gyr et al 1984, Singer et al 1985) (Table 24.1). Only long-term observation of pancreatic duct morphology permits differentiation between acute pancreatitis, chronic progressive pancreatitis and chronic obstructive (non-progressive) pancreatitis.

Few studies are available which document the frequency of chronic pancreatitis. In one prospective Danish study the incidence was 8.2 new cases per 1 million inhabitants per year and the prevalence was 27.4 cases per 1 million (Copenhagen Pancreatitis Study 1981). The average incidence collected from retrospective studies in Europe and North America is about 3–10 per million (Sato 1951, Haemmerli et al 1962, O'Sullivan et al 1972). In areas where sequential data have been published the incidence has usually increased with time (Fig. 24.1). For example, in England and Wales the number of patients discharged from hospital with a diagnosis of chronic pancreatitis rises four-fold in men and two-fold in women when the periods 1960–1964 and 1980–1984 are compared (Johnson & Hosking 1991). The regional differences in incidence rates are striking and cannot be explained only by a different pattern of alcohol consumption. However, the recent data from England and Wales show a close correlation between alcohol consumption per head of population and number of hospital discharges with chronic pancreatitis 6 years later (Fig. 24.2, Johnson & Hosking 1991). Considerable differences in patient referral patterns, the clinical diagnostic approach used and the level of local awareness of the disease must also be considered when interpreting such epidemiological data.

Table 24.1 Revised classification of pancreatitis: Marseilles 1984 (Singer M V et al 1985 Gastroenterology 89:693–690)

Acute pancreatitis
Chronic pancreatitis
  – with focal necrosis
  – with segmental or diffuse fibrosis
  – with or without calculi
  obstructive chronic pancreatitis

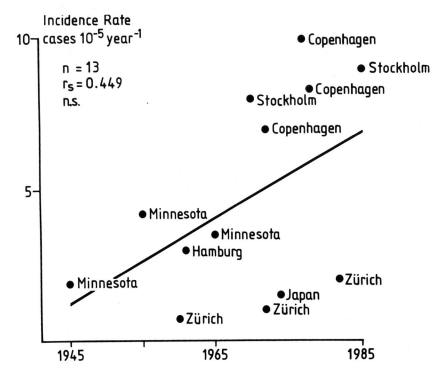

Fig. 24.1 Incidence of chronic pancreatitis during the years 1945 to 1985. (Reproduced from Worning H 1990 Incidence and prevalence of chronic pancreatitis. In: Beger H G, Büchler M, Ditschuneit H, Malfertheiner P (eds) Chronic pancreatitis, Springer-Verlag, Berlin, p 8–14 with permission of the publishers.)

In the majority of patients, chronic pancreatitis is caused by nutritional factors. Chronic alcohol consumption, often in connection with a diet rich in fat and protein, is a common aetiological factor in industrialized countries. In areas with endemic protein deficiency, a diet lacking in various macronutrients or micronutrients may be associated with chronic pancreatitis in childhood. Other forms of chronic pancreatitis are caused by or associated with metabolic disorders (notably hypercalcaemia), ductal obstruction or ill-defined hereditary factors; in many patients a specific causal factor is not identified (Table 24.2). Pancreatic insufficiency occurs in a substantial number of patients with cystic fibrosis; however, the pancreatic findings in this disease should not be classified as chronic pancreatitis.

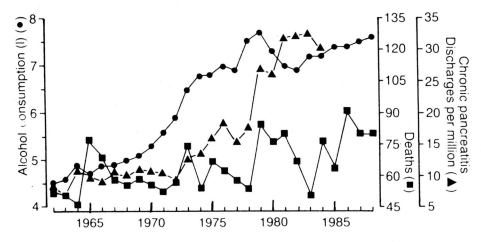

Fig. 24.2 Changes in annual alcohol consumption (litres per head of population), hospital discharges for chronic pancreatitis per million population, and total number of deaths from chronic pancreatitis in England and Wales, 1960–1988. (Reproduced from Johnson C D, Hosking S 1991 National statistics for diet, alcohol consumption and chronic pancreatitis in England and Wales, 1960–1988. Gut 32: 1401–1405, with permission of the publishers.)

Table 24.2 Aetiology of chronic pancreatitis

Nutritional factors	Alcohol Deficiency in protein and trace elements Dietary toxins
Metabolic causes	Hypercalcaemia
Pancreatic duct obstruction	Pancreas divisum Scarring, strictures Tumours
Miscellaneous causes	Hereditary Idiopathic

ALCOHOLIC CHRONIC PANCREATITIS

Alcohol is the dominant aetiological factor in chronic pancreatitis in Western medicine. As noted earlier, the significant increase in the incidence of chronic pancreatitis in industrialized countries parallels a marked increase in alcohol consumption (Table 24.3). This connection is characterized by the linear relationship which exists between alcohol consumption and the logarithmic risk of developing chronic pancreatitis (Fig. 24.3). Depending on regional intake of alcohol, the relative importance of alcoholic pancreatitis as a form of chronic pancreatitis ranges from 40–50% in Northern Europe to 90% in Southern Europe (Sarles 1985, Singer & Goebell 1985). Men are more often affected than women because of their larger alcohol consumption.

Alcoholic chronic pancreatitis normally becomes clinically manifest about the middle or end of the fourth decade of life (Durbec & Sarles 1978, Andersen et al 1982, Sarles 1986b). The interval between the beginning of regular alcohol consumption in substantial quantities and the first clinical manifestation averages 17–18 years in men and 10–12 years in women (Durbec & Sarles 1978). Numerous studies have shown that the appearance of calcification increases with the duration of the disease, and after about 15 years, pancreatic calcification is evident in more than 90% of patients (Bernades 1983, Ammann 1989). Although only a minority of alcoholics develop clinically apparent pancreatic disease, distinct morphological changes in the pancreas are found at autopsy in 19–58% of cases (Pitchumoni et al 1980, Stigendahl & Olsson 1984, Renner et al 1985).

Table 24.3 Changing pattern of alcohol consumption in various countries (litres of pure ethanol per person per year). (From Worning H 1990 Incidence and prevalence of chronic pancreatitis. In: Beger H G, Büchler M, Ditschuneit H, Malfertheiner P (eds) Chronic pancreatitis, Springer-Verlag, Berlin, p 8–14.)

	1950	1960	1970	1980
Denmark	3.6	4.2	6.8	9.2
France	17.6	17.3	15.6	16.2
Japan	0.2	2.4	4.7	5.1
Sweden	3.6	3.7	5.7	5.9
Switzerland	7.9	9.8	10.5	10.3
USA	5.0	4.8	6.3	8.1

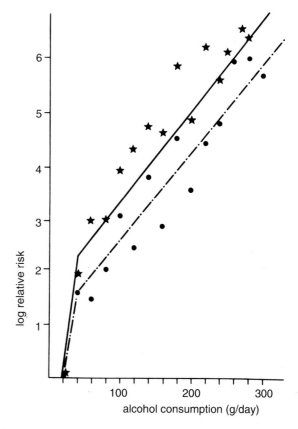

Fig. 24.3 Linear relationship between alcohol consumption and the logarithmic risk of chronic pancreatitis. (Reproduced from Durbec J P, Sarles H 1978 Multicenter survey of the etiology of pancreatic disease, Digestion 18: 337–350, with permission of the publishers.)

In contrast to studies on the liver, no threshold toxic dose of daily alcohol consumption could be demonstrated in the development of chronic pancreatitis. However, the average daily intake of pure alcohol usually exceeds 60–80g. Thus, the quantity of pure alcohol rather than the quality of the alcoholic beverage appears to play the decisive role. In a recent French controlled study, Bourliere et al (1991) suggested that tobacco is also a risk factor for chronic pancreatitis, although there is clearly a strong correlation between daily consumption of alcohol and tobacco use.

Individuals who develop chronic pancreatitis on a lower intake of alcohol may be genetically more sensitive to its noxious effects; conversely, those who do not develop pancreatitis in spite of consuming higher amounts may be less sensitive. In general, women (who represent some 15% of patients with chronic alcoholic pancreatitis) seem to have a lower threshold for developing the disease but are affected earlier than men (Sarles et al 1979a, b).

Nutritional factors associated with chronic alcoholic pancreatitis

Some epidemiological data suggest that the risk of

developing alcoholic pancreatitis may increase with a diet high in protein and fat (Durbec & Sarles 1978). However, in other studies patients did not have a higher consumption of calories (Voirol et al 1980), or even had a significantly lower intake of calories, fat and protein, relative to controls (Pitchumoni et al 1980). Both findings could be reconciled by the notion that nutritional factors are additive and that the absence of one factor can be compensated by an increased role for one or several other factors. However, the relationship between chronic pancreatitis and protein and fat consumption is much weaker than that for alcohol, and there are indications that an insufficient supply of zinc and other trace elements such as copper or selenium also plays a role (Fell et al 1982, Dutta et al 1983).

Pathogenesis of chronic alcoholic pancreatitis

The mechanism by which alcohol induces chronic pancreatitis is still a matter of dispute. Three theories are under discussion. The first proposes that the initial step is a primary effect of alcohol on pancreatic exocrine secretion, with protein plug formation and obstruction of intrapancreatic ductules. The second proposes that an intracellular effect of alcohol on tissue integrity causes secondary alteration of pancreatic secretion. The third suggests that alcohol-induced dysfunction of hepatic mixed-function oxidases releases products which are toxic to the pancreas.

Theory of primary intraductal obstruction

Clinical and experimental evidence indicates that chronic alcohol uptake decreases pancreatic bicarbonate and water secretion, followed by an increase in protein secretion (Planche et al 1982). Both actions increase the concentration of intraductal proteins and juice viscosity. Several other factors, such as oversaturation, activation of enzymes, and reduction in the amount of substances which keep proteins soluble, may further contribute to the formation of protein plugs and their calcification within the pancreatic ductules. Some data support the concept that a specific 'pancreatic stone protein', known as PSP or lithostatine, plays a central role in preventing precipitation of calcium salts (predominantly calcium carbonate in the form of apatite). PSP is thought to be an acinar cell product and has been characterized as a glycosylated acidic phosphoroprotein of 14 kD in size. According to Sarles and his group it is a major constituent of pancreatic stones in chronic pancreatitis (De Caro et al 1979). PSP appears to be able to prevent the nucleation and growth of calcium carbonate crystals, and its concentration in the pancreatic juice of patients with chronic pancreatitis has been reported to be decreased, particularly in those with pancreatic calcifications (Multigner et al 1985). Low PSP levels could therefore favour the formation of intraductal calcification, with subsequent focal obstruction and the patchy lobular distribution of inflammation which characterizes chronic pancreatitis.

Intraductal eosinophilic protein precipitates have been found in the pancreatic juice and acini before ultrastructural or histopathological damage to acinar and ductal cells becomes manifest or marked (Giorgi et al 1985, Multigner et al 1985). Such precipitates were found in the pancreatic juice in 10% of normal controls, in 21% of asymptomatic alcoholics, but in 65% of patients with chronic calcific pancreatitis. They are uncommon in the juice of patients with obstructive chronic pancreatitis (see below). Once formed, the precipitates may trigger a pathological process which leads to damage of the ductal basement membranes, atrophy of the epithelium and a variety of other pathological lesions, including stenosis, cyst formation and parenchymal atrophy (Sarles et al 1989, 1990).

According to Sarles' group the formation of these calcium precipitates due to decreased synthesis of PSP is the key initial lesion in the pathogenesis of chronic pancreatitis (Sarles et al 1990). The theory is supported by the observation that the amount of messenger RNA encoding for PSP is lower in the juice and acini of patients with chronic calcific pancreatitis than in controls, regardless of whether the disease is alcoholic, hereditary, tropical or idiopathic in origin (de Caro et al 1979, Giorgi et al 1985, 1989). It is conceivable that hereditary predisposition to decreased PSP secretion, nutritional factors and ill-defined noxious agents may combine in the pathogenesis of chronic pancreatitis.

It must be stressed that not everyone accepts the central significance of PSP in pathogenesis. Some workers have failed to find any difference in PSP concentrations between groups of patients with chronic pancreatitis, pancreatic cancer and non-pancreatic disease, and have even questioned the independent existence of PSP (Schmiegel et al 1990). Nevertheless, the hypothesis provides an extremely useful platform from which to elucidate the process of protein plug formation and calcification in chronic pancreatitis.

Besides PSP, there are other factors which in alcoholics may favour calcification of protein in the pancreatic ductules. These include increased viscosity of pancreatic juice due to increased protein secretion, increased secretion of calcium by acinar cells (Lohse & Pfeiffer 1984) and a decreased concentration of citrate in pancreatic juice (Lohse et al 1983) (Fig. 24.4).

Theory of intracellular toxic metabolic actions of alcohol

In contrast to Sarles' hypothesis, which considers acinar cell damage to be primarily due to ductular obstruction by protein precipitates, others have suggested that these changes are secondary to fatty degeneration of pancreatic cells, associated with loss of zymogen content and periacinar fibrosis (Noronha et al 1981, 1984, Bordalo et

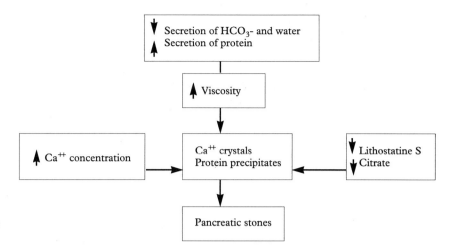

Fig. 24.4 Factors which contribute to pancreatic calcification.

al 1984). It has been postulated that overstimulation of the acinar cells could derange intracellular transport of secretory proteins, with abnormal admixture of digestive enzymes and lysosomal hydrolases and/or storage of zymogens in acid compartments. It has also been suggested that alcohol may lead to the production of toxic metabolites of lipid metabolism in pancreatic cells and so trigger the development of chronic pancreatitis.

Theory of primary disordered hepatic 'detoxification'

Another hypothesis is that disordered hepatic detoxification is the prime initiator of chronic pancreatitis (Braganza 1983). This concept is based on the finding that alcohol can induce hepatic mixed function oxidases. The process may be facilitated by an abundant intake of unsaturated fatty acids and could depend on individual genetic disposition. According to this hypothesis, products of hepatic 'detoxification', such as oxygen free radicals and reactive toxic intermediates, are then excreted into the bile and could cause damage to the pancreas after regurgitation into the duct system.

All these hypotheses regarding the development of chronic alcoholic pancreatitis are still speculative. The hypothesis put forward by Sarles and co-workers is based on firmer evidence than the others although many questions remain. It seems most likely that the cause of alcoholic pancreatitis is multifactorial, with an interaction of metabolic-toxic factors accompanied by secretory changes in the acini and juice on the basis of a genetically determined sensitivity to alcohol.

CHRONIC PANCREATITIS ASSOCIATED WITH DEFICIENCY OF MACRONUTRIENTS AND MICRONUTRIENTS

Tropical chronic pancreatitis

The term 'tropical pancreatitis' describes a type of calcific pancreatic disease which has been reported from several countries, all within 15 degrees of the equator. The major clinical features are abdominal pain and pancreatic calcification, diabetes mellitus, steatorrhoea due to exocrine insufficiency and death 'at the prime of life' (Nwokolo & Oli 1980, GeeVarghese 1986). The clinical picture and the histological appearance closely resemble the alcoholic type of chronic pancreatitis of industrialized countries; however, none of the patients have a history of alcohol abuse.

The major aetiological factor in the disease was once thought to be protein-energy malnutrition or childhood kwashiorkor (Shaper 1960). This association was strongly suggested by the high incidence of the disease in children and young adults in impoverished developing nations who consume a low-protein diet, show clinical signs of malnutrition, and have no other known causes of calcific pancreatitis. However, recent observations indicate that tropical pancreatitis may not be a consequence of kwashiorkor in that a history of childhood kwashiorkor is not obligatory for patients with tropical pancreatitis. Indeed, it has been suggested that the malnutrition in patients with tropical pancreatitis is the result rather than the cause of the disease. Furthermore, the fact that the disease is not seen in areas where protein-energy malnutrition is prevalent, has raised further doubts whether malnutrition is truly an initiating factor in the pathogenesis of tropical pancreatitis (GeeVarghese et al 1969).

It seems more likely that other factors, such as dietary substances, trace elements or nutritional toxins (perhaps in combination with a protein-deficient diet), are implicated. Based on epidemiological studies, cyanide-yielding natural food products such as cassava (*Manihot esculenta*) have been suggested as possible aetiological factors (Tropical Diabetes Workshop 1988), although at first sight their primary effect is more likely to be on the endocrine pancreas, with production of diabetes mellitus (McMillan & GeeVarghese 1979). However, cyanogens could play an important role in pancreatic injury by impairing enzymes such as superoxide dismutase which are important scavengers of free radicals, agents capable of causing pancreatic cell damage. Malnutrition may impair detoxification of cyanogens and thus favour generation of free radicals. This effect appears largely to be caused by a lack of methionine and trace elements such as selenium, zinc and copper; the cassava-rich diet, consumed in large quantities in countries with a high prevalence of tropical pancreatitis is not only deficient in protein, but also in methionine and trace elements.

Thus, at present the exact cause of tropical pancreatitis remains a matter of debate. It seems likely that the pathogenesis is explained by deficiency of macronutrients and micronutrients (such as trace elements) which are necessary to counteract the effects of toxic agents such as cyanogen-promoted free radicals.

Chronic pancreatitis and kwashiorkor

Adequate nutrition does not reverse the disease process in tropical pancreatitis. However, there is a specific form of pancreatitis which is strongly associated with juvenile kwashiorkor, which is reversible and which can be differentiated form tropical pancreatitis. Children suffering from juvenile kwashiorkor may develop atrophy of the pancreas and minor inflammatory lesions. The disease is further characterized by secretory insufficiency, abdominal pain (infrequent), and preservation of the pancreatic duct system (Barbezat & Hanson 1968, Blackburn & Vinijchaikul 1969, Pitchumoni 1984). Pancreatic calcifications are rare. Treatment with an adequate diet rapidly reverses pancreatic atrophy and restores secretion, provided that the parenchymal fibrosis produced by longstanding disease is not too extensive.

OBSTRUCTIVE CHRONIC PANCREATITIS

A form of chronic pancreatitis has been described which is secondary to ductal obstruction due to congenital or acquired strictures, congenital anomalies (such as pancreas divisum), tumours and inflammation of the papilla of Vater. This form of the disease is now known as 'chronic obstructive pancreatitis'. The epithelium of the obstructed ducts is usually preserved and the obstructed pancreas shows uniform inflammatory changes rather than the patchy lesion formation which characterizes alcoholic chronic pancreatitis. Intraductal protein plugs are found only occasionally in obstructive pancreatitis and do not appear to progress to calcification and stone formation.

Pancreas divisum

Pancreas divisum (see Ch. 34) is the most frequent ductal anomaly of the pancreas. In this condition the dorsal and ventral pancreatic ducts fail to fuse and the two independent duct systems draining the ventral and dorsal pancreas reach the duodenum separately via two distinct orifices. The larger part of the gland, the dorsal part, thus drains its secretion through the lesser papilla, whereas the smaller section of the gland, the ventral part, drains through the major papilla together with the main bile duct. Autopsy studies have shown that the frequency of pancreas divisum in the population ranges from 4 to 14%, while endoscopic retrograde cholangiopancreatography (ERCP) studies have shown a prevalence of up to 7% (Berman et al 1960, Seifert 1977, Rösch et al 1976, Richter et al 1981, Agha & Williams 1987). In some studies the incidence of pancreatitis in patients with pancreas divisum is higher than expected, and the hypothesis has been advanced that pancreatitis develops because of relative outflow obstruction since the minor papilla is not normally capable of handling such large volumes of pancreatic juice. This hypothesis is supported by recent studies showing that the dorsal intraductal pressure is significantly higher in pancreas divisum than in the normal pancreas (Staritz & Meyer-zum-Büschenfelde 1988).

While the clinical relevance of pancreas divisum remains controversial, most studies suggest a relationship between pancreas divisum and recurrent acute pancreatitis (Bernard et al 1990). Careful examination reveals pancreas divisum in up to 50% of patients with idiopathic recurrent pancreatitis and in a smaller proportion of patients with biliary pancreatitis.

The relationship between pancreas divisum and chronic pancreatitis is unclear. Although a number of patients with pancreas divisum and histological changes consistent with chronic pancreatitis in the dorsal part of the pancreas have been reported, epidemiological data now show that chronic pancreatitis is not more common in this group of patients (Sahel et al 1982, Bernard et al 1990). This suggests that ethanol or other factors may have been involved in the pathogenesis of the disease in such cases.

Chronic pancreatitis due to congenital or acquired strictures of the pancreatic duct or to neoplasia

Strictures are most often due to scarring after trauma or pancreatitis. Chronic obstructive pancreatitis has been reported after the healing of pseudocysts in acute pancreatitis due to a variety of causes, such as blunt abdominal trauma or gallstones (Laugier et al 1973).

In patients with ductal obstruction from pancreatic cancer, focal (Cubilla & Fitzgerald 1978) and, less often, extensive (Howard & Jordan 1977) areas of chronic pancreatitis may be found at operation. Diffuse pancreatic calcification and pancreatic duct stones are, however, rare.

CHRONIC PANCREATITIS AND BILIARY DISEASE

Biliary disease in the form of choledocholithiasis is the most frequent cause of acute pancreatitis in many industrialized countries. Whether recurrent episodes of acute pancreatitis due to biliary disease can proceed to chronic pancreatitis is not clear, but most observers agree that this virtually never happens (Ammann 1989). However, about one-half of patients with gallstone disease have abnormal findings on pancreatography, and one in six have changes suggestive of chronic pancreatitis (see Misra & Dwivedi 1991). Nonetheless, the relevance of these abnormal findings is not clear; in general the patients were asymptomatic and it remains doubtful whether the ductal changes represent clinically relevant chronic pancreatitis. Due to increased awareness of the need to avoid further attacks of gallstone pancreatitis by eradicating gallstones surgically or endoscopically, recurrent biliary pancreatitis should now occur only exceptionally.

While biliary tract disease does not appear to be an important cause of chronic pancreatitis, intermittent cholestasis is sometimes found in association with acute pancreatitis, regardless of cause, and may be seen in acute exacerbations of chronic pancreatitis. Cholestasis in such cases is usually secondary to oedematous swelling of the pancreatic head. More prolonged cholestasis may complicate chronic pancreatitis where it reflects fibrosis in the head of the pancreas.

CHRONIC PANCREATITIS ASSOCIATED WITH METABOLIC DISORDERS

Hypercalcaemia syndromes

Hypercalcaemic syndromes, notably primary hyperparathyroidism, can be associated with acute and chronic pancreatitis. In the majority of cases the hypercalcaemic crises appear to precipitate the acute attacks of pancreatitis (Kelly & Falor 1968). The pathophysiological basis for the association is not fully understood, but the most likely mechanism is cellular damage due to elevated serum calcium levels and increased calcium diffusion into pancreatic ducts, favouring calcified plug formation (Layer et al 1982).

It should be stressed that pancreatitis is now a rare complication of hyperparathyroidism, accounting for no more than 1–2% of cases (Bess et al 1980). The importance of hyperparathyroidism as a cause of chronic pancreatitis has probably decreased because of early detection of increased serum calcium levels by routine blood examinations.

Hyperlipidaemia

Hyperlipidaemia is known to be associated with acute pancreatitis. There is no proof, however, that it is involved in the pathogenesis of chronic pancreatitis, although elevated levels of blood lipids are often found in association with acute exacerbations of chronic alcoholic pancreatitis.

IDIOPATHIC CHRONIC PANCREATITIS: JUVENILE AND SENILE FORM

Idiopathic chronic pancreatitis in which alcohol or other known aetiological factors are not implicated accounts for about 10–20% of all cases of chronic pancreatitis. The *juvenile* form of idiopathic pancreatitis is characterized by a median age of onset of about 20 years, a painful clinical course, and an equal sex distribution. The main clinical features of the *senile* form of idiopathic chronic pancreatitis are its onset after the age of 50 years, prevalence in men, painless clinical course, marked weight loss associated with diarrhoea (steatorrhoea) or diabetes mellitus, and pancreatic calcific deposits (Ammann 1989). In some series, idiopathic senile chronic pancreatitis accounts for about two-thirds of the cases of non-alcoholic chronic pancreatitis, but it is rare when compared with the incidence of alcoholic chronic pancreatitis. The relationship of idiopathic senile chronic pancreatitis to normal age-related functional abnormalities of the exocrine pancreas is unknown. It has been suggested that the main pathogenetic factor is arteriosclerosis of pancreatic vessels (Ammann & Sulser 1976).

HEREDITARY CHRONIC PANCREATITIS

Hereditary chronic pancreatitis is a rare condition which usually becomes manifest between 5 and 15 years. The disease is inherited through an autosomal dominant gene of incomplete penetrance. The diagnosis should be suspected if several members of a family develop chronic pancreatitis without reason. Occasionally the diagnosis is made for the first time in adults. The pathogenetic mechanism responsible is not clear. There is no evidence that specific HLA haplotypes are involved. Recently, low concentrations of pancreatic stone protein have been described in the pancreatic juice of these patients (Sarles 1986a, b) but the significance of this observation is uncertain. Associated conditions include hyperlipidaemia and aminoaciduria. (Dalton-Clarke et al 1985). Hereditary chronic pancreatitis may increase the risk of developing pancreatic cancer (see Ch. 35), the risk being reported to be as high as 25% in some families.

REFERENCES

Agha F P, Williams K 1987 Pancreas divisum: incidence, detection, and clinical significance. American Journal of Gastroenterology 82:315–320

Ammann R 1989 Klinik, Spontanverlauf und Therapie der chronischen Pankreatitis, unter spezieller Berücksichtigung der Nomenklaturprobleme. Schweizerische Medizinische Wochenschrift

Ammann R, Sulser H 1976 Die 'senile' chronische Pankreatitis – eine nosologische Einheit? Schweizerische Medizinische Wochenschrift 106:429–437

Andersen B N, Thorsgaard Pedersen N, Scheel J, Worning H 1982 Incidence of alcoholic chronic pancreatitis in Copenhagen. Scandinavian Journal of Gastroenterology 17:247–252

Barbezat G O, Hansen J D L 1968 The exocrine pancreas and protein calorie malnutrition. Pediatrics 42:77

Berman L G, Priot J T, Abramow S M, Ziegler D D 1960 A study of the pancreatic duct system in man by the use of vinyl acetate casts of postmortem preparations. Surgery, Gynecology and Obstetrics 110:391–401

Bernard J P, Sahel K, Giovannini M, Sarles H 1990 Pancreas divisum is a probable cause of acute pancreatitis: a report of 137 cases. Pancreas 5 (3):248–254

Bernardes P 1983 Histoire naturelle de la pancréatique chronique. Étude de 120 cas. Gastroentérologie Clinique et Biologique 7:8–13

Bess M A, Edis A J, van Heerden J A 1980 Hyperparathyroidism and pancreatitis: chance or causal association? Journal of the American Medical Association 243:246–247

Blackburn W R, Vinijchaikul L 1969 The pancreas in kwashiorkor. An electron microscopic study. Laboratory Investigation 20:305–318

Bordalo O, Bapista A, Dreiling D, Noronha M 1984 Early pathomorphological pancreatic changes in chronic alcoholism. In: Gyr K E, Singer M V, Sarles H (eds) Pancreatitis – concepts and classification. Excerpta Medica, International Congress Series No. 642, Elsevier, Amsterdam

Bourliere M, Barthet M, Berthezene P, Durbec J P, Sarles H 1991 Is tobacco a risk factor for chronic pancreatitis and alcoholic cirrhosis? Gut 32:1392–1395

Braganza J M 1983 Pancreatic disease: a casualty of hepatic 'detoxification'? Lancet 2 1000–1003

Copenhagen Pancreatitis Study 1981 An interim report from a prospective epidemiological multicenter study. Scandinavian Journal of Gastroenterology 16:305–312

Cubilla A, Fitzgerald P J 1978 Pancreas cancer. I. Duct adenocarcinoma. A clinical-pathologic study of 380 patients. Pathology Annual 13(1):241

Dalton-Clarke H J, Lewis M H, Levi A J, Blumgart L H 1985 Familial chronic calcific pancreatitis: a family study. British Journal of Surgery 72:307–308

De Caro A, Lohse J, Sarles H 1979 Characterization of a protein isolated from pancreatic calculi of men suffering from chronic calcifying pancreatitis. Biochemical and Biophysiological Research Communication 87:1176–1182

Durbec J P, Sarles H 1978 Multicenter survey of the etiology of pancreatic diseases. Relationship between the relative risk of developing chronic pancreatitis and alcohol, protein, and lipid consumption. Digestion 18:337–350

Dutta S K, Miller P A, Greenberg L B, Lavander O A 1983 Selenium and acute alcoholism. American Journal of Clinical Nutrition 38:713–718

Fell B F, King T P, Davies N T 1982 Pancreatic atrophy in copper-deficient rats: histochemical and ultrastructural evidence of a selective effect on acinar cells. Histochemical Journal 14:665–680

GeeVarghese P J 1986 Calcific pancreatitis. Causes and mechanisms in the tropics compared with those in the subtropics. St Joseph's Trivandrum. Varghese, Bombay

GeeVarghese P J, Pitchumoni C S, Nair S R 1969 Is protein malnutrition an initiating cause of pancreatic calcification? Journal of the Association of Physicians of India 17:417–419

Giorgi D, Bernard J P, De Caro A, Multinger L, Lapointe R, Sarles H, Dagorn J C 1985 Pancreatic stone protein. I. Evidence that it is encoded by a pancreatic messenger ribonucleic acid. Gastroenterology 89:381–6

Giorgi D, Bernard J P, Ranquir S, Iovanna J, Sarles H, Dagorn J C 1989 Secretory pancreatic stone protein messenger RNA. Nucleotide sequence and expression in chronic calcifying pancreatitis. Journal of Clinical Investigation 84:100–106

Gyr K E, Singer M V, Sarles H 1984 Pancreatitis – concept and classification. Excerpta Medica, International Congress Series No. 642, Elsevier, Amsterdam,

Haemmerli U O, Hefti M L, Schmid M 1962 Chronic pancreatitis in Zürich 1958 through 1962. Bibl-Gastroenterol. 7:58–74

Howard J M, Jordan G L Jr 1977 Cancer of the pancreas. Current Problems in Cancer 2(3):11

Johnson C D, Hosking S 1991 National statistics for diet, alcohol consumption and chronic pancreatitis in England and Wales, 1960–1988. Gut 32:1401–1405

Kelly T R, Falor W H 1968 Hyperparathyroid crises associated with pancreatitis. Annals of Surgery 168:917–926

Laugier R, Camatte R, Sarles H 1973 Chronic obstruction of the pancreatic duct at the duodenum: a report of two cases in adulthood. Annals of Surgery 178:194

Layer P, Hotz J, Schmitz-Moormann H P, Goebell H 1982 Effects of experimental chronic hypercalcemia on feline exocrine pancreatic secretion. Gastroenterology 82:309–316

Lohse J, Pfeiffer A 1984 Duodenal total and ionised calcium secretion in normal subjects, chronic alcoholics, and patients with various stages of chronic alcoholic pancreatitis. Gut 25:874–880

Lohse J, Schmid D, Sarles H 1983 Pancreatic citrate and protein secretion of alcoholic dogs in response to graded doses of caerulein. Pflügers Archiv (European Journal of Physiology) 397:141–143

McMillan E E, GeeVarghese P J 1979 Dietary cyanide and tropical malnutrition diabetes. Diabetes Care, 2:202

Misra S P, Dwivedi M 1991 Do gallstones cause chronic pancreatitis? International Journal of Pancreatology 10:97–102

Multigner I, Sarles H, Lombardo D, De Caro A 1985 Pancreatic stone protein. II. Implication in stone formation during the course of chronic calcifying pancreatitis. Gastroenterology 89:387–391

Noronha M, Bordalo O, Dreiling D A: 1981 Alcohol and the pancreas. II. Pancreatic morphology of advanced alcoholic pancreatitis. American Journal of Gastroenterology 76:120–124

Noronha M, Bapista A, Bordalo O 1984 Sequential aspects of pathology in chronic alcoholic disease of the pancreas. In: Gyr K E, Singer M V, Sarles H (eds) Pancreatitis – concepts and classification. Excerpta Medica, International Congress Series No. 642, Elsevier, Amsterdam

Nwokolo C, Oli J 1980 Pathogenesis of juvenile tropical pancreatitis syndrome. Lancet 1:456-9

O'Sullivan J N, Noberga F T, Morlock C G, Brown A, Jr Bertholmew L G 1972 Acute and chronic pancreatitis in Rochester Minnesota 1940 to 1969. Gastroenterology 62:373–379

Pitchumoni C S 1984 Special problems in tropical pancreatitis. Clinical Gastroenterology 13:941–959

Pitchumoni C S, Sonneshein M, Candido F M, Panchacharam P, Cooperman J M (1980) Nutrition in the pathogenesis of alcoholic pancreatitis. American Journal of Clinical Nutrition 33:631–636

Planche N E, Palasciano G, Meullenet J, Laughier R, Sarles H: 1982 Effects of intravenous alcohol on pancreatic and biliary secretion in man. Digestive Diseases and Sciences 27:449–453

Renner I G, Savage W T, Pantoja J L, Renner V J 1985 Death due to acute pancreatitis: a retrospective analysis of 405 autopsy cases. Digestive Disease and Sciences 30:1005–1018

Richter J M, Shapiro R H, Mulley A G, Warshaw A L 1981 Association of pancreas divisum and pancreatitis, and its treatment by sphincteroplasty of the accessory ampulla. Gastroenterology 81:1104–1110

Rösch W, Koch H, Schaffner O, Demling L 1976 The clinical significance of pancreas divisum. Gastrointestinal Endoscopy 22:206–207

Sahel J, Cros R C, Bourry J, Sarles H 1982 Clinico-pathological conditions associated with pancreas divisum. Digestion 23: 1–8

Sarles H 1985 Chronic calcifying pancreatitis. Scandinavian Journal of Gastroenterology 20:651

Sarles H 1986a Etiopathogenesis and definition of chronic pancreatitis. Digestive Diseases and Sciences 31:91–107

Sarles H 1986b Chronic pancreatitis: etiology and pathophysiology. In:

Go V L W et al (eds) The exocrine pancreas. Raven Press, New York, p 527–540

Sarles H, Cros R C, Bidart J M 1979a A multicenter inquiry into the etiology of pancreatic disease. Digestion 19:110–125

Sarles H, Sahel J, Staub L, Bourry J, Laugier R 1979b Chronic pancreatitis. In: Howat H T, Sarles H (eds) The exocrine pancreas. W B Saunders, London

Sarles H, Bernard J P, Johnson C D 1989 Pathogenesis and epidemiology of chronic pancreatitis. Annual Review of Medicine 40:453–468

Sarles H, Bernard J P, Gullo L 1990 Pathogenesis of chronic pancreatitis. Gut 31:629–632

Sato T 1951 The annual report of the Ministry of Health and Welfare Chronic Pancreatitis Committee, Japan 1951. Ministry of Health and Welfare, Tokyo (in Japanese)

Schmiegel W, Buchert M, Kalthoft H et al 1990 Immunochemical characterization and quantitative distribution of pancreatic stone protein in sera and pancreatic secretions in pancreatic disorders. Gastroenterology 99:1421–1430

Seifert E 1977 Endoscopic retrograde cholangiopancreatography; evaluation based on experience with 805 examinations. American Journal of Gastroenterology 68:542–549

Shaper A G 1960 Chronic pancreatic disease and protein malnutrition. Lancet 1:1223–1224

Singer M V, Goebell H 1985 Acute and chronic actions of alcohol on pancreatic exocrine secretion in humans and animals. In: Seitz H K, Kommerell B (eds) Alcohol related diseases in gastroenterology. Springer-Verlag, Berlin

Singer M V, Gyr K E, Sarles H 1985 Revised classification of pancreatitis. Report of the Second International Symposium on the Classification of Pancreatitis in Marseille, France, March 28–30. Gastroenterology 89:683–690

Stigendahl L, Olsson R 1984 Alcohol consumption pattern and serum lipids in alcoholic cirrhosis and pancreatitis. A comparative study. Scandinavian Journal of Gastroenterology 19:582–587

Staritz M, Meyer-zum-Büschenfelde K H 1988 Elevated pressure in the dorsal part of pancreas divisum: the cause of chronic pancreatitis? Pancreas 3(1):108–110

Tropical Diabetes Workshop 1988 Proceedings of the meeting held in June 30–July 2. Wellcome Tropical Institute, London.

Voirol M, Infante F, Brahime-Reteneo O, Raymond L, Hollenweger V, Loizeau E 1980 Consommation d'alcool, de tabac et de nutriments dans les affections pancréatiques. Schweizerische Medizinische Wochenschrift 110:854–855

Worning H 1990 Incidence and prevalence of chronic pancreatitis. In: Beger H G, Büchler M, Ditschuneit H, Malfertheiner P (eds) Chronic pancreatitis. Springer-Verlag, Berlin, p 8–14

25. Conservative management of chronic pancreatitis

D.C. Carter   M. Trede

Assessment and management of patients with chronic pancreatitis is both difficult and time-consuming, and demands considerable skill and experience on the part of the clinicians concerned. It must be emphasized from the outset that not all patients developing the disease require surgery and that in many reported series about 50% of patients have been managed conservatively (Ammann et al 1984, Levy et al 1989). Successful management of this complex disease requires a multidisciplinary approach, with care often extending over many years. The team of clinicians usually includes a surgeon, gastroenterologist and radiologist, and may include a diabetologist and psychiatrist in addition to supporting services such as dieticians, counsellors and social workers. Although this multidisciplinary approach is essential to success in this complex disease, the distribution of responsibility within the team varies from centre to centre. Whichever pattern of care is adopted, it is important that the patient is not allowed to drift into 'committee management' with all of its attendant shortcomings. In many centres, the gastroenterologist is the clinician principally concerned with the initial assessment and conservative management, but close continued collaboration with the surgeon is essential if appropriate decisions are to be made regarding the need for, and timing of, surgery. In other centres, the surgeon assumes the central role in management, but works closely with his colleagues in other disciplines. Given the relative rarity of chronic pancreatitis, management of such patients should ideally be concentrated in specialist referral centres so that the necessary expertise and experience can be aquired and maintained.

Before embarking on conservative management of chronic pancreatitis it is essential to:

1. confirm that the patient does indeed have chronic pancreatitis
2. establish the cause and, if possible, eradicate it
3. stage the severity of the disease, define morphological and functional changes, and detect any complications, and

4. exclude the presence of accompanying disease, notably pancreatic cancer.

A decision can then be made as to the most appropriate form of management, bearing in mind that the natural history of chronic pancreatitis is extremely variable and that the decision to continue with conservative as opposed to surgical management often requires frequent reappraisal.

DIAGNOSIS OF CHRONIC PANCREATITIS

No single test can confirm the diagnosis of chronic pancreatitis with absolute certainty. Much depends on a careful history and clinical examination, supplemented by selective use of the methods of investigation now available.

History and clinical examination

Evaluation of pain

Pain is the outstanding symptom in the great majority of patients with chronic pancreatitis. A careful history is important not only to analyse the nature of this pain, but also as a first step in getting to know the patient and so establish the rapport which is so essential for long term success. The site of the pain depends to some extent on the main focus of the disease and may be the epigastrium and/or the right or left subcostal region. The pain frequently radiates through to the back, either centrally or to one side. In some patients back pain predominates while in others the pain is more diffuse, with no particular region of the upper abdomen or lower chest being affected more than any other. Occasionally, the pain radiates to the shoulder, radiation which is more common on the left side. Many patients find that adopting a certain position brings some relief; some lean forwards and avoid lying flat on their backs, while others curl up and find that lying on a particular side is less painful. In extreme cases the patient may kneel on all fours in an attempt to gain relief. Nausea is common during attacks of pain and vomiting may occur although it rarely relieves the pain.

The pain is usually described as a dull gnawing ache and is seldom colicky. There are often no clear precipitating factors, although some patients find that pain may be triggered by meals or certain foods such as those high in fat. In others, bouts of pain are associated with drinking alcohol. However, it must be emphasized that in the majority of patients there is no clear relationship between oral intake and pain, although most patients tend to reduce their intake substantially during a bad attack.

There is great variation in the pattern and periodicity of the pain of chronic pancreatitis. The attacks may be intermittent, lasting for hours or days, while some patients consider that they are never really free of pain. Loss of sleep, time off work, and the need for admission to hospital are useful pointers to severity. It is important to establish whether the pain is a 'background' problem which does not significantly impair the patient's quality of life, or whether, at the other end the spectrum, it is leading to devastating destruction of the quality of his existence. The need for analgesics to control the pain is also a useful index of severity. By the time of referral, many patients are already taking opiates for relief, and in some cases addiction may already be established. Assessment of pain can be one of the most difficult aspects of management, and never more so than in patients who are also addicted to alcohol or who have developed manipulative personalities in their search for powerful analgesics. As a general rule, all patients with chronic pancreatitis should be fully evaluated on an inpatient basis on at least one occasion so that their pain can be assessed comprehensively in the light of their compliance with medical advice and treatment.

Evaluation of other symptoms

Steatorrhoea usually means that pancreatic lipase output has fallen to less than 10% of normal (Di Magno 1982). It is not an invariable feature of chronic pancreatitis and many patients have severe pain in the absence of troublesome steatorrhoea. Indeed, there is some evidence that marked functional impairment and calcification is associated with relief from pain as the years pass (Ammann et al 1984). The patient should be questioned specifically about bowel habit, noting whether the stool is pale, bulky, oily and particularly offensive in smell, and whether it floats on the surface and is difficult to flush away. The stool frequency may be increased but it is unusual to have more than five or six movements a day. Watery diarrhoea is unusual in chronic pancreatitis (see below). Some patients have no evidence of steatorrhoea at any stage of their disease; indeed, in some cases constipation results from the high intake of analgesics.

Diabetes mellitus is also variable and tends to be a relatively late manifestation of chronic pancreatitis, developing after overt exocrine insufficiency. In time, many patients show gradual decline in pancreatic endocrine function, and dietary control of diabetes then has to be supplemented by the use of oral hypoglycaemic drugs and then by insulin. Contrary to earlier beliefs, the risks of complications such as diabetic retinopathy, and the timing of their onset, is no different from that in patients with idiopathic diabetes (Gullo et al 1990).

Other symptoms that may be present include weight loss, jaundice due to biliary tract obstruction, nausea and vomiting due to duodenal stenosis, and gastrointestinal bleeding due to splenic vein thrombosis and the development of gastric and oesophageal varices, or to erosion of pancreatic and peripancreatic arteries by inflammation.

Clinical examination

There are no pathognomonic physical signs in chronic pancreatitis. Malnutrition and weight loss may be a sign of reduced oral intake (due to the pain), exocrine insufficiency, and underlying chronic alcoholism. Burn marks on the abdomen and back may indicate repeated use of heat pads and hot water bottles in an attempt to relieve pain. In complicated disease, the patient may have jaundice (common bile duct obstruction), a visible or palpable abdominal mass (Fig. 25.1) or an enlarged spleen (splenic vein thrombosis and left-side portal hypertension). Stigmata of chronic liver disease and hepatic decompensation are relatively uncommon. On rare occasions, a patient may present with pancreatic ascites or pleural effusions as a consequence of rupture of the duct system or a pseudocyst.

Investigations

The investigations used to establish the diagnosis of

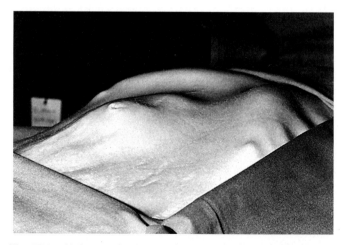

Fig. 25.1 Abdomen of a 42-year-old woman with chronic pancreatitis showing a visible painful mass in the region of the head of the pancreas.

pancreatic disease have been discussed at length in Section 2. As indicated earlier, no single test is sufficiently sensitive and specific to establish the diagnosis of chronic pancreatitis unequivocally, so that a combination of tests is needed (Niederau & Grendell 1985, Table 25.1). When chronic pancreatitis is suspected clinically, ultrasonography is a valuable first step to outline the pancreas and define its size, contour and texture. Ultrasonography may also reveal calcification, duct dilatation, cysts, pseudocysts and abscesses, and disease affecting neighbouring organs such as the liver, biliary tree and spleen. Opinions vary as to whether CT scanning should be carried out as well as, or instead of, ultrasonography. CT scanning is the best method of detecting pancreatic calcification and should be regarded as complementary to ultrasonography in its ability to detect chronic pancreatitis and pancreatic cancer. In practice, few patients with chronic pancreatitis are assessed and managed without at least one CT scan, but considerations of cost and the potential hazards of ionizing radiation mean that the investigation should be used sparingly. When pancreatic cancer is suspected, either ultrasound or CT can be used for targeted percutaneous fine-needle aspiration or biopsy.

Endoscopic retrograde pancreatography (ERP) is the single most effective method of detecting chronic pancreatitis and differentiating it from pancreatic cancer. ERP can be used to complement ultrasonography or CT scanning, in each case increasing the sensitivity and specificity of the combination to over 90%. When all three investigations are combined, a sensitivity of 95–97% and a specificity of 100% have been reported for the diagnosis of both chronic pancreatitis and pancreatic cancer (see Niederau & Grendell 1985).

Given the accuracy of imaging, it is doubtful whether tests of pancreatic exocrine function are of value in diagnosis. Although there is evidence from earlier studies that direct function tests can improve the sensitivity of individual imaging tests by up to 10% (Di Magno et al 1977, Braganza et al 1982), few centres now use such direct tests in routine practice. Similarly, despite the relative simplicity of the indirect (tubeless) tests discussed in Chapter 13, these too are now rarely used in diagnosis. Most surgeons dealing with chronic pancreatitis rely on the patient's history of steatorrhoea as an index of exocrine insufficiency rather than on the results of tests of exocrine function. However, a case can still be made for using such tests to establish a baseline when attempting to document the effect of surgery.

Endocrine function tests are usually restricted to those normally used to establish the presence of diabetes mellitus.

CONSERVATIVE MANAGEMENT OF CHRONIC PANCREATITIS

Treatment of pain

Pain mechanisms

The mechanism of pain production in chronic pancreatitis is still far from clear (see Ch. 32), and in many cases the pain has to be treated empirically in the absence of a defined cause. Acute exacerbations of inflammation are often troublesome but in most patients the major problem is chronic pain. Chronic pancreatitis is characterized by dense fibrosis, but the suggestion that this might cause nerve entrapment and so contribute to pain production has been questioned. Alternative explanations include neural invasion by inflammatory cells, including eosinophils (Keith et al 1989), and changes in the perineurial sheath which might affect pain thresholds (Bockman et al 1989). There is little doubt that obstruction of the pancreatic duct system is a major factor in the pathogenesis of chronic pancreatitis, and increased ductal or interstitial pressure is a further plausible explanation for the pain. However, the relationship between morphological changes, ductal pressures and pain is very variable, and other factors must be implicated (Leahy & Carter 1991, see Ch. 28). Pseudocysts are common in chronic pancreatitis. They may be asymptomatic, but the pain relief experienced by some patients after surgical or percutaneous drainage suggests that the pseudocyst was responsible, at least in part, for the pain. As will be discussed in Chapter 28, about two-thirds of patients with chronic pancreatitis have cholangiographic evidence of stenosis of the intrapancreatic common bile duct. However, pain cannot be assumed to be due to biliary obstruction in this context unless there is cholangitis, and alternative causes of pain (e.g. pseudocysts, inflammation in the head of pancreas) should be sought in patients who present with obstructive jaundice. Stenosis of the duodenum is less common than biliary obstruction, but can be a source of pain, nausea and

Table 25.1 Methods used to diagnose and assess chronic pancreatitis

History and clinical examination	Hypotonic duodenography (to evaluate duodenal stenosis)
Ultrasonography	Barium enema and colonoscopy (to evaluate colonic obstruction)
CT scan (nuclear magnetic resonance imaging)	Angiography (to locate source of bleeding and evaluate portal and splenic thrombosis)
Endoscopic retrograde pancreatography (ERP)	Doppler ultrasonography (to evaluate portal and splenic thrombosis)
Laboratory investigation:	
Endocrine function tests	
Exocrine function tests (direct and indirect)	
Percutaneous fine-needle cytology/histology	

vomiting. It should be borne in mind that patients with chronic pancreatitis have a higher than expected incidence of duodenal ulceration and cholelithiasis.

Acute exacerbations

Acute exacerbations of chronic inflammation may produce episodes of severe abdominal pain and tenderness. The diagnosis is supported by elevations of serum amylase and lipase, although not usually to the degree seen in acute pancreatitis, and by CT scan evidence of active inflammation and oedema. Pancreatic necrosis is said to be rare in chronic pancreatitis as the gland may not have enough function for a full-blown attack of acute necrotizing inflammation. However, in some series, as many as 10% of patients undergoing surgery for chronic pancreatitis have had acute necrosis requiring debridement (Machado et al 1984). Episodes of acute inflammation require admission to hospital, intravenous fluids, cessation of oral intake and prescription of appropriate analgesics (see Ch. 32). The surgeon should resist any temptation to abandon conservative treatment in favour of operation in the face of such acute exacerbations. In the great majority of cases, symptoms can be brought under control by conservative means. Opinions vary as to the role of total parenteral nutrition (TPN) during such exacerbations; although TPN may be well tolerated, it has been difficult to show significant clinical benefit and there is some evidence that these patients are at increased risk of catheter sepsis (Grant et al 1984). Nevertheless, when symptoms fail to settle promptly and a period of assessment is required, it seems reasonable to maintain nutritional status by parenteral feeding for a trial period of some 10–14 days (Banks 1989).

Chronic pain

Analgesics. Treatment of the pain of chronic pancreatitis is one of the most difficult areas of clinical medicine, and inability to control pain remains the outstanding indication to abandon conservative treatment in favour of surgery. The non-opioid drugs aspirin and paracetamol are more effective in the relief of musculoskeletal pain than in the treatment of visceral pain, so that opioid analgesics are often required, with all of their attendant problems of dependence and tolerance. Dihydrocodeine (DF 118) and codeine are suitable for patients with mild to moderate pain and are usually given orally (30 mg every 6 hours). In common with all opioid analgesics, they can cause constipation, nausea and dizziness, and when taken in large quantities may produce respiratory depression. Buprenorphine (Temgesic) is used to treat moderate to severe pain and is normally given sublingually (200–400 µg every 6–8 hours). Relative to morphine, it has less marked side-effects, a lower risk of dependence, and a longer duration of action (8–12 hours). However, it has both opioid agonist and antagonist properties and may produce withdrawal symptoms, including pain, in patients dependent on other opioids. Dipipanone hydrochloride is combined with an antiemetic in Diconal (dose 1–3 tablets every 6 hours) and like pethidine hydrochloride (50–150 mg every 4 hours) can be used orally for moderate to severe pain. Both give rise to less constipation than morphine. For severe pain, morphine (5–20 mg every 4 hours) can be given orally, and although it may produce more nausea it is generally preferred to diamorphine (heroin). MST Continus is a slow-release preparation which is useful for chronic severe pain (starting dose 10–20 mg twice daily).

It must be emphasized that great care must be exercised in the prescription of powerful opioid analgesics, given the risk of dependence. At the same time, appropriate analgesics must not be withheld in patients experiencing the often agonizing pain of chronic pancreatitis. As will be discussed in Chapter 32, attempts to obtain pain relief by alternative methods, such as percutaneous coeliac blockade, have proved extremely disappointing, and it remains to be seen whether other non-operative methods, such as endoscopic stenting with extracorporeal lithotripsy to disrupt pancreatic stones (Sauerbruch et al 1992, see Ch. 27), will be of long-term value. Analgesic use should be kept under close surveillance and the patient admitted to hospital if this is considered necessary. The possibility that exacerbations of pain may be due to remediable causes (e.g. pseudocysts) should be borne in mind, and the case for surgical intervention must be periodically reviewed. In some patients, anxiety or depression may be severe enough to necessitate referral for psychiatric appraisal; the use of self-help groups and support social services may also be of immense value. Although all avenues must be explored, there can be no doubt that the key to successful management remains the development of a strong relationship between the patient and his principal clinician. The relationship has to be built on trust and a sympathetic but firm handling of the difficulties that may arise, and is often emotionally demanding and time-consuming for both parties.

There has been considerable debate about whether the pain of chronic pancreatitis can be expected to diminish with time. Ammann et al (1984) observed 145 patients with alcoholic chronic pancreatitis for a median of 10.4 years and found that 85% experienced lasting pain relief within a median of 4.5 years from the time of onset. Pain relief was accompanied by a marked increase in the incidence of pancreatic calcifications and in exocrine and endocrine insufficiency, and the proportion of patients experiencing lasting pain relief was similar in operated and non-operated patients. Such studies have promoted the concept that in a substantial number of patients chronic pancreatitis will eventually 'burn itself out', with lasting pain relief, and that surgery is of questionable value in the management of chronic pain. As Warshaw (1984) has pointed out, the patients coming to surgery in the study by Ammann et al (1984) are a selected group in that they represent failures of conservative management, and that some of the operations performed would no longer be considered appropriate in this condition. In our view, many patients with chronic pancreatitis can indeed be managed without recourse to surgery, but there are many with severe intractable pain in whom it is unjustifiable to persist with conservative management in the forlorn hope that relief will occur spontaneously. In many ways, the clinical decision to abandon conservative management is simpler in patients with a pancreatic duct system which is so dilated that a drainage operation offers a good prospect of pain relief. In patients without such dilated ducts, some form of resection represents the only real alternative, and anxieties about operative risk and long-term morbidity may mean that there is greater reluctance to abandon conservative treatment.

Abstinence from alcohol. There is general agreement that abstinence is a crucial factor in long-term prognosis, and that it is a major determinant of outcome whether or not the patient has surgery. Abstinence may be extremely difficult to maintain and its importance should be emphasized repeatedly to the patient and his relatives. Every assistance should be invoked, including counselling, social review, psychiatric consultation and the use of self-help groups such as Alcoholics Anonymous. Much depends on the rapport established between the patient and his gastroenterologist or surgeon, and a great deal of time has to be spent providing the emotional support so necessary for success. Unfortunately, determination of blood alcohol levels at outpatient visits reveals that many patients are failing to abstain, despite vigorous assurances to the contrary. At this point it is worth emphasizing that alcohol as a cause of chronic pancreatitis must be kept in perspective. As many as one-third of patients in our practice have disease due to other causes or do not have a clear-cut history of alcohol abuse. Such patients are often labelled inappropriately as suffering from alcoholic chronic pancreatitis and understandably resent the stigma that is attached.

Although all would recommend abstinence to these patients, it must be freely admitted that there is still debate about whether alcohol withdrawal leads to pain relief and arrest of functional deterioration (Banks 1989). A major difficulty experienced by some patients is that they have continuing severe pain despite total abstinence. This undoubtedly reflects the fact that the 'damage has already been done' and that permanent fibrosis, scarring and stricture formation has taken place during the period of alcohol abuse. In chronic alcoholic pancreatitis, serial endoscopic retrograde pancreatography has shown that ductal changes may progress despite abstinence or reduction in alcohol consumption, a progression which may not occur in those with non-alcoholic disease (Nagata et al 1981). The experienced clinician, anticipating these difficulties, must remain sympathetic while at the same time stressing the need to avoid further damage to the gland or the other long-term consequences of alcohol abuse. In the experience of Ammann et al (1984) the cumulative survival rate was some 20% higher in patients with non-alcoholic disease, and the 50% survival time for patients with alcoholic pancreatitis was only 20–24 years from the onset of the disease. Other studies have confirmed the poor prognosis for patients with alcoholic chronic pancreatitis; about 20% of the deaths can be attributed directly to the disease and its complications, while other common causes of death include cancer, alcoholic liver disease, cardiovascular disease and complications of diabetes mellitus (Levy et al 1989, Miyake et al 1989). In their continuing study of the natural history of chronic pancreatitis, Ammann et al (1992) have recently highlighted the late complication of pancreatic and hepatic abscesses. Although the pathogenesis of such late abscesses is uncertain, it is of interest that nine of the 10 patients with alcoholic pancreatitis had previously undergone a pancreaticojejunostomy. Smoking has been implicated as a potentially important factor in the pathogenesis of chronic pancreatitis and it may be a particulary unfavourable prognostic factor in patients with alcohol-associated disease.

Dietary considerations. In theory, patients with chronic pancreatitis should avoid a high-fat, high-protein diet in order to reduce stimulation of the pancreas by cholecystokinin (CCK) release from the duodenum. In practice, the patient should be advised to avoid any foods that he feels may give rise to pain, avoid a diet that is rich in fat, and avoid eating large meals. Elemental diets were once advocated in the hope that they would stimulate less pancreatic enzyme secretion, but they are now known to release as much CCK as conventional diets (Watanabe et al 1986) and their use is no longer recommended. It has been suggested that pancreatic exocrine supplements may contribute to pain relief by reducing the pancreatic secretory response to food (see Ch. 3). There is evidence that luminal proteases may govern pancreatic exocrine function by a negative feedback mechanism (Slaff et al 1984, Layer et al 1990), but the existence of this mechanism and the role of CCK in its mediation is disputed; indeed, there is other evidence that pancreatic enzyme extracts actually stimulate pancreatic secretion through release of CCK (Mössner et al 1989). Similarly, there is debate about whether patients experience less pain while taking oral pancreatic enzyme supplements (Isaksson & Ihse 1983, Larvin et al 1992).

Treatment of steatorrhoea

The progressive loss of pancreatic exocrine function leads to excessive losses of fat (steatorrhoea) and protein (creatorrhoea) in the stool, and makes a major contribution to the weight loss and muscle wasting of chronic pancreatitis. In practice, the clinical picture is dominated by fat loss rather than protein loss, and it is the steatorrhoea which proves so troublesome to the patient and his doctors.

Under normal circumstances, the first step in fat digestion is the partial hydrolysis of dietary fat, a process which is commenced in the stomach by gastric and salivary lipase. This step is unaffected by pancreatic insufficiency, but the second step, namely completion of lipolysis in the duodenum, depends on adequate secretion of pancreatic bicarbonate and lipase. Failure of alkalinization of the duodenum also impairs lipid solubilization, with a resultant fall in mucosal lipid absorption. Furthermore, lipid solubilization and micelle formation depends on the presence of adequate concentrations of appropriate bile acids in the duodenum, and the postprandial concentration of such bile acids is reduced in alcoholic pancreatitis (for discussion, see Zentler-Munro & Northfield 1987).

All of the currently available pancreatic enzyme supplements consist of crude extracts of porcine pancreas known in many countries as pancreatin. Originally, pancreatin was not available in enteric-coated form and some 90% of the enzyme activity was lost before entry into the duodenum (Di Magno et al 1977), the enzymes being rapidly and irreversibly inactivated below pH 5. Preparations then became available in which tablets or granules were coated in an enteric coating designed to dissolve above pH 6, although there was little evidence to suggest that they improved efficacy. More recently, enteric-coated microspheres have been developed in which hundreds of individually coated microspheres are contained in a gelatin capsule. The particles are released within the stomach, pass readily into the duodenum because of their small size (less than 2 mm), and then lose their enteric coating when exposed to pH values of around pH 6. Unfortunately, conditions in the upper gastrointestinal tract in chronic pancreatitis may not be ideal for rapid enzyme release, and steatorrhoea is sometimes difficult to abolish, despite increasing doses of pancreatic enzyme supplements. Pancrease and Creon are preparations of pancreatin in which enteric-coated microspheres are used. Creon contains more lipase, and over 80% of this is liberated at pH 5.6 in less than 30 minutes. The capsules are swallowed whole with meals, or opened to allow the granules to be taken with fluid or soft food. One or two capsules are taken with meals in the first instance, the dose being increased as necessary, usually to some 10–15 capsules daily. Patients with no pancreatic exocrine function frequently need three or four times this intake to control steatorrhoea. The preparations should not be used in acute pancreatitis, and their high purine content means that hyperuricosuria and hyperuicaemia have been reported occasionally when very high doses have been taken. Newer formulations may enable the same amount of enzyme to be given daily in a smaller number of capsules.

If steatorrhoea does not respond to oral pancreatic enzyme supplements, measures designed to raise duodenal pH should be used. Although in theory this can be achieved by antacids, in practice an H_2 receptor antagonist such as cimetidine (400 mg two or three times a day) is usually prescribed (Zentler-Munro & Northfield 1987). If steatorrhoea is still troublesome, fat intake may have to be reduced to approximately 50 g per day and consideration given to supplementing the diet with medium chain triglycerides.

Treatment of diabetes mellitus

Diabetes is by no means inevitable in chronic pancreatitis and, as indicated above, usually develops after exocrine insufficiency has become manifest. It may be controlled by diet alone, oral hypoglycaemic drugs or insulin. In patients requiring insulin, the accompanying lack of endogenous glucagon secretion may give rise to insulin sensitivity and a greater risk of hypoglycaemia. Conversely, the risk of diabetic ketoacidosis is minimal in that there is usually enough insulin secretion to prevent the release of fatty acids from adipose tissue and their subsequent metabolism to ketone bodies in the liver (Banks 1989).

Treatment of malnutrition

Malnutrition, weight loss and muscle wasting are common in chronic pancreatitis. The patient may be afraid to eat because of pain, may have steatorrhoea and creatorrhoea because of pancreatic dysfunction, and may have the nutritional problems associated with chronic alcoholism. Vitamin deficiency may occur, particularly in alcoholics, and supplementation may be needed. Deficient fat intake or excessive fat loss can be countered by increased protein and carbohydrate intake, although the dietary management of diabetes mellitus can make for difficulties. Regular involvement of a dietician is advisable, and nutritional status should be monitored by regular weight measurements, anthropometry (mid-arm muscle circumference and triceps skinfold thickness), and serum albumin determinations. However, anthropometry may be inaccurate in patients with subcutaneous oedema and lack the precision needed to assess the effects of nutritional intervention. Similarly, serum albumin measurements are frequently affected by factors other than nutritional status. Bioelectrical impedance analysis is a new method of measuring body composition which can be applied at the patient's bedside and, by measuring total body potassium, provides a useful index of body cell mass (Fearon et al 1992).

Treatment of complications

Some of the complications of chronic pancreatitis demand that conservative management be abandoned in favour of operative intervention, and these will be discussed further in Chapter 26. Haemorrhage is almost always an indication for operation, whereas duodenal and colonic obstruction can often be treated conservatively (Fig. 25.2) unless it is obvious that a fibrotic stricture has developed. Biliary tract obstruction is rarely an isolated indication for surgery (Aranha et al 1984) but should be undertaken if there is persistent obstructive jaundice or cholangitis. The serum alkaline phosphatase levels are a useful means of monitoring the effect of biliary obstruction on liver function in patients being treated conservatively. Elevation of alkaline phosphatase levels to more than twice the normal value on two occasions is an indication for ultrasonography, and possibly liver biopsy, as a means of determining the need for surgery (Wilson et al 1989).

The management of pseudocysts in chronic pancreatitis remains controversial. Persistent pseudocysts are liable to complications such as bleeding and rupture, so that operative intervention is usually recommended when the pseudocyst fails to resolve within 6 weeks of conservative management (Bradley & Clements 1975). Size is an important predictor of outcome, and most surgeons are reluctant to defer operation in patients with pseudocysts larger than 6 cm in diameter (Bradley 1990). Percutaneous drainage offers an alternative to surgical and endoscopic drainage of persistent pseudocysts, but precise definition of its role is still hampered by a lack of prospective controlled studies and by the fact that most reports deal with a mixture of patients with acute and chronic pancreatitis. In a recent retrospective study, Adams & Anderson (1992) found that, although percutaneous drainage had no mortality, the mean duration of catheter drainage was 42 days and the drain track infection rate 48%. Furthermore, the frequency of further operations to deal with the complications of chronic pancreatitis was greater in patients having percutaneous drainage (19%) than in those having surgical drainage (9.5%), although this difference was not statistically significant. They consider that the drawbacks of drainage (creation of an external pancreatic fistula and track infection) are balanced by its low mortality rate, the ability to avoid operation, and the fact that the operative field is not violated if duct drainage surgery is subsequently required.

A number of authors have advocated selective non-operative, non-interventional management of pseudocysts, using an expectant approach in patients without significant pain, gastrointestinal obstruction or other

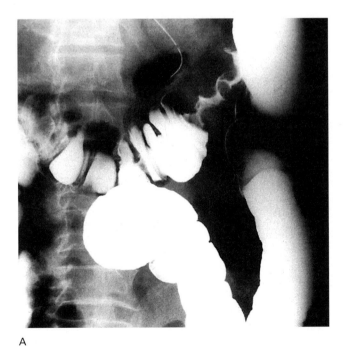

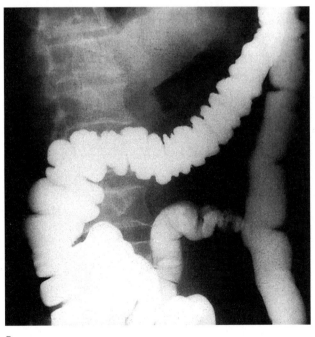

A

B

Fig. 25.2 Barium enema in a 68-year-old man. **A** Severe stenosis of the transverse colon during an acute exacerbation of chronic pancreatitis. **B** The stenosis had resolved spontaneously 7 weeks later.

complications necessitating surgery, and a pseudocyst which appears mature on imaging and which has no features of a cystic neoplasm (Yeo et al 1990, Vitas & Sarr 1992). Vitas & Sarr (1992) treated 68 of their 114 patients, 69 of whom had chronic pancreatitis, expectantly. After a mean follow-up of 46 months, severe life-threatening complications had occurred in only 6 (9%) of the patients treated expectantly. The pseudocyst resolved in 57% of the patients followed radiologically, and although patients eventually coming to operation tended to have larger pseudocysts than those who did not (mean diameter 6.9 vs. 4.9 cm), it is of interest that no serious complications developed in the seven patients with pseudocysts larger than 10 cm who were treated expectantly. Despite these encouraging reports of selective non-operative management or percutaneous drainage, we would still normally advocate operation if the pseudocyst is larger than 6 cm in diameter and has failed to resolve within 6 weeks from the onset of symptoms.

Pancreatic ascites and pleural effusions are relatively rare spontaneous complications of chronic pancreatitis that frequently escape prompt diagnosis. A high index of suspicion must be entertained in any patient developing ascites or pleural effusion (unilaterally or bilaterally) on a background of pancreatic inflammation. The diagnosis is confirmed by the finding of high amylase and protein (more than 30 g/l) levels in peritoneal or pleural aspirates, and ERP is invaluable in demonstrating the site of leakage from the pancreatic duct. In some patients, an external pancreatic fistula is the consequence of attempts to treat pancreatic pseudocysts by percutaneous means. Conservative management, consisting of nil by mouth, repeat paracentesis and TPN, is instituted, and the long-acting somatostatin analogue octreotide (50–100 μg two or three times a day, by subcutaneous injection) is now usually prescribed. While there is little doubt that this regimen reduces pancreatic output and may cure fistulas which have followed pancreatic trauma or necrosectomy for acute pancreatitis, healing is much less likely in malnourished patients with the scarred fibrotic pancreas of chronic pancreatitis. For these reasons, early surgery is usually recommended in patients with chronic pancreatitis when the fistula fails to heal promptly (Parekh & Segal 1992).

REFERENCES

Adams D B, Anderson M C 1992 Percutaneous catheter drainage compared with internal drainage in the management of pancreatic pseudocyst. Annals of Surgery 215: 571–576

Ammann R W, Akovbiantz A, Largiader F, Schueler G 1984 Course and outcome of chronic pancreatitis. Longitudinal study of a mixed medical-surgical series of 245 patients. Gastroenterology 86: 820–828

Amman R, Munch R, Largiader F, Akovbiantz A, Marincek B 1992 Pancreatic and hepatic abscesses: a late complication in 10 patients with chronic pancreatitis. Gastroenterology 103: 560–565

Aranha G V, Prinz R A, Freeark R J, Greenlee H B 1984 The spectrum of biliary tract obstruction from chronic pancreatitis. Archives of Surgery 119: 595–600

Banks P A 1989 Medical strategy in chronic pancreatitis. In: Carter D C, Warshaw A L (eds) Pancreatitis. Churchill Livingstone, Edinburgh, p 133–147

Bockman D E, Büchler M, Malfertheiner P, Beger H G 1989 Analysis of nerves in chronic pancreatitis. Gastroenterology 94: 1459–1469

Bradley E L III 1990 Pseudocysts in chronic pancreatitis: development and clinical implications. In: Beger H G, Büchler M, Ditschuneit H, Malfertheiner P (eds) Chronic pancreatitis. Springer-Verlag. Berlin, p 260–268

Bradley E L III, Clements L J Jr 1975 Spontaneous resolution of pancreatic pseudocysts: implications for timing of operative intervention. American Journal of Surgery 129: 23–28

Braganza J M, Hunt L P, Warwick F 1982 Relationship between pancreatic exocrine function and ductal morphology in chronic pancreatitis. Gastroenterology 82: 1341–1347

Di Magno E P 1982 Controversies in the treatment of exocrine pancreatic insufficiency. Digestive Diseases and Sciences 27: 481–484

Di Magno E P, Malagelada J R, Taylor W F L, Go V L W 1977 A prospective comparison of current diagnostic tests for pancreatic cancer. New England Journal of Medicine 297: 737–742

Fearon K C H, Richardson R A, Hannan J, Cowan S, Watson W, Shenkin A, Garden O J 1992 Bioelectrical impedance analysis in the measurement of the body composition of surgical patients. British Journal of Surgery 79: 421–423

Grant J P, James S, Grabowski V, Trexler K M 1984 Total parenteral nutrition in pancreatic disease. Annals of Surgery 200: 627–631

Gullo L, Parenti M, Monti L, Pezzilli R, Barbara L 1990 Diabetic retinopathy in chronic pancreatitis. Gastroenterology 98: 1577–1581

Isaksson G, Ihse I 1983 Pain reduction by an oral pancreatic enzyme preparation in chronic pancreatitis. Digestive Diseases and Sciences 28: 97–102

Keith R G, Saibil F G, Sheppard R H 1989 Treatment of chronic alcoholic pancreatis by pancreatic resection. American Journal of Surgery 157: 156–162

Larvin M, McMahon M J, Pumtis M C A, Thomas W E G 1992 Marked placebo responses in chronic pancreatitis: final results of a controlled trial of Creon therapy. British Journal of Surgery 79: 457 (Abstract)

Layer P, Jansen J B M J, Cherian L, Lamers C B H W, Goebell H 1990 Feedback regulation of human pancreatic secretion. Effects of protease inhibition on duodenal delivery and small intestinal transit of pancreatic enzymes. Gastroenterology 98: 1311–1319

Leahy A L, Carter D C 1991 Pain and chronic pancreatitis. European Journal of Gastroenterology and Hepatology 3: 425–433

Levy P, Milan C, Pignon J P, Baetz A, Bernardes P 1989 Mortality factors associated with chronic pancreatitis. Unidimensional and multidimensional analysis of a medical-surgical series of 240 patients. Gastroenterology 96: 1165–1172

Machado M C, Da Cunha J E M, Bachella T, Mott C de B, Duarte I, Bettarello A 1984 Acute pancreatic necrosis in chronic alcoholic pancreatitis. Digestive Diseases and Sciences 29: 709–713

Miyake H, Harada H, Ochi K, Kunichika K, Tanaka J, Kimura I 1989 Prognosis and prognostic factors in chronic pancreatitis. Digestive Diseases and Sciences 34: 449–455

Mössner J, Wresky H P, Kestel W, Zeeh J, Regner U, Fischbach W 1989 Influence of treatment with pancreatic extracts on pancreatic enzyme secretion. Gut 30: 1143–1149

Nagata A, Homma T, Tamai K et al 1981 A study of chronic pancreatitis by serial endoscopic pancreatography. Gastroenterology 81: 884–891

Niederau C, Grendell J H 1985 Diagnosis of chronic pancreatitis. Gastroenterology 88: 1973–1995

Parekh D, Segal I 1992 Pancreatic ascites and effusion. Archives of Surgery 127: 707–712

Sauerbruch T, Holl J, Sackmann M, Paumgartner G 1992 Extracorporeal lithotripsy of pancreatic stones in patients with chronic pancreatitis and pain: a prospective follow-up study. Gut 33: 969–972

Slaff J, Jacobson D, Randall Tillman C, Curington C, Toskes P 1984 Protease-specific suppression of pancreatic exocrine secretion. Gastroenterology 87: 44–52

Vitas G J, Sarr M G 1992 Selected management of pancreatic pseudocysts: Operative versus expectant management. Surgery 111: 123–130

Warshaw A L 1984 Pain in chronic pancreatitis. Patients, patience and the impatient surgeon. Gastroenterology 86: 987–987

Watanabe S, Shiratori K, Takeuchi T, Chey W Y, You C H, Chang T M 1986 Release of cholecystokinin and exocrine pancreatic secretion in response to an elemental diet in human subjects. Digestive Diseases and Sciences 31: 919–924

Wilson C, Auld C D, Schlinkert R et al 1989 Hepatobiliary complications in chronic pancreatitis. Gut 30: 520–527

Yeo C J, Bastidas J A, Lynch-Nyhan A, Fishman E K, Zinner M J, Cameron J L 1990 The natural history of pancreatic pseudocysts documented by computed tomography. Surgery, Gynecology and Obstetrics 170: 411–417

Zentler-Munro P L, Northfield T C 1987 Review: pancreatic enzyme replacement – applied physiology and pharmacology. Alimentary Pharmacology Therapeutics 1: 575–591

26. Preoperative assessment and indications for operation in chronic pancreatitis

M. Trede   D. C. Carter

Chronic pancreatitis is not primarily a surgical disease. It is, in fact, difficult to envisage this malady as a single disease at all. Rather it presents itself as 'multiple diseases with multiple causes and varying natural histories' (Howard 1987a). Nevertheless, surgeons will find themselves confronted by patients referred to them in the hope that there is some surgical solution for the problem of chronic pancreatitis. However, before any operative procedure is even considered, it is wise to assess the patient with the aims defined in Chapter 25:

1. to confirm the diagnosis of chronic pancreatitis
2. to find the cause and, if possible, eradicate it
3. to stage the severity of the disease, its morphology and its complications
4. to exclude other accompanying diseases.

The diagnostic methods at our disposal for the clarification of these four points have been discussed in detail in Section 2 and in Chapter 25. Here, we intend merely to analyse their practical value as applied to the surgical management of chronic pancreatitis.

DIAGNOSIS AND ASSESSMENT

History and clinical examination

The patient will usually present with one main symptom: pain. A careful history is important not only to analyse the nature of this pain, but also as a first step in really getting to know the patient. Questions will concern:

1. the location of the pain: is it epigastric, radiating to the left or to the right or centred in the back (depending on the main focus of disease)?
2. the nature of the pain: it will usually be a dull, gnawing ache and less frequently colicky.
3. its timing and severity: is the pain precipitated by dietary excesses; is it permanent or intermittent, and how many attacks occur per year; how much time has been lost off work or spent in hospital; are analgesics

required for pain control; and is there already addiction to these drugs?

This leads on to the question of alcohol consumption. In most series of chronic pancreatitis, alcoholism accounts for about 60% of cases and an unknown number of patients with alcohol-associated disease are probably concealed in the so-called 'idiopathic' group (Williamson & Cooper 1987, Hollands & Little 1989, Marks 1990). Above all, the surgeon must find out if the patient is really 'dry' or whether he remains an unrepentant alcoholic. The answer to this question will never be completely reliable. Involving relatives and friends in this part of the problem early on is probably more effective than involving a psychiatrist. Nevertheless, proper care of the patient over the long course of this chronic disease will necessitate an interdisciplinary approach with participation of the gastroenterologist, endocrinologist, radiologist, surgeon and psychiatrist (Creutzfeldt 1987). While it would be unethical to exclude alcoholics completely from an operation that is positively indicated, there can be no doubt that continued alcohol abuse plays a bigger part in the final outcome than does the operation itself (Block 1983, Adson & McIlrath 1986, Little 1987, Trede 1987).

Characteristic physical signs may be missing altogether in uncomplicated chronic pancreatitis. However, depending on the duration and severity of the disease, the patient will usually show signs of malnutrition and weight loss. There will often be the burns of innumerable hot water bottles applied to the abdomen for pain relief and possibly the scars of previous and ineffective operations (Fig. 26.1). Some of the complications of chronic pancreatitis, such as an inflammatory mass in the pancreatic head or a large pseudocyst may be palpable or even visible.

Ultrasonography

Ultrasonography is included as part of the physical examination; the portable high-resolution real-time scanner is developing into the 'second stethoscope' of the surgeon.

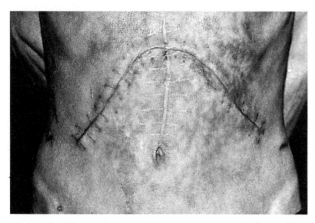

Fig. 26.1   43-year-old man with chronic pancreatitis demonstrating loss of weight, hot-water-bottle 'burns' and three scars of operations (appendicectomy, partial gastrectomy and left hemipancreatectomy).

Sonography will discover fluid collections, inflammatory masses, cysts, calculi and dilatation of the pancreatic duct with an overall sensitivity of around 60–70% (Bolondi et al 1989). It is particularly useful in the cachectic or pregnant patient and whenever repeated follow-up examinations are called for. However, as long as it remains dependent on the experience of the examiner and as long as false negative findings are reported in some 25% of cases (Bolondi et al 1989), ultrasonography will retain second place after computed tomography (CT) in assessment.

Computed tomography

Particularly when used in conjunction with dynamic bolus contrast enhancement, CT will provide clear and reproducible findings with a false negative rate of only 7% as far as detection of chronic pancreatitis is concerned (Luetmer et al 1989). It frequently provides valuable information about morphological changes in the gland and the presence of complications which may influence both the decision to operate and the type of operation performed. In this regard, CT should be viewed as complementary to ultrasonography and endoscopic retrograde cholangiopancreatography (ERCP) in the decision making process.

Magnetic resonance imaging has so far not been able to add anything that CT cannot provide and so plays no role in the assessment of chronic pancreatitis at present (Freeny 1990).

Endoscopic retrograde cholangiopancreatography

(ERCP) may reveal the typical findings of pancreatic and biliary ductal dilatation, define filling defects caused by calculi, and detect cysts and collections, provided these communicate with the pancreatic duct system (see Ch. 10). The examination may be of crucial importance in deter-

mining whether resection or drainage is appropriate, and may help to determine whether additional procedures, such as biliary drainage or pseudocyst drainage, will be required at the time of pancreatic surgery. Furthermore, the investigation can help to exclude other causes of epigastric pain such as peptic ulcer and gastric cancer. On the other hand, ERCP fails to outline the duct system in some 5–10% of patients and gives a correct diagnosis of chronic pancreatitis in only 90% of the remainder (Swobodnik et al 1983). This is why some surgeons occasionally still have recourse to intraoperative pancreatography (Cooper & Williamson 1983). Like other diagnostic methods, even ERCP may fail to detect early changes of the disease (Caletti et al 1982) and the morphological changes found correlate neither with impaired pancreatic function (Braganza et al 1982) nor with the severity of the symptoms (Malfertheiner et al 1986).

Other examinations

Hypotonic duodenography and barium enema

An upper gastrointestinal barium study, once the mainstay of diagnosis, has been largely superseded by endoscopy. Hypotonic duodenography may still have a place when it comes to assessing the functional significance of duodenal stenosis and the need (rare) for surgical intervention. Similarly, a barium enema is called for in those rare cases of colonic obstruction complicating chronic pancreatitis.

Selective angiography

Upper abdominal angiography fulfills three functions in the assessment of potential candidates for surgery. In the arterial phase it can discover pseudoaneurysms and the source of bleeding in cases with haemorrhage into the pancreatic duct (Stanley et al 1976). In the portal venous phase, various degrees of obstruction ranging from slight stenosis to complete thrombosis of the splenic, superior mesenteric and/or portal vein with oesophageal varices may be detected (Rignault et al 1968, Warshaw et al 1987, Williamson & Cooper 1987). Finally, angiography will give forewarning of congenital vascular anomalies that occur in some 20% of cases and which might complicate any operative procedure, especially those involving the region of the pancreatic head.

Cytological examination

Cytological examination of an inflammatory mass of the head of the pancreas by means of fine-needle aspiration is indicated mainly in patients with a possible carcinoma who are not fit for operation. Clearly only the unequivocal detection of malignant cells is of any consequence (Hollands & Little 1989) (Ch.12).

Laboratory

Laboratory tests of pancreatic function, both endocrine and exocrine, come at the end of this list, since their results have little influence on the indication for or against any operation. In fact, many experienced pancreatic surgeons do not include these tests in their preoperative work-up (Rossi et al 1985). In the authors' view, function studies may nevertheless have a place in providing a baseline for postoperative follow-up and assessment of the disease (Frey & Braasch 1984, Lankisch 1990, Toskes 1990).

INDICATIONS FOR OPERATION

It bears repeating, that chronic pancreatitis is not a surgical disease – it belongs primarily in the domain of the gastroenterologist. Chronic pancreatitis causes progressive loss of pancreatic function both endocrine and exocrine and there is no surgical intervention that can reverse this process. In spite of some reports to the contrary (Nealon et al 1988, Beger & Büchler 1990) it seems improbable that any operation can even slow down the progress of the underlying disease (Moossa 1981, Warshaw 1990).

Unfortunately, as discussed in Chapter 25, the same applies to most conservative medical measures available at this time. Even complete abstinence from alcohol has no influence on progressive pancreatic duct changes (Nagata et al 1981) and will reduce pain in only 50% of patients (Ihse & Lankisch 1988). Furthermore, the pain-relieving effect of pancreatic enzyme medication, based on the hypothesis of a negative feedback regulation of pancreatic secretion by intraduodenal protease levels (Ihse et al 1977, Isaksson & Ihse, 1983, Slaff et al 1984) has not been regularly confirmed in clinical practice (Fölsch 1989, Halgren et al 1986), especially when pain is severe and constant (Warshaw 1990).

It is when this medical treatment fails, based as it mainly is on dietary restriction, analgesics and substitution therapy for loss of function, that many of these patients are finally referred to the surgeon. Over the past 19 years, more than 700 patients were referred to the Surgical Clinic in Mannheim with the diagnosis of chronic pancreatitis and with the express purpose of having an operation. After careful assessment from the surgical point of view, it seemed that in 42% of these patients there was no compelling indication for surgery, as yet (Fig. 26.2). The remaining 58% did have surgery directed at one or more of three main objectives:

- to bypass or remove the complications of the disease
- to rule out any suspicion of carcinoma
- to ameliorate intractable pain.

One final objective accompanied all the others: to preserve as much functional pancreatic tissue as possible.

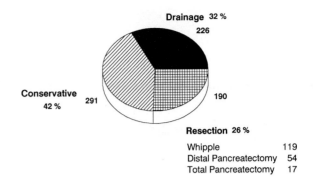

Fig. 26.2 The spectrum of conservative and operative treatment for chronic pancreatitis, as seen in 707 patients at the University Surgical Clinic at Mannheim, October 1972 to January 1992.

Table 26.1 lists the indications for operation in chronic pancreatitis. The list is headed by the so-called 'mechanical' complications. If any one of these forms of mechanical obstruction is irreversible and resistant to conservative measures, then the only solution will be a 'mechanical', i.e. a surgical one.

Erosion of either the pancreatic duct or peripancreatic vessels may require emergency intervention.

The inability to exclude the suspicion of carcinoma accounts for some 15% of operations in patients presenting with chronic pancreatitis, in spite of all modern diagnostic procedures directed at this very question.

Finally, the chief indication that underscores all of the others is intractable pain. Although its exact cause may not be known in each case, it does respond to operations designed to relieve mechanical obstruction. Each of these indications will now be dealt with in turn.

Biliary stenosis

Stenosis of the common bile duct is not as rare in chronic pancreatitis as was once thought. It occurs in 30–65% of patients in most series (Sarles & Sahel 1978, Morel & Rohner 1987, Hollands & Little 1989, Wilson et al 1989, Beger & Büchler 1990). This stenosis involves the retropancreatic portion of the common duct. It is usually of the tapering type – not an abrupt cut-off as in malignant obstruction – and it is seldom complete. That is why prestenotic dilatation of the biliary tree is usually not very

Table 26.1 Indications for operation

Biliary obstruction
Duodenal stenosis (colonic stricture)
Pancreatic duct stenosis
Pseudocysts
Pancreatic ascites (pleural effusion)
Portal venous compression (splenic/mesenteric venous thrombosis)
Pancreatic haemorrhage
Suspicion of pancreatic carcinoma
Intractable pain

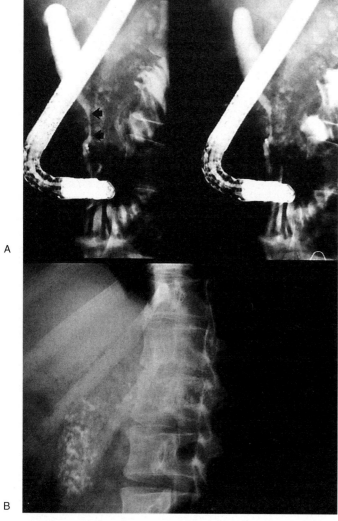

Fig. 26.3 32-year-old man with **A** common duct stenosis (arrows) shown on endoscopic retrograde cholangiopancreatography and **B** extensive calcification (by plain abdominal X-ray).

marked and bilirubin values seldom exceed 85–170 μmol/l (5–10 mg%) (Fig. 26.3).

Biliary obstruction can be accompanied by pain in chronic pancreatitis (Warshaw 1990) although it is not clear whether it is directly painful or whether the pain is the result of the pancreatic inflammation. The jaundice may wax and wane in the early stages of chronic pancreatitis, making it difficult to distinguish this from biliary pancreatitis (Ch. 21).

Although 16% of patients with chronic pancreatitis also have bile duct stones (Aranha et al 1984), cholelithiasis plays no significant role in the aetiology of this disease. Once severe chronic pancreatitis is established, fibrotic changes in the head of the pancreas will extend directly into the wall of the duct causing permanent obstruction (Singh & Reber 1990) that can lead to cholangitis and, rarely, even to biliary cirrhosis (Warshaw et al 1976, Wilson

et al 1989). Simple decompression by partial resection of the pancreatic head is unable to influence such strictures of the common duct wall.

Bornman et al (1990) found that some 20% of patients with asymptomatic common duct stenosis on ERCP had raised alkaline phosphatase levels. These patients may be followed conservatively since no deterioration of liver function was found after a mean follow-up of 4 years. However, if biliary obstruction is symptomatic (i.e. causes jaundice and pain), relief should be sought before hepatic sequelae occur. Endoscopic transpapillary drainage by means of a stent is indicated only as a temporary measure in this benign condition, since the prolonged course of the disease would mean an inordinate number of stent changes.

If biliary obstruction is the only complication of chronic pancreatitis, (which it rarely is) then some form of bilioenteric bypass is indicated. Bradley & Salam (1979) advocated a choledochoduodenostomy since this would cause the least problems should a subsequent resection be necessary. However, this anastomosis depends on a well-dilated duct for long-term patency, a condition that seldom applies in chronic pancreatitis. Hollands and Little (1989) had satisfactory results with cholecystojejunostomy whereas most authors, fearing cholangitis, prefer a hepatico-jejunostomy utilizing a long Roux-en-Y-loop (Bornman et al 1990).

It is interesting that the symptom of pain is improved along with the jaundice following bypass in some of the patients so treated (Hollands & Little 1989, Warshaw et al 1976). Usually, however, biliary obstruction is only one aspect of the disease centred in the head of the pancreas, and for this situation some form of resection is then required.

Duodenal stenosis

Some degree of duodenal obstruction is commonly found in chronic pancreatitis during endoscopy or on upper gastrointestinal radiology. This must be distinguished from stenosis due to a peptic ulcer and from transient compression caused by an acute exacerbation of recurrent pancreatitis. Fibrotic, and possibly ischaemic (Bockman 1988), changes in the duodenal wall, leading to irreversible stenosis with vomiting and inanition are relatively rare (Fig. 26.4). Only five out of 19 patients in a series reported by Bradley & Clements (1981) actually required a bypass. This is best achieved by gastrojejunostomy combined with some form of vagotomy to avoid peptic ulceration. However, this also is rarely a solitary complication so that here too, pancreatoduodenectomy will provide the final and optimal solution in many cases.

Colonic stricture

A colonic stricture that may mimic carcinoma, rarely

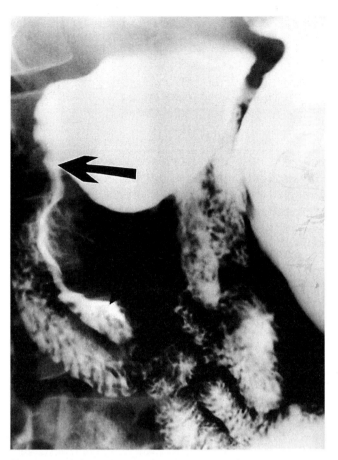

Fig. 26.4 37-year-old man with severe stenosis of the second part of the duodenum (arrows).

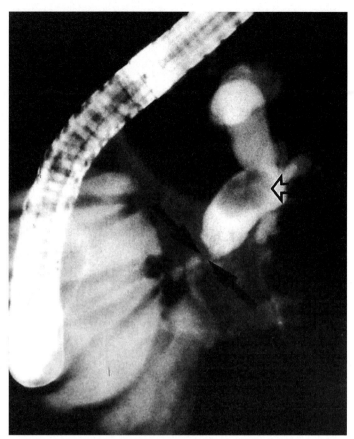

Fig. 26.5 44-year-old man with stenosis (black arrows), dilatations and calculi (white arrow) in the pancreatic duct at endoscopic retrograde pancreatography (ERP).

complicates chronic pancreatitis (Hancock et al 1973, Hoffmeister & Trede 1977). Once a carcinoma has been excluded by colonoscopy, an expectant conservative strategy will usually be rewarded by spontaneous resolution of the stenosis. Bradley (1982a) collected 34 patients with colonic strictures primarily involving the transverse colon and splenic flexure. When fibrotic and ischaemic involvement of the colonic wall causes irreversible changes and chronic ileus, this can only be relieved by segmental resection of the affected colon.

Pancreatic duct stenosis/obstruction

Regarding pancreatic duct pathology, patients can be divided into two numerically equal groups: those with a dilated duct system and those with so-called small-duct-disease (Warshaw 1990). So far, there is no aetiological explanation for this difference. In small-duct-disease the pancreatic duct may appear quite normal on ERCP, whereas duct dilatation is associated with stenoses, protein precipitates and calculi often appearing as a so-called 'chain of lakes' (Figs 26.5 & 26.6).

Both forms of chronic pancreatitis are associated with pain and it is the pain that therapeutic endeavours are aimed at. In dilated-duct-disease pain could be explained by stenoses causing raised intraductal pressure due to pancreatic secretion, particularly after meals. In fact, duct pressure has been measured both during operation and percutaneously and found to be elevated to above 20–30 cmH$_2$O which is 3–4 times the level in normal controls (Bradley 1982b, Sato et al 1986, Ebbehoj et al 1990, see Leahy & Carter 1991). On the other hand, it is remarkable to observe the ease with which these dilated ducts are cannulated and filled and how rapidly the contrast medium empties away following ERCP.

Nevertheless, with duct dilatation of at least 8 mm in diameter, some drainage procedure is indicated (Fig. 26.6). Procedures involving resection of the pancreatic tail, splenectomy and retrograde drainage of the duct into a Roux-en-Y-loop of jejunum (Du Val 1954) have been largely abandoned because pain relief was disappointing (possibly due to multiple proximal stenoses preventing complete drainage), or because of a reduction of pancreatic functional reserve (by resection of the tail), and because of the hypothetical sequelae of splenectomy (sepsis). The latter two disadvantages also apply if the anastomosis is extended toward the right by unroofing the pancreatic duct (Puestow & Gillesby 1958).

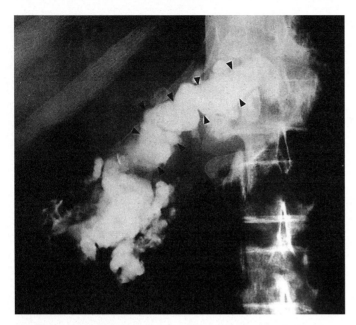

Fig. 26.6 48-year-old man with massively dilated pancreatic duct at ERP.

Currently a long side-to-side pancreaticojejunostomy reaching as far as possible into the head of the pancreas and avoiding any loss of spleen and pancreatic parenchyma is the method of choice (Partington & Rochelle 1960). Pain relief can be expected in 60–75% of patients and it will last for several years provided the patient stops drinking (Cuilleret & Guillemin 1990). In others, pain returns even though the anastomosis remains patent.

It remains to be seen whether interventionist methods of duct drainage, e.g. by an endoscopically inserted trans-papillary stent (Soehendra et al 1986) provide more than temporary relief. The same applies to the endoscopic extraction of pancreatic duct calculi, or their fragmentation by external shock wave lithotripsy or laser energy transmitted along the quartz fibre of a miniscope (Ell et al 1988, Kozarek 1990).

The endoscopic occlusion of the pancreatic duct by means of Ethibloc with the aim of producing fibrosis of exocrine pancreatic tissue (Gebhardt & Stolte 1978) has not produced encouraging results in clinical practice (Rösch 1983).

Pancreatic cysts and pseudocysts

True cystic dilatations of the pancreatic duct as well as pseudocysts outside the confines of the pancreas, complicate chronic pancreatitis in some 25% of patients (Aranha et al 1983). Pseudocysts of less than 6 cm in diameter can be safely observed for a period of up to 6 weeks, particularly if they are asymptomatic. Spontaneous resolution of cysts larger than 6 cm is rare and simple observation carries a risk of complications (leak or rupture,

compression of adjacent structures and haemorrhage) that is greater than that of elective surgery (Bradley 1990).

Today, few patients reach the surgeon before some form of interventionist drainage has been at least attempted. While appealing to the patient at first sight, these methods are not without risk and the rate of recurrence is high. Percutaneous cyst aspiration is followed by recurrence in almost 70% of cases (Bradley 1982c). Results are better if prolonged drainage is employed. Another alternative is endoscopic transgastric cyst drainage by means of a stent (Hancke & Henriksen 1986). However, this assumes an adherence between the stomach and cyst wall that may not be present in up to 60% of cases (Bradley 1990). Apart from the dangers of leakage and haemorrhage that these interventionist manoeuvres carry, there is the risk of draining an unrecognized neoplastic cyst that should, in fact, be radically removed (Fig. 26.7). Biopsy of the cyst wall which is part of every operation on pseudocysts is, of course, not possible during percutaneous or endoscopic drainage.

Operative treatment is indicated as a rule for all pseudocysts of more than 6 cm in diameter that show no sign of resolution within a 6-week observation period. Depending on cyst location, drainage will be achieved by anastomosing the stomach, duodenum or a Roux-en-Y-loop of jejunum to the lowest point of the cyst wall. In Europe, the last-mentioned method has priority (Zirngibl et al 1983). For cysts situated near the tail of the pancreas resection is often the best solution. One must remember, however, that simple cyst drainage, or even resection, may not solve the underlying problems of chronic pancreatitis. Thus, biliary or pancreatic duct obstruction and intractable pain will require additional drainage procedures or even resection (Prinz 1990, Roscher 1990).

Pancreatic ascites and pleural effusion

Ascites and pleural effusion are rare but ominous complications of both chronic and acute pancreatitis. Occurring in only 1% of patients they carry a mortality of 20–30% if not treated (Fielding et al 1989, Neoptolemos & Winslet 1990). This particular form of ascites is due to a leak either from the pancreatic duct or a pseudocyst. The diagnosis depends on ultrasonography, aspiration of ascites (showing raised amylase and protein levels >30 g/l) and ERCP to localize the leak. Conservative treatment including repeated paracenteses, parenteral alimentation and somatostatin to minimize pancreatic secretion, should be given a chance for 2–3 weeks. If that does not lead to improvement, then operative treatment is indicated. This depends on an accurate localization of the leak (by ERCP) and consists either of a resection or internal drainage of the fistula into a Roux-en-Y-loop of jejunum. Pleural effusions will dry out once the abdominal cause has been eradicated (Cameron 1978).

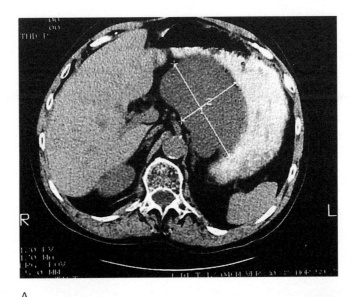

Fig. 26.7 **A** 57-year-old man with presumed pseudocyst of the pancreas. Because of severe cardiopulmonary insufficiency an endoscopic cystogastrostomy was attempted. This led to perforation, peritonitis and the need for emergency removal of the 'cyst'. **B** The resection specimen shows the spleen (S) and cyst (C) that turned out to be a dermoid cyst with solid teratomatous components.

Portal venous obstruction

Some involvement of the portal vein and its two main tributaries is encountered in 10% of patients presenting with chronic pancreatitis (Beger & Büchler 1990). It ranges from mild compression to complete occlusion with thrombosis, portal hypertension, cavernous transformation of peripancreatic veins and oesophageal varices which may bleed (Rignault et al 1968). Quite apart from the therapeutic implications, portal venous stenosis on angiography may pose differential diagnostic problems since it mimics neoplastic compression (Saeger et al 1990) (Ch. 42).

Whereas mild to moderate degrees of portal venous stenosis may be an indication for decompression (usually as part of an operation also directed against other mechanical complications), such an operation would be prohibitively haemorrhagic once there is complete thrombosis of the vein. For this reason, portal or superior mesenteric venous thrombosis with portal hypertension and cavernous transformation of the peripancreatic veins is considered to be a contraindication to any procedure on the pancreas itself (Braasch 1987, Warshaw 1990) (Fig. 26.8).

This does not apply to thrombosis confined to the splenic vein as occurs in patients with predominantly left-sided pancreatitis (Moossa & Gadd, 1985). This may lead to so-called segmental portal hypertension with bleeding

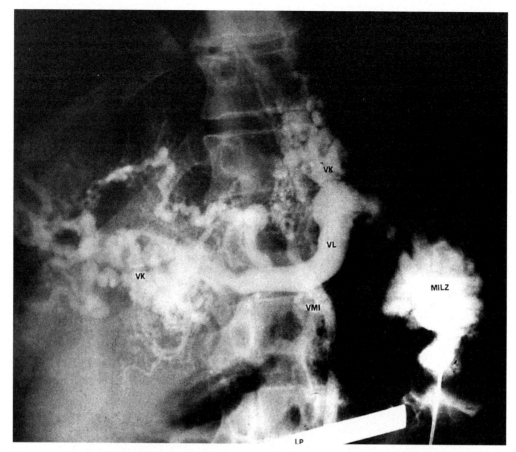

Fig. 26.8   Direct splenoportography (via a laparoscope, LP) in a patient with portal vein thrombosis due to chronic pancreatitis. Milz, spleen; VK, varicose veins; VL, splenic vein; VMI, inferior mesenteric vein.

from gastric and oesophageal varices. Here the best solution is splenectomy and resection of the pancreatic tail (Salam et al 1973).

Pancreatic haemorrhage

Changes in the peripancreatic arteries (splenic, hepatic, gastroduodenal and gastroepiploic) are rarely seen in chronic pancreatitis on preoperative angiography. They range from increased tortuosity to pseudoaneurysms and erosion with massive haemorrhage (Boijsen & Tylen 1972, Stanley et al 1976). Bleeding may take the form of 'haemosuccus pancreaticus' when a fistula between one of the above arteries and the pancreatic duct occurs (Sandblom 1970). More commonly bleeding occurs into a pseudocyst (Hoffmeister & Reiter 1980) and this may be fatal. Emergency angiography is indispensable to locate the source of haemorrhage and if possible, obliterate this through the same catheter (Börjesson et al 1981) (Fig. 26.9). Once the patient has recovered, this is usually followed by resection of the offending part of the pancreas.

Suspicion of pancreatic cancer

The inability to exclude carcinoma in a patient supposedly suffering from chronic pancreatitis is a dilemma that continues to confront experienced diagnosticians and surgeons even in the last decade of this century (Carter, 1992). In spite of the fact that sophisticated radiological methods, fine-needle cytology and endoscopic ultrasonography are at our disposal, there will be some 15% of cases in whom it may be impossible to say whether a symptomatic mass in the head of the pancreas is inflammatory or malignant (Hunt & Blumgart 1982, Trede 1987, Hollands & Little 1989). This can be difficult even for the experienced surgeon at the operating table. And even frozen section examination of needle biopsies may not be helpful in this situation (Harbrecht 1979). Thus, in a report by Gall et al (1982) on resection for chronic pancreatitis, inability to rule out the possibility of carcinoma was part of the indication for operation in 30% of patients. Suspicion of cancer was one additional indication in 34% of patients operated upon for chronic pancreatitis in the Mannheim Surgical Clinic (Saeger et

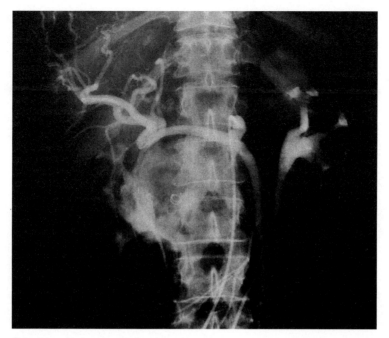

A

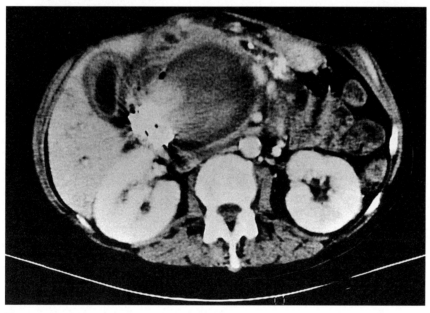

B

Fig. 26.9 A Selective mesenteric arteriography showing bleeding into the false aneurysm of an eroded totally aberrant common hepatic artery in a 57-year-old patient with chronic pancreatitis. **B** Contrast CT demonstrates contrast medium entering the false aneurysm. The aneurysm was obliterated using Gianturco coils.

al 1990). Table 26.2 shows that out of a total of 136 patients, in whom chronic pancreatitis was finally and histologically proven by pancreatic resection, suspicion of carcinoma could not be completely excluded preoperatively in 47 (Fig. 26.10).

It is a sobering thought that in a series of patients operated upon for chronic pancreatitis by White, some 16% turned out to have carcinoma of the pancreas on subsequent follow-up (White & Hart 1979). And conversely, of the 16 'small cancers' resected by Moossa, four were found incidentally by microscopic examination of the specimen resected with the presumptive diagnosis of chronic pancreatitis (Moossa & Levin 1981) (Fig. 26.11).

These observations raise the perennial question of whether there is any cause-and-effect linkage between

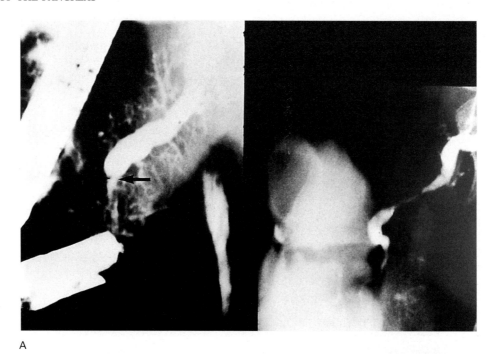

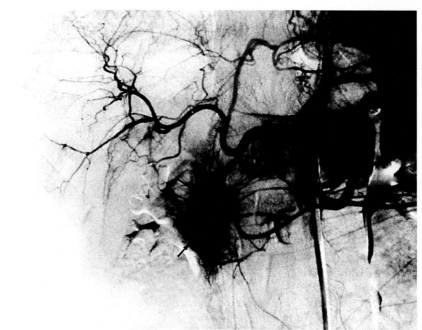

Fig. 26.10 A Pancreatic duct stenosis in a 19-year-old girl presenting with epigastric pain and weight loss. **B** Coeliac arteriography shows flush due to an apparently vascular tumour of the head of the pancreas.

chronic pancreatitis and pancreatic cancer. In spite of the observation that pancreatic carcinoma is always accompanied by some inflammation (Becker 1978) and in spite of very suggestive but anecdotal cases (see Fig. 37.3), there is no clear evidence supporting such a link (Pour 1990).

That leaves us with the conclusion that the surgeon confronted with a symptomatic mass of the pancreas

should remove this by radical resection even if proof of malignancy is lacking, provided the resection can be done with a reasonable risk (Moossa et al 1979, Trede et al, 1990).

Intractable pain

The symptom of pain underscores each of the other

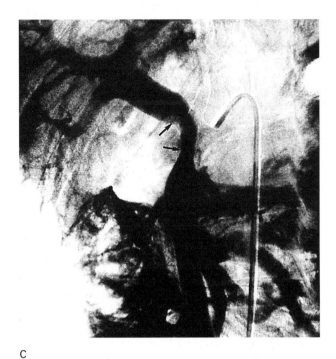

C

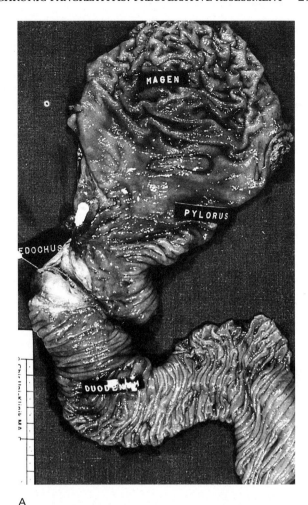

A

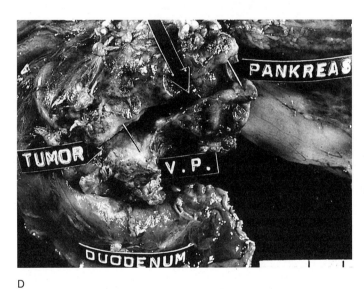

D

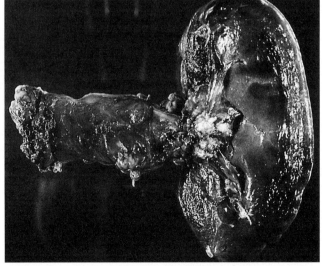

B

Fig. 26.10 (*continued*)   **C** In the portal venous phase doubts as to the operability of this 'tumour' were raised due to constriction of the portal vein. **D** Dissection of the Whipple resection specimen revealed a firm white tumour which led to a dilated pancreatic duct (arrow). V.P., retropancreatic groove in which the portal vein was encased. In spite of these suggestive signs, no malignancy was found on histological examination. The patient is symptom-free 3 years later.

Fig. 26.11   **A** Operative specimen of a Whipple resection performed for presumed chronic pancreatitis in a 36-year-old alcoholic with a 4-year history of recurrent attacks of pancreatic pain. The pathologist unexpectedly found carcinoma of the head of the pancreas reaching up to the line of resection. **B** Operative specimen of remaining pancreas and spleen that were resected 7 days later. The patient died of recurrent cancer 6.5 years later. (With permission of C.V. Mosby Co., St. Louis, from Trede 1985 Surgery 97: 28–35)

Table 26.2 Chronic pancreatitis or carcinoma? Difficulties of preoperative differentiation between pancreatic cancer and chronic pancreatitis in 439 patients seen in the University Surgical Clinic at Mannheim, between October 1972 and January 1992

Preoperative diagnosis	Postoperative diagnosis (histology)	
	Pancreatic carcinoma	Chronic pancreatitis
Pancreatic carcinoma (n = 333)	286	47 (14%)
Chronic pancreatitis (n = 106)	17 (16%)	89
Total	303	136

indications for operation listed in Table 26.2. Intractable pain that significantly affects quality of life, that leads to drug addiction and inanition from fear of eating, is an indication for operation by itself. Neither patients nor their doctors will have the patience to wait for such incapacitating pain to 'burn itself out' (Warshaw 1984).

Ammann et al (1984) first postulated the possiblity that the disease of chronic pancreatitis 'burns itself out' after a median time of 4.5 years from onset, leaving the patient free of pain albeit largely without pancreatic exocrine and endocrine function. However, Ammann (1990) has made it clear that this did not apply to those 50% of patients with persistently severe pain usually due to some complication of pancreatitis. Physicians and surgeons agree that operation is the only hope for these particular patients.

SURGICAL OPTIONS IN CHRONIC PANCREATITIS

Table 26.3 lists the surgical procedures that have been used in the treatment of chronic pancreatitis. While some of the indirect procedures are still used in conjunction with other procedures, none are now advocated in isolation and many are seldom performed (e.g. total denervation). Most of the direct procedures will be dealt with in the subsequent chapters of this section. Therefore in closing this introduction, it seems appropriate to summarize some principles of the surgical treatment of chronic pancreatitis.

● Chronic pancreatitis is not primarily a surgical disease.

● The disease causes a progressive loss of pancreatic exocrine and endocrine function and no surgical operation can reverse this process.

● However, when medical treatment fails or complications occur, surgical treatment is indicated and has to be directed at three main objectives:
1. to bypass or remove the complications of the disease
2. to rule out any suspicion of carcinoma
3. to ameliorate intractable pain.

● Surgical intervention must also aim at preserving as much functioning pancreatic paranchyma as possible.

● Operations for chronic pancreatitis may be divided into indirect and direct procedures. The indirect approach is largely obsolete since none of these methods have been consistently successful: gastric resections or vagotomy have not reduced hormonal stimulation of pancreatic secretion (Stone et al 1985, Moossa 1987); cholecystectomy cannot alter the course of chronic pancreatitis since cholelithiasis rarely causes this disease; and denervation procedures have not shown any reproducible effect (Mallet-Guy 1983, Hiraoka et al 1986, Cuilleret & Guillemin 1990).

● Direct operations on the pancreas are divided into drainage and resection procedures. There should be no 'rivalry' between the two. Quite apart from the fact that every resection implies some drainage as well, both have their distinct indications.

● Drainage is indicated for pseudocysts, biliary obstruction and for pancreatic ducts dilated to a diameter of more than 8 mm. Currently, optimal drainage is provided by a long parenchyma-sparing, side-to-side pancreatico-jejunostomy (Rossi et al 1985, Frey 1990).

● The theoretical advantages of simple drainage notwithstanding, whenever mechanical obstruction involves

Table 26.3 Surgical treatment of chronic pancreatitis

Indirect procedures	Direct procedures
Gastric	Drainage
Billroth II gastrotectomy	External cyst drainage
Selective proximal vagotomy (SPV)	Internal cyst drainage (to stomach, duodenum or jejunum)
Gastrojejunostomy	Pancreaticojejunostomy
Biliary	Retrograde drainage with splenectomy
Cholecystectomy	Lateral side-to-side drainage
Sphincteroplasty	Resection
Bilioenteric anastomosis	Distal pancreatectomy (40–95%)
Denervation	Pancreatoduodenectomy
Splanchnicectomy + coeliac ganglionectomy	Standard Whipple
Total denervation of pancreas	Pylorus-preserving
Denervated pancreatic flap	Total pancreatectomy
	Duodenum preserving resections
	Partial resection of head of pancreas
	Total resection of pancreas
	Resection with autotransplantation

several structures (e.g. duodenum, biliary and pancreatic ducts) the principle of drainage is overextended. Triple drainage procedures (gastrojejunostomy, choledocho-duodenostomy plus pancreaticojejunostomy) seem more complicated and less effective than resection (i.e. of the head of the pancreas) (Prinz 1985, Warshaw 1985).

● Drainage is at a disadvantage compared to resection in that the diseased parenchyma, including possibly a malignant lesion, is left behind.

● Resection procedures are indicated for localized complications, for painful small-duct-disease and whenever carcinoma is suspected and cannot be excluded.

● As a rule, chronic pancreatitis involves the entire gland. Frequently, however, the 'pacemaker' is situated in the head of the pancreas causing pain and stenoses of some or all of the structures meeting there, namely the pancreatic and bile ducts, duodenum and portal vein (Traverso et al 1979).

● Isolated pancreatitis of the tail of the gland is rare. Distal pancreatectomy (resecting 40% of the gland up to the portal vein) is indicated for lesions centred in the left half of pancreas (cysts, splenic vein thrombosis). Subtotal 90% resections from the left have fallen into disrepute since poor long-term pain relief is coupled with a high rate of diabetes (Frey 1981).

● The standard Whipple pancreatoduodenectomy is the preferred resection procedure for most cases of painful complicated pancreatitis centred in the pancreatic head (Gall et al 1982, Morel & Rohner 1987, Trede 1987, Carter 1990, Howard 1990). Various pylorus- and duodenum-preserving alternatives provide equally good results Frey & Smith 1987, Beger & Büchler 1990). But

so far none of the claims of theoretical advantages of these partial resections of the pancreatic head have been substantiated in clinical practice.

● Total pancreatectomy with or without duodenum-preservation is indicated in rare cases of end-stage disease, when all else has failed (Russell 1990, Williamson & Cooper 1987). Surprisingly perhaps, the rate of pain relief is no higher than after partial resection and the ensuing diabetes is particularly difficult to control, if the patient continues to drink.

● Total or subtotal pancreatic resection combined with segmental pancreatic autotransplantation, has not so far been a convincing solution (Rossi et al 1990). Both the rates for pain relief and independence from insulin have been disappointing.

● There is no single ideal operation for the various problems of chronic pancreatitis.

● More important than any particular operative technique is the selection of an appropriate method of management for any particular patient.

● Comparisons between different operative techniques are invidious so long as they are not based on controlled trials. At the very least, the preoperative state of the patient, intraoperative measurements and postoperative follow-up must be comparable and recorded (Frey & Braasch 1984).

● Finally, the long-term results of surgical treatment in chronic alcoholic pancreatitis depend more on the drinking habits of the patient than on the type of surgery performed (Block 1983, Adson & McIlrath 1986, Little 1987). ˙

REFERENCES

Adson M A, McIlrath D C 1986 Surgical treatment of chronic pancreatitis. In: Go V L W et al (eds) The exocrine pancreas: biology, pathobiology, and diseases. Raven Press, New York, p 587–599

Ammann R W 1990 Natural history of chronic (progressive) pancreatitis: A life experience. In: Beger H G, Büchler M, Ditschuneit H, Malfertheiner P (eds) Chronic pancreatitis. Springer-Verlag, Berlin, p 47–62

Ammann R W, Akovbiantz A, Largiader F, Schueler G 1984 Course and outcome of chronic pancreatitis. Longitudinal study of a mixed medical-surgical series of 245 patients. Gastroenterology 86:820–828

Aranha G V, Prinz R A, Esguerra A C, Greenlee H B 1983 The nature and course of cystic pancreatic lesions diagnosed by ultrasound. Archives of Surgery 118:486–488

Aranha G V, Prinz R A, Freeark R J, Greenlee H B 1984 The spectrum of biliary tract obstruction from chronic pancreatitis. Archives of Surgery 119:595–600

Becker V 1978 Carcinoma of the pancreas and chronic pancreatitis a possible relationship. Acta – Hepato-Gastroenterologica 25:257–259

Beger H G, Büchler M 1990 Duodenum-preserving resection of the head of the pancreas in chronic pancreatitis with inflammatory mass in the head. World Journal of Surgery 14:83–87

Block G E 1983 Selection of the appropriate operation for chronic pancreatitis. In: Delaney J P, Jarco R L (eds) Controversies in surgery II. W B Saunders, Philadelphia, p 319–325

Bockman D E 1988 Systems underlying involvement of the duodenum in pancreatic disease. Pancreas 3:592

Boijsen E, Tylen U 1972 Vascular changes in chronic pancreatitis. Acta Radiologica Scandinavica 12:34

Bolondi L, Bassi S L, Gaiani S et al 1989 Sonography of chronic pancreatitis. Radiological Clinics of North America 27:815–833

Börjesson B, Evander A, Ihse I, Joelsson B, Lunderquist A 1981 Gastrointestinal bleeding caused by haemosuccus pancreaticus. Acta Chirurgica Scandinavica 147:299–301

Bornman P C, Kalvaria I, Girdwood A H, Marks I N 1990 Clinical relevance of cholestasis syndrome in chronic pancreatitis – the Cape Town experience. In: Beger H G, Büchler M, Ditschuneit H, Malfertheiner P (eds) Chronic pancreatitis. Springer-Verlag, Berlin, p 256–259

Braasch J W 1987 Discussion of Warshaw 1987. Archives of Surgery 122:410

Bradley E L III 1982a Enteropathies. In: Bradley E L III (ed) Complications of pancreatitis, medical and surgical management. W B Saunders, Philadelphia

Bradley E L III 1982b Pancreatic duct pressure in chronic pancreatitis. American Journal of Surgery 144:313–316

Bradley E L III (ed) 1982c Pseudocysts in complications of pancreatitis. W B Saunders, Philadelphia, p 125

Bradley E L III 1990 Pseudocysts in chronic pancreatitis: development and clinical implications. In: Beger H G, Büchler M, Ditschuneit H,

Malfertheiner P (eds) Chronic pancreatitis. Springer-Verlag, Berlin, p 260–268

Bradley E L III, Clements J L Jr 1981 Idiopathic duodenal obstruction. An unappreciated complication of pancreatitis. Annals of Surgery 193:638–643

Bradley E L III, Salam A A 1979 Hyperbilirubinaemia in inflammatory pancreatic disease. Annals of Surgery 188:620–629

Braganza J M, Hunt L P, Warwick F 1982 Relationship between pancreatic exocrine function and ductal morphology in chronic pancreatitis. Gastroenterology 82:1341–1347

Caletti G, Brocchi E, Agostini D et al 1982 Sensitivity of endoscopic retrograde pancreatography in chronic pancreatitis. British Journal of Surgery 69:507–509

Cameron J L 1978 Chronic pancreatic ascites and pancreatic pleural effusion. Gastroenterology 74:134–140

Carter D C 1990 Pancreatico-duodenectomy for chronic pancreatitis. In: Trede M, Saeger H D (eds) Aktuelle Pankreaschirurgie. Springer-Verlag, Berlin, p 149–157

Carter D C 1992 Cancer of the head of pancreas or chronic pancreatitis? A diagnostic dilemma. Surgery 111:602–603

Cooper M J, Williamson R C N 1983 The value of operative pancreatography. British Journal of Surgery 70:577–580

Creutzfeldt W 1987 Chirurgische Therapie der chronischen Pankreatitis. Langenbecks Archiv für Chirurgie 372:373–378

Cuilleret J, Guillemin G 1990 Surgical management of chronic pancreatitis on the continent of Europe. World Journal of Surgery 14:11–18

Du Val M J Jr 1954 Caudal pancreaticojejunostomy for chronic relapsing pancreatitis. Annals of Surgery 140:775–785

Ebbehoj N, Borly L, Bülow et al 1990 Pancreatic tissue fluid pressure in chronic pancreatitis. Relation to pain, morphology, and function. Scandinavian Journal of Gastroenterology 25:1046–1051

Ell C H, Lux G, Hochberger J et al 1988 Laser lithotripsy of common bile duct stones. Gut 29:746–751

Fielding G, McLatchie G R, Wilson C, Imrie C W, Carter D C 1989 Acute pancreatitis and pancreatic fistula formation. British Journal of Surgery 76:1126–1128

Fölsch U R 1989 Indikationen und Erfolge Operativer und Konservativer Therapie: chronische Pankreatitis. Ergebuisse der Gastroenterologie 24:104–106

Freeny P C 1990 Imaging of chronic pancreatitis: a synopsis. In: Beger H G, Büchler M, Ditschuneit H, Malfertheiner P (eds) Chronic pancreatitis. Springer-Verlag, Berlin, p 303–341

Frey C F 1981 Invited commentary. World Journal of Surgery 5:273–274

Frey C F 1990 Why and when to drain the pancreatic ductal system. In Beger H G, Büchler M, Ditschuneit H, Malfertheiner P (eds) Chronic pancreatitis. Springer-Verlag, Berlin, p 415–425

Frey C F, Braasch J 1984 Surgical management of chronic pancreatitis: the need to improve our observations and assessment of results. American Journal of Surgery 147:189–190

Frey C F, Smith G J 1987 Description and rationale of a new operation for chronic pancreatitis. Pancreas 2:701–707

Gall F P, Gebhardt C, Zirngibl H 1982 Chronic pancreatitis – results in 116 consecutive, partial duodenopancreatectomies combined with pancreatic duct occlusion. Hepatogastroenterology 29:115–119

Gebhardt C, Stolte M 1978 Pankreasgangokklusion durch Injektion einer schnellhärtenden Aminosäurelösung. Langenbecks Archiv für klinische Chirurgie 346:149–166

Halgren H, Pedersen N T, Worning H 1986 Symptomatic effect of pancreatic enzyme therapy in patients with chronic pancreatitis. Scandinavian Journal of Gastroenterology 3:104–108

Hancke S, Henriksen F W 1986 Percutaneous pancreatic cystogastrostomy guided by ultrasound scanning and gastroscopy. British Journal of Surgery 72:916–917

Hancock R J, Christensen R M, Osler T R, Cassim M M 1973 Stenosis of the colon due to pancreatitis and mimicking carcinoma. Canadian Journal of Surgery 16:393

Harbrecht P J 1979 Discussion of Wilson S M. Archives of Surgery 108:539

Hiraoka T, Watanabe E, Katoh T, Hayashida N, Mizutani J, Kanemitsu K, Miyauchi Y 1986 A new surgical approach for control of pain in chronic pancreatitis: complete denervation of the pancreas. American Journal of Surgery 152:549–551

Hoffmeister A, Reiter J 1980 Arrosionsblutungen in Pankreaszysten. 20 Tagung der Österreichischen Gesellschaft für Chirurgie, Demeter Verlag, Gräfelfing, p 411

Hoffmeister A, Trede M 1977 Pankreatische Kolonstenosen. Fortschritte der Medizin 95:1034

Hollands M J, Little J M 1989 Obstructive jaundice in chronic pancreatitis. Hepatobiliary Surgery 1:263–270

Howard J M 1987a Pancreatitis: multiple diseases with multiple causes and varying natural histories. A progress report based on a clinical review. In: Howard J M, Jordan G L, Reber H A (eds) Surgical diseases of the pancreas. Lea & Febiger, Philadelphia, p 171–228

Howard J M 1987b Surgical treatment of chronic pancreatitis. Principles, applications, results. In: Howard J M, Jordan G L, Reber H A (eds) Surgical diseases of the pancreas. Lea & Febiger, Philadelphia, p 496–521

Howard J M 1990 Pancreaticoduodenectomy (Whipple resection) in the treatment of chronic pancreatitis: indications, techniques, and results. In: Beger H G, Büchler M, Ditschuneit H, Malfertheiner (eds) Chronic pancreatitis. Springer-Verlag, Berlin, p 467–480

Hunt D R, Blumgart L H 1982 Preoperative differentiation between carcinoma of the pancreas and chronic pancreatitis: the contribution of cytology. Endoscopy 14:171–173

Ihse I, Lilja P, Lundquist I 1977 Feedback regulation of pancreatic enzyme secretion by intestinal trypsin in man. Digestion 15:303–308

Ihse I, Lankisch P G 1988 Treatment of chronic pancreatitis – current status. Acta Chirurgica Scandinavica 154:553–558

Isaksson G, Ihse I 1983 Pain reduction by an oral pancreatic enzyme preparation in chronic pancreatitis. Digestive Diseases and Sciences 28:97–103

Kozarek R A 1990 Direct cholangiopancreatoscopy and use of pancreatic duct stents and drains in the treatment of pancreatitis. In: Beger H G, Büchler M, Ditschuneit H, Malfertheiner P (eds) Chronic pancreatitis. Springer-Verlag, Berlin, p 371–382

Lankisch P G 1990 Value of indirect pancreatic function tests. In: Beger H G, Büchler M, Ditschuneit H, Malfertheiner P (eds) Chronic pancreatitis. Springer-Verlag, Berlin, p 291–301

Leahy A L, Carter D C (1991) Pain and chronic pancreatitis. European Journal of Gastroenterology and Hepatology 3:425–431

Little J M 1987 Alcohol abuse and chronic pancreatitis. Surgery 101:357–360

Luetmer P H, Stephens D H, Ward E M 1989 Chronic pancreatitis: reassessment with current CT. Radiology 171:353–357

Malfertheiner P, Büchler M, Stanescu A et al 1986 Exocrine pancreatic function in correlation to ductal and parenchymal morphology in chronic pancreatitis. Hepatogastroenterology 33:110–114

Mallet-Guy P A 1983 Late and very late results of resections of the nervous system in the treatment of chronic relapsing pancreatitis. American Journal of Surgery 145:234–238

Marks I N 1990 Alcohol, the alimentary tract and pancreas: facts and controversies. In: Beger H G, Büchler M, Ditschuneit H, Malfertheiner P (eds) Chronic pancreatitis. Springer-Verlag, Berlin, p 26–34

Moossa A R 1987 Surgical treatment of chronic pancreatitis: an overview. British Journal of Surgery 74:661–667

Moossa A R, Gadd M 1985 Isolated splenic vein thrombosis. World Journal of Surgery 9:384–390

Moossa A R, Levin B 1981 The diagnosis of 'early' pancreatic cancer: the University of Chicago experience. Cancer 47:1688–1697

Moossa A R, Lewis M H, Mackie C R 1979 Surgical treatment of pancreatic cancer. Mayo Clinic Proceedings 54:468–474

Morel P, Rohner A 1987 Surgery for chronic pancreatitis. Surgery 101:130–135

Nagata A, Homma T, Tamai K et al 1981 A study of chronic pancreatitis by serial endoscopic pancreatography. Gastroenterology 81:884–891

Nealon W H, Townsend C M Jr, Thompson J C 1988 Operative drainage of the pancreatic duct delays functional impairment in patients with chronic pancreatitis. Annals of Surgery 208:321–329

Neoptolemos J P, Winslet M C 1990 Pancreatic ascites. In: Beger H G, Büchler M, Ditschuneit H, Malfertheiner P (eds) Chronic pancreatitis. Springer-Verlag, Berlin, p 269–279

Partington P F, Rochelle R E L 1960 Modified Puestow procedure for retrograde drainage of the pancreatic duct. Annals of Surgery 152:1037–1043

Pour P M 1990 Is there a link between chronic pancreatitis and pancreatic cancer? In: Beger H G, Büchler M, Ditschuneit H, Malfertheiner P (eds) Chronic pancreatitis. Springer-Verlag, Berlin, p 106–112

Prinz R A 1985 Combined pancreatic duct and upper gastrointestinal and biliary tract drainage in chronic pancreatitis. Archives of Surgery 120:361–366

Prinz R A 1990 Pseudocyst drainage in chronic pancreatitis. In: Beger H G, Büchler M, Ditschuneit H, Malfertheiner P (eds) Chronic pancreatitis. Springer-Verlag, Berlin, p 426–432

Puestow C B, Gillesby W J 1958 Retrograde surgical drainage of pancreas for chronic relapsing pancreatitis. Archives of Surgery 76:898–905

Rignault D, Mine J, Moine D 1968 Splenoportographic changes in chronic pancreatitis. Surgery 63:571

Rösch W 1983 The value of endoscopic occlusion of the pancreatic duct. Endoscopy 15:173–177

Roscher R 1990 What type of pseudocyst should undergo surgery? In: Beger H G, Büchler M, Ditschuneit H, Malfertheiner P (eds) Chronic pancreatitis. Springer-Verlag, Berlin, p 439–453

Rossi R L, Heiss F W, Braasch J W 1985 Surgical management of chronic pancreatitis. Surgical Clinics of North America 65:79–101

Rossi R L, Soeldner J S, Braasch J W, Heiss F W, Shea J A, Watkins Jr. E, Silverman M L 1990 Long-term results of pancreatic resection and segmental pancreatic autotransplantation for chronic pancreatitis. American Journal of Surgery 159:51–58

Russell R C G 1990 Preservation of the duodenum in total pancreatectomy for chronic pancreatitis. In: Beger H G, Büchler M, Ditschuneit H, Malfertheiner P (eds) Chronic pancreatitis. Springer-Verlag, Berlin, p 539–550

Saeger H D, Schwall G, Trede M 1990 Dilemma: Pankreatitis/Pankreaskarzinom. In: Trede M, Seager H D (eds) Aktuelle Pankreaschirurgie. Springer-Verlag, Berlin, p 22–127

Salam A A, Warren W D, Tyras D H 1973 Splenic vein thrombosis: a diagnosable and curable form of portal hypertension. Surgery 74:961–972

Sandblom P 1970 Gastrointestinal haemorrhage through the pancreatic duct. Annals of Surgery 171:61–63

Sarles H, Sahel J 1978 Progress report: cholestasis and lesions of the biliary tract in chronic pancreatitis. Gut 19:851

Sato T, Miyashita E, Matsuno S, Yamauchi H 1986 The role of surgical treatment for chronic pancreatitis. Annals of Surgery 203:266–271

Singh S M, Reber H A 1990 The pathology of chronic pancreatitis. World Journal of Surgery 14:2–10

Slaff J, Jacobson D, Tillman C R, Curlington C, Toskes P 1984 Protease-specific suppression of pancreatic exocrine secretion. Gastroenterology 87:44–52

Soehendra N, Grimm H, Schreiber H W 1986 Endoskopisch

transpapilläre Drainage des Ductus Wirsungianus bei der chronischen Pankreatitis. Deutsche Medizinische Wochenschrift 111:727

Stanley J L, Frey C F, Miller A, Lindenbauer S M, Child C G 1976 Major arterial hemorrhage – a complication of pancreatic pseudocysts and chronic pancreatitis. Archives of Surgery 111:435

Stone H H, Mullins R J, Scovill W A 1985 Vagotomy plus Billroth II gastrectomy for the prevention of recurrent alcohol induced pancreatitis. Annals of Surgery 201:684–689

Swobodnik W, Meyer W, Brecht-Kraus D et al 1983 Ultrasound, computed tomography and endoscopic retrograde cholangiopancreatography in the morphologic diagnosis of pancreatic disease. Klinische Wochenschrift 61:291–296

Toskes P P 1990 How to position exocrine and endocrine function tests in the diagnostic approach to chronic pancreatitis. In: Beger H G, Büchler M, Ditschuneit H, Malfertheiner P (eds) Chronic pancreatitis. Springer-Verlag, Berlin, p 302–308

Traverso L W, Tompkins R K, Urrea P T, Longmire W P 1979 Surgical treatment of chronic pancreatitis. Twenty-two years experience. Annals of Surgery 190:312–319

Trede M 1987 Therapie der chronischen Pankreatitis – Schulßkommentar. Langenbecks Archiv für Chirurgie 372:379–382

Trede M, Schwall G, Saeger H D 1990 Survival after pancreatoduodenectomy. 118 consecutive resections without an operative mortality. Annals of Surgery 211:447–458

Warshaw A L 1984 Pain in chronic pancreatitis: patients, patience, and the impatient surgeon. Gastroenterology 86:987–989

Warshaw A L 1985 Conservation of pancreatic tissue by combined gastric, biliary, and pancreatic duct drainage for pain from chronic pancreatitis. American Journal of Surgery 149:563–569

Warshaw A L 1990 Indications for surgical treatment in chronic pancreatitis. In: Beger H G, Büchler M, Ditschuneit H, Malfertheiner P (eds) Chronic pancreatitis. Springer-Verlag, Berlin, p 395–399

Warshaw A L, Schapiro R H, Ferrucci J T Jr 1976 Persistent obstructive jaundice, cholangitis, and biliary cirrhosis due to common bile duct stenosis in chronic pancreatitis. Gastroenterology 70:562–567

Warshaw A L, Jin G, Ottinger L W 1987 Recognition and clinical implications of mesenteric and portal vein obstruction in chronic pancreatitis. Archives of Surgery 122: 410–415

White T T, Hart M J 1979 Pancreaticojejunostomy versus resection in the treatment of chronic pancreatitis. American Journal of Surgery 138:129

Williamson R C N, Cooper M J 1987 Resection in chronic pancreatitis. British Journal of Surgery 74:807–812

Wilson C, Auld C D, Schlinkert R et al 1989 Hepatobiliary complications in chronic pancreatitis. Gut 30:520–527

Zirngibl H, Gebhardt C, Fassbender D 1983 Drainagebehandlung von Pankreaspseudocysten. Langenbecks Archiv für Chirurgie 360:29

27. Endoscopic interventional techniques in chronic pancreatitis

A. Maydeo   H. Grimm   N. Soehendra

Chronic inflammation of the pancreas is a clinical entity which has always eluded precise characterization. In spite of the tremendous expansion of knowledge and experience gained over the past three decades, effective treatment of the unrelenting pain and deteriorating function continues to be one of the major therapeutic challenges in medicine. The numerous surgical procedures devised stand testimony to the inadequacy of any single procedure in this multifaceted disease. Differing opinions and lack of exact knowledge about the cause of pain and progress of the disease have added to the confusion (Leahy & Carter 1991).

With the belief that functional impairment of the gland cannot be halted or reversed, treatment of the severe and disabling pain has been the main indication of all therapeutic modalities. Some reports have even shown an inclination towards only expectant, conservative management in the hope that the pain would ultimately disappear after total gland destruction over the years (Levrat et al 1970, Ammann et al 1973). This theory is however of little value for the individual patient who actually suffers from the debilitating recurrent pain and is at risk of narcotic addiction. Surgery has therefore formed the mainstay of therapy for chronic pancreatitis. Theoretically, this pain-producing so-called hopeless disease can be treated surgically in one stroke i.e by removing or denervating the gland which is causing pain. However, the results of major resections are usually not worth the severe metabolic price paid by the patient who may already be surviving on marginal pancreatic function (Leger et al 1974, Braasch et al 1978) while denervation procedures are of temporary benefit at best (Smith 1973). Thus, procedures such as ductal drainage which conserve pancreatic tissue and simultaneously provide good pain relief have been preferred whenever the ductal anatomy is suitable. The striking immediacy of pain relief after ductal drainage (Taylor et al 1981, Holmberg & Isaksson 1985), the relatively high mortality and morbidity of resection operations (Cuilleret & Guillemin 1990), and the difficulties and complications sometimes associated with operations for pseudocysts or abscesses (Becker et al 1968, Miller et al 1974) has led to the emergence of non-surgical approaches such as endoscopy in the last decade (Fuji et al 1985, Soehendra et al 1986a, b, Huibregtse et al 1988, McCarthy et al 1988, Cremer et al 1989, Grimm et al 1989, Kozarek et al 1989). Since the majority of the patients with chronic pancreatitis in the western world are alcoholics (Durbec & Sarles 1978) with a poor compliance and poor general condition, emerging endoscopic techniques have been embraced enthusiastically.

BASIC CONCEPTS LEADING TO DEVELOPMENT OF THE ENDOSCOPIC APPROACH

Encouraged by the excellent results of endoscopic methods in the treatment of biliary tract disorders, endoscopists have extended their techniques to treat chronic pancreatitis. When dealing with this disease we believe that the ideal therapeutic modality is that which:

1. provides the best pain relief with a low mortality and post-procedure morbidity
2. treats associated complications such as pseudocysts and biliary obstruction at the same time
3. preserves or even improves the exocrine and islet cell function as much as possible.

The pain relief which can follow surgical drainage of the duct has been confirmed by numerous reports, indicating that ductal obstruction and the resultant increase in intraductal pressure is one of the important causes of the pain. Additionally, some reports (although not all) on endoscopic (Okazaki et al 1986) or operative measurement (Bradley 1983) of intraductal pressure have shown abnormally high pressure in patients having chronic pancreatitis with a dilated duct (see Leahy & Carter 1991). Thus, selecting an adequate and safe drainage procedure for releasing the stagnant pancreatic secretion seems to be a logical approach. However, this is not possible if the disease is too advanced to be drained and/or the gland has become completely fibrotic with a narrow ductal system.

As opposed to metabolic complications such as diabetes and steatorrhoea which occur late in the course of the disease (Levrat et al 1970), pseudocysts usually form in the first 5 years after onset (Gastard et al 1973). The incidence of such pseudocysts in chronic pancreatitis is about 10–30% (Strum & Spiro 1971, Ammann et al 1984) and complications such as infection, rupture, haemorrhage, jaundice and intestinal obstruction occur in around 40% of patients, a majority of them needing active management (Bradley et al 1979). In this context, surgery has been the mainstay of treatment to date, internal drainage of the pseudocyst being the most effective therapy. However even internal drainage is associated with a recurrence rate of around 5% and postoperative mortality rates of up to 7% (Becker et al 1968). The mortality and the difficulty of the operation is increased if the pseudocyst is infected.

From the proceedings of the 2nd Marseille Symposium (Sahel & Sarles 1984) there is a general consensus of opinion that chronic pancreatitis is basically of two distinct types. One is the chronic calcifying pancreatitis where the disease starts in the smaller ducts, causing a lobular distribution of lesions with later calcification. Further attacks of inflammation lead to involvement of the main duct and the entire gland is ultimately fibrotic. The other entity recognized is obstructive pancreatitis which begins with obstruction in the main pancreatic duct leading to stasis, stone formation and a diffuse distribution of the lesions. It has been pointed out that chronic pancreatitis is perhaps pathogenetically related in some cases to acute pancreatitis and the starting point is an attack of acute pancreatitis due to any cause with autodigestive tissue necrosis. In those cases with predominant tissue necrosis (like some patients with alcoholic acute pancreatitis) there is advancing perilobular fibrosis and stricture formation in the duct. This leads in turn to a reduced flow of pancreatic juice, increased viscosity, and plugs of protein upstream. These protein plugs later calcify causing stones, and aggravate the obstruction with further acute attacks and ductal alteration (Klöppel 1986). This view provides an explanation for the following observations:

- 60% of patients with acute alcoholic pancreatitis go on to develop chronic pancreatitis over 10 years (Reid & Kune 1980).
- Non-calcifying and calcifying pancreatitis are often two stages of the same disease, patients who are without calcification going on to develop calcification over a period of years (Gastard et al 1973).
- Pancreatic calculi are almost always intraductal and proximal to an obstruction in the duct (Konishi et al 1981, Nagai & Ohtsubo 1984).

Our clinical experience is fully in accordance with the pathological observation that partial ductal obstruction originating from an acute attack is the main cause of recurrent pancreatitis (Stolte 1984, Klöppel 1986). The recurrent attacks lead in turn to further scarring, stone formation and increased ductal obstruction. This vicious cycle ultimately leads to the development of chronic pancreatitis, ductular destruction and total gland atrophy. Thus, interrupting this cycle by relieving obstruction may not only eliminate the pain but if done in the early stage might even halt progression of the disease. This has been supported recently by a prospective, controlled study which showed that surgical drainage of the pancreatic duct, especially if done in the early stage, did halt if not reverse progression of the disease (Nealon et al 1988).

As well as accurately outlining the ductal anatomy, endoscopic therapy today also allows treatment of ductal strictures and intraductal stones and even permits effective and safe treatment of complications such as pseudocysts, abscesses and gastric varices.

ENDOSCOPIC FINDINGS IN CHRONIC PANCREATITIS

Chronic pancreatitis is morphologically a multifaceted disease. The most commonly observed finding at endoscopic retrograde cholangiopancreatography (ERCP) is stricturing of the main pancreatic duct which often occurs at multiple sites. Peripheral ductal changes are also frequently seen but are of little or no significance as far as endoscopic therapy in concerned. In our experience of more than 200 endoscopically treated patients with chronic pancreatitis, 90% had ductal obstruction with stricture as the main cause, the predominant location being in the pancreatic head; 35% of them had intraductal calculi. In 25% of cases, cysts were demonstrated at ERCP and 35% of patients showed distal bile duct stenosis; 20% of patients had associated pancreas divisum.

PANCREATIC SPHINCTEROTOMY

Endoscopic incision of the pancreatic sphincter is usually performed as a prerequisite before stone extraction, dilatation or stenting of the main pancreatic duct. As a form of treatment in its own right, sphincterotomy is indicated for a localized benign stenosis at the papilla. Technically, it is performed in a similar way to biliary sphincterotomy, using a modified Erlangen sphincterotome with a short cutting wire of less than 1 cm and with a tilt towards the 2 o'clock position. After selective cannulation of the main pancreatic duct, the incision is made in a step by step manner using a predominantly cutting current and during withdrawal of the the papillotome. Normally, the length of the cut should not exceed 1 cm. By cutting in a step-by-step fashion and using the short-wire papillotome, complications like bleeding or perforation are relatively rare, having an incidence of less than 1%. The commonly feared complication of acute pancreatitis should not occur if a clean cut is made and if this is followed by proper drainage of pancreatic secretions. In principle, except for the direction of the cut and the length of the incision, the technique of endoscopic pancreatic sphincterotomy does not differ from that of biliary sphincterotomy.

PANCREATIC DUCT STENTING

Since stricture of the main pancreatic duct is the most frequently observed pathology in chronic pancreatitis, stenting is the most commonly practised endoscopic therapy. However, as in any other drainage procedure this method is only beneficial if a distinct ductal dilatation is present. In our experience pancreatic stenting is successful in around 80% of patients presenting with ductal stenosis, the most common cause of failure being tight and multiple strictures. Stenting may also be indicated in pancreas divisum patients having pancreatitis-like pain without any significant dilatation of the dorsal duct, as a therapeutic trial to prove that there is inadequate drainage through the minor papilla.

The technique of pancreatic duct stenting is similar to that of biliary stenting and is based on the Seldinger principle. Strictures of the pancreatic duct however may be more difficult to stent than those of the bile duct due to their notoriously fibrotic, tight and tortuous nature. A small endoscopic incision of the pancreatic duct orifice should be performed to facilitate further manipulation. The 0.032 inch curved or straight, radiofocus hydrophilic glide wire (Terumo Corp., Tokyo) is most suitable and is preferred because of its atraumatic and slippery property. For guiding and manipulating the wire through the stricture, we prefer to use the universal catheter from Wilson Cook Inc (USA) which is made from a 7 French Teflon, radio-opaque material having a 4 Fr tapered tip. Once the wire is across the stricture, the narrowed area is first dilated using the same catheter. After dilatation, a 7–10 Fr Teflon or polyethylene stent is pushed over the wire. The stent should have side holes along its length for adequate drainage of side branches of the duct and a side flap to prevent dislocation. The length of the stent is governed by the number and length of the strictures and that of the dilated portion of the duct. Usually, the stent is placed along the entire length of the duct, bypassing all the strictures and draining all of the dilated parts of the system (Fig. 27.1). Adequate placement of the stent is usually evident from the flow of clear pancreatic juice.

Stenting has proved to be a safe and effective method of draining the duct in chronic pancreatitis, complete or partial pain relief being achieved initially in around 85% of patients, with complication rates of 6–22% and mortality rates of 0–3%. The figure for pain relief drops to around 70% during follow-up, mainly due to intermittent stent blockage (Table 27.1). As long as the problem of stent blockage and fear of causing ductal epithelial changes due to the stent remain (Kozarek 1990), stenting cannot be

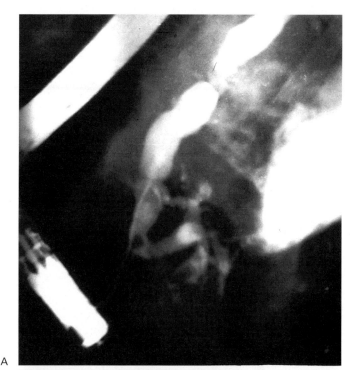

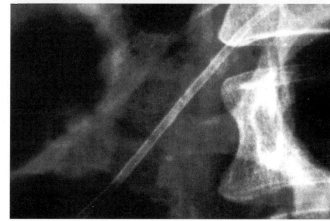

Fig. 27.1 **A** A guide-wire being passed prior to stenting in a patient with multiple strictures and a dilated pancreatic duct. **B** A 7 Fr Teflon endoprosthesis has been placed in the duct bypassing all of the strictures.

considered as permanent therapy. However, due to its relative safety even in the treatment of poor risk patients and its efficacy in achieving pain relief, stenting can be considered as a primary method of ductal drainage. This may not only help to tide over a crisis but may also serve as a therapeutic trial before surgical drainage. With improvement in stent material or design, and resolution of the problem of stent blockage, endoscopic stenting could become a useful and permanent form of therapy for patients with obstructive pancreatitis and a dilated duct. Even though self-expanding metal stents have been used effectively for biliary drainage, their use in the pancreas is not advisable. The reason for this is the possible danger of the

Table 27.1   Results of endoscopic treatment in chronic pancreatitis

Authors	Cases (n)	Procedures	Success rate %	Improved initially %	Improved during follow-up %	Follow-up period (months)	Complication rate %	Mortality %
Mc Carthy et al (1988)	37	Ductal stenting only	89		76	6–36 (mean = 14)	14	0
Grimm et al (1989)	70	Ductal stenting, Cyst drainage, Stone removal etc.	87	82	57	2–36 (mean = 19)	6 (all 4 required surgery)	3
Huibregtse et al (1988)	32	Ductal stenting Cyst drainage Stone removal etc.	94	89	78	2–69 (mean = 11)	22 3/7 required surgery	3

stent getting blocked due to tissue hyperplasia and the inability to remove or replace it.

TREATMENT OF PANCREATIC STONES

Pancreatic duct stones which are always intraductal, cause symptoms and need therapy only if they cause ductal obstruction. Like bile duct stones however, pancreatic duct stones cannot be extracted easily as they are usually located behind an area of ductal stenosis. In addition, some stones are impacted in the duct and therefore cannot be caught. These patients thus need additional procedures such as endoscopic stenting or shock wave lithotripsy. If stones are present without an associated stricture, they can be extracted in the usual manner using either the Dormia basket or the balloon catheter (Fig. 27.2). A sphincterotomy of the pancreatic orifice has to be made first, its length depending upon the size of the stones to be ex-

tracted. It is better to catch the stones in the Dormia basket first before pulling them out, but if they are soft and not well formed, they can be extracted only by fishing them out with an open basket. If the stones are too large and hard to be pulled out and the duct is sufficiently dilated, electrohydraulic lithotripsy (EHL) using the mother–babyscope can be employed. Mechanical lithotripsy if needed should be used with extreme caution and only if the basket is impacted and the stone can be pulled up to the prepapillary region.

Stones which are impacted or situated proximal to a stricture have to be crushed first before attempting extraction. This can be effectively achieved with extracorporeal shock wave lithotripsy (ESWL) (Cremer et al 1988, Neuhaus et al 1989, Soehendra et al 1989, Sauerbruch et al 1989). Calcified stones which can be seen on plain X-ray can be crushed directly using the X-ray guided ESWL machines. If however the stones are

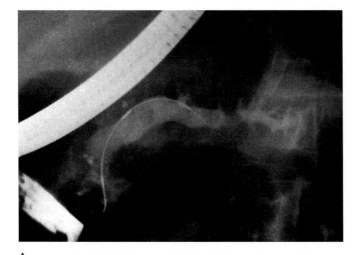

A

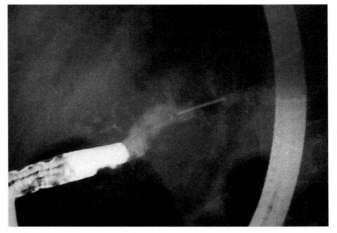

B

Fig. 27.2   **A** Endoscopic pancreatic stone extraction using a Dormia basket. **B** Endoscopic stone extraction using a balloon catheter.

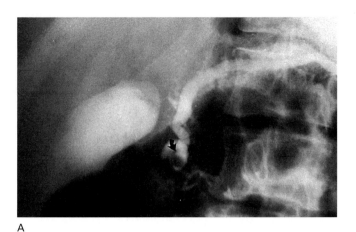

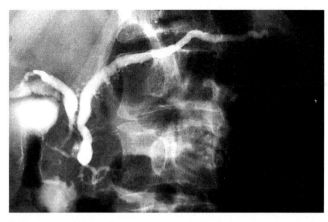

A   B

Fig. 27.3   **A** Endoscopic retrograde pancreatogram (ERP) showing an impacted pancreatic stone in the prepapillary region (arrow).
B Spontaneous passage of the pulverized stone after disruption by extracorporeal shock wave lithotripsy (ESWL).

not calcified enough to be seen on X-ray, a nasopancreatic catheter has to placed first for contrast instillation. ERCP should be repeated after the ESWL sessions to check for ductal clearance. In some situations, the crushed stones pass out of the duct on their own and do not need further extraction (Fig. 27.3). If this is not the case, then extraction with a Dormia basket should be attempted again. In patients who have stones associated with strictures, a stent or a nasopancreatic catheter should be inserted if possible before subjecting them to ESWL therapy. The nasopancreatic catheter can then be used for irrigation as well as fluoroscopic monitoring. It is likely that the pulverized stone will pass through the stent itself. Shock wave lithotripsy is well tolerated by these patients and is not associated with any significant complications. Fragmentation of stones can be achieved in 88–100% of cases with pain relief in 50–90% of cases (Table 27.2). In our experience of treating 76 patients with pancreatic stones, basket stone extraction was possible after a sphincterotomy alone in 16 cases, whereas 60 required prior ESWL because of stone impaction or associated stricture. A total of 40 patients had to be stented subsequently for ductal stenosis. Removal of the stones was ultimately successful in 70 patients. Once again as with stenting of the duct, stone extraction and procedures like EHL or ESWL have proved to be effective and safe methods of therapy in patients of chronic pancreatitis.

ENDOSCOPIC TREATMENT OF PANCREATIC PSEUDOCYSTS

Pancreatic pseudocysts which occur with an incidence of around 10–30% in chronic pancreatitis (Strum & Spiro 1971, Ammann et al 1984) need treatment either because they produce symptoms like pain, nausea and vomiting or because they produce complications such as gastric outlet obstruction, biliary obstruction, abscess formation, rupture or erosion. Pseudocysts occurring in chronic pancreatitis spontaneously resolve less frequently than those found in acute pancreatitis and have a tendency to develop complications especially if treatment is delayed (Bradley et al 1979). Symptomatic pseudocysts, which are usually larger than 6 cm in diameter, can now be treated effectively and safely by endoscopic methods. This can be achieved using the transpapillary approach if the cyst communicates with the main pancreatic duct (Fig. 27.4) or by a transmural approach if they have direct contact with the gastric or duodenal wall and produce a recognizable bulge in the lumen. The proximity of the cyst to the wall and its thickness can be assessed precisely by computed tomography (CT) or endoscopic ultrasonography. However, a relatively simpler and cheaper method of confirming the position of the collection is to puncture the most prominent part of the visible bulge with an injection needle and instil contrast medium. This not only helps to select

Table 27.2   Extracorporeal shock wave lithotripsy (ESWL) of pancreatic stones for pain relief

Authors	Cases n	% Fragmentation	% Complete clearance	% Improved	Mortality
Cremer et al (1988)	31	90	52	90	0
Sauerbruch et al (1989)	8	88	88	50	0
Neuhaus et al (1989)	8	100	88	88	0
Soehendra (present series)	60	100	90	90	0

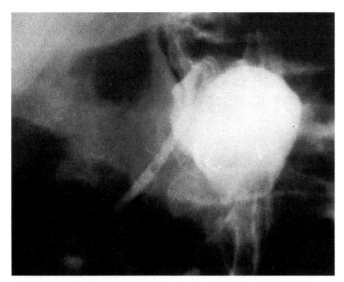

Fig. 27.4 Transpapillary placement of a stent for drainage of a communicating pancreatic pseudocyst.

the proper site for the drainage but even rules out presence of blood vessels in the wall which can bleed if punctured. In fact in daily practice, in spite of obtaining a preprocedure CT scan we prefer to routinely confirm the position of the cyst again with the injection needle before carrying out drainage. For thinning the site of puncture in the wall prior to injection, we use blended current delivered through a blunt probe. In our experience, if the distance between the cyst cavity and the gastric/duodenal wall is more than 1 cm, endoscopic drainage can be risky. After confirming the position of the cyst, the wall is punctured using the same probe. Thereafter a 10 Fr pigtail endoprosthesis is inserted into the cyst over a guide wire for maintaining the drainage (Fig. 27.5).

Endoscopic cystogastrostomy or cystoduodenostomy can also be done by extending the site of puncture with a regular papillotome. However this technique does not have any added advantage and is associated with a morbidity rate of 15% and mortality as high as 6% (Sahel 1990). It is our experience that with the endoprosthesis inside, even

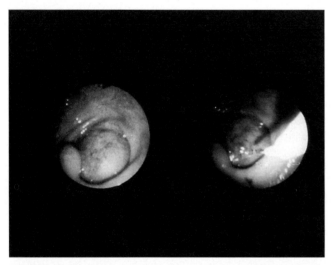

A & B

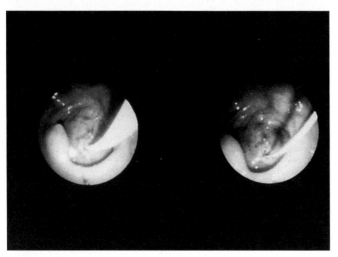

C & D

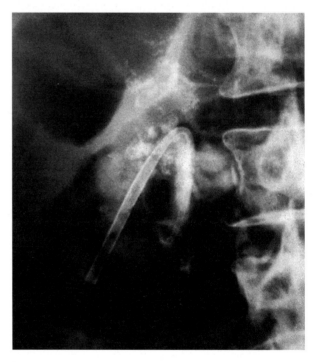

E

Fig. 27.5 **A** Endoscopic appearance of an easily recognizable bulge in the duodenum due to a pseudocyst in the pancreatic head. **B** Needle puncture of the most prominent part of the bulge to allow instillation of contrast medium prior to initiating drainage. **C** A puncture being made with the coagulation probe at the selected site. **D** Guide-wire placed in the cyst over which the stent can be pushed. **E** Plain film of the transduodenally placed stent in the pseudocyst. Figures 27.5 **A–D** are reproduced in colour in the plate section at the front of the volume.

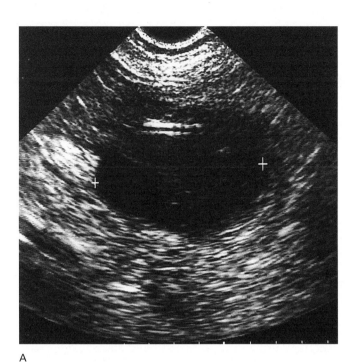

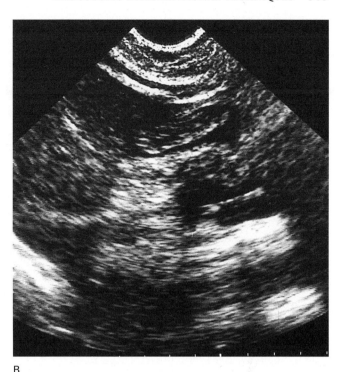

A   B

Fig. 27.6   A Ultrasonographic picture of a 7 cm pseudocyst drained with a 10 Fr transgastrically placed pigtail endoprosthesis. **B** Disappearance of the cyst following 7 days endoscopic transgastric drainage.

large pseudocysts usually disappear within 2 weeks and the stent will be discarded spontaneously into the gastric or duodenal lumen (Fig. 27.6).

Of the 52 drainage procedures carried out by us in 48 patients, 31 were transpapillary, 15 transduodenal and 6 transgastric. The procedure-related complication rate was 10% (5 out of 48) which included one case of pancreatitis, one puncture of the gallbladder, one case of bleeding, and two abscesses, with a mortality rate of zero. In 42 out of 45 patients (93%) the cyst disappeared.

Similar long-term results have been reported by other authors (Table 27.3). The technique of pseudocyst drainage is also eminently suitable for treating pancreatic abscess, a condition which usually carries a high operative mortality (Shi et al 1984). Here, in addition to the endoprosthesis, a naso-abscess catheter is inserted to maintain effective irrigation (Brückner et al 1990). Concomitant pancreatic fistulae can be occluded by using a two-component fibrin glue after the abscess cavity is clean (Fig. 27.7).

ENDOSCOPIC TREATMENT IN CASES OF PANCREAS DIVISUM

Endoscopic therapy for chronic pancreatitis in patients with pancreas divisum may prove to be difficult as most of the procedures have to be carried out though the minor papilla. For stenting the dorsal duct through the minor papilla, we prefer to begin directly with a tapered dilator and a 0.035 inch straight glide wire (Terumo Corp., Japan) instead of carrying out a prior papillotomy. In our experience, incision of the minor papilla is more easily done with a wire-guided papillotome or with a needle knife over a preplaced stent. If it has to be done with a regular short-wire Erlangen papillotome, it is better to dilate the papillary orifice first. With increased experience, endoscopic therapeutic procedures through the minor papilla can be carried out with an overall success rate of 90% (Soehendra et al 1986a, b, McCarthy et al 1988).

Table 27.3   Endoscopic drainage of pseudocysts

Author	Patients n	% Success rate	% Complication rate	% Mortality	Follow-up (months)
Sahel (1990)	33	90	15	6	1–37
Cremer et al (1989)	33	82	6	0	3–84
Soehendra (present series)	48	93	10	0	1–60

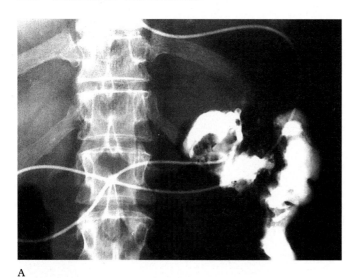
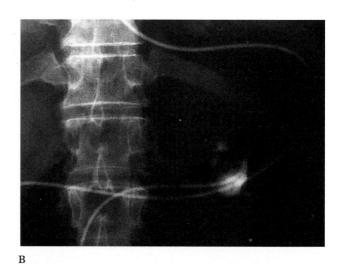

A   B

Fig. 27.7 Pancreatic abscess with colonic fistula following acute gallstone pancreatitis. **A** 7 Fr nasopancreatic catheter is placed in the abscess for irrigation. **B** Near-total disappearance of the abscess and closure of the fistula after treatment with two-component fibrin glue.

ENDOSCOPIC BILIARY DRAINAGE FOR CHRONIC PANCREATITIS

It is known that around 30% of patients with chronic pancreatitis, especially those with predominant disease in the pancreatic head develop a tubular stenosis of the distal bile duct. However, only less than half of them present with jaundice and require therapy (Sarles & Sahel 1978, Deviere et al 1990). Endoscopic transpapillary stenting can be done here in the same manner as that used for malignant biliary obstruction (see Ch. 44). However, for benign stenoses like those due to chronic pancreatitis, stenting is unable to achieve permanent dilatation. Therefore it should be used only for inoperable patients. When used over a long period in such patients, a regular and strict follow-up is mandatory due to possible clogging of the stent after an average of 3–4 months.

OBLITERATION OF GASTRIC VARICES

Gastric varices are one of the dreaded complications of chronic pancreatitis and occur due to splenic or portal vein thrombosis. Their treatment in the acute stage as well as in the interval thereafter seems to be ineffective and unsatisfactory with all known therapeutic modalities. Endoscopic obliteration of these varices with the tissue adhesive (n-butyl-2-cyanoacrylate) offers some hope of therapeutic improvement in this regard. The tissue adhesive which is a watery substance, hardens immediately when in contact with blood and thus causes an effective and permanent obliteration of the varix irrespective of its size and mode of presentation. Varices can be eliminated safely, with a recurrence rate of 2%. When used for acute bleeding, haemostasis can be achieved in many patients, obviating the

need for emergency surgery or balloon tamponade (Soehendra et al 1990).

CURRENT STATUS OF NON-SURGICAL INTERVENTIONAL TECHNIQUE FOR CHRONIC PANCREATITIS

Of the various non-operative interventional techniques used to treat chronic pancreatitis, the radiologically- or ultrasonographically-guided procedures have mainly been used to treat pancreatic pseudocysts. There is no doubt that simple percutaneous aspirations are associated with a high recurrence rate of nearly 70% (MacErlean et al 1980, Hancke & Henriksen 1985, Torres et al 1986). Percutaneous cystogastrostomy using the double pigtail endoprosthesis has therefore been recommended and practised so far with a success rate of 80–90% without any significant complication (Hancke & Henriksen 1985, Heyder et al 1988).

Endoscopic transpapillary or transmural pseudocyst drainage can be carried out effectively and safely with encouraging initial as well as long-term results. Additionally endoscopic stone extraction from a dilated pancreatic duct without stenosis, has shown promising results as far as pain relief is concerned. Treatment of pancreatic strictures by endoscopic stenting however is associated with poor long-term results, the nature of the strictures making permanent and efficient long-term dilatation difficult. In addition, the propensity of the currently used plastic stents to block prevents them from being useful in the long-term. Pancreatic stenting as long-term therapy should therefore be considered only for inoperable patients and must involve a regular follow-up. Temporarily, stents are useful even in operable patients either to tide over a crisis or as a therapeutic trial before surgical drainage. According to our hypothesis regarding the vicious cycle involved in the development of chronic pancreatitis, procedures such as stenting would be best utilized in early stage disease where relief of obstruction could conceivably prevent further progress to advanced disease. Distal biliary obstruction in chronic pancreatitis can also be effectively treated with endoscopic stenting, but here also the problem of clogging persists. With the use of tissue adhesives, treatment of gastric varices has become safe, and may prove definitive.

REFERENCES

Ammann R W, Hammer B, Fumagalli J 1973 Chronic pancreatitis in Zurich, 1963–1972 Clinical findings and followup studies of 102 cases. Digestion 9:404–415

Ammann R W, Akovbiantz A, Largiader F, Schueler G 1984 Course and outcome of chronic pancreatitis. Longitudinal study of a mixed medical-surgical series of 245 patients. Gastroenterology 86:820–828

Becker W F, Pratt H S, Ganji H 1968 Pseudocysts of the pancreas. Surgery Gynecology and Obstetrics 127:744–747

Braasch J W, Vito L, Nugent F W 1978 Total pancreatectomy for end stage chronic pancreatitis. Annals of Surgery 188:317–322

Bradley E L III 1983 Pancreatic duct pressure in chronic pancreatitis. American Journal of Surgery 144:313–316

Bradley E L III, Clements J L Jr, Gonzalez A C 1979 The natural history of pancreatic pseudocysts. A unified concept of management. American Journal of Surgery 137:135–141

Brückner M, Grimm H, Nam V Ch, Soehendra N 1990 Endoscopic treatment of pancreatic abscess originating from biliary pancreatitis. Surgical Endoscopy 4:227–229

Cremer M, Vandermeeren A, Delhaye M 1988 Extracorporeal shock wave lithotripsy (ESWL) for pancreatic stones. Endoscopy 20 (Suppl 2):A23

Cremer M, Deviere J, Engelholm L 1989 Endoscopic management of cysts and pseudocysts in chronic calcifying pancreatitis: long-term follow-up after 7 years of experience. Gastrointestinal Endoscopy 35:1–9

Cuilleret J, Guillemin G 1990 Surgical management of chronic pancreatitis on the continent of Europe. World Journal of Surgery 14:11–18

Deviere J, Devaere S, Baize M, Cremer M 1990 Endoscopic biliary drainage in chronic pancreatitis. Gastrointestinal Endoscopy 36:96–100

Durbec J P, Sarles H 1978 Multicenter survey of the etiology of pancreatic diseases. Relationship between the relative risk of developing chronic pancreatitis and alcohol protein and lipid consumption. Digestion 18:337–350

Fuji T, Amano H, Harima K, Albe T, Asagami F, Kinukawa K, Ariyama S, Takemoto T 1985 Pancreatic sphincterotomy and pancreatic endoprosthesis. Endoscopy 17:69–72

Gastard J, Joubaud F, Farbos T, Looussouaarn J, Marion J, Pannier M, Renaudet F, Valdazo R, Gosselin M 1973 Etiology and course of primary chronic pancreatitis in western France. Digestion 9:416–428

Grimm H, Meyer W H, Nam V Ch, Soehendra N 1989 New modalities for treating chronic pancreatitis. Endoscopy 21:70–74

Hancke S, Henriksen F W 1985 Percutaneous pancreatic cystogastrostomy guided by ultrasound scanning and gastroscopy. British Journal of Surgery 27:916–917

Heyder N, Fluegel H, Domschke W 1988 Catheter drainage of pancreatic pseudocysts into the stomach. Endoscopy 20:75–77

Holmberg J T, Isaksson G 1985 Long term results of pancreaticojejunostomy in chronic pancreatitis. Surgery Gynecology and Obstetrics 160:339–346

Huibregtse K, Schneider B, Vrij A A, Tytgat G N J 1988 Endoscopic pancreatic drainage in chronic pancreatitis. Gastrointestinal Endoscopy 34:9–15

Klöppel G 1986 Pathomorphology of chronic pancreatitis. In: Malfertheiner P and Ditschuneit M (eds) Diagnostic procedures in pancreatic diseases. Springer-Verlag, Berlin, p 135

Konishi K, Izumi R, Kato O, Yamaguchi A, Miyaazaki I 1981 Experimental pancreatolithiasis in the dog. Surgery 89:687–691

Kozarek R A 1990 Pancreatic stents can induce ductal changes consistent with chronic pancreatitis. Gastrointestinal Endoscopy 36:93–95

Kozarek R A, Patterson D J, Ball T J, Traverso L W 1989 Endoscopic placement of pancreatic stents and drains in the management of pancreatitis. Annals of Surgery 209:261–266

Leahy A, Carter D C 1991 Pain and chronic pancreatitis. European Journal of Gastroenterology and Hepatology 3:425–431

Leger L, Lenriot J P, Lemaigre G 1974 Five to twenty year follow-up after surgery for chronic pancreatitis in 148 patients. Annals of Surgery 180:185–191

Levrat M, Descos L, Moulinier B, Pasquier J 1970 Evolution au long cours des pancréatites chroniques. Archives Françaises des Maladies de l'Appareil Digestif 59:305–314

MacErlean D P, Bryan P J, Murphy J J 1980 Pancreatic pseudocyst. Management by ultrasound-guided aspiration. Gastroentestinal Radiology 5:255–257

McCarthy J, Geenen J E, Hogan W J 1988 Preliminary experience with endoscopic stent placement in benign pancreatic disease. Gasrointestinal Endoscopy 34:16–18

Miller T A, Lindenauer S M, Fry C F, Stanley J C 1974 Pancreatic abscess. Archives of Surgery 108:545–551

Nagai H, Ohtsubo K 1984 Pancreatic lithiasis in the aged. Its clinopathology and pathogenesis. Gasroenterology 86:331–338

Nealon W H, Townsend C M Jr, Thompson J C 1988 Operative drainage of the pancreatic duct delays functional impairment in patients with chronic pancreatitis. A prospective analysis. Annals of Surgery 208:321–329

Neuhaus H, Hagenmüller F, Brandstetter K, Gerhard K, Classen M 1989 Extrakorporale Stosswellen-Lithotripsie (ESWL) von Pankreassteinen. Zeitschrift für Gastroenterologie 27:A526

Okazaki K, Yamamoto Y, Ito K 1986 Endoscopic measurement of papillary sphincter zone and pancreatic main ductal pressure in patients with chronic pancreatitis. Gastroenterology 91:409–418

Reid B G, Kune G A 1980 Natural history of acute pancreatitis. A long term study. Medical Journal of Australia 2:555–558

Sahel J, Sarles H 1984 Chronic calcifying pancreatitis and obstructive pancreatitis – Two entities. In: Gyr K E, Singer M V, Sarles H (eds), Pancreatitis concepts and classification – Proceedings of the second international symposium on the classification of pancreatitis, Marseille, France, March 28–30, Excerpta Medica, Amsterdam, p 47

Sahel J 1990 Endoscopic cysto-enterostomy of cysts of chronic calcifying pancreatitis. Zeitschrift für Gastroenterologie 28:170–172

Sarles H, Sahel J 1978 Progress report. Cholestasis and lesions of the biliary tract in chronic pancreatitis. Gut 19:851–857

Sauerbruch T, Holl J, Sackmann M, Paumgartner G 1989 Extrocorporeal shock wave lithotripsy of pancreatic stones. Gut 30:1406–1411

Shi E C, Yeo B W, Ham J M 1984 Pancreatic abscesses. British Journal of Surgery 71:689–691

Smith R 1973 Progress in the surgical treatment of pancreatic disease. American Journal of Surgery 125:143–153

Soehendra N, Grimm H, Schreiber H W 1986a Endoskopische transpapilläre Drainage des Ductus Wirsungianus bei der chronischen Pankreatitis. Deutsche Medizinische Wochenschrift 111:727–731

Soehendra N, Kempeneers I, Nam V C, Grimm H 1986b Endoscopic dilatation and papillotomy of the accessory papilla and internal drainage in pancreas divisum. Endoscopy 18:129–132

Soehendra N, Grimm H, Meyer H W, Schreiber H W 1989 Extrakorporale Stosswellenlithotripsie bei chronischer Pankreatitis. Deutsche Medizinische Wochenschrift 114:1402–1406

Soehendra N, Grimm H, Maydeo A, Nam V Ch, Eckmann B, Brückner M 1990 Endoscopic obliteration of fundal varices. Canadian Journal of Gastroenterology 4:643–646

Stolte M 1984 Chronische Pancreatitis. Morphologie-Pancreatographie-Differentialdiagnose. Perimed, Erlangen

Strum W B, Spiro H M 1971 Chronic pancreatitis. Annals of Internal Medicine 74:264–277

Taylor R H, Bagley F H, Braasch J W, Warren J W 1981 Ductal drainage or resection for chronic pancreatitis. American Journal of Surgery 141:28–33

Torres W E, Evert M B, Baumgartner B R, Bernardino M E 1986 Percutaneous aspiration and drainage of pancreatic pseudocysts. American Journal of Roentgenology 147:1007–1009

28. Surgical drainage procedures in chronic pancreatitis

D. C. Carter

INTRODUCTION

Pain is the cardinal symptom of chronic pancreatitis and in the great majority of surgical patients it is the outstanding indication for operation. There are two principal forms of surgery in chronic pancreatitis, namely resection of the gland or operations designed to improve the drainage of exocrine secretions. A number of forms of resection, such as the Whipple operation of partial pancreaticoduodenectomy and its variants, may also improve the drainage of the remaining pancreatic tissue. However, resection of diseased pancreas is the primary objective of such operations and they will be considered in detail elsewhere (Ch. 30). This chapter will be confined to consideration of drainage operations which are not accompanied by resection of significant amounts of the pancreas. Drainage operations are clearly less hazardous than resection and have a lower operative mortality and morbidity. Furthermore, drainage does not involve loss of pancreatic parenchyma with is attendant risk of precipitating or exacerbating exocrine or endocrine insufficiency. Drainage operations can be classified into three types: those involving anastomosis between the pancreas and the jejunum (pancreaticojejunostomy), those involving anastomosis between the pancreas and the stomach (pancreaticogastrostomy), and those designed to improve drainage into the duodenum (sphincterotomy and sphincteroplasty). Of the three, pancreaticojejunostomy is the most frequently employed and will be the main subject for discussion.

RATIONALE FOR THE USE OF DRAINAGE OPERATIONS IN CHRONIC PANCREATITIS

Drainage operations in chronic pancreatitis are based on the concept that ductal obstruction leads to distension and that this in turn gives rise to pain. Accordingly, any measure which improves drainage, either by improving flow into the duodenum or by allowing flow into the jejunum or stomach, might be expected to relieve pain.

As many patients with chronic pancreatitis do not have a pancreatic duct system which is distended, other factors undoubtedly contribute, and the mechanism of pain production is still far from clear. In our own practice, only a minority of patients coming to surgery for chronic pancreatitis have ducts which are deemed to be sufficiently enlarged to allow a drainage procedure to be performed.

Direct measurements made at the time of laparotomy initially suggested that patients with chronic pancreatitis and dilated ducts or pseudocysts had raised intraduct pressures (Du Val 1958, Anderson & Hagstrom 1962, White & Bourde 1970, Christofferson et al 1981, Bradley 1982). A variety of methods were employed to measure duct pressure in these studies and the pressures recorded ranged from 15 to 57 cmH₂O (Table 28.1). In general, these pressures were higher than those measured by endoscopic cannulation of the pancreatic duct in patients who were not found to have pancreatic disease in the course of investigation of abdominal pain (Rosch et al 1976, Bar-Meier et al 1979, Carr-Locke & Gregg 1981, Novis et al 1985). Okazaki et al (1988) have demonstrated increased pancreatic duct pressure at endoscopic retrograde cholangiopancreatography (ERCP) in patients with chronic pancreatitis due to a variety of causes, half of whom were thought to have early stage disease. Patients with minimal or moderate change disease on pancreatography had higher mean ductal pressures than those with more advanced disease (Table 28.2). However,

Table 28.1 Pancreatic duct pressure measured by direct puncture in patients with chronic pancreatitis and duct dilatation or pseudocysts

Reference	Number of patients	Pancreatic duct pressure (cmH₂O)	
		Mean	Range
Du Val (1958)	9	28	16–37
Anderson & Hagstrom (1962)	1	24	16–31
White & Bourde (1970)	1	19	15–22
Christofferson et al (1981)	3	40	30–59
Bradley (1982)	19	36	23–57

Table 28.2   Pancreatic duct pressure measured in patients with 'normal' pancreas and in patients with chronic pancreatitis. Pressures measured directly via traumatic fistula (Du Val, 1958) or by endoscopic cannulation (all other series). (SD, standard deviation; SE, standard error)

Reference	Controls		Chronic pancreatitis	
	Number of patients	Mean pressure (cmH$_2$O)	Number of patients	Mean pressure (cmH$_2$O)
Du Val (1958)	4	10.3 (range 9–13)		
Rosch et al (1976)			2	16 (14 and 18)
Bar-Meier et al (1979)	15	14.8 (SD = 4.2)		
Carr-Locke et al (1981)	12	20.4 (SE = 1.4)	13*	17
Bradley (1982)	25	15.5 (SD = 4.1)		
Novis et al (1985)	6	31.3 (range 5–54)	15	30.6 (range 12–60)
Okazaki et al (1988)	22	21.1 (SD = 11.8)		
			12 (minimal change)	61.1 (SD = 28)
			14 (moderate change)	76.0 (SD = 48)
			5 (advanced change)	43.8 (SD = 23)

* Patients thought to have idiopathic recurrent pancreatitis

it must be emphasized that the duct pressures recorded in this Japanese study are much greater than those found by others using similar techniques.

A number of other studies have cast doubt on the relationship between pain in chronic pancreatitis and pancreatic duct size and pressure. Bar-Meier et al (1979) found that patients with normal calibre ducts and chronic pancreatitis had duct pressures at ERCP which were similar to those of normal controls. Similarly, Novis et al (1985) found no difference between patients and controls in terms of pressures measured at ERCP, indeed, there were no significant differences between patients with and without pain, with and without ductal strictures and obstruction, and with and without calcification. These negative studies may be explained in part on technical grounds, as it may not be possible to advance endoscopically introduced catheters beyond an area of duct narrowing.

Stenosis of the pancreatic duct system is a frequent finding in chronic pancreatitis but its importance in the genesis of pain is uncertain. Bornman et al (1980) carried out ERCP in 39 patients with chronic pancreatitis, 20 of whom had experienced pain in the preceding year. The incidence of pancreatic duct stricture was similar in the patients with 'painless' disease (65%) and 'painful' disease (79%). This group also found no difference between patients with chronic pancreatitis and controls in terms of pressure at the sphincter of Oddi or frequency of papillary contraction, reinforcing the current view that disordered papillary motility is unlikely to have a significant role in the pathogenesis of chronic pancreatitis.

Calculi may also contribute to duct obstruction and the production of pain in chronic pancreatitis, and a number of studies have reported pain relief in the short-to-medium term in patients having stones removed by transduodenal or endoscopic sphincterotomy (Schneider & Lux 1985, Hansell et al 1986). As has been discussed in Chapter 27, endoscopic procedures including sphincterotomy, balloon dilatation and pancreatic duct stenting are now being applied cautiously in chronic pancreatitis,

sometimes in conjunction with destruction of pancreatic calculi by extracorporeal shock wave lithotripsy. All of these measures are designed to improve or restore the flow of pancreatic juice and the encouraging results reported to date support the contention that impaired ductal drainage is a major factor in pain production. Similarly, the success of surgical measures such as longitudinal pancreaticojejunostomy (see below) underlines the importance of ductal obstruction in the pathogenesis of pain.

In a proportion of patients, chronic pancreatitis is said to 'burn itself out' over a period of years (Ammann et al 1984). Although this view has aroused controversy (Warshaw 1984), patients who become pain-free often have marked pancreatic exocrine dysfunction (Girdwood et al 1981) and it is tempting to speculate that decreased pancreatic function does lead to reduction in ductal pressure and consequent relief of pain. In the Japanese study referred to earlier, ductal pressures were lower in patients with advanced disease (Okazaki et al 1988). It has also been suggested that oral pancreatic enzyme supplements such as Creon may diminish pain by lowering postprandial cholecystokinin (CCK) release and so lowering pancreatic duct pressure (Isaksson & Ihse 1983, Ihse & Lankisch 1988; Leahy & Carter 1991). Although this is an attractive hypothesis, it must be emphasized that the existence of a feedback loop based on intraduodenal concentrations of trypsin remains controversial (see Ch. 3), and recent studies suggest that any benefits attributable to enzyme supplements may be simply a placebo effect (Larvin et al 1992).

Pancreatic tissue pressure as measured by intraoperative needling by Ebbehøj et al (1986) has been shown to correlate with intraduct pressure and is elevated in patients with chronic pancreatitis and dilated ducts or pseudocysts. Following surgical drainage, tissue pressure decreased to normal, and this was associated with pain relief at the time of discharge from hospital. However, longer-term relief was not related to the fall in tissue pressure recorded at surgery, the type of drainage operation performed or anastomotic patency as assessed at ERCP. Similary, Holmberg et al (1985) found that long-term patency following drainage surgery did not necessarily correlate with pain relief, suggesting that duct decompression is not the only factor involved in eradicating or relieving pain. However, as will be discussed, the majority of patients do obtain substantial or complete relief of pain following effective drainage procedures such as longitudinal pancreaticojejunostomy (Warshaw et al 1980, Greenlee et al 1990) and it is difficult to believe that relief of ductal obstruction is not implicated. At the same time it is clear that pain production in chronic pancreatitis is multifactorial, and other agencies such as perineural inflammation and infiltration, cysts and pseudocysts, and biliary obstruction may all make major contributions.

PANCREATICOJEJUNOSTOMY

Cattell in 1947 first described the use of a Roux loop of jejunum to bypass the obstructed pancreatic duct in a patient with pancreatic cancer. Given the manifest shortcomings of operations such as biliary diversion and sphincterotomy in relieving the pain of chronic pancreatitis, it is not surprising that surgeons began to explore the concept in patients with this disease. Accordingly, Du Val (1954) employed retrograde drainage of the pancreas into a Roux loop following amputation of the tip of the pancreatic tail and splenectomy (Fig. 28.1). Although pain relief was reported in 80% of cases and the operation was endorsed by others (Leger et al 1974), it soon became apparent that relief was short-lived. Surgeons began to realize that chronic pancreatitis is not the result of a single stricture close to the papilla of Vater, and that multiple strictures are frequently present. Furthermore, long-term patency of the pancreaticojejunal anastomosis in the Du Val procedure could not be assured given the small calibre of the duct when sectioned in the tail of the pancreas. Puestow & Gillesby (1958) recognized the importance of multiple strictures and the so-called 'chain of lakes' changes in the pancreatic duct system, and extended the Du Val procedure by unroofing the main pancreatic duct from the tail to the right of the portal and superior mesenteric vein (Fig. 28.2). The tip of the gland was still amputated in this operation and the spleen was removed prior to 'implanting' the body and tail of the pancreas into the open *end* of the Roux loop. Partington & Rochelle (1960) extended the concept further by creating a side-to-side anastomosis between the open pancreatic duct system and the *side* of the Roux loop (Fig. 28.3), their operation having the added advantage that it was not necessary to remove the spleen or resect the tail of the pancreas. It should be emphasized that this was not a mucosa-to-mucosa anastomosis and that the opened jejunum was simply sutured to the

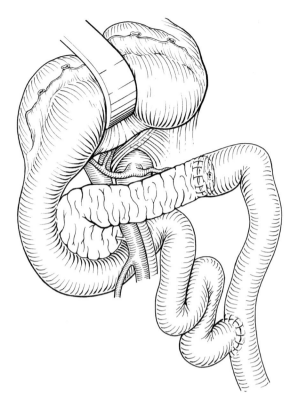

Fig. 28.1 The Du Val operation in which the tip of the pancreas is transected and the spleen removed prior to creating an end-to-end anastomosis between the cut end of the pancreatic remnant and a Roux loop of jejunum.

pancreatic capsule on the front of the gland. Indeed, it was stressed that mucosa-to-mucosa anastomosis should be avoided so as to ensure that the side branches of the main pancreatic duct were not occluded by the sutures. It is this operation of side-to-side pancreaticojejunostomy which forms the basis of the modern operation.

Technical considerations

Whenever possible the morphology of the duct should be defined before surgery by ERCP so as to detect all strictures and calculi, and any communicating pseudocysts which may be dealt with at the same operation. If ERCP fails to define the duct, useful information regarding duct size may be obtained from ultrasonography and CT scanning; otherwise percutaneous antegrade pancreatography can be carried out in expert hands under radiological or ultrasound guidance. If all else fails, pancreatography can still be carried out at the time of operation using direct needle puncture or transduodenal cannulation of the papilla of Vater (Cooper & Williamson 1983).

It is now generally accepted that pancreaticojejunostomy should only be performed in patients with a distended duct system and that the longer the

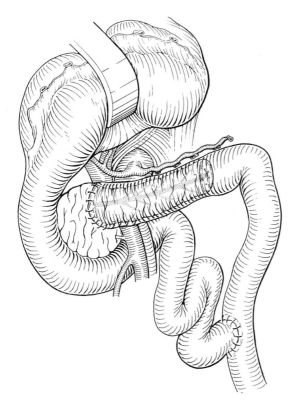

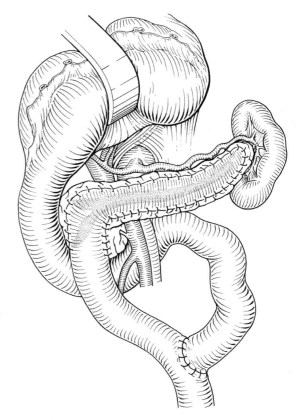

Fig. 28.2 Pancreaticojejunostomy as described by Puestow & Gillesby (1958). As in the Du Val procedure, the tail of the pancreas is first resected and the spleen removed. The main pancreatic duct is then unroofed from the tail to just beyond the neck of the pancreas. The body and tail of the gland are then implanted into the open end of a Roux loop of jejunum.

Fig. 28.3 Pancreaticojejunostomy based on the operation described by Partington & Rochelle (1960). None of the pancreas is resected and the spleen remains in place. The pancreatic duct system is opened as widely as possible, with extension of the incision into the head and uncinate process if possible. A side-to-side pancreaticojejunal anastomosis is then created between the open pancreas and a Roux loop of jejunum. Note that the blind end of the Roux loop is directed towards the tail of the pancreas.

anastomosis, the greater the long-term prospects for pain relief. Most authorities agree that the pancreatic duct should have a diameter of at least 7–8 mm, and the bigger the duct, the easier the operation technically. It is important to open the pancreatic duct as widely as possible, and the incision must start within 1–2 cm of the hilus of the spleen and extend to open the duct system in the head of the gland and, if possible, in the uncinate process as well (see Fig. 28.3).

The abdomen is entered by an upper midline or transverse incision and a thorough laparotomy is performed, paying particular attention to the liver, biliary system and pancreas. It must always be borne in mind that pancreatic cancer can masquerade as chronic pancreatitis and that many large series of patients undergoing pancreatic drainage procedures contain at least one patient in whom pancreatic cancer subsequently became manifest. It is our practice to use intraoperative ultrasonography routinely to scan both liver and pancreas prior to performing the drainage procedure, and we also routinely obtain a Trucut biopsy of the liver at the time of surgery to assess structural changes in the liver.

The anterior surface of the pancreas is exposed widely by dividing the gastrocolic omentum completely. Adhesions between the pancreas and the back of the stomach are divided carefully, staying close to the anterior surface of the gland. Once the pancreas has been fully exposed, its anterior surface is palpated so as to detect any duct enlargement. Needling of the body of the gland is also a useful way of localizing the duct and ultrasonography may also prove helpful in this regard. Significant difficulty in localizing the duct system probably means that it is not large enough to justify pancreaticojejunostomy, but if uncertainty remains it can be found by making an oblique incision across the front of the gland in the mid-body region. Once the duct has been entered it is opened widely with diathermy or by cutting down with a scalpel onto a probe placed within it; in some cases the pancreatic tissue in front of the duct is so thinned that it can be opened with scissors. A specimen of duct fluid is sent for cytological examination and a sliver of pancreatic tissue is obtained for histological examination. As indicated above, the duct is opened as widely as possible and all calculi within it are removed meticulously. Despite the extensive incision into the pancreas, bleeding is rarely difficult to control, given the fibrosis and thickening that characterizes the disease.

Once the pancreas has been prepared, the jejunum is traced downwards and divided some 20–30 cm distal to the ligament of Treitz. It is convenient to employ a linear stapler for this purpose and advisable to oversew the distal end of the jejunum before bringing it through a window in an avascular portion of the transverse mesocolon to serve as a Roux loop. The Roux loop is then opened along its antimesenteric border and anastomosed to the open anterior surface of the pancreas using delayed absorbable sutures. Opinions vary as to whether the anastomosis should be constructed in one or two layers and whether a mucosa-to-mucosa anastomosis is advisable. The argument against mucosa-to-mucosa apposition is that the side branches of the duct may be inadvertently occluded by sutures. It is my practice to use one layer of interrupted sutures and to pick up the mucosa of the pancreatic duct if the gland overlying the anterior aspect of the duct is thinned. It is essential to orientate the Roux loop so that its blind end is toward the tail of the pancreas, allowing the possibility of using the same loop for anastomosis to the biliary system (see below). Pseudocysts can also be drained into the same Roux loop without any increase in morbidity or mortality (Munn et al 1987).

On completion of the pancreaticojejunal anastomosis the window in the mesocolon is closed snugly around the Roux loop and intestinal continuity is restored beneath the mesocolon by an end-to-side anastomosis. Opinions vary as to the correct distance that should be left between the pancreaticojejunal anastomosis and the end-to-side enteric anastomosis; in the absence of objective data, a distance of some 40 cm seems reasonable in that reflux of intestinal content does not appear to constitute the same hazard after this type of surgery as after biliary-enteric anastomosis or revisional surgery for reflux gastritis. On completion of the anastomoses, the abdomen is closed without drainage.

Frey & Smith (1987) have argued that if the head of the pancreas is more than 3–4 cm thick, it is unlikely to be drained adequately by the standard longitudinal pancreaticojejunostomy. In the Frey procedure the main duct in the body and tail of the gland is opened widely as described above, the incision being carried as close to the duodenum as possible. If the head of the pancreas is not adequately decompressed, as shown by the persistence of impacted calculi and retention cysts, then the head is cored out to remove cysts and any areas of necrosis and scarring. Damage to the superior mesenteric vein and portal vein is avoided by keeping these structures in view throughout and retaining a thickness of some 4–5 mm of

pancreatic tissue between the veins and the coring-out incision. Similarly, a rim of pancreatic tissue 4–5 mm thick is preserved along the inner aspect of the duodenum to protect its blood supply. Posteriorly, a shell of pancreatic tissue must also be preserved to prevent leakage into the retroperitoneum. The risk of damage to the common bile duct can be reduced by inserting a metal dilator into the duct at the outset. Once the coring-out process is complete, all of the opened pancreas is anastomosed to a Roux loop as described above.

The Beger operation (Beger & Büchler 1990) also cores out tissue from the pancreatic head but in this case the entire head of the gland is removed, apart from a cuff of tissue on the inner aspect of the duodenum (see Ch. 30). Although the remaining body and tail of pancreas are subsequently anastomosed to a Roux loop of jejunum, the anastomosis is constructed in an end-to-end fashion and the operation should be regarded as a resection rather than as a drainage procedure.

Biliary tract drainage and pancreatico-jejunostomy

Chronic pancreatitis may be associated with a spectrum of hepatobiliary disorders. Oedema in the head of the gland and pseudocysts can give rise to transient obstructive jaundice and disturbed liver function tests, while fibrosis and scarring following chronic inflammation can cause frank stenosis of the intrapancreatic portion of the common bile duct. Cholangiographic evidence of such stenosis has been reported in as many as two-thirds of patients with chronic pancreatitis (Sarles et al 1965, Wilson et al 1989) but in most cases this produces no symptoms or gives rise to only transient episodes of jaundice or elevations in the serum alkaline phosphatase levels. Pain is not usually a feature of common bile duct obstruction in chronic pancreatitis in the absence of cholangitis (Frey et al 1990). Cholangitis is however rare in unoperated patients, and although long-standing obstruction can produce secondary biliary cirrhosis, this is also an extremely rare complication (Wilson et al 1989).

It follows that relatively few patients with chronic pancreatitis require surgery for biliary stenosis alone, and the literature suggests that biliary surgery is needed for this complication in only some 4–16% of cases (Scott et al 1977, Ammann et al 1984, Aranha et al 1984). Most surgeons now agree that the radiological or ultrasonographic demonstration of a dilated bile duct proximal to a stricture and/or elevation of the alkaline phosphatase levels are not sufficient grounds for surgical intervention, but should be an indication for close followup with monitoring of liver function, repeat ultrasonography (or cholangiography) and liver biopsy (Stahl et al 1988, Wilson et al 1989). Absolute indications for surgical intervention are the development of acute cholangitis, formation of bile duct stones, secondary biliary cirrhosis, and jaundice which persists for more than 1 month. In the absence of absolute indications, biliary drainage should still be considered in patients with a biliary stricture and past history of cholangitis who are undergoing pancreatic surgery for other reasons, such as intractable pain.

In general, biliary drainage is best achieved by a hepaticojejunostomy using a Roux loop. As mentioned earlier, the Roux loop used for side-to-side pancreaticojejunostomy can also be used to drain the obstructed biliary tree in patients requiring drainage of both systems. Less desirable alternatives include choledochoduodenostomy or use of a second Roux loop of jejunum which can be brought up to the biliary system. Use of the gallbladder for drainage is not acceptable as the anastomosis seldom provides effective drainage in the long term; indeed, many surgeons prefer to remove the gallbladder if biliary surgery is required and so avoid problems arising from it. Similarly, sphincterotomy or sphincteroplasty are of no value as drainage operations in the present context in that they fail to decompress the biliary tree effectively. In the presence of severe disease in the head of the pancreas, the Whipple operation may prove to be a better option than complex drainage surgery. As will be discussed, the fear of occult pancreatic cancer is always present in patients undergoing pancreatic drainage procedures, and resection undoubtedly dispels any lingering doubts. Interestingly, it is now recognized that prior pancreaticojejunostomy does not necessarily prevent the subsequent development of biliary stricture, a complication that has been recorded in 5–30% of patients, with most authors reporting an incidence of less than 10% (Frey et al 1990).

Duodenal obstruction and pancreaticojejunostomy

Nausea and vomiting are common features of chronic pancreatitis, and exacerbations of inflammation in the head of the gland can give rise to frank duodenal obstruction and delayed gastric emptying. In most cases, such duodenal hold-up is transient, but if it persists for more than 3–4 weeks, operation is indicated. It should be emphasized that duodenal obstruction is rarely the sole indication for surgery; most of these patients also have long-standing pain which in itself is sufficient to merit operation. When pancreaticojejunostomy is being undertaken in patients who also have duodenal obstruction, gastrojejunostomy can be used to drain the stomach. 'Triple bypass' has been described in which a Roux loop is used to drain the pancreas, biliary system and stomach, but it can be argued that a Whipple procedure is a less complicated and more satisfactory solution in these circumstances. To my mind, the same arguments apply to the use of separate Roux loops to drain the

pancreas and stomach, and to the use of an isolated loop of jejunum to drain the pancreas and bile duct before being anastomosed to the duodenum (Frey et al 1990).

Results of pancreaticojejunostomy

The reported results of pancreaticojejunostomy are difficult to interpret. Many reports have incomplete follow-up, lack objective assessment of patients by an independent observer, and include patients dealt with by forms of drainage surgery which are now considered to be inadequate. The problem is further complicated by the fact that the indications for operation vary from centre to centre. Much depends on the degree of dilatation of the pancreatic duct, the extent of calcification, and the underlying cause of the pancreatic inflammation. In general, the results of all forms of pancreatic surgery deteriorate with time and particularly poor results can be anticipated in patients who cannot abstain from alcohol or who have become dependent on narcotic analgesics.

Operative mortality

As might be expected, pancreaticojejunostomy carries an appreciably lower risk of operative mortality and morbidity than operations involving resection of the pancreas (Table 28.3). The thickened fibrosed pancreas holds sutures well, bleeding is seldom troublesome in the absence of splenic vein thrombosis and segmental portal hypertension (complications which usually mean that distal pancreatectomy and splenectomy is more appropriate than drainage surgery), and leakage from the anastomosis should not occur in skilled hands. Many recent series, including our own series of 46 patients, have no operative mortality for this operation.

Pain relief

Relief of pain is the primary objective of pancreatic drainage procedures (Table 28.4). Although the pancreas is conserved, improved exocrine and endocrine function should not be expected; it is more realistic to hope that the procedure will arrest or at least slow the development of exocrine and endocrine insufficiency (see below). Way et al (1974) initially reported good or fair results in 19 (90%) of 21 patients undergoing longitudinal pancreaticojejunostomy, but by 5 years this proportion had fallen to 80%. Leger et al (1974) in a study involving follow-up of 5–20 years found that only 63% of their patients had good or fair results, while Jordan et al (1977) found that although 79% of their 24 patients had excellent or improved results on assessment within a year of operation, this figure fell to 74% with increasing follow-up. In one of the largest series, Greenlee et al (1990) report complete or substantial pain relief in 82% of their

Table 28.3 Comparison of pancreaticojejunostomy and resection in the treatment of chronic pancreatitis (from Eckhauser et al 1984)

	Pancreaticojejunostomy	Distal pancreatectomy	Pancreaticoduodenectomy
Number of patients	228	102	276
% Operative mortality	4.3	8.2	5.3
% Insulin-dependent diabetes diabetes			
Preoperative	26	11	28
Postoperative	50	62	64
% Satisfactory pain control	74	72	68
% Late mortality	39	36	30
% Reoperation rate	22	9.5	Unknown

patients undergoing side-to-side pancreaticojejunostomy with a follow-up of 1–25 years (mean 7.9 years). Their study also highlights the less satisfactory result obtained with earlier operations of the type described by Du Val (Table 28.5). Sato et al (1986) from Japan have reported results which are greatly superior to those of other centres; no less that 91% of their 43 patients undergoing side-to-side pancreaticojejunostomy were said to have complete pain relief at a mean follow-up interval of 9.1 years. These results must be regarded as atypical; in general, patients being considered for pancreaticojejunostomy can be told that their chances of complete or substantial relief of pain at 5 years are of the order of 70% (see Table 28.3).

It is widely accepted that the prospects for pain relief are poor if the pancreatic duct is not dilated, and the importance of an extensive unroofing of the pancreatic duct has already been emphasized. Failure to abstain from alcohol is a major obstacle to achieving pain relief as well as dramatically reducing long-term survival (Prinz & Greenlee 1981). It has been argued that extensive pancreatic calcification denotes marked exocrine dysfunction and that this can lead to spontaneous diminution in pain (Ammann et al 1984). If this were true then one might anticipate better results from pancreatic drainage in patients with extensive calcification; unfortunately, this hope does not appear to be borne out in practice (Prinz & Greenlee 1981, Holmberg et al 1985).

Exocrine and endocrine function

Early hopes that fat absorption would improve following pancreaticojejunostomy have not been sustained. While ERCP has confirmed continued anastomotic patency

Table 28.4 Pain relief after longitudinal/side-to-side pancreaticojejunostomy

Reference	Number of patients	Duration of follow-up (months)	% Obtaining pain relief	Definition used
Jordan et al (1977)	13	58* (12–123)	39	Excellent
			35	Improved
Taylor et al (1981)	18	60		
Prinz & Greenlee (1981)	87	91*	56	Complete/significant relief
			37	Complete relief
			45	Substantial relief
Sarles et al (1982)	30	60	55	Complete relief
			30	Incomplete relief
Brinton et al (1984)	39	24–180	67	Total relief; only transient
Morrow et al (1984)**	46	48–156	46	Asymptomatic
			35	Occasional pain
Warshaw (1985)	17	42* (6–120)	77	Excellent (no pain) or good (no narcotics, able to work despite some pain).
Noguiera & Dani (1985)	36	57*	58	Total relief/considerable improvement
Sugerman et al (1986)	20	35*	55	Complete pain relief; no narcotics
Sato et al (1986)	4.3	109*	30	Partial relief; occasional narcotics (less than once/twice per week)
			91	Pain disappeared
			9	Pain alleviated
Bradley (1987)	46	69* (10–144)	28	Good; pain eliminated
			38	Fair; pain decreased and no narcotics required
Pain & Knight (1988)	19	48	25	Good; pain free, minor discomfort, no interference with life
			34	Fair, episodic pain needing analgesia but no hospitalization
Carter personal series (1992)	32	46	45	Complete relief
			28	Substantial relief

* Denotes mean duration of follow-up (months): value estimated from figure rather than text. ** Includes some patients having Du Val procedure

Table 28.5 Comparison of the results of various pancreatic drainage operatons (Greenlee et al 1990)

	Side-to-side pancreaticojejunostomy	Longitudinal pancreaticojejunostomy	Du Val procedure
Number of patients	53	43	8
Operative deaths (%)	1 (2%)	1 (2%)	1 (13%)
Pain relief			
Complete (%)	21/50 (42%)	10/36 (28%)	1/5 (20%)
Substantial (%)	20/50 (42%)	18/36 (50%)	1/5 (20%)
Unsuspected carcinoma	1/53	1/43	1/8
Lost to follow-up	1/53	4/43	1/8

after side-to-side pancreaticojejunostomy (in contrast to the Du Val procedure), pancreatic exocrine function does not improve and usually continues to decline (Kugelberg et al 1976, Warshaw et al 1980, Bradley & Nasrallah 1984). There is some evidence that the rate of functional decline may be slowed by timely drainage surgery, regardless of whether the patient abstains from alcohol (Nealon et al 1988). However, it is quite common for patients to develop frank steatorrhoea for the first time in the years following an apparently successful drainage operation. Similarly, operation does not protect against the progression of endocrine insufficiency and a proportion of patients develop insulin-dependent diabetes after a drainage procedure. However, diabetes is generally less common, less brittle, and easier to manage than that which may follow pancreatic resection (see Table 28.3).

Development of cancer

Most large series of patients having undergone drainage surgery eventually turn out to contain patients who have pancreatic cancer. For example, of the 100 patients reported by Greenlee et al (1990), three died from metastatic cancer within a year of operation, while 9 (16%) of the 55 patients described by White & Slavotinek (1979) were found to have pancreatic cancer at eventual autopsy. The main problem is undoubtedly the difficulty of detecting cancer in a chronically inflamed pancreas at the time of surgery (Carter 1992) and it is well recognized that pancreatic cancer may cause marked ductal distension and inflammation. However, a number of series, including our own, contain patients who were diagnosed as having pancreatic cancer some years after their drainage operation. While there is little hard evidence incriminating chronic pancreatitis as a risk factor for pancreatic cancer (Haddock & Carter 1990), a causal role for inflammation cannot be completely discounted. It is also well recognized that patients with chronic pancreatitis have a significantly reduced life expectancy, and that smoking and alcohol make a major contribution to their demise. Common causes of death in these patients include cardiovascular disease, chronic lung diseases, cirrhosis and chronic alcoholism, and various forms of cancer, including oropharyngeal and lung cancer (Greenlee et al 1990).

Pancreaticojejunostomy in specific situations

Tropical pancreatitis

Tropical pancreatitis is a form of chronic pancreatitis encountered in parts of Asia, Africa and South America which is characterized by onset in childhood or early adult life. There is a high incidence of diabetes mellitus, marked pancreatic calcification, malnutrition and recurrent abdominal pain. At one time it was believed that protein–calorie malnutrition was responsible for the condition but it is now recognized that this may be the result rather than the cause of the disease. Biliary tract disease and alcohol are not implicated and there is now evidence that dietary toxins such as the cyanogenetic glycosides found in cassava are involved (see Ch. 24).

As the majority of patients with tropical pancreatitis have dilated ducts, pancreatic drainage procedures rather than resection have been advocated should surgery become necessary. The southern Indian state of Kerala has a particularly high incidence of tropical pancreatitis, and Thomas & Augustine (1988) have reported good relief of pain in 13 of 15 patients surviving drainage surgery, which in all but one case took the form of side-to-side pancreaticojejunostomy. The authors emphasize that the body and tail of the pancreas may be so shrunken and diseased that distal resection may be appropriate in addition to a drainage procedure. Many of these patients are grossly undernourished and it is hardly surprising that the operative mortality approaches 10% (Ramesh & Augustine 1992).

Tropical pancreatitis is not exempt from major anxieties about the presence of pancreatic cancer. Ramesh & Augustine (1992) have reported that no fewer than 19 (21%) of their 91 patients diagnosed initially as having tropical pancreatitis turned out to have malignancy. It is not clear whether tropical pancreatitis predisposes to malignant change. Although patients with carcinoma in this series were significantly older than those with benign disease, they all had calculi in areas remote from the tumour or changes suggestive of chronic pancreatitis in the ductal system downstream of the tumour. Exocrine pancreatic cancer is an uncommon form of cancer in Southern India (accounting for just over 1% of all malignancies), and the possibility that tropical pancreatitis predisposes to cancer is strengthened by reports of coexistence of the two conditions in siblings (Thomas & Augustine 1987).

Pancreaticojejunostomy in childhood

Chronic pancreatitis in childhood is an extremely rare disease. The pancreatic manifestations of cystic fibrosis are not usually classified as chronic pancreatitis but recurrent attacks of pancreatitis can be associated with hyperparathyroidism, hyperlipidaemia and ductal obstruction (due to lesions such as choledochal cysts and ampullary stenosis). Hereditary pancreatitis is the commonest form of chronic pancreatitis in children away from areas affected by tropical pancreatitis. Comfort & Steinberg (1952) were the first to describe a kindred with this autosomal dominant trait and at least 40 affected families have now been identified with a total of some 200 individual patients (Scott et al 1984). The aetiology of hereditary pancreatitis is unknown but dilatation of the pancreatic duct system is usual and stone formation may be marked. Pancreaticojejunostomy gives excellent results (Scott et al 1984), although all reported series are small. Uncertainty also surrounds the association between this condition and pancreatic cancer in that approximately one-third of affected patients in some series have developed cancer, although family members without pancreatitis also appear to be at increased risk (Castleman et al 1972).

Repeat pancreaticojejunostomy

As indicated above, some 30% of patients fail to obtain long-lasting relief of pain after pancreaticojejunostomy. Before proceeding to pancreatic resection, other causes of abdominal pain, such as biliary tract disease or peptic ulcer, must first be excluded. If the pain is still thought to be pancreatic, ERCP should be carried out to determine whether the pancreatic duct system is dilated and draining adequately. In some cases, the drainage will be found to be inadequate or non-existent, particularly when the initial operation was a caudal or longitudinal pancreaticojejunostomy. In these circumstances, redrainage may well prove the best option, given that it carries a lower operative risk than resection and that it conserves rather than removes functioning pancreatic tissue. Prinz et al (1986) have reported 14 patients undergoing redrainage, 10 (71%) of whom achieved complete or substantial relief of pain.

PANCREATICOGASTROSTOMY

Pancreaticogastrostomy has been advocated by some authors as a better form of drainage procedure than pancreaticojejunostomy. Pain & Knight (1988) argue that the 'chain of lakes' appearance is relatively uncommon in chronic pancreatitis and that in their experience pan-creatic duct obstruction is usually due to one or two isolated strictures, often with associated calculi. After an encouraging initial experience, they adopted pancreaticogastrostomy as their standard operation in patients with dilated ducts and intractable pain, and report that it led to significantly better pain relief than pancreaticojejunostomy. Within 4 years of operation, no less than 35% of their pancreaticojejunostomy patients had required reoperation, as opposed to only 10% of those having pancreaticogastrostomy. These data must be interpreted in the light of their description of the technique of pancreaticojejunostomy, which states that in the absence of 'extensive stricturing throughout the pancreatic duct we have avoided longitudinal PJ and instead have used a limited mucosal to mucosal pancreaticoenteric anastomosis performed over a silastic T tube'. As argued above, this cannot be regarded as an adequate pancreaticojejunostomy and it comes as no surprise that it produced poor results. The authors also stress the importance of precise mucosa-to-mucosa anastomosis around a T tube in their description of pancreaticogastrostomy. Of interest, more of their patients had steatorrhoea following pancreaticogastrostomy, possibly because of the inactivation of pancreatic enzymes by gastric acid.

Ebbehøj et al (1989) have also employed pancreaticogastrostomy in a series of 45 patients with painful chronic pancreatitis. Good or fair results were achieved in 79% of cases following an operation similar to that used by Pain & Knight (1988). Pain relief was not related to duct patency in the 14 patients undergoing ERCP, and poor results were commoner in those using tranquillisers before operation and in those not abstaining from alcohol after surgery. It is difficult to know whether pancreaticogastrostomy has a place in the management of chronic pancreatitis; for the moment most surgeons still regard pancreaticojejunostomy as the drainage operation of choice.

SPHINCTEROTOMY AND SPHINCTEROPLASTY

Transduodenal (biliary) sphincterotomy was originally proposed by Doubilet & Mulholland (1956) for the treatment of chronic pancreatitis in the mistaken belief that the disease was caused by bile reflux. The operation did not prove effective and subsequent attempts to improve pancreatic drainage by dividing the septum between the bile duct and pancreatic duct (Bartlett & Nardi 1960) have not proved popular. In chronic pancreatitis it is unusual to find uniform dilatation of the pancreatic duct system resulting from localized obstruction at the termination of the main duct (Moossa, 1987, Ihse et al 1990). It follows that attempts to improve pancreatic drainage by transduodenal sphincterotomy or sphincteroplasty are unlikely to prove successful in the long term. Early success rates of around 50% when pain relief was assessed at 5 years (Doubilet & Mulholland 1956, Bartlett & Nardi 1960, Dreiling & Greenstein 1979, Bagley et al 1981) have not been sustained and may have been attributable in large measure to patient selection. For example, in the study by Bagley et al (1981) the 67 patients with disabling pain had only minimal evidence of duct change on pancreatography and minimal evidence of disease at operation. Although 66% of patients had pain relief at 6 months, by 5 years this figure had fallen to 43%; abstinence from alcohol appeared to be the major determinant of successful long-term outcome. Most surgeons no longer use sphincter operations in chronic pancreatitis although some believe that sphincteroplasty and formal septoplasty (Fig. 28.4) is still indicated in highly selected patients with a short stricture at or immediately adjacent to the papilla (Cooper & Williamson 1984).

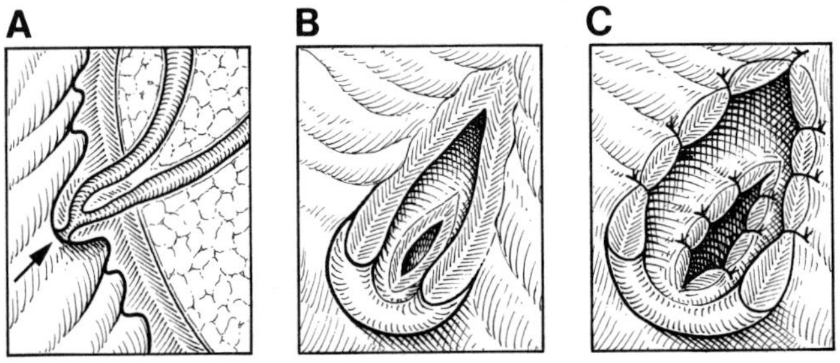

Despite the lack of surgical enthusiasm for sphincterotomy and sphincteroplasty, it must be admitted that the initial results of endoscopic and related measures to improve drainage through the papilla of Vater have proved encouraging. These approaches are discussed in detail elsewhere (Ch. 27) but the study reported by Grimm et al (1989) is illustrative. A total of 70 patients with painful chronic pancreatitis were reviewed of whom 61 were treated successfully. The basic procedure consisted of endoscopic papillotomy of the pancreatic duct, and additional procedures included extraction of calculi,

Fig. 28.4 A The intimate relationship between the common bile duct and pancreatic duct as they traverse the wall of the duodenum. **B** This allows the pancreatic duct to be opened through the posterior wall of the bile duct after preliminary sphincterotomy. **C** The operation is completed by placement of interrupted sutures to fashion a formal biliary sphincteroplasty and pancreatic sphincteroplasty or septoplasty.

insertion of an endoprosthesis and extracorporeal shock wave lithotripsy. Of the 61 patients 50 (82%) were initially pain-free but in the 2–36 month follow-up period, 15 patients suffered recurrence which in some cases necessitated surgery. The long-term place of such endoscopic measures to improve pancreatic drainage is at present uncertain but it may be that they will find a place in the armamentarium as an alternative to surgical drainage, at least in patients in whom surgery is contraindicated or has to be postponed.

REFERENCES

Ammann R W, Akovbiantz A, Largiader F, Schueler G 1984 Course and outcome of chronic pancreatitis. Longitudinal study of a mixed medical-surgical series of 245 patients. Gastroenterology 86: 820–828

Anderson M C Hagstrom W J 1962 A comparison of pancreatic and biliary pressures recorded simultaneously in man. Canadian Journal of Surgery 5: 461–468

Aranha G V, Prinz R A, Freeark R J, Greenlee H B 1984 The spectrum of biliary tract obstruction from chronic pancreatitis. Archives of Surgery 119: 595–600

Bagley F H, Braasch J W, Taylor R H, Warren K W 1981 Sphincterotomy or sphincteroplasty in the treatment of pathologically mild chronic pancreatitis. American Journal of Surgery 141: 418–421

Bar-Meier S, Geenen J E, Hogan W J, Dodds W J, Stewart E T, Arndorfer R C 1979 Biliary and pancreatic duct pressures measured by ERCP manometry in patients with suspected papillary stenosis. Digestive Diseases and Sciences 24: 209–213

Bartlett M K, Nardi G L 1960 Treatment of recurrent pancreatitis by transduodenal sphincterotomy and exploration of the pancreatic duct. New England Journal of Medicine 262: 643–648

Beger H G, Büchler M 1990 Duodenum-preserving resection of the head of the pancreas in chronic pancreatitis with inflammatory mass in the head. World Journal of Surgery 14: 83–87

Bornman P C, Marks I N, Girdwood A H et al 1980 Is pancreatic duct obstruction or stricture a major cause of pain in calcific pancreatitis? British Journal of Surgery 67: 425–428

Bradley E L 1982 Pancreatic duct pressure in chronic pancreatitis. American Journal of Surgery 144: 313–316

Bradley H L 1987 Long-term results of pancreaticojejunostomy in patients with chronic pancreatitis. American Journal of Surgery 153: 207–213

Bradley F L, Nasrallah S M 1984 Fat absorption after longitudinal pancreaticojejunostomy. Surgery 95: 640–643

Brinton M H, Pellergrini C A, Stein S F, Way L W 1984 Surgical treatment of chronic pancreatitis. Annals of Surgery 148: 754–760

Carr-Locke D L, Gregg J A 1981 Endoscopic manometry of pancreatic and biliary sphincter zones in man. Digestive Diseases and Sciences 26: 7–13

Carter D C 1992 Cancer of the head of pancreas or chronic pancreatitis? A diagnostic dilemma. Surgery 111: 602–603

Castleman B, Scully R, McNeeley B U 1972 Case records of the Massachusetts General Hospital, Case 25. New England Journal of Medicine 286: 1353

Cattell R B 1947 Anastomosis of the duct of Wirsung: its use in palliative operations for cancer of the head of the pancreas. Surgical Clinics of North America 27: 636–642

Christofferson I, Madsen P, Philbert A, Schmidt K 1981 Chronic obstructive pancreatitis treated by pancreaticogastrostomy. Gastroenterology 80: 1124–1127

Comfort M W, Steinberg A G 1952 Pedigree of a family with hereditary chronic relapsing pancreatitis. Gastroenterology 21: 53

Cooper M J, Williamson R C N 1983 The value of operative pancreatography. British Journal of Surgery 70: 577–580

Cooper M J, Williamson R C N 1984 Drainage operations in chronic pancreatitis. British Journal of Surgery 71: 761–766

Doubilet H, Mulholland J H 1956 Eight-year study of pancreatitis and sphincterotomy. Journal of the American Medical Association 160: 521–528

Dreiling D A, Greenstein R J 1979 State of the art: the sphincter of Oddi, sphincterotomy and biliopancreatic disease. American Journal of Gastroenterology 72: 665–670

Du Val M K 1954 Caudal pancreaticojejunostomy for chronic pancreatitis. Annals of Surgery 140: 775–785

DuVal M K 1958 The effect of chronic pancreatitis on pressure tolerance in the human pancreatic duct. Surgery 43: 798–803

Ebbehøj N, Borly L, Madsen P, Svendsen L B 1986 Pancreatic tissue pressure and pain in chronic pancreatitis. Pancreas 1: 556–558

Ebbehøj N, Klaaborg K-E, Kronborg O, Madsen P 1989 Pancreaticogastrostomy for chronic pancreatitis. American Journal of Surgery 157: 315–317

Eckhauser F E, Strodel W E, Knol J A, Harper M, Turcotte J G 1984 Near-total pancreatectomy for chronic pancreatitis. Surgery 96: 599–607

Frey C F, Smith G J 1987 Description and rationale for a new operation for chronic pancreatitis. Pancreas 2: 701–705

Frey C F, Suzuki M, Isaji S 1990 Treatment of chronic pancreatitis complicated by obstruction of the common bile duct or duodenum. World Journal of Surgery 14:59–69

Girdwood A H, Marks I N, Bornman P C, Kottler R E, Cohen M 1981 Does progressive pancreatic insufficiency limit pain in calcific pancreatitis with duct stricture or continued alcohol insult? Journal of Clinical Gastroenterology 3: 241–245

Greenlee H B, Prinz R A, Aranha G V 1990 Long-term results of side-to-side pancreaticocjejunostomy. World Journal of Surgery 14: 70–76

Grimm H, Meyer W-H, Nam V C h, Soehendra N 1989 New modalities for treating chronic pancreatitis. Endoscopy 21: 70–74

Haddock G, Carter D C 1990 Aetiology of pancreatic cancer. British Journal of Surgery 77: 1159–1166

Hansell D T, Gillespie G, Imrie C W 1986 Operative transampullary extraction of pancreatic calculi. Surgery, Gynecology and Obstetrics 163: 17–20

Holmberg T J, Isaksson G, Ihse I 1985 Long-term results in pancreaticojejunostomy in chronic pancreatitis. Surgery, Gynecology and Obstetrics 160: 339–346

Ihse I, Lankisch P G 1988 Treatment of chronic pancreatitis current status. Acta Chirurgica Scandinavica 154: 553–558

Ihse I, Borch K, Larsson J 1990 Chronic pancreatitis: results of operations for relief of pain. World Journal of Surgery 14: 53–58

Isaksson G, Ihse I 1983 Pain reduction by an oral pancreatic enzyme preparation in chronic pancreatitis. Digestive Diseases and Sciences 28: 97–102

Jordan G L, Strug B S, Crowder W E 1977 Current status of pancreaticojejunostomy in the management of chronic pancreatitis. American Journal of Surgery 133: 46–50

Kugelberg C H, Wehlin L, Arnesjö B, Tylén U 1976 Endoscopic pancreatography in evaluating results of pancreaticojejunostomy. Gut 17: 267–272

Larvin M, McMahon M J, Puntis M C A, Thomas W E G 1992 Marked placebo responses in chronic pancreatitis: final results of a controlled trial of Creon therapy. British Journal of Surgery 79, (in press)

Leahy A, Carter D C 1991 Pain and chronic pancreatitis. European Journal of Gastroenterology & Hepatology 3: 425–433

Leger L, Lenriot J P, Lemaigre G 1974 Five- to twenty-year followup after surgery for chronic pancreatitis in 148 patients. Annals of Surgery 180: 185–191

Moossa A R 1987 Surgical treatment of chronic pancreatitis: an overview. British Journal of Surgery 74: 661–667

Morrow C E, Cohen J I, Sutherland E R, Najarian J S 1984 Chronic pancreatitis: Long-term surgical results of pancreatic duct drainage, pancreatic resection, and near-total pancreatectomy and islet autotransplantation. Surgery 96: 608–615

Munn J S, Aranha G V, Greenlee H B, Prinz R A 1987 Simultaneous treatment of pancreatic pseudocysts and chronic pancreatitis. Archives of Surgery 122: 622–667

Nealon W H, Townsend C M, Thompson J C 1988 Operative drainage of the pancreatic duct delays functional impairment in patients with chronic pancreatitis. A prospective analysis. Annals of Surgery 208: 321–329

Nogueira C E D, Dani R 1985 Evaluation of the surgical treatment of chronic calcifying pancreatitis. Surgery, Gynecology and Obstetrics 161: 117–128

Novis B H, Bornman P C, Girdwood A W, Marks I N 1985 Endoscopic manometry of the pancreatic duct and sphincter zone in patients with chronic pancreatitis. Digestive Diseases and Sciences 30: 225–228

Okazaki K, Yamamoto Y, Kagiyama S et al 1988 Pressure of papillary sphincter zone and pancreatic main duct in patients with chronic pancreatitis in the early stage. Scandinavian Journal of Gastroenterology 1: 23–501–507

Pain J A, Knight M J 1988 Pancreaticogastrostomy: the preferred operation for pain relief in chronic pancreatitis. British Journal of Surgery 75: 220–222

Partington P F, Rochelle R E L 1960 Modified Puestow procedure for retrograde drainage of the pancreatic duct. Annals of Surgery 152: 1037–1043

Prinz R A, Greelee H B 1981 Pancreatic duct drainage in 100 patients with chronic pancreatitis. Annals of Surgery 194: 313–318

Prinz R A, Aranha G V, Greenlee H B 1986 Redrainage of the pancreatic duct in chronic pancreatitis. American Journal of Surgery 151: 150–156

Puestow C B, Gillesby W J 1958 Retrograde surgical drainage of the pancreas for chronic relapsing pancreatitis. Archives of Surgery 76: 898–907

Ramesh H, Augustine P 1992 Surgery in tropical pancreatitis: analysis of risk factors. British Journal of Surgery 79: 544–549

Rosch W, Koch H, Demling L 1976 Manometric studies during ERCP and endoscopic papillotomy. Endoscopy 8: 30–35

Sarles H, Sarles J C, Camatte R et al 1965 Observations on 205 confirmed cases of acute pancreatitis, recurring pancreatitis and chronic pancreatitis. Gut 6: 545–559

Sarles J, Nacchiero M, Garani F, Salasc B 1982 Surgical treatment of chronic pancreatitis. American Journal of Surgery 144: 317–321

Sato T, Miyashita E, Matsuno S, Yamauchi H 1986 The role of surgical treatment for chronic pancreatitis. Annals of Surgery 203: 266–271

Schneider M J, Lux G 1985 Floating pancreatic duct concrements in chronic pancreatitis. Pain relief by endoscopic removal. Endoscopy 17: 8–10

Scott J, Summerfield J A, Elias E, Dick R, Sherlock S 1977 Chronic pancreatitis: a cause of cholestasis. Gut 18: 196

Scott H W, Neblett W W, O'Neill J A, Sawyers J L et al 1984 Longitudinal pancreaticojejunostomy in chronic relapsing pancreatitis with onset in childhood. Annals of Surgery 199: 610–622

Stahl T J, Allen M O, Ansel H J, Vennes J A 1988 Partial biliary obstruction caused by chronic pancreatitis. Annals of Surgery 207: 26–32

Sugerman H J, Barnhart G R, Newsome H H 1986 Selective drainage for pancreatic, biliary and duodenal obstruction secondary to chronic fibrosing pancreatitis. Annals of Surgery 203: 558–567

Taylor R H, Bagley F H, Braasch J W, Warren K W 1981 Ductal drainage or resection for chronic pancreatitis. American Journal of Surgery 141: 28–31

Thomas P G, Augustine P 1987 Pancreatic cancer in siblings with tropical pancreatitis. Indian Journal of Gastroenterology 6: 185–186

Thomas P G, Augustine P 1988 Surgery in tropical pancreatitis. British Journal of Surgery 75: 161–164

Warshaw A L 1984 Pain in chronic pancreatits. Patients, patience, and the impatient surgeon. Gastroenterology 86: 987–989

Warshaw A L 1985 Conservation of pancreatic tissue by combined gastric, biliary and pancreatic duct drainage for pain from chronic pancreatitis. American Journal of Surgery 149: 563–569

Warshaw A L, Popp J W, Schapiro R H 1980 Long-term patency, pancreatic function, and pain relief after lateral pancreaticojejunostomy for chronic pancreatitis. Gastroenterology 79: 289–293

Way L W, Gadacz T, Goldman L 1974 Surgical treatment of chronic pancreatitis. American Journal of Surgery 127: 267–272

White T T, Bourde J 1970 A new observation on human intraductal pancreatic pressure. Surgery, Gynecology and Obstetrics 130: 275–278

White T T, Slavotinek A H 1979 Results of surgical treatment of chronic pancreatitis: report of 142 cases. Annals of Surgery 138: 129–133

Wilson C, Auld C D, Schlinkert R, Hasan A H et al 1989 Hepatobiliary complications in chronic pancreatitis. Gut 30: 520–527

29. Distal pancreatectomy in chronic pancreatitis

C. F. Frey

Distal pancreatectomy as described by Mayo in 1913 was used only infrequently in the operative management of patients with chronic pancreatitis until the 1960s. Although resection of the tail of the pancreas (and spleen) was an integral part of the drainage operations described by Zollinger et al (1954), Du Val & Enquist (1961) and Puestow & Gillesby (1958) (see Ch. 28), in all of these early descriptions of pancreaticojejunostomy, the distal pancreatectomy was performed to facilitate drainage of the pancreatic duct rather than with the intention of resecting diseased pancreatic tissue.

In 1958 Eliason & Welty described three patients with chronic calcific pancreatitis who were treated by distal resection of two-thirds of the pancreas. Two of the three patients were relieved of pain. A year earlier, 95% resection of the distal pancreas had been described by Barrett & Bowers (1957), and by 1965, Fry & Child had performed 26 such operations, removing 80–95% of the pancreas. During the 1960s and 1970s, distal pancreatectomy was the most commonly performed operation for the relief of pain in chronic pancreatitis (Frey 1981).

Distal pancreatectomy can be subdivided into 80–95% pancreatectomy (Fig. 29.1) and less-than-80% pancreatectomy (Fig. 29.2). In 80–95% pancreatectomy, major portions of the head and uncinate process are excised as well as the body and tail of the gland. In less-than-80% pancreatectomy, the greatest amount of pancreas that is removed is the neck, body and tail, and a small portion of the head. Before the widespread availability of CT scanning and endoscopic retrograde cholangiopancreatography (ERCP), the extent of pancreatic disease and ductal abnormalities was difficult to define. In many centres, duct size was not taken into account and 80–95% distal pancreatectomy was used in patients with diffuse disease and less-than-80% pancreatectomy in patients in whom disease seemed to be limited to the body and tail of the pancreas.

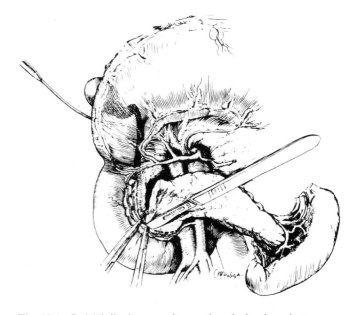

Fig. 29.1 In 95% distal pancreatic resection, the head, uncinate process, and body and tail of the pancreas are removed. Only a small rim of tissue is preserved along the inner aspect of the duodenum. (Reproduced with permission from Frey C F Distal subtotal pancreatectomy. In: Malt R A (ed) Surgical techniques illustrated 2nd ed. Little, Brown, p. 82.)

RESULTS OF DISTAL PANCREATECTOMY

Pain relief

Proximal and distal resection of the pancreas have in common that if the diseased portion of the pancreas is removed, the proportion of patients experiencing pain relief, at least initially, is about 80% (Frey et al 1976, Eckhauser et al 1984, Morrow et al 1984, Gall et al 1989). With resection, the fact that the diseased tissue is removed means that it does not matter whether the pain is due to distension of an obstructed duct or to some other cause such as perineural inflammation and fibrosis. In terms of pain relief, the results of distal pancreatec-

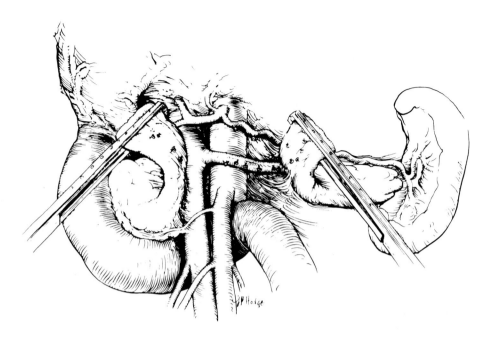

Fig. 29.2 Division of the pancreas in front of the superior mesenteric vein and portal vein results in removal of approximately 50% of the pancreas when distal pancreatectomy is performed. (Reproduced with permission from Frey C F Pancreaticoduodenectomy. In: Malt R A (ed) Surgical techniques illustrated, 2nd ed. Little, Brown, p. 95.)

tomy were comparable to those of pancreaticojejunostomy; opinions varied as to whether pancreaticoduodenectomy gave results which were better than (Traverso et al 1979, Taylor et al 1981, Gall et al 1989) or equivalent to those of 80–90% distal pancreatectomy (Frey et al 1976, Eckhauser et al 1984, Morrow et al 1984, Keith et al 1989).

As will be discussed later, distal pancreatectomy fell into disfavour in the 1980s, not because of failure to relieve pain but because of the high immediate incidence of endocrine and exocrine insufficiency, particularly after 80–95% pancreatectomy, and the development of alternative operations which dealt with disease in the pancreatic head (Warren et al 1984, Frey & Smith 1987, Beger & Büchler, 1990).

Operative mortality

When comparing the mortality and morbidity of the various operations performed for chronic pancreatitis, it is often difficult to disentangle the effects of the operation itself from those of continued alcohol and tobacco abuse and from the natural progression of the underlying disease process (Marks et al 1980, Sarles et al 1982, Frey et al 1989). As shown in Table 29.1, the various procedures (distal pancreatectomy, pancreaticoduodenectomy, pancreaticojejunostomy and total pancreatectomy) do have differing intrinsic risks. Although several recent reports suggest that the operative mortality of pancreaticoduodenectomy may now be as low as 1.3% (Koehler et al 1987, Mannell et al 1988, Gall et al 1989, Howard & Zhang 1990), no less than 172 of the 234 patients concerned were treated in the same centre (Gall et al 1989) which in an earlier report already had an operative mortality of only 1% (Gall et al 1982). While the low operative mortality rates reported from such specialized centres are impressive, it is doubtful whether they can be achieved by the wider surgical community unless the pancreatic operative experience is concentrated in the hands of one or two surgeons in each hospital. Pancreatic surgery is not for the occasional operator.

Diabetes and steatorrhoea

In most series, diabetes mellitus is already present in some 10–30% of patients who come to operation with chronic pancreatitis. As might be expected, patients subjected to 80–95% pancreatectomy have a higher immediate incidence of postoperative diabetes (72%) than those undergoing less-than-80% pancreatectomy (32%), and as many as one-half to two-thirds of these patients will require insulin (Frey et al 1976, see Table 29.2). Insulin-dependent diabetes mellitus can pose major

Table 29.1 Operative mortality rates in procedures for chronic pancreatitis in series published between 1972 and 1988. References listed in full in Frey et al (1989)

Procedure	Number of patients	Number of deaths	% Operative mortality
Pancreaticojejunostomy	1194	41	3.4
Distal pancreatectomy	1625	66	4.1
Pancreaticoduodenectomy	1108	66	5.9
Total pancreatectomy	324	31	9.6

Table 29.2   Effects of operations for chronic pancreatitis on exocrine and endocrine function in representative series. Figures in parentheses refer to patients requiring insulin to control diabetes mellitus

Procedure	n	% Incidence of clinical steatorrhoea			% Incidence of clinical diabetes mellitus		
		Preoperative	Postoperative		Preoperative	Postoperative	
			'Early'	'Late'		'Early'	'Late'
< 80% distal pancreatectomy							
Frey et al (1976)	53	4		19	17 (4)		32 (19)
80–95% distal pancreatectomy							
Frey et al (1976)	77	9		38	28 (19)		72 (58)
Eckhauser et al (1984)	87				28 (12)		? (62)
Pancreaticoduodenectomy							
Frey et al (1976)	19	5		55	15 (11)		26 (11)
Rossi et al (1987)	73	26	57	75	25 (15)	45 (38)	69 (66)
Gall et al (1989)*	289			94	46 (14)	64 (34)	66 (40)
Pancreaticojejunostomy							
Prinz & Greenlee (1981)	87	17		33	34 (10)		52 (28)
Beger procedure							
Beger & Büchler (1990)	114			33	41 (20)	39 (21)	52 (27)

* Pancreaticoduodenectomy in this series was accompanied by injection of Ethibloc into the pancreatic duct system to ablate exocrine function

problems following operation, and severe hypoglycaemic episodes with diabetic coma and brain damage are reported in 2–4% of all patients after distal pancreatectomy. The risk of such potentially lethal complications is highest in alcoholics who indulge in binge drinking and mismanage their diet or insulin needs. In the Michigan experience, pancreaticoduodenectomy was associated with insulin-dependent diabetes in 26% of cases (Frey et al 1976), a figure which is actually lower than that recorded in some series following longitudinal pancreaticojejunostomy using the Partington-Rochelle modification of the original Puestow procedure (Prinz & Greenlee 1981).

Steatorrhoea is usually apparent when more than 20% of ingested fat is lost in the stool. Following 80–95% distal pancreatectomy, measured loss averages 25–30% and twice as many patients have steatorrhoea as after less than 80% pancreatectomy. Representative figures for the incidence of steatorrhoea after pancreaticoduodenectomy and pancreaticojejunostomy are 55% and 33% respectively (Table 29.2).

It is generally accepted that all resections for chronic pancreatitis are followed by progressive deterioration in exocrine and endocrine function with time. This is not surprising in that such deterioration also occurs in patients with chronic pancreatitis not subjected to surgery. Of 145 patients followed for a median of 5.7 years by Ammann et al (1984), 74% eventually had evidence of diabetes while 93% developed exocrine insufficiency. Alcohol is generally regarded as an important determinant of the rate of functional deterioration, and those who abstain have a slower decline, regardless of whether they have had a resection (Gullo et al 1988).

Most patients subjected to pancreaticoduodenectomy also show progressive loss of endocrine and exocrine function. Interestingly, surgeons who have used Ethibloc injection to destroy exocrine function after pancreatico-

duodenectomy have claimed that endocrine function does not deteriorate significantly after the immediate postoperative period. However, in the 289 patients undergoing this type of surgery in two major series (Gall et al 1989, Gebhardt 1990), the incidence of clinical diabetes rose from an immediate postoperative level of 37–53% at 36 months. While it is true that the number of patients with normal carbohydrate metabolism only decreased from 35 to 34% in the 36-month follow-up period, the severity of endocrine dysfunction in those with disordered metabolism increased appreciably. It is pertinent to ask whether injection of Ethibloc into the pancreatic remnant after pancreaticoduodenectomy might not result in a higher immediate incidence of diabetes than resection followed by end-to-side drainage of the remnant into the jejunum.

While it is generally acknowledged that exocrine and endocrine function also deteriorates after pancreaticojejunostomy (Sato et al 1981, Bradley 1987), there is some evidence that effective drainage may slow the rate of deterioration. Presumably, ductal hypertension, in addition to causing pain (Okazaki et al 1988), may injure the acinar cells, perhaps irreversibly, depending on the duration of the obstruction and the degree of elevation of pressure. In a series of 87 patients followed by Prinz & Greenlee (1990) for an average of 7.9 years after longitudinal pancreaticojejunostomy, the incidence of diabetes rose from 39% to 52%, an incidence lower than that which might have been expected from Ammann's experience with patients who never came to operation (Ammann et al 1984). In patients treated by longitudinal pancreaticojejunostomy prior to the development of severe morphological or functional changes, there appears to be a slowing of functional deterioration, whether or not the patient abstains from alcohol (Nealon et al 1988). Corroboration of these findings is needed in view of the relatively short follow-up period (14 months).

Late mortality

A major reason for the decline in the use of distal pancreatectomy during the 1980s has been the effect of loss of exocrine and endocrine function on quality of life and life expectancy. The number of late deaths which can be attributed to functional impairment after pancreatic surgery is difficult to define and depends in large part on the 'brittleness' of the diabetes, the competence of the patient to look after himself (a factor markedly influenced by whether the patient continues to drink) and the rate of progression of the disease that remains. As indicated above, some operations, as well as removing pancreatic mass, may hasten exocrine and endocrine deterioration (e.g. Ethibloc injection) while others may ameliorate the natural progression of the disease (e.g. longitudinal pancreaticojejunostomy). Perhaps surprisingly, some reports show that distal pancreatectomy is associated with a lower late mortality rate than other forms of resection or pancreaticojejunostomy. However, variability of follow-up probably invalidates these apparent differences and Frey et al (1989) could find no significant differences between the various operations on review of the literature (Table 29.3).

In the experience of Eckhauser et al (1984) only half of the patients who had undergone near-total distal pancreatectomy were alive 10 years later. The causes of death were almost equally distributed between those related to complications of pancreatic insufficency or continued dependence on alcohol and narcotics, and those unrelated to such factors. Nearly two-thirds of the patients who died from causes unrelated to alcohol or diabetes had non-alcoholic chronic pancreatitis. In contrast, 53% of those dying from causes related to alcohol or diabetes had alcohol-related disease. Frey et al (1976) have also emphasized the importance of alcohol as a determinant of long-term suvival; in their series less than 60% of alcoholics undergoing 80–95% distal pancreatectomy were alive at 10 years. Diabetes mellitus and malnutrition probably account for about 30% of all late deaths after surgery for chronic pancreatitis, and distal pancreatectomy appears to fare no worse than other operations in this regard (Frey et al 1976, Rossi et al 1987, Gall et al 1989, Prinz & Greenlee 1990). The remaining 70% of late deaths are largely attributable to the effects of alcoholism and its almost invariable accompaniment, smoking. Important individual causes of death include cirrhosis, diabetic complications, sepsis, pulmonary disease, cardiovascular disease, carcinoma, cachexia, suicide and trauma.

PRESENT STATUS OF DISTAL PANCREATECTOMY

General considerations

Before embarking on any operation for chronic pancreatitis, full preoperative assessment must be undertaken;

1. The diagnosis of chronic pancreatitis is confirmed, and it is established with as much certainty as possible that this is indeed the cause of the patient's pain.

2. The suitability of the patient for operation is evaluated, including assessment of addiction to drugs and alcohol, and presence of other major disease processes.

3. Pancreatic exocrine and endocrine function are measured.

4. The structural pathology of the pancreas is defined, including: duct size; location of strictures; number and location of pseudocysts; degree of obstruction of the common bile duct and duodenum; presence of pseudoaneurysms in the pancreatic and peripancreatic vasculature; presence of splenic and portal vein thrombosis, and the presence and location of pancreatic fistulas with associated ascites and pleural effusions.

5. Extrapancreatic causes of pancreatitis are excluded. (Operations on the pancreas should be avoided if possible until underlying biliary tract disease and peptic ulceration have been dealt with.)

6. Nutritional status is assessed, as many patients are malnourished and will benefit from parenteral or enteral nutrition prior to operation.

Assessment of structural changes

CT scanning, ERCP and angiography are key investigations to detect the structural changes outlined and so determine whether distal pancreatectomy will provide an appropriate solution for the patient's disease. Angiography can have a particularly important influence on the choice of operation. It may demonstrate tumour vessels or collateral venous flow in patients with neoplasms masquerading as pancreatitis. It may also reveal pseudoaneurysms of the splenic or gastroduodenal artery, usually in association with pseudocyst. Such pseudoaneurysms may rupture into the pseudocyst and present with ductal bleeding (Stanley et al 1976, Frey et al 1982). Angiographic embolization should be employed if the patient presents with active bleeding; if this is not feasible then proximal control of the splenic artery and distal pancreatectomy may be needed. If this cannot be

Table 29.3 Late mortality rates following surgery for chronic pancreatitis in series published between 1972 and 1988. References listed in full in Frey et al (1989)

Procedure	Number of patients	Number of deaths	% Late mortality
Pancreaticojejunostomy	639	185	28.9
Distal pancreatectomy	934	170	18.2
Pancreaticoduodenectomy	805	171	21.2
Total pancreatectomy	250	62	24.8

accomplished, then the pseudocyst should be opened and an attempt made to oversew the bleeding vessel. Angiography may also reveal splenic vein thrombosis with left-sided portal hypertension and gastric varices, in which case splenectomy should be included in any operation planned for the pancreas.

Choice of operation

Ideally, the operation should:
1. correct or deal with all structural abnormalities
2. provide long-term pain relief
3. have a low mortality and morbidity
4. not depend on ability to abstain from alcohol
5. minimize subsequent long-term exocrine and endocrine insufficiency

The operations available can be divided into those whose only purpose is to relieve pain and those designed to deal with the complications of chronic pancreatitis (e.g. pseudocysts, ascites, pleural effusions, pericardial tamponade, duodenal or common bile duct obstruction, bleeding from pseudoaneurysms, splenic vein thrombosis and left-sided portal hypertension), which may or may not be associated with pain. No one operation can provide an optimal solution to the operative management of pain or these diverse complications. At present, distal pancreatectomy still has an important, although diminished role in management.

The expectations of patient and surgeon regarding the risks and benefits of operation must be the same. The patient must be fully aware of the effects of distal pancreatectomy on exocrine and endocrine function, and of the consequences of splenectomy with regard to reduced immune competence and risk of infection. Reluctance to proceed on the part of the patient after being fully informed is an absolute indication to desist; many patients who initially refuse surgery reconsider it if their pain worsens.

Choice of surgeon

The surgeon should have a clear understanding of the natural history of chronic pancreatitis and its complications, and be fully conversant with the operative solutions available. The surgeon is in the best position to monitor the patient's endocrine and exocrine function and nutritional status, and to provide the emotional support which may be needed over many years. Those lacking experience of, and commitment to, pancreatic surgery, would be well advised to refer the patient to a qualified colleague. Operations for chronic pancreatitis are not for surgeons who seldom operate on the pancreas.

Contraindications to distal pancreatectomy

Patients with terminal disease or addiction to narcotics are not suitable for distal pancreatectomy. Addicted patients must go through a drug withdrawal programme before being considered for surgery. Pain is a subjective symptom and may be exaggerated by patients who present with manipulative behaviour, and it may be difficult to avoid making some mistakes in management. The illiterate, mentally subnormal and binge drinkers are not suitable candidates for distal pancreatectomy as they are often unable to regulate their insulin requirements and diet reliably.

Disease in the head and uncinate process is a contra-indication to distal pancreatectomy. With less-than-60% pancreatectomy, the resection fails to remove the diseased part, leaving behind problems such as a bulky inflamed and thickened head of pancreas, intrapancreatic stricture of the common bile duct, pancreas divisum, retention cysts and pseudocysts. Near-total (80–95%) distal pancreatectomy does remove parts of the head and uncinate process, but is now rarely indicated in view of the high risk of precipitating functional insufficiency and its undesirable effect on the quality of life, if not its duration. The recent development of alternatives to pancreatico-duodenectomy, such as the Beger procedure (Beger et al 1990) and the Frey procedure (Frey & Smith 1987) which deal with a diseased head of pancreas, means that 80–95% distal pancreatectomy is now virtually obsolete.

Indications for less-than-80% distal pancreatectomy

Some surgeons feel that there is still a role for distal resection of less than 80% of the pancreas. One recent study (Keith et al 1989) found that after an average of 4 years 16 of 31 patients (52%) were pain-free and nine (29%) were appreciably improved, while three had undergone subsequent total pancreatectomy because of recurrent pain. The incidence of diabetes had increased from 9–45% following operation, and more rapid progression of diabetes was noted in those continuing to drink. These results with regard to pain relief are comparable to the 80% incidence of pain relief after an average of 7.8 years in patients undergoing 80–95% distal pancreatectomy in the University of Michigan experience (Frey et al 1976). In both series, patients with both large and small pancreatic ducts underwent resection, and it is noteworthy that Keith and his associates perform pancreaticojejunostomy only when the pancreatic duct diameter exceeds 1 cm.

At present our group perform distal pancreatectomy only:

1. When the patient has pain but the pancreatic duct is too small for pancreaticojejunostomy (i.e. 4 mm in

diameter or less) and disease is located predominantly in the distal pancreas on CT scanning and ERCP;

2. In the presence of a pseudocyst(s) limited to the body and tail of the pancreas behind strictures in the main duct or tributary ducts;

3. When disease is limited to the distal pancreas but decompression of a pseudocyst or pancreaticojejunostomy has failed to relieve pain;

4. When a pseudocyst of the body or tail of the pancreas is associated with a pseudoaeneurysm;

5. When 'small-duct-disease' is associated with pain and left-sided portal hypertension with gastric, colonic or oesophageal varices (in this case, distal pancreatectomy must be accompanied by splenectomy); or

6. When cancer of the body and tail of the gland cannot be ruled out.

The exclusion of cancer remains problematic because neither negative aspiration cytology nor intraoperative frozen section analysis is totally reliable. These techniques both have a 15% sampling error, and in the case of frozen section, there is an additional 15% interpretation error (Campanale et al 1985). The decision to resect often comes down to the surgeon's judgement based on the preoperative and operative findings. Errors can be made even by experienced surgeons. For example, Keith et al (1989) reported one death from undetected pancreatic cancer occurring 6 months after distal pancreatectomy, while White & Slavotinek (1979) reported that nine of their 55 patients subjected to longitudinal pancreaticojejunostomy were later found to have cancer of the pancreas.

Technical considerations

While preservation of spleen during distal pancreatectomy is desirable, this is often not technically feasible because inflammation and fibrosis of the splenic artery and vein may make dissection of the tail of pancreas from the splenic hilum virtually impossible (Fig. 29.3). Warshaw (1988) has described a technique in which the splenic artery and vein are divided distal to the tip of the pancreas, so that splenic viability is preserved through the short gastric vessels (Fig. 29.4). However, we have seen one patient who developed left-sided portal hypertension and massive gastric variceal bleeding after this approach and who required splenectomy for cure. Although this complication is reported infrequently, it does sound a note of caution about preserving the spleen at distal pancreatectomy.

While there can be arguments about the extent of distal resection of the pancreas in chronic pancreatitis, there are situations in which distal pancreatectomy is the only option available. We believe that distal resection should be limited to those portions of the body and tail which have been shown to be diseased by ERCP and CT scanning. Unfortunately, much of the discussion in the literature about the advantages and disadvantages of distal pancreatectomy is based on the results of operations which were performed before the widespread availability of CT and ERCP enabled the definition of structural abnormalities so that therapy could be tailored to the needs of the individual (Morrow et al 1984, Morel & Rohner 1987, Williamson & Cooper 1987, Moossa 1987, Rossi et al 1987, Cuillert & Guillemin 1990; Ihse

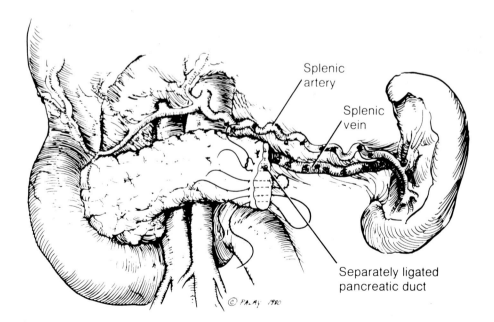

Fig. 29.3 It may be possible to preserve the spleen during distal pancreatectomy as long as the splenic artery and vein are not involved in dense inflammation and fibrosis. (Reproduced with permission from Frey C F. Partial and subtotal pancreatectomy for chronic pancreatitis. In: Nyhus, Baker (eds) Mastery of surgery, update, vol. c2. Little, Brown, p. 1038.)

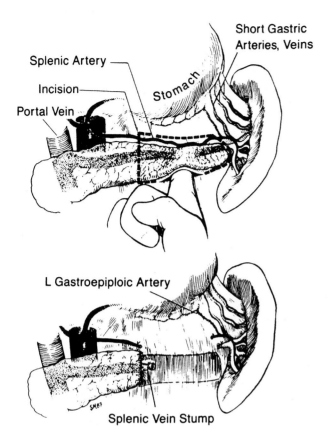

Fig. 29.4 Warshaw's technique conserves the spleen during distal pancreatectomy by preserving its blood supply through the short gastric vessels. (With permission, from Warshaw 1988, Surgery 123: 550–553)

as 5 mm. Eggink et al (1983) undertook distal pancreatic resections despite ERCP evidence of main duct 'dilatation' in 16 of their 29 patients. Pain relief was judged to be good in three-quarters of their patients undergoing 95% pancreatectomy, although exocrine and endocrine insufficiency was more difficult to manage than in patients undergoing more limited resection.

One final technical point should be mentioned. After distal resection, the cut end of the pancreas is usually oversewn with mattress sutures or stapled. If the pancreatic duct is identified it should be oversewn separately. There is no useful purpose in bringing up a Roux-en-Y limb of jejunum to drain the cut end of the pancreas provided drainage via the papilla is known to be adequate (Shankar et al 1990).

CONCLUSIONS

There is no single ideal operation for chronic pancreatitis. The surgeon, with his knowledge of the patient, understanding of the natural history of chronic pancreatitis and its complications, and awareness of the operative solutions available, must make a judgement as to the operation most appropriate to the patient's needs. We believe that there is still a place for limited distal resection in chronic pancreatitis. This belief is based on the fact that there are few other options in patients with disease limited to the body and tail of the gland (as assessed by ERCP and CT scan) and a main pancreatic duct which is 4 mm or less in diameter, and it has been supported by our more recent experience in 15 patients treated by distal resection. Eight of these patients underwent 60% distal pancreatectomy on the basis of ERCP and CT demonstration of disease confined to the body and tail; seven of the eight did well, as far as pain relief and maintenance of pancreatic function were concerned, after follow-up averaging 3.5 years. Another seven patients (four of whom were operated on elsewhere) underwent 60% distal pancreatectomy when disease was either predominant in the head of the gland or spread diffusely throughout the pancreas. All but two of these seven patients had recurrence of pain which required reoperation within a year.

et al 1990, Ihse & Gasslander, 1990). In the University of Michigan, operations for chronic pancreatitis in the 1960s and 1970s were limited to proximal and distal pancreatic resection. With present day indications, many of the 80–95% resections performed in patients with ducts more than 5 mm in diameter could be regarded as unnecessary. However, not all surgeons share this view. As indicated earlier, Keith et al (1989) do not perform pancreaticojejunostomy unless the diameter of the pancreatic duct exceeds 1 cm and so undoubtedly perform more distal resections than surgeons who would drain ducts as small

REFERENCES

Ammann R W, Akovbiantz A, Largiader F, Schueler G 1984 Course and outcome of chronic pancreatitis: Longitudinal study of a mixed medical-surgical series of 245 patients. Gastroenterology 86: 820–828

Barrett O Jr, Bowers W F 1957 Total pancreatectomy for chronic relapsing pancreatitis and calcinosis of the pancreas. USAF Medical Journal 8: 1037–1045

Beger HG, Büchler M 1990 Duodenum-preserving resection of the head of the pancreas in chronic pancreatitis with inflammatory mass in the head. World Journal of Surgery 14: 83–87

Beger H G, Büchler M, Bittner R, Uhl W 1990 Duodenum-preserving resection of the head of the pancreas: an alternative to Whipple's

procedure in chronic pancreatitis. Hepatogastroenterology 37: 283–289

Bradley E L III 1987 Long-term results of pancreatojejunostomy in patients with chronic pancreatitis. American Journal of Surgery 153: 207–213

Campanale R P II, Frey C F, Farias L R, Twomey P L, Guernsey J M, Keehn R, Higgins G 1985 Reliability and sensitivity of frozen section pancreatic biopsy. Archives of Surgery 120: 283–288

Cuilleret J, Guillemin G 1990 Surgical management of chronic pancreatitis on the continent of Europe. World Journal of Surgery 14: 11–18

Drake D H, Fry W J 1989 Ductal drainage for chronic pancreatitis. Surgery 105: 131–140

Du Val M K Jr, Enquist I F 1961 The surgical treatment of chronic pancreatitis by pancreaticojejunostomy: an 8 year old reappraisal. Surgery 50: 965–969

Eckhauser F E, Strodel W E, Knol J A, Harpier M, Turcotte J G 1984 Near-total pancreatectomy for chronic pancreatitis. Surgery 96: 599–607

Eggink W F, Bauer F L, Schattenkerk M, Obertop H, Bruining H A, Jeekel J, van Houten H 1983 Surgical treatment of chronic pancreatitis by distal pancreatectomy. Netherlands Journal of Surgery 35: 184–187

Eliason E L, Welty R F 1958 Pancreatic calculi. Annals of Surgery 127: 150–157

Frey C F 1981 Role of subtotal pancreatectomy and pancreaticojejunostomy in chronic pancreatitis. Journal of Surgical Research 31: 361–370

Frey C F, Smith G T 1987 Description and rationale of a new operation for chronic pancreatitis. Pancreas 2: 701–707

Frey C F, Child C G, Fry W 1976 Pancreatectomy for chronic pancreatitis. Annals of Surgery 184: 403–413

Frey C F, Eckhauser F, Stanley J 1982 Hemorrhage. In: Bradley E F (ed) Complications of pancreatitis. W B Saunders, Philadelphia, p 96–123

Frey C F, Suzuki M, Isaji S, Zhu Y 1989 Pancreatic resection for chronic pancreatitis. Surgical Clinics of North American 69: 499–528

Frey C F, Suzuki M, Isaji S, 1990 Treatment of chronic pancreatitis complicated by obstruction of the common bile duct or duodenum. World Journal of Surgery 14: 59–69

Fry W J, Child C G III 1965 Ninety-five percent distal pancreatectomy for chronic pancreatitis. Annals of Surgery 162: 543–549

Gall F P, Gebhardt C, Zirngibl H 1982 Chronic pancreatitis: results of 116 consecutive, partial duodenopancreatectomies combined with pancreatic duct occlusion. Hepatogastroenterology 29: 115–119

Gall F P, Gebhardt C, Meister R, Zirngibl H, Schneider M U 1989 Severe chronic cephalic pancreatitis: use of partial duodenopancreatectomy with occlusion of the pancreatic duct in 289 patients. World Journal of Surgery 13:809–816, discussion 816–817

Gebhardt C 1990 Surgical treatment of pain in chronic pancreatitis: Role of the Whipple procedure. Acta Chirurgica Scandinavica 156: 303–306, discussion 307

Gullo L, Barbara L, Labo G 1988 Effect of cessation of alcohol use on the course of pancreatic dysfunction in alcoholic pancreatitis. Gastroenterology 95: 1063–1068

Howard J M, Zhang Z 1990 Pancreaticoduodenectomy (Whipple resection) in the treatment of chronic pancreatitis. World Journal of Surgery 14: 77–82

Ihse I, Borch K, Larsson J 1990 Chronic pancreatitis: results of operation for relief of pain. World Journal of Surgery 14: 53–58

Ihse I, Gasslander T 1990 Surgical treatment of pain in chronic pancreatitis: the role of pancreaticojejunostomy. Acta Chirurgica Scandinavica 156: 299–301

Keith R G, Saibil F G, Sheppard R H 1989 Treatment of chronic alcoholic pancreatitis by pancreatic resection. American Journal of Surgery 157: 156–162

Koehler H, Schafmayer A, Peiper H J 1987 Follow-up results of surgical treatment in chronic pancreatitis. Digestive Surgery 4: 67–75

Mannell A, Adson M A, McIlrath D C, IIstrup D M 1988 Surgical management of chronic pancreatitis: long term results in 141 patients. British Journal of Surgery 75: 467–472

Marks I N, Girdwood A H, Bank S, Louw J H 1980 The prognosis of alcohol-induced calcific pancreatitis. South African Medical Journal 57: 640–643

Mayo W J 1913 The surgery of the pancreas. Annals of Surgery 58: 145–150

Moossa A R 1987 Surgical treatment of chronic pancreatitis: an overview. British Journal of Surgery 74: 661–667

Morel P, Rohner A 1987 Surgery for chronic pancreatitis. Surgery 101: 130–135

Morrow C E, Cohen J I, Sutherland D E, Najarian J S 1984 Chronic pancreatitis: long-term surgical results of pancreatic duct drainage, pancreatic resection and near-total pancreatectomy and islet autotransplantation. Surgery 96: 608–616

Nealon W H, Townsend C M Jr, Thompson J C 1988 Operative drainage of the pancreatic duct delays functional impairment in patients with chronic pancreatitis. Annals of Surgery 208: 321–329

Okazaki K, Yamamoto Y, Kagiyama S, Tamura S, Sakamoto Y, Nakazawa Y, Morita M, Yamamoto Y 1988 Pressure of papillary sphincter zone and pancreatic main duct in patients with chronic pancreatitis in the early stage. Scandinavian Journal of Gastroenterology 23: 501–507

Partington P F, Rochelle R E 1960 Modified Puestow procedure for retrograde drainage of the pancreatic duct. Annals of Surgery 152: 1037–1043

Prinz R A, Greenlee H B 1981 Pancreatic duct drainage in 100 patients with chronic pancreatitis. Annals of surgery 194: 313–320

Prinz R A, Greenlee H B 1990 Pancreatic duct drainage in chronic pancreatitis. Hepatogastroenterology 37: 295–300

Puestow C B, Gillesby W J 1958 Retrograde surgical drainage of pancreas for chronic relapsing pancreatitis. Archives of Surgery 76: 898–907

Rossi R L, Rothschild J, Braasch J W, Munson J L, ReMine S G 1987 Pancreatoduodenectomy in the management of chronic pancreatitis. Archives of Surgery 122: 416–420

Rossi R L, Soeldner J S, Braasch J W, Heiss J W, Shea J A, Watkins E Jr, Silverman M L 1990 Long-term results of pancreatic resection and segmental pancreatic autotransplantation for chronic pancreatitis. American Journal of Surgery 159: 51–57, discussion 57–58

Sarles J C, Nacchiero M, Garani F, Salasc B 1982 Surgical treatment of chronic pancreatitis: Report of 134 cases treated by resection or drainage. American Journal of Surgery 144: 317–321

Sato T, Noto N, Matsuno S, Miyakawa K 1981 Follow-up results of surgical treatment for chronic pancreatitis: Present status in Japan. American Journal of Surgery 142: 317–323

Shankar S, Theis B, Russell R C G 1990 Management of the stump of the pancreas after distal pancreatic resection. British Journal of Surgery 77: 541–544

Stanley J C, Frey C F, Miller T A, Lindenauer S M, Child C G III 1976 Major arterial hemorrhage; a complication of pancreatic pseudocysts and chronic pancreatitis. Archives of Surgery 111: 435–440

Taylor R H, Bagley F H, Braasch J W, Warren K W 1981 Ductal drainage or resection for chronic pancreatitis. American Journal of Surgery 141: 28–33

Traverso L W, Tompkins R K, Urrea P T, Longmire W P Jr 1979 Surgical treatment of chronic pancreatitis. Annals of Surgery 190: 312–319

Warren W D, Millikan W J Jr, Henderson J M, Hersh T 1984 A denervated pancreatic flap for control of chronic pain in pancreatitis. Surgery, Gynecology and Obstetrics 159: 581–583

Warshaw A L 1988 Conservation of the spleen with distal pancreatectomy. Archives of Surgery 123: 550–553

White T T, Slavotinek A H 1979 Results of surgical treatment of chronic pancreatitis: Report of 142 cases. Annals of Surgery 189: 217–224

Williamson R C N, Cooper M J 1987 Resection in chronic pancreatitis. British Journal of Surgery 74: 807–812

Zollinger R M, Keith L M Jr, Ellison E H 1954 Pancreatitis. New England Journal of Medicine 251: 497–502

30. Partial pancreatoduodenectomy for chronic pancreatitis

J. W. Braasch   R. L. Rossi

Chronic pancreatitis is a descriptive term denoting changes in the pancreas produced by a diverse group of causes that have a variety of mechanisms of action. Other than the prevention or treatment of contributing factors, such as alcoholism, biliary calculous disease, hyperlipidaemia, hyperparathyroidism, or operative or external trauma to the ampulla of Vater or the pancreas, no rational treatment is available for patients with this condition other than drainage of obstructed pancreatic ducts or partial or total resection.

A substantial number of patients with chronic pancreatitis would benefit from resection of the head and uncinate process of the pancreas. The amount of pancreas to be removed has been determined in the past by trial and error. Preservation of the duodenum and the distal bile duct requires preservation of a portion of the uncinate process because the posterior pancreatico-duodenal arcade is the principal blood supply to these organs (Michels 1951, Thomas 1990), and these vessels are associated with the uncinate process. A varied amount of the neck and body of the pancreas can be removed in addition to removing the head of the gland. Whether a more conservative or more radical resection is beneficial will have to be settled by the test of time and experience.

Patients with chronic pancreatitis present several problems when being evaluated for any surgical procedure. Depending on the patient population served by the institution, an appreciable number of patients with chronic pancreatitis are addicted to alcohol, and some are addicted to narcotics. In some patients, cessation of the use of alcohol is more important for the result than the treatment used (Bagley et al 1981). The accuracy of the assessment of the result by the patient can be influenced by the patient's continuing use of alcohol or addiction to narcotics.

The natural history of chronic pancreatitis is also of great importance in evaluating the indications for and the results of treatment. Ammann et al (1984) reported their experience with long-term follow-up of a group of patients with chronic pancreatitis caused by alcoholism. Their study indicated that a number of patients eventually have 'burn out' of their disease and some relief of pain after 5 years and that, especially in alcoholics, the incidence of diabetes resulting from the disease rises to about 45% at this time. These points should be recognized when decisions are made relative to the type of operation used in treatment and indeed, whether any surgical treatment should be performed.

INDICATIONS

Of the various indications for operative treatment, pain is the most prominent. It should be present at a level of intensity that causes serious disruption to the patient's lifestyle as evidenced by loss of considerable time from work, extensive hospitalizations, and the requirement of major amounts of narcotics for relief. Correctable causes of pancreatitis, such as alcoholism, biliary tract calculous disease, and hyperparathyroidism, should have been sought and eliminated.

Complying with these guidelines can be difficult, especially with regard to alcoholism and the patient's compliance with advice to abstain. Likewise, predicting the length of time until 'burn out' of pancreatitis and subsequent relief of pain is also a problem. Destruction of the pancreas with calcification and fibrosis is more likely in patients with alcohol-related disease than with other causes. However, the exact time needed to complete these changes cannot be predicted. It is unusual for secondary problems such as biliary obstruction or obstruction of the duodenum, to require surgical treatment.

The major indications for partial pancreatoduodenectomy are disease that is appreciably more advanced in the head of the gland than in the body and tail (Fig. 30.1) and absence of dilatation of the pancreatic duct that would be suitable for pancreaticojejunostomy. Endoscopic retrograde cholangiopancreatography and computed tomography of the pancreas are invaluable in making this assessment.

Secondary indications for resection of the right half of

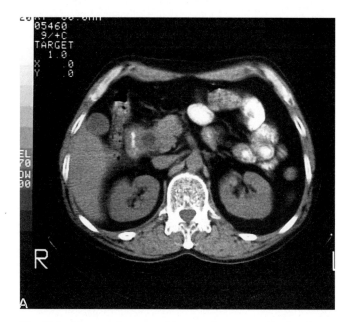
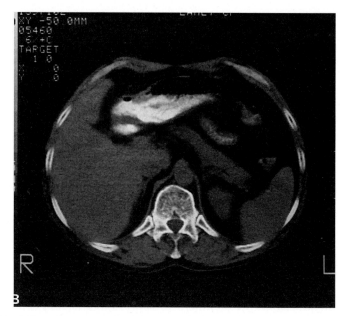

Fig. 30.1   Computed tomographic scan of pancreas with chronic pancreatitis. **A** Scan shows cyst and calcifications in the pancreatic head. **B** Scan shows normal pancreatic body and tail.

the pancreas, duodenum, and distal bile duct include obstruction of the bile duct and/or duodenum. The presence of diabetes mellitus, with or without exocrine pancreatic insufficiency and steatorrhoea means that it is less important to avoid resection in favour of islet-sparing operations. An important issue is the personality and stability of the patient as the probability of the development of diabetes is high after resection of half of the pancreas. In our experience (Rossi et al 1987), partial pancreatoduodenectomy has been followed by an increase in the incidence of diabetes from about 20% preoperatively to about 60% in the years that follow. The natural history of alcoholic pancreatitis suggests that with time, the incidence of diabetes is around 40% (Ammann et al 1984). Thus, a 20–25% increase in the incidence of diabetes may be attributed to removal of half of the islet cell population. The decision-making process involved in choosing the appropriate operation for patients with chronic pancreatitis is depicted in Figure 30.2.

The pylorus- and gastric-preserving variant of the Whipple operation was first performed in 1944 by Watson and reported subsequently by Traverso and Longmire in 1978. A similar procedure was used early in this century in the initial attempts at resection of the head of the pancreas, but was always embellished by oversewing the proximal duodenum and construction of a gastro-jejunostomy (Whipple et al 1935). The advantage of preserving the stomach and pylorus was thought to be preservation of the normal gastric functions of storage, mixing, and digestion of fats and proteins. It was hoped

that better nutrition would follow and that the incidence of dumping, small stomach syndrome, and afferent loop syndrome would be decreased. Furthermore, it was hoped that the pylorus would continue to function and prevent bile reflux gastritis, and that the incidence of jejunal ulceration or jejunitis would be minimal. It was obvious immediately that the operation of pancreato-duodenectomy would be simplified by the omission of partial gastrectomy and, possibly, truncal vagotomy.

TECHNICAL CONSIDERATIONS

Partial pancreatoduodenectomy can be a relatively easy procedure because the residual pancreas is usually suitable for anastomosis. On the other hand, it also can be extraordinarily difficult, either because of splenic vein obstruction and the presence of high-pressure venous collaterals or because of a fibrosing inflammatory change that destroys the natural planes of dissection and makes it difficult to dissect the head and neck of the pancreas from the superior mesenteric and portal veins.

Our preference is for the pylorus-preserving type of pancreatoduodenectomy which permits a technically easier procedure by avoiding partial gastrectomy (and truncal vagotomy) (Fig. 30.3). The techniques of standard and pylorus-preserving pancreatoduodenectomy are basically the same, except for the treatment of the antrum, pylorus, and duodenum. In each procedure, four planes must be established before the head of the pancreas can be resected.

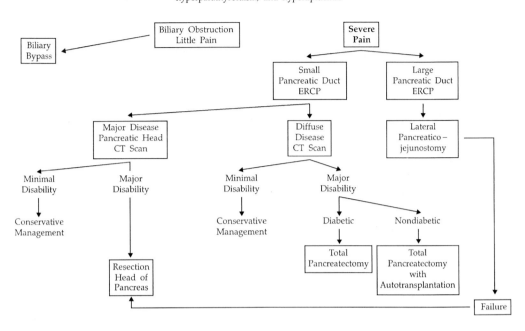

CHRONIC PANCREATITIS
Stop alcohol, treat biliary calculi,
hyperparathyroidism, and hyperlipidemia

Fig. 30.2   The decision-making process for partial pancreatoduodenectomy.

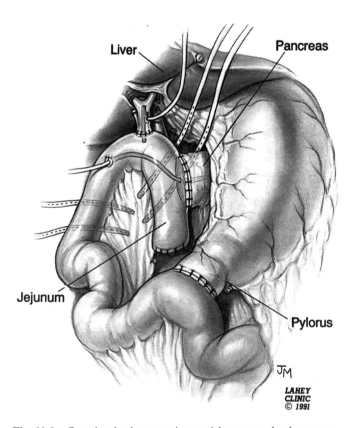

Fig. 30.3   Completed pylorus-sparing partial pancreatoduodenectomy with end-to-side pancreaticojejunostomy. (Reprinted by permission of Lahey Clinic.)

Plane I is opened by the extended Kocher manoeuvre (Fig. 30.4), which should mobilize the head of pancreas and duodenum as far as the left side of the aorta and the ligament of Treitz. Care must be exercised with the left renal vein, which can adhere to the underside of the pancreas and can be damaged. Control of haemorrhage from this vein can be exceedingly difficult.

Anomalous origin of the right hepatic artery, part of the right hepatic arterial blood supply, or even the entire hepatic arterial supply is possible. The anomalous hepatic artery (Fig. 30.5) usually originates from the superior mesenteric artery, ascends to the liver behind the head of the pancreas, portal vein, and distal common bile duct, and proceeds lateral to the bile duct to the liver. In establishing plane II (Fig. 30.6), which is lateral to the hepatic artery and anterior to the portal vein, great care must be taken to avoid damaging such anomalous arteries. Cholecystectomy is carried out routinely and before the common duct is severed usually distal to its cystic duct junction, careful palpation of the duodeno-hepatic ligament can reveal pulsation of an anomalous artery either behind or lateral to the common bile duct. If this anomalous artery is large, pulsation in the normal hepatic artery will be reduced. Plane II dissection proceeds down to the gastroduodenal artery. After ligation of this artery, dissection is carried down to the superior edge of the pancreas.

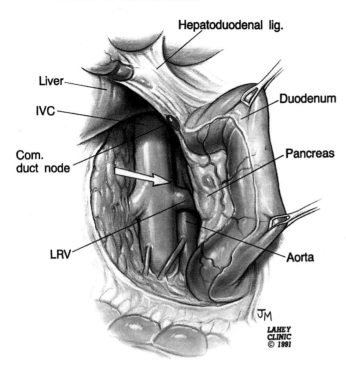

Fig. 30.4   Plane I is the Kocher manoeuvre. (Reprinted by permission of the Lahey Clinic.)

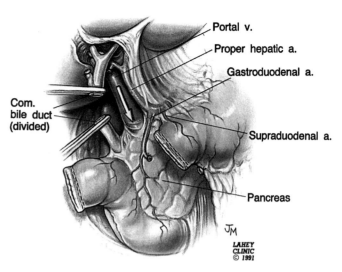

Fig. 30.6   Plane II is lateral to the hepatic artery and anterior to the portal vein. (Reprinted by permission of the Lahey Clinic.)

Plane III lies behind the neck of the pancreas, anterior to the portal and superior mesenteric veins (Fig. 30.7). This plane is usually easily dissected because no blood vessels traverse this space.

Plane IV lies lateral to the superior mesenteric vein between it and the head and uncinate process of the pancreas (Fig. 30.8). At this point in the operation, it is necessary to sever the jejunum distal to the ligament of Treitz or to sever the duodenum just proximal to the mesenteric vessels so as to dissect plane IV. If the latter point of division is chosen, it is not necessary to remove the retroperitoneal fourth portion of the duodenum and duodenojejunal junction. This short cut simplifies this portion of the operation.

When the pylorus-preserving procedure is chosen, the duodenum should be divided approximately 1–2 cm distal to the pylorus (Fig. 30.9). Great care must be taken with the vagal innervation of the pylorus and antrum in

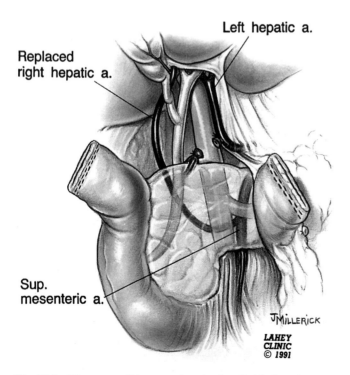

Fig. 30.5   The course of the anomalous (replaced) right hepatic artery. (Reprinted by permission of the Lahey Clinic.)

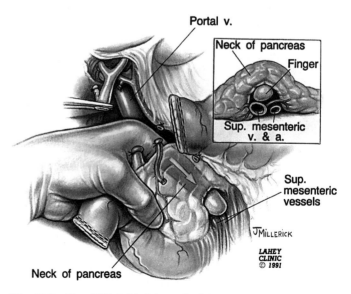

Fig. 30.7   Plane III is behind the neck of the pancreas. (Reprinted by permission of the Lahey Clinic.)

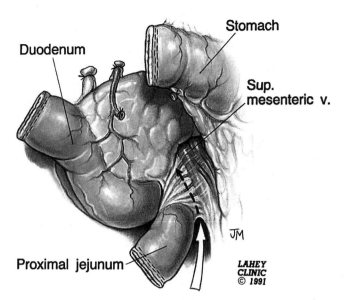

Fig. 30.8 Plane IV is to the right of the superior mesenteric vein. (Reprinted by permission of the Lahey Clinic.)

approaching the proximal duodenum. It is possible that gastric emptying will be impaired if vagotomy is performed.

The arterial supply to the first portion of duodenum comes from the supraduodenal artery, which arises from the hepatic artery. At times, it is possible to preserve this artery and its blood supply to the pylorus and duodenum; at other times it cannot be preserved because of angulation of the subsequent anastomosis of the duodenum to the jejunum. In these circumstances, as much as 1 cm of proximal duodenum cannot be preserved because of compromise of its arterial supply, and the subsequent anastomosis to the jejunum has to be made closer to the pylorus.

After the upper gastrointestinal tract has been disconnected and the four planes have been established, the neck of the pancreas can be divided, and the attachments of the head of the pancreas and the uncinate process to the pancreaticoduodenal arteries and the superior mesenteric and portal veins are dissected and divided.

Reconstruction of the gastrointestinal tract is begun with the pancreatico-jejunal anastomosis (Fig. 30.10). In patients with chronic pancreatitis, a two-layer anastomosis is used, the inner layer uniting the pancreatic duct with a stab wound in the first portion of the jejunum, end-to-side. The anastomosis is then reinforced with sutures that approximate the serosa-muscularis of the jejunum to the capsule of the pancreas. This anastomosis should be stented with a small tube that is brought out through the jejunum, through the abdominal wall, and placed on suction postoperatively.

Choledochojejunostomy is accomplished with a single layer of interrupted fine sutures and the anastomosis is stented with a T tube. The duodenojejunostomy is performed using two layers of sutures in the usual fashion.

Placement of a gastrostomy tube is optional. The operative area is drained by four subhepatic drains placed behind the biliary and pancreatic anastomoses. Figure 30.3 depicts the completed procedure.

In the standard Whipple procedure, partial gastrectomy with vagotomy is performed. A little less than a 50% gastric resection is performed in the usual fashion and

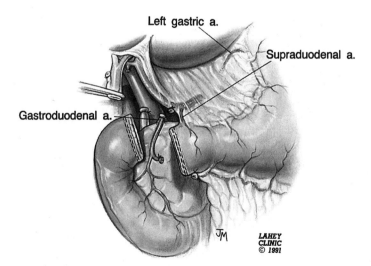

Fig. 30.9 The point of severance of the proximal duodenum for pylorus-preserving resection is shown. Note origin of the supraduodenal artery from the hepatic artery and lack of right gastric artery. (Reprinted by permission of the Lahey Clinic.)

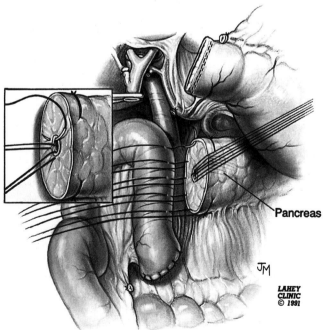

Fig. 30.10 Initial steps in reconstruction by end-to-side pancreaticojejunostomy. Sutures are placed in the posterior lip of the pancreatic duct before suturing the posterior pancreatic capsule to the serosa-muscularis of the jejunum. (Reprinted by permission of the Lahey Clinic.)

standard truncal vagotomy is performed before the resection or after, depending on individual preference. The vagotomy should include a search for branches of the vagus nerve other than the two main trunks. The reconstruction is achieved by gastrojejunostomy, again placed distal to the pancreatic and biliary anastomoses, and usually antecolic in position.

Three unusual situations can be encountered at times when performing partial pancreatoduodenectomy for chronic pancreatitis. The first arises when a Puestow pancreaticojejunostomy has been performed previously but has failed to relieve pain. The usual planes are established as described previously, and the head of the pancreas is resected just to the right of the end of the pancreaticojejunostomy anastomosis. In reconstruction, the jejunum used for the previous anastomosis can be continued around the divided neck of the pancreas, and the whole cut edge of the pancreas can be anastomosed in one layer to an incision in the jejunum. The pancreas in these instances is almost always firm, and a watertight anastomosis can be performed.

In the second situation, when no plane can be established behind the neck of the pancreas and anterior to the major veins, it is sometimes necessary to cut down through the neck of the pancreas from the anterior aspect without defining the anterior surface of the portal vein. Before this is accomplished, of course, the head of the pancreas and the portal vein must be elevated so that any untoward bleeding can be controlled by pressure between the fingers and the thumb. Sectioning of the pancreatic neck should proceed carefully under excellent vision with suction control of secretions and blood. In this manner, the neck of the gland can be divided, usually without undue haemorrhage.

In the third situation where obstruction of the splenic vein has occurred because of the pancreatitis or unsuspected carcinoma of the pancreas, dissection of the planes can be difficult and massive transfusion may be needed. Auxiliary techniques in this situation include use of hypotensive anesthaesia, use of a cell saver, and expeditious dissection because bleeding subsides after the planes have been established and the head of the pancreas is removed.

POSTOPERATIVE CARE

The three basic groups of complications after pancreatoduodenectomy are complications common to all major abdominal procedures (such as myocardial infarction, pneumonia, pulmonary embolism, wound infection, and wound dehiscence); complications related to leakage at the various anastomoses (which may lead to subhepatic and subphrenic infection, septicaemia, and erosive haemorrhage from arterial stumps and major retroperitoneal veins), and multiorgan failure involving the liver, lung, and kidneys. Most of the last two groups of problems stem from leakage at the pancreatico-jejunal anastomosis, which is the most difficult anastomosis and the one that permits pancreatic, biliary, and jejunal contents to bathe the retroperitoneum.

Every effort is directed at preventing retroperitoneal infection, sepsis, and organ failure by careful construction of the pancreatico-jejunal anastomosis. In the presence of chronic pancreatitis, leakproof anastomoses should be possible because the pancreas can be sutured readily. Suction is applied to all drains and to the pancreatic stent so as to remove pancreatic juice from the retroperitoneum should leakage occur. The drainage from the drains is monitored for major elevations in amylase. If such elevation occurs, the retroperitoneum can be bathed with Ringer's lactate solution by infusing 1 litre a day into one of the four drains and continuing suction to the other three. This routine tends to remove infected fluids and amylaserich fluids from the retroperitoneal area and so protect this region from their erosive effects. It also prolongs patency of the drains.

Gastric emptying can be a problem after operation. In our experience with the pylorus-preserving operation (Braasch et al 1986), more than one-half of these patients required nasogastric suction for longer than 7 days postoperatively. Our impression is that this problem is caused in part by minor pancreatic leakage and in part by preservation of the duodenopyloric mechanism. Conservative management by nasogastric suction and intravenous alimentation almost always manages the situation. The establishment of gastrostomy suction at the time of resection is an option.

The administration of broad-spectrum antibiotics perioperatively and postoperatively is important. Careful survey of the patient for subhepatic, subphrenic, and other intra-abdominal complications by CT is obligatory. Maintenance of the patient's natural resistance to infection by nutritional assistance before and after operation is likewise important.

Some questions arise as to the indications for reoperation. Major leakage at the pancreatic anastomosis requires prompt surgical intervention to control the effects and to correct the leakage. This can be accomplished in some patients by a few sutures, but in other situations, complete total pancreatectomy is required.

In the unusual event that gastric outlet obstruction is prolonged beyond 20–30 days, reoperation is necessary to resect the distal stomach, pylorus, and first portion of the duodenum and to convert to a Billroth II anastomosis. Before carrying out this resection, care must be taken to ascertain that the obstruction is at the gastric outlet and not in the upper small bowel or elsewhere.

The development of abscesses within the abdominal cavity can frequently be treated by percutaneous drainage with the use of two catheters. It is likely that open drainage will be required for multiple abscess sites or interloop abscesses.

Long-term follow-up requires surveillance to detect the development of diabetes and pancreatic exocrine insufficiency and institute appropriate treatment. H_2-blocking agents should be given on a long-term basis to prevent jejunal ulceration, and administration should begin immediately after operation.

RESULTS AND DISCUSSION

It is difficult to evaluate the results of pancreato-duodenectomy for chronic pancreatitis, and especially the results relative to relief of pain and return to societal living. Ideally, follow-up assessment should be carried out by individuals who have not been involved in the previous care of the patient. The effect of avoidance of alcohol should be ascertained. The differentiation between narcotics taken because of addiction and narcotics taken because of pain should be made. Follow-up for at least 5 years is important because reduction in the initial number of good results is common after all operations for chronic pancreatitis (Taylor et al 1981). Postoperative and late deaths should be recorded, identifying late related and unrelated causes. The severity of diabetes and steatorrhoea that requires insulin and pancreatic enzymes is also vital information for assessment of the operation.

The world results with partial pancreatoduodenectomy for chronic pancreatitis are summarized in Tables 30.1 and 30.2. Table 30.1 contains information from reports in which the operations performed were largely or exclusively the standard Whipple resection of part of the stomach, head of the pancreas, duodenum, and distal bile duct. Table 30.2 contains data comparing the results of the standard Whipple procedure with the pylorus-preserving procedure in a smaller number of patients reported by Morel et al (1990) and collected from the Lahey Clinic experience (Gagner et al 1991 unpublished data, Rossi et al 1987). These tables concentrate on five main issues, namely, postoperative mortality, relief of pain, development of diabetes, late mortality, and information on the length of observation. Postoperative mortality ranged from 0 or 1% to 5% in the most recent series, reflecting the advantage of a firm pancreas in constructing the pancreaticojejunostomy anastomosis. It also reflects the advantage of experience afforded by the larger series of patients.

Relief of pain was good to excellent in 64–94% of patients. A 'satisfactory' result was seen in 79% (median) of patients. Of course, no uniformity exists in defining a 'satisfactory' or a 'good to excellent' result, nor is uniformity apparent in the calculations relative to patients lost to follow-up or lost to late mortality. In addition, the judgment as to relief of pain is clouded by the continuing use of lesser amounts or strengths of narcotics and by unresolved questions concerning work disability and other insurance problems.

Islet cell function (Table 30.1) decreased following resection, and the postoperative rate of diabetes ranged from 26 to 64%, with a median level of 53%. All series showed a deterioration of carbohydrate metabolism when comparing preoperative rates with postoperative rates of diabetes. As indicated earlier, patients with chronic alcoholic pancreatitis develop diabetes without surgical treatment in up to 40–45% of cases (Ammann et al 1984). Most patients whose islet cell function deteriorates require insulin for the management of their diabetic state; only a few patients can control their diabetes by diet or oral hypoglycaemic medication.

It is possible that management of diabetes after partial pancreatectomy is easier than management after total

Table 30.1 Results of partial pancreatoduodenectomy for chronic pancreatitis. (Adapted from Braasch J W 1988 Pancreatoduodenal resection. Current Problems in Surgery 25: 323–363 with permission.)

Authors	Total cases (n)	% Operative mortality	Pain relief Mean follow-up (years)	% Good to excellent	Incidence of diabetes % Preoperative	% Post-operative (%)	Late mortality Follow-up (years)	(%)
Leger et al (1974)	16	6	5 +	75				
Frey et al (1976)	19	5	5 +*	64	15	26	1–20	14
Sarles et al (1982)	23	9	5	71				50
Gall et al (1982)	116	1	1	93	54	56		3.5
Moreaux (1984)	50	2	10.7	73			5–18	50
Hanyu et al (1985)	43	5		79		33		12
Sato et al (1985)	14	21		76				
Rossi et al (1987)	73	3	4.9*	79	25	64	1–20	26
Stone et al (1988)	15	0	6.2	80			6	20
Gall et al† (1989)	289	1	8	88	17	53	8	19
Howard & Zhang (1990)	16	0	5 +	94			10	0

* Range 1–20
† Occlusion of pancreatic duct with Ethibloc

pancreatectomy because some glucagon secretion is also preserved (Warshaw 1987).

Late mortality in patients who have had partial pancreatoduodenectomy ranged from 0 to 50%. The median figure in Table 30.1 is 19%. The majority of these patients did not die of the direct effects of pancreatitis or of the operation, but many died because of the ravages of alcohol, tobacco, or narcotic abuse. A small number of patients could not manage their diabetes satisfactorily and died of acidosis or hypoglycaemia.

The incidence of exocrine insufficiency after pancreatoduodenectomy is difficult to estimate because many patients are given pancreatic enzymes routinely after operation. Often the use of this medication cannot be assessed due to the lack of faecal fat estimations and body weight measurements before and after the onset of enzyme therapy.

Data with regard to the results of pancreatoduodenectomy when the standard Whipple procedure is compared with the pylorus-preserving procedure are shown in Table 30.2. No studies have been reported that compare the two operations when a blinded prospective method of case selection was used. In both series of patients in Table 30.2, the operative mortality is low for both techniques and the incidence of postoperative complications is about the same. Improvement in the severity of pain is similar, as is the development of diabetes postoperatively. In patients who underwent the pylorus-preserving procedure, points of difference included an increased requirement for nasogastric suction postoperatively, a decrease in dumping and the full stomach syndrome, and an increase in the number of patients who noted an increase in body weight postoperatively.

Postoperative gastric emptying does appear to be delayed with preservation of the pylorus (Newman et al 1983). The reason for this delay is not entirely clear, but it has occurred in other series (Itani et al 1986, Warshaw & Torchiana 1985). Interestingly, in our patients who had total pancreatectomy and pylorus preservation, the rate of delay in gastric emptying is not nearly as great (Gagner et al 1991, unpublished data).

The incidence of jejunal ulcer varies between 6 and 20% after the standard Whipple procedure. In Table 30.2, it is seen that in the series of Morel et al (1990), 20% of patients with pylorus-preservation developed jejunal ulceration or its consequences and were treated with long-term H_2-blocking agents. In a discussion of the Morel paper, Traverso (1990) suggested that the ulcers might be the result of the shortness of the duodenal stump anastomosed to the jejunum in reconstruction. Certainly the buffering power of the exocrine secretion of the pancreas is greatly reduced in patients with chronic pancreatitis, especially after hemipancreatectomy, and this could be exacerbated if there is any obstruction of the pancreaticojejunal anastomosis. Studies of the function of the preserved pylorus in our experience (Braasch et al 1986) and that of Patti et al (1987) have suggested that there may be some deficiency of the preserved pyloric sphincter. The role played by other gastric and duodenal hormones that are affected by duodenal resection is unknown (Inoue et al 1987, Kim et al 1987). Whether preservation of more duodenum would influence the incidence of jejunal ulcer is unknown.

Other variants of the Whipple operation being advocated in the treatment of chronic pancreatitis include the use of Ethibloc to occlude the pancreatic duct system at the time of surgery and so induce complete atrophy of the exocrine pancreas (Gall et al 1989), and the duodenum-preserving resection introduced by Beger and his group in 1972 (Beger et al 1985, Beger & Büchler 1990). Gall et al (1989) began to use Ethibloc injection because of their dissatisfaction with the results of total pancreatico-

Table 30.2 Comparison of standard Whipple procedure with pylorus-preserving partial pancreatoduodenectomy for chronic pancreatitis

	Morel et al (1990)		Lahey Clinic	
	Standard	Pylorus-preserving	Standard (Rossi et al 1987)	Pylorus-preserving (Gagner et al, In preparation)
Number of cases [†]	15/18	19/20	41	45
Mean follow-up (years)	8.5	2.8	7.7	5
% Operative mortality	7	0	5	2
% Major postoperative complication	7	37	20	22
Gastric suction postoperatively (mean days)	4.5*	7*		
% Pain improved	78	85	86	90
Number of significant jejunal ulcers	0	4	1	6
Number of stools per day	4*	2*		
% Diabetes, postoperatively [‡]	47	26	64	31
Increase in body weight postoperatively, number of patients	9*	19*	13/31 (42%)	15/23 (65%)

[†] Numerator denotes patients having partial pancreatoduodenectomy; denominator also includes patients undergoing total pancreatectomy
* Statistically significant difference
[‡] Patients who had total pancreatectomy have been omitted

duodenectomy and the desire to minimize the postoperative morbidity and mortality associated with leakage from the pancreaticojejunal anastomosis following the conventional Whipple operation. In a series of 289 patients they experienced an operative mortality of 1% and documented pancreatic or biliary fistulas in eight cases. They concluded that Ethibloc occlusion was highly effective in inducing complete exocrine atrophy, but at the same time, claim that endocrine function may be preserved. Few other centres have adopted this approach, given that operative mortality and morbidity is now acceptably low following operations which do not ablate pancreatic exocrine function.

The Beger operation is designed to deal with patients who have an inflammatory mass in the head of the gland as a consequence of severe chronic pancreatitis. Subtotal resection of the head is carried out, conserving the duodenum and common bile duct, and leaving a rim of 5–8 mm of pancreatic tissue within the C loop of the duodenum. The posterior 'capsule' behind the head of the pancreas is preserved. A Roux loop of jejunum is used for anastomosis to the remaining body and tail of the pancreas, and an end-to-end or side-to-side anastomosis is constructed according to the state of the pancreatic duct within the remnant. The authors believe that the procedure provides satisfactory decompression of the bile duct in the majority of cases, but in 17% of their patients, it was deemed advisable to also perform an anastomosis between the common bile duct and the jejunal loop. In a recent series of 141 patients, the hospital mortality was 0.7% and the late mortality was 5%. A total of 77% of the patients were completely free of abdominal pain and two-thirds returned to their former occupation. After a median follow-up period of 3.6 years, glucose metabolism was unchanged in 82% of cases, worse in 10% and improved in 8%. A number of centres are in the process of assessing the Beger operation and it will be of interest to see whether the operation sustains any advantage over the Whipple procedure and its pylorus-preserving variant.

SUMMARY

With careful patient selection, 80% of patients who undergo resection of the head of the pancreas for chronic pancreatitis can expect some improvement in their pain. Patients undergoing this operation have a reasonable long-term life expectancy at a cost of a less-than-5% postoperative mortality and an increase of 20% in the anticipated development of diabetes. Preservation of the pylorus and the stomach makes for a simpler operation with the added advantage that the patients may have greater weight gain and fewer postgastrectomy symptoms, but at the possible expense of an increased incidence of jejunal ulceration. It remains to be seen whether other variants of the Whipple operation will command a permanent place in the management of chronic pancreatitis.

REFERENCES

Ammann R W, Akovbiantz A, Largiader F, Schueler G 1984 Course and outcome of chronic pancreatitis: longitudinal study of a mixed medical-surgical series of 245 patients. Gastroenterology 86: 820–828

Bagley F H, Braasch J W, Taylor R H, Warren K W 1981 Sphincterotomy or sphincteroplasty in the treatment of pathologically mild chronic pancreatitis. American Journal of Surgery 141: 418–422

Beger H G, Büchler M 1990 Duodenum-preserving resection of the head of the pancreas in chronic pancreatitis with inflammatory mass in the head. World Journal of Surgery 14: 83–87

Beger H G, Krautzberger W, Bittner R, Büchler M, Limmer J 1985 Duodenum-preserving resection of the head of the pancreas in patients with severe chronic pancreatitis. Surgery 97: 467–473

Braasch J W, Deziel D J, Rossi R L, Watkins E Jr, Winter P F 1986 Pyloric and gastric preserving pancreatic resection: experience with 87 patients. Annals of Surgery 204: 411–418

Frey C F, Child C G, Fry W 1976 Pancreatectomy for chronic pancreatitis. Annals of Surgery 184: 403–413

Gall F P, Gebhardt C, Zirngibl H 1982 Chronic pancreatitis: results in 116 consecutive, partial duodenopancreatectomies combined with pancreatic duct occlusion. Hepatogastroenterology 29: 115–119

Gall F P, Gebhardt C, Meister R, Zirngibl H, Schneider M U 1989 Severe chronic cephalic pancreatitis: use of partial duodenopancreatectomy with occlusion of the pancreatic duct in 289 patients. World Journal of Surgery 13: 809–817

Hanyu F, Nakamura M, Suzuki M 1985 Surgical treatment of chronic pancreatitis: with special reference to pancreatectomy. In: Soto T, Yamauchi H (eds) Pancreatitis: its pathophysiology and clinical aspects. University of Tokyo Press, Tokyo, Japan, p 425–431

Howard J M, Zhang Z 1990 Pancreaticoduodenectomy (Whipple resection) in the treatment of chronic pancreatitis. World Journal of Surgery 14:77-82

Inoue K, Tobe T, Suzuki T, Hosotani R, Kogire M, Fuchigami A, Miyashita T, Tsuda K, Seino Y 1987 Plasma cholecystokinin and pancreatic polypeptide response after radical pancreatoduodenectomy with Billroth I and Billroth II type of reconstruction. Annals of Surgery 206: 148–154

Itani K M F, Coleman R E, Meyers W C, Akwari O E 1986 Pylorus-preserving pancreatoduodenectomy: a clinical and physiologic appraisal. Annals of Surgery 204: 655–664

Kim H C, Suzuki T, Kajiwara T, Miyashita T, Imamura M, Tobe T 1987 Exocrine and endocrine stomach after gastrobulbar-preserving pancreatoduodenectomy. Annals of Surgery 206: 717–727

Leger L, Lenriot J P, Lemaigre G 1974 Five to twenty year follow-up after surgery for chronic pancreatitis in 148 patients. Annals of Surgery 180: 185–191

Michels N A 1951 Hepatic, cystic and retroduodenal arteries and their relations to biliary ducts, with samples of entire celiacal blood supply. Annals of Surgery 133: 503–524

Moreaux J 1984 Long-term follow-up study of 50 patients with pancreaticoduodenectomy for chronic pancreatitis. World Journal of Surgery 8: 346–353

Morel P, Mathey P, Corboud H, Huber O, Egeli R A, Rohner A 1990 Pylorus-preserving duodenopancreatectomy: long-term complications and comparison with the Whipple procedure. World Journal of Surgery 14: 642–647

Newman K D, Braasch J W, Rossi R L, O'Campo-Gonzales S 1983 Pyloric and gastric preservation with pancreatoduodenectomy. American Journal of Surgery 145: 152–156

Patti M G, Pellegrini C A, Way L W 1987 Gastric emptying and small bowel transit of solid food after pylorus-preserving pancreaticoduodenectomy. Archives of Surgery 122: 528–532

Rossi R L, Rothschild J, Braasch J W, Munson J L, ReMine S G 1987 Pancreatoduodenectomy in the management of chronic pancreatitis. Archives of Surgery 122: 416–420

Sarles J C, Nacchiero M, Garani F, Salasc B 1982 Surgical treatment of chronic pancreatitis: report of 134 cases treated by resection or drainage. American Journal of Surgery 144: 317–321

Sato T, Yamauchi H, Miyashita E, Matsuno S 1985 Long-term follow-up study on surgical treatment for chronic pancreatitis. In: Soto T, Yamauchi H (eds) Pancreatitis: its pathophysiology and clinical aspects. University of Tokyo Press, Tokyo, Japan, p 449–456

Stone W M, Sarr M G, Nagorney D M, McIlrath D C 1988 Chronic pancreatitis: results of Whipple's resection and total pancreatectomy. Archives of Surgery 123: 815–819

Taylor R H, Bagley F H, Braasch J W, Warren K W 1981 Ductal drainage or resection for chronic pancreatitis. American Journal of Surgery 141: 28–33

Thomas 1990 Use of ultrasound dissection in pancreatic surgery. Presented at the 3rd World Congress on Hepato-Pancreato-Biliary Surgery, London

Traverso L W 1990 Commentary on Morel P, Mathey P, Corboud H, Huber O, Egeli R A, Rohner A 1990 Pylorus-preserving duodenopancreatectomy: long-term complications and comparison with the Whipple procedure. World Journal of Surgery 14: 646–647

Traverso L W, Longmire W P Jr 1978 Preservation of the pylorus in pancreaticoduodenectomy. Surgery, Gynecology and Obstetrics 146: 959–962

Warshaw A L 1987 Discussion of Rossi R L, Rothschild J, Braasch J W, Munson J L, ReMine S G 1987 Pancreatoduodenectomy in the management of chronic pancreatitis. Archives of Surgery 122: 420

Warshaw A L, Torchiana D L 1985 Delayed gastric emptying after pylorus-preserving pancreaticoduodenectomy. Surgery, Gynecology and Obstetrics 160: 1–4

Watson K 1944 Carcinoma of ampulla of Vater: successful radical resection. British Journal of Surgery 31: 368–373

Whipple A O, Parsons W B, Mullins C R 1935 Treatment of carcinoma of the ampulla of Vater. Annals of Surgery 102: 763–779

31. Total pancreatoduodenectomy

R. C. G. Russell

INTRODUCTION

The last procedure in a section describing surgical options in the management of chronic pancreatitis should be total pancreatectomy, for this is the final ablation of pancreatic tissue in an attempt to cure symptoms. This position for total pancreatectomy is not only logical, but proven by experience to be the correct point at which a clinician considers this operation. Indeed, the procedure can create as many problems as the clinician hoped that it would solve. The reputation of this procedure frequently suffers from it having been performed too early or too late in the course of the disease. If surgery is performed too early, the patient or physician may cast doubt on the need for the operation, which helps little in the discipline required if the pancreatectomized patient is to control the metabolic effects of the procedure; it is frequently not appreciated that this is a lifelong discipline and that the problems posed by the metabolic consequences of the operation do not decrease with time. In contrast, postponing the operation until the patient is metabolically crippled by weight loss and the consequences of the complications of pancreatic disease, as well as being dependent on narcotics, will create psychological problems of such magnitude that the patient can never be fully rehabilitated. Great emphasis has been laid on the technical aspects of the surgery of chronic pancreatitis, but the skill in achieving good results lies in the careful overall management of patients who suffer from this disease. The results depend largely on the timing of operative intervention, and it is this question of timing which requires careful consideration.

HISTORICAL BACKGROUND

The first authenticated report of total pancreatectomy was that of Rockey in 1943. The patient survived 15 days, succumbing to a 'blow out' of the ligated end of the common bile duct. Of historical interest are two cases culled from the literature by Sauve (1908) in which near total pancreatectomy was performed. The first case was credited to Billroth by Mayo Robson in 1901, the operation having been done in 1884. Since this case was never fully reported the exact extent of resection and end result are not adequately documented. The second case was reported by Franke in 1900. This operation was undertaken for cancer of the pancreas, but the duodenum was not removed and some pancreas was preserved; the patient survived 6 months before dying of recurrent cancer. The first successful total pancreatectomy was performed by Priestley on July 14, 1942 at St Mary's Hospital, Rochester, in a patient with hypoglycaemia in whom no tumour could be palpated at operation. A total pancreatectomy was performed for what proved to be an 8 mm by 5 mm islet adenoma. The patient survived for 29 years (van Heerden 1986). By 1948, Gaston reported one case of total pancreatectomy and reviewed 16 others, 11 of which had been performed for cancer with only 3 survivals, and 6 for benign disease, 3 of whom died. Over the next decade, advances were made with the technical aspects of the operation in patients who were undergoing resection for cancer. Reports occasionally emphasized the difficulty of distinguishing chronic pancreatitis from cancer (Gourevitch & Whitfield 1952), and this was the reason for some patients with chronic pancreatitis undergoing total pancreatectomy. Technical improvement meant that more than 150 successful procedures had been reported in the literature by 1966.

Warren et al in 1966 reported eight patients who had had a resection for advanced chronic relapsing pancreatitis; emphasis was laid on reserving this procedure for those with disabling symptoms and marked destruction of pancreatic parenchyma associated with innumerable points of intraductal obstruction. Six patients were followed closely, and good results obtained in five. The drawbacks of performing the procedure too late in the course of the disease, when debilitation and addiction to drugs and alcohol made rehabilitation to a useful life difficult or impossible, were emphasized by ReMine et al in 1970. Review of their results from the Mayo Clinic showed that only three of their series of 36 patients had undergone total pancreatectomy for benign disease. These patients did badly, two dying within a year, of hypoglycaemic problems, and the third dying 8 years later with massive gastrointestinal haemorrhage. In a subsequent report dealing with a further 4 years' experience, only two more patients had been operated on for chronic pancreatitis (Pliam & ReMine 1975). This experience in a unit dealing with large numbers of patients with chronic pancreatitis reflects the reluctance to perform this procedure for benign disease, and explains why it has taken so long to assess this procedure as an option in the management of chronic pancreatitis.

Experience with total pancreatectomy for benign disease has remained limited. In 1978, Braasch et al were able to find only 53 instances of total pancreatectomy performed for pancreatitis. To this they added the Lahey Clinic experience of 26 patients, indicating a changing attitude to the operation and an increased willingness to perform it in specialist centres. For the first time, data were provided in this report which enabled an assessment of the role of total pancreatectomy in the management of chronic pancreatitis. Operative mortality was nil, but morbidity, both in-hospital and delayed, was considerable. All the patients were subject to insulin reactions, and there were 12 late deaths. Of significance, and at variance with subsequent experience, was the relief of the severe epigastric pain, yet three of the 14 surviving patients still took narcotics. The authors considered that the results showed an improvement over the preoperative state in general, but there was a failure to normalize the life of the majority of patients; this has proved to be a key factor in the subsequent analysis of this operation.

The rather cautious approach to total pancreatectomy as advocated by the American school of surgery was not adopted in Europe where a number of groups, particularly in France and Germany, were gaining considerable experience in the management of chronic pancreatitis, as a consequence of an increase in the incidence of the disease due to changed socioeconomic circumstances. During the 1970s a large experience was acquired by Gall and his colleagues in Erlangen (1981), who reported 63 total pancreatectomies performed between 1972 and 1977. In 75% of cases the pancreatitis was attributed to alcohol abuse with consumption in excess of 80 g/day. Their operative mortality was high (21%) compared to that of pancreatoduodenectomy (8%). Their morbidity was also high with 75% of patients having difficulty in stabilizing their blood sugar, and their late mortality of 19% was similar to the 20% late mortality rate after pancreatoduodenectomy. After total pancreatectomy, 11% fewer patients were alive at the end of the follow-up period than after partial pancreaticoduodenectomy. These deaths were accounted for by continued alcohol abuse and/or hypoglycaemia.

The varied mortality of the operation in different centres can probably be explained by differences in selection criteria, but the late morbidity and high mortality found in both the Lahey and Erlangen experiences was confirmation that the fears voiced in the early reports were justified. Nevertheless, the high late mortality must be considered in the light of the natural history of the disease, a subject about which little was known until relatively recently. According to Strum & Spiro (1971), the non-operative treatment of severe pancreatitis is associated with a late mortality rate of 30%. This indicates that the complications of the disease, and the personality of the patient may be associated with a poor outcome. The question remains whether surgery improves this outcome, and is justified for such a high risk group of patients with benign disease. Many health care organizations now consider that chronic pancreatitis has a very low priority and that the cost of care or surgical intervention is difficult to justify in a period of diminishing health care resources (British Medical Journal 1991).

INDICATIONS

To justify the operation of total pancreatectomy, it is necessary to fulfil criteria that are strict and agreed by a team who have experience in managing patients with pancreatic disease, and who are prepared to continue caring for these patients for a long time postoperatively.

Firstly, medical therapy must have failed after an adequate trial which must include a prolonged period of pancreatic rest with nil by mouth and parenteral nutrition. Such inpatient treatment enables the team to acquaint themselves with the patient, assess the determination to get better, and willingness to comply with therapy and abstain from alcohol and narcotics. The role of drugs in this assessment is indeterminate, but H_2 receptor antagonists and somatostatin analogues may be of value. Specific psychotherapy has not been helpful, but support from staff dedicated to the care of these patients has proved useful.

Secondly, the pain must be intractable and unrelieved by conservative therapy; it may be intermittent or continuous, but when present it must be severe enough to prevent the patient pursuing his normal life. It is doubtful if total pancreatectomy is ever indicated in the absence of pain.

Thirdly, operations of lesser severity, such as a drainage procedure or partial resection, must have been undertaken previously and deemed to have failed, as a result of the persistence or recurrence of the symptoms. These symptoms are frequently worse than before the original operation and the threshold for total pancreatectomy must be higher than that used by most surgeons for a drainage procedure or partial resection. It is doubtful if total pancreatectomy should ever be performed in a patient who has neither overt endocrine nor exocrine insufficiency.

Fourthly, the complications of pancreatitis may precipitate total excision in patients who have already had a resection of the head or tail of the pancreas. This is particularly the case when an abscess or phlegmon develops in the pancreatic remnant after pancreatoduodenectomy; such patients frequently become diabetic, and so the long-term risks posed by the complications of diabetes are not increased (Fig. 31.1). Similarly, if the patient has had a distal pancreatectomy (often inappropriately if disease was located predominantly in the head of the pancreas) and develops an acute exacerbation of pancreatitis in the head of the pancreas with formation of phlegmon, fistula or abscess, then early completion pancreatectomy is greatly to the patient's long term advantage (Fig. 31.2).

Fifthly, in patients with parenchymatous disease of the pancreas (often related to multiple calculi in the smaller ducts) who are already insulin-dependent and enzyme-deficient, total pancreatectomy is preferable to a partial procedure in that preservation of some pancreas can confer no advantage (Fig. 31.3).

Finally, there are a few patients in whom there is no ductal abnormality, but who suffer from repeated episodes of pain of pancreatic origin. These patients inevitably develop recurrent pain after lesser procedures, and can be appropriately managed by total pancreatectomy, but only after most careful assessment.

Thus, the principle underlying resection for total pancreatectomy is that it is a last resort procedure, but the

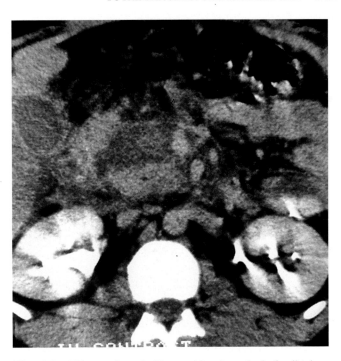

Fig. 31.2 CT scan of a male 35-year-old patient who had a distal pancreatectomy for a pancreatic abscess with good result. He was readmitted 10 months later with severe pancreatitis. The scan shows disruption of the head of the pancreas.

option to operate should not be taken when severe personality changes have intervened with dependence on narcotics, loss of family support and physical deterioration. Narcotic dependence is a topic that has to be faced by the clinical care team in charge of a patient with unremitting pain. A clinical judgment, with or without the aid of a psychiatric assessment, must be made on whether the narcotic usage is part of primary drug dependence or whether the drugs are being used primarily to relieve the pain. This is a fine decision because many patients in this position have an addictive personality with a background of heavy alcohol consumption. Nevertheless, a major contraindication to total pancreatectomy is continued alcohol and narcotic abuse. Before embarking on the operation it is advisable to try to relieve the pain, or treat the complication precipitating the need for total pancreatectomy, by conservative management. Once the pain is controlled, the narcotic can be reduced in a stepwise manner with complete cessation before the planned operation. If the disease is under control, but narcotic requirement cannot be reduced, the care team should carefully reconsider the indication for total pancreatectomy, as it is these patients who are often unreliable and experience the hypoglycaemic complications which can follow total pancreatectomy. If it is the considered opinion of the team that the pain has not been totally relieved, then, and only after much thought, a coeliac plexus block can be undertaken. If this does not relieve the pain, or if narcotics cannot be with

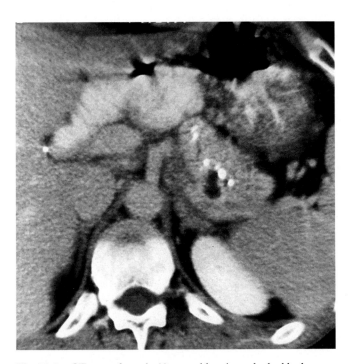

Fig. 31.1 CT scan of a male 42-year-old patient who had had a pancreatoduodenectomy for chronic pancreatitis. He had initial freedom from pain, but after 2 years developed intractable pain and diabetes with inflammation around a small cystic space in the pancreas. His progress was good after a distal pancreatectomy.

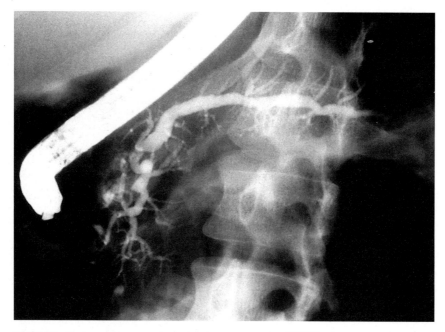

Fig. 31.3   Endoscopic retrograde cholangiopancreatogram (ERCP) of a 30-year-old man with changes in the head of the pancreas and an abnormal duct in the body and tail of the pancreas. A total ablation of the pancreas was performed with excellent results.

drawn, then that patient is unsuitable for total pancreatectomy.

In the assessment of the patient, emphasis is laid on the social background and the environment to which the patient will return. This procedure should not be performed on patients who do not have ready access to adequate medical support. A secure home and secure personal relationships are an advantage, although lack of either is not a contraindication. Age over 65 years and major impairment of cardiovascular, renal, pulmonary or central nervous system are contraindications. Finally, it must be stressed that some doubt the logic of total pancreatectomy in the sensible management of chronic pancreatitis (Imrie 1990).

PREOPERATIVE PREPARATION

Once a decision has been made to offer the patient total pancreatectomy, it is necessary to provide full information regarding the implications of the procedure. If the patient has neither pancreatic enzyme deficiency nor the need for insulin, it is essential to start enzyme replacement therapy to ensure that the rather unpalatable capsules can be taken with good compliance. It is also essential for the patient to see the diabetologist and the liaison sister to discuss the management of the inevitable diabetes, and the details concerning the injection of insulin – a cavalier approach to this discussion is a warning of impending problems. Because many of these patients are malnourished, it is preferable to improve their nutrition by means of parenteral feeding, as postoperative rehabilitation is

hastened by an adequate lean body mass. Further, the intestinal rest associated with parenteral nutrition enables the dose of narcotics to be reduced and hopefully stopped. It cannot be overemphasized that narcotic abuse must be stopped preoperatively rather than postoperatively.

Before operation it is advisable to repeat the CT scan of the pancreas and to obtain a pancreatic ductogram and cholangiogram. This will alert the surgeon to technical problems, ensure that a lesser procedure is not appropriate, and determine whether a traditional total pancreatectomy or duodenal- or pyloric-preserving procedure is indicated. An angiogram is not essential, but ultrasonography with Doppler flow studies will ensure that there are no varices and that the portal vein is patent if the CT scan has not clearly visualized the portal vein.

Infection, bleeding and peptic ulceration are major complications associated with the procedure; these problems should be excluded and prevented by the appropriate therapy. Because patients requiring these operations are a high risk group, it is important to ensure that cardiac, pulmonary and renal function are within normal limits.

CHOICE OF PROCEDURE

This is largely dictated by the previous surgery, and it is rare to undertake this operation in the absence of previous pancreatic surgery. Only 14% of patients in the combined British experience (Cooper et al 1987) had not had a previous operation. Thus, for those patients who have had a pancreatoduodenectomy, a distal pancreatectomy is necessary; this should be splenic-preserving, if technically possible. For those who have had a distal pancreatectomy or a drainage procedure there is a wider choice in that the surgeon can undertake a duodenal-preserving procedure (Lambert et al 1987), a pylorus-preserving procedure (Traverso et al 1979) or the traditional pancreatoduodenectomy including partial gastrectomy. At present there is probably little to choose between these procedures (Stone et al 1988), and thus technical ease and avoidance of complications is the prime consideration of the surgeon.

THE OPERATION

The choice of incision will be influenced by the approach used by the previous surgeon. The principle is that wide exposure is essential to achieve adequate exposure of the body and tail of the pancreas. My own preference is for a transverse incision in the skin crease to ensure a good cosmetic result, particularly as this procedure is performed for benign disease in young people (median age 35 years). On opening the abdomen, it is important to assess the residual pancreas to confirm that the disease is as outlined in the preoperative investigations.

Previous pancreatoduodenectomy

This completion pancreatectomy is often considered to be the easier option, but experience suggests that the previous surgery can make this a formidable procedure if not approached with care. A formal approach to the body and tail of the pancreas through the lesser sac is undertaken. The right gastroepiploic artery will already have been divided, and the left gastroepiploic vessels will be divided during the operation; hence, in order to preserve the omentum which is useful for packing the cavity left by the pancreas, the epiploic arcade has to be maintained. Therefore, the omentum is separated from the transverse colon and splenic flexure, and lifted off the posterior abdominal wall and pancreas on to the stomach, so exposing the lesser sac. Frequently the lesser sac is obliterated and the anterior surface of the pancreas has to be exposed by sharp dissection to separate it from the posterior wall of the stomach. To improve exposure, the splenic flexure of the colon should be separated from the spleen and packed inferiorly, with the mesocolon. The entire front surface of the pancreas should be exposed down to the original pancreaticojejunal anastomosis. The lower border of the pancreas is dissected from the meso-colon, identifying the inferior mesocolic artery. The superior border of the pancreas is dissected carefully from the left gastric artery and vein. The splenic artery must be dissected at its origin from the coeliac artery, and tied early in the procedure to facilitate further dissection.

A decision is made whether or not the spleen can be preserved. If it is to be removed then the short gastric vessels are divided and the spleen and pancreas mobilized; if it is to be preserved, the tail of the pancreas is dissected from the spleen with division of the splenic artery and vein. The short gastric arteries and veins are left undisturbed, and as little dissection as possible is undertaken in the hilum of the spleen so that the anastomoses between the short gastric vessels and the branches of the splenic artery and vein can dilate to maintain an adequate splenic blood flow. Once the tail of the pancreas is mobilized, there is usually a good plane of cleavage which passes behind the splenic vein to the portal vein, but beware, for it is easy, because of the previous surgery, to tear a major tributary of the portal vein and produce bleeding which can be difficult to control. Once the body of the pancreas is well mobilized, it is wise to divide the pancreatojejunal anastomosis, separate the jejunum from the portal vein on which it will be lying, and dissect out and side clamp the splenic vein at its junction with the portal vein. The splenic vein is then divided, so releasing the remaining pancreas. The jejunum requires formal closure without further disturbance of the previous reconstruction.

Previous distal pancreatectomy

After survey of the pancreas and assessment of the extent of previous surgery, the surgeon will determine the procedure to be performed. If the head of the pancreas is markedly inflamed, then duodenal preservation is inappropriate, while if it is a fibrosed and the seat of end-stage pancreatitis with much calcification, a duodenal preserving pancreatectomy can be ideal. During assessment it is particularly important to be aware of the position of the portal vein as, if the previous procedure was an extended distal pancreatectomy, the portal vein is exposed and more anterior than anticipated. Defining its location is therefore the first stage of the operation. Apart from this, the procedure is undertaken in an identical manner to the Whipple operation outlined in Chapter 30, except that at the time of reconstruction there is no pancreatic anastomosis. If a Roux loop has been constructed previously for use in a pancreatojejunostomy, it is probably better to sacrifice this segment of bowel in the reconstruction of the intestine and biliary tree so as to ensure freedom from subsequent fibrosis or stasis due to altered motility.

Duodenum-preserving total pancreatectomy

During assessment of the pancreas, it is important not to mobilize the duodenum by a Kocher manoeuvre as the duodenum draws some blood supply from the peritoneal vessels. The first step in the operation is to expose the front of the pancreas by dissecting the hepatic flexure of the colon away from the pancreas and dividing the right gastroepiploic artery between ligatures. The portal vein is then exposed. In order to simplify the dissection, if the body and tail of the pancreas are still present, it is appropriate to mobilize them first; the mobilized body and tail serve as a useful retractor during subsequent dissection (Fig. 31.4).

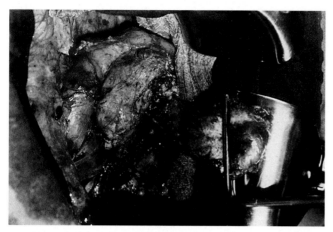

Fig. 31.4 The body and tail of the pancreas have been mobilized, and dissected sufficiently to expose the portal vein. This figure is reproduced in colour in the plate section at the front of the volume.

The portal vein and superior mesenteric vein are cleared of branches down to the fourth part of the duodenum. The uncinate process at the junction of the duodenum and mesenteric vessels is lifted forward with a pair of tissue-holding forceps. Using mosquito forceps each vessel between the pancreas and duodenum or mesenteric vessels is dissected out and tied as near to the pancreas as possible; ties are preferred to Ligaclips as they are less prone to be brushed off during handling (Fig. 31.5). The dissection is then continued upwards for 3 cm along the mesenteric vessels and to the right along the fourth part of the duodenum so that the tip of the uncinate process can be mobilized and a finger inserted on to the posterior surface of the uncinate process.

Once this step has been achieved, dissection of the small vessels between the duodenum and pancreas is easier and preservation of the inferior pancreatoduodenal artery

more secure, for the main trunk of this vessel should not be tied although its branches will be eventually tied one by one. With careful dissection, 3–4 cm of this vessel can be preserved and a good blood supply to the fourth part of the duodenum maintained. The dissection along the fourth and third parts of the duodenum is continued tying each vessel individually and with great care until the papilla of Vater is reached. The plane between the pancreas and the inferior vena cava is developed at this stage so that the pancreas can be lifted further forward away from the vessels on the posterior wall of the duodenum. The duodenum is not mobilized, and the peritoneum on the outer border of the duodenum should not be divided. Near the fourth part of the duodenum there is a good plane of cleavage between the duodenum and the pancreas, but as the dissection nears the third part of the duodenum, this plane becomes less defined and is absent 1 cm from the papilla (Fig. 31.6).

The absence of this plane of cleavage is a warning of the increasing proximity of the papilla and the more profuse blood supply. It is preferable at this point to turn attention to the attachment of the pancreas to the superior mesenteric artery and vein to reduce the bleeding from the pancreas. Therefore, with the finger behind the pancreas lifting it forward, the vessels from the superior mesenteric vein and artery are dissected out individually, tied and divided until the first part of the duodenum is reached. In the triangle between the first part of the duodenum, the pancreas and the portal vein lies the bile duct, which, lying posterior to the pancreas, can easily be seen and dissected out at this point, great care being taken not to destroy its blood supply. The pancreatoduodenal artery is next dissected and its branches to the first part of the duodenum preserved before tying the vessel as it enters the pancreatic substance.

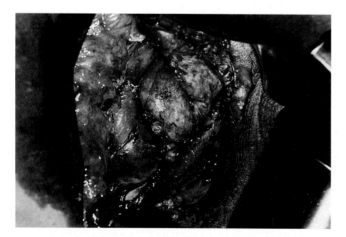

Fig. 31.5 Dissection of the portal vein has been completed and the uncinate process of the pancreas mobilized from the fourth part of the duodenum. This figure is reproduced in colour in the plate section at the front of the volume.

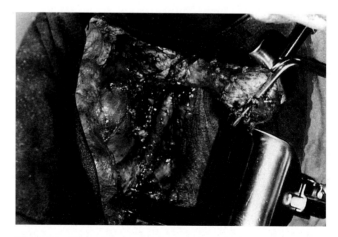

Fig. 31.6 Dissection around the ampulla is difficult because of the lack of a clear plane of dissection, and numerous small vessels. This figure is reproduced in colour in the plate section at the front of the volume.

The dissection is then continued along the first and second parts of the duodenum until the probable site of the papilla of Vater is reached. Great care is necessary at this point to dissect the bile and pancreatic duct. Attention is next turned to the third part of the duodenum, and the region of the ampulla of Vater is dissected. Occasionally, if the bile duct is easily identified on the posterior aspect of the pancreas, dissection from behind can lead to the ampulla of Vater, which then enables the bile duct to be dissected away from the pancreas. It is usually easier to define the bile duct as it enters the duodenum and in a plane of cleavage on the posterior surface to dissect the bile duct away from the pancreas and free it completely, by lifting the pancreas forward and to the right.

On the inferior border of the bile duct the main pancreatic duct is seen, dissected out and divided. The cut duct end is oversewn with a non-absorbable suture of 6-0 Prolene. Interestingly, removing the pancreas from the second part of the duodenum is the most difficult part of the dissection, for here there is no plane of cleavage between the pancreas and duodenum, and the operator occasionally has to develop a false plane, tying the vessels as he dissects them off the duodenum and ensuring that he does not damage the duodenal muscle. As he proceeds down from the first to the second part of the duodenum, the accessory duct is dissected out, divided and oversewn with a non-absorbable suture of 6-0 Prolene. Once this has been done, further dissection between the major and minor papillae releases the rest of the pancreatic substance.

The C loop should now be empty apart from the bile duct coursing across the upper part. The colour of the C loop varies from a dusky blue to pink but should show active peristalsis (Fig. 31.7). Oversewing the inner border of the C loop with interrupted sutures is advised, so that the serosa at the front of the pancreas is brought down to the posterior border of where the pancreas used to be. Once meticulous haemostasis has been achieved, a drain is placed within the C loop.

POSTOPERATIVE CARE

The trend in pancreatic surgery has been towards simplification in care. Thus in recent years, emphasis has been laid on precision in operative technique with a decrease in blood loss, more careful replacement of fluid loss, and improved intraoperative monitoring so that the patient is fitter when returned to the recovery area. It is not our practice to ventilate these patients postoperatively, and the majority are returned to the ward within 6 hours of surgery. The greatest problem in the first 48 hours is the control of pain. Many of these patients have developed tolerance, and require frequent large doses of opioids. Infusions have not proved successful, as these patients have grown used to the bolus effect. Similarly, the use of epidural opioids has been unhelpful in our practice. Adequate

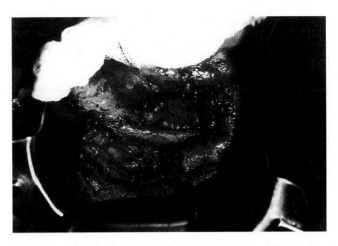

Fig. 31.7 The completed dissection with the common bile duct lying free of attachment. The typical dusky hue of the duodenum at the end of the dissection is seen. This figure is reproduced in colour in the plate section at the front of the volume.

analgesia has been best achieved with 2-hourly injections of an opioid, in conjunction with diazepam and a non-steroidal anti-inflammatory drug such as diclofenac, preferably given as a daily suppository. It is essential to control pain, to mobilize quickly to decrease the incidence of the complications of immobility, and to rest the intestine by a nil-by-mouth regimen until gastric emptying returns to normal. Delayed gastric emptying is frequent following extensive retroperitoneal dissection.

In order to inspire confidence regarding the ease of control of diabetes, it is essential to maintain a stable blood sugar level in the perioperative period. This is preferably achieved by the use of a constant infusion pump, to which is attached a 50 ml syringe containing 50 ml of normal saline and 50 units of soluble insulin. The rate of the syringe pump is adjusted to maintain the blood glucose level between 5 and 8 mmol/l as determined by the fingerprick blood glucose strip. Once oral intake is recommended, insulin should be given as an injection on a twice daily basis; at this stage it is essential to involve the diabetologist so that the patient becomes fully acquainted with the diabetic team. When food is introduced, enzyme replacement capsules should be prescribed at the same time to ensure that the patient accepts these as a necessary part of his replacement therapy. Some diarrhoea can be expected in the early postoperative period; the patient must be taught to balance enzyme replacement therapy according to his diet and the consistency of his stool. It frequently takes longer to convince the patient of the need for this balance than of the need to control diabetes, but without regular and reproducible absorption of food, the diabetes becomes well-nigh impossible to manage accurately. Few, even amongst medically qualified personnel, are aware of the fundamental importance of reproducible absorption, and avoidance of diarrhoea in the management of diabetes. It is this which accounts for many of the hypoglycaemic episodes which characterize the reports of series of patients who have undergone total pancreatectomy.

Once postoperative wound pain has disappeared, opioid analgesics are withdrawn, and the patient managed without addictive drugs. A careful support and education programme is undertaken to ensure that the patient can cope with his diabetes, exocrine deficiency and absence of pancreatic pain. Until the patient is stable and beginning to gain weight he should be kept in hospital. Time spent in the establishment of these habits will decrease the number of subsequent admissions.

RESULTS

Recent data on total pancreatectomy for chronic pancreatitis are sparse, and there are few large series from which to glean information. The review by Frey and colleagues (1989) which includes all published cases between 1972 and 1988, provides limited information as the original papers lack vital detail. The largest recent review is a retrospective study describing collected data on 83 patients from six centres in the United Kingdom (Cooper et al 1987) but this article included little information on follow-up. The largest series from Mannheim describes 52 patients who had a total pancreatectomy, but only 17 of these operations were performed for chronic pancreatitis (Trede & Schwall 1988). In my own series, there are now 58 patients who have had a total pancreatectomy for chronic pancreatitis, 32 of whom were included in the paper by Cooper et al (1987). Smaller experiences from Kiviluoto et al (1985, 10 patients), Keith et al (1989, 7 patients) and McAfee et al (1989, 4 patients) support the general conclusions reached from the larger studies.

Chronic alcoholism appears to have been the commonest indication for total pancreatectomy, but accounts for only half the patients. Gallstones, congenital anomalies, trauma, minimal-change pancreatitis and idiopathic pancreatitis are the other named causes. The symptom necessitating the operation is invariably pain, with most patients requiring narcotics to control the pain, and nearly half were thought to be addicted. Most patients are well below their ideal body weight, and much of the weight loss occurs in the period immediately before the operation. The length of history prior to operation has been variable with a median of about 6 years.

Operation

Between 80 and 90% of patients coming to total pancreatectomy have undergone previous pancreatobiliary procedures, often on more than one occasion; distal pancreatectomy has been the most common prior procedure. Perhaps surprisingly, 14% of the patients in the series reported by Cooper et al (1987) and 22% of the patients in my own series underwent total pancreatectomy as their first pancreatic procedure.

Most patients have had a traditional resection which has included removal of one-third to one-half of the stomach. Pylorus preservation is as yet of unproven advantage due to limited experience, and the value of duodenal preservation has yet to be proved. Nevertheless, the original contraindication to gastric preservation, gastric haemorrhage, is a rare complication (Trede & Schwall 1988), and if it does occur it can be controlled with one of the effective acid secretory inhibitors.

Major intraoperative complications are relatively uncommon (approximately 10% of cases) the most notable complication being haemorrhage from the portal vein, with or without associated portal hypertension.

Mortality

In the review by Frey and colleagues (1989), 31 of 324 (9.6%) patients died. More recent publications have shown a lower mortality (Kiviluoto et al 1985, Cooper et al 1987, Stone et al 1988, Keith et al 1989, McAfee et al 1989) varying from zero to 6%. I have lost three patients in 58 operations, and in each fatal case death followed emergency total pancreatectomy performed for either bleeding or sepsis. However the morbidity of the operation is high with as many as 40% of cases developing complications in the postoperative period (Trede & Schwall 1988). Sepsis was the most common complication, a biliary or enteric leak next, and a delayed haemorrhage occurred in a small number. Those who develop complications, particularly sepsis, tend to develop multiple complications. Infection in the pancreatic bed is particularly difficult to eliminate and a left subphrenic abscess is a pitfall for the unwary; even on CT scanning the subdiaphragmatic gas can be indistinguishable from the splenic flexure of the colon which occupies the space vacated by the spleen. Late complications are rare, but readmissions are frequent due to the metabolic effects of the operation.

Outcome

Details regarding long-term outcome are sparse, but early experience suggested that there was an increased early mortality, and major complications from diabetes (Warren et al 1966). In my own series there were two early deaths (one from sepsis and the other from an unsuspected malignancy in a man of 30 years), four deaths from the combined effects of alcohol and diabetic instability at 24, 29, 54 and 72 months respectively, and one death from a gastrointestinal perforation at 72 months. At 1 year there are 49 evaluable patients in this series, 26 of whom have no significant pain, take no analgesics and are fit for work. At 3 years follow-up, there are 41 evaluable patients, of whom 17 have no significant pain or other problem, and at 5 years there are 26 evaluable patients of whom 16 have no pain, 15 take no analgesics and 14 are fit for work. Nevertheless at 5 years there are still eight with severe pain, seven taking opioids and six undertaking minimal activity only.

The outcome of such patients appears to be that approximately 50% will be completely rehabilitated and require little medical care, but the remainder require constant support with frequent admissions to hospital.

Diabetes mellitus

Management of diabetes after total pancreatectomy is a troublesome problem, and the most serious complications is hypoglcaemic shock. Pliam and ReMine (1975) reported that in approximately 24% patients who had undergone total pancreatectomy, diabetes was managed with difficulty. In addition, they reported that 38% of the patients experienced hypoglycaemia and more than half of them required hospitalization. Furthermore, McCullagh et al (1958) and Ihse et al (1977) reported cases of hypoglycaemic shock that resulted in death. As a consequence of this experience, it became fashionable to restrict the dose of insulin relative to caloric intake, with the consequent risk of malnutrition, hyperosmolar coma and other diabetic complications. In our own experience (Linehan et al 1988), the dose of insulin required varies from 14 to 96 units per day with a median at 1, 3 and 5 years of 35.5, 39 and 40 units per day respectively. The patients who had a duodenum-preserving pancreatectomy required more insulin than those who had a standard procedure (at 3 years, 43 units/day compared to 34 units/day). This is interpreted as indicating a more normal dietary intake in the duodenum-preserving group, a suggestion which is borne out by the greater weight of that group of patients.

The slight increase in the dose of insulin after the first year indicates a better diet, rather than the development of insulin antibodies, a response which is uncommon in the pancreatectomized patient using synthetic human insulin (Ishikawa et al 1989). Diabetes should present no great problem after total pancreatectomy, provided that compliance is good.

Enzyme replacement

The role of exocrine replacement in the control of diabetes and steatorrhoea has already been mentioned, but it is worthy of emphasis, for the symptoms which make patients uncomfortable after this procedure relate to exocrine insufficiency with diarrhoea, flatulence and abdominal discomfort amounting is some patients to an irritable bowel syndrome. The standard doses of enzyme consumption are inadequate. Using the capsules containing enteric-coated microspheres, the daily requirement is a median of 60 capsules per day with a range of zero to 150 capsules per day. The correct dose for an individual can only be determined by trial and error, but those patients who do well achieve a steady state around the median requirement.

CONCLUSIONS

Total pancreatectomy is an operation of last resort; it is a procedure for patients who have not responded to medical management and in whom previous operative approaches have failed. Therefore, it is not surprising that the clinical results are poor, and it must be considered as a salvage procedure after which half the patients are returned to a relatively normal existence. On this basis it is an appropriate procedure to undertake, but only after careful assessment, and due recognition that the patient will need lifelong monitoring.

REFERENCES

Braasch J W, Vito L, Nugent F W 1978 Total pancreatectomy for end-stage chronic pancreatitis. Annals of Surgery 188:317–322

British Medical Journal 1991 Oregon revises Health Care priorities. 302:549

Cooper M J, Williamson R C N, Benjamin I S et al 1987 Total pancreatectomy for chronic pancreatitis. British Journal of Surgery 74:912–915

Frey C F, Suzuki M, Isaji S, Zhu Y 1989 Pancreatic resection for chronic pancreatitis. Surgical Clinics of North America 69:499–528

Gall F P, Mühe E, Gebhardt C 1981 Results of partial and total pancreaticoduodenectomy in 117 patients with chronic pancreatitis. World Journal of Surgery 5:269–275

Gaston E A 1948 Total pancreatectomy. New England Journal of Medicine 238:345–354

Gourevitch A, Whitfield A G W 1952 Total pancreatectomy. British Journal of Surgery 40:104–107

Ihse I, Lilja P, Arnesjo B, Bengmark S 1977. Total pancreatectomy for cancer. An appraisal of 65 cases. Annals of Surgery 186:675–680

Imrie C W 1990. Management of recurrent pain following previous surgery for chronic pancreatitis. World Journal of Surgery 14:88–93

Ishikawa O, Ohnigashi, Sasakuma F, Imaoka S, Hasegawa K, Okishio T, Sasaki Y, Koyama H and Iwanaga T 1989 Insulin antibodies and management of diabetes after total pancreatectomy. Surgery 105:57–64

Keith R G, Saibil F G, Sheppard R H 1989 Treatment of chronic pancreatitis by pancreatic resection. American Journal of Surgery 157:156–162

Kiviluoto T, Shröder T, Lempinen M 1985 Total pancreatectomy for chronic pancreatitis. Surgery, Gynecology and Obstetrics 160:223–227

Lambert M A, Linehan I P, Russell R C G 1987 Duodenum preserving total pancreatectomy for end stage chronic pancreatitis. British Journal of Surgery 74:35–39

Linehan I P, Lambert M A, Brown D C, Kurtz A B, Cotton P B, Russell R C G 1988 Total pancreatectomy for chronic pancreatitis. Gut 29:358–365

McAfee M K, van Heerden J A, Adson M A 1989 Is proximal

pancreatoduodenectomy with pyloric preservation superior to total pancreatectomy? Surgery 105:347–351

McCullagh E P, Cook J R, Shirley E K 1958 Diabetes following total pancreatectomy: clinical observations of ten cases. Diabetes 7:298–307

Pliam M B, ReMine W H 1975 Further evaluation of total pancreatectomy. Archives of Surgery 110:506–512

ReMine W H, Priestley J T, Judd E S, King J N 1970 Total pancreatectomy. Annals of Surgery 172:595–604

Rockey E W 1943 Total pancreatectomy for carcinoma: a case report. Annals of Surgery 118:603–611

Sauve L 1908 Des pancréatectomies et spécialement de la pancréatectomie céphalique. Revue de Chirurgie 37: 113–152

Stone W M, Sarr M G, Nagorney D M, McIlrath D C 1988 Chronic pancreatitis – result of Whipple's resection and total pancreatectomy. Archives of Surgery 123:815–819

Strum W B, Spiro H M 1971 Chronic pancreatitis. Annals of Internal Medicine 74:264–277

Traverso L W, Tomkins R K, Urrea P T, Longmire W P 1979 Surgical treatment of chronic pancreatitis: 22 years' experience. Annals of Surgery 190:312–319

Trede M, Schwall G 1988 The complications of pancreatectomy. Annals of Surgery 207:39–47

van Heerden J A 1986 The first total pancreatectomy. American Journal of Surgery 151:197–199

Warren K W, Poulantzas J K, Kune G A 1966 Life after total pancreatectomy for pancreatitis. Annals of Surgery 164:830–834

32. Pain-relieving procedures in chronic pancreatitis

L. F. Hollender   B. Laugner

PAIN AND CHRONIC PANCREATITIS

Painful stimuli from the pancreas are transmitted by sympathetic fibres which travel along the hepatic, splenic and superior mesenteric arteries to the coeliac ganglion. From there, pain impulses are thought to travel by the greater and lesser splanchnic nerves to segments 5 to 10 of the thoracic spinal cord (Mallet-Guy 1943a, b). The great splanchnic nerve is primarily responsible for autonomic innervation of the viscera of the upper compartment of the abdomen and is the principal target for neurectomy operations in patients with intractable pancreatic pain.

Chronic pancreatitis is characterized by progressive perilobar fibrosis, acinar atrophy and peripancreatic fibrosis, the dense fibrosis making for extreme difficulty when attempting to resect the gland. Entrapment of sensory nerves is one mechanism that has been suggested for the pain of chronic pancreatitis, and it is well recognized that pain may persist even after total pancreatectomy (Cooper et al 1987, Stone et al 1988, Linehan et al 1988). However, Bockman et al (1988) have questioned whether nerve entrapment is a significant factor in the pain of chronic pancreatitis, and have reported that the mean diameter of the nerves increased in chronic pancreatitis while the area served by each nerve decreased. Keith et al (1989) found no correlation between perineural fibrosis or inflammation and severity of pain in chronic pancreatitis, but noted eosinophilic infiltration, suggesting that the eosinophils and their products might be implicated in the production of pain. Bockman et al (1988) also noted invasion of neural tissue by inflammatory cells in some patients with chronic pancreatitis and found ultrastructural changes suggesting that the perineural sheath might serve less effectively as a barrier between the connective tissues and the internal neural components. It was considered likely that both sensory and motor nerves are affected by these histological and ultrastructural changes in chronic pancreatitis.

In addition to neural and perineural changes, there are other mechanisms which may contribute to the pain of chronic pancreatitis, including raised pancreatic duct pressure, raised interstitial pressure, pseudocyst formation, and biliary tract obstruction (Leahy & Carter 1991).

Pain is undoubtedly the principal clinical feature of chronic pancreatitis. It may be chronic or intermittent, is often associated with intake of food, and frequently disrupts sleep. The pain may be felt in the epigastrium and/or either hypochondrium, and frequently radiates to the back and around the lower chest wall. Pain referred to the thoracolumbar region is often indistinguishable from root pain with muscle contractures, neuralgia and pain on movement of the spinal apophyses. Much less commonly the pain is referred to the shoulder. The pain is variously described as gnawing, biting or burning and is frequently sufficiently severe to destroy the patient's quality of life. Although classified as non-neoplastic pain, it may be very similar to the pain of pancreatic cancer, and in some series the 5-year survival rate of patients with chronic pancreatitis is not dissimilar to that of patients with colon cancer.

Patients with chronic pancreatitis tend to be relatively young, the average age in most series ranging from 38 to 45 years. In as many as 80–90% of cases alcohol abuse is implicated in the pathogenesis and may be a major complicating factor in management. The abdominal pain of chronic pancreatitis often has a more marked emotional component than other types of chronic pain. Many patients harbour a hidden fear of cancer, and problems at home and at work can have further adverse repercussions. The personality changes associated with the disease are often expressed through multiple complaints, a general feeling of being unwell, and anxiety and/or depressive states. Alcohol abuse also predisposes the patient to addictive behaviour in the constant search for powerful analgesics, and self-medication is common. Exocrine and endocrine insufficiency due to progressive failure of the pancreas may complicate matters further by producing nutritional and metabolic deficiencies, problems which may be particularly troublesome in alcoholic individuals.

Pain relief can be provided by non-surgical or surgical means. Both approaches will be discussed here, with particular reference to their relative indications.

NON-SURGICAL TREATMENT OF THE PAIN OF CHRONIC PANCREATITIS

The treatment of pain is one of the key aspects of the overall management of chronic pancreatitis. The first is to persuade the patient to abstain totally from alcohol, while the second is to institute effective treatment for any exocrine and/or endocrine insufficiency.

The concept of suppressing pancreatic secretion as a means of obtaining pain relief has in practice proved very disappointing (see Ch. 25). Although anticholinergic compounds are reputed to reduce pancreatic secretions in experimental animals, they do not appear to contribute to pain relief in patients with chronic pancreatitis. Similarly, there is no clinical evidence that histamine H_2 receptor antagonists such as cimetidine contribute to analgesia despite their ability to inhibit gastric secretion and thereby reduce duodenal acidity – effects which in turn lead to diminished stimulation of pancreatic secretion by reducing duodenal release of secretin. Pancreatic exocrine supplements such as Pancrex V and Creon may reduce pancreatic exocrine secretion by providing intraluminal trypsin and thereby inhibiting cholecystokinin secretion (Ihse et al 1977, see p. 39). Although there is persuasive physiological and experimental evidence to underpin this hypothesis, recent studies suggest that much of the benefit attributed to supplements such as Creon may be a placebo effect (Larvin et al 1992).

Thus, the control of pain by analgesics and co-analgesics remains the only effective medical method of management.

Oral analgesic therapy

Analgesic treatment of patients with chronic pancreatitis is particularly difficult because of their frequently compulsive search for analgesics and the inherent risk of drug addiction. The most difficult problem is to determine when it may be permissible to prescribe oral morphine or its derivatives. A major concept in prescription is that of dividing analgesic treatment into three stages, the principal analgesic in each stage being aspirin or paracetamol, codeine, and morphine respectively.

Stage 1 analgesics

Mild to moderate pain may respond to non-opioid or peripherally acting analgesics such as aspirin or paracetamol. Aspirin itself may cause gastric irritation or other adverse reactions which limit its effectiveness, whereas paracetamol has fewer side-effects (digestive, haematological and allergic) and has become the drug of choice. Nevertheless, paracetamol must only be taken in strict accordance with medical instructions. The recommended adult dose is 500–600 mg every 4 hours (taken in regular divided doses), up to a maximum of 3–4 g a day. Paracetamol diffuses freely across the blood–brain barrier and thus also has a direct central action. This distinguishes it from analgesics with a purely peripheral action and explains why the undesirable side-effects of non-steroidal anti-inflammatory drugs such as aspirin (which are due to inhibition of peripheral prostaglandin synthesis) do not occur with paracetamol.

It should be noted that both aspirin and paracetamol are particularly effective for the relief of musculoskeletal pain and are of only limited value for the visceral pain of chronic pancreatitis.

Stage 2 analgesics

Once stage 1 analgesics fail to provide adequate pain relief, centrally acting weak opioids such as those containing codeine or dextropropoxyphene may have to be considered. It should be noted, however, that although dextropropoxyphene when given in combination with codeine or paracetamol provides excellent pain relief, it must be prescribed with caution because of the increasing problem of drug abuse with such compound preparations and the risk of respiratory depression in debilitated alcoholic patients. The combination of codeine with paracetamol provides an additive analgesic effect and may even potentiate the effect of each compound. (It should be noted here that there has been increasing debate about the advisability of using compound analgesics and many clinicians now prefer single-ingredient preparations). In order to achieve the desired effect it is essential to adhere to a strict pharmacokinetic schedule of dosage, using 500 mg of paracetamol and 30 mg of codeine. It is in the patient's best interest to have a precise plan of treatment, with medication being taken at set times and regular intervals, rather than to allow treatment on demand with its attendant risks of addiction.

An intermediate stage 2B has recently been interposed between stage 2 (codeine/dextropropoxyphene) and stage 3 (morphine). This modification is based on the proven benefit of a new class of opiates called morphine agonists/antagonists because of their dual polarity of action. This means that if the dose is increased, the risk of side-effects (notably respiratory depression) decreases while the analgesic effect does not increase further; the so-called plateau phenomenon. Buprenorphine (Temgesic) is one example of a stage 2B analgesic and is available in injectable form (as 1 ml ampoules containing 0.3 mg) and in tablet form (0.2 mg). The normal dose is one tablet taken sublingually every 8–12 hours.

Nalbuphine (Nubain) also belongs to the group of morphine agonists/antagonists. At the moment it is available only in injectable form (as 1 or 2 ml ampoules containing 10 or 20 mg of the active ingredient respectively). Tramadol, which is at present available only in some countries, is a particularly interesting agonist/antagonist in that it provides excellent pain relief but has only minor side-effects, and in particular does not cause constipation. It can be given either by injection or orally (as 50 mg tablets).

All of the above analgesics can be combined with co-analgesics. Indeed, anxiolytics and antidepressants can increase the efficacy of analgesics proper because they relieve some of the personality problems associated with chronic pancreatitis.

Stage 3 analgesics

In chronic pancreatitis one is often dealing with persistent pain which can no longer be controlled by stage 1 and stage 2 analgesics, even in combination with co-analgesics. Some patients may already have undergone neurolytic procedures at the level of the splanchnic nerve or coeliac plexus (see below) yet despite all this continue to suffer. Is it permissible to prescribe oral morphine in such cases? This is a difficult question not only because of the risk of tolerance but also because of the personality changes seen in many of these patients. Yet, as mentioned earlier, chronic pancreatitis cannot be regarded as a wholly benign disorder since in many series survival rates at 5 years are similar to those of cancer of the colon. Thus, prescription of oral morphine, either as a syrup or as slow-release tablets, is an acceptable and effective means of controlling the chronic pain of this distressing disorder when other analgesics have failed.

Infiltrative techniques

When a stable analgesic regimen cannot be established with the analgesics mentioned above, infiltrative techniques may be indicated, not only to elucidate the basis of the pain, but also in an attempt to control it effectively.

Using a catheter inserted at the level of T11–T12, epidural injection of sympathoplegic doses of local anaesthetic (15–20 ml 0.25% lignocaine or 0.125% bupivacaine) allows the effect of highly selective interruption of afferent sympathetic fibres to be assessed. One can thus determine precisely the visceral origin of the alleged pain, the degree and duration of pain relief that might be achieved by infiltrative techniques, and the possible circulatory side-effects.

Most authors are unwilling or reluctant to recommend alcoholization of the splanchnic nerves as a first step in the treatment of the pain of chronic pancreatitis. On the other hand, percutaneous injection of 50% or 70% alcohol into the coeliac plexus is a technique which has been well described for the relief of pain due to inoperable supracolic neoplasms, notably cancers of the pancreas (Leung et al 1983). Provided that the pain is exclusively of visceral origin, injection of 40 ml 50% alcohol at the level of the anterolateral part of the body of L1, either behind the diaphragmatic crura (to ablate the splanchnic nerves) or

in front of them as close as possible to the coeliac trunk (to ablate the coeliac plexus), gives complete or partial relief in up to 80% of such patients, most of whom have a limited life expectancy. All of these procedures are carried out under radiographic or ultrasonographic control after prior injection of contrast material and observation of its diffusion. The duration of pain relief obtained is variable, and in the case of pancreatic cancer is related to the often rapid growth of the tumour. There are so far only few studies which have attempted to quantify the efficacy of neurolytic block of the coeliac plexus and the degree and duration of pain relief afforded.

Neurolysis of the coeliac plexus for the pain of chronic pancreatitis has been particularly disappointing. Myrhe et al (1989) studied six patients with chronic pancreatitis who underwent injection/infusion of 40 ml of 25% alcohol and found only transient pain relief of several days' duration in four cases and no effect in the other two. Similarly, Leung et al (1983) found that only 12 of 23 patients with chronic pancreatitis had complete pain relief after coeliac plexus block and that the mean pain-free period was 2 months, with a maximum of 4 months. The ineffectiveness of neurolysis in these patients contrasts with the more satisfactory results obtained in patients with cancer of the pancreas, and may reflect the longer duration of survival of those with chronic pancreatitis. In addition, the anatomical relationships may be altered by the restrictive fibrosis of pancreatitis, making diffusion of the alcohol solution more difficult. Finally, it may be that the lysed sympathetic fibres regenerate. Use of a more concentrated solution (75% alcohol) appears to give slightly better results, but at the expense of more complications (Leung et al 1983).

The side-effects of neurolysis include orthostatic hypotension, diarrhoea, intercostal neuritis and root pain, and problems with ejaculation. The technique can therefore be recommended only very cautiously, if at all, and then only as an option after other methods of pain control have been explored.

Technique. A posterior unilateral right approach is preferred. The needle is placed in front of the diaphragmatic crura and 40 ml of 25% or 50% alcohol is injected, under ultrasonographic control if possible, taking care to avoid its diffusion towards the lumbar sympathetic chain. More recently, Evans (1990) has recommended infiltration of the coeliac plexus according to the technique described above, but with the addition of 160 mg methylprednisolone and 60 ml of 0.125% bupivacaine. The early results appear to be satisfactory but the completed study has yet to be published.

With regard to other pain-relieving techniques, intrapleural injection of local anaesthetic solutions or neurolytics is of anecdotal interest only and should now be proscribed. On the other hand, continuous or bolus injection of local anaesthetic into the epidural space (using an implanted pump), or injection of morphine intrathecally, may be of benefit in patients who are incapacitated by their pain and in whom there is no other alternative.

SURGICAL TREATMENT FOR THE PAIN OF CHRONIC PANCREATITIS: NEUROTOMY

Based on the fact that in chronic pancreatitis there are inflammatory foci centred on neural tissues within the gland, Mallet-Guy (1943a, b) proposed that the splanchnic nerves should be sectioned, with simultaneous resection of the horn of the semilunar ganglion, in order to achieve pain relief. The splanchnicectomy can be performed retroperitoneally or intraperitoneally.

Extraperitoneal left splanchnicectomy using the lumbar approach

The patient is placed on the contralateral side in the lateral semidecubitus position, using a firm bolster to exaggerate the lordosis and thus open the costoiliac space as widely as possible. The uppermost thigh is well flexed to relax the psoas muscle. An incision is made between the 11th and 12th rib, starting from the middle of the 12th rib and running parallel to it towards the outer border of the rectus sheath. It should be about 15 cm long. Some authors advocate resection of the 12th rib along its entire length, but we do not consider this necessary.

The three superficial muscular layers are divided, preferably with cutting diathermy. The aponeurosis of the transversalis is incised 1 cm below the rib, allowing the perirenal fat to protrude. Together with the parietal peritoneum it is then detached from the muscle layers and pushed back towards the middle of the abdomen with a mounted swab. Then, and only then, is the entire thickness of the muscle layer incised fully, up to the anterior angle of the incision.

After division of the ligament of Henle and freeing of the diaphragm, the thin and fragile pleural cul-de-sac is easily located towards the top of the operating field; its integrity must be carefully respected.

The mass of perirenal fat is now freed and the kidney is pushed forward (Fig. 32.1). This opening-up of the retroperitoneal space must be continued to about the middle of the vertebral bodies. The dissection remains in contact with the posterior muscle mass and then the psoas major, taking care not to damage their aponeurotic sheaths. The diaphragm, its arcades and crura are easily identified. Reflection of the tissues of the pancreatic and renal region reveals the cellular tissue which occupies a plane on the left lateral aspect of the lumbar spine.

Two nerves traverse the region: the greater and the lesser splanchnic nerve. The greater splanchnic nerve appears as a thin filament emerging from the diaphragmatic crus, lying almost in a line continued from the arcade of the

quadratus lumborum and turning forward before spreading out into the posterior peritoneum. The fact that it is the only structure which runs horizontally from the diaphragmatic crus to the semilunar ganglion makes it easy to identify.

The procedure does not need to be limited to resection of the splanchnic nerve alone. The nerve, which is divided after infiltration with lignocaine, serves as a guide to the semilunar ganglion and as a means of retracting it. The ganglion is freed after section of its posterior attachments, taking care to spare the adjacent venules, as bleeding from these vessels can be difficult to control. The posterior border of the semilunar ganglion is then resected (see Fig. 32.1).

Intraperitoneal splanchnicectomy

Right splanchnicectomy

The easiest way to do this is by a retroduodenopancreatic approach at laparotomy (Fig. 32.2). The peritoneum is incised along the external border of the second part of the duodenum. The duodenum together with the head of pancreas is then retracted forwards and towards the left. The detachment is continued to the midline to reveal the left border of the inferior vena cava (which is widely freed with a mounted swab) and its confluence with the left renal vein. Alternatively, the duodenopancreatic mobilization can be carried out through an infracolic approach,

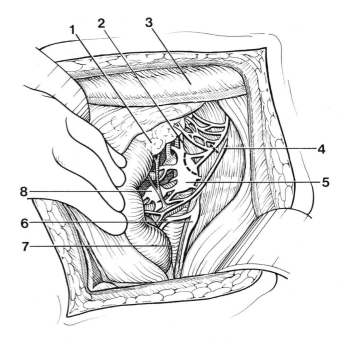

Fig. 32.1 Extraperitoneal splanchnicectomy using a left lumbar approach. 1, left adrenal gland; 2, coeliac branch of Posterior vagus nerve; 3, 11th rib; 4, lesser splanchnic nerve; 5, left semilunar ganglion; 6, sympathetic chain; 7, abdominal aorta; 8, mesenteric ganglion. The two dotted lines denote the point of division of the greater splanchnic nerve and the posterior border of the semilunar ganglion.

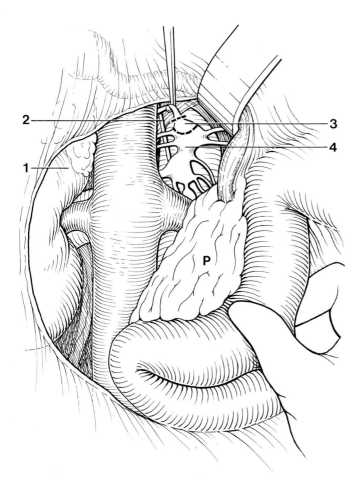

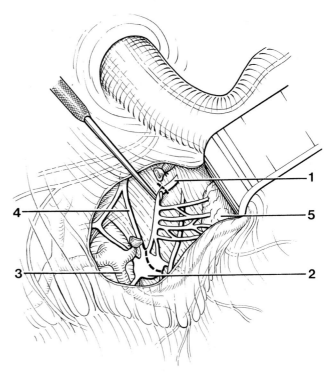

Fig. 32.3 Left splanchnicectomy using a laterogastric transperitoneal approach. 1, Left greater splanchnic nerve. 2, left semilunar ganglion. 3, right gastric artery. 4, coeliac branch of posterior vagus nerve. 5, left adrenal gland.

Fig. 32.2 Right splanchnicectomy using a retroduodenal transperitoneal approach. 1, Right kidney; 2, right lesser splanchnic nerve; 3, right greater splanchnic nerve; 4, right semilunar ganglion.

with elevation of the transverse mesocolon and incision of the right leaf of the mesocolon along the infracolic part of the second part of the duodenum.

The right crus of the diaphragm appears between the inferior vena cava on the right, the aorta on the left, the left renal vein below and the liver above. It is dissected out for 3–4 cm, respecting the small vessels which cross it horizontally. The right greater splanchnic nerve is found at the left border of the inferior vena cava, above its junction with the left renal vein. It appears as a white flattened ribbon which passes almost transversely to emerge between the right crus and the inferior vena cava. The nerve is lifted with a nerve hook and freed with blunt scissors. After infiltration with lignocaine it is divided between two clips.

Left splanchnicectomy

Two approaches are possible.

Laterogastric approach (Fig. 32.3). The left lobe of the liver is turned towards the right after division of the left triangular ligament. The peritoneum in front of the lower oesophagus is then incised and the oesophagus is retracted towards the left. The lesser omentum is divided along its hepatic attachment, and the lesser curvature of the stomach is pulled towards the left and downwards using a Langenbeck retractor. This manoeuvre puts the left gastric pedicle under tension. Ligation and section of the left gastric vessels gives access to the left crus of the diaphragm. This is widely exposed, if necessary after mobilization of the posterior aspect of the stomach with a mounted swab, in relation to the plane in which the inferior diaphragmatic artery and vein lie.

The posterior parietal peritoneum is then incised and the inferior diaphragmatic vessels are tied and divided since they block access to the dehiscence between the principal and accessory fascicles of the diaphragmatic crus at the level at which splitting of the muscular fibres allows one to dissect out the left greater splanchnic nerve. The nerve runs along the anterior border of the spine and descends vertically along the side of the aorta (see Fig. 32.5). After infiltration of lignocaine the nerve is divided between two clips. The only precaution necessary in this approach to the left splanchnic nerve is to avoid too high a cleavage of the crus as this endangers the left pleural cul-de-sac. The approach allows easy access to the left splanchnic nerve at the level at which it traverses the

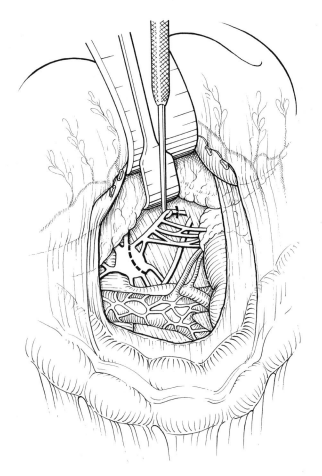

Fig. 32.4 Left splanchnicectomy using a subpancreatic transperitoneal approach.

left suprarenal vessels can occur, hence the importance of previous control.

The horn of the semilunar ganglion leads to the left splanchnic nerve, which emerges from it. The nerve is divided 2 cm above the ganglion, and the external horn is resected after clipping.

Bilateral splanchnicectomy using a transhiatal approach

This method was described by Dubois (1977), Michotey et al (1983) and Sastre et al (1992) (Fig. 32.5). The abdomen is opened through a midline laparotomy. A Fruchaud retractor is recommended to facilitate elevation of the chondrocostal margin, as well as specially designed slender, very long and rigid splanchnicectomy rectractors with which to retract the oesophagus and aorta. Use of a subcostal bolster, resection of the xiphoid process and mobilization of the left liver by division of the left triangular ligament all facilitate this procedure, which is carried out in four stages:

1. Isolation of the abdominal oesophagus is carried out as in the treatment of hiatus hernia. The peritoneum in front of and to the sides of the oesophagus is incised and pushed back with a mounted swab to free the oesophagus, taking care to protect the oesophagogastric vessels and vagus nerves. Dissection of the hiatus allows good separation of the right and left diaphragmatic crura, which can then be retracted in turn.

2. The arcuate ligament is incised in order to mobilize the aorta fully. The pleura is then detached with a small mounted swab, starting on the anterior aspect of the aorta, which must be carefully 'peeled' and denuded. The dissection is continued downwards along the vertebral plane, where a looser plane of dissection allows the pleura to be retracted easily. A small pleural breach may occur during the aortic dissection (more often on the left than on the right) but is without consequence provided the air is expelled at the end of the procedure and the pleural hole closed with an absorbable suture.

3. Isolation of the greater splanchnic nerve is easier on the right than on the left. An easily visible, small prespinal transverse vein running at right angles to the nerve (which is always paravertebral) helps to identify it. Bleeding from small veins is avoided and controlled by the use of small clips. The right greater splanchnic nerve appears as a wide greyish-white band or ribbon lying flat against the fibrous spinal covering. The nerve is isolated using a nerve dissector and a 2–3 cm length is resected between two clips.

Isolation of the left greater splanchnic nerve is slightly more difficult because of the aortic prominence. A retractor is used to reflect first the oesophagus and then the aorta to the right so as to allow access to the left paravertebral region where the nerve, now readily visible, descends as on the right. Again, a 2–3 cm length is resected.

diaphragm, and at a relatively safe distance from the pancreas.

Subpancreatic approach (Fig. 32.4). The lesser sac is opened by dividing the gastrocolic ligament along the greater curvature of the stomach. The stomach is reflected upwards and to the right. The superior leaf of the transverse mesocolon is then incised along the inferior border of the body of the pancreas. Using a mounted swab, the retropancreatic tissue is freed to allow the pancreas to be carefully reflected upwards with a Langenbeck retractor. The transverse mesocolon is pulled downwards.

The left semilunar ganglion can be found in the depth of the dissection. It lies between the splenic artery above and the renal vein below; on the right it is flanked by the left border of the aorta and on the left by the left adrenal gland. The anterior aspect of the left renal vein is freed carefully along its superior border to reveal the left suprarenal vessels, which must be controlled as they may give rise to troublesome bleeding when mobilizing the adrenal gland towards the left. The structures around the semilunar ganglion are then reflected so that its external horn can be dissected out. It is at this stage that damage to the

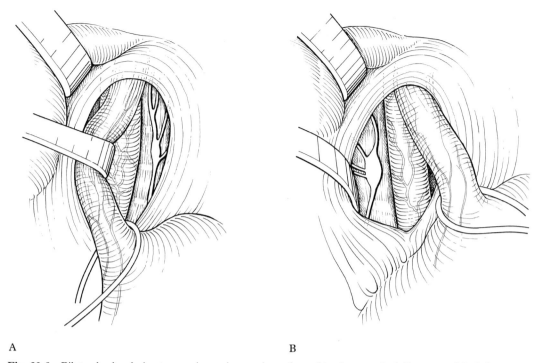

A   B

Fig. 32.5   Bilateral splanchnicectomy using an intraperitoneal transhiatal approach. **A** Exposure of the left greater splanchnic nerve. **B** Exposure of the right greater splanchnic nerve.

4. The muscular crura of the diaphragm are then approximated behind the oesophagus with one or two absorbable sutures, taking care not to close the hiatus too tightly. The angle of His must be restored to prevent gastro-oesophageal reflux.

Neurotomy according to a Japanese technique

In view of the fact that certain sympathetic fibres do not follow the course of the splanchnic nerves, Yoshioka and Wakabayashi (1958) recommended division of the postganglionic fibres, which lie in stages between the semilunar ganglion proximally and the pancreas distally, in order to achieve certain pain relief (Fig. 32.6).

After division of the gastrocolic ligament the stomach is reflected upwards and the root of the transverse mesocolon is lowered. Freeing of the inferior border of the pancreas at the level of its neck gives access to the superior mesenteric pedicle. The vein lies to the right of the artery, but in a more anterior plane, and is progressively dissected out. Once dissected, it is retracted to the left or right (Fig. 32.6A, B) to allow access to the plane of the uncinate process of the pancreas, which comes into view deeper down, to the right of and behind the artery. Between the superior mesenteric artery and the uncinate process lies a dense cellular mass containing the nerve fibres which run from the left semilunar gang-

lion to the uncinate process. This pedicle is divided with extreme care. Division of the corresponding nerve fibres on the right necessitates extension of the mobilization of the second part of the duodenum and head of the pancreas. Bringing the duodenum and pancreatic head forwards puts under tension a fibrous tissue band which, on the left of the inferior vena cava, joins the plane of the right semilunar ganglion to the uncinate process. This fibrous band, which is situated on the right of the superior mesenteric artery, is progressively dissected out and then divided.

Choice of operative technique

Which of these procedures should one choose? The extraperitoneal lumbar approach is the simplest but gives access only to the left splanchnic nerve. The transperitoneal approach has the advantage of allowing, in addition to neurotomy, a thorough exploration of the pancreas and biliary tree. It also permits bilateral splanchnicectomy to be carried out. It will be of interest to set whether thoracoscopic splanchnicectomy will find a place in pain management. With regard to the Japanese technique, apart from its proponents very few surgeons have experience of it.

Patients with chronic pancreatitis who have peripheral calcifications and signs of compression and dilatation of

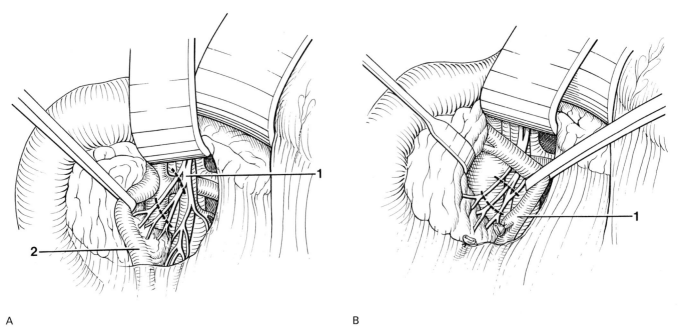

A   B

Fig. 32.6 Resection of postganglionic sympathetic fibres using the transperitoneal Japanese approach. **A** Retraction of the superior mesenteric vein to the right exposes the nerve fibres passing to the uncinate process. 1, Mesenteric plexus; 2, superior mesenteric vein. **B** Alternatively, the superior mesenteric vein can be retracted to the left. 1, Superior mesenteric vein.

the biliary tree generally respond poorly to this type of intervention. Neurotomy, of whatever type, is contra-indicated in patients with chronic pancreatitis who have ductal lithiasis and sphincter stenosis, as well as in those in whom the disease is secondary to gallstones.

Patients most likely to benefit from neurotomy are those with primary parenchymatous pancreatitis, whether localized or diffuse, in whom there is no dilatation of the pancreatic duct (which would make them suitable candidates for treatment by pancreaticojejunostomy or some other form of drainage procedure).

Results of neurotomy

Since the different types of neurotomy have been used in different ways, the results of collective reviews tend to be variable and difficult to interpret. Mallet-Guy (1980), who performed 215 neurotomies (splanchnicectomies or left coeliac gangliectomies), reported an operative mortality of 4.7% and a failure rate of 16.9%. The late results are based on follow-up of 5–34 years and refer to 127 patients, of whom 90% made a lasting recovery. The rate of late recurrence was low at 2.5%. However, it is important to note that these findings refer primarily to patients with chronic pancreatitis who underwent surgery in the very early stages of the disease and in whom neurotomy might have been expected to have a beneficial effect.

In our own experience of 27 procedures (20 left and 7 bilateral splanchnicectomies) only three patients obtained pain relief lasting beyond 3 years. On the other hand,

Michotey et al (1983) reported lasting pain relief in all 14 of their patients treated by bilateral splanchnicectomy using a transhiatal approach.

Results of the Japanese technique (resection of the postganglionic plexus) are more difficult to assess since this method has been used only very rarely. The excellent early results of the Japanese authors (35 good results in 36 patients) lack follow-up and have not been confirmed by others; indeed, Hoffmann & Jensen (1986) found no relief or only transient relief of pain in their six patients treated by selective pancreatic denervation in this way. Similarly, the results of complete denervation of the pancreas as described by Hiraoka et al (1986) and of trans-thoracic left splanchnicectomy combined with truncal vagotomy as described by Stone & Chawin (1990) require confirmation by others.

Because of the unpredictable results of neurotomy, surgical relief of the pain of chronic pancreatitis is now rarely contemplated. It might be considered in patients in whom conservative treatment has failed or who have not obtained pain relief from surgical drainage procedures or resection (Ihse et al 1990). The deep anatomical position of the nerves concerned, together with the local changes brought about by the chronic pancreatitis, make identification of the splanchnic nerves extremely difficult, particularly when attempting section in the immediate vicinity of the gland. Although the extraperitoneal lumbar approach permits section of the nerve well away from the gland, thus allowing complete division, the long-term results also remain unpredictable.

REFERENCES

Bockman D E, Büchler M, Malfertheiner P, Beger H G 1988 Analysis of nerves in chronic pancreatitis. Gastroenterology 94:1459–1469

Cooper M J, Williamson R C N, Benjamin I S et al 1987 Total pancreatectomy for chronic pancreatitis. British Journal of Surgery 74:912–915

Dubois F 1977 Splanchnicectomie par voie abdominale trans-hiatale. Nouvelle Presse Médicale 6:2069–2070

Evans P J D 1990 Steroid coeliac plexus block for chronic pancreatitis. Pain (Suppl 5):176, S9

Hiraoka T, Watanabe E, Katom T et al 1986 A new surgical approach for control of pain in chronic pancreatitis: complete denervation of the pancreas. American Journal of Surgery 152:549–551

Hoffmann J, Jensen H E 1986 Selective denervation of the pancreas for the pain of chronic pancreatitis. Journal of the Royal College of Surgeons of Edinburgh 31:37–39

Ihse I, Lilja P, Lundquist I 1977 Feedback regulation of pancreatic secretion by intestinal trypsin in man. Digestion 15:303–308

Ihse I, Borch K, Larsson J 1990 Chronic pancreatitis: results of operations for relief of pain. World Journal of Surgery 14:53–58

Keith R G, Saibil F G, Sheppard R H 1989 Treatment of chronic alcoholic pancreatitis by pancreatic resection. American Journal of Surgery 157:156–162

Larvin M, McMahon M J, Puntis M C A, Thomas W E G 1992 Marked placebo responses in chronic pancreatitis: final results of a controlled trial of Creon therapy. British Journal of Surgery 79:457 (abstract)

Leahy A L, Carter D C 1991 Pain and chronic pancreatitis. European Journal of Gastroenterology and Hepatology 3:425–433

Leung J, Bowen-Wright M, Aveling W, Shorvon P, Cotton P B 1983 Coeliac plexus block for pain in pancreatic cancer and chronic pancreatitis. British Journal of Surgery 70:730–732

Linehan I P, Lambert M A, Brown D C C, Kurtz A B, Cotton P B, Russell R C G 1988 Total pancreatectomy for chronic pancreatitis. Gut 29:358–365

Mallet-Guy P 1943a La splanchnicectomie gauche dans le traitement des pancréatites chroniques. Presse Médicale 51:145–146

Mallet-Guy P 1943b Splanchnicectomie gauche pour pancréatite chronique. Lyon Chirurgical 38:481–483

Mallet-Guy P 1980 Bilan de 215 opérations nerveuses, splanchnicectomies ou gangliectomies coeliaques gauches, pour pancréatite chronique et récidivante. Lyon Chirurgical 76:361–372

Michotey G, Sastre B, Argeme M, Mannara P, Crespy B 1983 La splanchnicectomie par voie transhiatale de Dubois. Technique, indications et résultats. A propos de 25 sections nerveuses pour algies viscérales abdominales. Journal de Chirurgie 120:487–491

Myrhe J, Hilsted J, Tronier B, Philipsen E et al 1989 Monitoring of coeliac plexus block in chronic pancreatitis. Pain 38:269–274

Sastre B, Carabalona B, Crespy B, Delpero J R, Sielezneff I, Michotey G (1992) Transhiatal bilateral splanchnicectomy for pain control in pancreatic cancer: basic anatomy, surgical technique and immediate results in fifty-one cases. Surgery 111:640–646

Stone W M, Sarr M G, Nagorney D M, McIlrath D C 1988 Chronic pancreatitis. Results of Whipple's resection and total pancreatectomy. Archives of Surgery 123:815–819

Stone H H, Chawin E J 1990 Pancreatic denervation for pain relief in chronic alcohol associated pancreatitis. British Journal of Surgery 77:303–305

Yoshioka H, Wakabayashi T 1958 Therapeutic neurotomy on the head of the pancreas for relief of pain due to chronic pancreatis. A new technical procedure and its results. Archives of Surgery 76:546–554

33. Late results of surgical treatment of chronic pancreatitis

J. Horn

INTRODUCTION

Many different procedures have been proposed and practised in the surgical treatment of chronic pancreatitis and it would be desirable to be able to assess the results of each procedure individually so that an informed and objective decision could be made regarding the most appropriate operation for each patient or group of patients. Unfortunately, this is not possible from the results reported in the literature as these provide only general pointers in an overall appraisal of therapy (Horn 1985). Some of the factors complicating assessment of long-term results will be discussed in this chapter.

FACTORS COMPLICATING ASSESSMENT OF RESULTS

Differences in aetiology and pathogenesis

The Marseilles classification of chronic pancreatitis revolves around the most common form of the disease, namely alcohol-induced chronic pancreatitis (Singer et al 1985). However, there are many other causes and patterns of progression which must be considered when assessing long-term results (Ammann & Sulser 1976, Aldrete et al 1980, Ammann et al 1984, Ammann 1985, Lowes et al 1988). Instead of providing detailed information about aetiology, all too often published series use only a general diagnosis of 'chronic pancreatitis', an approach which undoubtedly clouds the interpretation of long-term results.

Disease course and timing of operation

Irrespective of the particular aetiology, the course of the disease varies from patient to patient. For example, in those with alcohol-induced chronic pancreatitis it depends on the rate of progression of fibrosis and on the pattern of complications. Once fibrosis is complete the patient may become pain-free (Ammann et al 1979), and one early study comparing patients treated conservatively with those treated surgically showed no difference with regard to freedom from pain and late mortality (Ammann et al 1973). These results, although not necessarily representative, highlight the difficulties which can occur when assessing the long-term results of surgery.

Diversity of morphological change

The differences in disease course and the wide spectrum of symptoms are due primarily to the different patterns of morphological change in different patients. Apart from peripancreatic complications (such as stenosis of the common bile duct, duodenum or transverse colon, cysts, and thrombosis of major vessels), which are often treated surgically, the morphological changes in the inflamed pancreas itself often vary widely. For example, obstruction of the pancreatic duct system may be the result of stenosis, calculi or compression by a cyst, all of which can disturb secretion dynamics while carrying differing implications for treatment and long-term outcome. The choice of operation must therefore take into account the particular morphological changes that are present and results must be assessed in relation to the specific aims of treatment (Horn 1985, Nogueira & Dani 1985).

Compliance with conservative treatment

Patient compliance and persistence with conservative treatment (diet, endocrine and exocrine replacement therapy, pain-relieving measures) are crucial in determining the course of the disease (Sarles & Sarles 1976, Ammann et al 1984). The importance of diet is well established and failure to abstain from alcohol is a highly significant obstacle to a successful outcome (White & Keith 1973, Leger et al 1974, Prinz et al 1978, Holmberg et al 1985). Any meaningful evaluation of the results of surgery must therefore take into account the effect of both pre- and postoperative medical treatment and the patient's dietary habits, including continuing alcohol consumption.

Aims of treatment

Although relief of pain is the most frequent aim of operation (Sarles et al 1982, Gooszen et al 1988), a number of other factors, notably body weight, diabetes, ability to work, number of 'relapses' and late mortality, must be considered when evaluating late results. For example, while total pancreatectomy removes the inflamed pancreas in its entirety, subsequent problems are by no means obviated, and diabetes mellitus often presents difficulties in management (Braasch et al 1978; Kümmerle et al 1978, McConnell et al 1980, Kiviluoto et al 1985, Linehan et al 1988). Simply describing late results as 'good' or 'satisfactory' is therefore not helpful, as this gives no indication of problems which may persist and require medical therapy.

Type of operation

While it may be reasonable to classify the operations used in terms of the type of procedure performed, i.e. resection, drainage or combined procedure, this classification is inappropriate as a basis for the long-term assessment of results (Proctor et al 1979, White & Hart 1979, Rosenberger et al 1980, Taylor et al 1981). The varying morphological nature of chronic pancreatitis means that there can be no simple debate as to whether resection of drainage represents the 'best' operation; on the contrary, we need to establish when, under defined conditions, drainage or resection constitutes the appropriate method of operation. The problem is complicated further by the fact that resection of the head of the pancreas (the Whipple procedure) is frequently classified as a resection operation (Proctor et al 1979, Traverso et al 1979, Rosenberger et al 1980) when in reality the operation usually also includes drainage of the remaining pancreas (Guillemin 1972). The question 'resection or drainage' implies that these are competing methods of management whereas it is really a matter of selecting the more appropriate option in defined circumstances.

It also makes little sense to include drainage of cysts under the heading of 'drainage operations' (Traverso et al 1979, Rosenberger et al 1980, Gooszen et al 1988). This practice precludes correct evaluation of the results of drainage operations and ignores the actual aim of such surgery, namely restoration of flow of secretions from the pancreatic duct system to the intestine.

These preliminary remarks emphasize that the results of surgery in chronic pancreatitis must be subjected to critical analysis before they can be translated into guidelines for therapeutic decisions. So far, however, hardly any studies have taken into consideration all of the criteria mentioned above so that the results mentioned in the following discussion must be interpreted with caution and only used as an aid to decision-making in individual patients after careful consideration.

LATE RESULTS OF SURGICAL TREATMENT

Resection versus drainage

Although the two methods cannot be directly compared for the reasons just outlined, important conclusions can still be drawn from careful analysis of published results (Table 33.1). Good long-term results can be obtained with either method if appropriate indications are present. Failure of therapy is more likely to be due to incorrect choice of operation rather than inherent shortcomings in the operation itself (Aldrete et al 1980, Taylor et al 1981).

Drainage surgery has the advantage that the pancreas is preserved morphologically and functionally whereas resection inevitably means some loss of organ substance and function. The long-term effect of this loss following resection is as important a consideration as the potential benefit of maintaining function after drainage surgery. Indeed, some have claimed that endocrine and exocrine function may improve after drainage surgery (Partington & Rochelle 1960, Cox & Gillesby 1967, Lankisch et al 1975) although most surgeons now doubt whether improvement occurs and have the more modest aim of preventing any further decline in pancreatic function.

The more clearly the indication for drainage surgery is established on the basis of morphological and pathogenetic criteria, the better the late results. The pancreatic duct must be sufficiently dilated (see Ch. 28), the anastomosis must be sufficiently long, and all duct segments affected by stenosis must be drained. Drainage of a non-dilated pancreatic duct inevitably fails, as does incomplete drainage of segmental duct dilatations. Such technical considerations have a major effect on the long-term results of drainage surgery (Way et al 1974, Jordan et al 1977, White & Hart 1979, Taylor et al 1981, Brinton et al 1984).

Estimates of the late mortality following resection or drainage operations vary widely. Some authors report roughly equal late mortality (Leger et al 1974, Nogueira & Dani 1985) whereas others have found a higher mortality after drainage surgery (White & Slavotinek 1979). Analysis of this last series underlines the difficulty of trying to

Table 33.1 Comparison of the long-term results of resection and drainage surgery in chronic pancreatitis

Authors	% Satisfactory late results	
	Resection	Drainage
Leger et al (1974)	79	63
Prinz et al (1978)	50	83
Proctor et al (1979)	76	88
White & Hart (1979)	51	80
Sato et al (1981)	80	77
Sarles et al (1982)	67	85
Brewer & Proctor (1983)	60	85
Nogueira & Dani (1985)	62	58
Gooszen et al (1988)	48	68

formulate general guidelines on the basis of a single set of observations. Of the 21 deaths, 9 were due to carcinoma, and the dangers of failing to detect pancreatic cancer at the time of drainage are well recognized. However, several other series show no greater incidence of carcinoma among patients who have had drainage surgery (Leger et al 1974, Prinz & Greenlee 1981, Sarles et al 1982; Morrow et al 1984). Many studies show that a large number of deaths in patients with chronic pancreatitis are attributable less to the disease itself than to the effects of continued alcohol abuse, lifestyle and concomitant disease (Kümmerle et al 1978, Rossi et al 1987).

Diabetes mellitus has particular significance in the appraisal of the long-term results of surgery. Although resection always entails additional loss of function, the development of diabetes depends in large measure on the disease process itself. Thus, assessment of the condition of the pancreas may help to determine the risk of insulin-dependent diabetes developing after resection, a risk which must be evaluated for each patient individually in the light of knowledge regarding his ability to manage diabetes effectively after operation (Cooper et al 1987). However, despite these considerations, the choice of surgical method will always be influenced primarily by the initial morphological findings (Rossi et al 1985).

Overall comparisons of 'resection' and 'drainage' fail to take into account that each category contains a large number of surgical variants, each of which really requires evaluation in its own right (Proctor et al 1979, Horn & Hohenberger, 1987). Ideally, the different procedures should be used in the same morphological situation and their results then compared, an ideal which is almost certainly unattainable. In general terms, the short- and long-term results of drainage surgery indicate that this approach is appropriate when the pancreatic duct is dilated and the flow of secretions abnormal. Raised pressure in the dilated segments of the pancreatic duct system confirms that flow of secretion is disturbed (Sápy et al 1983, Okazaki et al 1988). As indicated earlier, good long-term results can be obtained if attention is paid to technical detail (Castiglioni et al 1984), and the avoidance of resection means that any remaining function in the pancreas is conserved (Creutzfeld & Lankisch 1980). According to Greenlee (1983) a drainage operation is feasible and indicated in about 80% of patients coming to surgery, although most would regard this figure as a significant overestimate (see Ch. 28).

Resection is indicated when surgery is required but the pancreatic duct is not dilated or when there is a localized focus of the disease. In general, subtotal resection and total pancreatectomy are regarded as last-resort procedures when all else has failed, whereas partial pancreatectomy gives good long-term results provided that the indications are correct and the surgery is of a high technical standard.

Surgery on the papilla of Vater

Surgery on the papilla of Vater has also been recommended in chronic pancreatitis, either on its own (Doubilet & Mulholland 1956, Farrell et al 1963, Bagley et al 1981, Nardi et al 1983) or as part of a combined procedure (Rumpf & Pichlmayr 1983). The aim is to improve drainage of pancreatic secretions but the poor long-term results suggest that the indications for this approach have not been adequately established. In alcohol-induced chronic pancreatitis the papillary region is usually not involved in the process of sclerosis, so that it is no surprise that operations confined to the papilla have failed to produce the desired outcome. Only primary disease processes located in the region of the papilla with subsequent development of chronic obstructive pancreatitis are therapeutically accessible to this approach (Sutherland et al 1983, Rossi et al 1985). In such cases, good long-term results can only be obtained when the actual cause of the disease is eliminated by papillary surgery.

Side-to-side pancreaticojejunostomy

The precondition for long-term success with this operation is dilatation of the pancreatic duct to a diameter of at least 7–8 mm in patients with alcohol-induced calcifying chronic pancreatitis (Leger et al 1974, Way et al 1974, Traverso et al 1979, Taylor et al 1981, Adloff et al 1985, Holmberg et al 1985, Mannell et al 1988). Great care must be taken to ensure that the anastomosis is at least 10 cm long and that all stenosed parts of the duct system are drained adequately (White & Keith 1973, White & Hart 1979, White & Slavotinek 1979, Sarles et al 1982). The more consistently the indication criteria are fulfilled and all technical factors are observed, the more likely will be long-term success (Table 33.2). Long-term patency and efficacy of such anastomoses has been confirmed (Warshaw et al 1980, Adloff et al 1985) and the operation does not appear to lead to a significant additional increase in the incidence of diabetes mellitus (Warshaw et al 1980, Sarles et al 1982, Cooper & Williamson 1984).

Combined operations

Following the description of the Du Val procedure (1954), a variety of operations have been described which combine elements of resection and drainage. The Du Val operation involved resecting the tail of the pancreas and constructing an end-to-end pancreaticojejunostomy. Later variants include the Puestow procedure, in which resection of the tail is combined with side-to-side pancreatico-jejunostomy (Puestow & Gillesby 1958), and the operation of 'split' pancreaticojejunostomy (James 1967, Beger et al 1984). Because of the great variation in methods it is not possible to present uniform data on late results; however,

Table 33.2   Long-term results of side-to-side pancreaticojejunostomy in chronic pancreatitis

Authors	Number of patients	Duration of follow up (years)	% Good results	% Late mortality
White & Keith (1973)	50	4.4	81	30
Leger et al (1974)	45	12	60	36
Way et al (1974)	15	5	80	20
White & Slavotinek (1979)	55	9.6	49	38
Warshaw et al (1980)	10	3	89	0
Sarles et al (1982)	64	5	85	26
Gebhardt and Gall (1983)★	246	5–20	69	26
Brinton et al (1984)	39	2–15	85	—
Cooper & Williamson (1984)	11	2.5	91	0
Morrow et al (1984)	35	6	80	9
Adloff et al (1985)	81	5.4	70	10
Nogueira & Dani (1985)	36	20	58	47
Mannell et al (1988)	23	8.5	80	30

★Collected data from literature

the indifferent late results of the Du Val and original Puestow operations (Gillesby & Puestow 1961) emphasize the importance of establishing strict indication criteria and adhering to meticulous technique.

The modern combined operations all aim to eliminate foci of inflammation by resection and to ensure adequate drainage of the remaining pancreas. As discussed earlier, the Whipple operation must be regarded as a form of combined operation; it is incomprehensible that it continues to be assigned to the resection group in debates about the relative merits of 'resection' and 'drainage'. Although resection of the head of the gland undoubtedly carries a greater risk of operative mortality than a drainage procedure alone (Holmberg et al 1985), mortality should be minimal in specialist hands, and good long-term results can be obtained with the Whipple operation with appropriate establishment of the indications for surgery (Table 33.3).

Distal resection

Resection of the distal pancreas is of proven value in patients with inflammatory lesions in the body and tail of the gland (Table 33.4). Drainage of the residual pancreas is not necessary when the duct system is not dilated, but when transpapillary drainage is impaired a retrograde

drainage procedure must be carried out at the time of distal resection. Preoperative endoscopic retrograde pancreatography is of great value in determining the need for a drainage procedure, and intraoperative pancreatography may be indicated if a pancreatogram has not been obtained prior to operation and where there is any doubt about the free flow of pancreatic secretions into the duodenum. The frequency of diabetes after distal resection depends on the extent of the resection and the degree of sclerosis in the remaining pancreas (Gebhardt et al 1981, Morrow et al 1984).

Subtotal resection

Subtotal 'left-to-right' resection as recommended by Fry and Child (1965) had the objective of removing almost all of the parenchyma and seat of inflammation while at the same time avoiding the need for total pancreaticoduodenectomy and preserving some endocrine function. The initial wave of enthusiasm was soon supplanted by disillusion in view of the relatively poor long-term results (Table 33.5). Diabetes mellitus was detected in about 40–60% of patients after this operation and posed significant therapeutic problems which did not dissipate with time (Gebhardt et al 1981, Prinz & Greenlee 1981, Morrow et al 1984). Furthermore, it soon became clear

Table 33.3   Long-term results following duodenopancreatectomy (Whipple procedure) in chronic pancreatitis

Authors	Number of patients	Duration of follow up (years)	% Good results	% Late mortality
Guillemin et al (1971)	63	5	89	26
Frey et al (1976)	19	8.7	69	11
Mangold et al (1977)	37	1.5	73	8
Gall et al (1981a, b)	49	8	56	20
Sarles et al (1982)	23	5	71	31
Gebhardt & Gall (1983)	539	6.5–30	81	19
Moreaux (1984)	50	5	80	34
Flautner et al (1985)	48	4	50	29
Rossi et al (1987)	73	5	79	6
Stone et al (1988)	15	1.5–12	80	20

Table 33.4   Long-term results of distal resection in chronic pancreatitis

Authors	Number of patients	Duration of follow up (years)	% Good results	% Late mortality
Leger et al (1974)	71	12	79	44
Frey et al (1976)	53	6	89	21
Mangold et al (1977)	35	3.5	60	12
White & Slavotinek (1979)	16	6.3	56	25
Gebhardt et al (1981)	42	7	62	9
Sarles et al (1982)	17	5	67	45
Gebhardt & Gall (1983)*	386	9–30	69	17
Brinton et al (1984)	20	2–15	80	—
Williamson & Cooper (1987)	16	5	66	6
Mannell et al (1988)	23	8.5	83	19

*Collected data from literature

Table 33.5   Long-term results of subtotal resection in chronic pancreatitis

Authors	Number of patients	Duration of follow up (years)	% Good results	% Late mortality
Fry & Child et al (1965)	20	5	90	10
Frey et al (1976)	77	7.8	73	29
Mangold et al (1977)	14	3	83	14
White & Slavotinek (1979)	9	5.3	89	0
Gebhardt et al (1981)	65	7	67	13
Morrow et al (1984)	21	7	43	15
Rückert & Frick (1987)	18	10	—	53
Mannell et al (1988)	22	8.5	68	14

that the operation carried a significant late mortality (Frey et al 1976).

Total pancreatectomy

Total pancreatectomy should only be considered when all other methods have failed (White & Slavotinek, 1979, McConnell et al 1980, Flautner et al 1985, Horn 1985, Linehan et al 1988, Kiviluoto et al 1985), and many patients will already have undergone one or more operations on the pancreas (Braasch et al 1978, Cooper et al 1987). The total loss of endocrine and exocrine pancreatic function has a major adverse effect on prognosis, and a particularly positive and cooperative attitude on the part of the patient is imperative for effective medical management (Kiviluoto et al 1985, Stone et al 1988). The high late mortality of total pancreatectomy (Table 33.6) has been stressed repeatedly and is related principally to the difficulties of managing brittle diabetes, continuing alcohol abuse and diseases affecting organs other than the pancreas (Braasch et al 1978, Gall et al 1981a, b).

CONCLUSIONS

The long-term results of surgery in chronic pancreatitis cannot be presented without referring to the importance of the initial indications for operation. In general it is not simply a question of whether to undertake 'resection' or 'drainage' but of an appraisal of the individual situation in which good late results may be obtained by either approach. Analysis of the available literature shows that late results do indeed depend on the presence of the correct indication (Silen et al 1963). As a general rule, it

Table 33.6   Long-term results of total pancreatectomy in chronic pancreatitis

Authors	Number of patients	Duration of follow up (years)	% Good results	% Late mortality
Mangold et al (1977)	13	3	91	15
Braasch et al (1978)	26	4	79	46
McConnell et al (1980)	5	<38	80	20
Gall et al (1981a, b)	68	8	32	19
Kiviluoto et al (1985)	10	3.5	90	10
Cooper et al (1987)	83	1.5	72	13
Williamson & Cooper (1987)	12	4.5	70	25
Mannell et al (1988)	17	8.4	76	44
Stone et al (1988)	15	2.1–13.1	67	40

is an advantage to preserve as much parenchyma (and thus function) as possible. However, the prognosis also depends in large measure on the attitude of the patient and on disease-specific criteria which cannot be influenced by the operation itself.

REFERENCES

Adloff M, Ollier J C, Schloegel M 1985 Les opérations de drainage dans le traitement des pancréatites chroniques. Chirurgie 111:371–377

Aldrete J S, Jimenez H, Halpern H B 1980 Evaluation and treatment of acute and chronic pancreatitis. A review of 380 cases. Annah of Surgery 191:664–671

Ammann R W 1985 Diagnose und Therapie der alkoholischen chronischen Pankreatitis. Eine kritische Standortbestimmung. Schweizerische Medizinische Wochenschrift 115:42–51

Ammann R W, Sulser H 1976 Die 'senile' chronische Pankreatitis – eine neue nosologische Einheit? Schweizerische Medizinische Wochenschrift 106:429–437

Ammann R W, Hammer B, Fumagalli I 1973 Chronic pancreatitis in Zurich 1963–1972. Clinical findings and follow-up of 102 cases. Digestion 9:404–415

Ammann R W, Largiadèr F, Akovbiantz A 1979 Pain relief by surgery in chronic pancreatitis? Relationship between pain relief, pancreatic dysfunction and alcohol withdrawal. Scandinavian Journal Gastroenterology 14:209–215

Ammann R W, Akovbiantz A, Largiadér F, Schueler G 1984 Course and outcome of chronic pancreatitis. Longitudinal study of a mixed medical-surgical series of 245 patients. Gastroenterology 86:820–828

Bagley F H, Braasch J W, Taylor R H, Warren K W 1981 Sphincterotomy or sphincteroplasty in the treatment of pathologically mild chronic pancreatitis. American Journal of Surgery 141:418–421

Beger H G, Krantzberger W, Bittner R, Büchler M, Block S 1984 Die duodenumerhaltende Pankreaskopfresektion bei chronischer Pankreatitis – Ergebnisse nach 10jähriger Anwendung. Langenbecks Archiv für Chirurgie 362:229–236

Braasch J W, Vito L, Nugent F W 1978 Total pancreatectomy for end-stage chronic pancreatitis. Annals of Surgery 188:317–321

Brewer K F, Proctor H J 1983 Surgery for chronic pancreatitis: the tailored approach. Southern Medical Journal 76:1351–1353

Brinton M H, Pellegrini C A, Stein S F, Way L W 1984 Surgical treatment of chronic pancreatitis. American Journal of Surgery 148:754–759

Castiglioni G C, Doglietto G B, Cascini V, 1984 Considerazioni sul trattamento chirurgico della pancreatite cronica calcifica. Minerva Chirurgica 39:583–596

Cooper M J, Williamson R C N 1984 Drainage operations in chronic pancreatitis. British Journal of Surgery 71:761–766

Cooper M J, Williamson R C N, Benjamin I S et al 1987 Total pancreatectomy for chronic pancreatitis. British Journal of Surgery 74:912–915

Cox W D, Gillesby W J 1967 Longitudinal pancreatico-jejunostomy in alcohol pancreatitis. Archives of Surgery 94:469–475

Creutzfeldt W, Lankisch P G 1980 Totale Duodenopankreatektomie bei chronischer Pankreatitis. Zeitschrift für Gastroenterologie 18:641–643

Doubilet H, Mulholland J H 1956 8-year study of pancreatitis and sphincterotomy. Journal of the American Medical Association 160:521–528

Du Val M K 1954 Caudal pancreatico-jejunostomy for chronic relapsing pancreatitis. Annals of Surgery 140:775–783

Farrell J J, Richmond K C, Morgan M M 1963 Transduodenal pancreatic duct dilatation and curettage in chronic relapsing pancreatitis. American Journal of Surgery 105:30–34

Flautner L, Tihanyi T, Szecseny A 1985 101 pankreatoduodenekómia eredménye a krónikus pankreatitis kezelésében. Orvosi Hetilap 126:2943–2949

Frey C F, Child C G, Fry W J 1976 Pancreatectomy for chronic pancreatitis. Annals of Surgery 184:403–412

Fry W J, Child C G 1965 Ninety-five per cent distal pancreatectomy for chronic pancreatitis. Annals of Surgery 162:543–549

Gall F P, Gebhardt C, Zirngibl H 1981a Chronische Pankreatitis. Ergebnisse bei 116 konsekutiven, partiellen Duodenopankreatektomien mit Gangokklusion. Fortschritte der Medizin 99:1963–2014

Gall F P, Mühe E, Gebhardt C 1981b Results of partial and total pancreaticoduodenectomy in 117 patients with chronic pancreatitis. World Journal of Surgery 5:269–275

Gebhardt C, Gall F P 1983 Prooperative Behandlung der chronischen Pankreatitis. Zeitschrift für Gastroenterologie 21:182–184

Gebhardt C, Zirngibl H, Gossler M 1981 Pankreaslinksresektion zur Behandlung der chronischen Pankreatitis. Langenbecks Archiv für Chirurgie 354:209–220

Gillesby W J, Puestow C B 1961 Surgery for chronic recurrent pancreatitis. Surgical Clinics of North America 41:83–90

Gooszen H G, Schmidt J M, van Heurn W E, Jansen J B M J, Lamers C B H W, Terpstra J L 1988 Surgical treatment for pain relief in chronic pancreatitis. Scandinavian Journal of Gastroenterology 23 (Suppl 154):98–102

Greenlee H B 1983 The role of surgery for chronic pancreatitis and its complications. Surgery Annual New York 15:283–305

Guillemin G 1972 Duodenopankreatektomie in der Behandlung der chronischen Pankreatitis mit Steinbildung. Chirurg 43:263–266

Guillemin G, Cuilleret J, Michel A, Berard P, Feroldi J 1971 Chronic relapsing pancreatitis. Surgical management including sixty-three cases of pancreaticoduodenectomy. American Journal of Surgery 122:802–807.

Holmberg J T, Isaksson G, Ihse I 1985 Long term results of pancreaticojejunostomy in chronic pancreatitis. Surgery, Gynecology and Obstetrics 160:339–345

Horn J 1985 Therapie der chronischen Pankreatitis. Individualisierte Verfahrenswahl, chirurgische Technik. Springer, Berlin p 275–304

Horn J, Hohenberger P 1987 Chronische Pankreatitis – Drainage und Resektionsverfahren: Standortbestimmung. Chirurg 58:14–24

James M 1967 Treatment of pancreatic duct obstruction by 'split' pancreaticojejunostomy. American Surgeon 33:1–6

Jordan G L, Strug B S, Crowder W E 1977 Current status of pancreaticojejunostomy in the management of chronic pancreatitis. American Journal of Surgery 133:46–51

Kiviluoto T, Schröder T, Lempinen M 1985 Total pancreatectomy for chronic pancreatitis. Surgery, Gynecology and Obstetrics 160:223–227

Kümmerle F, Mangold G, Rückert K 1978 Leben und Lebenserwartung nach Eingriffen an der Bauchspeicheldrüse. Lebensversicherungsmedizin 30:34–38

Lankisch P G, Fuchs K, Schmidt H Peiper H-J, Creutzfeldt W 1975 Ergebnisse der operativen Behandlung der chronischen Pankreatitis mit besonderer Berücksichtigung der exokrinen und endokrinen Funktion. Deutsche Medizinische Wochenschrift 100:1048–1060

Leger L, Lenroit J P, Lemaigre G 1974 Five to twenty year follow-up after surgery for chronic pancreatitis in 148 patients. Annals of Surgery 180: 185–191.

Linehan I P, Lambert M A, Brown D C, Kurtz A B, Cotton P B, Russell R C G 1988 Total pancreatectomy for chronic pancreatitis. Gut 29:358–365

Lowes J R, Rode J, Lees W R, Russell R C G, Cotton P B 1988 Obstructive pancreatitis: unusual causes of chronic pancreatitis. British Journal of Surgery 75:1129–1133

McConnell D B, Sasaki T M, Garnjobst W, Vetto R M 1980 Experience with total pancreatectomy. American Journal of Surgery 139:646–649

Mangold G, Neher M, Oswald B, Wagner G 1977 Ergebnisse der Resektionsbehandlung der chronischen Pankreatitis. Deutsche Medizinische Wochenschrift 102:229–234

Mannell A, Adson M A, McIlrath D C, Ilstrup D M 1988 Surgical management of chronic pancreatitis: long-term results in 141 patients. British Journal of Surgery 75:467–472

Moreaux J 1984 Long-term follow-up study of 50 patients with pancreaticoduodenectomy for chronic pancreatitis. World Journal of Surgery 8:346–353

Morrow C E, Cohen J I, Sutherland D E R, Najarian J S 1984 Chronic pancreatitis: long-term surgical results of pancreatic duct drainage, pancreatic resection, and near-total pancreatectomy and islet autotransplantation. Surgery 96:608–616

Nardi G L, Michelassi F, Zannini P 1983 Transduodenal sphincteroplasty. 5–25 year follow-up of 89 patients. Annals of Surgery 198:453–459

Nogueira C E D, Dani R 1985 Evaluation of the surgical treatment of chronic calcifying pancreatitis. Surgery, Gynecology and Obstetrics 161:117–128

Okazaki K, Yamamoto Y, Nishimori I et al 1988 Motility of the sphincter of Oddi and pancreatic main ductal pressure in patients with alcoholic, gallstone-associated and idiopathic chronic pancreatitis. American Journal of Gastroenterology 83:820–826

Partington P F, Rochelle R F 1960 Modified Puestow procedure for retrograde drainage of the pancreatic duct. Annals of Surgery 152:1037–1043

Prinz R A, Bruce H, Frank F A, Greenlee H B 1978 Pancreaticojejunostomy. Archives of Surgery 113:520–525

Prinz R A, Greenlee H B 1981 Pancreatic duct drainage in 100 patients with chronic pancreatitis. Annals of Surgery 194:313–318

Proctor H J, Mendes O C, Thomas C G, Herbst C A 1979 Surgery for chronic pancreatitis. Drainage versus resection. Annals of Surgery 189:664–671

Puestow C B, Gillesby W J 1958 Retrograde surgical drainage of pancreas for chronic relapsing pancreatitis. A.M.A. Archives of Surgery 76:898-907

Rosenberger J, Stock W, Altmann P, Pichlmaier H 1980 Spätergebnisse nach organerhaltenden und resezierenden Eingriffen wegen chronischer Pankreatitis. Leber Magen Darm 10:22–27

Rossi R L. Heiss H W. Braasch J W 1985 Surgical management of chronic pancreatitis. Surgical Clinics of North America 65:79–100

Rossi R L, Rothschild J, Braasch J W, Munson J L, ReMine S G 1987 Pancreatoduodenectomy in the management of chronic pancreatitis. Archives of Surgery 122:416–420

Rückert K, Frick S 1987 Linksresektion. In: Gall P, Hermanek P (eds) Chronische Pankreatitis. Chirurgische Gastroenterologie 3:93–99

Rumpf K D, Pichlmayr R 1983 Eine Methode zur chirurgischen Behandlung der chronischen Pankreatitis: die transduodenale Pankreaticoplastik. Chirurg 54:722–728

Sápy P, Asztalos L, Mikó I, Tarsoly E, Furka I 1983 Intraductal pressure in experimental chronic pancreatitis and the management of decompression after different types of operation. Acta Chirurgica Hungarica 24:155–160

Sarles J-C, Sarles H 1976 Konservative und chirurgische Therapie der chronischen Pankreatitis. Leber Magen Darm 6:294–299

Sarles J-C, Nacchiero M, Garani F, Salasc B 1982 Surgical treatment of chronic pancreatitis. Report of 134 cases treated by resection or drainage. American Journal of Surgery 144:317–321

Sato T, Noto N, Matsuno S, Miyakawa K 1981 Follow-up results of surgical treatment for chronic pancreatitis. Present status in Japan. American Journal of Surgery 142:317–323

Silen W, Baldwin J, Goldman L 1963 Treatment of chronic pancreatitis by longitudinal pancreaticojejunostomy. American Journal of Surgery 106:243–248

Singer M V, Gyr K, Sarles H 1985 Revidierte Klassifikation der Pankreatitis – Marseille 1984. Innere Medizin 12:242–245

Stone W M, Sarr M G, Nagorney D M, McIlrath D C 1988 Chronic pancreatitis. Results of Whipple's resection and total pancreatectomy. Archives of Surgery 123:815–819

Sutherland C M, Muchmore J H, Browder I W, Vega P J 1983 Chronic calcific pancreatitis with pancreatic duct lithiasis due to stenosing papillitis. Southern Medical Journal 76:1318–1319

Taylor R H, Bagley F H, Braasch J W, Warren K W 1981 Ductal drainage or resection for chronic pancreatitis. American Journal of Surgery 141:28–31

Traverso L W, Tompkins R K, Urrea P T, Longmire W P 1979 Surgical treatment of chronic pancreatitis. Twenty-two years' experience. Annals of Surgery 190:312–319

Warshaw A L, Popp J W, Schapiro R H 1980 Long-term patency, pancreatic function and pain relief after lateral pancreaticojejunostomy for chronic pancreatitis. Gastroenterology 79:289–293

Way L W, Gadacz T, Goldmann L 1974 Surgical treatment of chronic pancreatitis. American Journal of Surgery 127:202–209

White T T, Keith R G 1973 Long-term follow-up study of fifty patients with pancreaticojejunostomy. Surgery 136:353–358

White T T, Hart M J 1979 Pancreaticojejunostomy versus resection in the treatment of chronic pancreatitis. American Journal of Surgery 138:129–134

White T T, Slavotinek A H 1979 Results of surgical treatment of chronic pancreatitis. Annals of Surgery 189:217–224

Williamson R C N, Cooper M J 1987 Resection in chronic pancreatitis. British Journal of Surgery 74:807–812

Congenital anomalies of the pancreas

34. Congenital anomalies of the pancreas

F. G. Moody   J. R. Potts III

INTRODUCTION

Pancreas divisum, a relatively common anatomical configuration of the pancreatic duct in man (5–10% of the population), can hardly be considered an infrequent deviation from the normal and thereby classified as an anomaly (Moody 1990). Annular pancreas, a rare anomaly, may not in a strict sense of the word be a congenital birth defect, inasmuch as there is evidence that it may derive from an autosomal dominant gene (MacFadyen & Young 1987). It is convenient, however, to classify these two entities along with pancreatic heterotopia as congenital anomalies, in that each represents an aberration in developmental anatomy, which may be associated with digestive symptoms either in infancy or adult life (McLean 1979).

ANNULAR PANCREAS

Developmental anatomy

The encirclement of the duodenum by pancreatic tissue was first described by Tiedman in 1818 and was ascribed its descriptive name, annular pancreas, by Ecker in 1862. The first successful treatment of duodenal obstruction in a neonate by gastrojejunostomy in 1904 antedated the preoperative diagnosis of annular pancreas (about 1914) by a decade. Experience with this relatively uncommon anomaly increased exponentially over the subsequent decades to the point where 287 cases had been reported in the English literature by 1981 (Brandow et al 1987).

The incidence and prevalence of annular pancreas can be reflected in several ways. It is estimated to be present in 2.5–10 of 100 000 live births. The prevalence is reflected in the finding of an annular pancreas in 3 of 20 000 post-mortems, 1 in 22 000 laparotomies, and in approximately 1 in 200 endoscopic pancreatograms. The frequency of clinical manifestations is reflected in the fact that it accounts for 1% of the cases of intestinal obstruction in children. Assessing prevalence from the point of view of the pancreas, Synn et al (1988) encountered 13 patients with annular pancreas out of 79 under the age of 18 who had pancreatic disease. Because the entity is asymptomatic in most people who have it, the true prevalence and clinical significance is not known.

Aetiology and pathogenesis

Annular pancreas is presumed to represent a failure of rotation of the ventral endodermal bud during the 8th week of gestation as the foregut makes its ninety-degree clockwise rotation to accommodate to the confines of the coelomic cavity (Lloyd-Jones et al 1972). As described above, this is the point in gestation when the ventral and dorsal endodermal buds fuse to form the head and body of the pancreas and the dominant configuration of the drainage system of the pancreas, where the ventral duct (duct of Wirsung) becomes the major outlet for secretions from the gland. Failure of dorsal rotation of the ventral pancreas appears to be a reasonable explanation for encirclement of the duodenum.

It is important to recognize that annular pancreas is associated with numerous other congenital defects, the most relevant being those that relate to the duodenum and gut in general (Kiernan et al 1980). This provides an explanation for its relatively frequent implication in duodenal obstruction in the perinatal period when duodenal stenosis, atresia, duplication, and malrotation of the gut are commonly recognized. If these anomalies or other problems that require laparotomy are not present, then annular pancreas is likely to remain a curiosity only to be found by chance during radiological imaging or exploratory laparotomy in later life, or by autopsy after death.

Clinical manifestations

The clinical manifestations of annular pancreas are best considered at two periods, in infancy and in middle age. Abdominal pain and vomiting, both as a consequence of duodenal obstruction, are the usual features of its presentation in the infant, whereas episodic upper abdominal pain with nausea is a presumptive manifestation of annular pancreatitis in the adult. The vomiting that occasionally accompanies this clinical entity may be related to a local duodenal or generalized ileus that commonly accompanies acute pancreatitis. There are case reports, however, that attest to mechanical obstruction of the duodenum by associated anomalies or from fibrotic constriction of the duodenum as a consequence of chronic inflammation within the annular pancreas (Akers et al 1972, Gilinsky et al 1987). Of special note is the high incidence of peptic ulcer in association with annular pancreas (about 25% of adults who have the anomaly).

The preoperative diagnosis of annular pancreas can be made with a high level of precision with contemporary tools of radiographic imaging. In fact, the diagnosis of duodenal obstruction can now be made by ultrasonography in the third trimester of pregnancy through the detection of a 'double-bubble' sign (Pachi et al 1989). The 'double-bubble' sign is also the way in which duodenal obstruction is identified in the perinatal period and in infancy by plain abdominal radiography as well as ultrasonography, but it must be kept in mind that this sign is not specific for annular pancreas. Computed tomographic radiography (CT) offers the most precise information as to the presence and the status of the pancreas and its annular component (Itoh et al 1989). An example of the 'double-bubble' image as detected by a plain roentgenogram of the abdomen and ultrasonography in infancy is shown in Figure 34.1. The frequent use of endoscopic retrograde pancreatography in the evaluation of upper abdominal pain in the adult has led to a presumptive diagnosis of annular pancreas in 1 in 150–300 cases in two reported series (Chevillotte et al 1984, Yogi et al 1987). Does this mean that the anomaly is in some way a causative factor in the patient's pain? This finding in the absence of objective signs of biliary, pancreatic, or acid-peptic disease poses a diagnostic dilemma. Our opinion, based on inexperience with such patients, can best be classified as 'curiously sceptical'. It is possible that the anomaly in some way contributes to biliary or pancreatic ductal hypertension, a condition that can induce upper abdominal pain. There have been no reports to date, however, that provide manometric or radiographic evidence that the flow of bile or pancreatic juice is impeded by an annular pancreas.

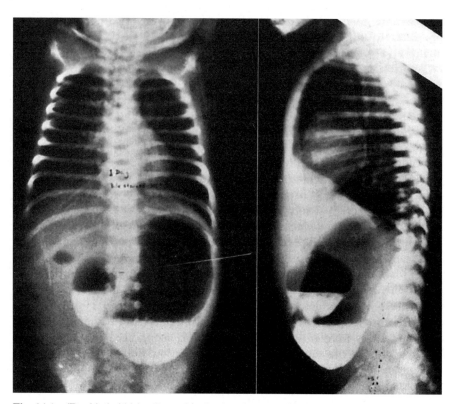

Fig. 34.1 'Double-bubble' radiographic sign in a neonate with duodenal obstruction from an annular pancreas. (Reproduced from Ravitch 1973, Anomalies of the Pancreas, In Carey L C (ed) The Pancreas, p 412, with permission of Mosby–Year Book Inc.)

The evaluation of an infant, either at birth or during its early development, for annular pancreas, should include a plain film of the abdomen and an ultrasound examination after a thorough physical examination. The latter is especially important in view of the high incidence of associated anomalies. Contrast radiography of the upper or lower gastrointestinal tract may be helpful in the differential diagnosis of associated anomalies within the gastrointestinal tract that may be the cause of duodenal obstruction. CT scan is neither practical nor indicated, in that treatment requires laparotomy.

The adult with an annular pancreas presents a different clinical challenge (Lloyd-Jones et al 1972, Thomford et al 1972). The patient is usually a middle-aged female who presents with unexplained episodic upper abdominal pain. If gallstones, pancreatitis, or peptic ulcer is found, then the annular pancreas may be an incidental finding. Ultrasonography of the upper abdomen and an upper gastrointestinal barium study is the simplest and most cost-effective way to pursue these diagnoses. If these tests are negative and the pain persists, an upper gastrointestinal endoscopic examination is indicated. If this is negative, we obtain a CT scan for it represents the best way to detect acute and chronic pancreatitis and the presence of an annular pancreas in the adult. Endoscopic retrograde cholangiopancreatography should be reserved for those patients whose painful episodes persist in spite of symptomatic treatment of irritable bowel or dyspeptic complaints. A diagnostic laparoscopy or laparotomy may be indicated as a procedure of last resort. Although the yield is low, there is in those patients who are incapacitated by their pain and are entering an addictive phase of their illness, an appropriate time for a thorough examination of the abdomen and its retroperitoneum.

Treatment

The treatment for annular pancreas and duodenal obstruction in infancy is bypass of the obstructing lesion by duodenojejunostomy or duodenoduodenostomy (Ravitch & Woods 1950, Merrill & Raffensberger 1976). Inasmuch. as the lesion usually occurs just above the papilla in the second part of the duodenum, the flow of bile and pancreatic juice is usually unimpeded. There is general agreement that no attempt should be made to resect or divide the annular pancreas. Operation in the adult should be directed towards not only bypassing the duodenum, but also reducing the acid secretory capacity of the stomach. A proximal gastric vagotomy with a gastrojejunostomy serves both these ends without interfering with the normal motor function of the antrum and the innervation of the gut distally. Otherwise, peptic ulcer disease, gallstones and biliary tract disease, and acute and chronic pancreatitis should be treated as they would be in patients with a normal anatomical configuration of their pancreas.

HETEROTOPIC PANCREAS

Pancreatic tissue not attached to the pancreas has been reported in a variety of sites within the gut wall, including Meckel's diverticulum and the papilla of Vater as well as the gallbladder, umbilicus, Fallopian tubes, mediastinum, and a gastric duplication (Lai & Tompkins 1986). In the majority of cases, however, there is equal distribution between the stomach, duodenum, and upper jejunum (Feldman & Weinberg 1952). Because the heterotopic pancreas is usually small (0.5 cm on the average) and within the submucosal layer of the gut, it is rarely symptomatic (Dolan et al 1974). Since heterotopic pancreas contains all the elements of normal pancreas, it is not surprising that on rare occasions the ectopic tissue becomes the site of inflammation, neoplasia, or endocrinopathy (insulinoma). Whereas larger lesions that obstruct the duodenal or jejunal lumen have been reported, the majority of even those greater than 0.5 cm are asymptomatic.

The discovery of a submucosal tumour during the work-up of a patient who presents with vague gastrointestinal complaints represents a diagnostic dilemma. Gastric and duodenal pancreatic ectopic foci are best identified by contrast barium radiography (Martinez et al 1958). Rarely, the lesion will present with an umbilicated centre or reveal its fluid-filled ducts as 'the spokes of a wheel' in a thin barium coating. Upper gastrointestinal endoscopy usually does not further elucidate the nature of the lesion but should be done to establish that it is not of epithelial origin.

There is a consensus that submucosal lesions that are small and asymptomatic should not be removed unless they present as a polyp that can be removed transendoscopically. Patients who present with occult gastrointestinal bleeding or vague complaints may benefit from local resection of the submucosal lesion in the duodenal wall (most occur on the mesenteric or pancreatic border of the duodenum), or full thickness excision if on the antimesenteric wall of the duodenum or within the stomach. Such lesions should not be excised when encountered incidentally during the palpation of the gut wall in the course of exploration of the abdominal contents prior to another operative procedure. The relatively frequent occurrence of pancreatic heterotopia (0.5–14% of the population) means that it may be found by digestive and trauma surgeons who carefully inspect the wall of the gastrointestinal tract whenever they enter the abdomen.

PANCREAS DIVISUM

The anatomical configuration of the ductal system that

delivers the pancreatic effluent to the duodenum has been the subject of extensive study (Millbourn 1950). It has been well documented that the most common relationship of the ducts that drain the dorsal and ventral lobes of the pancreas is one in which they join within the neck of the gland. The duct of Wirsung enters the duodenum along with the bile duct by passing through the papilla of Vater, and is usually the dominant route for pancreatic exocrine secretion. The duct of Santorini, which enters through a separate opening cephalad to the papilla of Vater, is of variable diameter and importance as a conduit for the delivery of pancreatic secretion to the gut (Baldwin 1911). In 5–10% of people, the ducts of Santorini and Wirsung have no identifiable communication within the gland. In this situation, the duct of Santorini is the major route for secretion from the dorsal pancreas. The duct of Wirsung in this case drains only the ventral lobe of the pancreas and thereby represents a minor route for pancreatic secretion. This arrangement, termed 'pancreas divisum' by Opie in 1913, has been suspected of being a potential cause of pancreatic disease, especially in cases where the opening of the duct of Santorini was too small to handle the flow of secretion from the body of the pancreas. These two arrangements have been commented upon (Baldwin 1911) and are shown from the ventral or anterior surface of the gland in Figure 34.2. The following discussion reviews the developmental anatomy of the pancreas, and the evidence for and against whether pancreas divisum per se can produce signs and symptoms of pancreatic disease.

Developmental anatomy

The pancreas derives form two separate endodermal buds from the foregut during the 4th and 6th weeks of gestation. The ventral lobe of the pancreas is shared with that of the biliary tree, and it is for this reason that its duct, first described by Wirsung, empties into the duodenum with the bile duct within the papilla of Vater. The dorsal pancreas has a direct communication with the duodenum and its accessory or minor papilla through the duct of Santorini (Berman et al 1960). During gestation, the duodenum rotates clockwise on its long axis in order to accommodate to the confines of the coelomic cavity, and in doing so brings the bile duct and ventral lobe of the pancreas posterior to the dorsal lobe of the pancreas and the duct of Santorini (Fig. 34.3). In about 90% of people (autopsy studies), the duct of Wirsung fuses with the dorsal pancreatic duct and becomes the major outflow tract for the pancreas. Although a minor or accessory papilla is always present, its communication with the dorsal pancreas through the duct of Santorini is either too small to identify or not present in about 50% of autopsy specimens. Pancreas divisum, a situation in which the dorsal and ventral ducts fail to fuse, occurs in about 10% of the population of patients whose pancreas was studied after autopsy and found to be free of pancreatic disease. The fact that only 5% of patients without demonstrable pancreatic disease have non-fused ducts at the time of retrograde endoscopic pancreatography remains an unexplained curiosity (Mitchell et al 1979).

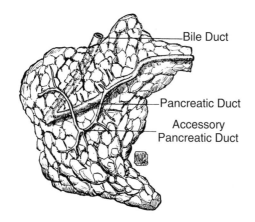

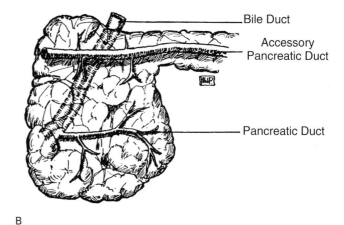

A

B

Fig. 34.2 **A** Anterior view of the head of the pancreas demonstrating the relationships between the fused dorsal and ventral (accessory) pancreatic ducts to the bile duct. **B** In pancreas divisum, the ductal system (pancreatic duct) in the ventral lobe of the pancreas fails to join the dorsal (accessory) ductal system. In this anatomical configuration, the dorsal duct drains the major portion of the head and body of the pancreas through the duct of Santorini that enters the duodenum at the minor papilla. (From Baldwin, The Anatomical Record 5:213, copyright © 1911 American Association of Anatomists. Reprinted by permission of Wiley-Liss, a division of John Wiley and Sons, Inc.)

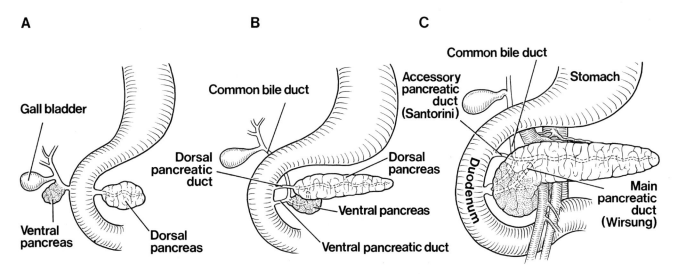

Fig. 34.3 This schematic diagram reveals **A** the development early in gestation of endodermal buds that will ultimately become the pancreas from the ventral and dorsal surfaces of the foregut; **B** the ventral lobe rotates behind the evolving duodenum to join the dorsal lobe; **C** the subsequent fusion of the ductal systems leads to continuity of the drainage of both lobes of the pancreas through the primordial ventral duct (duct of Wirsung). Failure to fuse leads to the variant called pancreas divisum, whereby the dorsal duct (Santorini) becomes the dominant outflow track for pancreatic secretion. (Reproduced with permission from Leese et al 1989 Pancreatitis caused by congenital anomalies of the pancreatic ducts, Surgery 105:127, Mosby-Year Book Inc.)

Baldwin (1911), in an extensive review of autopsy studies, found that the accessory duct or duct of Santorini was absent in 62 of 209 specimens examined by injection techniques. A junction between the dorsal and ventral systems was not observed in 32 of 349 studies, whereas the accessory duct was longer than the major duct in 24 of 310 studies. Unfortunately, the important point of whether the accessory or duct of Santorini was present or absent in patients with non-fusion was not commented upon. It must be assumed however that the minor duct was of sufficient size to allow instillation of the injectant used to visualize the dorsal system.

Pancreas divisum and pancreatic disease

Because pancreas divisum is a common anatomical configuration of the pancreatic ductal system, it would be expected that it would be recognized with equal or increased frequency in patients who undergo pancreatography for presumed pancreatic disease. As pointed out above, the prevalence of the entity as assessed by pancreatography (5%) is only half that identified by anatomical cadaveric studies (10%). Whether pancreas divisum is in fact an aetiological factor in pancreatic disease is therefore a statistical problem. Endoscopic visualization of the major as well as minor pancreatic ductal systems has allowed an approach to the question of whether the entity occurs with increased frequency in patients with pancreatic disease. Mitchell et al (1979) in Leeds, in fact, did not find an increased incidence of pancreas divisum

in patients with pancreatitis in a review of 449 endoscopic retrograde pancreatograms. Cotton (1980), however, observed an increased frequency of pancreas divisum in patients with pancreatitis who had successfully undergone endoscopic retrograde pancreatography. In 877 patients in whom pancreatography was indicated and successful, 47 were found to have pancreas divisum (5.8%). The variant was present in 3.6% of patients with biliary tract disease and 16.4% of 188 patients with acute or chronic pancreatitis. Unfused ducts were found most frequently in patients with 'idiopathic recurrent pancreatitis' (20 of 78 patients whose duct(s) were visualized). This report in 1980 drew attention to the possibility that pancreas divisum itself might have pathogenetic significance in pancreatic disease.

A more comprehensive study by Delhaye et al in Belgium (1985) of 5357 patients who had successful endoscopic pancreatography revealed that there was no statistical difference between patients with non-pancreatic disease (5.5%), or chronic (6.4%), or acute pancreatitis (7.5%), as shown in Table 34.1. Others, however, have observed a higher incidence of pancreas divisum in patients with acute pancreatitis (Cotton 1980, Gregg 1977). The issue of clinical significance has not yet been resolved (Cotton 1982). It has been recognized, however, that acute and chronic pancreatitis can lead to a discontinuity of the dorsal and ventral ductal systems and therefore account for an acquired pancreas divisum at the time of pancreatography. Clearly, in this situation the disease would be the cause of the variant anatomy, rather than the reverse.

Table 34.1 Prevalence of pancreas divisum in pancreatic and nonpancreatic diseases. (Reproduced with permission from Delhaye et al 1985, Gastroenterology 89: 955.)

Disease	Number of patients	Number with pancreas divisum	% Incidence	$p^{\star}$
Chronic pancreatitis	406	26	6.4	NS
Acute pancreatitis	335	25	7.5	NS
Pancreatic carcinoma	291	16	5.5	NS
Papillary carcinoma	68	2	2.9	NS
Nonpancreatic diseases	4257	235	5.5	NS
Total	5357	304	5.7	

χ^2 analysis; $\star$ NS not significant.

Therapeutic outcomes

A second approach to defining the clinical relevance of pancreas divisum derives from attempts to improve drainage of the dorsal duct by sphincteroplasty of the duct of Santorini, the duct of Wirsung, or both ducts. The operative indications and approach will be discussed below. Let us here examine the evidence for a role of pancreas divisum in the causation of pain of presumed pancreatic origin. Heiss and Shea (1978) reported their experience with four patients with recurrent episodes of abdominal pain and hyperamylasaemia who were found at endoscopic retrograde pancreatography to have a non-fused ductal system. One patient, a male, was found to have advanced chronic cicatricial pancreatitis and underwent a subtotal distal pancreatectomy. A second patient (36-year-old female) with recurrent episodes of abdominal pain underwent sphincteroplasty of the minor papilla with interruption of her episodic pain for the 6-month follow-up period. The third patient underwent a dual sphincteroplasty without discussion of the outcome, and the fourth was not operated upon. The authors speculated from this experience that the pancreatitis in this group of patients might have been the consequence of inadequate flow through the minor papilla. The brief nature of the case studies in this report provided little support for this tenable but undocumented speculation.

The Gastrointestinal Unit at the Middlesex Hospital in London has made important contributions to our understanding of the relationship between non-fusion of the ventral and dorsal ducts and pancreatitis. Cotton and Kizu (1977) reported on 24 patients with pancreas divisum whose anatomical variant was recognized at the time of endoscopic retrograde cholangiopancreatography (ERCP). Three of these patients had a dilated dorsal duct. An endoscopic papillotomy was performed on one of these patients with a good 'short-term' result. This experience was expanded upon to the point (Cotton 1980) whereby 20 of 78 patients were shown to have pancreas divisum by endoscopic pancreatography who otherwise had no identifiable factors (gallstones, alcohol, trauma) as a cause for their presumed pancreatitis. Eight of 19 patients in whom alcohol was not implicated underwent specific treatment, six surgically and two by endoscopic accessory sphincteroplasty. Unfortunately, the outcomes from these procedures were not reported. The analysis of this patient population stressed the critical role that chronic alcohol ingestion might play in patients with pancreas divisum. The clinical stratification of 47 patients with pancreas divisum is shown in Table 34.2.

Gregg (1977) identified 33 patients with pancreas divisum in his first 1100 ERCP examinations. A total of 15 were considered to have pancreatitis by clinical and laboratory criteria. Secretin stimulation of pancreatic exocrine secretion in six patients revealed a mean flow of pancreatic juice of 0.2 ml/min from the ventral pancreas and 3.4 ml/min from the dorsal duct. The diagnosis of pancreas divisum was made by this technique in four patients in whom neither the ventral nor dorsal ducts were visualized. Gregg (1977) speculated that the small size of the duct of Santorini that provides the only drainage for the relatively large dorsal gland may be the cause of pancreatitis in this condition. Gregg et al (1983) subsequently reported on 19 patients with pancreatitis and pancreas divisum, who underwent a standardized surgical approach that included exploratory laparotomy, cholecystectomy (if not previously performed), and a

Table 34.2 Clinical grouping of 47 patients with pancreas divisum. (Reproduced by permission of the British Medical Association from Cotton (1980) Gut 21: 108.)

Group	Total	Clinical status	Anomaly relevance
A	9	Definite non-pancreatic pain	Nil
B	19	Idiopathic recurrent pancreatitis	Probable
C	10	Alcohol-associated pancreatitis	Possible
D	9	Pancreatic-type pain without definite evidence of pancreatitis	Probable

sphincteroplasty of the major and minor ducts. One patient died of acute pancreatitis. Initially, 13 patients gained pain relief during an interval of follow-up of 6–12 months. Four had a recurrence of symptoms within 6 months, and five had an unsatisfactory result early after operation. Six of these eight failures were reoperated upon in a variety of ways, with only a 50% improvement rate. This early study paralleled the relative success rate reported by others who attempted to interrupt episodes of pancreatitis or relieve abdominal pain by surgical means.

Richter et al (1981) at the Massachusetts General Hospital reported on nine patients with pancreas divisum who also underwent a surgical enlargement of the accessory papilla as well as cholecystectomy and sphincteroplasty of the major papilla and the duct of Wirsung, if these procedures had not previously been performed. Five of six patients with documented episodes of acute pancreatitis had no further attacks over 9–42 months follow-up. The one failure was in a patient with chronic pancreatitis. Three patients with recurrent episodes of abdominal pain but no documented evidence of pancreatitis did not benefit from dual duct sphincteroplasty.

Warshaw et al (1990) reported on the long-term follow-up of 100 patients surgically treated at the Massachusetts General Hospital for symptomatic pancreas divisum. Patients with chronic pancreatitis were excluded from the study. There were 77 females and 23 males; none were known to be alcoholics. It is of interest that only one patient had a dilated dorsal duct on pancreatography, and only 'a few' had delayed emptying of contrast after the study. The majority (66 of 88 patients undergoing accessory sphincteroplasty) had evidence of stenosis at the mucosal level. The overall results during a 6-month to 4- or more years follow-up (93% of patients operated upon) revealed that approximately 59% were totally free of pain during the period of observation. The authors ascribed their improved results to their selection criteria; these included ultrasonographic evidence of dorsal duct dilatation as an indicator of ductal hypertension, following stimulation of pancreatic exocrine secretion by the intravenous administration of secretin in a dose of 1 mg/kg body weight. Over 90% of patients with a positive ultrasound–secretin test obtained benefit. In view of these extraordinary results, Warshaw et al (1990) have suggested that the therapeutic focus should be on the accessory papilla and the efficiency of emptying of the dorsal duct rather than the non-fusion of the ductal systems in pancreas divisum.

In spite of enthusiastic reports of the benefits of accessory sphincteroplasty by Warshaw et al (1990) and others (Keith et al 1982, Madura 1986, Marshall & Eckhauser 1985) with similar experience and shorter follow-up, there are also reports of only modest success with this approach (Britt et al 1983, Russell et al 1984, Traverso et al 1982). A critical analysis of reported outcomes is difficult because many patients in all series have undergone concomitant cholecystectomy or procedures on the papilla of Vater. Furthermore, the presence of pancreatitis is hard to document unless the patient has evidence of fibrosis or fluid accumulation in or around the gland.

There is a suggestion, however, in the results thus far reported that there is a subset of patients with pancreas divisum who have recurrent episodes of upper abdominal pain, with or without hyperamylasaemia, on the basis of a restriction in the rate of excretion of pancreatic juice through the duct of Santorini and the accessory papilla. The gastrointestinal group at the Middlesex Hospital (Blair et al 1984) has come to a similar conclusion in their study of over 300 patients with pancreas divisum. This group has also provided histological evidence that the dorsal pancreas is the likely source of pancreatic pain, in that the pancreas of nine of 14 patients with pancreas divisum who underwent pancreatectomy (10 Whipple procedures and four total pancreatectomies), revealed histological evidence of chronic inflammation. In two pancreaticoduodenectomy specimens, the ventral portion of the gland was normal, whereas the dorsal pancreas revealed the typical histological characteristics of chronic pancreatitis. It is of note that eight of the 10 patients undergoing pancreaticoduodenectomy were improved by this approach to their debilitating and painful illness. There were no deaths and minimal early and late morbidity. The authors suggest that proximal resection (Whipple procedure) of the pancreas is the procedure of choice in patients with pancreas divisum and well-established chronic pancreatitis and narcotic addictive pain. On the basis of this experience, Blair et al (1984) are less enthusiastic about accessory sphincteroplasty alone when performed either endoscopically or by a transduodenal surgical approach. Endoscopic accessory sphincteroplasty was accomplished in five of 12 patients but only one patient gained pain relief.

Personal views

Our experience of the surgical treatment of paients with symptomatic pancreas divisum is limited. We have attempted to present the results as they have been reported, without making a value judgment as to their validity. A surgical experience with 12 patients with pancreas divisum has, however, provided us with an opportunity to experience many of the findings described in the literature with regard to anatomical variations as well as clinical outcomes. From this experience and that reported in the literature, we do not believe that pancreas divisum per se is a major factor in pancreatic inflammation or in the episodic abdominal pain experienced by some patients who are subsequently shown to have an unfused ductal system on endoscopic pancreatography. Warshaw et al (1990) are on the right track. Some patients who have the duct of Santorini as the major pancreatic outflow tract have an opening at the accessory papilla that is too small to allow free flow of pancreatic juice during the stimulated state. The submucosal vestibule that he describes is present in some patients but not in others. A dilated dorsal duct in the absence of chronic pancreatitis is a rare finding. It is conceivable that endoscopic ultrasonography of the duodenum in the region of the papilla may, in future, offer a useful way to identify patients with outflow resistance at the level of the mucosal opening of the minor papilla, a situation in which pancreatic juice accumulates within a submucosal vestibule.

We have preformed transduodenal sphincteroplasty of the major papilla and transampullary septectomy of the atretic duct of Wirsung in the 12 patients whom we have treated surgically for pancreas divisum. Of these patients, 11 had previously undergone cholecystectomy and were presumed to have pain from stenosing papillitis secondary to the chronic passage of gallstones. Seven underwent a concurrent accessory duct sphincteroplasty. The outcome in this small number of patients was the same with or without accessory sphincteroplasty.

Madura (1986) has reported a 75% success rate with dual sphincteroplasty in patients with gallstone disease. Unfortunately, a large number of patients who underwent concomitant cholecystectomy had abnormal gallbladders (12 of 14). In this situation, it is difficult to ascribe pain relief solely to sphincteroplasty of the ductal systems. Most reported studies have a similarly large percentage of patients who have undergone concomitant cholecystectomy, and in some, the pathological state of the gallbladder is not mentioned.

Patient selection for treatment

The above discussion reveals the confusion surrounding the question of which patients with pancreas divisum should be treated, and by what means. Warshaw et al (1990) have had the largest and most successful experience with the problem. The patients in the series who derived the most benefit from sphincteroplasty of the accessory ducts were those with a positive ultrasound–secretin study, who were non-alcoholic, and did not have an abnormal pancreas at operation. Warshaw emphasizes the importance of the resistance at the mucosal opening of the accessory duct, rather than the calibre of the duct of Santorini or the duct draining the dorsal pancreas. Unfortunately, the role of the gallbladder or the papilla of Vater and duct of Wirsung is de-emphasized in their reports; therefore, it is difficult to discern the role that gallstone disease might play in the patients' episodic pain and hyperamylasaemia. In order to prove the hypothesis that the pain is due to hypertension

in the dorsal duct, it will be necessary for the studies to include a cohort of patients without gallstones or pancreatic disease, who undergo only an accessory papillotomy, and who have dilatation of the duct with secretin stimulation.

There is no reason to remove a normal gallbladder when sphincteroplasty is not performed on the papilla of Vater. The random selection of a major versus minor sphincteroplasty might be hard to justify on ethical grounds, but further perfection of endoscopic enlargement of the minor as well as the major papilla and the opening of the duct of Wirsung, may help to clarify whether the episodic pain experienced by some patients with pancreas divisum is due to a problem in the dorsal or the ventral pancreas. One must remain sceptical as to whether either the dorsal or ventral ductal systems, or their openings, play any role in the episodic pain of pancreatitis associated with pancreas divisum; the variant is common, whereas the incidence of those who have symptoms in its presence is exceedingly low. Furthermore, the prevalence is equally distributed between males and females, whereas those who have symptoms with pancreas divisum are for the most part females and in their middle age.

We agree with Russell et al (1984) that patients with pancreas divisum and chronic pancreatitis should be treated as other patients with chronic addictive pain are treated. Pancreaticoduodenectomy appears to be well suited to this purpose, as their results show, because the operation removes the defective ventral lobe and allows preservation of the majority of the body and tail of the gland.

Patients with gallstones and pancreas divisum should undergo cholecystectomy and removal of common duct stones if found at operation, as their initial treatment. Usually, a preoperative endoscopic cholangiogram will have identified the presence of duct stones and led to their transpapillary removal following endoscopic papillotomy. Transduodenal sphincteroplasty with transampullary septectomy should be reserved for patients who have a well established unrelenting episodic post-cholecystectomy pain. The visualization of a dilated dorsal duct requires, in addition, an enlargement of the opening of the duct of Santorini, a procedure that will be described below. As has been described so clearly by Warshaw et al (1990), we attempt to identify patients who have a mucosal stenosis and a normal dorsal duct by stimulating the pancreas to secrete at a maximal rate during exploration of the duodenal lumen. The slow intravenous administration of secretin in a dose of 1 mg/kg body weight will identify a submucosal swelling of the minor papilla in such patients. The prominence of the accessory papilla and exudation of pancreatic juice through its pinpoint ostium allows cannulation with a small diameter lacrimal probe. The mucosal web is excised in the direction of the maximal extent of the papillary swelling, thereby unroofing the opening of the duct of Santorini as it exits the muscularis of the duodenal wall. This technique will also be described below. We believe that patients with normal accessory papillae and dorsal ducts should not be subjected to either transendoscopic or transduodenal sphincteroplasty. Furthermore, neither the minor nor major pancreatic ducts should be stented, because injury or fibrosis of either duct may lead to stenosis and acute and chronic pain or subsequent pancreatitis in an otherwise normal organ. All surgical reports describe a normal-appearing pancreas at exploratory laparotomy, except in cases in which clinical pancreatitis is suspected following preoperative evaluation. Probably the signs of mild acute pancreatitis found at exploration in some patients are secondary to the performance of a pancreatogram prior to operation.

Operative technique

We will not describe how one should perform cholecystectomy. This procedure has been well standardized over the past 100 years and now is being modified by a less invasive laparoscopic approach. The convenience and, hopefully, safety of the procedure in the future will reduce the temptation to do concurrent procedures on the major or minor papillae that house the termination of the ducts of Santorini and Wirsung respectively. As mentioned above, cholecystectomy, when gallstones are present, is the first step in the treatment of patients with episodic upper abdominal pain and pancreas divisum.

We have standardized the transduodenal approach to sphincteroplasty of the papilla of Vater and the transampullary septectomy to enlarge the opening of the duct of Wirsung. The operative approach is similar in patients with pancreas divisum except for two important points. First, the opening of the duct of Wirsung may be small and difficult to identify. It was present in the 12 cases we have operated upon, but secretin stimulation and vascular loupes are required to find it. Second, the duct of Wirsung is small and short, and in some patients, the ventral lobe is remarkably deficient. Manipulation of the duct therefore must be gentle in order to avoid penetration outside its lumen.

Accessory sphincteroplasty must be carried out with great precision, because injury or occlusion of the orifice could compromise the patient's major outflow tract. A thorough exploration of the abdominal cavity and its lesser sac is required prior to either procedure. We fully mobilize the duodenum and the head of the pancreas in patients with pancreas divisum so that the major and accessory papilla are in full view following a 2 cm longitudinal anterior duodenotomy. Only experienced pancreatic surgeons should undertake this procedure. A long (2 cm) anterior sphincteroplasty of the papilla of

Vater should be performed prior to embarking upon manipulation of the minor papilla. The accessory papilla usually lies approximately 2–4 cm cephalad and to the left of the major papilla. It sometimes can be more easily palpated than seen, especially when secretion has been administered and a submucosal cistern is present. It is not always possible to insert even the smallest lacrimal probe when mucosal stenosis is present. In this situation, we carefully incise the point of efflux of pancreatic juice, a manoeuvre that allows free flow of pancreatic juice and the insertion of the probe which can then be used as a guide for a deeper division. In patients with a dilated duct, it is possible to approximate the mucosa of the enlarged duct of Santorini to the duodenal mucosa with 7–0 polyglycolic acid sutures placed in interrupted fashion. In cases with mucosal stenosis and a submucosal cistern, there is usually little ductal mucosa to approximate. In this situation, we place sutures at each quadrant of the small orifice of the duct of Santorini to reduce the possibility of scar formation. A headlight and at least ×2.5 magnification is required to perform this procedure. We do not advocate the placement of a stent or the performance of a pancreatogram at its completion. Rather, we sound the duct with a 5 or 3 Fr infant feeding tube to ensure its patency. Figure 34.4 depicts the essential steps in the procedure of enlarging the opening of the minor duct as it enters the duodenum.

A meticulous closure of the duodenotomy is an essential part of the procedure. The duodenotomy is best closed longitudinally with an inner continuous fine absorbable suture to approximate all layers of the duodenal wall, which is then reinforced by fine non-absorbable sutures placed in an interrupted serosubmucosal (Lembert) fashion. The suture line should be covered with adjacent omentum to prevent contact with a single active drain that is placed in the subhepatic space and removed in 36–48 hours.

The procedure is usually followed by 48–72 hours of duodenal dysfunction. The patient will benefit form nasogastric suction during this period. Diet progression therafter is tailored to the patient's tolerance.

Long-term follow-up is essential and should be scheduled at appropriate intervals. We advise patients to keep a symptom diary and to call us between visits if they experience severe episodes of pain. The most difficult aspect of pain management is the process of detoxification. Patients must be formally detoxified within the confines of a facility designed for management of the complex problem of medical addiction. Most patients, however, want to go home and attempt weaning from narcotics on an ambulatory basis. This is difficult if not impossible to achieve if the patient lives at a distance. Fortunately, only very few patients with pancreas divisum have clinical symptoms or signs of pancreatic disease, and an even smaller number need a surgical approach to their problem.

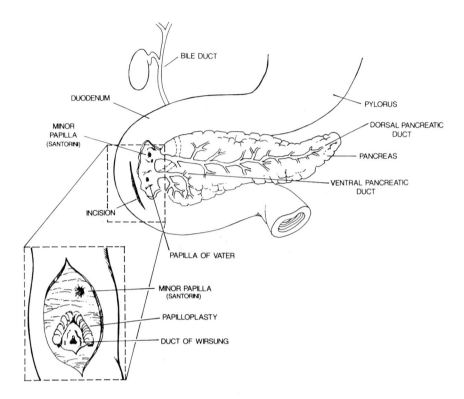

Fig. 34.4 The dorsal and ventral pancreatic ducts in pancreas divisum enter the duodenum through separate openings in the second part of the duodenum. As shown schematically in the insert, the surgical treatment of outflow obstruction to pancreatic secretion entails the enlargement of the minor and major papillae by precise incision and reconstruction of each opening. Division of the papilla of Vater requires a complete division of the sphincter of Oddi and excision of the transampullary septum at the ostium of the duct of Wirsung. This procedure should be performed on highly selected patients who have evidence of recurrent pancreatitis and an abnormality of the minor or major papilla.

CONCLUSION

Annular pancreas, pancreatic heterotopia, and pancreas divisum are well recognized developmental abnormalities of the pancreas. Although these anomalies may remain undetected during infancy or even adult life, they each have unique and clinically identifiable manifestations. Annular pancreas may present as duodenal obstruction in infancy or as abdominal pain from acute or chronic pancreatitis in the adult. Duodenal stenosis is a commonly associated anomaly in the former population, and duodenal ulcer is often a presenting complaint in the latter. A duodenojejunal bypass of the obstructing duodenal stenosis is the treatment of choice. Division or resection of an annular pancreas should be avoided except when it is the site of a neoplastic process.

Pancreatic heterotopia is usually a diagnostic curiosity that is manifested as a shadow on a barium roentgenogram of the upper gastrointestinal tract or by palpation as a small intramural (submucosal) lesion of the stomach or small intestine at the time of laparotomy. Small lesions rarely cause symptoms. When large, they can lead to intestinal obstruction or upper gastrointestinal bleeding. In this situation, the involved portion of the bowel should be resected or the lesion removed by local excision.

Pancreas divisum is a common anomaly of the pancreatic ductal system whereby the ventral duct of Wirsung fails to join with the dorsal or dominant duct of the pancreas. In this situation, the duct of Santorini becomes the major outflow port for pancreatic secretion. Whether pancreas divisum can per se lead to pancreatic pain or inflammation is unclear. The incidence of pancreatic disease does not appear to be higher than that experienced by those individuals who have a normally fused ductal system. However, some patients with recurrent episodes of abdominal pain from presumed pancreatitis have pancreas divisum, and they are relieved of their symptoms by enlargement of the opening of the duct of Santorini. Patients with gallstone disease also may develop stenosing papillitis and stenosis of the opening of the already atretic duct of Wirsung. These patients appear to benefit from a combined enlargement of the opening of the minor and major papillae and the ostium of the duct of Wirsung.

REFERENCES

Akers D R, Favara B E, Franciosi R A, Nelson J M 1972 Duplications of the alimentary tract: Report of three unusual cases associated with bile and pancreatic ducts. Surgery 71: 817–823

Baldwin W M 1911 The pancreatic ducts in man, together with a study of the microscopical structure of the minor duodenal papilla. The Anatomical Record 5: 197–228

Berman L G, Prior J T, Abramow S M, Ziegler D D 1960 A study of the pancreatic duct system in man by the use of vinyl acetate casts of postmortem preparations. Surgery, Gynecology and Obstetrics 110: 391–403

Blair A J III, Russell C G, Cotton P B 1984 Resection for pancreatitis in patients with pancreas divisum. Annals of Surgery 200: 590–594

Brandow K R, Neville R, Fielding L P 1987 Clinical relevance of an exploratory laparotomy: general principles derived from a singular instance of annular pancreas. Current Surgery 44: 98–101

Britt L G, Samuels A D, Johnson J W Jr 1983 Pancreas divisum: is it a surgical disease? Annals of Surgery 197: 654–662

Chevillotte G, Sahel J, Raillat A, Sarles H 1984 Annular pancreas: Report of one case associated with acute pancreatitis and diagnosed by endoscopic retrograde pancreatography. Digestive Diseases and Sciences 29: 75–77

Cotton P B 1980 Congenital anomaly of pancreas divisum as cause of obstructive pain and pancreatitis. Gut 21: 105–114

Cotton P B 1982 Pancreas divisum. Gastroenterology (Correspondence) 82: 1001

Cotton P B, Kizu M 1977 Malfusion of dorsal and ventral pancreas; a cause of pancreatitis? Gut (Correspondence) 18: A400

Delhaye M, Engelholm L, Cremer M 1985 Pancreas divisum: congenital variant or anomaly? Gastroenterology 89: 951–958

Dolan R V, ReMine W H, Dockerty M B 1974 The fate of heterotopic pancreatic tissue. Archives of Surgery 109: 762–765

Feldman M, Weinberg T 1952 Aberrant pancreas: A cause of duodenal syndrome. Journal of the American Medical Association 148: 893–898

Gilinsky N H, Lewis J W, Flueck J A, Fried A M 1987 Annular pancreas associated with diffuse chronic pancreatitis. American Journal of Gastroenterology 82: 681–684

Gregg J A 1977 Pancreas divisum: its association with pancreatitis. American Journal of Surgery 134: 539–543

Gregg J A, Monaco A P, McDermott W V 1983 Pancreas divisum results of surgical intervention. American Journal of Surgery 145: 488–492

Heiss F W, Shea J A 1978 Association of pancreatitis and variant ductal anatomy. American Journal of Gastroenterology 770: 158–162

Itoh Y, Hada T, Terano A, Itai Y, Harada T 1989 Pancreatitis in the annulus of annular pancreas demonstrated by the combined use of computed tomography and endoscopic retrograde cholangiopancreatography. American Journal of Gastroenterology 84: 961–964

Keith R G, Shapero T F, Saibil F G 1982 Treatment of pancreatitis associated with pancreas divisum by dorsal duct sphincterotomy alone. Candian Journal of Surgery 25: 622–626

Kiernan P D, ReMine S G, Kiernan P C, ReMine W H 1980 Annular pancreas: Mayo Clinic experience from 1957–1976 with review of the literature. Archives of Surgery 115: 46–50

Lai E C S, Tompkins R K 1986 Heterotopic pancreas. American Journal of Surgery 151: 697–700

Leese T, Chiche L, Bismuth H 1989 Pancreatitis caused by congenital anomalies of the pancreatic ducts. Surgery 105: 125–130

Lloyd-Jones W, Mountain J C, Warren K W 1972 Annular pancreas in the adult. Annals of Surgery 176: 163–170

MacFadyen U M, Young I D 1987 Annular pancreas in mother and son. American Journal of Medical Genetics (Correspondence) 27: 987–988

Mchean J M 1979 Embryology of the pancreas. In: Howarth T, Sarles H (eds) The exocrine pancreas. W B Saunders, Philadelphia, p 3–14

Madura J A 1986 Pancreas divisum: Stenosis of the dorsally dominant pancreatic duct. American Journal of Surgery 742–745

Marshall J B, Eckhauser M L 1985 Pancreas divisum a cause of chronic relapsing pancreatitis. Digestive Diseases and Sciences 30: 582–587

Martinez N S, Morlock C G, Dockerty M B, Waugh J M, Weber H M 1958 Heterotopic pancreatic tissue involving the stomach. Annals of Surgery 147: 1–12

Merrill J R, Raffensberger J G 1976 Pediatric annular pancreas: Twenty years' experience. Journal of Pediatric Surgery 11: 921–925

Millbourn E 1950 On the excretory ducts of the pancreas in man, with special reference to their relations to each other, to the common bile duct and to the duodenum. Acta Anatomica IX: 1–34

Mitchell C J, Lintott D J, Ruddell W S J, Losowsky M S, Axon A T R 1979 Clinical relevance of an unfused pancreatic duct system. Gut 20: 1066–1071

Moody F G 1990 Pancreas divisum and other surgical anomalies of the pancreatic ducts. In: Najarian J S, Delaney J P (eds) Progress in Hepatic, Biliary and Pancreatic Surgery. Mosby-Year Book, Chicago, p 260–268

Pachi A, Maggi E, Giancotti A, Torcia F, De Prosperi V 1989 Ultrasound diagnosis of fetal annular pancreas. Journal of Perinatal Medicine 17: 361–364

Ravitch M M 1973 Anomalies of the pancreas. In: Carey L C (ed) The Pancreas. Mosby, St. Louis, 404–416

Ravitch M M, Woods A C 1950 Annular pancreas. Annals of Surgery 132: 1116–1127

Richter J M, Schapiro R H, Mulley A G, Warshaw A L 1981 Association of pancreas divisum and pancreatitis, and its treatment by sphincteroplasty of the accessory ampulla. Gastroenterology 81: 1104–1110

Russell R C G, Wong N W, Cotton P B 1984 Accessory sphincterotomy (endoscopic and surgical) in patients with pancreas divisum. British Journal of Surgery 1984: 954–957

Synn A Y, Mulvihill S J, Fonkalsrud E W 1988 Surgical disorders of the pancreas in infancy and childhood. American Journal of Surgery 156: 201–205

Thomford H R, Knight P R, Pace W G, Madura J A 1972 Annular pancreas in the adult: selection of operation. Annals of Surgery 176: 159–162

Traverso L W, Perry W W, Musser G, Frey C F, Tompkins R K 1982 Pancreas divisum: the role of pancreatic duct drainage. Surgical Gastroenterology 1: 11–16

Warshaw A L, Simeone J F,. Schapiro R H, Flavin-Warshaw B 1990 Evaluation and treatment of the dominant dorsal duct syndrome (pancreas divisum redefined). American Journal of Surgery 159: 59–66

Yogi Y, Shibue T, Hashimoto S 1987 Annular pancreas detected in the adult diagnosed by endoscopic retrograde cholangiopancreatography: Report of four cases. Gastroenterologia Japonica 22: 92–99

Tumours of the exocrine pancreas and periampullary region

35. Aetiology and epidemiology of pancreatic and periampullary cancer

D. C. Carter

AETIOLOGY OF PANCREATIC CANCER

The cause of pancreatic ductal adenocarcinoma is unknown. Animal models have as yet shed little light on the factors that initiate the disease in man and much of our imperfect understanding of the aetiology of human pancreatic cancer has been derived from demographic and epidemiological studies. The disease continues to have an appalling prognosis with less than 1% of patients surviving for more than 5 years from diagnosis (Gudjonsson 1987), so that mortality rates and annual incidence are virtually identical.

INCIDENCE AND MORTALITY RATES

The incidence of pancreatic cancer appears to have increased steadily in many countries over the past 50–60 years. For example, in the United States the age adjusted mortality rate rose from 2.9 per 100 000 population to 9 per 100 000 in the period 1920 to 1970 (American Cancer Society 1977). There is evidence that its annual incidence is now levelling off at approximately 10 new cases per 100 000 of the population (Gordis & Gold 1984), the plateau effect being most marked in males (Fontham & Correa 1989). It has been estimated that the disease accounts for 24 500 deaths each year in the USA alone (American Cancer Society 1988), making it the fifth leading cause of death after cancer of the lung, large intestine, breast and prostate, and second only to colorectal cancer as a cause of death from cancer of the digestive tract. In the United Kingdom the mortality of pancreatic cancer doubled between 1930 and 1970 (Office of Population Censuses and Surveys 1975) and some 6520 cases have been registered annually in recent years (Cancer Research Campaign 1989). In British men in 1987, pancreatic cancer was surpassed as a cause of death only by cancer of the lung, prostate and bladder, colorectum and stomach, whereas in women it was the sixth commonest form of cancer death after cancer of the breast, lung, colorectum, ovary and stomach (Cancer Research Campaign 1989). In Japan, the mortality rate attributed to pancreatic cancer in 1950 was one per 100 000 population but by 1974 this had risen to nearly six per 100 000 population (Aoki & Ogawa 1978).

Some caution must be exercised in interpretation of these data. Of 5881 cases of pancreatic cancer registered in England and Wales in 1979, two-thirds of the patients had no surgical operation (Allen-Mersh & Earlam 1986) and presumably histological confirmation was lacking in the majority. Similarly, four studies examining the accuracy of cancer registration in the United States showed a frequency of histological verification of pancreatic cancer of 38–62% (Gudjonsson et al 1978, Gudjonsson 1981). Modern techniques of ultrasonographic and radiological localization of pancreatic cancer now allow targeted fine-needle aspiration cytology or biopsy before operation, and allow the diagnosis to be confirmed in patients being treated by non-operative means such as endoscopic stenting. In addition, when the diagnosis has not yet been confirmed in patients coming to operation, surgeons now routinely seek diagnostic confirmation by direct sampling of the primary cancer or secondary tumour deposits for cytological and/or histological assessment. There seems little doubt that some of the apparent increase in the incidence of pancreatic cancer may reflect earlier under-reporting and misdiagnosis (Levin & Connelly 1973), and despite the recent emphasis on diagnostic confirmation, we still fail to obtain histological/cytological proof of the diagnosis in a significant number of patients.

DESCRIPTIVE EPIDEMIOLOGY

The incidence of pancreatic cancer varies with age, sex and race. Age-specific incidence rates show that the disease is uncommon before the age of 45 years but incidence rates increase steadily thereafter so that more than 80% of cases occur in the 60- to 80-year-old age group (Morgan & Wormsley, 1977, Gordis & Gold 1984). This is not to say, that pancreatic cancer never affects children and young adults, and the disease has been reported in children as young as 3 months of age (Tsukimoto et al 1973, Taxy 1976). Pancreatic cancer is commoner in males with an overall male to female ratio which is usually between 1.5:1 and 2:1 (Aoki & Ogawa 1978, Muir et al 1987). The ratio before the menopause in the United States is approximately 2:1 but declines thereafter to approach unity, leading Wynder et al (1973) to postulate that oestrogens may exert some protective effect.

Carcinoma of the pancreas is in general more common in Western or idustrialized countries, but the highest incidence rates in men have been found in New Zealand Maoris and native Hawaiians. In women, Hawaiians, Latins and Maoris, have the highest incidence. India, Singapore and Kuwait all have a low reported incidence and in Madras the incidence is 20 times lower than that reported in the black population of Alameda, California (Table 35.1). Black Americans, regardless of their gender, generally appear to have higher incidence rates than their white counterparts although in Connecticut, the incidence rate in both blacks and whites is eight per 100 000 (Muir et al 1987). Age-standardized incidence rates from a number of selected countries are shown in Table 35.1.

Table 35.1 Age-Standardized incidence rates of pancreatic cancer in 1978–1982 in selected countries. (From Muir C, Waterhouse J, Mack T (eds) Cancer incidence in five continents, IARC Scientific Publication No. 88, International Agency for Research on Cancer, 1987)

| | Age-standardized incidence | |
	Male	Female
Canada	8.6	5.5
Colombia, Cali	5.2	3.6
Finland	10.0	6.3
France, Calvados		
Urban	6.2	2.8
Rural	4.1	2.2
Hong Kong	3.5	2.4
India, Madras	0.9	0.4
Israel		
All Jews	8.9	5.9
Non-Jews	3.1	2.1
Japan, Osaka	7.7	4.5
Kuwait		
Kuwaitis	1.2	1.3
Non-Kuwaitis	2.5	3.5
New Zealand		
Maori	12.1	5.0
Non-Maori	7.5	4.7
Puerto Rico	4.9	3.4
Sweden	8.7	6.3
Singapore		
Chinese	4.5	2.8
Indian	2.6	2.4
Malay	1.9	2.2
US, Alameda		
White	8.4	6.2
Black	16.3	9.4
US, New Mexico		
Hispanic	9.3	7.4
Other White	8.0	5.4
American Indian	5.0	3.9
US, New Orleans		
White	9.8	5.3
Black	12.0	7.0

It remains uncertain whether such geographic and racial differences reflect differing genetic susceptibility to pancreatic cancer or whether environmental and socioeconomic factors are also involved. Migrant studies have been relatively unhelpful in unravelling these influences. For example, Japanese migrants to the United States have a higher incidence of pancreatic cancer than native Americans or Japanese remaining in Japan. The American-born offspring of these immigrants have an incidence which lies between that of the native populations of the two countries (Smith 1956, Bueli & Dunn 1968, Haenszel et al 1968). It is not clear whether these apparent changes in incidence reflect undercertification of pancreatic cancer in Japan and it is possible that some deaths from this cancer were wrongly attributed to the more common Japanese problem of gastric cancer (Jablon et al 1966, Bueli & Dunn 1968). Confusion also surrounds the situation in the Northern American state of Ohio where Negro migrants from the Southern States appear to assume a higher incidence of pancreatic cancer than Negroes born in Ohio (Mancusco & Sterling 1974). Migrants from various European countries to Australia also had higher mortality rates than those of their country of origin or of native Australians, but the suggestion that this might reflect increased pancreatic exocrine activity due to changes in dietary habits (McMichael et al 1980) is unsubstantiated.

Socioeconomic status, income and level of education have shown an inconstant relationship with the risk of developing pancreatic cancer, but some religious groups appear to have an increased susceptibility. For example, in New York City, pancreatic cancer had an increased frequency in Jews as opposed to Catholics or Protestants (MacMahon 1960, Newill 1961), an increase which was particularly marked in women (Seidman 1970). Similarly, Utah Mormons had a lower incidence of pancreatic cancer than non-smoking white American men (Enstrom 1978), although pancreatic cancer has a low incidence in Utah in both Mormons and non-Mormons (Lyon et al 1976).

RISK FACTORS

Tobacco smoking

Cigarette smoking is the most consistent risk factor in epidemiological studies of pancreatic cancer. The relative risk ranges from 1.6:1 in male British doctors (Doll & Peto 1976) to 3.1:1 in Swedish males (Cederlof et al 1975). Although the prospective study in male British doctors did not demonstrate an overall statistically significant association, the authors concluded that higher rates of cigarette consumption did confer increased risk. Other studies have shown that there is a dose relationship between the number of cigarettes smoked and risk (Best 1966, Hammond 1966, Hirayama 1977, Mack et al

1986, Falk et al 1988, Ghadirian et al 1991) and the rising incidence of pancreatic cancer in the USA appears to have paralleled the increase in cigarette smoking (Krain 1970, Weiss & Bernarde 1983). A number of studies have attempted to dissect out the risk attributable to cigarette smoking from that of other potentially confounding variables, notably alcohol and coffee consumption. In general, the increased risk attributable to cigarette smoking persists after controlling for these other putative risk factors (Gold et al 1985, Mack et al 1986, Norell et al 1986a), although in one case–control study, alcohol emerged as the more important association (Durbec et al 1983). Binstock et al (1983) found that per capita consumption of coffee, dietary fat and saturated fat in the period 1957–1965 had a significant positive correlation with pancreatic cancer mortality rates in 1971–1974 while the relationship with cigarette smoking was weak and not statistically significant. A retrospective analysis of US male college students (Harvard University 1916–1950, University of Pennsylvania, 1931–1940) found that cigarette smoking during college was associated with a relative risk of 2.6:1 for the subsequent development of pancreatic cancer but failed to find a relationship with coffee consumption (Whittemore et al 1983). There is debate as to whether smoking pipes or cigars affects risk (Kahn 1966, Best 1966, Krain 1970, Wynder et al 1973, Ghadirian et al 1991).

The mechanism(s) by which cigarette smoking may increase the risk of developing pancreatic cancer remain obscure. Autopsy studies have shown that hyperplastic changes in the pancreatic duct mucosa are commoner in smokers and more marked in heavy smokers (Fraumeni 1975), and Wynder (1975) suggested that carcinogens in tobacco smoke might cause cancer by being excreted in bile and refluxing into the pancreatic duct, by reaching the pancreas via the bloodstream, or by increasing blood lipid concentrations which might in turn influence the development of cancer. Reflux of bile from the bile duct into the pancreatic duct undoubtedly occurs in some individuals, particularly in those with a long functional common channel (Armstrong & Taylor 1986) and reflux of carcinogens in this way might help to explain why cancer most frequently arises in the head of the pancreas (Cubilla & Fitzgerald 1979). However, Di Magno et al (1982) found that pancreatic ductal epithelial abnormalities were commoner in patients who did not have a prominent common channel between the two duct systems. While nitrosamines are undoubtedly carcinogenic in animal models (Pour et al 1981, Howatson & Carter 1985), none of the nitrosamines in cigarette smoke have yet been shown unequivocally to cause pancreatic cancer.

Diet

The demographic differences in the incidence of pancreatic cancer in various countries suggest that diet might play a role in its aetiology. Consumption of a 'Western diet' with its relatively high fat and meat intake has been implicated, and Doll & Peto (1981) suggested that as many as one-third of all cancer deaths in the US might be related to dietary factors. A number of studies have shown a positive correlation between per capita consumption of fat and oils and the mortality rate from pancreatic cancer (Lea 1967, Segi et al 1969, Maruchi 1973). Similarly in a large Japanese cohort study, Hirayama (1981) found that daily or more frequent consumption of meat was associated with a 50% increased risk of developing pancreatic cancer. Indeed it has been suggested that the increased incidence of pancreatic cancer in Japan could reflect changes in the Japanese diet with greater fat and protein consumption (Wynder et al 1973, Hirayama 1975). However, Durbec et al (1983) found that while the risk of developing pancreatic cancer increased with increasing dietary fat consumption in a French study, dietary protein intake did not appear to affect risk. In a case–control study from Baltimore, Gold et al (1985) found no significant association between pancreatic cancer and intake of meat or deep-fried foods, while risk decreased with consumption of raw fruit, vegetables and diet soda. Fruit also appeared to give some protection in a large study based in Louisiana (Falk et al 1988) but pancreatic cancer was associated with consumption of pork products and rice, the association with pork being particularly strong in Cajuns. From Sweden, Norell et al (1986a) in a case–control study found a very strong association with intake of fried and grilled meat; in this study margarine intake exceeding 15 G increased risk fourfold while butter intake reduced risk.

Mills et al (1988) found a lower than expected mortality rate from pancreatic cancer in a large study of 34 000 Californian Seventh Day Adventists whose religion proscribes smoking, drinking alcohol and eating pork. Also of interest is the fact that some 50% of these individuals eat a lacto-ovo-vegetarian diet. The observed reduction in mortality rate did not prove to be statistically significant, and the increased risk due to consuming meat, eggs and coffee disappeared when the data were controlled for cigarette smoking. A high consumption of vegetables (beans, lentils and peas) and fruit appeared to exert some protective effect in this study, this observation being supported by other workers (Gold et al 1985, Norell et al 1986a Mack et al 1986). Vitamin consumption may be implicated in these findings and could play an important role in risk determination. For example, vitamins C and E can inhibit nitrosation in various experimental conditions (Mirvish 1986) and this could help to explain the inverse association between risk of pancreatic cancer and the consumption of fruit and vegetables, particularly when eaten fresh and raw. It is of interest that while dietary fat and protein increase susceptibility to nitrosamine-induced pancreatic cancer in animal models (Birt et al 1981, 1983, Longnecker et al 1985), retinoids appear to inhibit carcinogenesis (Longnecker et al 1982, 1986). Low serum levels of vitamin A (retinol) have been linked to an increased cancer risk (Wald et al 1980) although such low levels could be a result of cancer metabolism rather than a cause of its development (Wald et al 1980).

The importance of micronutrients in pancreatic carcinogenesis has also been examined in a detailed long-term study from Maryland, USA (Burney et al 1989). Between 1974 and 1975 blood samples were stored from over 25 000 individuals, representing approximately 30% of the adult residential population. Over the subsequent years 22 patients developed pancreatic cancer and their original serum levels of micronutrients were compared with those of matched non-cancer controls. Levels of lycopene and selenium were lower at the time of sampling in individuals destined to develop pancreatic cancer. Lycopene is a carotenoid not dissimilar to B-carotene, which has antioxidant but not retinoid or preretinoid activity. Diets rich in fruit may provide a high lycopene intake, in keeping with suggestions that such diets protect against pancreatic cancer. Selenium, by virtue of its presence as the active centre of the enzyme glutathione peroxidase, is a key natural antioxidant. It is known to protect against carcinogenesis in animal models and a link between low serum selenium levels and various forms of cancer has been suggested in man. In this study an association between selenium and pancreatic cancer was found in men, but, inexplicably, low serum levels of the lipid antiperoxidant vitamin E appeared to have a protective effect.

The mechanisms whereby dietary factors might increase the risk of developing pancreatic cancer remain speculative. It is well recognized that exogenous cholecystokinin and secretin can cause pancreatic hypertrophy and potentiate cancer development in some animal models (Mainz et al 1973, Barrowman & Mayston 1974, Howatson & Carter 1985) while a diet rich in trypsin inhibitor (raw soya flour) promotes the effect of the carcinogen, azaserine, in rats (Morgan et al 1977). It may be postulated that diets rich in fat and protein stimulate the release of hormones such as cholecystokinin which increase pancreatic cell turnover and so increase susceptibility to the actions of carcinogens. The effect of raw soya flour can be explained by enhanced cholecystokinin release as a consequence of high intraluminal concentrations of trypsin inhibitors. In hamster models, nitrosamines are particularly effective carcinogens, and it is worth noting that these agents can form during cooking or be manufactured in the stomach from nitrites and nitrates used in the preservation of meats (Weisbeger et al 1975, Miller & Miller 1986).

Consumption of beverages (Tables 35.2–35.4)

Considerable controversy has surrounded the putative link between coffee drinking and pancreatic cancer. Stocks (1970) correlated the age-adjusted mortality rates from various forms of cancer in the years 1964–1965 with cigarette smoking and tea and coffee consumption in 20 countries. A positive correlation with coffee consumption emerged but only in males. Bernarde and Weiss (1982) also found a significant correlation ($r = 0.59$) in a study involving 13 countries, but major inconsistencies caused the authors to doubt whether the association was one of cause and effect. In the United States, Lin & Kessler (1981) conducted a case–control study covering the years 1972–1975 and reported a significant association between pancreatic cancer risk and drinking decaffeinated coffee. No association emerged in the case of 'regular' (i.e. non-decaffeinated) coffee and the authors hypothesized that the use of solvents such as trichloroethylene in the extraction process until the mid-1970s might have explained the increased risk linked to decaffeinated coffee. On the other hand, Wynder et al (1986) found that drinking decaffeinated coffee was associated with an odds ratio of less than unity in men (0.7; 95% confidence limits 0.4–1.9) and women (0.9; 95% confidence limits 0.4–1.9). Of interest in this study, an association appeared to exist in females when one or two cups a day were consumed, but the link was lost with higher levels of consumption.

In 1981, MacMahon et al reported a large case–control study which showed a strong association between coffee consumption and pancreatic cancer. Risk appeared to be dose-related in that relative risk increased from 1.8 with one or two cups a day to approximately three–fold with greater intake. This dose–response relationship was significant only in women but remained when males and females were combined and persisted after adjustment for

Table 35.2   Epidemiological studies examining the relationship between coffee consumption and pancreatic cancer

Authors	Number of countries	Findings
Stocks et al (1970)	20	Strong association in males only
Cuckle & Kinlen (1981)	16	Positive correlation (lost when Japan excluded)
Bernarde & Weiss (1982)	13	Positive but unimpressive correlation
Binstock et al (1983)	22	Positive correlation

Table 35.3 Case–control studies examining the relationship between coffee consumption and pancreatic cancer

Authors	Country	Findings
Lin & Kessler (1981)	US	Significant association (with decaffeinated coffee)
MacMahon et al (1981)	US	Significant association (with dose relationship)
Jick & Dinan (1981)	US	No association
Kinlen & McPherson (1984)	UK	No association
Gold et al (1985)	US	No association (dose relationship noted in women)
Wynder et al (1986)	US	No association
Mack et al (1986)	US	Significant association (with dose relationship)
MacMahon et al (1981)	US	Slight increase only with >5 cups/day
Norell et al (1986a)	Sweden	No association
La Vecchia et al (1987)	Italy	No association
Gorham et al (1988)	US	Association only in smokers
Falk et al (1988)	US	No association
Ghadirian et al (1991)	Canada	No association (non-significant reductions in risk)

the effects of cigarette smoking. MacMahon (1982) subsequently urged caution in interpretation of this study and shortcomings in the choice of the control group have been higlighted (Feinstein et al 1981). In a more recent case–control study, MacMahon's group (Hseih et al 1986) reported only a slight increase in risk in those who consumed more than five cups of coffee a day.

In a study of mortality data from 22 countries, Binstock et al (1983) found a significant positive correlation between per capita coffee imports and pancreatic cancer mortality rate on univariate analysis. This relationship persisted when the data were controlled on bivariate analysis for intake of total dietary fat, saturated fat and cholesterol, cigarette smoking and national income. Cuckle & Kinlen (1981) also found a significant positive correlation between per capita coffee imports in the periods 1945–1949 and 1960–1964 and pancreatic cancer mortality rates in 16 countries. However, exclusion of Japan from this analysis eliminated the significant association.

Other case–control studies have failed to show a consistent relationship between coffee drinking and pancreatic cancer. In a large Los Angeles study involving 490 matched pairs Mack et al (1986) found that relative risk increased significantly to 1.6 with one to four cups a day, and to 2.0 with five or more cups. However, when controlled for tobacco smoking, the dose-related link to coffee consumption disappeared in male smokers and in

females, regardless of their smoking habits. This study also failed to find a link between pancreatic cancer and previous levels of consumption of tea, carbonated drinks, beer or spirits. In contrast, in rural California, Gorham et al (1988) did report a positive association between coffee consumption and pancreatic cancer which was restricted to smokers only. In Baltimore, Gold et al (1985) studied 201 matched pairs, reporting no significant association with coffee drinking although a dose–response effect was observed in women. Jick & Dinan (1981), using questionnaires to analyse data from pancreatic cancer patients and a mixture of hospital controls and cancer controls drawn from several countries, found no significant association. In a recent population based case–control study from Quebec, Ghadirian et al (1991) found that coffee drinkers were collectively at lower risk than nondrinkers particularly when coffee was consumed with meals and not on an empty stomach. In Britain, Kinlen & McPherson (1984) studied 216 patients with pancreatic cancer and 432 controls with other forms of cancer, failing to find any relationship between coffee drinking and pancreatic cancer. Wynder et al (1983) also failed to find an association, and controlling the data for cigarette smoking did not alter relative risk. In a Swedish study, Norell et al (1986a) also found no significant association with coffee consumption when using both a hospital control group and a population control group. In northern Italy, La Vecchia et al (1987) compared 150 patients with

Table 35.4 Prospective cohort studies examining the relationship between coffee consumption and pancreatic cancer

Authors	Population	Findings
Nomura et al (1981)	8004 ethnic Japanese, 28 cases pancreatic cancer	Suggestive association
Heuch et al (1983)	16 713 Norwegians, 63 cases pancreatic cancer	No association
Whittemore et al (1983)	50 000 male US college students 126 cases pancreaticcancer	No association
Mills et al (1988)	34 000 Californian Seventh Day Adventists 40 cases pancreatic cancer	Suggestive association (lost after controlling for cigaratte smoking)
Hiatt et al (1988)	122 894 healthcare plan subscribers 49 cases pancreatic cancer	No association

pancreatic cancer with 605 hospital controls with acute non-neoplastic disease. Coffee consumption was associated with a small increase in the relative risk of pancreatic cancer, but increasing consumption led to reduction in risk, and the authors stress the further reduction in relative risk when other possible aetiological factors such as cigarette smoking were taken into account. In Louisiana, coffee drinking had no association with pancreatic cancer after adjustment for smoking, alcohol, diet and demographic factors (Falk et al 1988). In this study, heavy coffee consumption was associated with low fruit consumption, underlining the potential role of other dietary factors in risk previously attributed to coffee drinking.

Prospective cohort studies have also failed to find a consistent relationship between coffee drinking and risk of pancreatic cancer. In the study of US male college graduates referred to earlier (Whittemore et al 1983) no association was found between pancreatic cancer and coffee drinking habits while in college. Similarly, in the study of 34 000 Californian Seventh Day Adventists (Mills et al 1988), coffee consumption had no significant association, while Hiatt et al (1988) found no increased risk attributable to coffee drinking in an analysis involving 49 cases of pancreatic cancer drawn from a cohort of 122 894 individuals subscribing to a healthcare plan. In Norway, Heuch et al (1983) found no association in a prospective study of 16 713 subjects, 63 of whom developed pancreatic cancer. Finally, in a study involving 8004 men of Japanese ancestry living in Hawaii, Nomura et al (1981) found a suggestive association in that incidence rates adjusted for age and smoking were 2.4 per 1000 in those who did not drink coffee and 5.0 per 1000 in those drinking five or more cups a day. It should be stressed that this analysis was based on only 28 cases of pancreatic cancer developing during the 13 years of follow-up.

It can be concluded that while the possibility of a link between coffee consumption and pancreatic cancer cannot be disregarded, the available data do not prove a causal association. In the case of tea drinking, the overwhelming majority of studies have failed to find any association (MacMahon et al 1981, Whittemore et al 1983, Kinlen & McPherson 1984, Gold et al 1985, Mack et al 1986, La Vecchia et al 1987, Hiatt et al 1988).

Alcohol consumption

It is generally accepted that alcohol is implicated in the development of certain cancers such as those of the mouth, oesophagus and liver, but that the available data are equivocal. Burch & Ansari (1968) originally suggested that alcohol might be a risk factor for development of pancreatic cancer, based on their finding that 65% of 83 pancreatic cancer patients admitted to moderate-to-heavy consumption for at least 15 years, as opposed to less than

15% of a control group. Three case–control studies have also appeared to support an association between pancreatic cancer and alcohol consumption. Ishii et al (1968) reported that the risk of pancreatic cancer was twice as high in men drinking alcohol every day compared with those who did not. In a study of 69 pancreatic cancer patients and 199 normal controls, Durbec et al (1983) found that pancreatic cancer risk increased with a high fat diet and high alcohol intake; although tobacco smoking also increased risk, alcohol appeared to be a more important risk determinant. In Norway, Heuch et al (1983) found that frequent alcohol consumption was associated with a relative risk of 5.4. However, the majority of case–control studies have failed to demonstrate a consistent link (Lin & Kessler 1981, MacMahon et al 1981, Haines et al 1982, Wynder et al 1983, Gold et al 1985, Mack et al 1986, Norell et al 1986a, Falk et al 1988, Hiatt et al 1988, Ghadirian et al 1991).

Studies of alcoholics and of various communities have also failed to show a consistent relationship between alcohol consumption and pancreatic cancer risk (Hakulinen et al 1974, Monson & Lyon 1975, Robinette et al 1979, Klatsky et al 1981, Schmidt & Popham 1981, Heuch et al 1983). Velema et al (1986) aggregated the results of nine studies involving individuals with high alcohol intake. A total of 90 cases of pancreatic cancer were observed where 76.6 might have been expected, an observed: expected ratio of 1.17 which was not statistically significant (95% confidence limits 0.94–1.43). In contrast, three prospective general population cohort studies have suggested a significant increase in risk. In Japan risk was increased significantly only in male whisky drinkers (Hirayama 1978); in California relative risk increased threefold (6 pancreatic cancer deaths in drinkers as opposed to 2 in non-drinkers; Klatsky et al 1981), while in Norway, relative risk increased to 2.7 (95% confidence limits 1.2–6.0) in those drinking beer or spirits frequently (Heuch et al 1983).

As in the case of coffee drinking, the available data do not support a consistent relationship between alcohol consumption and the the risk of developing pancreatic cancer. Some studies have even suggested that moderate levels of wine consumption may exert a protective effect (Gold et al 1985, Ghadirian et al 1991) and the confounding effect of tobacco smoking remains difficult to disentangle when attempting to establish links to alcohol consumption.

Effects of disease

Diabetes mellitus

It has been recognized for many years that there may be a link between pancreatic cancer and diabetes mellitus, although in trying to define the nature of the link it has proved difficult to distinguish cause from effect. Carbohydrate metabolism is known to be abnormal in many patients with pancreatic cancer. As early as 1941, Berk, on the basis of collected statistics, reported that 9.4% of these patients had glycosuria while 19.4% had hyperglycaemia. More sophisticated studies assessing blood glucose, serum insulin and serum C-peptide levels after oral glucose showed abnormal carbohydrate tolerance in 81% of pancreatic cancer patients as opposed to 36% of controls, and a lower level of insulin secretion in cancer patients (Schwartz et al 1978).

There is a positive correlation between diabetes and pancreatic cancer when national incidences are compared (Waterhouse et al 1976), and both conditions have a declining sex ratio with increasing age, a pattern not seen with other digestive tract cancers or tobacco-related malignancy (Wynder et al 1973, Gordis & Gold, 1986). Bell (1957) reported that the incidence of diabetes in patients coming to autopsy with pancreatic cancer (38/587 or 6.5%) was twice that of the general autopsy population in men and 50% greater than in women. However, the average duration of diabetes in the pancreatic cancer patients was only 3.4 years and it was less than 1 year in 10 of the cases. When the 13 patients in whom the symptoms of pancreatic cancer preceded or coincided with onset of diabetes were excluded, the incidence of diabetes in pancreatic cancer patients fell to that of the general autopsy population. Green et al (1985) also reported an autopsy-based study in which nine (4.3%) of 209 pancreatic cancer patients had pre-existing diabetes, while 15% were found to have diabetes after developing symptoms of pancreatic cancer and a further 29% had glycosuria. Of the 65 pancreatic cancer patients reported by Clark and Mitchell (1961), 10 were diabetic and in all but one case the interval between the diagnosis of cancer and diabetes was less than 1 year. In a study of 265 patients admitted to Aberdeen Royal Infirmary with proven pancreatic cancer in the period 1955–1967, Karmody and Kyle (1969) found that 51 were diabetic. In 80% of cases diabetes had been present for less than 1 year while in six cases it exceeded 2 years. These authors concluded that the incidence of pancreatic cancer in diabetes was greater than that which might be attributed to chance.

Kessler (1970) examined the incidence of 15 types of cancer in 21 447 diabetic patients attending the Joslin Clinic, Boston over the years 1930–1956. A statistically significant excess of deaths in both men and women was observed for pancreatic cancer, with standardized mortality ratios of 1.47 and 2.13 respectively. When deaths were excluded where it could not be established that diabetes has preceded the cancer, the ratios fell to 1.27 for men and 1.82 for women, statistical significance being retained only in females. This study has been criticized on the basis of use of an inappropriate control group in calculating mortality ratios, and Kessler (1971) himself urged caution

in interpretation of the reported association between diabetes and pancreatic cancer, given the wide variation in study design and risk of bias in autopsy studies. He also proposed that animal insulins used to treat diabetics should be examined for carcinogenic effects in man given their antigenic and teratogenic properties in animals.

In a prospective cohort study, Green and Jensen (1985) followed all insulin-dependent diabetics in Fyn County, Denmark for 8.5 years, reporting a significant excess of pancreatic cancer (observed: expected ratio, 6 : 2.4 cases). However, exclusion of patients in whom diabetes might have been an early manifestation of cancer reduced the excess to levels (4 : 2.4) which caused them to question an association between the two conditions. A case–control study in three Swedish hospitals (Norell et al 1986b) found that patients with pancreatic cancer were much more likely than hospital-based or population-based controls to have diabetes (relative risks 19.7 and 3.3 respectively). Exclusion of patients in whom diabetes had been present for less than 5 years before development of pancreatic cancer reduced the relative risks to 6.9, compared with hospital controls, and 2.4, compared with population controls. In their study of Seventh Day Adventists, Mills et al (1988) reported a relative risk of 3.4 for development of pancreatic cancer in diabetics, although the diagnosis of diabetes was accepted on the basis of reports by the patients. Given the inconsistent findings from such studies, diabetes mellitus cannot be regarded as a proven risk factor in the development of pancreatic cancer. A major problem which has dogged interpretation of available data has been failure to distinguish between insulin-dependent and non-insulin-dependent diabetes. Endogenous insulin levels are low in the former and high in the latter condition and it might be postulated that the two subgroups would have different levels of cancer risk. Animal studies have failed to clarify the situation. Syrian hamsters made diabetic by injection of streptozotocin do not develop pancreatic cancer when exposed to carcinogen (Bell & Strayer 1983), while when genetically diabetic and non-diabetic Chinese hamsters were exposed to carcinogen, pancreatic cancers developed only in non-diabetic animals (Bell & Pour, 1987). However, in an apparent paradox, growth of a pancreatic cancer cell line in hamster cheek pouches was accelerated in the presence of streptozotocin-induced diabetes (Fisher et al 1988).

Pernicious anaemia

Borch et al (1988) have recently suggested that pancreatic cancer may be more common in patients with pernicious anaemia. A total of 361 patients followed over 7 years showed the expected increase in the incidence of gastric cancer (0.6%/year) but also revealed an increased incidence of pancreatic cancer (0.3%/year). Pancreatic cancer was the primary cause of death in five of the 134 patients who died during follow-up. Conversely, in 127 unselected patients with pancreatic cancer, four were known to have pernicious anaemia. While far from conclusive, these data suggest that further evaluation is indicated. Of the various mechanisms which could explain a link, high circulating levels of gastrin could have a trophic effect on the pancreas, and cholecystokinin levels may also be increased in pernicious anaemia.

Chronic pancreatitis

Familial chronic pancreatitis was first described in 1952 (Comfort & Steinberg 1952), and further families affected by what is now considered to be an autosomal dominant trait with incomplete penetrance have since been reported (Gross et al 1962, Whitten et al 1968, Appel 1974, Miller et al 1992). Up to one-third of affected family members develop cancer but the risk also appears to extend to family members who do not have chronic pancreatitis (Castleman et al 1972).

The relationship between pancreatic cancer and non-familial chronic pancreatitis is less certain. Common aetiological factors could be implicated in the development of the two conditions, the two not infrequently coexist, and it is well recognized that chronic ductal obstruction in pancreatic cancer may lead to pancreatic inflammation. Whether chronic pancreatitis increases the risk of developing pancreatic cancer is extremely doubtful. Gambill (1971) found histological evidence of chronic pancreatitis in 10% of 255 patients with pancreatic and periampullary cancer, but in an earlier report, none of 56 patients with chronic pancreatitis followed for 16–20 years developed cancer (Gambill et al 1960). Admittedly there have been reports of cancer developing in patients with long-standing chronic pancreatitis (Bartholomew et al 1958, Mohr et al 1975) and Rocca et al (1987) recently reported an increased incidence of both pancreatic and extrapancreatic cancers in a study of 172 patients with chronic pancreatitis. It seems likely that factors such as cigarette smoking may explain this apparent increase in cancer incidence in this patient population. Thus while the overall incidence of pancreatic cancer in patients with chronic pancreatitis has been estimated at around 3% (range in various reported series 0.8–25%; Lin et al 1988), it is doubtful whether chronic inflammation per se increases the risk of cancer development.

Cholelithiasis

In a large autopsy study of 609 patients dying with pancreatic cancer, Bell (1957) found that 14% of men and 38% of women also had gallstones. While the overall incidence of gallstones exceeded that found in the general autopsy population, it was concluded that there was no definite link between cholelithiasis and pancreatic cancer. Wynder et al (1973) in a case–control study involving 142 pancreatic cancer patients found that a previous history of cholecystectomy was more common than in controls (15 vs. 8%). This difference was originally regarded as 'suggestive' but was not statistically significant and was based on small numbers. In another case–control study, Haines et al (1982) found no association between pancreatic cancer and cholecystectomy carried out at least 5 years earlier, While Mack et al (1986) also failed to establish an association with cholecystectomy.

On the other hand, a review of 586 patients with abdominal malignancy in Finland showed a significantly increased frequency of previous cholecystectomy in pancreatic cancer, the peak incidence of pancreatic cancer falling some 5 years after gallbladder surgery (Hyvarinen & Partanen 1987). In a case–control study from Stockholm, Norell et al (1986a) reported a risk of developing pancreatic cancer in patients with gallstone disease that was 1.7 relative to hospital controls and 2.7 relative to population controls. When patients were excluded who reported gallstones in the 5 years before pancreatic cancer was diagnosed, the relative risk values become 1.2 and 2.9 respectively. These authors concluded that gallstones were associated with an increased risk of pancreatic cancer.

In experimental models, exogenous cholecystokinin and high fat diets are known to cause pancreatic hypertrophy and potentiate cancer development (Mainz et al 1973, Howatson & Carter 1985). It has been postulated that cholecystectomy could predispose to pancreatic cancer by resulting in increased circulating levels of cholecystokinin. In hamsters, cholecystectomy increases pancreatic hyperplasia and hypertrophy in association with increased circulating levels of cholecystokinin (Rosenberg et al 1983, Rosenbeg et al 1984), and cholecystectomy increases the yield of chemically induced pancreatic cancer when carried out 1 week before the first injection of carcinogen (Ura et al 1986). However, this increased incidence was not statistically significant unless cholecystectomy was combined with administration of the secondary bile acid, lithocholic acid. In rats, Stace et al (1987) showed that long term pancreaticobiliary diversion produced not only high circulating levels of cholecystokinin but also produced hyperplastic and adenomatous nodules in the pancreas. However, the relevance of these models to pancreatic cancer in man is uncertain and major molecular differences between human cancer and that produced in rats by pancreaticobiliary diversion have now been described. In the rat model, Hall et al (1991) found no evidence of Kirsten *ras* mutation, abnormal expression of C-erb-B-2 or abnormal expression of epidermal growth factor receptor, changes all well documented in human cancer.

It must be concluded that a link between previous cholecystectomy and pancreatic cancer, although plausible, is not supported by strong epidemiological or experimental evidence. The evidence in favour of an association with cholelithiasis is even less convincing.

Gastric surgery

In 1982, McLean–Ross et al reported on mortality rates and causes of death in 779 patients who had undergone various forms of peptic ulcer surgery in Edinburgh. Life expectancy was reduced in all age groups and much of the excess mortality was attributable to smoking-related disease. Somewhat surprisingly pancreatic cancer emerged as the third commonest cause of cancer death behind lung and colorectal cancer but ahead of gastric cancer. A total of 11 deaths were attributed to pancreatic cancer whereas 3.9 were expected, and this excess may well have been smoking-related. Caygill et al (1987) reviewed the cases of 5018 patients undergoing gastric surgery for peptic ulcer in London at least 25 years earlier. There was no increase in mortality from cancer during the first 15 years but from 20 years there was a fourfold excess risk of pancreatic cancer. In contrast to the Edinburgh group, Caygill et al considered that given the long latency period, the predisposition to pancreatic and other forms of cancer after gastric surgery was unlikely to be due to cigarette smoking and more likely to be related to an event occurring at the time of surgery.

In their Los Angeles case–control study, Mack et al (1986) found a higher than expected frequency of previous ulcer surgery (partial gastrectomy in most cases) in patients with pancreatic cancer. The relative risk of pancreatic cancer in non-smokers at least 10 years after gastrectomy was 7.4, in smokers following gastrectomy it was 8.1, while in smokers who had not undergone gastrectomy it was 2.3. Thus the effects of gastrectomy were independent of those of smoking status. Other workers have reported an increase in pancreatic cancer risk after partial gastrectomy when compared to control groups of patients with other diseases (Offerhaus et al 1987), although an association was not confirmed by a study involving 336 patients who had undergone surgery for benign peptic ulcer in Olmsted County, Minnesota, only one of whom developed pancreatic cancer (Marighini et al 1987).

Thus, it remains uncertain whether previous surgery for peptic ulcer and in particular, partial gastrectomy, increases the risk of developing pancreatic cancer. If a risk is established it may not simply reflect cigarette smoking habits; pancreatic cancer could conceivably result from increased production of carcinogenic nitroso-compounds in an achlorhydric or hypochlorhydric gastric remnant colonized by bacteria.

Other disease states

There is some evidence that allergic diseases may protect against development of pancreatic cancer. For example, Gold et al (1985) found that relative risk in patients with allergic disorders was 0.39 when compared with hospital controls. Similarly Mack et al (1986) found that a past history of any allergic disease, including asthma, gave a relative risk of 0.2; the protective effect of allergy appeared to be independent of smoking status.

Gold et al (1985) also reported a significantly reduced relative risk (0.3) of pancreatic cancer after tonsillectomy, although risk was not affected by tonsillectomy in the study by Mack et al (1986). In Seventh Day Adventists both tonsillectomy and a history of allergy had a slight non-significant protective effect on pancreatic cancer (Mills et al 1988). Further data are needed to establish the significance of these findings.

Physico-chemical agents

Exposure to potentially carcinogenic chemicals has long been implicated as a risk factor in pancreatic cancer. Mancusco & El-Attar (1967) reported a fivefold increase in mortality rate from pancreatic cancer in a study of 639 men employed in a chemical plant manufacturing B-naphthylamine and benzidine, who were followed for more than 25 years. Although pancreatic cancer accounted for almost one-third of the malignant gastrointestinal tumours recorded, this amounted to only six deaths. Li et al (1969) reviewed 3637 of 4644 death certificates of members of the American Chemical Society who died between 1948 and 1967. They recorded 56 deaths from pancreatic cancer as opposed to 35 deaths which might have been expected. Other studies have failed to find an excess mortality in chemists (Searle et al 1981, Hoar & Pell 1981), while increased mortality rates have been reported in workers involved in coke plants (Redmond et al 1976), the oil and petrochemical industry (Thomas et al 1980), dry cleaning (Lin & Kessler 1981) and paper manufacture (Pickle & Gottlieb 1980), and in those exposed to coal tar pitch derivatives (Turner & Grace 1938). In one recent report where pancreatic cancer developed almost simultaneously in both a husband and wife, the husband worked in a factory producing and storing chlorinated insecticides, including the putative carcinogen lindane, and both lived in an apartment at the factory (Rubio & Rodriguez 1989). However, simultaneous pancreatic cancer in husband and wife has been attributed in another report to shared dietary idiosyncrasy rather than occupational exposure (Ferguson & Watts 1980). In general case–control studies have failed to implicate occupational risk factors in pancreatic carcinogenesis (Wynder et al 1973, Gold et al 1985, Mack et al 1986), and reports which have suggested an association have usually been unable to implicate any particular chemical as a potential carcinogen. The incidence of pancreatic cancer in a rural setting, namely the Faroe Islands, is as high as elsewhere in Scandinavia, making it unlikely that urban and industrial pollution is a major risk factor in this context (Jacobsen et al 1985).

Radiation has also received attention as a potential risk factor. An increased number of deaths have been reported in workers exposed to irradiation in US atomic plants (Mancusco et al 1977, Anderson 1978, Hutchinson et al 1979), among patients irradiated as treatment for ankylosing spondylitis (Court-Brown & Doll 1965), and in British radiologists (Smith & Doll 1981). However, these associations have been called into question given the lack of increase in pancreatic cancer in the British atomic industry (Smith & Douglas 1986), the lack of excess incidence in Japanese survivors of the atomic bomb (Cohen 1980), and the marginal nature of the increase in British radiologists. However, the significance of irradiation cannot be diminished and sporadic cases of pancreatic adenocarcinoma have been reported in patients previously irradiated for other abdominal malignancies (Rokkas et al 1989).

GENETIC FACTORS

Pancreatic cancer is one of the malignancies known to occur in 'cancer family syndromes' (Lynch 1967, Li & Fraumeni 1969). Inherited conditions such as familial chronic pancreatitis, ataxia telangiectasia and diabetes mellitus (Katz & Spiro 1966) may predispose to its development, and a number of reports of familial pancreatic cancer have appeared in recent years. For example MacDermott & Kramer (1973) reported four siblings who developed the disease between the ages of 59 and 72 years, Friedman and Fialkow (1976) reported four brothers who developed the disease in their seventh and eighth decades, and Ehrenthal et al (1987) report three women in one family who died of the disease at progressively younger ages. In the last study, the granddaughter died at the age of 29 years, and although two of the three women smoked cigarettes, familial predisposition seems likely. In some reports of familial pancreatic cancer, common exposure to risk factors such as cigarette smoking (Friedman & Fialkow 1976) or exposure to toxic chemicals (Reimer et al 1977) has been more strongly implicated. As discussed earlier, the simultaneous development of pancreatic cancer in a husband and wife (Ferguson & Watts 1980) underlines the problem of disentangling environmental factors from constitutional factors. However, it seems likely that a genetic predisposition may be present in some patients who develop pancreatic cancer.

Advances in molecular biology and human genetics may soon increase our understanding of the molecular events concerned with both the sporadic and familial forms of pancreatic cancer. Activation of protooncogenes by gene amplification, mutation or overexpression has been implicated in the initiation and progression of a number of human cancers. Ductal adenocarcinoma of the pancreas is known to overexpress the protooncogenes c-Kirsten-*ras* (c-Ki-*ras*) and c-*fos* (Wakita et al 1992), and the Ki-*ras* oncogene is activated by specific point mutations involving codon 12 in as many as 95% of cases. The fact that the same mutations are present in both the intraductal and invasive components of ductal adenocarcinoma suggests that *ras* activation is already associated with the preinvasive stage of tumorigenesis (LeMoine et al 1992). Mutations in Ki-*ras* codon 12 may also prove to be helpful in distinguishing pancreatic cancer with its high incidence of mutation, from bile duct and periampullary cancers with their much lower (< 20%) incidence (Motojima et al 1991).

Loss of tumour suppressor genes has also been implicated in the pathogenesis of human cancers, and this may be reflected in loss of heterozygosity on various chromosomes. Numerous chromosomal rearrangements, including deletions and unbalanced translocations, have been identified in some cases of pancreatic cancer (Johansson et al 1992), and loss of heterozygosity on chromosomes 1 and 11 has been reported recently in both exocrine and endocrine pancreatic cancer (Ding et al 1992). Loss or mutation of the p53 tumour suppressor gene at the locus 17p13 appears to be important in the development of a number of different cancers, and pancreatic cancer is no exception (Barton et al 1991).

AETIOLOGY OF PERIAMPULLARY CANCER

Periampullary tumours must be distinguished from those arising in the pancreas, duodenum or common bile duct, although in clinical practice, this can prove difficult. The distinction between the different types of neoplasm has important implications for management and prognosis, in that many periampullary tumours and some duodenal tumours are localized at the time of diagnosis and amenable to surgical cure. A pragmatic definition of periampullary tumours includes all neoplasms arising at, or within, 1 cm of the papilla of Vater, recognizing that this blurs the distinction between periampullary and duodenal tumours. In many ways, the tumours would be better termed 'papillary' than 'periampullary', but the latter term is hallowed by long usage and will be retained here. Given the relative rarity of periampullary cancer, little is known of its aetiology, but certain premalignant conditions have been identified and associations with other diseases have emerged.

Traditionally, periampullary tumours have been described as papillary or non-papillary, but the majority of tumours in surgical series appear to be of the intestinal type, that is, showing histological resemblance to adeno-carcinomas of the colon and rectum (Neoptolemos et al 1988). Benign adenomas of the papilla of Vater are rare, but there is persuasive evidence that they may be premalignant. Neoptolemos et al (1988) found coexisting adenoma in 35% of their patients with carcinoma, while Kozuka et al (1981) found 'adenomatous residues' in 18 of their 22 (82%) Japanese patients. Increasing dysplasia in adenomas is associated with increasing frequency and density of staining for the tumour markers, carcinoem-bryonic antigen (CEA) and gastrointestinal cancer asso-ciated antigen CA 19–9 (Yamaguchi & Enjoji 1991), a finding consistent with the hypothesis that there is an 'adenoma–carcinoma sequence' analogous to that found in the large intestine. Kimura and Ohtsubo (1988) have examined the relationship between epithelial atypia and cancer of the papilla of Vater in material from 576 autopsies. Two-thirds of the patients had no abnormality, whereas mild atypia, borderline atypia, severe atypia (possibly malignant) and carcinoma were present in 30, 3.1, 0.9 and 0.2% of cases respectively. As shown in Table 35.5, borderline and severe atypia were most frequent in the common channel between bile duct and pancreatic duct, supporting the contention that most cancers of the papilla of Vater arise in this area.

Patients with familial adenomatous polyposis (FAP) and Gardner's syndrome are at a particularly high risk of developing duodenal or periampullary cancer. Jagelman et al (1988) found 39 patients with such cancers (36 of whom had periampullary cancer) in a series of 1255 FAP patients, a much higher incidence than would be expected in the general population. Spigelman et al (1989) carried out upper gastrointestinal endoscopy in 102 FAP patients to determine the incidence of adenomatous polyps and dysplasia in the stomach and duodenum. None of the patients had involvement of the duodenal bulb alone, 8 had involvement of the first three parts of the duodenum, and 80 had involvement of the second and third parts of the duodenum only (Fig. 35.1). Histological examination of duodenal biopsies revealed dysplasia in 94 cases and hyperplasia in 6, and biopsy of the periampullary area revealed abnormalities in 90% of cases. Non-adeno-matous fundic gland polyps were also seen in 56 patients,

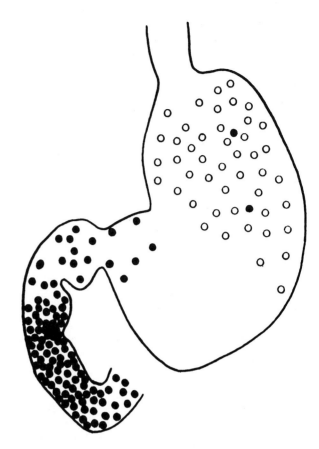

Fig. 35.1 Overall representation of sites affected by upper gastrointestinal polyposis in 102 patients with familial adenomatous polyposis undergoing upper gastrointestinal endoscopy. The open circles represent patients with fundic gland polyps; the closed circles represent patients with adenoma(s) (Reproduced with permission from Spigelman et al 1989, Lancet 783–785)

and although not regarded as premalignant, these lesions probably reflect the general tendency to gastrointestinal mucosal overgrowth in this condition.

The clustering of duodenal adenomas around the papilla of Vater and their relative rarity in the stomach in patients with FAP, has fuelled the suggestion that a car-cinogen or co-carcinogen in bile or pancreatic secretions may interact with genetically determined abnormalities in mucosal growth to cause neoplasia. Spigelman et al

Table 35.5 Incidence of atypical epithelium at various sites related to the papilla of Vater. (Data from Kimura W, Ohtsubo K 1988 Incidence, sites of origin, and immunohistochemical and histochemical characteristics of atypical epithelium and minute carcinoma of the papilla of Vater. Cancer 61: 1394–1402)

	Common channel	Bile duct	Pancreatic duct	Duodenum
Number of cases	451	531	531	481
Condition of epithelium (percentages)				
Normal	71.4	82.7	92.7	96.5
Mild atypia	24.6	14.9	6.2	2.9
Borderline atypia	2.9	1.7	0.6	0.4
Severe atypia	0.9	0.6	0.4	0.2
Malignant	0.2	0.2	0.2	

(1990) failed to find convincing evidence of mutagenic activity in bile from FAP patients relative to control bile, and it may be that bile has a non-specific effect in FAP by promoting the growth of cells already at high risk of malignant transformation. The association between periampullary cancer and FAP must be kept in perspective. Most surgical series of patients with periampullary cancer contain few patients who have undergone previous colorectal surgery for FAP, although this may change as more patients avoid death from colorectal cancer by timely bowel surgery. It should also borne in mind that Jagelman et al (1988) report a median interval of 22 years between the development of upper gastrointestinal cancer and prior colectomy for FAP.

Carcinoid tumours of the papilla of Vater are also extremely rare, but have a well-recognized association with von Recklinghausen's disease (VRD). Klein et al (1989) found less than 30 reported cases where such carcinoids occurred in the absence of VRD, and collected 37 cases where neoplasms of the duodenum, head of pancreas, distal bile duct or ampulla of Vater were associated with VRD. Of the 37 cases, 20 had periampullary tumours as defined in the opening paragraph in this section, and histological examination revealed 12 carcinoids, 4 neurofibromas, 2 paraganglionomas, 1 adenocarcinoma and 1 ganglioneuroma. It appears that patients with VRD should be regarded as at increased risk of developing malignancies in tissues not derived from the neural crest, as well as in those of neural crest origin. Although some of these lesions may appear to be benign, the propensity of tumours such as neurofibroma to undergo malignant transformation means that radical excision (e.g. the Whipple operation) is usually recommended.

Primary malignant lesions of the duodenum are also rare. Although duodenal carcinomas account for about 0.35% of all gastrointestinal cancers, 33–48% of all small bowel carcinomas occur in the duodenum, making it inch for inch the part of the small intestine most at risk (see Lillemoe & Imbembo, 1980). No aetiological factors have been identified for duodenal cancer, although it seems likely that some arise by malignant change in pre-existing adenomas. The prevalence of malignant change in villous tumours of the duodenum is between 25 and 63% (Ryan et al 1986). It is well recognized that biopsies may be unrepresentative and that malignancy may be overlooked unless the entire lesion is available for examination. In general, adenocarcinoma of the duodenum has a prognosis midway between that of periampullary cancer and pancreatic cancer, with less than 30% of patients surviving 5 years after resection. There is some evidence that adenocarcinomas arising from the third and fourth parts of the duodenum (midgut) may have a better outlook than adenocarcinomas arising from the first or second parts (foregut) (Lowell et al 1992), although the significance of this unconfirmed finding is uncertain.

Since completing this chapter, new evidence has emerged from a large multi-centre historical cohort study that the risk of pancreatic cancer in patients with chronic pancreatitis may be significantly elevated, the increased risk being independent of sex, country and type of pancreatitis (Lowenfels et al, 1993).

REFERENCES

Akoi K, Ogawa H 1978 Cancer of the pancreas: international mortality trend. World Health Statistics Quarterly 31: 2–26

Allen-Mersh T G, Earlam R J 1986 Pancreatic cancer in England and Wales: a surgeon's look at epidemiology. Annals of the Royal College of Surgeon of England 68: 154–158

American Cancer Society. Cancer facts and figures. American Cancer Society New York, 1977

American Cancer Society 1988 Cancer facts and figures – 1988. American Cancer Society New York

Anderson T W 1978 Radiation exposures of Hanford workers. A critique of the Mancuso, Stewart and Kneale report. Health Physics 35: 743

Appel M F 1974 Hereditary pancreatitis; review and presentation of additional kindred. Archives of Surgery 108: 63–65

Armstrong C P, Taylor T V 1986 Pancreatic-duct reflux and acute gallstone pancreatitis. Annals of Surgery 204 (1): 59–64

Barrowman J A, Mayston P D 1974 The trophic influence of cholecystokinin in rat pancreas. Journal of Physiology 238: 73P

Bartholomew L G, Gross J B, Comfort M W 1958 Carcinoma of the pancreas associated with chronic relapsing pancreatitis. Gastroenterology 35: 473–477

Bell E T 1957 Carcinoma of the pancreas I. A clinical and pathologic study of 609 necropsied cases. II. The relation of carcinoma of the pancreas to diabetes mellitus. American Journal of Pathology 33 (3): 499–523

Bell R H, Strayer D S 1983 Streptozotocin prevents development of nitrosamine-induced pancreatic cancer in the Syrian hamster. Journal of Surgical Oncology 24: 258–262

Bell R H, Pour P M 1987 Pancreatic carcinogenicity of N-nitrosobis (2-oxopropyl) amine in diabetic and non-diabetic Chinese hamsters. Cancer Letters 34: 221–230

Berk J E 1941 The diagnosis of carcinoma of the pancreas. Archives of Internal Medicine 68: 525–559

Bernarde M A, Weiss W 1982 Coffee consumption and pancreatic cancer: temporal and spatial correlation. British Medical Journal 284: (1) 400–402

Best E W 1966 A Canadian study of smoking and health. Department of National Health and Welfare, Ottawa

Binstock M, Krakow D, Stamler J 1983 Coffee and pancreatic cancer: an analysis of international mortality data. American Journal of Epidemiology 188 (8): 630–640

Birt D F, Salmosi S, Pour P M 1981 Enhancement of experimental pancreatic cancer in Syrian golden hamsters by dietary fat. Journal of the National Cancer Institute 71: 1327–1332

Birt D F, Stepan K R, Pour P M 1983 Interaction of dietary fat and protein on pancreatic carcinogenesis in Syrian golden hamsters. Journal of the National Cancer Institute 67: 355–360

Borch K, Kullman E, Hallhagen S, Ledin T et al 1988 Increased incidence of pancreatic neoplasia in pernicious anaemia. World Journal of Surgery 12: 866–870

Bueli P, Dunn J E 1968 Cancer mortality among Japanese Issei and Nisei of California. Cancer 18: 656–664

Burch E G, Ansari A 1968 Chronic alcoholism and carcinoma of the pancreas. Archives of Internal Medicine 122: 273–275

Burney P G J, Comstook G W, Morris J S 1989 Serologic percursors of cancer: Serum micronutrients and the subsequent risk of pancreatic cancer. American Journal of Clinical Nutrition 49: 895–900

Cancer Research Campaign 1989 Facts on cancer

Castleman B, Scully R, McNeeley B U 1972 Case records of the Massachusetts General Hospital, Case 25-1972, New England Journal of Medicine 286: 1353–1359

Caygill C P J, Hill M J, Hall N, Kirkham J S, Northfield T C 1987 Gastric surgery as a risk factor in human carcinogenesis. Gastroenterology 88: 1344

Cederlof R, Friberg L, Hrubec Z, Lorich U 1975 The relationship of smoking: a ten-year follow-up in a probability sample of 55000 Swedish subjects, age 18–69, Karolinska Institute, Stockholm, parts 1/2.

Clark C G, Mitchell P E G 1961 Diabetes mellitus and primary carcinoma of the pancreas. British Medical Journal 2: 1259–1262

Cohen B L 1980 The low-level radiation link to cancer of the pancreas. Health Physics 38: 712

Comfort M, Steinberg A G 1952 Pedigree of a family with hereditary chronic relapsing pancreatitis. Gastroenterology 21: 54–63

Court-Brown W M, Doll R 1965 Mortality from cancer and other causes after radiotherapy for ankylosing spondylitis. British Medical Journal 2: 1327

Cubilla A L, Fitzgerald P J 1979 Classification of pancreatic cancer (non-endocrine). Mayo Clinic Proceedings 54: 449–458

Cuckle S H, Kinlen L J 1981 Coffee and cancer of the pancreas. British Journal of Cancer 44: 760–761

Di Magno E P, Shorter R G, Taylor W F, Go V L W 1982 Relationships between pancreaticobiliary ductal anatomy and pancreatic ductal and parenchymal histology. Cancer 49: 361–368

Ding S F, Habib N A, Delhanty J D A, Bowles L, Greco L, Wood C, Williamson R C N, Dooley J S 1992 Loss of heterozygosity on chromosomes 1 and 11 in carcinoma of the pancreas. British Journal of Cancer 65: 809–812

Doll R, Peto R 1976 Mortality in relation to smoking: 20 years of observation on male British doctors. British Medical Journal 2: 1525–1536

Doll R, Peto R 1981 The causes of cancer, quantitative estimates of avoidable risks of cancer in the United States today. Journal of the National Cancer Institute 66: 1191–1308

Durbec J P, Chevillotte G, Bidart J M, Berthezene P, Sarles H 1983 Diet, alcohol, tobacco, and risk of pancreatic cancer: a case-controlled study. British Journal of Cancer 47: 463–470

Ehrenthal D, Haeger L, Griffin T, Compton C 1987 Familial pancreatic adenocarcinoma in three generations. Cancer 59: 1661–1664

Enstrom J E 1978 Cancer and total mortality among active Mormons, 1943–1951. Cancer 42: 1943–1951

Falk R T, Pickle L W, Fontham E T, Correa P, Fraumeni J F 1988 Lifestyle risk factors for pancreatic cancer in Louisiana: a case control study. American Journal of Epidemiology 128 (2): 324–336

Feinstein A R, Horwitz R I, Spitzer W O 1981 Coffee and pancreatic cancer. The problems of etiologic science and epidemiologic case control research. Journal of the American Medical Association 246: 957

Ferguson L J, Watts J M 1980 Simultaneous cancer of the pancreas occurring in husband and wife. Gut 21: 537–540

Fisher W E, McCullough P J, Ray M B, Rogers D H, Bell R H 1988 Diabetes enhances growth of pancreatic carcinoma cells. Surgery 104: 431–435

Fontham E T H, Correa P 1989 Epidemiology of pancreatic cancer. Surgical Clinics of North America 69 (3): 551–567

Fraumeni J F 1975 Cancers of the pancreas and biliary tract: epidemiological considerations. Cancer Research 35: 3437–3446

Friedman J M, Fialkow P J 1976 Familial carcinoma of the pancreas. Clinical Genetics 9: 463–469

Gambill E E 1971 Pancreatitis associated with pancreatic carcinoma: a study of 26 cases. Mayo Clinic Proceedings 46: 174–177

Gambill E E, Baggenstoss A H, Priestley J T 1960 Chronic relapsing pancreatitis: fate of fifty-six patients first encountered in the years 1939 to 1943, inclusive. Gastroenterology 39: 404–413

Ghadirian P, Simard A, Baillargeon J 1991 Tobacco, alcohol and coffee and cancer of the pancreas. A population-based case-control study in Quebec, Canada. Cancer 67: 2664–2670

Gold E B, Gordis L, Diener M D 1985 Diet and other risk factors for cancer of the pancreas. Cancer 55: 460–467

Gordis L, Gold E B 1984 Epidemiology of pancreatic cancer. World Journal of Surgery 8: 808–821

Gordis L, Gold E B 1986 Epidemiology and etiology of pancreatic cancer. In: Go V L W et al (eds) The exocrine pancreas: biology, pathobiology and diseases. Raven Press, New York

Gorham E D, Garland C J, Garland F C 1988 Coffee and pancreatic cancer in a rural California country. Western Journal of Medicine 148: 48

Green A, Jensen O M 1985 Frequency of cancer among insulin treated diabetic patients in Denmark. Diabctologia 28: 128–130

Green R C, Baggenstoss A H, Sprague R G 1958 Diabetes mellitus in association with primary carcinoma of the pancreas. Diabetes 7 (4): 308–311

Gross J B, Gambill E E, Ulrich J A 1962 Hereditary pancreatitis. Description of a fifth kindred and summary of clinical features. American Journal of Medicine 33: 358–364

Gudjonsson B, Livstone E M, Spiro H M 1978 Cancer of the pancreas. Diagnostic accuracy and survival statistics. Cancer 42: 2494–2506

Gudjonsson B 1981 Pancreatic carcinoma: diagnostic and therapeutic approach – a word of caution. Journal of Clinical Gastroenterology 3: 301–305

Gudjonsson B 1987 Cancer of the pancreas. 50 years of surgery. Cancer 60: 2284–2303

Haenszel W, Kurihara M 1968 Studies of Japanese migrants I. Mortality from cancer and other diseases among Japanese in the United States. Journal of the National Cancer Institute 40: 43–68.

Haines A P, Moss A R, Whittenmore A, Quivey J 1982 A case control study of pancreatic carcinoma. Journal of Cancer Research and Clinical Oncology 103: 93

Hakulinen T, Lethimaki L, Lehtonen M, Teppo L 1974 Cancer morbidity among two male cohorts with increased alcohol consumption in Finland. Journal of the National Cancer Institute 52: 1711–1714

Hall P A, Lemoine N R, Murphy G, Dowling R H 1991 Molecular differences between human and experimental pancreaticobiliary diversion induced rat pancreatic neoplasia. Gut 32: 533–535

Hammond E C 1966 Smoking in relation to the death rates of one million men and women. National Cancer Institute Monograph 19: 126

Heuch I, Kvale G, Jacobson B K, Bjelke E 1983 Use of alcohol tobacco and coffee, and risk of pancreatic cancer. British Journal of Cancer 48: 637–643

Hiatt R A, Klatsky A C, Armstrong M A 1988 Pancreatic cancer, blood glucose and beverage consumption. International Journal of Cancer 41: 794

Hirayama T 1975 Epidemiology of cancer of the stomach with special reference to its recent decrease in Japan. Cancer Research 35: 3460–3463

Hirayama T 1977 Changing patterns of cancer in Japan with special reference to the decrease in stomach cancer mortality. In: Hiatt H H, Watson J D, Winston J A (eds) Origins of human cancer. Cold Spring Harbor Laboratory, Cold Spring Harbor, vol 4 p 55

Hirayama T 1978 Prospective studies on cancer epidemiology based on census populations in Japan. In: Nienbrugs H E. (ed) Prevention and detection of cancer Volume 1: Etiology. Marcel Dekker, New York

Hirayama T 1981 A large-scale cohort study on the relationship between diet and selected cancer of digestive organs, In: Correa P, Kipkin M, Tannebaums S, Wilkins S (eds) Banbury Report No: 7. Gastrointestinal cancer: Endogenous factors, Cold Spring Harbor Laboratory, Cold Spring Harbor

Hoar S K, Pell S A 1981 A retrospective cohort study of mortality and cancer incidence among chemists. Journal of Occupational Medicine 23: 485

Howatson A G, Carter D C 1985 Pancreatic carcinogenesis enhancement by cholecystokinin in the hamster-nitrosamine model. British Journal of Cancer 51: 107–114

Hseih C, MacMahon B, Yen S, Trichopoulos D et al 1986 Coffee and pancreatic cancer (Ch. 2). New England Journal of Medicine 315 (9): 587–589

Hutchison G B, MacMahon B, Jablon S 1979 Review of reports by

Mancuso, Stewart and Kneale of radiation exposure of Hanford workers. Health Physics 37: 207

Hyvarinen H, Partanen S 1987 Association of cholecystectomy with abdominal cancers. Hepatogastroenterology 34: 280–284

Ishii K, Takeuchi T, Hirayama T 1968 Chronic calcifying pancreatitis and pancreatic carcinoma in Japan. Digestion 9: 429

Jablon S, Angevine D M, Matsumoto Y S, Ishida M 1966 On the significance of cause of death as recorded on death certificates in Hiroshima and Nagasaki. Japanese National Cancer Institute Monograph 19: 445

Jacobsen O, Winther Olsen S, Nielsen N A 1985 Pancreatic cancer in the Faroe Islands. An epidemiologic study of patients with pancreatic cancer in the Faroe Islands 1972–82. Scandinavian Journal of Gastroenterology 20: 1142–1146

Jagelman D G, Decosse J J. Bussey H J R 1988 Upper gastrointestinal cancer in familial adenomatous polyposis. Lancet 1: 1149–1151

Jick H, Dinan B J 1981 Coffee and pancreatic cancer. (Letter) Lancet 2: 92

Johansson B, Bardi G, Heim S, Mandahl N, Mertens F, Bak-Jensen E, Andren-Sandberg A, Mitelman F 1992 Nonrandom chromosomal rearrangements in pancreatic carcinomas. Cancer 69: 1674–1681

Kahn H A 1966 The Dorn study of smoking and mortality among US veterans: report on eight and one-half years of observation. National Cancer Institute Monograph 19: 1–125

Karmody A J, Kyle J 1969 The association between carcinoma of the pancreas and diabetes mellitus. British Journal of Surgery 56 (5): 362–364

Katz L A, Spiro H M 1966 Gastrointestinal manifestations of diabetes. New England Journal of Medicine 275: 1350–1361

Kessler I I 1970 Cancer mortality among diabetics. Journal of the National Cancer Institute 44 (3): 673–685

Kessler I I 1971 Cancer and diabetes mellitus: a review of the literature. Journal of Chronic Diseases 25: 579–600

Kimura W, Ohtsubo K 1988 Incidence, sites of origin, and immunohistochemical and histochemical characteristics of atypical epithelium and minute carcinoma of the papilla of Vater. Cancer 61: 1394–1402

Kinlen L J, McPherson K 1984 Pancreas cancer and coffee and tea consumption: a case control study. British Journal of Cancer 49: 93–96

Klatsky A L, Friedmann G D, Siegelaub A B 1981 Alcohol and mortality. A ten-year Kaiser-Permanente experience. Annals of Internal Medicine 95: 139–143

Klein A, Clemens J, Cameron J 1989 Periampullary neoplasms in von Recklinghausen's disease. Surgery 106: 815–819

Kozuka S, Isuboni M, Yamaguchi A, Hachisuka K 1981 Adenomatous residue in cancerous papilla of Vater. Gut 22: 1031–1034

Krain L S 1970 The rising incidence of carcinoma of the pancreas – real or apparent? Journal of Surgical Oncology 2: 115–124

La Vecchia, Liati P, Decarli A, Negri E et al 1987 Coffee consumption and risk of pancreatic cancer. International Journal of Cancer 40: 309–313

Lea A J 1967 Neoplasms and environmental factors. Annals of the Royal College of Surgeons of England 41: 432–438

LeMoine N R, Jain S, Hughes C M, Staddon S L, Maillet B, Hall P A, Kloppel G 1992 Ki-ras oncogene activation in preinvasive pancreatic cancer. Gastroenterology 102: 230–236

Levin D L, Connelly R R 1973 Cancer of the pancreas: available epidemiologic information and its implications. Cancer 31: 1231–1236

Li F P, Fraumeni J F 1969 Soft-tissue sarcomas, breast cancer, and other neoplasms: A familial syndrome? Annals of Intern Medicine: 71: 747–752

Li F P, Fraumeni J F, Mantel N, Miller R W 1969 Cancer mortality among chemists. Journal of the National Cancer Institute 43: 1159–1164

Lillemoe K, Imbembo A L 1980 Malignant neoplasms of the duodenum. Surgery, Gynecology and Obstetrics 150: 822–826

Lin R S, Kessler I I 1981 A multifactorial model for pancreatic cancer in man: epidemiologic evidence. Journal of the American Medical Association 245: 147–152

Lin J T, Wang T H, Chen D S 1988 Pancreatic carcinoma associated with chronic calcifying pancreatitis in Taiwan: a case report and review of the literature. Pancreas 3: 111–114

Longnecker D S, Curphey T J, Kuhlmann E T, Roebuck B D 1982 Inhibition of pancreatic carcinogenesis by retinoids in azaserine-treated rats. Cancer Research 42: 19–24

Longnecker D S, Roebuck B D, Kuhlmann E T 1985 Enhancement of pancreatic carcinogenesis by a dietary unsaturated fat in rats treated with saline or N-nitroso (2-hydroxypropyl) (2-oxopropyl) amine. Journal of the National Cancer Institute 74 (1): 219–222

Longnecker D S, Curphey T J, Kuhlmann E T, Roebuck B D, Neff R K 1986 Effects of retinoids in N-nitrosobis (2-oxopropyl) amine treated hamsters. Pancreas 3 (1): 241–244

Lowell J A, Rossi R L, Munson L, Braasch J W 1992 Primary adenocarcinoma of third and fourth portions of duodenum. Archives of Surgery 127: 557–560

Lowenfels A B, Maisonneuve P, Cavallini G et al 1993 Pancreatitis and the risk of pancreatic cancer. New England Journal of Medicine 328: 1433–1437

Lynch H T 1967 Hereditary factors in cancer. In: Lynch H T (ed) Recent results in cancer research, Springer-Verlag, New York, vol 23 p 125–142

Lyon J L, Klauber M R, Gardner J M, Smart C R 1976 Cancer incidence in Mormons in Utah. New England Journal of Medicine 294: 129–133

MacDermott R P, Kramer P 1973 Adenocarcinoma of the pancreas in four siblings. Gastroenterology 65: 137–139

MacMahon B 1960 The ethnic distribution of cancer mortality in New York City, 1955. Actol Unionis Internationalis Contra Cancrum 16: 1716

MacMahon B 1982 Risk factors for cancer of the pancreas. Cancer 50: 2676–2680

MacMahon B, Yen S, Trichopoulos D, Warren J et al 1981 Coffee and cancer of the pancreas. New England Journal of Medicine 304: 630–633

McLean-Ross A H, Smith M A, Anderson J R, Small W P 1982 Late mortality after surgery for peptic ulcer. New England Journal of Medicine 307 (9): 519–522

McMichael A J, McCall M J, Hartshorne J 1980 Patterns of gastrointestinal cancer in European migrants to Australia: the role of dietary change. International Journal of Cancer 25: 431

Mack T M, Yu M C, Hanisch R, Henderson B E N 1986 Pancreas cancer and smoking, beverage consumption, and past medical history. Journal of the National Cancer Institute 76 (1): 49–60

Mainz D L, Black O, Webster P D 1973 Hormonal control of pancreatic growth. Journal of Clinical Investigation 52: 2300–2304

Mancusco T F, El-Attar A A 1967 Cohort study of workers exposed to betanaphthylamine and benzidine. Journal of Occupational Medicine 9: 277–285

Mancusco T F, Sterling T D 1974 Relation of place of birth and migration in cancer mortality in the US: a study of Ohio residence (1959–1967). Journal of Chronic Diseases 27: 459–474

Mancusco T F, Stewart A, Kneale G 1977 Radiation exposure of Hanford workers dying from cancer and other causes. Health Physics 33: 369

Marighini A, Thiruvengadam R, Melton L J 1987 Pancreatic cancer risk following gastric surgery. Cancer 60: 245–247

Maruchi N 1973 An epidemiologic study of pancreatic cancer with special reference to US – Japanese comparison. Japanese Journal of Cancer Clinics 19: 73–82

Miller E C, Miller J A 1986 Carcinogens and mutagens that may occur in foods. Cancer 58: 1795–1803

Miller A R, Nagorney D M, Sarr M G 1992 The surgical spectrum of hereditary pancreatitis in adults. Annals of Surgery 215: 39–43

Mills P K, Beeson W L, Abbey D E, Fraser G E et al 1988 Dietary habits and past medical history as related to fatal pancreas cancer risk among adventists. Cancer 61: 2578–2585

Mikal S, Campbell J A 1950 Carcinoma of the pancreas: diagnostic and operative criteria based on one hundred consecutive autopsies. Surgery 28: 963–969

Mirvish S S 1986 Effects of vitamins C and E on N-nitroso compound formation, carcinogenesis, and cancer. Cancer 58: 1842–1850

Mohr P, Ammann R, Largiader F, Knoblauch M et al 1975 Pankreaskarzinom bei chronischer Pankreatitis. Schweizerische Medizinische Wochenschrift 105: 590–592

Monson R R, Lyon J L 1975 Proportional mortality among alcoholics. Cancer 36: 1077–1079

Morgan R G H, Wormsley K G 1977 Progress report: cancer of the pancreas. Gut 18: 580–596

Morgan R G H, Levinson D A, Hopwood D, Saunders J H B,

Wormsley K G 1977 Potentiation of the action of azaserine on the rat pancreas by raw soya bean flower. Cancer Letters 3: 87–90

Motojima K, Tsunoda T, Kanematsu T, Nagata Y, Urano T, Shiku H 1991 Distinguishing pancreatic carcinoma from other periampullary carcinomas by analysis of mutations in the kirsten-*ras* oncogene. Annals of Surgery 214: 657–662

Muir C, Waterhouse J, Mack T (eds) 1987 Cancer incidence in five continents. Volume V IARC Scientific Publication No. 88. International Agency for Research on Cancer, Lyons

Neoptolemos J P, Talbot I C, Shaw D C, Carr-Locke D L 1988 Long-term survival after resection of ampullary carcinoma is associated independently with tumor grade and a new staging classification that assesses local invasiveness. Cancer 61: 1403–1407

Newill V A 1961 Distribution of cancer mortality among ethnic subgroups of the white population of New York City. Journal of the National Cancer Institute 27: 459–474

Nomura A, Stemmermann G H, Heilburn L K 1981 Coffee and pancreatic cancer Lancet 2: 415 (letter)

Norell S E, Ahlborn A, Erwald R 1986a Diet and pancreatic cancer: a case-control study. American Journal of Epidemiology 124: 894–902

Norell S, Ahlborn A, Erwald R 1986b Diabetes, gallstone disease, and pancreatic cancer. British Journal of Cancer 54: 377–378 (letter)

Offerhaus J G A, Giardiello F M, Moore G W, Tersmette A C 1987 Partial gastrectomy: a risk factor for carcinoma of the pancreas? Human Pathology 18 (3): 285–288

Office of Population Censuses and Surveys 1975 Cancer mortality, England and Wales 1911–1970. In: Studies on Medical and Population Subjects. No. 29. HMSO, London

Osawa K, Ida T, Yamada T, Yamaoka Y, Takasan H, Honjo I 1975 Oral glucose tolerance in patients with jaundice. Surgery, Gynecology and Obstetrics 140: 582–588

Pickle L W, Gottlieb M S 1980 Pancreatic cancer mortality in Louisiana. American Journal of Public Health 70: 256

Pour P M, Runbe R G, Birt D 1981 Current knowledge of pancreatic carcinogenesis in the hamster and its relevance to human disease. Cancer 47: 1573–1587

Redmond C K, Strobino B R, Cypress R H 1976 Cancer experience among coke by-product workers. Annals of the New York Academy of Sciences 271: 102–115

Reimer R R, Fraumeni J F, Ozols R F, Bender R 1977 Pancreatic cancer in father and son. Lancet 1: 911–912 (letter)

Robinette C D, Hrubec Z, Fraumeni J F 1979 Chronic alcoholism and subsequent mortality in World War II veterans. American Journal of Epidemiology 109: 682–700

Rocca G, Gaia E, Juliano E 1987 Increased incidence of cancer in chronic pancreatitis. Journal of Clinical Gastroenterology 9: 175–179

Rokkas T, Palmer T J, Sladen G E 1989 Tumours of the pancreas as a sequel to abdominal radiation. Postgraduate Medical Journal 65: 493–496

Rosenberg L, Duguid W P, Brown R A, Greeley G et al 1983 The effect of cholecystectomy on plasma CCK and pancreatic growth in the hamster. Gastroenterology 84: 1289 (abstract)

Rosenberg L, Duguid W P, Brown R A 1984 Cholecystectomy stimulates hypertrophy and hyperplasia in the hamster pancreas. Journal of Surgical Research 37: 108–111

Rubio V, Rodriguez J I 1989 Near-simultaneous adenocarcinoma of the pancreas in husband and wife. Lancet 1: 166–167 (letter)

Ryan D P, Schapiro R H, Warshaw A L 1986 Villous tumors of the duodenum. Annals of Surgery 203: 301–306

Schmidt W, Popham R E 1981 The role of drinking and smoking in mortality from cancer and other causes in male alcoholics. Cancer 47: 1031–1041

Schwartz S S, Ziedler A, Moossa A R, Kuku S F et al 1978 A prospective study of glucose tolerance, insulin C-peptide and glucagon responses in patients with pancreatic cancer. Digestive Diseases 23 (12): 1107–1114

Searle C E, Waterhouse J A H, Henman B A, Bartlett D et al 1981 Epidemiological study of the mortality of British chemists. British Journal Cancer 38: 192–193

Seidman H 1970 Cancer death rates by site and sex for religions and socioeconomic groups in New York City. Environmental Research 3: 235

Segi M, Kurihara M, Matsuyama T 1969 Cancer Mortality for selected sites in 24 countries, No. 5 1964–65. Department of Public Health, Tohoku University School of Medicine, Sendai, Japan

Smith R L 1956 Recorded and expected mortality among Japanese of Hawaii and the States with special reference to cancer. Journal of the National Cancer Institute 17: 459–465

Smith P G, Doll R 1981 Mortality from cancer and all causes among British radiologists. British Journal of Radiology 54: 187–194

Smith P G, Douglas A J 1986 Mortality of workers at the Sellafield plant of British Nuclear Fuels. British Medical Journal 293:845–854

Spigelman A D, Williams C B, Talbot I C, Domizio P, Phillips R K S 1989 Upper gastrointestinal cancer in patients with familial adenomatous polyposis. Lancet 2: 783–785

Spigelman A D, Crofton-Sleigh C, Venitt S, Phillips R K S 1990 Mutagenicity of bile and duodenal adenomas in familial adenomatous polyposis. British Journal of Surgery 77: 878–881

Stace N H, Palmer T J, Vaja S, Dowling R H 1987 Long-term pancreaticobiliary diversion stimulates hyperplastic and adenomatous nodules in the rat pancreas: a new model for spontaneous tumour formation. Gut 28: 265–268

Stocks P 1970 Cancer mortality in relation to national consumption of cigarettes solid fuel, tea and coffee. British Journal of Cancer 24: 215–225

Taxy J B 1976 Adenocarcinoma of the pancreas in childhood. Cancer 37: 1508–1518

Thomas T L, Decowtle P, Mowe-Eraso R 1980 Mortality among workers employed in petroleum refinery and petrochemical plants. Journal of Occupational Medicine 22: 97

Turner H M, Grace H G 1938 An investigation into cancer mortality among males in certain Sheffield trades. Journal of Hygiene 38: 90–103

Tsukimoto I, Watanabe K, Lin J B, Nakayima T 1973 Pancreatic cancer in children in Japan. Cancer 31: 1203–1207

Ura H, Makino T, Ito S 1986 Combined effect of cholecystectomy and lithocholic acid on pancreatic carcinogenesis of N-nitrosobis (2-hydroxyproply) amine in Syrian golden hamsters. Cancer Research 46: 4782–4786

Velema J P, Walker A M, Gold E B 1986 Alcohol and pancreatic cancer: insufficient epidemiologic evidence for a casual·relationship. Epidemioligal Research 8: 28

Wakita K, Ohyanagi H, Yamamoto K, Tokuhisa T, Saitoh Y 1992 Overexpression of c-Ki-ras and c-**fos** in human pancreatic carcinomas. International Journal of Pancreatology 11: 43–47

Wald N, Idle M, Boreham J, Bailey A 1980 Low serum vitamin A and subsequent risk of cancer; preliminary results of a prospective study. Lancet 2: 813–815

Waterhouse J H, Muir C, Correa P (eds) 1976 Cancer incidence in five continents. Vol III. IARC Scientific Publication no. 45. International Agency for Research on Cancer, Lyons

Weisberger J H, Williams G M 1975 Metabolism of chemical carcinogens. In: Becker FF (ed) Cancer: a comprehensive treatise. Plenum Press, New York, vol 1 p 185

Weiss W, Bernarde M A 1983 The temporal relation between cigarette smoking and pancreatic cancer. American Journal of Public Health 74: 1403–1404

Whittemore A S, Paffenberger R S, Anderson K, Halpern J 1983 Early precursors of pancreatic cancer in college men. Journal of Chronic Diseases 365: 251–256

Whitten D M, Feingold M, Eisenklam E J 1968 Hereditary pancreatitis. American Journal of Diseases of Childhood 116: 426–428

Wynder E L 1975 An epidemiological evaluation of the causes of cancer of the pancreas. Cancer Research 35: 2228–2233

Wynder E L, Mabuchi K, Maruchi N, Fortner J G 1973 A case control study of cancer of the pancreas. Cancer 31: 641–648

Wynder E L, Hall N E L, Polansky M 1983 Epidemiology of coffee and pancreatic cancer. Cancer Research 43: 3900–3906

Wynder E L, Dieck S, Hall N E L 1986 Case-control study of decaffeinated coffee consumption and pancreatic cancer. Cancer Research 46: 5360–5363

Yamaguchi K, Enjoji M 1991 Adenoma of the ampulla of Vater: putative precancerous lesion. Gut 32: 1558–1561

36. Pathology and classification of tumours of the pancreas

V. Becker   P. Stömmer

INTRODUCTION

The pancreas is the topographical centre of man; the point of intersection of all areas of the body is situated in the head of the pancreas. In spite of its location and its phylogenetic age, it is the oldest salivary gland (Brunner 1987). Its function remained obscure till the experiments of Bernard (1856) clarified its role in digestion. Nowadays, inflammatory and neoplastic diseases of the pancreas are amongst the most challenging problems in surgery, oncology, internal medicine and modern diagnostics, as well as in pathology.

The first conclusive descriptions of human pancreatic tumours date back to Bigsby (1835) and Mondiere (1836), as the earlier communications of Morgagni & Bonetus (1661) are difficult to interpret. Up to the first decades of this century neoplasms of the pancreas were uncommon.

In Europe, pancreatic cancer is at present the seventh commonest form of cancer in men, after tumours of stomach, colon, rectum, lung, prostate and bladder (Boyle et al 1989). In the USA, pancreas neoplasms take fourth place as a cause of cancer mortality in men and fifth place as a cause of cancer mortality in women (Schottenfeld & Fraumeni 1982, Klöppel 1984). These rankings are not only determined by the availability of advanced diagnostic techniques in medical services; but also by the autopsy series of large institutes, the relative importance of pancreatic diseases having increased during the last few decades (Höpker 1987).

CLASSIFICATION

Human pancreatic tumours are commonly classified according to the WHO Classification Vol. 20 (Gibson & Sobin 1978) for exocrine tumours and the WHO Classification Vol. 23 (Williams 1980) for endocrine tumours. Some different classifications, largely because of new tumour types, were suggested by Becker (1973), Cubilla & Fitzgerald (1984), Klöppel & Fitzgerald (1986) and Morohoshi et al (1983) (Table 36.1). The detailed classification according to Cubilla & Fitzgerald (1984),

published by the American Forces Institute of Pathology is used here, with some minor deviations.

The recent UICC classification of tumour stage strictly distinguishes between malignant tumours of the exocrine pancreas, the ampulla of Vater and the distal bile duct. This strict separation of ampullary and pancreatic carcinomas causes problems in cases where carcinoma infiltrates the ampulla as well as the head of the pancreas; if such tumours are regarded as ampullary carcinomas they should be classified as pT_4; if they are looked upon as pancreatic carcinomas, the correct classification should be pT_2. Former classifications (Hermreck et al 1974, Pollard et al 1981, Klöppel et al 1984) are now obsolete (Table 36.2). Tumours with a diameter of less than 1 or 2 cm, without metastases or infiltration of peripancreatic tissue are sometimes classified as 'small' or 'early' cancers (Moossa 1980, Hermanek 1984, Ariyama 1990, Tashiro et al 1990). In another similar definition, early pancreatic cancer (Becker et al 1990, Tokuka et al 1990) comprises small pancreatic tumours in which the shape of the gland is preserved and endoscopic retrograde cholangiopancreatography (ERCP) is normal.

DUCTAL ADENOCARCINOMA OF THE PANCREAS

Epidemiology

The common pancreatic cancer is the ductal adenocarcinoma in the full range of its varieties. In contrast to all the other tumours of the pancreas, considerable epidemiological information is available concerning this particular neoplasm. From 1955 to 1985, the pancreatic cancer mortality rate doubled and pancreatic carcinomas formed an increasing proportion of all cancers (Table 36.3; Boyle et al 1989). After 1980 it is arguable whether the increase of deaths due to pancreatic cancer has diminished (Gordis & Gold 1984) or is still increasing (Boyle et al 1989). Little difference exists between European countries (Höpker 1987); in contrast, countries in the third world

Table 36. 1 Histological classification of exocrine pancreatic tumours. (AFIP, American Forces Institute of Pathology)

WHO/Gibson & Sobin 1978	Morohoshi et al 1983	AFIP/Cubilla & Fitzgerald 1984
Epithelial tumours	Duct cell origin	Ductule cell origin
Benign	Ductal adenoma	
Adenoma	Intraductal papilloma	
Cystadenoma	Serous cystadenoma	
	Mucinous cystic tumour	
Malignant		
Adenocarcinoma	Ductal adenocarcinoma	Ductal cell carcinoma
	Well differentiated	Giant cell carcinoma
	Poorly differentiated	Giant cell carcinoma
		Osteoclastoid
Squamous cell carcinoma	Adenosquamous carcinoma	Adenosquamous carcinoma
		Spindle cell carcinoma
		Microadenocarcinoma
Cystadenocarcinoma	Mucinous carcinoma	Mucinous carcinoma
		Mucinous cystadenocarcinoma
		Papillary cystic tumour
		Mucinous carcinoid carcinoma
		Carcinoid
		Oncocytic carcinoid
		Oncocytic carcinoma
		'Oat cell' carcinoma
		Ciliated cell carcinoma
	Pleomorphic carcinoma	
	Giant cell type	
	Osteoclast-like type	
	Acinar cell origin	Acinar cell origin
	Solid and cystic tumour	
Acinar cell carcinoma	Acinar cell carcinoma	Acinar cell carcinoma
	Acinar cystadenocarcinoma	Acinar cystadenocarcinoma
Undifferentiated carcinoma	Uncertain Histogenesis	Uncertain histogenesis
	Pancreatoblastoma	Pancreaticoblastoma (simple)
		Pancreaticoblastoma (mixed type)
	Pleomorphic carcinoma	Unclassified
	Small cell type	Small cell carcinoma
		Large cell carcinoma
		Clear cell carcinoma
		Mixed cell type
		Duct-islet-cell carcinoma
		Duct-islet-acinar-cell carcinoma
		Acinar-islet-cell carcinoma
		Carcinoid-islet-cell carcinoma
Tumours of islets		Connective tissue origin
Non-epithelial tumours		Leiomyosarcoma
Miscellaneous tumours		Malignant fibrous histiocytoma
Unclassified tumours		Haemangiopericytoma
Haemato/lymphatic neoplasms		Fibrosarcoma
Metastatic tumours		Malignant neurilemmoma etc
Epithelial abnormalities		
Tumour-like lesions		

show very low incidence rates (Muir et al 1988). The incidence rates for immigrants from the latter countries to the USA adjust to that of the host country (Lynch et al 1981).

Pancreatic adenocarcinoma is consistently reported to occur more commonly in blacks than in whites, and in urban rather than rural population groups. There is a male preponderance of pancreatic cancer all over the world (Klöppel 1984, Boyle et al 1989) and in our own series of 253 patients with ductal carcinoma there was a ratio of 1.25:1. This was influenced by the location of the neoplasm. Tumours of the pancreatic head showed a

male–female ratio of 1.68:1, those of the body 1.1:1, whereas tumours of the tail were exclusively seen in females. Ampullary carcinomas were slightly more common in women (1:1.06).

Correlation studies of mortality rates and consumption of cigarettes have shown a clear association between cigarette smoking and pancreatic cancer risk (Stocks 1970, Breslow & Enstrom 1974). A direct correlation with the number of cigarettes smoked has been observed (IARC Working Party 1986, Hiatt et al 1988).

The role of alcohol consumption in the development of pancreatic cancer is more controversial. Breslow and

Table 36.2 UICC classification of pancreatic tumours, pTNM (4th edition 1987). Regional lymph nodes are the peripancreatic nodes: superior, inferior, anterior, posterior and splenic.

pT1		No direct extension of the primary tumour beyond the pancreas
	pT1a	≤2 cm
	pT1b	>2 cm
pT2		Limited direct extension to duodenum, bile duct, peripancreatic tissue
pT3		Direct extension to spleen, stomach, colon, blood vessels
pN0		Regional lymph nodes not involved
pN1		Regional lymph nodes involved
pM0		No distant metastasis

Table 36.3 Pancreatic carcinomas in males, 1955 and 1985, as a percentage of all cancers in various countries. (Data according to Boyle et al 1989)

Country	1955	1985
Austria	3.3	5.1
Czechoslovakia	2.6	4.4
France	2.4	3.6
W Germany	2.5	4.5
Ireland	4.6	5.9
Greece	1.8	4.2
UK	3.8	4.2
Poland	2.0	4.1

Table 36.4 Success rates in diagnosing pancreatic neoplasms following the use of various methods of obtaining material for cytological examination

Method	% Success rates (true positives)
Duodenal aspirates (Kline et al 1978)	
Overall	66
Head	79
Body, tail	33
CT, fine-needle aspirates	Over 90 (Hajdu et al 1986, Mikuz et al 1987)
Endoscopic retrograde cholangiopancreatography, juice	50–85 (Smithies et al 1977)
Intraoperative fine-needle aspirates	94 (Mikuz et al 1987)

Enstrom (1974) reported significant positive correlation, whereas numerous case–control studies have found no significant increase (Lin & Kessler 1981, MacMahon et al 1981). The problem of alcoholic chronic pancreatitis and pancreatic cancer (Becker 1974) will be discussed later.

Daily consumption of coffee was found to correlate with increased pancreatic cancer risk (MacMahon et al 1981). However, other data have shown only a small effect in moderate and heavy coffee drinkers (Clavel et al 1989). The problem of bias with cigarette smoking is, however, still unresolved. The role of other dietary or other occupational factors remains controversial (Boyle et al 1989) and is discussed in Chapter 35. Familial pancreatic cancer was observed in 18 families by Lynch et al (1991).

General features

The clinical diagnosis of pancreatic cancer is difficult and in autopsy series, up to 47% of cases had received an incorrect clinical diagnosis (Connelly et al 1985, Höpker 1987).

The general features of the tumour are mainly the consequence of tumour extension; carcinomas of the head of the pancreas cause progressive jaundice and less commonly obstruction of the duodenum is found at the time of diagnosis. Tumours of the body and tail of the pancreas grow insidiously and usually show metastases by the time diagnosis is established. Apart from pain and weight loss, other general symptoms of pancreatic cancer are multiple thrombosis (Trousseau's sign) (Trousseau 1865, Lafler &

Hinerman 1961, Cruickshank 1986, Stömmer 1987), and symptomatic depression (Joffe & Adsett 1985, Stömmer 1987).

Morphologically the clinical diagnosis can be confirmed by intraoperative needle biopsy, fine-needle aspiration cytology under CT or ultrasonographic guidance; and duodenal aspiration cytology. The results of such procedures are encouraging (Table 36.4).

A novel method consists of endoscopy of the main pancreatic duct through the intact papilla using an endoscope with a diameter of less than 0.4 mm. Characteristic features of ductal carcinomas are a tent-wall-like compression of the lumen, coarse and irregular papillae, discolouration and large amounts of detritus. (Stömmer et al 1989, Foerster et al 1990). Biopsy and brush-cytology are feasible at the time of endoscopy.

Gross features

Ductal carcinomas are said to be located in the head of the pancreas in two-thirds of cases, the rest being found in the body and tail of the gland. In our own surgical specimens of 253 resected tumours of the pancreas, 81.7% of the ductal carcinomas were located in the head, 16% in the body, and only 2.3% in the tail of the gland (Stiegler 1990). The diameter of the tumours depended primarily on their location in that carcinomas of the head were usually smaller than tumours of body and tail (Table 36.5). Generally, pancreatic carcinomas are white on sectioning, with a slight green hue after formalin fixation (Fig. 36.1). They have a hard consistency because of their high content of collagenous fibres, and their borders are indistinct. Large tumour necroses are only seen in cases of duodenal infiltration with consequent infection. The diameter of the tumour does not correlate with the grade of malignancy and we have often seen features of high grade malignancy in small tumours.

Commonly, the tumours originate from the epithelium of large tributaries of the main pancreatic duct. Three types of tumour infiltration of the duct occur, namely, complete duct obstruction (Fig. 36.1), compression 'tapering' and irregular segmental strictures, often accompanied by

Table 36.5 Diameters of 253 pancreatic tumours in relation to their location, shown as percentage of total for each location. (Data according to Stiegler 1990)

Diameter	Head	Body	Tail	Ampulla	Bile duct
<1 cm	0	0	0	12.7	15.0
1–2 cm	15.0	0	0	14.5	45.0
2–3 cm	33.4	52.0	0	45.5	15.0
3–4 cm	23.3	26.3	0	18.8	5.0
>4 cm	27.8	21.1	100	9.1	20.0

Table 36.6 Infiltration of ventral and dorsal pseudocapsule, perineural sheaths, and blood vessels in relation to the location of small tumours (<2 cm). Data shown as percentages

	Tumour location		
Infiltration	Pancreas	Ampulla	Bile duct
Perineural	60	25	57
Blood vessel	75	33	66
Pseudocapsule			
Ventral	41	0	9
Dorsal	54	17	18

dilatation of the prestenotic duct and chronic obstructive pancreatitis. Even small tumours tend to infiltrate into the pseudocapsule and the peripancreatic soft tissue (Table 36.6) Infiltration and stenosis of the common bile duct are seen in 92% of all resected adenocarcinomas of the head of the pancreas and the stenosis usually shows a 'knickerbocker' phenomenon. Tumours of the body and tail never caused stenosis of the bile duct in our cases.

Lymph node metastases are common features, even in small pancreatic adenocarcinomas. Of tumours with a diameter of less than 2 cm (pT_1), 86% show lymph node metastases (Table 36.7). These metastases, in resectable carcinomas of the head of the pancreas, are found predominantly in the anterior and posterior duodenopancreatic lymph nodes and in the infrapancreatic nodes. Metastases to the splenic nodes are only observed in tumours of the pancreatic tail. Distant nodal metastases are commonly seen along the upper common bile duct (20%), the superior mesenteric artery (15%), and the lesser curvature of the stomach (10%). Less common are metastases around the coeliac trunk (6%) and the aorta (Hermanek et al 1987, Stiegler 1990). Interestingly, in ampullary carcinomas of the same diameters, lymph node metastases are much less

common than in the pancreatic ductal carcinomas, though there are no histological differences between pancreatic and periampullary carcinomas (Hermanek 1984, Klöppel 1987).

Microscopic features

The prototype of pancreatic carcinomas is classified as ductal pancreatic carcinoma. It is also called duct cell adenocarcinoma, as in Cubilla & Fitzgerald (1984).

This classification is based on the histological and submicroscopical appearance of the tumours, in particular, the absence of zymogen and neurosecretory granules in most of the tumour cells, the content of intracytoplasmic mucus and the tubular 'ductal' arrangement of the tumour cells (Cubilla & Fitzgerald 1986). It does not necessarily refer to the histogenesis of the tumours, though there is some evidence in that direction from experimental (Pour 1986), histological (Cubilla & Fitzgerald 1980) and submicroscopic studies (Kern et al 1986). The possibility of an origin from regressive acini, also forming ductal structures (Bockman et al 1983), cannot be completely excluded because of the very rare occurrence of ductal-acinar mixed tumours. However, in spite of this, the dedifferentiation of common acinar carcinomas never ends in a ductal carcinoma.

Their overall low-power appearance may be suggestive of malignancy, because of irregularities in the distribution and

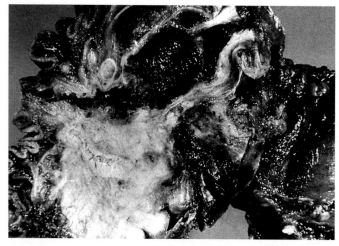

Fig. 36.1 Adenocarcinoma in the head of the pancreas. A white, hard tumour is seen in the lower part of the gland; destruction of the major pancreatic duct with complete occlusion and prestenotic dilatation; long stenosis of the choledochal duct, and the 'knickerbocker phenomenon'. × 1.5

Table 36.7 Tumour infiltration into the ventral and dorsal pseudocapsule of the pancreas and the pattern of lymph node metastasis, in relation to the diameter of ductal adenocarcinomas of head and body. Data are shown as percentages

	Tumour diameter		
Infiltration	<2 cm	<4 cm	>4 cm
Ventral pseudocapsule	42	48	70
Dorsal pseudocapsule	55	60	90
Lymph node metastasis			
Total	86	80	81
Suprapancreatic	38	30	33
Infrapancreatic	50	46	53
Anterior duodenopancreatic	37	38	58
Posterior duodenopancreatic	56	53	63
Bile duct	33	45	50

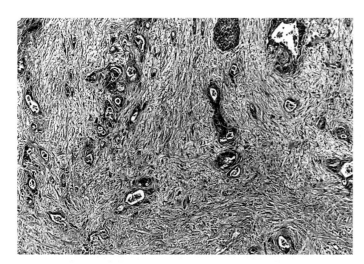

Fig. 36.2 Ductal adenocarcinoma with high grade desmoplastic reaction, surrounding irregular tubular and glandular tumour complexes. Haematoxylin–Eosin; × 50.

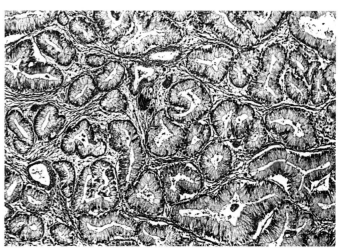

Fig. 36.4 Well differentiated ductal adenocarcinoma: irregular glands with single or double layered epithelium: basally located hypochromatic nuclei. Haematoxylin–Eosin; × 80.

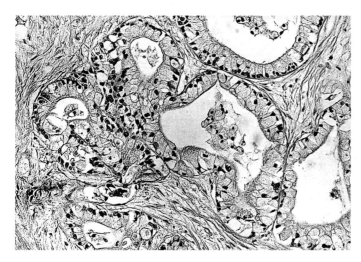

Fig. 36.3 Adenocarcinoma of the pancreas, biliary epithelial type: large tumour cells with clear cytoplasm, reminiscent of biliary epithelium. Haematoxylin–phloxin–safran; × 300.

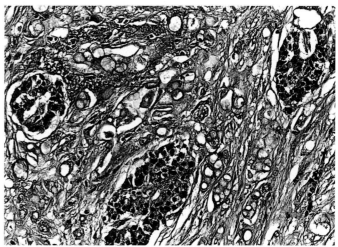

Fig. 36.5 Poorly differentiated adenocarcinoma with diffuse infiltration of the gland by mucinous tumour cells. Well preserved Langerhans islets amid the tumour cells ('Stobbe phenomenon'). PAS–alcian; × 325.

shape of the glands. Typically there is a highly desmoplastic reaction of the stroma (Fig. 36.2). Cellular characteristics of malignancy, seen at high power are loss of polarity, nuclear polymorphism, prominent nucleoli and enlarged nuclei. In comparison with non-neoplastic intestinal epithelia, the neoplastic cells may resemble either pancreatic ductal cells or epithelia from the gallbladder/bile ducts with clear, mucinous cytoplasm (Fig. 36.3) or, in some cases enterocytes. Usually there is an admixture with 'common mucinous carcinoma cells', which cannot be differentiated from other tumour cells in the gastrointestinal tract (Cubilla & Fitzgerald 1984).

Some hints for the differentiation of metastases may be given by immunocytochemistry in that ductal adenocarcinomas of the pancreas express cytokeratin 7 in contrast to tumours of the colon and stomach (Osborne et al 1986).

In our series, 7% of pancreatic carcinomas showed exclusively bile duct/clear-type epithelia (Fig. 36.3.) while a predominantly enterocytic type of tumour cells was seen in 7% of the pancreatic carcinomas reported by Stiegler (1990). Unusual types of metaplastic ductal cells (signet cells, squamous epithelia, or an admixture of endocrine cells) are regarded as separate entities.

Histologically, ductal adenocarcinoma of the pancreas may be classified according to UICC (1987) into G1, well-differentiated (Fig. 36.4), G2, moderately differentiated; G3, poorly differentiated (Fig. 36.5) and G4, undifferentiated (Hermanek et al 1987). Criteria defined by Klöppel (1984) are histological (formation of tubular/

Table 36.8 Histological and cytological criteria for the grading of ductal adenocarcinoma of the pancreas (based on Klöppel 1988)

Grade	Glandular differentiation	Mucin production	Mitoses (per 10 high-power fields)	Nuclear anaplasia
1	Duct-like glands	Intensive	1–5	Polar, monomorphic
2	Duct-like tubular	Irregular	6–10	Some polymorphism
3	Cribriform, pleomorphic	Abortive	>10	High pleomorphism
4	Solid	None	>10	Giant + sarcoid cell

glandular structures and amount of mucus) and cytological (polar arrangement, nucleoli, nuclear polymorphism and the number of mitoses) (Table 36.8). A different approach involves the differential grading of cytological and histological features. These two approaches do not show very good correlations and both could be included in a score which also comprised parameters of mitotic activity (Stiegler 1990).

Ultrastructural characteristics of ductal adenocarcinomas are dependent on their grade of differentiation. Cells of grade 1 adenocarcinomas of the pancreas are highly polarized with basally located nuclei, apical mucus granules with a diameter of about 100 mm and, in many cases, irregular microvilli located only at the apical cytoplasmic membrane. The basal membrane, which is the spatial organizer of these epithelia (Ingber et al 1986), is connected with the extracellular lamina basalis by numerous hemidesmosomes. Tight interconnections between the tumour cells contribute to their monodirectional secretion. Secretion products are located only at the apical cytoplasmic border and are shed by exocytosis and perhaps by apical expulsion.

The electron-microscopic features of high-grade malignancy are a decrease in laminin and basement membrane organization; loss of mucus granules; accumulation of small vesicles with central dense cores; loss of interdigitations, and a widened intercellular space. The microvilli of the tumour cells which are located at the apical cytoplasmic membranes in G1 tumours are distributed all over the luminal and basal cell surfaces in tumours of high-grade malignancy (Kern et al 1986a, b).

Immunocytochemistry

The normal ductal cells express gastrointestinal cancer-associated antigen, CA 19–9, and carcinoembryonic antigen (CEA) only at the apical surface membrane of the cells. This is also true for moderately differentiated (G1) tumours (Stömmer et al 1989c) (Fig. 36.6). In carcinomas with high-grade malignancy, CEA and CA 19–9 are distributed all over the cytoplasm (Makovitzky 1987, Schwenk & Makovitzky 1989a, b). In most cases the expression parallels the histological grading (Allum et al 1986, Ichihara et al 1988). The measurement of serum concentrations of CA 19–9 and CEA are clinical tests

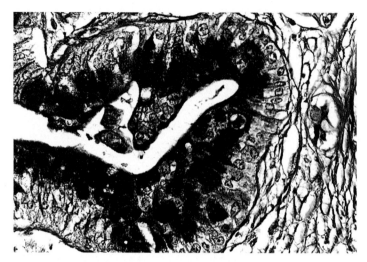

Fig. 36.6 Moderately differentiated ductal adenocarcinoma: Expression of carcinoembryonic antigen (CEA) only in the upper parts of the tumour cells. Anti-CEA-ABC Method; × 450.

for the presence of gastrointestinal and pancreatic carcinomas.

In the search for other tumour markers, a role for Lewis a and b antigens was postulated. These substances are chemically similar to CA 19–9. Patients without Lewis a antigen are not able to express CA 19–9 (Würmeling 1988, Schwenk & Makovitzky 1989a, b). The clinical consequence is that the evaluation of serum CA 19–9 should always be correlated with the Lewis status, because a lack of elevation of CA 19–9 can either result from the absence of pancreatic carcinoma or from the fact that the production of CA 19–9 (even in manifest tumours) is simply not possible. The role and importance of other monoclonal antibodies, such as C1p83 (Schmiegel et al 1985) or CA 50 (Schwenk & Makovitzky 1989b), are still the subject of investigation. Amylase, S-100, neuron specific enolase (NSE) or phospholipase are not expressed in duct cell adenocarcinoma although some endocrine cells are occasionally found in these tumours (Reid et al 1982, Pour 1986) (Table 36.9).

Macroscopic and surgical problems

Surgical problems of ductal adenocarcinomas of the pancreas include infiltration beyond the resection line, multicentricity of the neoplasm, and the presence of meta-

Table 36.9 Immunohistochemical reactivity of ductal carcinoma, acinar cell carcinoma, islet cell tumours and microadenocarcinoma

Antibody	Ductal carcinoma	Acinar carcinoma	Islet cell tumour	Microcarcinoma
Tissue peptide antigen (TPA)	+	−		+
α_1-antitrypsin	−	+	(+)	+
α_1-antichymotrypsin	−	+	(+)	+
Carcinoembryonic antigen (CEA)	+	−	−	−
Gastrointestinal cancer-associated antigen, CA 19–9	+	−	−	−
Neuron specific enolase (NSE)	−	−	+	+
S-100, hormones	−	−	+	−
Amylase	−	−	−	−
Phospholipase A_2	−	−	−	+
PAS	+	+	−	(+)

stases; the highly unfavourable prognosis with a median survival time after diagnosis of 2–3 months (Reber & Austin 1988) results from these problems. Most adenocarcinomas are located in the head of the pancreas, and examination of 108 pancreaticoduodenectomy (Whipple's procedure) surgical specimens, in Erlangen over the period 1984–1989, showed that gross or histological tumour residues were only rarely located at the transection line of the pancreas. The critical points were the ventral and dorsal pseudocapsules of the pancreas and the surrounding soft tissue (Table 36.6). Tumour infiltration was only loosely associated with the diameter of the tumour (Table 36.7).

The pancreaticojejunal anastomosis and the soft tissues surrounding the superior mesenteric artery are therefore an important site for tumour residues and recurrences (Nagai et al 1986, Guthoff et al 1987, Klöppel 1987). Multicentricity of tumour (Klöppel et al 1980) or residual tumour in the tail of the pancreas are uncommon causes of relapse (Klöppel et al 1987). Apart from this, even small ductal carcinomas shed malignant cells into the peritoneum and in one-third of technically resectable carcinomas, peritoneal lavage showed tumour cells (Warshaw 1990).

apparent chronic pancreatitis show a much lower incidence (0.2% of negative results (Hermanek 1986).

Hallmarks for the histological diagnosis of malignancy are the presence of irregular small glands surrounded by a dense desmoplastic stroma. Nuclear polymorphism, prominent nucleoli and (only sometimes seen) mitotic activity may help diagnosis. The tumour cells are positive for CEA and CA 19–9 as well as for human epithelial antigen (HEA), but non-cancerous duct cells may also express these antigens. Perineural invasion, seen in 60% of the pancreatic adenocarcinomas of our series and in 90% of cases according to Rosai (1989), is a strong indication of malignancy in these cases. In rare cases, acinar cells and islet cells can also be entrapped in the hypertrophied nerves of chronic pancreatitis and thus mimic malignancy (Costa 1977, Rosai 1989). Another hint of the presence of malignancy is the effect on the neighbouring pancreas; obstructive pancreatitis speaks in favour of carcinoma.

Other 'characteristic features' discriminating between chronic pancreatitis and carcinoma are of little value in diagnosis although the duodenal glands of Brunner are usually highly hypertrophied in chronic pancreatitis whereas

Histomorphological problems

In well differentiated ductal adenocarcinomas, the microscopic diagnosis may be extremely difficult (Heyland et al 1981, Rosai 1989) and sometimes, using small frozen sections, it may be impossible to decide whether tumour is present (Harris et al 1985). With needle biopsies, even at laparotomy, the centre of the tumour can be missed. The nodule palpated by the surgeon is composed of the tumour and the large perifocal desmoplastic reaction; the latter may be misinterpreted as scarring in chronic pancreatitis. Even when the biopsy includes tumour tissue, difficulties may result from the tumour itself. The similarities between ductal regenerative epithelia and ductal neoplastic cells are well-recognized pitfalls in histological diagnosis (Fig. 36.7), and the diagnosis made on small pancreatic biopsies may be ambiguous in up to 15% of cases. Frozen section biopsies in selected cases of clinically

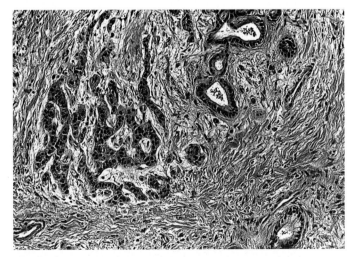

Fig. 36.7 Regressive pancreatic ducts and acinar cells in a case of chronic alcoholic pancreatitis. No adenocarcinoma present. Haematoxylin–phloxin–safran; × 80.

they are small (diameter below 2 mm) in cases of pancreatic carcinoma (Stolte 1987, Stiegler 1990).

Valuable hallmarks of malignancy in frozen section diagnosis are parapancreatic lymph node metastases or infiltration of the pseudocapsule and surrounding soft tissues.

Pancreatic tumours of high-grade malignancy pose no problems in frozen section diagnosis in terms of diagnosing malignancy. However, typing may be difficult and metastases from such tumours as malignant melanoma, large cell lung carcinoma or renal cell carcinoma have to be excluded to prevent unnecessary resection of the gland.

Location and histogenesis

The concept of ductal adenocarcinomas of the pancreas raises problems concerning the location and the histogenesis of these tumours. Although only 20% of pancreatic tissues are located in the pancreatic head, some 80% of ductal pancreatic carcinomas are found in this position and the pericholedochal part of the pancreatic head is the preferential site for the tumour (Stiegler 1990). What then are the special features of this region?

It was postulated that bile, containing carcinogenic substances, refluxes into the main pancreatic duct. Another suggestion is that carcinogenic substances, secreted by the pancreas, reach their highest concentrations in the main duct of the pancreatic head (Klöppel 1988). However, most carcinomas do not originate from the main pancreatic duct but may arise from the small pancreatic ducts surrounding the duct of Santorini. Older postulates that there were small connecting ducts between the bile duct and the pancreas (Loquvam & Russel 1950, Cross 1956) are incorrect. In our own experience, these ducts were not found, either in pancreatic cancer or in the 'normal' pancreas of 200 autopsy cases, despite the use of sophisticated radiographic methods.

In contrast to the body and tail of the pancreas which derive from the dorsal anlage of the pancreas, the head is formed by the ventral anlage as well. This ventral anlage has especially close connections to the matrix of bile duct and liver and seems to be less terminated than the dorsal anlage; less differentiated cells, especially in dislocation are more apt to form tumours (Cohnheim 1878). Histologically, the ductal carcinomas of the pancreatic head, the bile duct and the ampulla are so closely related, that they cannot be distinguished by their histological appearances alone (Hermanek 1984, Klöppel 1988).

A new aspect of histogenesis and prognosis in pancreatic cancers is the recognition of oncogenes. Their expression is the central point of regeneration and the differentiation of normal tissue, but also in the transformation of tumour tissue (Höfler et al 1987, Höfler 1988). The postulated role of oncogene K-*ras* (Bos 1989, Shibata et al 1990) has been questioned by Shimizu et al (1990).

VARIANTS OF DUCTAL PANCREATIC CARCINOMAS

Variants of ductal carcinomas are, in our opinion, tumours with predominant components which have counterparts in the cell population of normal pancreatic ducts or in benign metaplasia of duct cells. Five tumour entities will be discussed here, namely:

- carcinoma in situ of the pancreas
- ductal adenocarcinoma of the pancreas with predominant intraductal component
- papillary adenoma and papillary adenocarcinoma of the pancreas
- adenosquamous carcinoma of the pancreas and pure squamous carcinoma of the pancreas
- giant cell carcinoma and osteoclastoid giant cell carcinoma.

Carcinoma in situ of the pancreas

Pure carcinoma in situ or minimally invasive cancers have been observed in up to 8% of autopsy cases (Klöppel et al 1982, Mukada & Yamada 1982, Kishi 1990). Marked dysplasia or carcinoma in situ is seen in the small papillae and in flat areas found as concomitant phenomena in invasive ductal carcinoma in up to 24% of surgical specimens (Pour et al 1982, Fitzgerald & Cubilla 1986). These dysplasias show chronologically gradual transition towards distinct carcinoma (Klöppel et al 1982, Tsusumi & Konishi 1990) but have only been found in some tributaries in the vicinity of the carcinoma and never distributed all over the pancreatic ducts. We interpret them, in contrast to Klöppel et al (1980), not as precursors but as intraductal extensions of the invasive ductal carcinoma. Fitzgerald & Cubilla (1986) described five cases of intraductal carcinoma in situ which extended from the papilla of Vater to the tail of the pancreas, causing obstruction of the ducts and chronic obstructive pancreatitis. Ductal metaplasias and dysplasias are common features in chronic alcoholic pancreatitis (Kozuka et al 1979, Klöppel et al 1980, Volkholz et al 1982, Stolte 1987) and include squamous metaplasia, mucinous cell hypertrophy, papillary hyperplasia and epithelial atypia (Stolte 1987, Klöppel 1990, Wada 1990). Their transition to carcinoma in situ and invasive ductal carcinoma is suspected but has not been proved (Kozuka et al 1979, Schulz 1986). Alcoholism or chronic alcoholic pancreatitis are not regarded as important risk factors for pancreatic cancer.

Ductal adenocarcinoma with predominant intraductal component

In our series, there have been two cases of this peculiar variant; the tumours extended from the papilla of Vater to the tail of the pancreas. The main pancreatic duct and its

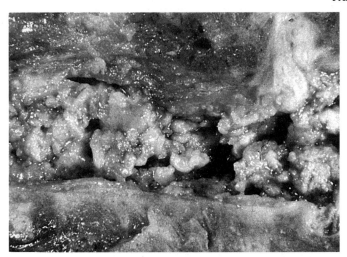

Fig. 36.8 Ductal adenocarcinoma with predominant intraductal component: close-up view of the major pancreatic duct narrowed by neoplastic epithelium and filled with detritus. × 6.5.

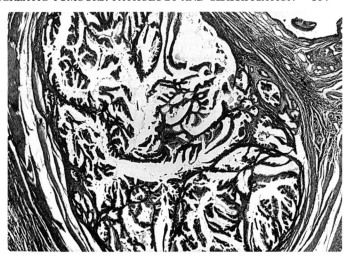

Fig. 36.9 Intraductal papilloma near the ampulla of Vater. Long, branching papillae with thin vascular core occlude the major pancreatic duct. Often combined with invasive ductal carcinoma. Haematoxylin–phloxin–safran; × 16.

tributaries were filled with granular detritus (Fig. 36.8) while the rest of the exocrine pancreas showed high-grade fibrosis with loss of acinar structures.

Histologically, Wirsung's duct and its large and medium-sized tributaries were linked with thick stratified tumour cell proliferations. The cells of the tumour were polygonal; they showed loss of nuclear polarity, large indented polymorphous nuclei with coarse chromatin, single nucleolus and an empty cytoplasm. The lymph nodes were free from metastases. Histochemical differences in relation to other ductal carcinomas were that the tumour cells contained high concentrations of α_1-antitrypsin and α_1-antichymotrypsin in the apical parts of the cytoplasm and in the detritus (Table 36.9; Stömmer et al 1988, 1989).

Intraductal papilloma and papillary carcinoma of Wirsung's duct

Intraductal papillomas and papillary carcinomas are discussed together because of their intimate relationship. All of our three cases of papillomas of the pancreatic duct had an unfavourable course with transition to, or concomitant, ductal adenocarcinoma.

Macroscopically, the tumours usually show obstruction of the pancreatic duct and obstructive pancreatitis, with dilatation of the duct and the formation of Virchow's ranulae. Benign papillomas are extremely rare tumours (Caroli et al 1975, Hivet et al 1975, Warshaw et al 1987). Histological hallmarks are the low degree of nuclear polymorphism, the preserved nuclear–cytoplasmic relations and the low number of mitoses (Ponsot et al 1989) although borderline features may be found (Morohoshi & Klöppel 1989, Seki 1990). The papillae are supported by little vascular stroma (Fig. 36.9). Intraductal papillomas should be differentiated from the more common papillary and pseudopapillary hyperplasias

in pancreatic obstruction ('permigration phenomenon' according to Kozuka et al 1979, Becker 1984) and papillary dysplasias in chronic pancreatitis (Hienert & Zeitlhofer 1956, Volkholz et al 1982).

Papillary adenocarcinomas of the pancreatic duct are more common, and some papillary features are commonly seen in 'typical' ductal carcinomas. The association of invasive ductal and papillary adenocarcinomas is well documented (Haban 1936, Place et al 1985, Conley et al 1987).

Adenosquamous carcinoma and squamous cell carcinoma of the pancreas

Adenosquamous carcinomas (mucoepidermoid tumours) of the pancreas are rare tumours and most publications are based on a few cases or even one case only (Shariff & Thomas 1989, Furukawa et al 1990, Matsuya 1990). In our series, the epidemiological data in patients with adenosquamous carcinomas did not differ from those of patients with other ductal carcinomas. However, the course of these patients was more protracted, in contrast to the observations of others (Wilczinsky et al 1984). The tumours were large and usually located in the pancreatic head and duodenal invasion occurred in two cases. Histologically, (Fig. 36.10) the hallmarks of diagnosis were squamous cells with broad intercellular bridges (desmosomes), and the amount of mucinous cells in the tumours varied greatly. In their three cases Ishikawa et al (1980) found squamous cells only in the periphery of the tumours, whereas Shariff & Thomas (1989) as well as ourselves found diffuse intermingling of both cell types, mucinous cells being in the minority. Metastases contained both cell types. Sometimes spindle cells can be found. Fine-needle aspiration may allow diagnosis (Gupta et al 1989).

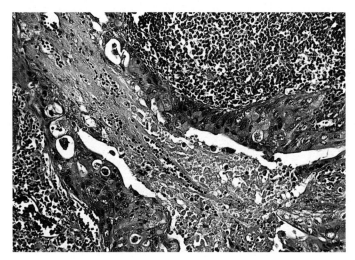

Fig. 36.10 Adenosquamous carcinoma of the pancreas: tumour cells featuring some characteristics of squamous cells, such as desmosomes and (perhaps) cornification, and some characteristics of glandular cells with intracytoplasmic mucous and tubular arrangement. Haematoxylin–phloxin–safran; × 240.

Pure squamous cell carcinomas of the pancreas have been regarded as adenosquamous carcinomas with an un-provably low content of mucus cells (Klöppel 1984, Rosai 1989); in one case, even in serial sections of the whole pancreas, no adenocomponent could be found (Matsuya 1990).

Theories of histogenesis (Chen et al 1985, Shariff & Thomas 1989) include: ductal adenocarcinoma undergoing malignant metaplasia; malignant transformation of meta-plastic squamous epithelium, and the differentiation of 'primitive cells' in two directions.

The first argument (Hanada et al 1986) seems improb-able, because in all cases, the squamous compartment greatly exceeds the glandular compartment. Ductal adenocarcinomas with small squamous metaplasias in the adjoining remnants of the pancreas should not be con-sidered as adenosquamous carcinomas, because squamous cell metaplasia (especially non-malignant metaplasia) is a common finding in chronic obstructive and chronic non-obstructive pancreatitis. Malignant transformation of primarily benign squamous metaplasia seems possible, but rather improbable, because in none of our cases, or in other published descriptions, was adenosquamous carcinoma associated with conditions inducing benign squamous metaplasia. We prefer the theory in which 'ductal stem cells' are potentially able to differentiate in two directions.

Giant cell carcinoma and giant cell carcinoma, osteoclastoid type

The position of giant cell and giant cell carcinoma, osteo-clastoid type, in the systematic classification of pancreatic tumours is not clear. Fitzgerald & Cubilla (1986) suggest a ductular cell origin and regard them as varieties of ductal adenocarcinomas, whereas the histogenetic classification of Morohoshi et al (1983), as well as that of Cruickshank (1986), subsumes these tumours into the category of pleomorphic carcinomas together with small cell carcinoma and anaplastic carcinoma.

Giant cell carcinoma of the pancreas is a rare tumour (if strict criteria are used). We define giant cell carcinoma as a malignant tumour having at least five mono- or multi-nuclear giant cells per 10 high-power fields. These large grey tumours (Fitzgerald & Cubilla 1986) show extended areas of necrosis and a soft consistency. Histologically they consist predominantly of mononuclear adenocarcinoma cells, in solid and glandular formations. There are, intermingled, malignant giant cells with broad, irregular acidophilic cytoplasm, and also found are one or two huge nuclei with a few nucleoli, intranuclear inclusions and ballooning of the nucleus. Besides these clear-cut malignant giant cells, benign histiocytic giant cells may occur (Kato 1990). Immunohistochemically, the malignant giant cells show expression of epithelial markers such as keratin, CEA and tissue peptide antigen (TPA). The formation of mucus in these tumours is variable. Sometimes, calcifi-cation, osteoid or metaplastic bone formation can be observed (Kaye & Harrison 1969). Cytophagocytosis has been seen in some of these giant cells (Silverman et al 1988). The prognosis with giant cell carcinoma is worse than in common ductal carcinoma, with a median survival time of less than 2 months (Morohoshi et al 1983).

Pancreatic carcinomas with osteoclastoid giant cells are said to have a better prognosis (Silverman et al 1989); histologically, in addition to the usual ductal features (and in some cases few malignant cells) these tumours show bland osteoclast-like cells characterized by a broad, acidophilic cytoplasm and up to 10 centrally located, benign-appearing nuclei; hyperchromasia and nucleoli are not found (Fig. 36.11). In contrast to the observations of Fischer et al (1988), which supported an epithelial origin of these osteoclast-like cells, in our experience, these cells show morphologically histiocytic features on immuno-histochemistry (expression of vimentin, antitrypsin and antichymotrypsin: no expression of keratins, CEA or human epithelial antigen, HEA) (Walts 1983, Silverman et al 1988). We regard their occurrence as a reactive phenomenon.

CYSTIC TUMOURS OF THE PANCREAS

Serous cystadenomas and cystadenocarcinomas

Serous cystadenomas are large, benign tumours in the body and tail of the pancreas in middle-aged women. They are uncommon, accounting for about 3% of exocrine pan-creatic tumours.

Macroscopically, they are well demarcated by a broad capsule and their cut surface shows multiple glistening

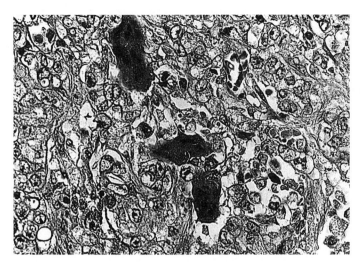

Fig. 36.11 Giant cell carcinoma with osteoclastoid features: large polymorphous tumour cells and intermingled (probably) benign osteoclastoid cells with characteristics of histiocytic origin: expression of antitrypsin, antichymotrypsin and negativity for epithelial markers. Haematoxylin-phloxin-safran; × 325.

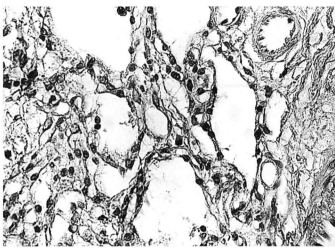

Fig. 36.13 Microcystic cystadenoma rich in glycogen: inconspicuous flat or cuboidal epithelia line the walls of the cysts. Haematoxylin–eosin; × 240.

cystic spaces, each with a diameter of up to 5 mm, a size which is smaller than in mucinous tumours. Compagno & Oertel (1978a,b) called this tumour entity 'microcystic cystadenoma rich in glycogen'. In the centre of the tumours, calcified nodules are sometimes found (Fig. 36.12) (Shorten et al 1986).

Histologically, the cysts are lined by flat, cuboidal or tall cells with inconspicuous centrally located nuclei and a clear cytoplasm containing some glycogen. The cysts contain clear fluid of low viscosity (Fig. 36.13). Not uncommonly, some mucinous cells are intermingled in the lining of the cysts (Alpert et al 1988). The prognosis of these tumours is excellent after complete resection.

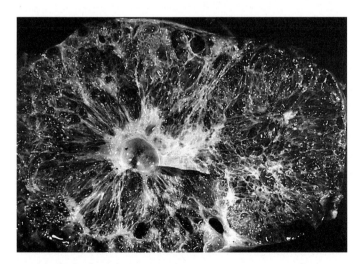

Fig. 36.12 Microcystic cystadenoma rich in glycogen: multiple glistening cystic spaces surrounded by a broad capsule. Calcified nodule in the centre of the tumour; × 2.

The prognosis is said to be less favourable only if there are large papillary formations (Glenner & Mallory 1956, Gearge et al 1989).

The matrix of these cystic neoplasms consists of ductular or centroacinar cells, which are also characterized by cytoplasm rich in glycogen. Differential diagnosis includes duct ectasia in chronic obstructive pancreatitis, congenital cysts (especially in Hippel–Lindau's disease) and, if the lining cells of the cysts are very small, lymphangioma of the pancreas (Rosai 1989). Coexistence of microcystic adenomas and pancreatic adenocarcinomas is not rare (Stömmer unpublished observations, Montag et al 1990).

Mucinous cystic tumours

Mucinous cystic tumours of the pancreas have a better prognosis than is usual for ductal carcinomas so that their strict separation from ductal carcinomas with high-grade intra- or extracellular mucous deposition is justified, although their matrix is formed by (metaplastic) mucus cells of large ducts. The average age of the patients is younger than in ductal carcinoma (54 years vs. 61 years in our series); a female preponderance (Rosai 1989) was not seen in our series.

The tumours are evenly distributed thoughout the pancreas and they show multiple cystic spaces with a larger diameter than microcystic serous adenomas. Sometimes the long axis of the cysts points towards a calcified or ossified common tumour centre. Unilocular tumours are rather uncommon.

The biological behaviour of the tumours is often unpredictable. In the case of malignancy they grow slowly and show only peritoneal implantation metastases. Compagno & Oertel (1978a,b) classified them as potentially malignant and they may also be regarded as mucinous

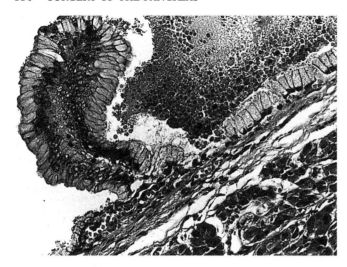

Fig. 36.14 Mucinous cystic tumour of the pancreas: large cysts lined by globlet cells. Small papillary folding (borderline tumour). Haematoxylin–eosin; × 95.

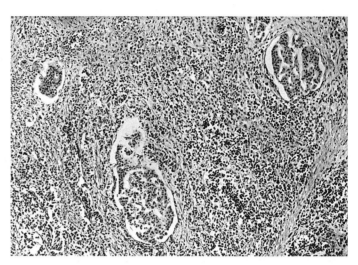

Fig. 36.15 Small cell carcinoma of the pancreas: diffuse infiltration and destruction of the gland by small, oat cell-like tumour cells. Well-preserved, non-infiltrated Langerhans islets in the tumour. Haematoxylin–phloxin–safran; × 65.

cystic tumours of low-grade malignancy (Hyde et al 1985, Riehl et al 1987).

By analogy to mucinous cystomas of the ovary, a subclassification as benign, borderline and frankly malignant may be applied (Rosai 1989). Histologically, benign mucinous tumours show cystic spaces with one layer of tall cylindrical cells, containing abundant mucus in the apical cytoplasm and basally located, bland nuclei. Sometimes, they are intermingled with serous cells or endocrine cells (Albores-Saavedra et al 1987). Borderline tumours show several layers of epithelia and papillary foldings (Fig. 36.14). In frankly malignant tumours there are anaplastic cells, irregular mitoses and infiltration of the walls. The vascularity of the tumours is higher (Yamaguchi & Nakayama 1990).

Differential diagnosis includes serous cystadenoma, pseudocysts (Warshaw et al 1987) and duodenal cysts. Aspiration cytology of the contents may be useful (Emmert & Bewtra 1986, Gupta et al 1989), but preoperative differentiation between benign and malignant tumours is difficult so that radical resection of a cystic tumour is favoured (Katoh et al 1989).

SMALL CELL CARCINOMA OF THE PANCREAS

Small cell carcinomas of the pancreas are classified by their peculiar cellular features. They represent about 1% of all pancreatic exocrine tumours (Klöppel 1988). In our series of eight cases, the average age was 52 years, with the youngest patient being 24 years old and the eldest 78 years. The course after resection of the tumours was unfavourable in that no patient survived longer than 1 year.

The firm white tumours were predominantly located in the pancreatic head and showed necroses, infiltration of the peripancreatic soft tissue and widespread metastases.

Histologically, the tumour cells were identical with the oat cells of other small cell carcinomas in that they had a centrally located round or oval nucleus and a small, sometimes invisible, cytoplasm. There was only a scant, thready fibrous stroma surrounding the sheets and nests of tumour cells. In spite of the destructive infiltration of adjoining tissue, Langerhans islets were well preserved in the tumour (Fig. 36.15).

Immunocytochemically, the tumour cells showed only slight expression of neuron specific enolase (NSE) and some CEA-positivity, but no hormones could be found in our cases. Rarely, ACTH was found in the tumour cells (Carrin et al 1973, Reyes & Wang 1981).

The histogenetic nature of the matrix of this tumour is far from clear. Undifferentiated ductal cells with the possibility of differentiating into ductal cells as well as endocrine cells (Iwafuchi et al 1987, Jones et al 1989) or malignant islet cells (Cruickshank 1986) could be the matrix. Another possible origin of these tumours is the diffuse endocrine system of Feyrter (1938), the so-called endocrine 'Gangsystem'. Morphologically, conditions to consider in differential diagnosis of small cell pancreatic carcinoma are:

1. Low grade malignant lymphomas in the pancreas. These are rare and seldom show desctruction of the acinar and ductal structures. Myoglandular complexes, characteristic of mucosa-associated lymphoid tissue (MALT) lymphomas, are extremely uncommon.

2. Lymphocytic chronic pancreatitis. This causes a destruction of pancreatic ducts and acini, but is associated with high-grade fibrosis of the gland. The expression of leucocyte common antigen (LCA) (True 1990) in lymphomas and lymphocytic pancreatitis separates them clearly from small cell carcinomas of the pancreas.

3. Metastasis of small cell lung cancer. Only the clinical or autopsy findings can exclude this possibility. If the tumour is connected with the superior or pericholedochal lymph nodes rather than the pancreas, metastasis should be considered.

MICROGLANDULAR ADENOCARCINOMAS OF THE PANCREAS

Microadenocarcinomas (Cubilla & Fitzgerald 1975, Stömmer et al 1989c) are rare pancreatic tumours with an uncertain histogenesis. They represent less than 1% of exocrine pancreatic neoplasms and show a male predominance (Kraus et al 1987). Apart from large extraductal compartments the tumours possess widespread intraductal compartments characterized by obstruction of the ducts and obstructive pancreatitis. In our cases, no lymph node metastases or distant metastases were found. In contrast to the observations of Cubilla & Fitzgerald (1984), the course of our cases was protracted in that the patients survived for at least 18 months before being lost to follow-up.

The tumour cells are uniform with little pleomorphism. Basally located nuclei are round or oval and situated in broad acidophilic cytoplasm. The tumour cells are arranged in glandular formations with a similar pattern in all glands. In the glands there are deposits of PAS-positive substances. Out of our three cases, two showed formation of osteoid and bone.

On electron microscopy the cytoplasm of the tumour cells contains vesicles with a diameter of 100–250 nm, surrounded partly by a single membrane and partly by a double membrane. These vesicles are extruded at the luminal membrane of the cytoplasm. Immunocytochemical features distinguish these tumours from ductal pancreatic cancer in that they show no expression of CEA or CA 19–9; S-100 and chromogranin, markers of endocrine cells, are also not expressed. There is, however, a strong reactivity with antitrypsin and antichymotrypsin as well as secretory phospholipase A_2, the markers of acinar cells. Neuron specific enolase is found in many tumour cells (Table 36.9). From this pattern of markers we presume that pluripotent undifferentiated ductular (Pour 1978) or intermediate cells (Melmed 1979, Cossel 1984) are resonsible for these neoplasms. This supposition contrasts with the opinion of Fitzgerald & Cubilla (1986) who postulated an acinar origin and of Rosai (1989), who considered that this tumour was a type of endocrine pancreatic carcinoma. Similarities with respect to acinar-endocrine tumours (Ulich et al 1982) or exo-endocrine tumours of the pancreas (Pedinelli et al 1975, Kamisawa et al 1990) are evident.

SOLID AND CYSTIC PANCREATIC TUMOURS

These are also described as solid and papillary tumours.

Cubilla & Fitzgerald (1975) described a tumour which can be distinguished from other pancreatic neoplasms by the fact that it is almost exclusively found in young women (Learmonth et al 1985) and by its favourable prognosis after complete resection. Rupture of the tumour with development of metastases has been observed (Lack et al 1983) but even in these rare cases, the course of disease is rather benign (Oertel et al 1982, Cubilla & Fitzgerald 1984, Matsuda et al 1987).

The large tumours (average diameter 10 cm) are evenly distributed throughout the pancreas. They are encapsulated and mostly cystic with large haemorrhagic necrosis (Figs 36.16, 36.17). In one of our 10 cases the tumour infiltrated into the spleen, whilst in another the rupture of a tumour cyst was followed by a lymph node and liver metastases. The patient is still alive 6 years after the first resection (Stömmer et al 1988a).

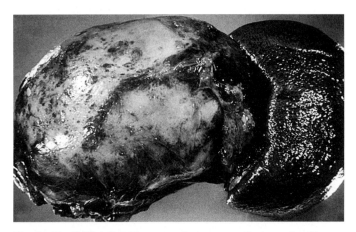

Fig. 36.16 Solid and cystic pancreatic tumour: well encapsulated large tumour in the body and the tail of the pancreas. Infiltration of adjacent structures is only very rarely seen. Natural size × 0.33.

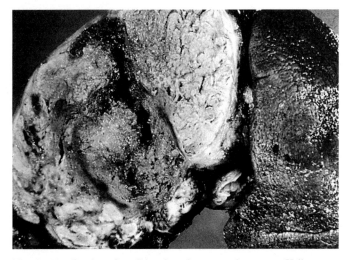

Fig. 36.17 Section of a solid and cystic pancreatic tumour. Yellow and white tumours with large necrotic, cystic and haemorrhagic areas. Natural size × 0.65.

Histologically, the tumour cells show round or oval nuclei and eosinophilic cytoplasm, which in some tumour cells contains PAS-positive granules, surrounded by single membranes (Fig. 36.18). Their diameters vary from cell to cell ranging from 50 to 2640 nm. Many granules show degeneration, forming round, small particles which are set free from the granules. The intensive positive reaction with antibodies indicates the presence of α_1-antitrypsin and α_1-antichymotrypsin. All of our solid and cystic pancreatic tumours showed at least focal presence of neuron specific enolase (Fig. 36.19), though no hormones or S-100 could be found. Staining for synaptophysin was intensely positive in 6 cases, whereas chromogranin A and B were not found in these tumours. In 6 cases, a few tumour cells exhibited production of phospholipase A_2, partly in the granules and partly distributed throughout the cytoplasm. Other tests for pancreatic enzymes such as amylase or lipase were constantly negative (Stömmer et al 1988, 1990).

Solid and cystic pancreatic tumours did not show the usual markers of pancreatic carcinomas, such as CEA, CA 19–9 or tissue peptide antigen, in all cases. CA 12.5 gave a weak reaction in 5 cases. All 5 solid and cystic tumours analysed showed the presence of progesterone receptors immunocytochemically (Ladanyi et al 1987).

The matrix of solid and cystic pancreatic tumours is unknown. An endocrine genesis (Schlosnagle & Campbell 1981, Murao et al 1983), acinar differentiation (Klöppel et al 1982, Klöppel 1984, Arai et al 1986, Ladanyi et al 1987) and an origin from centroacinar cells or small ducts (Boor et al 1979, Lieber et al 1987) have all been proposed. Compagno et al (1979) and Klöppel et al (1987) supported the thesis of small ductal origin and we also presume ductular cells to be the matrix for solid and cystic pancreatic tumours. These cells are supposed to differentiate predominantly via incomplete endocrine tumour cells but also into malformed acinar cells, so losing their ductular character.

Acinar differentiation is a lesser aspect of this tumour and its pluri-differentiation (Lack et al 1983, Matsuno & Konishi 1990) closely connects it with microglandular pancreatic carcinoma (Stömmer et al 1989), exo-endocrine pancreatic tumour (Schron & Mendelsohn 1984, Ordonez et al 1988) and carcinoma of embryonal type (Frable et al 1970). Cytological diagnosis is feasible (Foote et al 1986).

Morphologically, conditions to consider in the differential diagnosis of solid and cystic pancreatic tumours are endocrine neoplasms, pancreatoblastoma and, if there are large necrotic and cystic areas, pseudocysts in acute pancreatitis.

ACINAR CELL TUMOURS

Hyperplasia, adenomatous hyperplasia and adenoma

Adenoma of acinar cells is an exceedingly rare tumour in man. Only a few cases have been published until now, and in our series of 12 000 autopsy cases and 1450 surgical pancreatic specimens, we did not find a single case of this tumour.

Microadenomas and hyperplastic nodules (acinar cell focus) are incidental findings in pancreatic specimens.

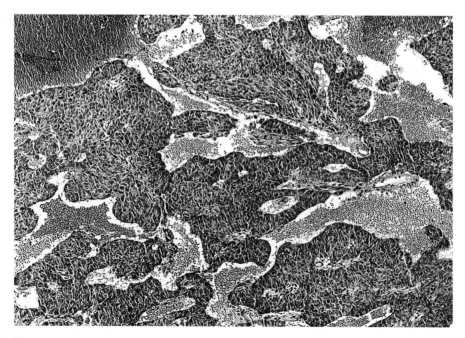

Fig. 36.18   Solid and cystic pancreatic tumour. Cystic papillary and haemorrhagic parts of the tumour: large tumour cells with glandular acidophilic cytoplasm and polymorphic nuclei. Haematoxylin–phloxin-safran; × 40.

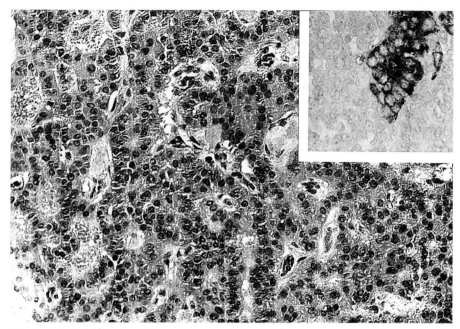

Fig. 36.19   Solid areas in solid and cystic pancreatic tumour. Uniform nuclei in the tumour cells. Hyalinization of the stroma. × 200. Inset: focal expression of neuron specific enolase (NSE) in the cytoplasm of the tumour cells. Anti-NSE-ABC-method; × 320.

Histologically, their nodular character causes confusion with Langerhans islets (Garcia et al 1975, Rosai 1989). These acinar cells are enlarged, their nuclei show prominent nucleoli and hyperchromasia and the apical cytoplasm is either pale and cloudy or shows enlarged zymogen granules (reminiscent of sialadenosis of other glands). Many cells lose their basal basophilia, centroacinar cells or ducts are missing, and no capsule surrounds the nodules. Kodama et al (1983a, b) and Shinozuka et al (1980) suggested that they might be precursors of acinar cell carcinomas. In rats treated with azaserine, Longnecker (1983, 1990) has described the transition of hyperplastic nodules to adenomas and acinar carcinomas. However, in our three cases of human acinar cell carcinomas, no adenomas could be found in the rest of the pancreas.

Acinar cell carcinoma

Carcinomas of the acinar cells are very rare in man. They comprise 1% (Klöppel 1988) to 2% (Cubilla & Fitzgerald 1975) of pancreatic neoplasms. In our own series of 1450 surgical pancreatic specimens and 302 tumours we observed two cases (0.66%) while one additional case showed acinar as well as ductal differentiations.

All patients are elderly and often suffer from distant metastases at the time of the admission. Their prognosis is no better than in the case of ductal carcinoma (Klöppel 1984). Associated findings include elevated serum lipase levels, non-suppurative panniculitis and a polyarthritis-like syndrome, due to periarticular fat necroses (Burns et al

1974, Schreiber & Probst 1977). Nephropathy, due to myeloma-like casts in the renal tubules may occur (Reducka et al 1988).

Well differentiated acinar adenocarcinomas of the pancreas (Fischer et al 1983) are large tumours, most often located in the body or tail of the pancreas. They are soft, yellow and, in contrast to ductal carcinomas, well circumscribed (Fig. 36.20). A predominantly cystic variety (acinar cell cystadenocarcinoma) was described by Stamm et al (1987).

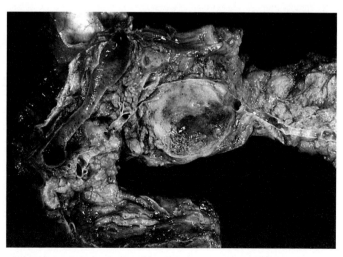

Fig. 36.20   Acinar cell tumour: soft, white and yellow tumour, sharply circumscribed, in the body of the pancreas. Note the displacement of the major pancreatic duct. Natural size.

Histologically, well differentiated acinar cell carcinomas are easily recognized by the fact that there are acinar cells with basally located nuclei and a broad apical cytoplasm full of small zymogen granules. Nuclear polymorphism and the number of mitoses are variable features (Klöppel 1984, Cruickshank 1986). The acinar arrangement of tumour cells is preserved (Figs 36.21, 36.22).

Problems in diagnosis may arise when dealing with anaplastic acinar tumours (Frantz 1959). The hallmark of diagnosis is the recognition of these cells as acinar cells. They are packed together, so that their contours are round or triangular. The presence of small PAS-positive granules is of little help in distinguishing these tumours from ductal carcinomas. On electron microscopy, some zymogen-like granules with enlarged diameters may be found. Well differentiated acinar cell carcinomas can be recognized by their intracytoplasmic expression of some secretory enzymes but the high molecular weight pancreatic amylase is almost never found, in contrast to parotid gland tumours. In our cases low molecular weight lipase and secretory phospholipase A_2 were more reliable markers of acinar structures (Stömmer 1989). Neuron specific enolase (NSE) staining is often positive, as is testing for α_1-antitrypsin and α_1-antichymotrypsin (Klöppel 1984, Stömmer 1988) (Table 36.9).

Important conditions to remember in the diagnosis of acinar cell carcinomas are:

1. endocrine tumours, which preferentially show ribbon and festoon formation, and positivity for NSE, synaptophysin and other neurosecretory markers and hormones
2. pleomorphic large cell duct adenocarcinoma, which shows expression of CEA and CA 19–9.

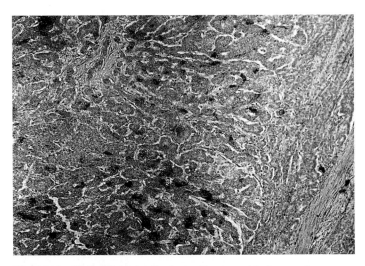

Fig. 36.22 Well differentiated acinar cell tumour: black areas show expression of exocrine enzymes such as phospholipase A_2 in some tumour cells. Amylase is very seldom (or never) expressed in these tumours. Anti-phospholipase-ABC method; $\times$ 40.

ENDOCRINE PANCREATIC TUMOURS

Endocrine tumours of the pancreas have a clinical incidence of less than 1/100 000 per year (Heitz 1987) while small, non-functional endocrine tumours are found in up to 1.5% of unselected autopsies.

The WHO classification (Williams 1980) strictly separates islet cell tumours (producing pancreatic hormones such as insulin or glucagon), carcinoids and poorly differentiated endocrine carcinomas. In accordance with others (Klöppel 1984), we prefer to use the term 'endocrine' tumour or 'islet cell' tumour in a broad sense and do not imply a specific histogenesis (Heitz & Klöppel 1987), as the cell of origin of Langerhans islets as well as carcinoids seems to be a stem cell belonging to the diffuse endocrine system of Feyrter (1938). The malignant endocrine cell, occasionally seen in exocrine pancreatic tumours (Eusebi et al 1981) causes many more problems in its interpretation.

Macroscopically, endocrine tumours show important differences in contrast to exocrine pancreatic carcinomas. They are found predominantly in the body and the tail of the pancreas. Desmoplasia is quite uncommon in these tumours and they are soft, white or yellow, and rarely haemorrhagic. They are sharply demarcated from the surrounding parenchyma and occasionally contain areas of calcification or ossification.

Histologically, the tumours can be classified in relation to their functional, histological and biological characteristics.

Functional characteristics. Hormones, produced by the tumours, such as insulin, glucagon, vasoactive intestinal peptide (VIP) and somatostatin form the basis of this classification. Commercially available antibodies for characterization allow a correct classification. The classification of the secretory granules by electron microscopy is less

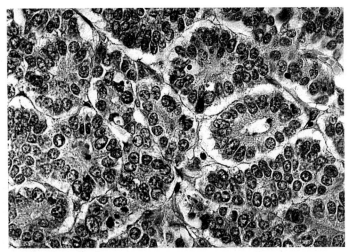

Fig. 36.21 Well differentiated acinar cell tumour: arrangement of the tumour cells in acinar-like structures; small basally located nuclei; small exocrine granules in some tumour cells. Haematoxylin–eosin; $\times$ 490.

definitive because, in contrast to normal endocrine cells, tumour cells show a greater variability of these granules (Creutzfeldt 1977). Other unsolved problems for this classification are multihormonality ('Facettentumoren', according to Becker et al 1976) and a changing pattern of hormone production with time. The most common endocrine tumours of the pancreas are non-secreting tumours (32%), followed by insulinomas (30%), gastrinomas (16%) and VIPomas (9%).

Histological characteristics. Endocrine tumours display generally accepted growth patterns, usually designated as insular, trabecular, glandular, and undifferentiated, or referred to as Type I – IV (Martin & Potet 1974), or A – D (Soga 1976). Rosai (1989) and Mukai et al (1982) classified pancreatic endocrine tumours as solid, gyriform, glandular and nondescript. The correlations between functional and histological characteristics are not strong: insulinomas and glucagonomas more often show a gyriform pattern, whereas VIPomas and gastrinomas more often display glandular structures (Rosai 1989). Somatostatinomas are often well characterized by psammoma body formation (Stömmer et al 1986, 1987).

Biological characteristics. Johnson et al (1983) showed a significant correlation between histological pattern and survival of patients with endocrine tumours. The worst prognosis is associated with undifferentiated tumours and the best prognosis with mixed (insular plus glandular) tumours. In a given patient, however, these generalizations are of less help. In contrast to other tumours, invasion of small veins, perineural spaces or the tumour capsule is no proof of malignancy and large areas of necrosis may be a more reliable marker. Only metastases in lymph nodes or distant organs confirm malignancy. Expressions of choriogonadotropin (Kahn et al 1977), or its alpha unit, are markers of malignancy with high specificity but rather low sensitivity (Heitz 1987).

Multiple endocrine neoplasia syndromes

Endocrine pancreatic tumours are common in patients with the autosomal dominant hereditary multiple endocrine neoplasia (MEN) I syndrome (Wermer 1974); but they may also occur in patients with MEN II or variants thereof (Heitz & Klöppel 1987) (Table 36.10). All of our three cases were patients with MEN I syndrome. Parathyroid adenomas, hyperparathyroidism and, in one case, hypophyseal adenoma preceded the diagnosis of a pancreatic tumour. Predominant syndromes were hyperinsulinism and hyperglucagonism.

The pancreatic tumours in MEN syndrome are similar to other endocrine tumours. However, in contrast, they are often multiple and associated with hyperplasia of the endocrine cells. Nesidioblastosis and disseminated microadenomas are common findings in patients with these tumours and sometimes are the first manifestation of the

Table 36.10 Occurrence of endocrine tumours in various types of multiple endocrine neoplasia (MEN). Data show the percentage of cases with benign or malignant endocrine tumours in given organ

	MEN I	MEN IIa	MEN IIb
Endocrine pancreas	50–80	(+)	(+)
Parathyroid	90	60	
Hypophysis	30–60	0	0
Thyroid C cells	0	90	0
Phaeochromocytoma	0	20–40	85–90

disease (Grimley & De Lellis 1986). The tumours are multihormonal and pancreatic polypeptide, gastrin and insulin are the most commonly secreted substances (Klöppel 1984). Malignancy of these tumours is said to be low.

MISCELLANEOUS TUMOURS AND TUMOUR-LIKE CONDITIONS

Infantile pancreatic carcinoma and pancreatoblastoma

Ductal pancreatic carcinomas are occasionally observed (Tsukimoto & Tsuchida 1982) in children and show the same features as these tumours in the adult (Benjamin & Wright 1980, Kühn 1887). A peculiar type is the infantile pancreatic carcinoma; this tumour usually has a large diameter and extends beyond the pancreas (Frable et al 1970). Histologically it is characterized by solid tumour cell complexes, predominantly of acinar cells with centrally located nests, exhibiting squamoid features or necroses. The presence of lipase, trypsinogen, chymotrypsinogen and α_1-antitrypsin (Iseki et al 1986, Morohoshi et al 1987) has been shown in the tumour, but the electron microscopic findings with regard to the presence of secretory granules in the cytoplasm are inconsistent (Kissane 1982, Rosai 1989). Besides the exocrine cells, an admixture of endocrine cells expressing NSE, synaptophysin, somatostatin and insulin has been found (Buchino et al 1984).

Because of their striking similarities Kissane (1982) classified this pancreatoblastoma and the solid and cystic neoplasms of the pancreas as pancreatoblastoma (pleomorphic type), pancreatoblastoma (solid and cystic type) and pancreatoblastoma (intermediate type). However, the differences in age, sexual preponderance, prognosis and histological/histochemical features have caused us to view solid and cystic tumours and pancreatoblastoma as separate entities.

Mesenchymal tumours of the pancreas

Mesenchymal tumours of the pancreas are uncommon tumours, which display the same features as in other organs. Neurinomas (schwannomas) are the most common, followed by malignant schwannomas, malignant fibrous histiocytomas, pancreatic lymphomas, granular cell tumours (probably arising in the retropancreatic bile duct) and nodular amyloidosis of the pancreas (Table 36.11).

CONCLUSIONS

The pancreas may be the site of a large variety of different tumours, perhaps more so than other organs, because of its dual role in endocrine and exocrine secretion. The vast majority of these tumours, however, are ductal adenocarcinomas with a worse prognosis than most of the other tumours. From a morphologist's view the predominant surgical problem is that resectability is limited by the ventral and dorsal tumour infiltration of the pseudocapsule. The predominant diagnostic problems are the correct classification of ductal and non-ductal tumours as well as the discrimination between regenerative and neoplastic processes (anaplasia of repair). In the future the contemporary histophenomenological classification should be replaced by a natural classification which considers the

Table 36.11 Mesenchymal tumours and tumour-like lesions of the pancreas. Data are based on the Erlangen files 1972–1989, and relative frequency is expressed as a percentage of all pancreatic tumours in those files

Type	Number of cases	Relative frequency
Neurinoma	4	1.3
Neurosarcoma	3	1.0
Malignant fibrous histiocytoma	2	0.65
Lymphoma, (excluding generalized lymphoma)	2	0.65
Granular cell tumour	2	0.65
Nodular amyloidosis	1	0.32

matrix as well as the proliferative, infiltrative and metastatic potential of the tumour.

Acknowledgement

The authors are greatly indebted to Ms Ingrid Bayer, MTA, Augsburg, for her skilful and dedicated assistance.

REFERENCES

Albores-Saavedra J, Angeles-Angeles A, Nadji M, Henson D E, Alvarez L 1987 Mucinous cystadenocarcinoma of the pancreas – morphologic and immunocytochemical observations. American Journal of Surgical Pathology 11:11–20

Allum W H, Stokes J J, McDonalds F, Fielding J W L 1986 Demonstration of carcinoembryonic antigen (CEA) expression in normal, chronically inflamed and malignant pancreatic tissue by immunohistochemistry. Journal of Clinical Pathology 39:610–614

Alpert L C, Truong L D, Bossart M I, Spjut H J 1988 Microcystic adenoma (serous cystadenoma) of the pancreas. A study of 14 cases with immunohistochemical and electronmicroscopic correlations. American Journal of Surgical Pathology 12:251–263

Arai T, Kino I, Nakamura S, Koda K 1986 Solid and cystic acinar cell tumors of the pancreas. A report of two cases with immunohistochemical and ultrastructural studies. Acta Pathologica Japonica 36:1887–1889

Ariyama J 1990 The diagnosis of small pancreatic carcinoma. Proceedings of the 4th Meeting International Association for Pancreatology & 3rd Symposium International Pancreatic Cancer Study Group, Nagasaki, vol 1

Becker V 1973 Bauchspeicheldrüse. Inselapparat ausgenommen. Springer-Verlag, Berlin

Becker V 1974 Carcinoma of the pancreas and chronic pancreatitis – a possible relationship. Acta Hepato-gastroenterology 25:269–287

Becker V 1984 Chronische Pankreatitis. Klinische Morphologie. In: Bartelheimer H, Kühn H A, Becker V, Stelzner F (eds): Gastroenterologie und Stoffwechsel. Ferdinand Enke Verlag, Stuttgart, vol 23

Becker V, Kümmerle J, Schier J, Lenner V, Londong W 1976 Tumoren des Pankreas. In: Forell M M, (ed): Handbuch der Inneren Medizin Vol. III: 6 Springer Publ, Berlin, p 1007–1104

Becker V, Stolte M, Stömmer P 1990 Funktionelle Morphologie der Bauchspeicheldrüse. In: Ottenjann R, Classen M (eds) Gastroenterologische Endoskopie und Biopsie. Thieme Verlag, Stuttgart

Beger H G, Bittner R (eds) 1986 Das Pankreaskarzinom. Frühdiagnostisches und therapeutisches Dilemma. Springer-Verlag, Berlin

Benjamin E, Wright D H 1980 Adenocarcinoma of the pancreas of childhood: a report of two cases. Histopathology 4:87–104

Bernard C 1856 Mémoire sur le pancréas. Académie des Sciences Supplément aux Comptes Rendues 1:472

Bigsby J 1835 Observations, pathological and therapeutic on diseases of the pancreas. Edinburgh Medical and Surgical Journal 44:85–102

Bockman D E 1986 Beziehungen zwischen chronischer Pankreatitis und Pankreaskarzinom. In: Beger H G, Bittner R (eds) Das Pankreaskarzinom. Springer-Verlag Berlin, p 16–24

Bockman D E, Boydston W R, Parsa J 1983 Architecture of human pancreas: implications for early changes in pancreatic disease. Gastroenterology 85:61

Bonetus T 1661 Sepulchretum, sive anatomia practica ex cadaveribus morto denatis. Cramer et Perachon, Genf

Boor P J, Swanson M R 1979 Papillary-cystic neoplasm of the pancreas. American Journal of Surgical Pathology 3:69–75

Bos J L 1989 ras Oncogenes in human cancer: a review. Cancer Research 49:4682–4689

Boyle P, Hsieh C C, Maisonneuve P, LaVecchia C, Macfarlane G J, Walker A M, Trichopoulos D 1989 Epidemiology of pancreas cancer. International Journal of Pancreatology 5:327–346

Breslow N E, Enstrom J E 1974 Geographic correlates between cancer mortality rates and alcohol-, tobacco-consumption in the United States. Journal of the National Cancer Institute 53:631–639

Brunner P 1987 Vergleichende Pankreaspathologie. Verhandlungen der Deutschen Gesellschaft für Pathologie 71:11–15

Buchino J J, Castello F M, Nagaraj H S 1984 Pancreatoblastoma. A histochemical and ultrastructural analysis. Cancer 53:963–969

Burns W, Mathews M J, Hamosh M, Vanderweide G, Blum R, Johnson F B 1974 Lipase secreting acinar cell carcinoma of the pancreas with polyarthropathy – a light and electron microscopic, histochemical and biochemical study. Cancer 33: 1002–1009

Caroli J, Hadchouel P, Marcardier M, Langeron A 1975 Papillome bénin du canal de Wirsung. Diagnostic par catheterisme retrograde. Médecine et Chirurgie Digestives 4:163–166

Carrin B, Gilby E D, Jones N F, Patrick J 1973 Oat cell carcinoma of the pancreas with ectopic ACTH secretion. Cancer 31:1523–1527

Chen J, Baithun S J 1985 Morphological study of 391 cases of exocrine pancreatic tumours with special reference to the classification of exocrine pancreatic carcinomas. 146:17–29

Chen J, Baithun S J, Ramsay M A 1985 Histogenesis of pancreatic carcinomas: a study based on 248 cases. Journal of Pathology 146:65–76

Clavel F, Benhamou E, Auquier A, Tarayre M, Flamant R 1989 Coffee, alcohol, smoking and cancer of the pancreas: a case control study. International Journal of Cancer 43:17–21

Cohnheim J 1878 Vorlesungen über allgemeine Pathologie. Berlin

Compagno J, Oertel J E 1978a Microcystic adenomas of the pancreas (glycogen-rich cystadenomas). A clinicopathologic study of 34 cases. American Journal of Clinical Pathology 69:289–298

Compagno J, Oertel J E, 1978b Mucinous cystic neoplasms of the pancreas with overt and latent malignancy (cystadenocarcinoma and cystadenoma). A clinicopathologic study of 41 cases. American Journal of Clinical Pathology 69:573–580

Compagno J, Oertel J E Kremzar M 1979 Solid and papillary epithelial neoplasm of the pancreas, probably of small duct origin; a clinico-pathologic study of 52 cases. Laboratory Investigations 40:248–249

Conley C R, Scheithauer B W, Van Heerden J A, Weiland L H 1987 Diffuse intraductal papillary adenocarcinoma of the pancreas. Annals of Surgery 205:393–398

Connelly R R, Levin D L 1985 Epidemiologie des Pankreaskarzinoms. In: Beger H. G, Bittner R (eds) Das Pankreaskarzinom. Frühdiagnostisches und therapeutisches Dilemma. Springer-Verlag, Berlin p 1–15

Connolly M M, Dawson P J, Michelassi F, Moossa A R, Lowenstein F 1987 Survival in 1001 patients with carcinoma of the pancreas. Annals of Surgery 206:366–373

Cossel L 1984 Intermediate cells in the adult human pancreas. Virchows Archiv B Cell Pathology 47:313–328

Costa J 1977 Benign epithelial inclusions in pancreatic nerves. American Journal of Clinical Pathology 67:306–307

Creutzfeldt W 1977 Endocrine tumours of the pancreas. In: Volk B W, Wellmann K F (eds) The diabetic pancreas. Bailliére Tindall, London, p 551–590

Cross K P 1956 Accessory pancreatic ducts. Archives of Pathology 61:434–440

Cruickshank A H 1986 Pathology of the pancreas. Springer-Verlag, Heidelberg

Cubilla A L, Fitzgerald P F 1975 Morphological patterns of primary nonendocrine human pancreas carcinoma. Cancer Research 35:2234–2240

Cubilla A L, Fitzgerald P J 1980 Surgical pathology of tumors of the exocrine pancreas. In: Moossa A R (ed) Tumors of the pancreas. Williams and Wilkins, Baltimore

Cubilla A L, Fitzgerald P F 1984 Tumors of the exocrine pancreas. In: Atlas of tumor pathology, Second series. American Forces Institute of Pathology, Washington DC

Cubilla A L, Fitzgerald P J 1986 Chirurgische Pathologie der Tumoren des exokrinen Pankreas. In: Beger H G, Bittner R (eds) Das Pankreaskarzinom. Springer-Verlag, Berlin p 73–80

Emmert G, Bewtra C 1986 Fine needle aspiration biopsy of mucinous cystic neoplasm of the pancreas. A case study. Diagnostic Cytopathology 2:69–71

Eusebi V, Capella C, Bondi A, Sessa F, Vezzadini P, Mancini A M 1981 Endocrine-paracrine cells in pancreatic exocrine carcinomas. Histopathology 5:599–613

Feyrter F 1938 Über diffuse endokrine epitheliale Organe. Barth-Verlag, Leipzig

Fischer H P, Doppl W, Stambolis C 1983 Azinuszelltumor des Pankreas. Zentralblatt für allgemeine Pathologic und Pathologische Anatomic 128:189–196

Fischer H P, Altmannsberger M, Kracht J 1988 Osteoclast type giant cell tumour of the pancreas. Virchows Archiv Pathologie Anatomie 412:247–253

Fitzgerald P J, Cubilla A L 1986 Pancreas. In: Henson D E, Albores-Saavedra J (eds) The pathology of incipient neoplasia. W B Saunders Philadelphia p 217–231

Foerster E C, Stommer P, Matek W, Gerner G, Domschke W 1990 Transpapillary miniscopy and minibiopsy of the pancreatic duct. Endoscopy 22:78–80

Foote A F, Simpson J S, Stewart R J, Wakefield S J, Buchanan A J, Gupta R K 1986 Diagnosis of the rare solid and papillary epithelial neoplasm of the pancreas by fine needle aspiration cytology. Light and electron microscopic study of a case. Acta Cytologica 30:519–522

Frable W, Still W, Kay S 1970 Carcinoma of the pancreas, infantile type. Cancer 27: 667–673

Frantz V K 1959 Tumors of the pancreas. Atlas of tumor pathology. American Forces Institute of Pathology, Washington DC

Furukawa T, Takahashi T, Kobari M, Matsuno S 1990a The mucin producing tumor of the pancreas - its development and extension visualized by 3-D computerized mapping. Proceedings. 4th Meeting International. Assoc.of the Pancreatology. and 3rd Symposium International. Cancer Study Group 1:110

Furukawa T, Takahshi T, Kobari M, Matsuno S 1990b Adenosquamous/mucoepidermoid carcinoma of the pancreas. Proceedings of the 4th Meeting International Association of Pancreatology and 3rd Symposium International Cancer Study Group. 1:179

Garcia H, Pelfrene A, Love L A 1975 Pancreatic acinar cell adenomas (Letter) Archives of Pathology 99:621

Gearge D H, Murphy F, Michalski R 1989 Serous cystadenocarcinoma of the pancreas: a new entity? American Journal of Surgical Pathology 13:61–66

Gibson J B, Sobin L H 1978 Histological typing of tumours of the liver, biliary tract and pancreas. WHO International Classification of tumours. World Health Organization, Geneva vol 20

Glenner G G, Mallory G K 1956 The cystadenoma and related nonfunctional tumours of the pancreas. Cancer 9:980–996

Gordis L, Gold E B 1984 Epidemiology of pancreatic cancer. World Journal of Surgery 8:808–821

Grimley P M, De Lellis R A 1986 Multisystem neuroendocrine neoplasms. In: Earl Henson D, Albores-Saavedra J. (eds) The pathology of incipient neoplasia. W B Saunders Co, Philadelphia, p 425–455

Gupta R K, Scally J, Stewart R J 1989 Mucinous cystadenocarcinoma of the pancreas: diagnosis by fine needle aspiration cytology. Diagnostic Cytopathology 5:408–411

Guthoff A, Rothe B, Klapdor R, Klöppel G 1987 Rezidivdiagnostik des Pankreaskarzinoms. Klinische Wochenschrift 65: Abstract 106

Haban G 1936 Papillomatose und Karzinom des Gangsystems der Bauchspeicheldrüse. Virchows Archiv 297:207–220

Hajdu E, Kumari-Subaiya S, Phillips G 1986 Ultrasonically guided percutaneous aspiration of the pancreas. Seminars in Diagnostic Pathology 3:166–175

Hanada M, Shimizu H, Takami M 1986 Squamous cell carcinoma of the gallbladder associated with squamous metaplasia and adenocarcinoma in situ of the mucosal columnar epithelium. Acta Pathologica Japonica 36:1879–1886

Harris P L, Rumley T O, Lineweaver W C, Copeland E M 1985 Pancreatic cancer: unreliability of frozen section in diagnosis. Southern Medical Journal 78:1053–1056

Heitz P U 1987 Neuroendocrine tumor markers. In: Seifert G (ed) Morphological tumor markers – general aspects and diagnostic relevance. Springer-Verlag, Berlin

Heitz P U, Klöppel G 1987 Endokrine Tumoren des Pankreas und des Duodenum. Verhandlungen der Deutschen Gesellschaft für Pathologic 71:202–221

Hermanek P 1984 Pankreastumoren. In: Gebhardt C (ed) Chirurgie des exokrinen Pankreas. Thieme, Stuttgart

Hermanek P 1986 Intraoperative histologische Diagnostik. In: Beger H G, Bittner R (eds) Das Pankreaskarzinom. Springer-Verlag, Berlin, p 255–260

Hermanek P, Giedl J 1986 Lymphogene Metastasierung des Pankreas-und periampullären Karzinoms, Häufigkeit, Topographie. In: Beger H G, Bittner R (eds) Das Pankreaskarzinom. Springer-Berlin, Heidelberg, New York p 114–119

Hermanek P, Scheibe O, Spiessl B, Wagner G 1987 TNM Klassifikation maligner Tumoren. Springer-Verlag, Berlin, 4 Aufl

Hermreck A S, Thomas C Y, Friesen S R 1974 Importance of pathologic staging in the surgical management of adenocarcinoma of the exocrine pancreas. American Journal of Surgery 12:653–657

Heyland C, Kheir S M, Kashlan N B 1981 An evaluation of pancreatic biopsy with the Vim–Silverman needle. American Journal of Surgical Pathology 5:179–191

Hiatt R A, Klatsky A L, Armstrong M A 1988 Pancreatic cancer, blood glucose and beverage consumption. International Journal of Cancer 41:794–797

Hienert G, Zeitlhofer J 1956 Chronische Pankreatitis mit Papillomatose des Ausführungsganges. Klin. Med. Wien 11:504–510

Hirayama T 1988 Epidemiology of pancreatic cancer in Japan International Journal of Pancreatology 3:203–204

Hivet M, Maisel A, Horiot A, Conte J 1975 Carcinome villeux diffus du Wirsung. Pancréatectomia totale. Médecine et Chirurgie Digestives 4:159–162

Höfler H 1988 Onkogenexpression als prognostischer Faktor maligner Tumoren. Verhandlungen der Deutschen Gesellschaft für Pathologic 72:174–187

Höfler H, Ruhri C, Pütz B, Wirnsberger G 1987 Oncogenexpression in endokrinen Pankreastumoren. Verh.Dtsch.Ges.Pathol. 71:300–310

Höpker W W 1987 Epidemiologie der Pankreaserkrankungen. Verhandlungen der Deutschen Gesellschaft für Pathologic 71:144–160

Hyde G L, Davies J B, McMillin R D, McMillin M 1985 Mucinous neoplasm of the pancreas with latent malignancy. American Surgeon 50:225–229

Hyland C, Kheir S M, Kashlan M B 1981 Frozen section diagnosis of pancreatic carcinoma. A prospective study of 64 biopsies. American Journal of Surgical Pathology 5:179–191

Ichihara T, Nagura H, Nakao A, Sakamoto J, Watanabe T, Takagi H 1988 Immunohistochemical localisation of CA 19–9 and CEA in pancreatic carcinoma and associated diseases. Cancer 61:324–333

Ingber D E, Madri J A, Jamieson J D 1986 Basement membrane as a spatial organizer of polarized epithelia. Exogenous basement membrane reorients pancreatic epithelial tumour cells in vitro. American Journal of Pathology 122:129–139

International Agency for Research on Cancer 1986 Monograph on tobacco smoking. IARC, Lyons

Iseki M, Suzuki T, Koizumi Y, Hirose M, Laskin W B, Nakazawa S, Ohaki Y 1986 Alpha-fetoprotein producing pancreatoblastoma. A case report. Cancer 57:1833–1835

Ishikawa O, Matsui Y, Aoki I, Iwanaga T, Terasawa T, Akirawada S 1980 Adenosquamous carcinoma of the pancreas: a clinicopathologic study and report of three cases Cancer 46:1192

Iwafuchi M, Watanabe H, Ishihara N 1987 Neoplastic endocrine cells in carcinomas of the small intestine: Histochemical and immunhistochemical studies of 24 tumors. Human Pathology 18: 185–194

Joffe R T, Adsett C A 1985 Depression and carcinoma of the pancreas. Canadian Journal of Psychiatry 30:117–118

Johnson L A, Lavin P, Moertel C G 1983 Carcinoids: The association of histologic growth pattern and survival. Cancer 51:882–889

Jones M A, Griffith L M, West A B 1989 Adenocarcinoid tumor of the periampullary region: a novel duodenal neoplasm presenting as biliary tract obstruction. Human Pathology 20:198–200

Kahn R, Rosen S W, Weintraub B D, Fajans S S, Gordon P 1977 Ectopic production of chorionic gonadotropin and its subunits by islet cell tumours. New England Journal of Medicine 297:565–569

Kamisawa T, Tabata I, Isawa T, Egawa N, Tsuruta K, Okamoto A, Fukuyama M, Koike M 1990 Endocrine differentiation in pancreatic exocrine carcinoma with special emphasis on duct-endocrine cell carcinoma of pancreas. Proceedings of the 4th Meeting of the International Association of Pancreatology 1:56

Kato Y 1990a Classification of pancreatic tumors. Japan experience. Proceedings of the 4th Meeting of the International Association for Pancreatology, and 3rd Symposium of the International Cancer Study Group 1:173

Kato Y 1990b A case of intraductal papillary adenoma of the pancreas. Proceedings of the 4th Meeting of the International Association for Pancreatology, and 3rd Symposium of the International Cancer Study Group 1:174

Katoh H, Rossi R L, Braasch J W, Monson J L, Shimozawa E, Tanabe T 1989 Cystadenoma and Cystadenocarcinoma of the pancreas Hepato-gastroenterology 36:424–430

Kaye S, Harrison J M 1969 Unusual pleomorphic carcinoma of the pancreas featuring production of osteoid. Cancer 23:1158–1162

Kern H F, Rausch U, Mollenhauer J 1986a Fine structure of human pancreatic adenocarcinoma. In: Go V L W, Gardner J D, Brooks F P, Lebenthal E, DiMagno E P, Scheele G A (eds) The exocrine pancreas. Raven Press, New York, p 637–647

Kern H F, Bülow M V, Röher H D, Klöppel G 1986b Feinstruktur des menschlichen Pankreas. In: Beger H G, Bittner R (eds) Das

Pankreaskarzinom. Springer-Verlag Berlin, p 81–93

Kishi K 1990 Preneoplastic lesions in autopsy pancreas. Proceedings of the 4th Meeting of the International Association for Pancreatology, and the 3rd Symposium of the International Pancreatic Cancer Study Group 1:191

Kissane J M 1982 Tumours of the exocrine pancreas in childhood. In: Humphrey G B, Grinday G B, Dehner L P (eds): Martinus Nijhoff, Boston, p 99–129

Kline T S, Joshi L P, Goldstein F 1978 Preoperative diagnosis of pancreatic malignancy by the cytologic examination of duodenal secretions. American Journal of Clinical Pathology 70:851–854

Klöppel G 1984 Pancreatic non-endocrine tumours. In: Klöppel G, Heitz P U (eds): Pancreatic pathology. Churchill Livingstone, Edinburgh p 79–113

Klöppel G 1987 Pankreaskarzinom. Verhandlungen der Deutschen Gesellschaft für Pathologic 71:187–201

Klöppel G 1988 Pancreatic carcinoma: structural features and biological behaviour In: Becker V, Hübner K (eds) The pancreas in connection with the epigastric unit. Gustav Fischer Verlag, Stuttgart, New York

Klöppel G 1990a Classification of pancreatic tumors – European experience. Proceedings of the 4th Meeting of the International Association for Pancreatology, and the 3rd Symposium of the International Pancreatic Cancer Study Group 1:172

Klöppel G 1990b Preneoplastic lesions of the pancreas – European experience. Proceedings of the 4th Meeting of the International Association for Pancreatology, and the 3rd Symposium of the International Pancreatic Cancer Study Group 1:189

Klöppel G, Fitzgerald P J 1986 Pathology of nonendocrine pancreatic tumors. In: Go V L W, Gardner J, Brooks P, Lebenthal E, Di Magno E P, Scheele G A The exocrine pancreas. Raven Press, New York, p 649–672

Klöppel G, Bommer G, Rückert K, Seifert G 1980a Intraductal proliferation in the pancreas and its relationship to human and experimental carcinogenesis Virch. Arch. A Pathol. Anat. Histol. 387:221–233

Klöppel G, Schneider H M, Volkholz H, Stolte M 1980b Zur multitopen Entstehung von Pankreaskarzinomeno Verhandlungen der Deutschen Gesellschaft für Pathologic 64:602

Klöppel G, Held H, Morohoshi T, Seifert G 1982 Klassifikation exokriner Pankreastumoren. Histologische Untersuchungen an 167 autoptischen und 96 bioptischen Fällen. Pathologe 2:319–328

Klöppel G, Lohse T, Bosslet K, Rückert K 1987 Ductal adenocarcinoma of the head of the pancreas: incidence of tumor involvement beyond the Whipple resection line. Analysis of 37 total pancreatectomy specimens. Pancreas 2:170–175

Kodama T, Mori W 1983a Morphological lesions of the pancreatic ducts: significance of pyloric gland metaplasia in carcinogenesis of exocrine and endocrine pancreas. Acta Pathologica Japonica 33:645–660

Kodama T, Mori W 1983b Atypical acinar cell nodules of the human pancreas. Acta Pathologica Japonica 33:701–714

Kozuka S, Sassa R, Taki T, Masamoto K, Nagasawa S, Saga S, Hasegawa B, Takeuch M 1979 Relation of pancreatic duct hyperplasia to carcinoma. Cancer 43:1418–1424

Kraus J, Langer E, Stömmer P 1987 Mikroglanduläre Pankreaskarzinomeseltene Tumoren mit ungeklärter Matrix. Virchows Archiv Abteilung A: Pathologische Anatomic und Histologic 71:327

Kühn A 1887 Über primäres Pankreaskarzinom im Kindesalter. Berliner Klinische Wochenschrift 24:494–496

Lack E E, Cassidy J R, Lever R, Vawter F 1983 Tumours of exocrine pancreas in children and adolescents: a clinical and pathological study of 8 cases. American Journal of Surgical Pathology 7:319–327

Lack E E, Cassidy J R, Lever R, Vawter F 1983 Tumours of exocrine pancreas in children and adolescents: a clinical and pathological study of 8 cases. American Journal of Surgical Pathology 7:319–327

Ladanyi M, Mulays, Arsenau J, Bettez P 1987 Estrogen and progesteron receptor determination in the papillary cystic neoplasm of the pancreas. Cancer 60:160–161

Lafler C J, Hinerman D L A 1961 A morphologic study of pancreatic carcinoma with reference to multiple thrombi. Cancer 14:944–952

Laszik Z, Pap A, Farkas G, Ormos J 1989 Endocrine pancreas in chronic pancreatitis: a qualitative and quantitative study. Archives of

Pathology and Laboratory Medicine 113:47–51

Learmonth G M, Price S K, Visser A E, Emms M 1985 Papillary and cystic neoplasm of the pancreas – an acinar cell tumour? Histopathology 9:63–79

Lieber M R, Lack E E, Roberts J R, Merino M J, Patterson K, Restrepo C, Solomon D, Chandra R, Triche T J 1987 Solid and papillary epithelial neoplasm of the pancreas. An ultrastructural and immunochemical study of six cases. American Journal of Surgical Pathology 11:85–93

Lin R S, Kessler I I 1981 A multifactorial model for pancreatic cancer in man. Journal of the American Medical Association 245:147–152

Longnecker D S 1983 Carcinogenesis in the pancreas. Archives of Pathology and Laboratory Medicine 107:54–58

Longnecker D S 1990 Preneoplastic lesions: USA experience. Proceedings of the 4th Meeting of the International Association for Pancreatology, and the 3rd Symposium of the International Pancreatic Cancer Study Group

Loquvam G S, Russel W O 1950 Accessory pancreatic ducts of the major duodenal papilla. American Journal of Clinical Pathology 20:305

Lynch H T, Fitzsimmons M L, Smyrk T C, Lanspa S J, Watson P, McClellan J, Mack J, Paganini-Hill A 1981 Epidemiology of pancreas cancer in Los Angeles. Cancer 47:1474–1483

MacManon B, Yen S, Trichopoulos D, Warren K, Nardi G 1981 Coffee and cancer of the pancreas. New England Journal of Medicine 304:630–633

Makovitzky J 1987 The localisation and distribution of the carbohydrate antigen 19-9 (CA 19-9) in chronic pancreatitis and pancreatic carcinoma. In: Klapdor R (ed) New tumour markers and their monoclonal antibodies. Thieme Verlag, Stuttgart, p 359–33

Martin E D, Potet F 1974 Pathology of the endocrine tumours of the GI tract. Clinics in Gastroenterology 3:511–532

Matsuda Y, Imai Y, Kawata J, Nishikawa M, Miyoshi S, Saito R, Minami Y, Tarui S 1987 Papillary cystic neoplasm of the pancreas with multiple hepatic metastases: a case report. Gastroent. Jpn. 22:379–384

Matsuya S 1990 A case of squamous cell carcinoma of the pancreas. Proceedings of the 4th Meeting of the International Association for Pancreatology, and the 3rd Symposium of the International Pancreatic Cancer Study Group 1:180

Matsuno H, Konishi H 1990 Papillary cystic neoplasm of the pancreas. Cancer 65:283–291

Melmed R N 1979 Intermediate cells of the pancreas. Gastroenterology 76:196–201

Mitchell M L, Carney C M 1985 Cytologic criteria for the diagnosis of pancreatic carcinoma. American Journal of Clinical Pathology 83:171–176

Mikuz G, Weger H, Graf A H 1987 Feinnadelbiopsie tumoröser Pankreasveränderungen Verhandlungen der Deutshen Gesellschaft für Pathologie 71:466

Miyakawa M, Watanabe M, Sato T, Natsui K, Koito K, Imamura A, Yaosaka T 1990 Peroral pancreatoscopy for mucin producing pancreatic tumor. Proceedings of the 4th Meeting of the International Association for Pancreatology, and the 3rd Symposium of the International Pancreatic Cancer Study Group 1:108

Mondiere J T 1836 Récherches pour servir à l' histoire pathologique du pancréas. Archives Générales de Médecine (2me séries) 3:133–164

Montag A G, Fossati N, Michelassi F 1990 Pancreatic microcystic adenoma coexistent with pancreatic ductal carcinoma. American Journal of Surgical Pathology 14:352–355

Moossa R A 1980 Tumors of the pancreas. Williams and Wilkins, Baltimore

Morgagni 1973 Cited in Becker V (1975)

Morohoshi T, Held G, Klöppel G 1983 Exocrine pancreatic tumours and their histological classification. A study based on 167 autopsy and 97 surgical cases. Histopathology 645–661

Morohoshi T, Kanda M, Horie A, Chott A, Dreyer A, Klöppel G, Heitz P U 1987 Immunocytochemical markers of uncommon pancreatic tumors. Cancer 59:739–747

Morohoshi T, Klöppel G et al 1989 Intraductal papillary neoplasms of the pancreas. A clinicopathologic study of six patients. Cancer 64:1329–1335

Mukada T, Yamada S 1982 Dysplasia and carcinoma in situ of the exocrine pancreas. Tohoku Journal of Experimental Medicine 137:115–124

Muir C S, Waterhouse J A H, Mack T, Powell J, Whelan S 1988 Cancer incidence in five continents. IARC Scientific Publication No. 88. IARC, Lyon, vol 5

Mukai K, Grotting J C, Greider M H, Rosai J 1982 Retrospective study of 77 pancreatic endocrine tumours using the immunoperoxidase method. American Journal of Surgical Pathology 6:387–399

Murao T, Toda K, Tokiyama Y 1983 Papillary and solid neoplasm of the pancreas in a child: report of a case in which acinar differentiation was demonstrated by immunohistochemistry and electron microscopy. Acta Pathologica Japonica 33:565–575

Nagai H, Kuroda A, Morioka Y 1986 Lymphatic and local spreading of T1 and T2 pancreatic cancer. Annals of Surgery 204:65–71

Oertel J E, Mendelsohn G, Compagno J 1982 Solid and papillary epithelial neoplasms of the pancreas. In: Humphrey G B, Grindey G B, Dehner L P, Acton R T, Pysher T J (eds) Pancreatic tumors in children. Martinus Nijhoff, The Hague, p 167–171

Oertel J E, Heffess C S, Oertel Y C 1989 Pancreas. In: Sternberg S S (ed): Diagnostic surgical pathology. Raven Press, New York, p 1057–1093

Ordonez N G, Balsaver A M, Mackay B 1988 Mucinous islet cell (amphicrine) carcinoma of the pancreas associated with watery diarrhea and hypokalemia syndrome. Human Pathology 19:1458–61

Osborne M, van Lessen G, Weber K, Klöppel G, Altmannsberger M 1986 Differential diagnosis of gastrointestinal carcinomas by using monoclonal antibodies specific for individual keratin polypeptides. Lab. Invest. 55:497–504

Pollard H M 1981 Staging of cancer of the pancreas. Pancreas task force. Cancer 47:1631–1637

Ponsot P, Molas G, Vilgrain V, Gayet B, Fékété F, Paolaggi J A 1989 Adénomes, adénomatoses et adénocarcinomes pancréatiques intracanalaires. Gastroentérologie Clinique et Biologique 13:663–670

Pour P 1978 Islet cells as a component of pancreatic ductal neoplasms. American Journal of Pathology 90:295–316

Pour P M 1986a Das experimentelle Pankreaskarzinom. In: Beger H G, Bittner R, (eds) Das Pankreaskarzinom. Springer-Verlag, Berlin, p 31–43

Pour P M 1986b Das Pankreaskarzinom des Menschen: Rückschlüsse aus experimentellen Beobachtungen. In: Beger H G, Bittner R, (eds) Das Pankreaskarzinom. Springer-Verlag, Berlin, p 59–70

Pour P M, Sayed S, Sayed S 1982 Hyperplastic, preneoplastic and neoplastic lesions found in 83 human pancreases. American Journal of Clinical Pathology 77:137–152

Pedinelli L, Quilichini R, Futsch D 1975 Les tumours pancréatiques à double composante endocrine et exocrine avec syndrome carcinoïde. Chirurgie (Paris) 101:42–51

Place S, Lovel A, Farhi J P, Chapuis Y 1985 Ductal papillary adeno-carcinoma of the pancreas. Gastroenterol. Clin. Biol. 9:361–364

Reber H A, Austin J L 1988 Cancer and other neoplastic disorders of the exocrine pancreas. In: Gitnick G, Hollander D, Kaplowitz N, Samloff L M, Schoenfield L J (eds) Principles and practice of gastroenterology and hepatology. Elsevier, New York, p 816–828

Reducka K, Gardiner G W, Sweet J, Vandenbroucke A, Bear R 1988 Myeloma-like cast nephropathy associated with acinar cell carcinoma of the pancreas. American Journal of Nephrology 8:421–424

Reid J D, Yuh S L, Petrelli M, Jaffe R 1982 Ductuloinsular tumors of the pancreas. Cancer 49:908–915

Reyes C V, Wang T, 1981 Undifferentiated small cell carcinoma of the pancreas. A report of five cases. Cancer 47:2500–2502

Riehl K A, Hahn D, Nathrath W, Kortmann H 1987 Muzinöses Cystadenom des Pankreas mit Carcinoma in situ – eine Fallbeschreibung. Chirurg 58:293–295

Rosai J 1989 Pancreas and periampullary region. In: Rosai J, Ackerman's surgical pathology. Mosby Co. St Louis, p 757–788

Safi F, Bittner R, Büchler M, Malfertheiner P, Beger H G 1985 Die Wertigkeit des monoclonalen Antikörpers CA 19–9 in der Differentialdiagnose der Pankreaserkrankungen. In: Beger H G, Bittner R (eds) Das Pankreaskarzinom. Springer, Berlin p 145–153

Schottenfeld D, Fraumeni J F 1982 Cancer epidemiology and prevention. Saunders Co, Philadelphia 598–823

Schlosnagle D C, Campbell W G 1981 The papillary and solid neoplasm of the pancreas: a report of two cases with electron microscopy, one containing neurosecretory granules. Cancer 47:2603–2610

Schmiegel W H, Kalthoff H, Arndt R, Gieseking J, Greten H, Klöppel G, Kreiker C, Ladak A, Lampe V, Ulrich S 1985 Monoclonal antibody-defined human pancreatic cancer associated antigens. Cancer Research 45:1402–1407

Schreiber D, Probst H 1977 Sekretorisch aktives Karzinom des exokrinen Pankreas. Fallbericht und Literaturübersicht. Zentralblatt für allgemeine Pathologic und Pathologische Anatomic 12:114–121

Schron D S, Mendelsohn G 1984 Pancreatic carcinoma with duct, endocrine and acinar differentiation: a histologic, immunocytochemical and ultrastructural study. Cancer 54:1766–1770

Schulz H J 1986 Dysplasie und Carcinoma in Situ des Pankreasgangepithels. Zentralblatt für allgemeine Pathologic und Pathologische Anatomic 134:3–14

Schwenk J, Makovitzky J 1989a Tissue expression of the cancer associated antigens CA 19–9 and CA 50 in chronic pancreatitis and pancreatic carcinoma. International Journal of Pancreatology 5:85–98

Schwenk J, Makovitzky J 1989b Comparative study on the expression of the blood group antigens Le a, Le b, Le x, Le y and the antigens CA 19–9 and CA 50 in chronic pancreatitis and pancreatic carcinoma. Virchows Archiv Abteilung A: Pathologische Anatomic und Histologic 414:465–476

Seki M 1990 Intraductal papillary tumor with borderline and atypia. Proceedings of the 4th Meeting of the International Association for Pancreatology and 3rd Symposium International Cancer Study Group 1:194

Shariff S, Thomas J A 1989 Adeno-squamous carcinoma pancreas – a case report with literature review. Indian Journal of Pathology and Microbiology 32:62–65

Shibata D, Almoguera C, Forrester K, Dunitz J, Martin S E, Cosgrove M M, Perucho M, Arnheim N 1990 Detection of c-K-ras mutations in fine aspirates from human pancreatic adenocarcinomas. Cancer Research 50:1279–1281

Shimizu M, Saitoh Y, Itoh H 1990 Immunohistochemical staining of Ha-ras oncogene product in normal, benign and malignant human pancreatic tissues. Human Pathology 21:607–612

Shinozuka H, Lee R E, Dunn I L, Longnecker D S 1980 Multiple atypical acinar cell nodules of the pancreas. Human Pathology 11:389–391

Shorten S D, Hart W R, Petras R E 1986 Microcystic adenomas (serous cystadenomas) of pancreas. A clinicopathologic investigation of eight cases with immunohistochemical and ultrastructural studies. American Journal of Surgical Pathology 10:365–372

Silverman J F, Dabbs D J, Finley J L, Geisinger K M 1988 Fine needle aspiration biopsy of pleomorphic (giant cell) carcinoma of the pancreas. Cytologic, immunocytochemical and ultrastructural findings. American Journal of Clinical Pathology 89:8–14

Silverman J F, Finley J L, Berns L, Unverferth M 1989 Significance of giant cells in fine needle aspiration biopsies of benign and malignant lesions of the pancreas. Diagnostic Cytopathology 5:388–391

Smithies A, Hatfield A R W, Brown B E 1977 The cytodiagnostic aspects of pure pancreatic juice obtained at the time of endoscopic retrograde cholangiopancreaticography (ERCP). Acta Cytologica (Baltimore) 21:191–195

Soga J 1976 Neoplasms of GEP endocrine cells: the present-day concept of carcinoids. In: Fujita T (ed) Endocrine gut and pancreas. Elsevier, Amsterdam, p 387–394

Stamm B, Burger H, Hollinger A 1987 Acinar cell cystadenocarcinoma of the pancreas. Cancer 60:2542–2547

Stiegler G 1990 Morphologische Untersuchungen zum Pankreaskarzinom. Inaugural Dissertation, University of Erlangen

Stocks P A 1970 Cancer mortality in relation to national consumption figures of cigarettes, solid fuel, tea and coffee. British Journal of Cancer 24:215–225

Stolte M 1987 Chronische Pankreatitis. Verhandlungen der Deutschen Gesellschaft für Pathologic 71:175–186

Stömmer P, 1986 Somatostatin-immunreaktive Zellen der Vater schen Papille und des peripapillären Duodenum, Leber-Magen-Darm 5:307–311

Stömmer P 1987 Pankreaserkrankungen und andere Organe. Hauptreferat d' Deutschen Gesellschaft für Pathologic 1987. Verhandlungen der Deutschen Gesellschaft für Pathologic 71:68–76

Stömmer P 1988 Pancreatic diseases and other organs. In: Becker V, Hübner K (eds) The pancreas in connection with the epigastric unit. Fischer Verlag, Stuttgart, p 56–65

Stömmer P 1990 Tumours of the human exocrine pancreas: EULEP Meeting on Exocrine Pancreas and Salivary Glands, Munich, October

Stömmer P, Stolter M, Seifert E 1987 Somatostatinoma of Vater's papilla and the minor papilla. Cancer 80:232–235

Stömmer P, Giedl J, Stolte M, Kraus J 1988a Solid papillary tumour of the pancreas: immunocytochemical and EM features in seven new cases. XVIIth International Congress of the International Academy of Pathology and Environmental Pathology p 153

Stömmer P, Kraus J, Gebhardt C, Schultheiss K 1988b Adenokarzinom des Pankreas mit prädominierender intraduktaler Komponente: eine Sonderform des ductalen Pankreaskarzinoms. Verhandlungen der Deutschen Gesellschaft für Pathologie 72:395

Stömmer P, Kraus J, Foerster E C, Domschke W 1989a Endoskopie und Biopsie im Ductus pancreaticus: eine neue Methode der Pankreasdiagnostik. Leber Magen Darm 6:311–318

Stömmer P, Kraus J, Foerster E C, Domschke W 1989b Endoskopie und Biopsie im Ductus Wirsungianus. Verhandlungen der Deutschen Gesellschaft für Pathologie 73

Stömmer P, Kraus J, Langer E 1989c Mikroglanduläre Pankreaskarzinome Pathologe 10:354–358

Stömmer P, Gebhardt C, Pliess M, Gentsch H, Schultheiss K 1989d Histomorphological investigation in immunoreactivity of MAb494/32–2–4 Behring with ductal pancreatic cancer. Sektion Experimentelle Krebsforschung. Book of Abstracts, Cancer Research 10.4.89, Heidelberg

Stömmer P, Gebhardt C, Schultheiss K H 1990a Adenocarcinoma of the pancreas with a predominant intraductal component: a special variety of ductal adenocarcinoma. Pancreas 5:114–118

Stömmer P, Kraus J, Stolte M, Giedl J 1990b Solid and cystic pancreatic tumours: clinical, histochemical and electron microscopic features in ten cases. Cancer 67:1635–1641

Stömmer P P, Stolte M, Seifert E 1986 Malignes Somatosatatinom der Vater schen Papille. Verhandlungen der Deutschen Gesellschaft für Pathologie 69:459

Stömmer P, Stolte M, Seifert E 1987 Somatostatinoma of Vater's papilla and the minor papilla. Cancer 60:232–235

Tannenbaum H, Anderson L, Schur P H 1975 Association of polyarthritis, subcutaneous nodules, and pancreatic disease. Journal of Rheumatology 2:15–20

Tashiro S, Hiraoka T, Uchino R, Kanemitsu K et al 1990 Clinicopathologic study of small ductal cell carcinomas of the pancreas. Proceedings of the 4th Meeting of the International Association for Pancreatology, and the 3rd Symposium of the International Pancreatic Cancer Study Group 1:67

Tokuka A, Hosotani R, Kajiwara T 1990 Five year survivors of pancreatic cancer and histological findings. Proceedings of the 4th Meeting of the International Association for Pancreatology, and the 3rd Symposium of the International Pancreatic Cancer Study Group 1:68

Trede M 1985 The minimal treatment of pancreatic carcinoma. Surgery 97:28–35

Trede M, Kerstin K H, Hofmeister A 1977 Das Pankreaskopfkarzinom. Münchener Medizinische Wochenschrift 119:617–622

Trousseau A 1865 Phlegmasia alba dolens. Clinique Medicale de l'Hotel de Dieu de Paris. Bailliére, Paris, vol 3, p 652–664

True L D 1990 Atlas of diagnostic immunohistopathology. Lippincott-Gower Medical Publishing, New York

Tsukimoto I, Tsuchida M 1982 Pancreatic carcinoma in children in Japan: review of the Japanese literature. In: Humphrey G B, Grindey G B, Dehner L P Pancreatic tumours in children. Martinus Nijhoff, Boston, p 149–157

Tsusumi M, Konishi Y 1990 Early pancreatic duct adenocarcinoma. Proceedings of the 4th Meeting of the International Association for Pancreatology, and the 3rd Symposium of the International Pancreatic Cancer Study Group 1:193

Ulich T, Cheng L, Lewin K J 1982 Acinar-endocrine cell tumour of the pancreas. Report of a pancreatic tumor containing both zymogen and neuroendocrine granules. Cancer 50:2099–2105

Volkholz H, Stolte M, Becker V 1982 Epithelial dysplasias in chronic pancreatitis. Virchows Archiv Abteilung A: Pathologische Anatomic und Histologic 396:331–334

Wada Y 1990a Preneoplastic lesion of the pancreas in surgical specimen; the significance of duct epithelial proliferation and its relation to duct obstruction. Proceedings of the 4th Meeting of the International Association for Pancreatology, and the 3rd Symposium of the International Pancreatic Cancer Study Group 1:190

Wada, Y 1990b Mucinous cystadenocarcinoma of the pancreas. Proceedings of the 4th Meeting of the International Association for Pancreatology, and the 3rd Symposium of the International Pancreatic Cancer Study Group 1:766

Walts A E 1983 Osteoclast-type giant cell tumor of the pancreas Acta Cytologica 27:500–504

Warshaw A L 1990 Implications of peritoneal cytology for staging of early pancreatic cancer. Proceedings of the 4th Meeting of the International Association for Pancreatology, and the 3rd Symposium of the International Pancreatic Cancer Study Group 1:622

Warshaw A L, Berry J, Gang D I 1987 Villous adenoma of the duct of Wirsung. Digestive Diseases and Sciences 32:1311–1313

Wermer P 1974 Multiple endocrine adenomatosis; multiple hormone-producing tumours, a familial syndrome. Clinics in Gastroenterology 3:671–684

Wilczynski S P, Velente P T, Atkinson B F 1984 Cytodiagnosis of adenosquamous carcinoma of the pancreas. Use of intraoperative finc needle aspiration. Acta Cytologica (Baltimore) 28:733

Williams E D (ed) 1980 Histological typing of endocrine tumours. WHO International Histological Classification of Tumours, Vol 23. World Health Organization, Geneva

Würmeling M J 1988 Über den immunhistochemischen Nachweis von Blutgruppenantigenen des ABO-Systems an der gesunden, entzündlich veränderten und malignen Bauchspeicheldrüse Inaugural Dissertation, University of Erlangen

Yamaguchi K, Nakayama F 1990 Mucinous cystic neoplasm of the pancreas: estimation of grade of malignancy with imaging techniques and its surgical implications. Proceedings of the 4th Meeting of the International Association for Pancreatology, and the 3rd Symposium of the International Pancreatic Cancer Study Group 1:114

Yamaguchi K, Miyagahara T, Tsuneyoshi M, Enjoji M, Horie A, Nakayama I, Suda N T, Fujii H, Takahara O 1989 Papillary cystic tumour of the pancreas: an immunohistochemical and ultrastructural study in 14 patients. Japanese Journal of Clinical Oncology 19:102–111

37. Clinical evaluation and preoperative assessment

M. Trede   D. C. Carter

The chief problem in the management of pancreatic cancer is the diagnosis. Due to its hidden location in the retroperitoneum, this tumour has usually grown and spread beyond the confines of the gland before symptoms appear. And when these do appear, they are for the most part vague and non-specific. To compound the problem further, there is a 'fatal delay' of some 4 months on average, between the onset of symptoms and the diagnosis, with a range of 2–18 months (Moossa & Levin 1981). The patients take little note of the vague and initially intermittent nature of their complaints. The doctors are reassured by negative findings on routine examination or they are misled by some irrelevant pathology (cholelithiasis, peptic ulcer or hepatitis). Thus, 14 of 283 patients with resectable periampullary carcinoma had had a cholecystectomy for gallstones within the previous 6 months (Trede, unpublished data).

There is also the widespread belief amongst physicians, that once symptoms appear in this particular disease it is too late for any meaningful treatment anyway. Unfortunately, they will be right most of the time. However, there are exceptions to this melancholy rule as exemplified by the following case report.

Case report: A 62-year-old radiologist noticed some epigastric pain and 3 kg loss in weight over a period of only 3 weeks before he had a CT scan done in his own practice. Disturbed by what

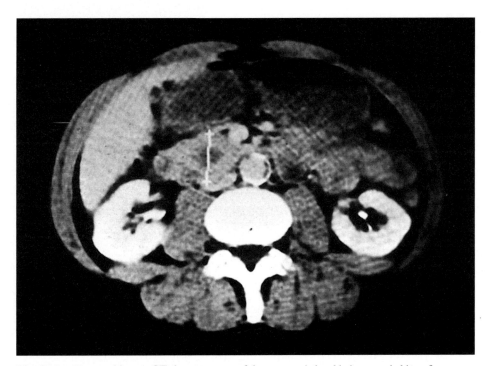

Fig. 37.1 62-year-old man. CT shows tumour of the pancreatic head being sampled by a fine needle for cytology.

he saw, a fine-needle cytology was performed on the suspicious mass in the head of the pancreas (Fig. 37.1). This was positive and within another 2 weeks a total pancreatectomy was carried out for a $T_2 N_0 M_x$ adenocarcinoma of the pancreas. This colleague is still alive and free of recurrence 10 years later.

Unfortunately, there are no effective screening tests for this cancer that are sensitive and specific enough and even if there were, there is no group at risk that would be worth screening (see Ch. 35). Therefore, patients who seek medical advice will be those with symptoms.

CLINICAL FINDINGS

The three main symptoms of pancreatic cancer are pain, loss of weight and jaundice (Table 37.1).

The pain is usually described as a dull intermittent ache in the epigastrium. Depending on the site and spread of the tumour it may radiate to the left (e.g. in tumours of the pancreatic body and tail) or to the right subcostal area (e.g. if there is significant distension of the gallbladder). A gnawing backache, initially present only at night time, is a grim sign usually signifying infiltration of the retroperitoneum and therefore incurability.

Weight loss may be quite severe, averaging 10 kg. The bigger the loss and the more rapidly it occurs, the less likely is the tumour to be resectable (Perez et al 1983, Petrek et al 1985).

Jaundice is the one symptom characteristic of pancreatic cancer, particularly if it occurs without any colicky pain. It is rarely intermittent and frequently accompanied by severe pruritus. Jaundice draws attention to periampullary tumours at a relatively early stage. That is why the resectability and cure rates are much higher for these tumours than they are for tumours further from the papilla (see Fig. 38.1). Conversely, jaundice in a patient with carcinoma of the body or tail of the pancreas is usually caused by hepatic or hilar metastases and therefore connotes inoperability.

Some 5% of patients with diagnosed pancreatic cancer have developed diabetes mellitus within the previous 2 years (Moossa & Levin 1981). Whereas the exact mech-anism of glucose intolerance in these patients is under debate (the possibilities are ductal obstruction or direct islet destruction; see also Ch. 35), diabetes of recent onset can serve as a warning sign.

The same applies to acute and chronic pancreatitis. Some 5% of cancer patients present with an atypical attack of acute or subacute pancreatitis (Gambill 1971). Such an episode, in a patient who neither abuses alcohol nor has gallstones, should alert one to the possibility of an underlying cancer.

Case report: A 57-year-old woman had spent 6 weeks in a medical intensive care unit with so-called 'atypical pancreatitis'. When she had recovered, was symptom-free and had gained 3 kg in weight, endoscopic retrograde cholangio-pancreatography (ERCP) was performed showing an abrupt cut-off of the pancreatic duct (Fig. 37.2). This was due to a genuine 'early' cancer of the pancreas that was removed by a Whipple operation. The patient lived for another 6.5 years.

On occasion a pancreatic cyst may be the harbinger of cancer (Itai et al 1982, Talamini et al 1992). Even more

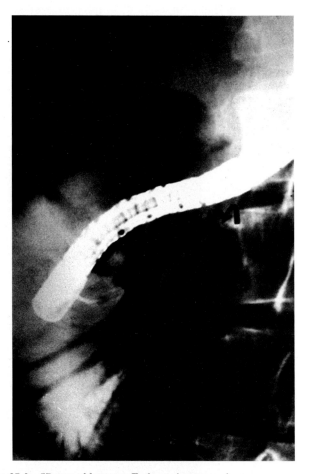

Fig. 37.2 57-year-old woman Endoscopic retrograde cholangiopancreatography (ERCP) shows suspicious cut-off of an otherwise normal pancreatic duct. (Reproduced with permission of C V Mosby Co, from Trede 1985, Surgery 97:28–35).

Table 37.1 Presenting symptoms in 303 consecutive patients with pancreatic or periampullary cancer. (Surgical clinic, University of Mannheim 1.10.72–1.1.92)

Symptom	Number of patients	%
Weight loss	272	91
'Pain'	251	83
Jaundice	219	71
Anorexia, nausea	134	44
Malaise	104	34
Vomiting	42	13

problematic is the interrelation between chronic pancreatitis and carcinoma. Although there is no evidence that chronic pancreatitis is a precancerous condition, there are remarkable cases suggesting some connection between the two.

Case report: A 39-year-old patient had suffered from attacks of abdominal pain since the age of 16. These had increased in frequency during the past 10 years and were labelled as recurrent attacks of pancreatitis. Five different ERCP examinations confirmed this diagnosis (Fig. 37.3). In between attacks, the patient was symptom-free; he had an excellent appetite and was 14 kg overweight. Finally, a duodenal ulcer was diagnosed and treated as such. Two months later, this ulcer proved to be a carcinoma of the head of the pancreas ulcerating into the duodenum. A 7 cm mucinous adenocarcinoma of the pancreas with surrounding chronic pancreatitis (pT_2 pN_1 pM_x-G2) was removed by duodenopancreatectomy and the patient

discharged 15 days later. He finally died of metastases 2 years later.

The diagnostic dilemma – 'pancreatitis or carcinoma' – has been discussed in Chapter 26. Suffice it to say that this problem of differential diagnosis cannot be completely solved, preoperatively or even at operation, in up to 15% of patients (Saeger et al 1990, Carter 1992).

Migratory thrombophlebitis (as a 'paraneoplastic' phenomenon) and persistent sciatica (due to retroperitoneal nerve infiltration) are rarely the first symptoms of the disease. These and most of the other complaints listed in Table 37.1 are, of course, non-specific for pancreatic cancer.

The same applies to the physical signs. Apart from jaundice with a palpable gallbladder (Courvoisier's sign)

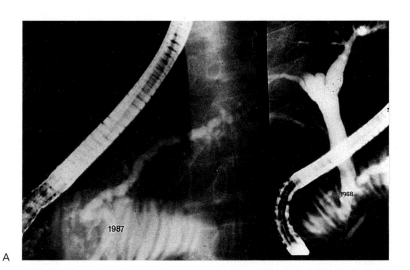

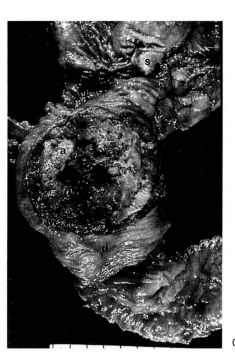

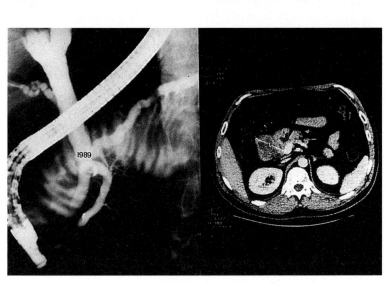

Fig. 37.3 39-year-old man. **A** Five different ERCP examinations in the course of 10 years only showed chronic pancreatitis; in 1987 (left) and in 1988 (right). **B** In 1989 a carcinoma of the head of the pancreas was finally diagnosed by ERCP ('double-duct' sign) (on left) and CT (on right). **C** Operative specimen showing mucinous adenocarcinoma of pancreas; a, eroding into duodenum, d; s, stomach. The patient died of metastases 2 years later.

other findings are conspicuous by their absence, or equivocal. A palpable and fixed epigastric mass, ascites or an enlarged supraclavicular lymph node (Virchow's node) are signs of inoperability.

LABORATORY FINDINGS

In the jaundiced cancer patient, bilirubin levels (reaching up to 500 μmol/l or some 30 mg%) will often exceed those normally seen with biliary obstruction due to chronic pancreatitis or common duct stones (Pellegrini et al 1982). Sometimes a raised alkaline phosphatase is the only pathological finding.

Elevated blood sugar (in up to 80% of cases) and serum amylase (in 5% of cases) as well as lowered haemoglobin levels (60%), possibly with occult blood in the stool, complete the list of equivocal laboratory findings (Warren et al 1983).

The hopes placed in new tumour markers have not been realized in clinical practice. Among the many antigens available (gastrointestinal cancer-associated antigen (CA 19-9), carcinoembryonic antigen (CEA), CA-50, alpha-fetoprotein (AFP), pancreatic oncofetal antigen (POA)) only the first, CA 19-9, has been of some use in clinical practice (Haglund et al 1989) given that there is some correlation with tumour burden. Whereas CA 19-9 levels are of little help in diagnosing early cancers, high values usually denote a large tumour or disseminated disease. Overall, the predictive value of this marker in the detection of recurrence following resection of pancreatic cancer is unreliable.

The yield from similar examinations using monoclonal antibodies against other antigens, enzymes, isoenzymes or hormones is disappointingly low, even when they are applied in combination (Greenway et al 1983; see Ch. 13).

In analysing this dearth of specific clinical symptoms and signs, one is nevertheless left with a group of patients in whom there is enough circumstantial evidence to start a determined diagnostic programme. This must then be pursued until pancreatic carcinoma has been either excluded or confirmed. According to Moossa and Levin, the following four criteria should raise suspicion since one can expect to detect pancreatic cancer in up to 50% of patients so afflicted (Moossa & Levin 1981):

1. persistent upper abdominal pain or backache of recent onset in patients over the age of 35, in whom cholelithiasis or peptic ulcer disease has been excluded by ultrasound or endoscopy
2. unexplained weight loss, greater than 5% of normal body weight, particularly if it is associated with anorexia and vague dyspepsia
3. an attack of acute or subacute pancreatitis, unexplained by cholelithiasis or alcohol abuse
4. recent onset of diabetes mellitus associated with

dyspepsia, in a patient who lacks predisposing factors such as obesity or family history.

SPECIAL DIAGNOSTIC PROCEDURES

Confronted some 20 years ago with patients fulfilling Moossa and Levin's criteria, described above, the diagnostic options available were limited to upper gastrointestinal barium studies, possibly laparoscopy, and finally, exploratory laparotomy. Diagnostic accuracy and the rate of resectability were correspondingly low. Since then a whole armamentarium of special diagnostic tests has been developed. These have been discussed in detail in Section 2. It is up to the surgeon, for the good of his patient, to channel and control the various diagnostic efforts and to sift the information obtained. Way (1987) formulated this nicely when he pleaded for earlier testing of patients with subtle findings, and less extensive testing of patients with advanced findings.

The step-by-step approach to the patient referred with suspicion of pancreatic cancer is outlined in the algorithm shown in Figure 37.4. The prime aim is to separate the operable from the inoperable patients, so as to save the latter an unnecessary laparotomy.

It is good practice to begin with the innocuous, non-invasive procedures and to use the other invasive modalities sparingly or not at all. Tempting as it may be in an academic setting to employ all of the diagnostic tools listed in Figure 37.4 (because they are there!), this is often unnecessary, unsafe, costly, and time-consuming (Olen et al 1989). In most institutions not all of these tools will indeed be available.

Evaluation of the patient begins by spending sufficient time on the history and clinical examination. This will not, perhaps, provide many clues pointing to the diagnosis but will help the surgeon to get acquainted with the patient, his fears, his motivation and his stamina. If at the end of this diagnostic process, the patient is to be subjected to pancreatic resection, we must have the appropriate information to assess the risk and to balance this against any potential benefits of operation. Whereas neither old age, arteriosclerotic risk factors, or even obesity, are by themselves insuperable obstacles to pancreatectomy today, they may tip the scales against resection if the chance for cure or at least meaningful palliation is smaller than the risk.

Valuable as the somewhat subjective 'clinical impression' of the senior surgeon in the unit may be, it is helpful to bolster this by more objective data obtainable in Mannheim by means of a simple 'student test'. In this, the youngest medical student on the unit takes the patient up three flights of stairs, measuring pulse and respiratory rate as well as blood pressure before and after the exercise. This, together with a good history of the patient's daily activities (gardening, sports etc.) contributes more to the question

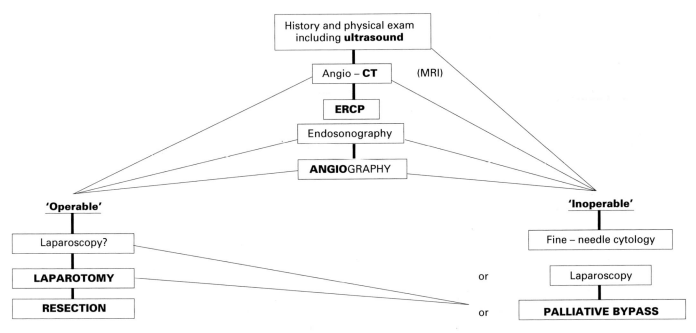

Fig. 37.4   Diagnostic algorithm followed in a patient with suspicion of pancreatic cancer.

of whether the patient is operable than a whole battery of sophisticated cardiopulmonary function studies.

Ultrasonography is included as part of the physical examination, because as we near the end of the twentieth century it has evolved into the 'stethoscope of the surgeon'. It is able to identify the pancreatic tumour as well as dilated bile ducts with or without stones. Furthermore, it can save considerable time and inconvenience, if liver metastases are found at this preliminary ultrasound examination. The main drawbacks of ultrasonography lie in its dependence on the skill and experience of the investigator and in the high rate of failure for technical reasons (e.g. obesity and intestinal gas).

It remains to be seen if endoscopic ultrasonography with the possibility of biopsy, can add specific information. So far, it is possible to detect enlarged lymph nodes, but not to distinguish between inflammatory or metastatic involvement (see Ch. 11).

Computerized tomography (CT), in combination with contrast medium given both orally and intravenously, can show up not only the tumour but extrapancreatic spread as well (e.g. hepatic metastases, and coeliac or paracaval lymph node involvement). In our experience and that of others, magnetic resonance imaging (MRI) has not been able to add any information on pancreatic cancer that cannot be provided by other methods, and especially by CT (Warshaw & Del Castillo 1992).

Endoscopic retrograde cholangiopancreatography (ERCP) can, of course, reveal a papillary carcinoma by direct visualization and biopsy. All other pancreatic tumours are detectable only if they impinge on the pancreatic duct.

Thus, small early cancers and those situated in the uncinate process may elude detection by this examination.

The well-known 'double-duct' sign signifies a large and often inoperable tumour. This phenomenon can also be produced by chronic pancreatitis (Fig. 37.5), but if there is the slightest doubt, laparotomy should be advised. A discrete stenosis, particularly if the remaining duct and its branches are normal, must also be taken seriously (Fig. 37.6).

In a patient presenting with jaundice, ERCP rates as the diagnostic procedure of choice, provided that an experienced endoscopist is readily available. Following clinical examination, ultrasonography and laboratory tests (above all to exclude hepatitis), ERCP is performed as the next step, usually within 1 or 2 days of admission.

The algorithm of decision-making that follows in patients with malignant biliary obstruction is outlined in Figure 37.7. If there is biliary obstruction, it can be localized and, if there happens to be an impacted gallstone, removed. If a tumour is seen it is biopsied and whatever its location, we aim to relieve the obstruction by passing a transpapillary stent across it while the endoscope is in position. Stenting will succeed in 80% of patients, allowing bile to flow once more into the gut (Manegold et al 1990).

The risks of operating on a deeply jaundiced patient are well recognized (Blamey et al 1983) but the pros and cons of preoperative biliary drainage are still under discussion. Suffice it to say that the postoperative course of these jaundiced patients appears to us smoother, particularly as regards avoiding haemorrhage and infection, if biliary obstruction is relieved before pancreatectomy is embarked

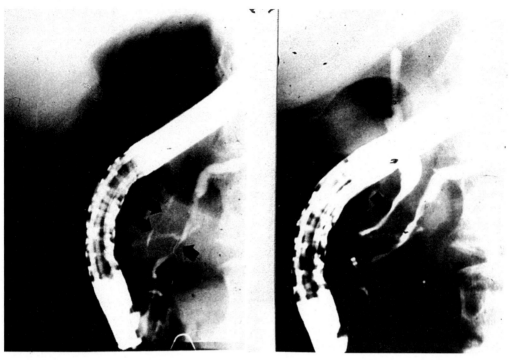

A   B

Fig. 37.5   72-year-old woman. **A** ERCP shows 'double-duct' stenosis. **B** 5 weeks later, the stenosis has partly resolved. The cause was chronic pancreatitis. The patient is alive and well 6 years later.

upon (Lygidakis et al 1987, Trede et al 1990). This is to say nothing of the preoperative course where in most cases jaundice fades, pruritus disappears and appetite returns. If drainage is successful, we allow the patient to recover for 1 or 2 weeks, using this time to stage the tumour and ascertain its operability. Indeed some patients are discharged home temporarily and are then often reluctant to return for the operation because they feel so much better already.

If endoscopic drainage fails, assessment of both the patient's operability and the tumour's resectability are completed expeditiously so that the attempt at resection

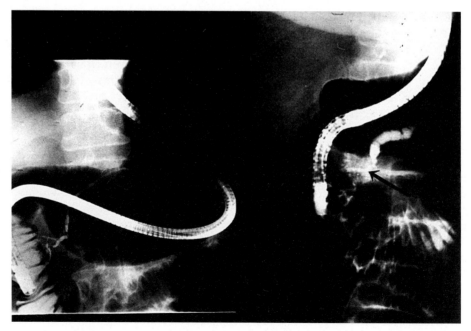

Fig. 37.6   45-year-old man presenting with 'lumbago'. ERCP shows only a very discrete stenosis (left); 4 months later, the patient returned with jaundice and an obvious tumour stenosis (right). The tumour was inoperable.

can follow within a few days (Fig. 37.7). Patients who for general medical reasons are unlikely to tolerate a major pancreatic resection, can be stented by the percutaneous transhepatic route or rendezvous technique (see Ch. 45), if the symptoms of jaundice and pruritus are severe. Some patients in this group may, however, be fit enough for a laparotomy and surgical bilioenteric anastomosis. The latter is certainly preferably to any form of interventionalist drainage in fit patients and it provides the best chance to assess resectability of the tumour itself. If the tumour appears to be easily resectable and if the patient makes a smooth and speedy recovery from this 'test-operation', then definitive resection as a second-stage operation may be carried out after all (Fig. 37.7).

Finally, the tumour may appear irresectable in an otherwise operable patient. In this case, an operative biliary bypass is performed after irresectability has been confirmed at operation.

It is worth stressing that the algorithm shown in Figure 37.7 demonstrates the close interdependence of the en-

doscopic, radiological and surgical approaches to diagnosis and treatment of pancreatic cancer. Each patient is seen by all three members of the team. This ensures that no patient is diagnosed, stented and then sent home without any further assessment of resectability.

Following the first algorithm (Fig. 37.4), we should now discuss angiography. Until recently, coeliac and superior mesenteric arteriography together with evaluation of the portal venous phase was an indispensable part of preoperative assessment. Not only did it provide the surgeon with a road map of any vascular anomalies, it also gave warning of irresectability, if tumour infiltration of the major retropancreatic vessels was demonstrated (Trede 1985). In a recent evaluation in Edinburgh, selective angiography revealed significant vascular anomalies in 16 of 46 (35%) patients with pancreatic or periampullary cancer. However, it is well recognized that angiography can mislead as far as vascular invasion is concerned (see Ch. 42). In Edinburgh, of 13 patients reported to have irresectable disease on angiography, two proved to have resectable

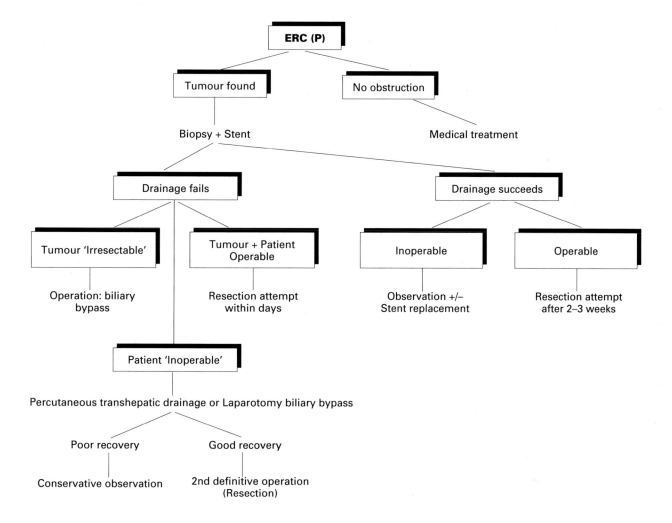

Fig. 37.7   Diagnostic and therapeutic algorithm for patients with malignant biliary obstruction. ERC(P), endoscopic retrograde cholangio (pancreatography).

cancer and the overall predictive value of angiography with regard to resectability was only 61%. We now advocate the selective use of angiography (Trede et al 1990), and it is still valuable as a final confirmation of irresectability in patients believed to be inoperable on other counts. In addition to demonstrating liver metastases prior to laparotomy, the newly introduced technique of laparoscopic contact ultrasonography (Miles et al 1992) may also provide useful information about vascular involvement in pancreatic cancer, further reducing the need for angiography.

An upper gastrointestinal roentgenogram with barium or gastrografin was once the mainstay of imaging procedures for suspected pancreatic cancer. Today, it is restricted to an occasional hypotonic duodenography to confirm stenosis or infiltration of the duodenum, a finding that is usually discovered more directly by endoscopy. Marked duodenal changes usually mean that the tumour, though possibly still resectable, will rarely be curable. Fixed duodenal stenosis is one indication for adding a bypassing gastrojejunostomy in patients who require a palliative procedure for jaundice.

Fine-needle cytology (see Ch. 12) is confined to clearly inoperable patients as a means of confirming the diagnosis. If no palliative procedure is required because the patient is neither jaundiced nor vomiting, but radiotherapy or chemotherapy is planned, then cytological proof of cancer can be obtained by this percutaneous method in some 75% of patients. In patients still being considered for surgery, there are anxieties that puncture of the tumour may cause dissemination of malignant cells, as suggested by a recent study using peritoneal cytology (Warshaw 1991).

With the laudable intention of avoiding an unnecessary laparotomy, laparoscopy has been used by some as the final hurdle to be taken before embarking on surgical exploration (Cuschieri et al 1978, Warshaw et al 1986). The usefulness of laparoscopy lies in its undisputed ability to discover most (if not all) small but visible peritoneal or hepatic metastases, nodules that would be missed by all other available imaging procedures (Warshaw et al 1990). Such metastases were indeed discovered by Warshaw in 23 of 88 patients. Contact ultrasonography can now be carried out laparoscopically and the early experience in Edinburgh suggests that the technique may detect deep-seated hepatic metastases in some patients with negative CT scans, in addition to providing useful information about vascular invasion and displacement.

The authors certainly recognize the existence of hepatic and peritoneal nodules in patients with pancreatic cancers, but consider that such metastases are only rarely the decisive cause of inoperability in those patients with pancreatic cancer who are selected for an exploratory laparotomy (see Ch. 14). Indeed, there is a case to be made for palliative pancreatectomy in the rare patient with a small solitary hepatic nodule. If the primary tumour causes symptoms (jaundice, vomiting, weight loss and pain) and if it is readily resectable, then a solitary hepatic metastasis should not deter one from performing pancreatectomy in a low-risk patient.

Using a multimodal approach to staging (including contrast-enhanced CT, angiography and laparoscopy), Warshaw et al (1990) were able to demonstrate that 89% of unresectable cases could be identified preoperatively. However, there was a false-positive rate of 5% and it is these five patients out of 100 that justify an exploratory laparotomy, provided that the patient's general condition and the surgeon's expertise make pancreatic resection a realistic option, should the tumour turn out to be resectable at operation.

Finally, one indication for laparotomy in pancreatic cancer patients, that has little to do with scientific staging and assessment, needs mention. In every referral centre dealing with these patients, there will be some whose every hope, their last hope, in fact, is focused on the operation. If the course has not been set away from operation, as it should have been early on, it may be very difficult for the surgeon to do so, once the patient has entered the surgical ward. To label the patient as inoperable, to refuse him the small chance that a laparotomy could offer, may do more psychological harm than physical good. This is no plea for the placebo effect of a 'sham-operation'. It is understood, of course, that at best such an exploratory laparotomy will benefit the patient only by finalizing the diagnosis and, perhaps, providing better palliative relief, than that offered by other forms of treatment.

REFERENCES

Blamey S L, Fearon K C H, Gilmour W H et al 1983 Prediction of risk in biliary surgery. British Journal of Surgery 70:535–538

Carter D C 1992 Cancer of the head of pancreas or chronic pancreatitis? A diagnostic dilemma. Surgery 111: 602–603

Cuschieri A, Hall A W, Clark J 1978 Value of laparoscopy in the diagnosis and management of pancreatic carcinoma. Gut 19:672–677

Gambil E F 1971 Pancreatitis associated with pancreatic carcinoma: a study of 26 cases. Mayo Clinic Proceedings 46:174

Greenway B, Iqbal M J, Johnson P J, Williams R 1983 Low serum testosterone concentrations in patients with carcinoma of the pancreas. British Medical Journal 286:93

Haglund C, Kuusela P, Roberts P J 1989 Tumour markers in pancreatic cancer. Annales Chirurgiae et Gynaecologiae 78:41–53

Itai Y, Moss A A, Goldberg H I 1982 Pancreatic cysts caused by carcinoma of the pancreas: a pitfall in the diagnosis of pancreatic carcinoma. Journal of Computer Assisted Tomography 6:772

Lygidakis N J, van der Heyde M N, Lubbers M J 1987 Evaluation of preoperative biliary drainage in the surgical management of pancreatic head carcinoma. Acta Chirurgica Scandinavica 153:665–668

Manegold B C, Buschulte J, Jung M 1990 Pankreaskarzinom –

Interventionelle Endoskopie. In: Trede M, Saeger H D (eds) Aktuelle Pankreaschirurgie. Springer-Verlag, Berlin, p 27–40

Miles W F A, Paterson-Brown S, Garden O J 1992 Laparoscopic contact hepatic ultrasonography. British Journal of Surgery 79:419–420

Moossa A R, Levin B 1981 The diagnosis of 'early' pancreatic cancer: the University of Chicago experience. American Cancer Society 47:1688–1697

Olen R, Pickleman J, Freeark R J 1989 Less is better. The diagnostic workup of the patient with obstructive jaundice. Archives of Surgery 124:791–795

Pellegrini C A, Thomas M J, Way L W 1982 Bilirubin and alkaline phosphatase values before and after surgery for biliary obstruction. American Journal of Surgery 143:67–73

Perez M M, Newcomer A D, Moertel C G, Go V L W, Di Magno E P 1983 Assessment of weight loss, food intake, fat metabolism, malabsorption, and treatment of pancreatic insufficiency in pancreatic cancer. American Cancer Society 52:346–352

Petrek J A, Sandberg W A, Bean P K, Bradley E L III 1985 Can survival in pancreatic adenocarcinoma be predicted by primary size or stage? American Surgeon 51:42–46

Saeger H D, Schwall G, Trede M 1990 Dilemma: Pankreatitis/Pankreaskarzinom. In: Trede M, Saeger H D (eds) Aktuelle Pankreaschirurgie. Springer-Verlag, Berlin p 122–127

Talamini M A, Pitt H A, Hruban R H, Boitnott J K, Coleman J, Cameron J L 1992 Spectrum of cystic tumors of the pancreas. American Journal of Surgery 163:117–124

Trede M 1985 The surgical treatment of pancreatic carcinoma. Surgery 97:28–35

Trede M, Schwall G, Saeger H D 1990 Survival after pancreatoduodenectomy. 118 consecutive resections without an operative mortality. Annals of Surgery 211:447–458

Warren K W, Christophi C, Armendariz R, Basu S 1983 Current trends in the diagnosis and treatment of carcinoma of the pancreas. American Journal of Surgery 145:813–818

Warshaw A L, Tepper J E, Shipley W U 1986 Laparoscopy in the staging and planning of therapy for pancreatic cancer. American Journal of Surgery 151:76–80

Warshaw A L, Zhuo-yun G V, Wittenberg J et al 1990 Pre-operative staging and assessment of resectability of pancreatic cancer. Archives of Surgery 125:230–233

Warshaw A L 1991 Implications of peritoneal cytology for staging of early pancreatic cancer. American Journal of Surgery 161:26–30

Warshaw A L, del Castillo C F 1992 Pancreatic carcinoma. New England Journal of Medicine 326:455–465

Way L W 1987 Diagnosis of pancreatic and other periampullary cancers. In: Howard J M, Jordan G L, Reber H A (eds) Surgical diseases of the pancreas. Lea and Febiger, Philadelphia, p 641–656

38. The surgical options

M. Trede

The overall outlook for carcinoma of the pancreas is gloomy. It is in fact the cancer with the lowest 5-year survival rate (Warshaw & del Castillo 1992). One of the main reasons for this lies in the hidden location of the gland, making diagnosis difficult and 'early' diagnosis the exception. This has lead to a disappointingly low resectability rate of around 10–20%. In general, the chance of a curative resection depends on the location and stage of the tumour. The closer the tumour lies to the papilla, the more likely is its early detection due to obstructive jaundice (Cubilla & Fitzgerald 1978, Nix et al 1991). Conversely tumours of the body or tail are seldom resectable and hardly ever curable (Moossa & Levin 1981, Gordon-Taylor 1934).

The role played by size and stage of the tumour has been stressed repeatedly (Moossa & Levin 1981, Tsuchiya et al 1986, Hermanek 1990). True early carcinoma of the pancreas (T_{1a}, N_0 according to the UICC classification of 1987) is only found in some 5% of resectable tumours (Gall & Kessler 1987, Hermanek 1990). Often these tumours are found by chance and diagnostic methods have contributed little to their detection.

However, with the ubiquitous use of imaging modalities, more and more resectable (if not 'early') tumours are being detected today. This progress is exemplified by the improving resection rate in our institution over the past two decades (Fig. 38.1).

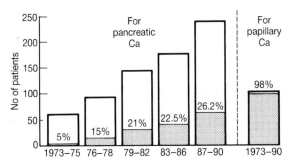

Fig. 38.1 Resectability for pancreatic and papillary carcinoma over two decades at the University Surgical Clinic, Mannheim

When analysing resectability, two things must be kept in mind: first, resectability depends not only on diagnostic excellence or surgical aggressiveness. It is even more dependent on referral practice. Thus, well-known pancreatic centres will have increasing numbers of 'difficult' (i.e. inoperable) cases referred to them, leading to an apparently lower resectability. Secondly, resectability rates for papillary tumours have always been above 90% for the reasons mentioned.

Confronted with the diagnosis of a resectable pancreatic carcinoma in an operable patient, the surgeon has three basic options: the nihilist, the activist and the realistic approaches (Fig. 38.2).

The 'nihilist' approach

The 'nihilists' advocate palliative procedures even for resectable lesions. They contend that an operative mortality of around 30% (Bernard 1987, Condie et al 1989) and dismal long-term survival rates (Herter et al 1982, Grace 1986b, Schouten 1986) make any radical resection valueless. They claim that following a palliative bypass more patients live longer and with better quality of life than after pancreatectomy (Crile 1970, Shapiro 1975, Gudjonsson et al 1978). Furthermore, in view of the high morbidity of resection as compared to palliation, the cost-effectiveness of the former is being questioned (Lea & Stahlgren 1987).

As a final touch, some surgeons are wondering – albeit with tongue in cheek – whether 'congress should pass a law making it illegal to do a Whipple operation' (Harken 1986).

This nihilist hypothesis is based largely on older and retrospective data. It has never been put to the test of a prospective, randomized and controlled trial. Today, such an experiment would not pass any ethics committee in any case.

Palliative procedures will be dealt with later on, and they certainly have their place in the management of unresectable lesions or inoperable patients. However, the

433

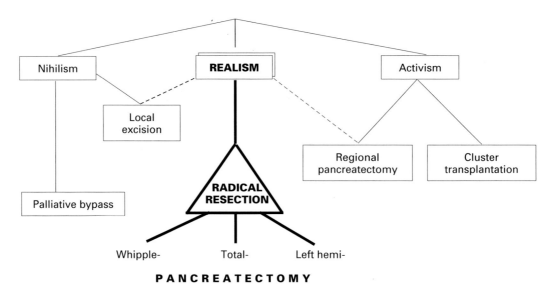

Fig. 38.2 The surgical options for periampullary and pancreatic carcinoma.

purely palliative approach will rob some few patients of their only chance for cure (Smith 1979), not to mention that in our experience, a resection often provides the best possible palliation, even if the lesion turns out to be incurable (Bailey et al 1991).

Local excision

In the treatment of some papillary tumours a case can be made for the more conservative (not nihilistic) approach of local excision. This is what Halsted did in February 1898 when he performed the transduodenal excision of a papillary carcinoma on a 60-year-old jaundiced lady. After a stormy course and a second operation the patient died of recurrent cancer 6 months later (Halsted 1899).

Today, local excision is recommended for benign villous adenomas of the papilla or duodenum, particularly in high-risk patients who might not tolerate any more radical resection (Knox & Kingston 1986, Tarazi et al 1986, Sharp 1990, Farouk et al 1991). It must be realized, however, that up to 50% of these apparently benign adenomas may recur as carcinomas, if indeed they do not harbour early malignant changes from the outset (Dupont-Lampert & Landmann 1989, Shutze et al 1990). That is why many surgeons, including the author, favour radical pancreatoduodenectomy even for (apparently) benign lesions, unless these are so small that they can be treated endoscopically, or unless the overall risk seems too high for that particular patient (Jones et al 1985, Robertson et al 1987, Sellner 1987, Schwall & Trede 1991).

Case report: A 51-year-old man presented with adenomatosis of the gallbladder, papilla of Vater and duodenum. In February

1972, a cholecystectomy and transduodenal polypectomy was performed. In August 1978, a recurrent villous adenoma of the papilla was removed by local transduodenal excision. In September 1982, a further recurrence was diagnosed endoscopically and the biopsy showed a severe cell metaplasia in an otherwise benign villous tumour. This time, a Whipple duodenopancreatectomy was performed. The villous adenoma was still completely benign but two gallstones were impacted in the common duct above it (Fig. 38.3). The patient was symptom-free at the last follow-up in 1991.

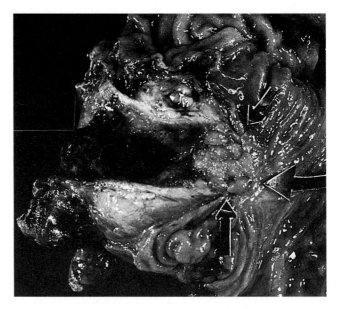

Fig. 38.3 Operative specimen of 51-year-old patient with pancreatoduodenectomy undertaken for recurrent villous adenoma and choledocholithiasis.

If radical resection is the best operation for benign papillary lesions, this applies even more to overt papillary carcinoma. In spite of a retrospective multicentre study apparently showing the superiority of local excision over radical resection both as regards operative mortality and 5-year survival (Knox & Kingston 1986, Koch et al 1991), the author would plead for the radical resection of these tumours, because these are the only carcinomas affecting this region with a realistically good chance for cure (Martin et al 1990, Shutze et al 1990, Trede et al 1990, Schwall & Trede 1991).

The 'activist' approach

At the other end of the spectrum, the 'activists' recommend an extensive so-called 'regional pancreatectomy', whenever possible (Fortner 1973). And if this seems impossible, due to hepatic metastases for example, then abdominal organ cluster transplantation could be the last resort (Starzl et al 1989).

The criticism of this approach was formulated by the late Mark Ravitch when he said that it represents 'the reductio ad absurdum of the idea that cancer is a surgical disease' (Ravitch 1974). True as this may be, it is equally true that up to this last decade of the twentieth century, surgery does provide the only chance for cure. It is on this last fact that all efforts at extending radicality are based (Sunada et al 1992). These efforts are not new: Brunschwig reported the case of a patient who survived total pancreatectomy, total gastrectomy, splenectomy, omentectomy and left renal adrenalectomy for ductal carcinoma of the pancreas (albeit for only $3\frac{1}{2}$ months) almost 50 years ago (Brunschwig et al 1945).

In the early 1950s there were isolated reports of portal or superior mesenteric vein resection together with pancreatectomy for tumour. In two cases, patients survived resection of the portal vein without any reconstruction whatsoever (Child et al 1952). Simple end-to-end anastomosis of the superior mesenteric vein (Moore et al 1951), or reconstruction by means of a mesocaval shunt (McDermott 1952, Hubbard 1958) or by interposition of homologous (Asada et al 1963) or autologous vein grafts (Sigel et al 1965), were further pioneer ventures in this field.

Credit must go to Fortner for pursuing this activist approach to its logical conclusion and giving it the name 'regional pancreatectomy' (Fortner 1984, 1989). The three variants of this operation are summarized in Table 38.1. The operative technique will be described later on in Chapter 42. The impartial reader will want to know, however, whether regional pancreatectomy has so far provided any benefit in comparison with other forms of resection. The answer is that up to now the results of regional pancreatectomy have not encouraged many others to follow Fortner's lead (Dardik et al 1975, Sindelar 1989). In

Table 38.1 Regional pancreatectomy. (Classification according to Fortner et al 1977)

Type 0	Total pancreatectomy (including hemigastrectomy cholecystectomy, splenectomy, retroperitoneal lymphadenectomy)
Type I	As above, plus: Resection of portal vein segment
Type II	
IIa	As above, plus: Resection of proximal superior mesenteric artery
IIb	As Type I, plus: Resection of coeliac axis and/or hepatic artery
IIc	As Type I, plus: Resection of coeliac axis and superior mesenteric artery

spite of improvements in the procedure and outcome of regional pancreatectomy (operating time is down from 31 to 9.5 hours; operative mortality is down from 23 to 9%, and the 5-year survival rate is estimated at 26%) (Fortner 1984, 1989, Dresler et al 1991), its results have not reached the standard set by the third option (below).

Therefore, it is not the policy of the editors to perform regional pancreatectomy on principle for every operable case of pancreatic cancer. We do, however, resort to these techniques out of necessity from time to time, if that is the only way to remove an otherwise operable tumour even though the chances of a cure are very slim.

The 'realistic' approach

The third option is the realistic approach of pancreatic resection: total, partial or pylorus-preserving pancreatoduodenectomy, or left hemipancreatectomy, for all patients with resectable tumours. It is based on the concept that many periampullary, and some early or small pancreatic carcinomas (T_{1a} or T_{1b} according to the UICC classification of 1987), can be cured by such procedures. On the other hand, tumour growth outside the confines of the gland and involving regional lymph notes (T_2 or N_1) is practically beyond the reach of the surgeon's knife.

Left hemipancreatectomy is reserved for those rare tumours of the tail of the pancreas that are discovered before they are inoperable. But even when the tumour has been operable, only a handful of long-term survivors has ever been reported (Gordon-Taylor 1934, Goyanes et al 1971, Nakase et al 1977, Tsuchiya et al 1988).

At first sight, total pancreatectomy would appear to be superior as a cancer operation (Table 38.2). One would expect it to be more 'radical', eradicating possible multicentric malignancy within the gland and permitting wider lymph node clearance without. The question of multicentricity is still under debate. Whereas in some series it was discovered in about 30% of cases (van Heerden et al 1988, Brooks et al 1989), others describe multicentricity in only 2.5% of resected specimens (Michelassi et al 1989, Hermanek 1990). If there really is true multi-

Table 38.2 Arguments in favour of total pancreatectomy for pancreatic carcinoma

Increased radicality	Removal of:	Improved long-term survival?
	Multicentric tumours	
	Diffuse carcinomatosis	
	Intraductal tumour cells	
	Tumour spread to Whipple resection line	
	Peripancreatic lymph nodes	
Decreased morbidity	Avoidance of:	Lower operative mortality?
	Any pancreatic anastomosis	

centricity of pancreatic carcinoma (as distinct from diffuse duct metaplasia or multifocal carcinoma in situ) then one would expect the long-term results of total (as distinct from partial) pancreatoduodenectomy to be better. In actual fact, they are not (Tables 38.3, 38.4).

The fact that survival after total pancreatectomy is no better than after less radical resection, has led erstwhile protagonists of the former to question the clinical significance of so-called multicentric tumour growth (van Heerden et al 1988). This discussion is reminiscent of a similar controversy concerning breast cancer (Carter 1980) where bilateral mastectomy (undertaken because of possible multicentricity) has been abandoned as treatment for unilateral cancer.

As for tumour extension to the plane of a potential Whipple resection, this was found in 14–18% of total pancreatectomy specimens (Mongé et al 1964, Forrest &

Longmire 1979, Brooks et al 1989). However, in spite of routine examination of this plane by frozen section in the course of 259 Whipple resections for cancer, we came across unexpected tumour infiltration at this site in only three cases, and total resection was then performed.

That leaves the contention that morbidity and therefore operative mortality should be lower following total pancreatectomy, since the potentially hazardous pancreatic anastomosis (the 'Achilles heel' of the Whipple procedure) is avoided. Again, clinical experience has shown that if anything, mortality after the total resection is higher (Tables 38.5, 38.6). The absence of postoperative pancreatic complications is apparently balanced by a larger retroperitoneal wound, loss of the spleen and need for insulin following total pancreatectomy.

For all these reasons, the editors reserve total pancreatectomy for those large pancreatic tumours that extend within 3 cm of the plane of a potential Whipple resection. On rare occasions, total removal may be preferable to anastomosis, if the pancreatic tail is very soft and friable and if it is drained by a very narrow duct. Finally, the decision for total pancreatectomy is taken more easily, if the patient already is an insulin-dependent diabetic. It should be added, however, that diabetes following total pancreatectomy for cancer is usually easily controlled, since these patients (in contrast to their counterparts with alcoholic chronic pancreatitis) are disciplined and motivated to comply with dietary instructions.

Pylorus-preserving pancreatoduodenectomy

The alternative of pylorus-preserving pancreatoduodenectomy (PPPD) was first described by Watson in 1944 for resection of an ampullary carcinoma (Watson

Table 38.3 Long-term survival after total pancreatectomy for carcinoma

Author	Institution	Number of patients	5-year survival (%)
Moossa 1979	Chicago University	33	4 (12)
Herter et al 1982	Columbia University	64	1 (1.5)
Andrén-Sandberg & Ihse 1983	Lund University	85	4 (4.6)
van Heerden et al 1988	Mayo Clinic	89	3 (3.4)
Brooks et al 1989	Harvard	48	6 (14)
Trede 1992 unpublished data	Mannheim	44	5 (11)

Table 38.4 Long-term survival after Whipple operation for cancer

Author	Institution	Number of patients	% 5-year survival rate
Cooperman 1981	Columbia, NY	70	7.1
van Heerden et al 1981	Mayo Clinic	44	2.3
Lerut et al 1984	Insel Spital Berne	25	6.0
Jones et al 1985	Toronto	28	7.0
Grace et al 1986b	UCLA	37	3.0
Connolly et al 1987	Chicago University	89	3.4
Crist & Cameron 1989	Johns Hopkins	50	18

Table 38.5 Operative mortality of total pancreatectomy for carcinoma

Author	Institution	Number of patients	Operative mortality (%)
Herter et al 1982	Columbia University	64	15 (23.4)
Andrén-Sandberg & Ihse 1983	Lund University	85	25 (29.0)
Connolly et al 1987	Chicago University	39	9 (23.1)
van Heerden et al 1988	Mayo Clinic	89	9 (10.1)
Brooks et al 1989	Harvard	48	4 (8.3)
Trede 1992 unpublished data	Mannheim	44	3 (6.8)

Table 38.6 Operative mortality of Whipple operation for cancer

Author	Institution	Number of patients	Operative mortality (%)
van Heerden 1984	Mayo Clinic	146	6 (4.1)
Jones et al 1985	Toronto	87	4 (4.6)
Siedeck et al 1985	St Elisabeth Krankenhaus, Köln	112	2 (1.8)
Braasch et al 1986	Lahey Clinic	87	2 (2.3)
Grace et al 1986b	UCLA	45	1 (2.2)
Tsuchiya et al 1986	Nagasaki	94	4 (4.2)
Bittner et al 1989	Ulm	55	3 (5.4)
Ceuterick et al 1989	Université Libre, Brussels	79	4 (5.0)
Lygidakis et al 1989	Amsterdam	78	3 (3.8)
Pellegrini et al 1989	University of California, San Francisco	51	1 (2.0)
Cameron (personal communication 1991)	Johns Hopkins	60	1 (1.7)
Trede 1992 unpublished data	Mannheim	259	7 (2.7)

1944). The operation was revived by Traverso and Longmire in 1978 (Traverso & Longmire 1978) and has found favour in many centres (Braasch et al 1986). The operation is described in detail in Chapter 30. In our view it has two advantages, one practical, one theoretical, and some drawbacks.

The practical advantage is the saving of some operating time, since antrectomy is avoided (Grace et al 1986a). The advantages of a 'more physiological' gastrojejunal food passage appear to be mainly theoretical (Itani et al 1986, Sato et al 1986, Kim et al 1987, Patti et al 1987, Takada et al 1989). In fact, the postgastrectomy dumping syndromes that are said to plague patients following standard Whipple resection could not be confirmed on careful examination (Linehan et al 1988). Most comparisons of PPPD with the conventional Whipple procedure are historical (Morel et al 1990) or retrospective (Fink et al 1988) and therefore of limited scientific value. The protagonists of the method themselves admit that 'the long-term benefit of PPPD remains unproven', since they found no significant differences in a clinical and bio-chemical comparison with standard pancreatoduo-denectomy (Fink et al 1988).

It is mainly the *disadvantages* of the new method that have prevented its acceptance world-wide. First, there is a delay in gastric emptying in 50% of patients for as long as several weeks postoperatively (Warshaw & Torchiana 1985, Braasch et al 1986). This means that a nasogastric tube had to be left in place for a mean of 14 days, a tube that is removed within 24 hours after a standard Whipple (Trede et al 1990). Furthermore, some patients required reoperation to relieve gastric outlet obstruction (Hunt & McLean 1989). This has also led to a significantly longer hospitalization after PPPD (Warshaw & Torchiana 1985).

The second problem concerns jejunal ulceration. On the one hand, pyloric and gastric preservation is designed to reduce the incidence of postoperative ulcers. These were previously thought to be a troublesome consequence the traditional Whipple operation, so that some surgeons had recommended the addition of vagotomy to reduce the ulcerogenic potential of partial or total pancrea-tectomy (Scott et al 1980). In the Mannheim experience with 378 Whipple operations, jejunal ulcers occurred post-operatively in only eight patients (2.3%), although vagotomy has never been part of the procedure. In a review of 339 PPPDs the rate of marginal ulceration was also a low 3.6% (Grace et al 1990). However, in comparing PPPD with the Whipple resection, the Mayo group found a much higher rate of marginal ulceration with the former (13% as against 5%) (McAfee et al 1989). In Erlangen, PPPD was abandoned after seven out of 18 patients developed marginal ulcers, requiring a secondary partial gastrectomy in 6 cases (Gebhardt et al 1982).

Finally, a note of caution is required when PPPD is applied to malignant tumours. This method may well have a place in the treatment of papillary or distal common duct neoplasms and the UCLA group have reported a remarkable 5-year survival rate of 25% even with

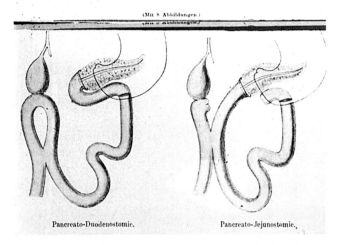

Fig. 38.4   Title and operative sketch in Kausch's original publication in 1912.

carcinomas of the head of the pancreas. (However, this was 'actuarial' survival in only 13 patients and of the two 5-year survivors, one had a carcinoma in situ while the other had stage I disease (Grace 1986b)). Other reports have shown that the potential chance for curative resection of pancreatic carcinoma was compromised by PPPD (Sharp et al 1989, Boerma & Coosemans 1990, Roder et al 1992). It is surely inappropriate to trade possible curability by a Whipple resection for the theoretical advantages of PPPD.

Whipple's pancreatoduodenectomy

We are left with Whipple's pancreatoduodenectomy as the optimal operation for the large majority of patients with a resectable periampullary or pancreatic carcinoma (Gall et al 1991).

The first successful en bloc resection of part of the pancreatic head, distal common duct and duodenum was actually performed by Kausch in the summer of 1909 (Kausch 1912) (Fig. 38.4). The patient was a 49-year-old messenger suffering from obstructive jaundice due to a papillary carcinoma. He survived the two-stage operation and went back to work, only to succumb 9 months later to septic cholangitis due to a stricture of the bilioenteric

anastomosis. At autopsy neither metastasis nor recurrent tumour was found.

Twenty-five years later, Alan O. Whipple performed his first pancreatoduodenectomy also as a two-stage procedure (Whipple et al 1935) (Fig. 38.5). It took another 7 years before the one-stage resection was perfected, much as we know it today (Whipple 1942). Towards the end of his life, Whipple could look back on a personal series of 37 of these procedures, 30 performed for periampullary tumours and seven for chronic pancreatitis (Whipple 1963, Peters & Carey 1991). In a 1951 review of the operation, the operative mortality was 31% and only one patient had survived more than 5 years (Loggan & Kleinsasser 1951).

Today, the operative mortality in centres experienced in pancreatic surgery has dropped to below 5% (Table 38.6) and indeed, there have been reports of long consecutive series of Whipple operations without any mortality at all (Table 38.7). But as if to remind us that even today this is one of the more formidable abdominal operations, some recently published mortality figures still reached 30% and more (Bernard 1987, Lea & Stahlgren 1987,

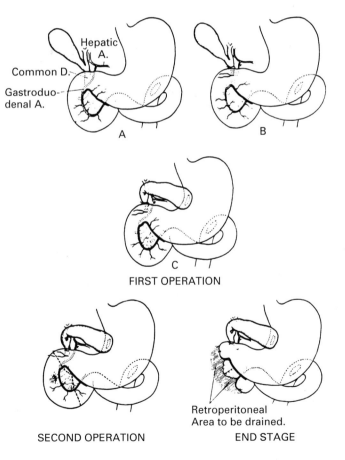

Fig. 38.5   Operative sketch of Whipple's first operation reported in 1935. (With permission of J B Lippincott Co, Philadelphia, from A O Whipple et al 1935 Annals of Surgery 102:763–779)

Table 38.7 Consecutive pancreatoduodenectomies without an operative mortality

Author	Institution	Number of resections
Howard 1968	Philadelphia	41
Warren 1973	Lahey Clinic	56
Warshaw 1985	Massachusetts General	88
Trede 1990	Mannheim	144
Cameron et al 1993	Johns Hopkins	145

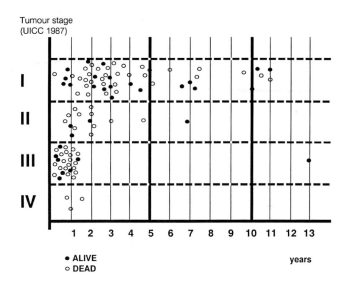

Fig. 38.7 Survival of 100 patients who had R_0 resections for pancreatic adenocarcinoma in the period 1.10.1972–1.1.1992 at the University Surgical Clinic, Mannheim. Survival in years is plotted against the stage of the disease.

Condie et al 1989), not to mention those that are not published.

With more patients surviving the operation, one would have expected that more of them would be long-term survivors. So far, however, these hopes have not materialized (Table 38.4). With the exception of a few series, the 5-year survival rate after pancreatoduodenectomy for adenocarcinoma of the pancreas stagnates at around 5%.

Nevertheless, in order to encourage the reader to go on to read the next section on the technique of pancreatoduodenectomy, it might be worthwhile to analyse the long-term results of this resection in more detail.

Late results can be viewed from three angles. First, the actuarial survival curve of 162 patients who had pancreatoduodenectomy for adenocarcinoma can be plotted according to Kaplan-Meier (Fig. 38.6). For those 62 patients with an R_1 or R_2 resection (i.e. those in whom microscopic or macroscopic residual tumour was left in the patient), the curve ends at 24 months. These were palliative resections, of course, but in most cases the palliation was worthwhile for at least 18 months. How-

ever, in 100 patients with R_0 resections (i.e. both surgeon and pathologist felt that the tumour was completely eradicated) the statistically estimated (actuarial) 5-year survival rate is 30%.

Another view of long-term results is provided by plotting survival against stage of the disease (according to the UICC classification of 1987) (Fig. 38.7). As one would expect, most of the long-term survivors belong to stage I ($T_1 N_0 M_x$). But it is worth noting that three patients

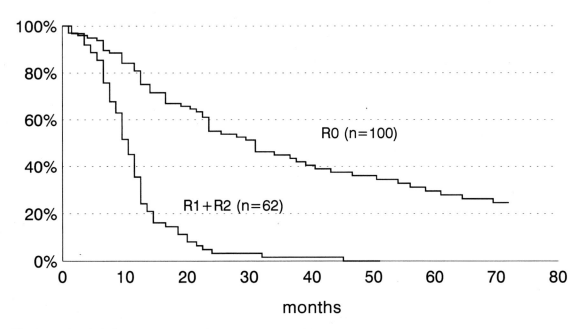

Fig. 38.6 Survival after pancreatectomy for adenocarcinoma of the pancreas (actuarial survival according to Kaplan-Meier). A total of 162 patients, R_0 (n = 100) or R_1/R_2 (n = 62) tumours, were treated at the University Surgical Clinic, Mannheim, in the period 1.10.1972–1.1.1992.

Table 38.8 Late results of pancreatectomy for pancreatic, papillary and periampullary carcinoma. (University Surgical Clinic, Mannheim, 1.10.72–1.1.1992)

	Number of patients operated before 1.1.1987	Number of 5-year survivors, 1.1.1992	
		Total	Died >5 years postoperatively
Head of pancreas	61	17	9
Papilla	51	30	6
Choledocus + duodenum	21	4	3
Total	133	51	18

survived for more than 3 years in spite of lymph node metastases and one of these is still alive 13 years after the resection.

Finally, without any statistical manipulation, one can look at the fate of 133 patients whose R_0 pancreatectomy for pancreatic or periampullary carcinoma took place more than 5 years ago (Table 38.8). Of these patients, 51 passed the 'magic' 5-year survival line, i.e. actual 5-year survival amounts to 38%. This series includes 51 patients with favourable papillary carcinoma carrying a 5-year survival of 58% as indeed has been reported in other series (Jones et al 1985, Chiappetta et al 1986, Shutze et al 1990). For those 61 patients with adenocarcinoma of the head of the pancreas, the actual 5-year survival is 28%, i.e. similar to the actuarial figures.

One of the main reasons for offering pancreatoduodenectomy to every operable patient with a periampullary tumour is the difficulty of distinguishing between a favourable papillary tumour that has invaded the pancreatic head, from a pancreatic carcinoma that has infiltrated the papilla. If this is difficult enough for the pathologist with the complete specimen before him, it may be impossible for the surgeon at the operating table (Harbrecht 1974).

By now, the attentive reader will have noticed that we are discussing survival not cure. The reason lies in the biological nature of these dread tumours; of the 17 patients who survived resection for pancreatic adenocarcinoma for more than 5 years in Mannheim, nine died subsequently of late recurrent and metastatic pancreatic cancer. Its biological nature is also such that there are a handful of patients who have survived histologically proven carcinoma of the pancreas for 9 years and more without any treatment at all! (see Everson & Cole 1955, Cattell & Young 1957, Howard et al 1987, Sanders & McBurney 1956, Hanna & Hastings 1968). So it is probably still fair to say that surgery alone, though it does provide the best chance for survival at present, is not really able to cure many patients with pancreatic carcinoma.

REFERENCES

Andrén-Sandberg A, Ihse I 1983 Factors influencing survival after total pancreatectomy in patients with pancreatic cancer. Annals of Surgery 198:605–610

Asada S, Itaya H, Nakamura K, Isohashi T, Masuoka S 1963 Radical pancreatoduodenectomy and portal vein resection. Report of two successful cases with transplantation of the portal vein. Archives of Surgery 87:609

Bailey I S, Johnson C D, Keating J 1991 Surgery offers the best palliation for carcinoma of the pancreas. Annals of the Royal College of Surgeons of England 73:243–247

Bernard H R 1987 Discussion of M M Connolly. Annals of Surgery 206:366–371

Bittner R, Roscher R, Safi F et al 1989 Der Einfluss von Tumorgrösse und Lymphknotenstatus auf die Prognose des Pankreaskarzinoms. Chirurg 60:240–245

Boerma E J, Coosemans J A R 1990 Non-preservation of the pylorus in resection of pancreatic cancer. British Journal of Surgery 77:299–300

Braasch J W, Deziel D J, Rossi R L et al 1986 Pyloric and gastric preserving pancreatic resection. Experience with 87 patients. Annals of Surgery 204:411–418

Brooks J R, Brooks D C, Levine J D 1989 Total pancreatectomy for ductal cell carcinoma of the pancreas. An update. Annals of Surgery 209:405–410

Brunschwig A, Ricketts H T, Bigelow R R 1945 Total pancreatectomy, total gastrectomy, total duodenectomy, splenectomy, left adrenalectomy and omentectomy in a diabetic patient, recovery. Surgery, Gynecology and Obstetrics 80:252–256

Cameron J L, Pitt H A, Yeo C J, Lillemoe K D, Kaufman H S, Coleman J 1993 One hundred and forty-five consecutive pancreaticoduodenectomies without mortality. Annals of Surgery 217:430–438

Carter D C 1980 Regular review: Surgery for pancreatic cancer. British Medical Journal 744–746

Cattell R B, Young W C 1957 Long survival in a case of carcinoma of the pancreas. Lahey Clinic Bulletin 10:131

Ceuterick M, Gelin M, Rickaert F et al 1989 Pancreaticoduodenal resection for pancreatic or periampullary tumors – a ten-year experience. Hepato-gastroenterology 36:467–473

Chiappetta A, Sperti C, Bonadimani B, Pasquall C et al 1986 Surgical experience with adenocarcinoma of the ampulla of Vater. American Surgeon 52:603–606

Child III C G, Holswade G, McClure R D, Gore A L, O'Neill E A 1952 Pancreaticoduodenectomy with resection of the portal vein in the macaca mulatta monkey and in man. Surgery, Gynecology and Obstetrics 94:31–45

Condie Jr J D, Nagpal S, Peebles S A 1989 Surgical treatment for ductal adenocarcinoma of the pancreas. Surgery, Gynecology and Obstetrics 168:437–445

Connolly M M, Dawson P J, Michelassi F, Moossa A R, Lowenstein F 1987 Survival in 1001 patients with carcinoma of the pancreas. Annals of Surgery 206:366–371

Cooperman A M 1981 Cancer of the pancreas: a dilemma in treatment. Surgical Clinics of North America 61:107–115

Crile Jr G 1970 The advantages of bypass operations over radical pancreatoduodenectomy in the treatment of pancreatic carcinoma. Surgery, Gynecology and Obstetrics 130:1049–1053

Crist D W, Cameron J L 1989 Current status of pancreaticoduodenectomy for periampullary carcinoma. Hepato-gastroenterology 36:478–485

Cubilla A L, Fitzgerald P J 1978 Pancreas cancer. 1. duct cell adenocarcinoma. Pathology Annual 13:241–287

Dardik H, Dardik II, Spreyregen S, Becker N, Gliedman M L 1975 Total pancreatectomy with primary mesenteric vascular reconstruction. American Journal of Surgery 129:691–693

Dresler C M, Fortner J G, McDermott K, Bajorunas D R 1991 Metabolic consequences of (regional) total pancreatectomy. Annals of Surgery 214:131–140

Dupont-Lampert V, Landmann J 1989 Tubulo-villöses adenom des duodenums: Fallvorstellung und Literaturübersicht. Schweizerische medizinische Wochenschrift 119:1057–1059

Everson T C, Cole W H 1955 Ten-year survival following pancreatoduodenectomy for carcinoma of the ampulla of Vater. Surgery 37:260

Farouk I, Niotis M, Branum G D, Cotton P B, Meyers W C 1991 Indications for and the technique of local resection of tumors of the papilla of Vater. Archives of Surgery 126:650–652

Fink A S, De Souza L R, Mayer E A, Hawkins R, Longmire Jr W P 1988 Long-term evaluation of pylous preservation after pancreatico duodenectomy. World Journal of Surgery 12:663–670

Forrest J F, Longmire Jr W P 1979 Carcinoma of the pancreas and periampullary region. Annals of Surgery 189:129–138

Fortner J G 1973 Regional resection of cancer of the pancreas: a new surgical approach. Surgery 73:307–320

Fortner J G 1984 Regional pancreatectomy for cancer of the pancreas, ampulla, and other related sites. Tumor staging and results. Annals of Surgery 199:418–425

Fortner J G 1989 'Radical' abdominal cancer surgery: current state and future course. Japanese Journal of Surgery 19:503–509

Fortner J G, Kim D K, Cubilla A et al 1977 Regional pancreatomy: en bloc pancreatic portal vein and lymph node resection. Annals of Surgery 186: 42–50

Gall F P, Kessler H 1987 Das Frühcarcinom des exokrinen Pankreas: Diagnose und Prognose. Der Chirurg 58:78–83

Gall F P, Kessler H, Hermanek P 1991 Surgical treatment of ductal pancreatic carcinoma. European Journal of Surgical Oncology 17:173–181

Gebhardt C, Gall F P, Rösch W, Schackert H K 1982 Anastomosenulkus nach Whipplescher Operation mit Magenerhaltung. Zentralblatt für Chirurgie 107:952–958

Gordon-Taylor G 1934 The radical surgery of cancer of the pancreas. Annals of Surgery 100:206–214

Goyanes Di A, Pack G T, Bowden L 1971 Cancer of the body and tail of the pancreas. Review of Surgery 28:153–175

Grace P A, Pitt H A, Longmire Jr W P 1986a Pancreatoduodenectomy with pylorus preservation for adenocarcinoma of the head of the pancreas. British Journal of Surgery 73:647–650

Grace P A, Pitt H A, Tompkins R K, DenBesten L, Longmire Jr W P 1986b Decreased morbidity and mortality after pancreatoduodenectomy. American Journal of Surgery 151:141–149

Grace P A, Pitt H A, Longmire Jr W P 1990 Pylorus preserving pancreatoduodenectomy: an overview. British Journal of Surgery 77:968–974

Gudjonsson B, Livstone E M, Spiro H M 1978 Cancer of the pancreas: diagnostic accuracy and survival statistics. Cancer 42:2494–2506

Halsted W S 1899 Contributions to the surgery of the bile passages, especially of the common bile-duct. Boston Medical and Surgical Journal 141:645–654

Hanna C B, Hastings Jr W D 1968 Carcinoma of the pancreas: Survival without resection. Journal of the South Carolina Medical Association 64:8

Harbrecht P J 1974 Discussion of Wilson S M. Archives of Surgery 108:539

Harken A H 1986 Presidential address: natural selection in university surgery. Surgery 100:129–133

Hermanek P 1990 Chirurgische Pathologie des Pankreaskarzinoms. In: Trede M, Saeger H D (eds) Aktuelle Pankreaschirurgie. Springer-Verlag Berlin, p 3–12

Herter F P, Cooperman A M, Ahlborn T N, Antinori C 1982 Surgical experience with pancreatic and periampullary cancer. Annals of Surgery 195:274–281

Howard J M 1968 Pancreatico-duodenectomy: forty-one consecutive Whipple resections without an operative mortality. Annals of Surgery 168:629–640

Howard J M, Jordan G L, Reber H A (eds) Surgical diseases of the pancreas. Lea & Febiger, Philadelphia

Hubbard Jr T B 1958 Carcinoma of the head of the pancreas: resection of the portal vein and portacaval shunt. Annals of Surgery 147:935–958

Hunt D R, McLean R 1989 Pylorus-preserving pancreatectomy: Functional results. British Journal of Surgery 76:173–176

Itani K M F, Coleman R E, Akwari O E, Meyers W C 1986 Pylorus-preserving pancreatoduodenectomy. A clinical and physiologic appraisal. Annals of Surgery 204:655

Jones B A, Langer B, Taylor B R, Girotti M 1985 Periampullary tumors: which ones should be resected? American Journal of Surgery 149:46–52

Jordan Jr G L 1987 Pancreatic resection for pancreatic cancer. In: Howard J M, Jordan Jr G L, Reber H A (eds) Surgical diseases of the pancreas. Lea and Febiger, Philadelphia, p 666–714

Kausch W 1912 Das Carcinom der Papilla duodeni und seine radikale Entfernung. Beiträge zur Klinischen Chirurgie 78:439–486

Kim H C, Suzuki T, Kajiwara T, Miyashita T, Imamura M, Tobe T 1987 Exocrine and endocrine stomach after gastrobulbar preserving pancreatoduodenectomy. Annals of Surgery 206:717–727

Knox R A, Kingston R D 1986 Carcinoma of the ampulla of Vater. British Journal of Surgery 73:72–73

Koch B, Hildebrandt U, Schüder G, Seitz G, Feifel G 1991 Eingeschränkte chirurgische Radikalität beim okkulten Karzinom der Papilla Vateri. Langenbecks Archiv für Chirurgie 376:195–198

Lea M S, Stahlgren L H 1987 Is resection appropriate for adenocarcinoma of the pancreas? A cost-benefit analysis. American Journal of Surgery 154:651–654

Lerut J P, Gianello P R, Otte J B, Kestens P J 1984 Pancreaticoduodenal resection. Surgical experience and evaluation of risk factors in 103 patients. Annals of Surgery 199:432–437

Linehan I P, Russell R C G, Hobsley M 1988 The dumping syndrome after pancreatoduodenectomy. Surgery, Gynecology and Obstetrics 167:114–118

Loggan P B, Kleinsasser L J 1951 Collective review of surgery of the pancreas; the results of pancreaticoduodenal resections reported in the literature. Surgery, Gynecology and Obstetrics 93:521

Lygidakis N J, van der Heyde M N, Houthoff H J et al 1989 Resectional surgical procedures for carcinoma of the head of the pancreas. Surgery, Gynecology and Obstetrics 168:157–165

Martin F M, Rossi R L, Dorrucci V, Silverman M L, Braasch J W 1990 Clinical and pathologic correlations in patients with periampullary tumors. Archives of Surgery 125:723–726

McAfee M K, van Heerden J A, Adson M A 1989 Is proximal pancreatoduodenectomy with pyloric preservation superior to total pancreatectomy? Surgery 105:347–351

McDermott Jr W V 1952 A one-stage pancreatoduodenectomy with resection of the portal vein for carcinoma of the pancreas. Annals of Surgery 136:1012

Michelassi F, Erroi F, Dawson P J, Pietrabissa A, Noda S, Handcock M, Block G E 1989 Experience with 647 consecutive tumors of the duodenum, ampulla, head of the pancreas, and distal common bile duct. Annals of Surgery 210:544–556

Mongé J J, Judd E S, Gage R P 1964 Radical pancreatoduodenectomy: a 22-year experience with the complications, mortality rate, and survival rate. Annals of Surgery 160:711–722

Moore G E, Sako Y, Thomas L B 1951 Radical pancreatoduodenectomy with resection and reanastomosis of the superior mesenteric vein. Surgery 30:550–553

Moossa A R 1979 Reoperation for pancreatic cancer. Archives of Surgery 114:502–504

Moossa A R, Levin B 1981 The diagnosis of 'early' pancreatic cancer: the University of Chicago experience. Cancer 47:1688–1697

Morel P, Mathey P, Corboud H, Huber O, Egeli R A, Rohner A 1990 Pylorus-preserving duodenopancreatectomy: long-term complications and comparison with the Whipple procedure. World Journal of Surgery 14:642–647

Nakase A, Matsumoto Y, Uchida K, Honjo I 1977 Surgical treatment of cancer of the pancreas and the periampullary region: cumulative results in 57 institutions in Japan. Annals of Surgery 185:52–57

Nix G A J J, Dubbelman C, Srivastava E D, Wilson J H P, Boender J, de Jongh F E 1991 Prognostic implications of the localization of carcinoma in the head of the pancreas. American Journal of Gastroenterology 86:1027–1032

Patti M G, Pellegrini C A, Way L W 1987 Gastric emptying and small bowel transit of solid food after pylorus-preserving pancreaticoduodenectomy. Archives of Surgery 122:528–532

Pellegrini C A, Heck C F, Raper S, Way L W 1989 An analysis of the reduced morbidity and mortality rates after pancreaticoduodenectomy. Archives of Surgery 124:778–781

Peters J H, Carey L C 1991 Historical review of pancreaticoduodenectomy. American Journal of Surgery 161:219–225

Ravitch M 1974 Discussion of Fortner J G et al. Archives of Surgery 109:153

Robertson J F R, Imrie C W, Hole D J, Carter D C, Blumgart L H 1987 Management of periampullary carcinoma. British Journal of Surgery 74:816–819

Roder J D, Stein H J, Hüttl W, Siewert J R 1992 Pylorus-preserving versus standard pancreatico-duodenectomy: an analysis of 110 pancreatic and periampullary carcinomas. British Journal of Surgery 79:152–155

Sanders L C, McBurney R P 1956 Carcinoma of the pancreas. American Journal of Gastroenterology 25:59

Sato T, Imamura M, Matsuro S, Sasaki I, Ohneda A 1986 Gastric acid secretion and gut hormone release in patients undergoing pancreaticoduodenectomy. Surgery 99:728–734

Schouten J T 1986 Operative therapy for pancreatic carcinoma. The American Journal of Surgery 151:626–630

Schwall G, Trede M 1991 Der Tumor der Papilla Vateri – eine diagnostische und therapeutische Herausforderung. Langenbecks Archiv für Chirurgie 376:193–194

Scott Jr H W, Dean R H, Parker T, Avant G 1980 The role of vagotomy in pancreaticoduodenectomy. Annals of Surgery 191:688–696

Sellner F 1987 Untersuchung zur Hypothese der Existenz einer Adenom-Karzinom-Sequenz im Dünndarm. Zeitschrift für Gastroenterologie 25:151–165

Shapiro T M 1975 Adenocarcinoma of the pancreas: a statistical analysis of biliary bypass vs Whipple resection in good risk patients. Annals of Surgery 182:715–721

Sharp K W, Ross C B, Halter S A, Morrison J G, Richards W O, Williams L F, Sawyers J L 1989 Pancreatoduodenectomy with pyloric preservation for carcinoma of the pancreas: a cautionary note. Surgery 105:645–653

Sharp K W 1990 Local resection of tumors of the ampulla of Vater. American Surgeon 56:214–217

Shutze W P, Sack J, Aldrete J S 1990 Long-term follow-up of 24 patients undergoing radical resection for ampullary carcinoma, 1953 to 1988. Cancer 66:1717–1720

Siedeck M, Birtel F, Mitrenga I 1985 Pankreasganganastomose und Pankreatojejunoplicatio nach Rechtsresektion. Langenbecks Archiv für Chirurgie 366:610

Sigel B, Bassett J G, Cooper D R, Dunn M R 1965 Resection of the superior mesenteric vein and replacement with a venous autograft during pancreaticoduodenectomy: case report. Annals of Surgery 162:941–945

Sindelar W F 1989 Clinical experience with regional pancreatectomy for adenocarcinoma of the pancreas. Archives of Surgery 124:127–132

Smith R 1979 Surgery of cancer of the pancreas. In: Taylor J H, Sarles H (eds) The exocrine pancreas. W B Saunders, London, p 520–535

Starzl T E, Todo S, Tzakis A, Podesta L, Mieles L, Demetris A, Teperman L, Selby R, Stevenson W, Stieber A, Gordon R, Iwatsuki S 1989 Abdominal organ cluster transplantation. Annals of Surgery 210:374–386

Sunada S, Miyata M, Tanaka Y, Okumura K, Nakamuro M, Kitagawa T, Shirakura R, Kawashima Y 1992 Aggressive resection for advanced pancreatic carcinoma. Japanese Journal of Surgery 22:74–77

Takada T, Yasuda H, Shikata J I, Watanabe S I, Shiratori K, Takeuchi T 1989 Postprandial plasma gastrin and secretin concentrations after a pancreatoduodenectomy. A comparison between a pylorus-preserving pancreatoduodenectomy and the Whipple procedure. Annals of Surgery 210:47–51

Tarazi R Y, Hermann R E, Vogt D P, Hoerr S O, Esselstyn Jr C B, Cooperman A M, Steiger E, Grundfest S 1986 Results of surgical treatment of periampullary tumors: a thirty-five-year experience. surgery 100:716–723

Traverso L W, Longmire Jr W P 1978 Preservation of the pylorus in pancreaticoduodenectomy. Surgery, Gynecology and Obstetrics 146:959–962

Trede M, Schwall G, Saeger H D 1990 Survival after pancreatoduodenectomy. 118 consecutive resections without an operative mortality. Annals of Surgery 211:447–458

Tsuchiya R, Tomioka T, Izawa K, Noda T, Yamamoto K, Tsunoda T, et al 1986 Collective review of small carcinomas of the pancreas. Annals of Surgery 203:77–81

Tsuchiya R, Harada N, Tsunoda T, Miyamoto T, Ura K 1988 Long-term survivors after operation on carcinoma of the pancreas. International Journal of Pancreatology 3:491–496

van Heerden J A, ReMine W, Weiland L, McIlrath D C, Ilstrup D M 1981 Total pancreatectomy for ductal adenocarcinoma of the pancreas. American Journal of Surgery 142:308–311

van Heerden J A, McIlrath D C, Ilstrup D M, Weiland L H 1988 Total pancreatectomy for ductal adenocarcinoma of the pancreas: an update. World Journal of Surgery 12:658–662

Warren K W 1973 Current concepts in management of periampullary carcinoma. American Surgeon 39:667–672

Warshaw A L, Torchiana D L 1985 Delayed gastric emptying after pylorus-preserving pancreaticoduodenectomy. Surgery, Gynecology and Obstetrics 160:1–4

Warshaw A L, del Castillo C 1992 Pancreatic carcinoma. New England Journal of Medicine 326:455–465

Watson K 1944 Carcinoma of ampulla of Vater. Successful radical resection. British Journal of Surgery 31:368

Whipple A O, Parsons W B, Mullins C R 1935 Treatment of carcinoma of the ampulla of Vater. Annals of Surgery 102:763–779

Whipple A O 1942 Present day surgery of the pancreas. New England Journal of Medicine 226:515–526

Whipple A O 1963 A reminiscence: pancreaticoduodenectomy. Review of Surgery 20:221–224

39. Local excision for tumours of the papilla

M. Trede

Optimal exposure is provided by a right subcostal incision.

Preliminary exploration is directed at the tumour itself, which is usually palpable through the duodenal wall, at the gallbladder which is distended in the 70% of patients with jaundice, and at the hepatoduodenal ligament where the lymph nodes are expected to be normal. If suspicious hepatic lesions or lymph nodes are found, these are removed for rapid frozen section examination before the operation enters a decisive phase.

A wide Kocher manoeuvre is performed to mobilize the second and third parts of the duodenum, from the hepatoduodenal ligament above to the mesenteric vessels crossing its third part below. The duodenum and pancreatic head can thus be elevated from the vena cava and aorta behind (Fig. 39.1).

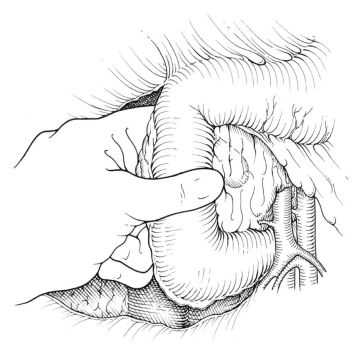

Fig. 39.1 Kocher manoeuvre to mobilize the duodenum and pancreatic head.

Now, the tumour can be palpated between thumb and fingers of the left hand and its relation to the head of the pancreas can be evaluated. Usually the pancreas will be of soft consistency and clearly demarcated from the small firm tumour situated in the medial duodenal wall. If the tumour exceeds 2–3 cm in diameter or if it infiltrates into the pancreatic head, local excision must be abandoned.

Two stay-sutures are placed close together on the free lateral wall of the duodenum exactly opposite the tumour. A longitudinal duodenotomy of about 5 cm is performed with the needle cautery. Using the stay-sutures and blunt retractors the duodenal edges are separated and the tumour can usually be delivered into the enterotomy (Fig. 39.2A). Avoid grasping the tumour or duodenal mucosa with forceps at this stage as both are friable and will bleed easily making subsequent orientation difficult.

A gentle squeeze on the gallbladder will help identify the papillary opening by producing a jet of bile squirting from it. The papilla is most often situated on the apex of the tumour and can now be cannulated by the soft tip of a Fogarty balloon catheter. With the balloon inflated one now has good control of the tumour because it can be moved in all directions without being touched directly. If there is difficulty in identifying the papilla, it can be cannulated from above by passing a Fogarty catheter through a small incision in the common duct (Fig. 39.2B).

Some surgeons recommend routine cholecystectomy as part of this operation, since, of course, the sphincter mechanism protecting the common duct from duodenal reflux will be destroyed and this is said to predispose to ascending cholangitis and possibly cholecystitis (Gertsch et al 1990).

Beginning some 5–10 mm clear of the tumour margin, the duodenal wall is infiltrated with dilute adrenaline solution, thus, elevating the mucosa circumferentially around the tumour (Fig. 39.2C).

Using fine-needle electrocautery, the duodenal mucosa is incised beginning well clear of the caudal margin of the tumour. This incision is deepened to include the whole of

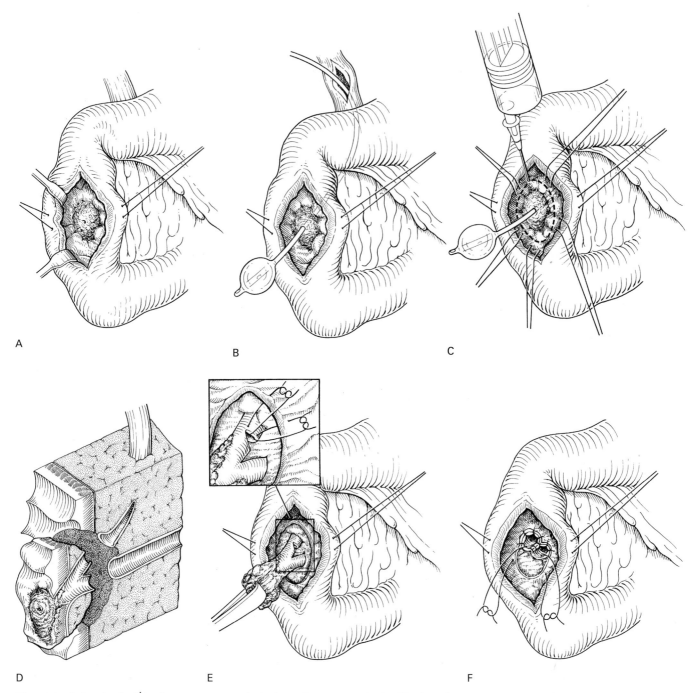

Fig. 39.2 **A** Longitudinal duodenotomy exposes the periampullary tumour. **B** Identification of the papilla by cannulation with a balloon catheter from a choledochotomy above. **C** Submucous infiltration of the duodenal wall with dilute adrenaline solution. **D** Schematic section through duodenal wall and head of pancreas to show extent of local excision for ampullary tumour. **E** Stepwise incision of the common bile duct while securing it with sutures. **E** Reimplantation of the openings of the bile and pancreatic ducts into the reconstructed duodenal wall.

the duodenal wall and then carried around the tumour on all sides. Slight bleeding is dealt with immediately by means of fine Dura forceps and cautery so as to keep the field dry.

Entering pancreatic tissue should be avoided, unless this is required to maintain adequate distance from the tumour (Fig. 39.2D).

In order to put the plane of dissection under tension, it is permissible to grasp the tumour with Allis forceps at this stage. The dissection now reaches the two ducts which form the 'stalk' on which the cherry-like tumour is situated. The larger and often dilated common bile duct is usually encountered first. It is easily identified by the indwelling balloon catheter and incised with a fine scalpel. Immediate-

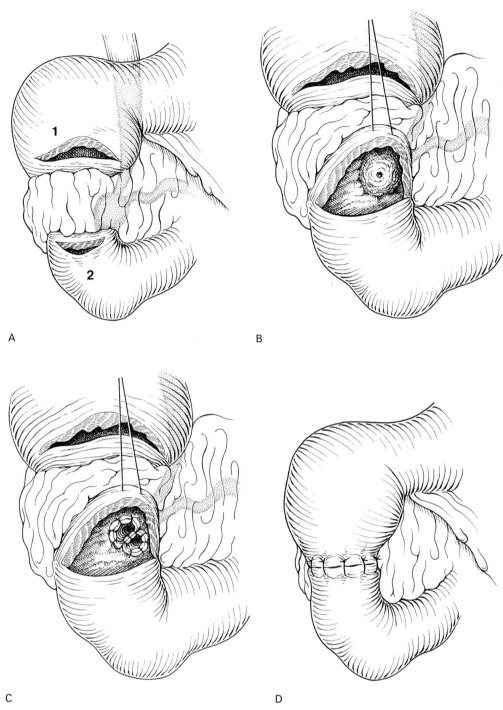

A

B

C

D

Fig. 39.3 **A** Operative sketch of a 40-year-old man with a periampullary tumour and annular pancreas. Two transverse duodenotomies are placed above and below the pancreatic ring. **B** The periampullary tumour is exposed through the lower duodenotomy. **C** Following excision of the periampullary tumour, the biliary and pancreatic duct openings are reimplanted into the posterior duodenal wall. **D** The annular pancreas is bypassed by anastomosing the two duodenotomies. No recurrence was reported after 1 year.

ly bile will gush out. A few millimetres caudally, the pancreatic duct will be entered. It carries clear pancreatic juice and can now also be cannulated by a fine catheter.

If there is any difficulty in identifying the fine pancreatic

duct opening, the intravenous injection of secretin (2 units/kg) may be helpful by stimulating a brisk flow of pancreatic juice (Kahn & Rush 1989).

At this stage it is helpful not to excise the tumour by

dividing both ducts too early. They will retract into the pancreatic tissue and may then be difficult to find. It is better to divide the ducts step by step while applying traction via the tumour and to catch the duct wall with several 4:0 resorbable sutures. These sutures are passed through the raw edge of the remaining posterior duodenal wall, but not tied as yet (Fig. 39.2E). Two similar sutures are placed to bring together the contiguous openings of the biliary and pancreatic ducts.

The openings of both ducts (particularly the common duct) are inspected to make sure that they are free of tumour. The specimen is marked by sutures and immediately examined by frozen section to be certain that the tumour has been removed completely. If this is confirmed by the pathologist (and this is no easy task for him (Harbrecht 1974)), then the sutures mentioned above are tied (Fig. 39.2F). Thus, the biliary and pancreatic ducts are reimplanted into the reconstructed posterior duodenal wall. Both ducts can be stented by tubes draining into the duodenum, but this is not necessary. Indeed it is surprising that serious complications, such as ascending cholangitis or acute pancreatitis are encountered but rarely.

The duodenotomy is closed either transversely or longitudinally by a single layer of resorbable sutures and a soft drain is placed nearby for 3–4 days.

Case report: A 40-year-old man presented with infrequent attacks of right upper abdominal pain without vomiting. Blood chemistry and tumour markers were normal. A papillary adenoma was diagnosed in another hospital and endoscopic removal was attempted on two occasions. Histology revealed a villous adenoma of the papilla with markedly atypical cells, but no malignancy.

Since the diagnosis was clear and all other investigations negative, laparotomy was performed with the aim of local excision, if possible, or a Whipple resection, if necessary. Surprisingly, a classic annular pancreas was found situated exactly at the level of the papillary tumour (and it was probably the main cause of the symptoms) (Fig. 39.3A).

With a view to relieving the obstruction by a duodenoduodenostomy two transverse incisions were made about 15 mm above and below the constricting pancreatic band. The papilla was accessible only through the lower incision (Fig. 39.3B). Through this, the tumour was excised as described above and both ducts were reimplanted (Fig. 39.3C). The two incisions were then anastomosed by 3:0 absorbable sutures (Fig. 39.3 D). Neither in frozen section analysis nor in the final histological assessment were signs of malignancy found. The patient was discharged 10 days later.

REFERENCES

Gertsch P, Baer H U, Lerut J, Blumgart L H 1990 Technik der Papilloduodenektomie. Langenbecks Archiv für Chirurgie 375:246–250

Harbrecht P J 1974 Discussion of Wilson S M. Archives of Surgery 108:539

Kahn M B, Rush B F 1989 The surgeon at work: the overlooked technique of ampullary excision. Surgery, Gynecology and Obstetrics 169:253–254.

40. Technique of Whipple pancreatoduodenectomy

M. Trede

This operation involves the en bloc removal of the following structures as shown in Figure 40.1:

- the distal one-third of the stomach with the right half of the greater omentum
- the gallbladder, cystic and common bile duct
- the duodenum and proximal 10 cm of the jejunum
- the head of the pancreas and varying amounts of its neck and body, depending on size and site of the tumour
- the peripancreatic and hepatoduodenal lymph nodes.

The operation has two phases: resection and reconstruction.

TECHNIQUE OF RESECTION

This can be subdivided into eight distinct steps (Trede 1985). The first two, incision and exploration, have already been dealt with in Chapter 14.

1. Incision

The author prefers a wide transverse subcostal approach.

2. Exploration

This is, of course, very much part of the actual resection. The aim must be to 'encircle' the tumour centripetally from the periphery, preferably without coming anywhere near it, assessing its resectability and mobilizing it at the same time. This preliminary exploration may be more time-consuming than the resection itself. The surgeon must proceed in a cautious step-by-step fashion, so that if the tumour turns out to be irresectable after all, an 'escape route' is still open, i.e. some form of palliative bypass.

Let us assume then, that the following steps have been completed as described in Chapter 14: a wide Kocher manoeuvre, detachment of the greater omentum from the right half of the colon and inspection of the root of the mesentery. Since the last-mentioned step is the most

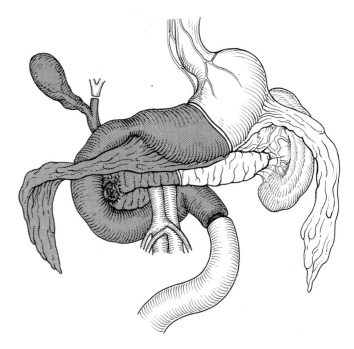

Fig. 40.1 The extent of resection in standard Whipple pancreatoduodenectomy.

dangerous and potentially haemorrhagic part of the whole operation, the author prefers just to 'inspect', leaving dissection of the large retropancreatic veins to a later stage, when control of bleeding is easier and safer.

3. Cholecystectomy and dissection of the hepatoduodenal ligament

There are three good reasons for removing the gallbladder in this operation:

1. Increasing radicality, particularly if the tumour lies in the distal common duct
2. avoidance of ischaemia of the biliary anastomosis by transecting the hepatic duct proximal to the cystic duct

447

3. avoidance of subsequent trouble with dyskinesia or stones in the gallbladder.

The gallbladder is grasped at the fundus and shelled out of its hepatic bed in a subserous, and hopefully, avascular plane. Any oozing from the hepatic bed is controlled by a pack and pressure from a retractor.

The cystic artery is divided so that now only the cystic duct tethers the gallbladder to the hepatoduodenal ligament. This is the guide to the common bile duct.

The peritoneal covering of the hepatoduodenal ligament and lesser omentum is divided close to the hepatic hilum and quadrate lobe, thus, exposing the structures within this ligament (Fig. 40.2).

Dissection of these structures proceeds from right to left and from above downwards. Blunt dissection behind the common hepatic duct will identify the large and bluish portal vein. Now, the hepatic duct can be freed and taped proximally to the cystic duct. Before dividing the duct, one must be sure that there are no aberrant biliary passages, i.e. a right hepatic duct entering the common duct lower down. (In two such cases the author has had to perform two separate biliary anastomoses).

Identification of the common hepatic duct is facilitated if an endoscopic drainage stent is inserted preoperatively. (On the other hand, these stents convert a nicely dilated, thin-walled bile duct into a shrunken, thickened and sometimes inflamed tube within a few days, making the subsequent anastomosis more tedious).

A small opening is next made in this duct, and bile gushes out under pressure enabling a bacteriological swab to be taken. A blunt probe is then introduced proximally to ascertain that both right and left hepatic ducts drain into the common hepatic. Only then is it divided.

Sometimes spurting bleeding in the wall of this duct (confirming the excellent blood supply) requires a 6:0 suture. The abundant blood supply to the proximal bile duct is derived from the right hepatic artery (Northover & Terblanche 1979, Traverso & Freeny 1989). This often courses in front of the common hepatic duct leaving less space for the biliary anastomosis.

To the right of the bile duct and portal vein there is a band of lymphoid tissue. This must be carefully palpated, because in 26% of cases it hides an aberrant or accessory right hepatic artery (Michels 1951). Whereas preoperative angiography usually provides warning of such an anomalous artery and its origin from the superior mesenteric, this is not invariably so; nor is angiography performed in every case. Therefore, it is important to think of this eventuality before dissecting the lymphoid tissue in the hepatoduodenal ligament.

With the bile duct divided and the portal vein identified, that leaves the hepatic artery and its right and left branches. In the dissection that now follows, the bile duct is peeled downwards together with all lymphoid tissue so that one is left with a clean portal vein and hepatic artery (Fig. 40.3).

The hepatic artery is mobilized in its horizontal course along the upper pancreatic border. Here, its two branches,

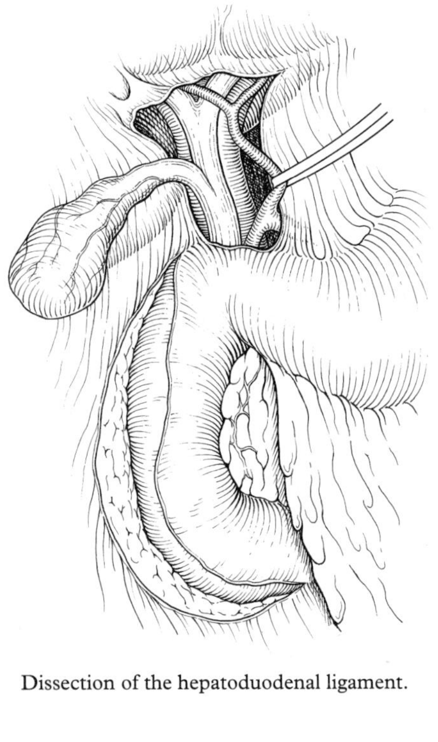

Fig. 40.2 Dissection of the hepatoduodenal ligament.

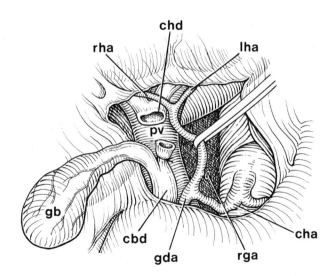

Fig. 40.3 Dissection of the hepatoduodenal ligament displaying divided common hepatic duct (chd), gallbladder (gb) shelled-out of its hepatic bed, the common bile duct (cbd), portal vein (pv), the common hepatic artery (cha) and its branches; gastroduodenal artery (gda), right gastric artery (rga), right (rha) and left hepatic artery (lha).

the small right gastric and the larger gastroduodenal artery, are divided (Fig. 40.3). With all but small periampullary tumours, dissection of the hepatic artery is continued right up to the trifurcation of the coeliac axis (the tripus Halleri). Rarely there are small branches entering the upper border of the pancreas. In any case, the latter has to be freed as far to the left as may be required for an adequate resection. There is a constant lymph node overlying the hepatic artery along this pancreatic border that has to be removed.

4. Mobilization of the pancreatic neck

As mentioned before, this is a most delicate manoeuvre and it is best begun from above. Before proceeding, however, it is wise to divide a constant pancreatic venous tributary, the posterior superior pancreatoduodenal vein, entering the portal vein on its lateral border, before subsequent manipulations tear it off.

Since almost all tributaries enter the large retropancreatic (portal and superior mesenteric) veins from the right or left side and hardly ever from the front, it is possible to mobilize and lift the pancreatic neck off these veins by careful blunt dissection. This is best done with an Overholt clamp or a very careful forefinger. By downward traction on the transverse mesocolon the tip of the finger can be met by a clamp at the lower pancreatic border and in front of the superior mesenteric vein (Fig. 40.4). This retropancreatic passage can then be carefully widened and a tape passed through it.

If resistance is encountered or the tunnel is too narrow due to tumour infiltration, it is wiser to retreat before haemorrhage occurs. In this case, or if the preoperative portogram shows discrete signs of venous compression, one gains control by dissecting and taping the superior mesenteric vein below, and the portal vein above the pancreas in preparation for step 6 (division of the pancreas).

If bleeding should occur, it is futile to attempt haemostasis by suturing in this tunnel. Tamponade with narrow gauze will often be sufficiently effective for the surgeon to go on to step 5 (partial gastrectomy). With the the stomach divided, one has far better control of the pancreas and the vessels behind it. Frequently, the bleeding will have stopped spontaneously anyway.

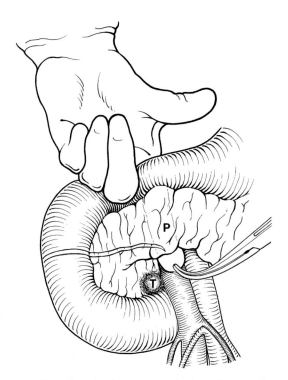

Fig. 40.4 Blunt dissection between portal vein and pancreatic neck. The clamp meets the fingertip at the lower border of the pancreas, P. T, tumour infiltration of the superior mesenteric vein from posterolaterally. Such infiltration would be missed by this finger.

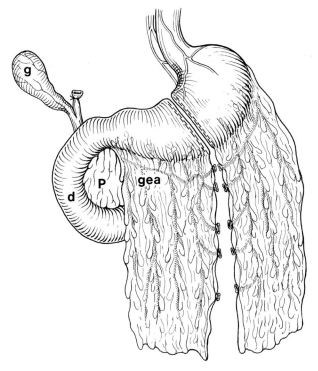

Fig. 40.5 Schematic drawing showing extent of gastric and omental resection; g, gallbladder; d, duodenum; P, pancreas; gea, gastroepiploic artery.

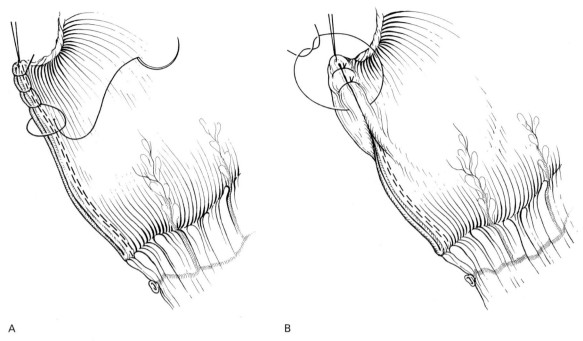

Fig. 40.6 **A, B** Two-layered closure of the right half of the transected stomach.

5. Partial gastrectomy

The right half of the greater omentum is mobilized up to the greater curve; the lesser omentum is dissected up to the lesser curve immediately proximal to the level of the nerve of Latarjet, and the stomach is divided with a stapler (Fig. 40.5).

Although no more than 40% of distal stomach is resected in this way and no formal vagotomy is performed, only eight patients with anastomotic ulcers have been observed postoperatively in 378 Whipple resections (2.3%).

The right half of the staple line is covered by two additional suture lines (an over-and-over locking stitch using 3:0 chromic catgut and an outer layer of interrupted sutures with 3:0 silk) (Fig. 40.6). This apparent 'belt-and-braces' policy is followed to prevent postoperative bleeding from this blindly closed section of the stomach. This had occurred in 19 out of 439 pancreatectomies (Whipple and total) – a rate of almost 5%.

With the distal stomach retracted towards the right, the pancreas, with its neck already taped, is freely exposed.

6. Division of the pancreas

Depending on the site of the tumour, the pancreas is divided well to the left of the large veins coursing through the retropancreatic tunnel and which were prepared in step 4.

This passage is gently widened to accommodate a broad sound (Fig. 40.7A). To keep blood loss to a minimum, a Satinsky clamp is used to control the resected part of the pancreas, whereas a soft non-crushing clamp is placed gently on the pancreatic tail (Fig. 40.7B). Between these two, the pancreas is divided with a scalpel, thus, displaying the confluence of superior mesenteric and splenic veins as well as the portal vein (Fig. 40.7C). While gently releasing the soft clamp on the pancreatic remnant, spurting bleeding is controlled by suture-ligature with 3:0 silk.

Alternatively, the pancreas can be transected by a stapler (Obertop & van Houten 1984) or the cut surface of the tail closed with a series of mattress sutures (Mercadier 1990). In both cases care is taken to free the opening of the pancreatic duct.

At this stage, a thin slice of pancreas is removed from the cephalad resection plane and examined immediately for microscopic tumour infiltration. If such tumour is indeed found (we have come across this only three times), total pancreatectomy is required.

7. Dissection of the retropancreatic vessels

The specimen as mobilized so far (gallbladder, common duct, distal stomach with omentum, pancreatic head and first three parts of the duodenum) is retracted towards the right and wrapped in a 'pack'. It remains fixed only by the fourth part of the duodenum, the proximal jejunum, ligament of Treitz and numerous vessels running into these

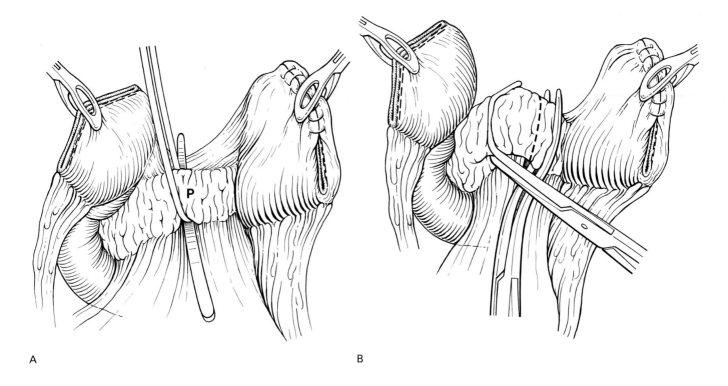

A   B

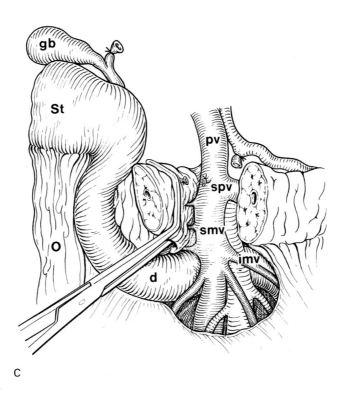

C

Fig. 40.7   A A broad (malleable) sound is passed under the taped pancreas, (P). **B** The pancreas is divided between the Satinsky clamp (to the right) and an atraumatic soft occlusion clamp (to the left). **C** Division of the pancreas displays portal vein (pv), splenic vein (spv) and superior mesenteric vein (smv); imv, inferior mesenteric vein; gb, gallbladder; St, stomach; d, duodenum; O, omentum.

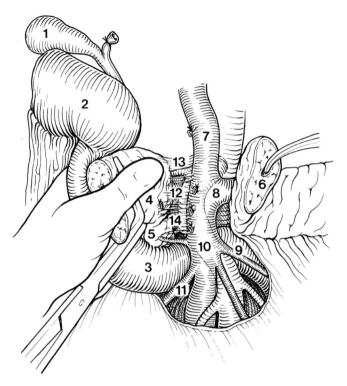

Fig. 40.8 Dissection of the retropancreatic vessels. 1, gallbladder; 2, stomach; 3, duodenum; 4, head of pancreas; 5, uncinate process; 6, pancreatic tail, retracted by blunt probe in duct opening; 7, portal vein; 8, splenic vein; 9, inferior mesenteric vein; 10, superior mesenteric vein; 11, middle colic vein; 12, superior mesenteric artery, appearing to the right of portal vein due to traction(!); 13, superior posterior pancreatoduodenal artery; 14, inferior posterior pancreatoduodenal artery. NB: The surgeon's left hand is grasping the pancreatic head and retracting to the right.

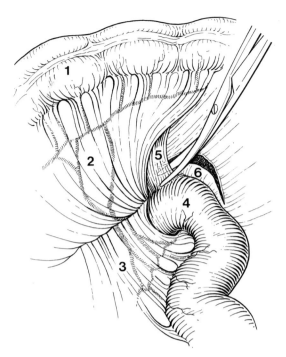

Fig. 40.9 Dissection of the duodenojejunal junction and division of ligament of Treitz (5); 1, transverse colon (retracted upwards); 2, transverse mesocolon; 3, mesentery; 4, duodenojejunal flexure; 6, inferior mesenteric vein.

structures and the pancreatic head from the proximal mesenteric vessels (Fig. 40.7C).

Traction on the specimen towards the right puts the lateral margin of the portal vein under gentle tension. By carefully 'rolling' this large vein off the posterior pancreatic surface by means of a peanut swab, a variable number of small veins (between two and five) come into view and are divided one by one between clips (Fig. 40.8). Should these clips 'swim away' on the portal venous side, the delicate venous stump is easily closed by a figure-of-eight suture (6:0 non-resorbable). If, however, these veins are torn out of the portal vein, a larger rent may result and the operative field is then flooded within seconds. Immediate control is obtained, if the operator grasps the pancreatic head with his or her left hand – fingers behind and thumb in front. A little traction and pressure from behind forwards will stop even the most torrential bleeding from these high-flow but low-pressure vessels. Now, the four chief veins (superior and inferior mesenteric, splenic and portal) can be clamped (in this order) and the damage repaired in a dry

field by a 6:0 suture.

With the portal vein freed from the back of the pancreatic head, there remains a dense sheet of fibrous tissue containing splanchnic nerves, lymphatics and at least two small arteries, the posterior pancreatoduodenal branches of the superior mesenteric artery (Fig. 40.8).

Useful as traction to the right on the pancreatic head may be, one must realize that this traction pulls the superior mesenteric artery from under the portal vein in a curve convex to the right. Since the artery is covered by the dense tissue mentioned above, it must be identified by palpation. The safest way to avoid damage to the superior mesenteric artery is to keep close to its lateral wall, tying branches as they are met, when dissecting the specimen clear off the mesenteric root.

Care must be taken not to skeletonize this artery for any distance below the inferior pancreatoduodenal artery, because here it gives off branches to the upper jejunum. If these are tied, more of the proximal jejunum may have to be sacrificed than necessary.

8. Division of the jejunum

With the transverse colon pulled upwards and the first jejunal loop retracted down, the duodenojejunal junction comes into view. This is freed by division of avascular adhesions including the ligament of Treitz, keeping close to the antimesenteric border of the gut. The inferior mesenteric vein will now be seen coursing to the left of the duodenojejunal junction (Fig. 40.9).

With this dissection, a wide communication to the upper abdomen along the duodenojejunal flexure is established. It is now possible to push the proximal jejunal loop behind the main mesenteric vessels and upwards to join the bulk of the resected specimen.

The jejunum is now carefully inspected for mesenteric pulsations and the most proximal part showing adequate blood supply is marked by a soft loop in preparation for transection at this point (Fig. 40.10A).

The mesentery proximal to this is skeletonized keeping quite close to the gut. Finally, the jejunum is divided by means of a stapler and the complete specimen can now be discarded en bloc (Fig. 40.10B).

THE TECHNIQUE OF RECONSTRUCTION

Among the 68 possible methods of re-establishing gastro-intestinal continuity (Léger 1969) (Fig. 40.11), the author prefers the reconstruction similar to that proposed by Child. The method, performed in three steps, is shown schematically in Figure 40.12.

1. Pancreatojejunostomy

The closed upper end of the jejunum is usually brought up behind the mesenteric vessels to lie tension-free against the cut surface of the pancreatic remnant. If the tumour involved the uncinate process, local recurrence at the mesenteric root has to be reckoned with. This has indeed occurred in seven of 411 cases in our experience causing jejunal obstruction with jaundice (see Fig. 53.9). Therefore, it is safer in these cases to pass the jejunum through an avascular gap in the mesocolon, i.e. some distance in front of the mesenteric vessels.

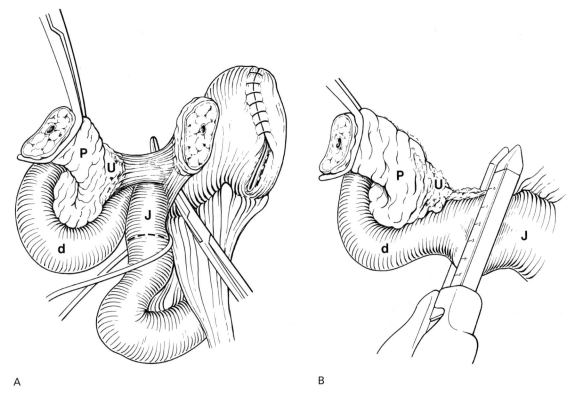

A   B

Fig. 40.10 A The proximal jejunum, J, has been passed behind the mesenteric root into the upper abdomen. The planned level of resection has been taped. The Overholt clamp marks the upper jejunal mesentery that will now be skeletonized; P, head of pancreas; U, uncinate process; d, duodenum. **B** Division of the jejunum with a stapler.

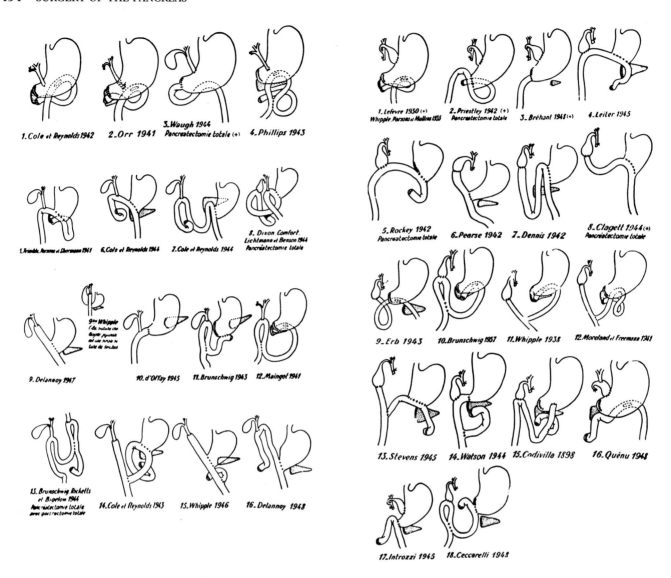

1. Cole et Reynolds 1942   2. Orr 1941   3. Waugh 1944 Pancréatectomie totale (+)   4. Phillips 1943

5. Trimble, Parsons et Sherman 1941   6. Cole et Reynolds 1944   7. Cole et Reynolds 1944   8. Dixon Comfort, Lichtmann et Benson 1944 Pancréatectomie totale

9. Delannoy 1947   10. d'Offay 1945   11. Brunschwig 1943   12. Maingot 1941

13. Brunschwig Ricketts et Bigelow 1944 Pancréatectomie totale avec gastrectomie totale   14. Cole et Reynolds 1943   15. Whipple 1946   16. Delannoy 1948

1. Lefevre 1930 (+) Whipple, Parsons et Mullins 1935   2. Priestley 1942 (+) Pancréatectomie totale   3. Bréhant 1948 (+)   4. Leiler 1945

5. Rockey 1942 Pancréatectomie totale   6. Pearse 1942   7. Dennis 1942   8. Clagett 1944 (+) Pancréatectomie totale

9. Erb 1943   10. Brunschwig 1937   11. Whipple 1938   12. Moreland et Freeman 1941

13. Stevens 1945   14. Watson 1944   15. Codivilla 1898   16. Quénu 1948

17. Introzzi 1945   18. Ceccarelli 1948

Fig. 40.11 68 variations in reconstructing gastrointestinal continuity. (From Léger 1969: Nouveau traité de technique chirurgicale, vol 12 (2), p 411, with permission of Masson et Cie, Paris).

The end-to-end invaginating telescope-type of anastomosis is performed in two layers (silk outside, chromic catgut inside) (Jordan 1987, Cameron 1990). Although this anastomosis can doubtless be done safely with a single row of absorbable sutures, the author feels reluctant to change a technique that has proved reliable in 91% of cases (32 complications have been experienced in connection with 350 Whipple pancreatojejunostomies).

More important than the suture material is probably the suture technique itself: placing each suture meticulously, avoiding any 'sawing' action as the thread is drawn through the tissue and tying knots with gentle, elastic compression. The outer posterior row consists of five or six 3:0 silk sutures, which take generous bites of jejunum about 2 cm from its cut end. Similar bites of the posterior pancreas are facilitated by tilting the cut pancreatic surface to the left with the blunt right-angled clamp introduced into the pancreatic duct opening (Fig. 40.13). When all are placed, these sutures are tied and cut except for the two corner sutures which are left as markers.

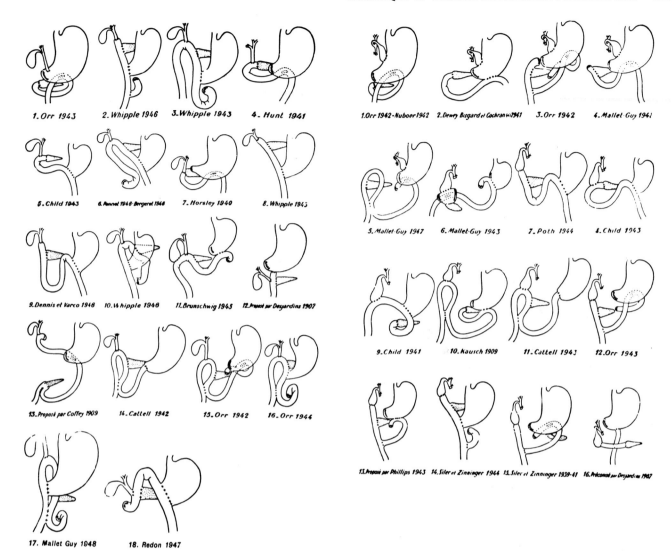

1. Orr 1943 *2. Whipple 1946* *3. Whipple 1943* *4. Hunt 1941*

5. Child 1943 *6. Pannet 1948·Bergeret 1946* *7. Horsley 1940* *8. Whipple 1945*

9. Dennis et Varco 1948 *10. Whipple 1946* *11. Brunschwig 1945* *12. Proposé par Desjardins 1907*

13. Proposé par Coffey 1909 *14. Cattell 1942* *15. Orr 1942* *16. Orr 1944*

17. Mallet Guy 1948 *18. Redon 1947*

1. Orr 1942·Nuboer 1942 *2. Dewey Bisgard et Cochran 1941* *3. Orr 1942* *4. Mallet·Guy 1941*

5. Mallet·Guy 1947 *6. Mallet·Guy 1943* *7. Poth 1944* *8. Child 1943*

9. Child 1941 *10. Kausch 1909* *11. Cattell 1943* *12. Orr 1943*

13. Proposé par Phillips 1943 *14. Siler et Zinninger 1944* *15. Siler et Zinninger 1939-41* *16. Préconisé par Desjardins 1907*

Fig. 40.11 cont'd

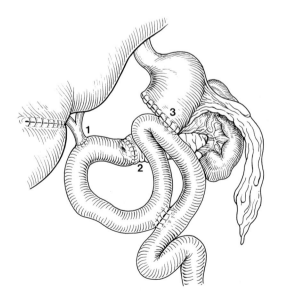

Fig. 40.12 Schematic drawing of current method of reconstruction after pancreatoduodenal resection, with hepaticojejunal (1), pancreatojejunal (2) and gastrojejunal (3) anastomoses.

Next the staple line is excised thus opening the jejunum. The second posterior row of sutures uses 3:0 chromic catgut. The right-angled clamp prevents the pancreatic duct opening from being obliterated by overlapping jejunal wall. We do not attempt mucosa-to-mucosa sutures with the duct unless this is dilated. Then it may be possible to place up to three such sutures, which splay the duct open for good drainage (Fig. 40.14).

The author has never used a pancreatic ductal drain, as advised by several surgeons (Manabe et al 1986, Warshaw & Swanson 1988, Howard 1990). It seems that either the duct is too narrow to accommodate a stent without obstruction or it is too widely dilated to require any sort of drainage.

The anterior suture begins with a row of inverting sutures placed inside-to-outside (jejunum) and outside-to-inside (pancreas), so that the chromic catgut knots come to lie within the lumen (Fig. 40.15).

The actual invaginating 'telescope effect' is produced by the outer anterior row of 3:0 silk sutures (Fig. 40.16A). Beginning at the upper and the lower borders, a wide bite of pancreas (2 cm from the cut edge) and an equally wide segment of jejunum is taken. By tying these sutures (first at the two corners and next in the midline), the jejunal wall is pulled over the pancreas, thus deeply invaginating some 2 cm of pancreas within the jejunal lumen (Fig. 40.16B).

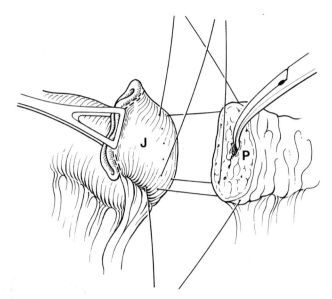

Fig. 40.13 Pancreatojejunostomy: three of six outer posterior sutures have been placed; J, jejunum; P, pancreatic remnant.

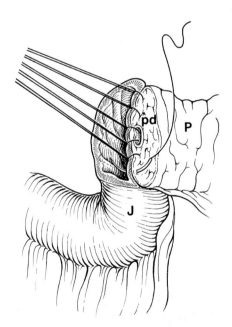

Fig. 40.14 Pancreatojejunostomy: the inner layer of posterior row of sutures (3:0 chromic catgut), two of which include the pancreatic duct, has been placed; P, pancreas; pd, pancreatic duct; J, jejunum.

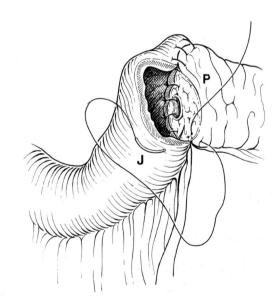

Fig. 40.15 Pancreaticojejunostomy: the inner layer of the anterior row of inverting sutures (3:0 chromic catgut) is being placed and tied with knots inside the lumen; P, pancreas; J, jejunum.

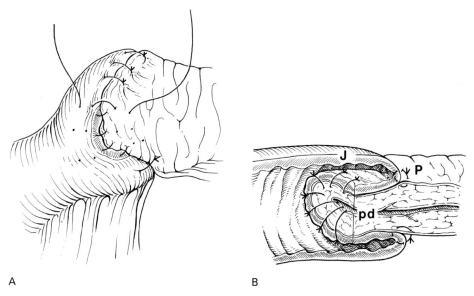

A   B

Fig. 40.16   A The outer invaginating layer of anterior sutures (3:0 silk) is being placed. **B** Schematic drawing demonstrating invagination of pancreatic stump into the jejunum; P, pancreas; pd, pancreatic duct; J, jejunum.

Occasionally the pancreatic remnant may be altogether too bulky to fit into the jejunum end-to-end. In this case, the blindly closed proximal jejunum is brought to lie with its antimesenteric border against the pancreas for an end-to-side anastomosis. The technique of this anastomosis is basically identical to the one described above, it is performed in two layers (3:0 silk outside, 3:0 chromic catgut within). Further variations of the pancreatic anastomosis are listed in Table 53.5).

2. Hepaticojejunostomy

The second anastomosis is placed as far 'down stream' from the pancreatic anastomosis as possible. But in order to avoid kinking (and therefore stasis) of jejunal loop, this distance will seldom exceed 12 cm.

The end-to-side anastomosis is fashioned with a single row of interrupted 4:0 resorbable sutures. First, the anterior wall of the common hepatic duct is suspended upwards by some five to seven sutures. These are placed (from within outwards) and fixed by light clamps for better exposure (Fig. 40.17A). Next, an opening is made in the antimesenteric border of the jejunum with a fine electrocautery. This should be made smaller than the hepatic duct opening to begin with, since in the course of subsequent manipulations it will tend to widen. The sutures of the posterior row are then placed and tied (Fig. 40.17B).

The author prefers to stent this anastomosis for four reasons. Firstly, it facilitates the construction of the anterior suture line if the hepatic duct happens to be narrow (which it usually is not in carcinoma cases). Secondly, it is hoped that this Völker-type drainage tube, with holes both in its intraductal and intrajejunal segment, will drain bile away from the endangered pancreatic anastomosis. Thirdly, it also serves to decompress the jejunal loop in case of stasis, thus, again protecting the pancreatic sutures. Fourthly, the stent serves as a port for postoperative radiographic control of both the biliary and pancreatic anastomoses should there be any suspicion of a leak there.

This silastic tube, of suitable size (3–5 mm), is drawn into the jejunum via a stab hole some 8 cm distal to the biliary anastomosis. It is then passed up one or other of the hepatic ducts and fixed by a 3:0 catgut suture (taking a bite of hepatic duct and stent). Without this fixation, the tube invariably dislodges before the anastomosis is even completed. The catgut suture will have disintegrated by the time the stent is withdrawn about 3 weeks later.

Now, the anterior suture line is completed by placing the sutures (that had suspended the hepatic duct from the outset) through the anterior jejunal wall from outside to inside. The sutures are tied with their (resorbable) knots inside (Fig. 40.17C).

This simple and tension-free anastomosis requires no further suspension sutures or covering with periportal tissue. The Völker tube is secured by a Witzel-type tunnel in the jejunal wall and brought to the outside by a stab wound (Fig. 40.17D).

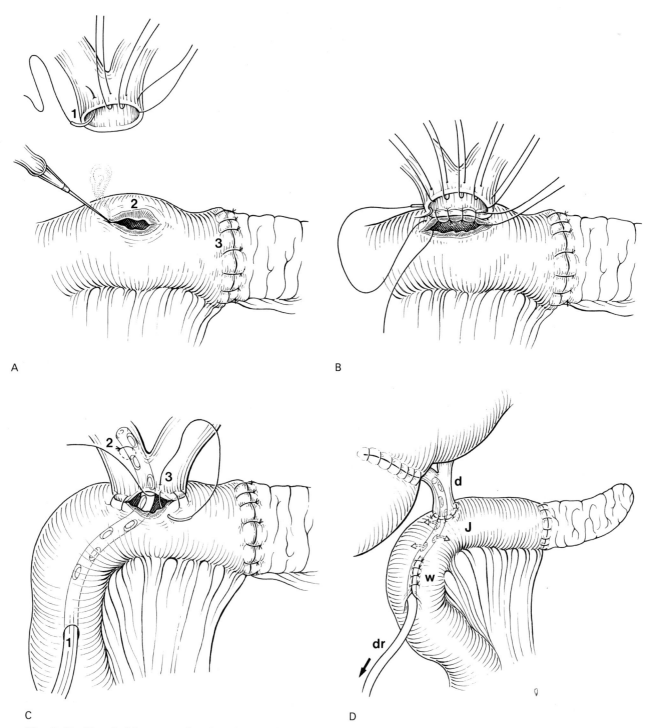

A

B

C

D

Fig. 40.17   Hepaticojejunostomy. **A** 1, Anterior row of sutures being placed in anterior wall of hepatic duct (4:0 absorbable);
2, opening is made in antimesenteric border of jejunum; 3, pancreatojejunal anastomosis (see text). **B** The posterior suture line is all
but completed (see text). **C** 1, Silastic drainage tube stents the anastomosis. 2, catgut suture (3:0) fixing the tube within the common
hepatic duct; 3, the anterior suture line is being completed (see text). **D** The hepaticojejunal anastomosis splinted by a Völker drain
(dr), brought out through the jejunal wall (J) by a Witzel-type canal (w); d, common hepatic duct.

3. Gastrojejunostomy

The final anastomosis is a partial end-to-side antecolic gastrojejunostomy (Fig. 40.12). This anastomosis lies a full 50 cm distal to the biliodigestive anastomosis. The loop of jejunum is brought up in front of the transverse colon to lie without tension or torsion against the transected proximal stomach. The right half of the latter has already been closed in layers (Fig. 40.6B). The left segment (some 6 cm in length) is then anastomosed to the antimesenteric apex of the jejunal loop (using 2:0 silk outside and 2:0 chromic catgut within). A final Braun jejunojejunostomy serves to ensure decompression of the proximal jejunal loop (carrying bile and pancreatic juice) and hopefully it also keeps jejunogastric reflux to a physiological minimum.

This antecolic anastomosis with a long jejunal loop is chosen deliberately to keep the gastric anastomosis well away from the other two. If there is any postoperative bleeding from the stomach and if the endoscopist fails to control it (he was successful 11 times out of 19), then it is very easy to perform a small gastrotomy and suture the bleeding point without disturbing the pancreatic or biliary anastomoses. If, however, there is need to intervene because of complications at or around the latter, there is more room to do this without disturbing the gastric anastomosis.

A single soft silastic drain is threaded behind the pancreatic and biliary anastomoses and is brought out through a stab wound some 5 cm away from the Völker drain in the right flank.

The abdominal wall is closed in layers; a posterior continuous suture line for peritoneum and posterior rectus sheath (catgut number 2); a heavy-duty continuous suture for the anterior rectus fascia (number 1 monofilament, resorbable); interrupted subcutaneous sutures (3:0 absorbable), and a continuous pull-out intracutaneous skin suture (2:0 Mirafil), which is removed after 2 weeks.

POSTOPERATIVE CARE

Postoperative care is kept as simple as possible and differs little from that after a partial gastrectomy. The anaesthetist will extubate the patient on the table, if possible. Thereafter, emphasis is placed on close-meshed clinical observation of the patient, including input–output records, on the surgical intensive care unit.

The nasogastric tube is removed on the morning after the operation, and the patient is encouraged to take a first few steps outside his bed at this time. Sips of tea are allowed as soon as peristalsis recommences (48–72 hours postoperatively). Thereafter, intravenous fluids are reduced until they are discontinued completely, usually on the 5th day after operation.

Postoperative medication is confined to perioperative antibiotic prophylaxis on the day of operation only, while stress ulcer, venous thrombosis and bronchopulmonary problems are countered by prophylaxis with omeprazole, heparin and physiotherapy.

The subhepatic drain is usually shortened on the 5th day and then removed on the 7th postoperative day. If drainage is copious, the fluid is examined for amylase (to exclude a pancreatic leak) or bile. On occasion, many litres of lymph fluid are drained daily, particularly after extensive retroperitoneal lymph node dissection. But this fluid loss invariably subsides spontaneously, even though it may take 2–3 weeks.

The Völker drain is clamped on the 5th postoperative day so that bile will now flow exclusively into the gut where it belongs. If all goes well, we no longer obtain a tubogram (using Angiografin-Ultravist) as a routine, since this has resulted in spikes of temperature (possibly signifying ascending cholangitis) in several patients. The Völker drain can be removed after 3 weeks. However, if the patient is discharged earlier (average postoperative hospitalization in our patients is 16 days), it is removed on an outpatient basis.

REFERENCES

Cameron J L 1990 Atlas of Surgery. B C Decker, Toronto, p 401

Howard J M 1990 Pancreaticoduodenectomy (Whipple resection) in the treatment of chronic pancreatitis: indications, techniques, and results. In: Beger H G, Büchler M, Ditschuneit H, Malfertheiner P (eds) Chronic pancreatitis. Springer-Verlag, Berlin, p 467–480

Jordan Jr G L 1987 Pancreatic resection for pancreatic cancer. In: Howard J M, Jordan Jr G L, Reber H A (eds) Surgical diseases of the pancreas. Lea and Febiger, Philadelphia, p 666–714

Léger L 1969 Nouveau traite de technique chirurgicale. Masson, Paris vol 12(2) p 411

Manabe T, Suzuki T, Tobe T 1986 A secured technique for pancreaticojejunal anastomosis in pancreaticoduodenectomy. Surgery, Gynecology and Obstetrics 163:379–380

Mercadier M 1990 Mattress suture for pancreatic closure and anastomosis. American Journal of Surgery 159:250–251

Michels N A 1951 The hepatic, cystic, and retroduodenal arteries and their relations to the biliary ducts. Annals of Surgery 133:503

Northover J M A, Terblanche J A 1979 A new look at the arterial blood supply of the bile duct in man and its surgical implications. British Journal of Surgery 66:379–384

Obertop H, van Houten H 1984 A new technique for pancreatojejunostomy. Surgery, Gynecology and Obstetrics 159:89–90

Traverso L W, Freeny P C 1989 Pancreaticoduodenectomy. The importance of preserving hepatic blood flow to prevent biliary fistula. American Surgeon 55:421–426

Trede M 1985 Technik der Duodenopankreateletomie nach Whipple. Chirurgische Praxis 34: 611–633

Trede M, Schwall G 1988 The complications of pancreatectomy. Annals of Surgery 207:39–47

Warshaw A L, Swanson R S 1988 Pancreatic cancer in 1988. Possibilities and probabilities. Annals of Surgery 208:541–553

41. Total pancreatectomy

M. Trede

Total duodenopancreatectomy involves the en bloc resection of: the whole of the pancreas, the spleen, the distal half of the stomach, the duodenum and proximal 10 cm of jejunum, the gallbladder, cystic and common ducts, as well as the retroperitioneal and peripancreatic lymph nodes (Fig. 41.1A, B).

The operation has two main indications. A one-stage procedure is performed if a pancreatic head carcinoma reaches too close to the plane of a possible Whipple resection, or if a carcinoma of the body or tail of the pancreas reaches too far to the right, i.e. into the pancreatic head.

Two-stage or 'completion-pancreatectomy' is performed, if following a Whipple operation, microscopic extension of carcinoma, that may have eluded frozen section examination at the first operation, is found to reach the plane of resection; or if dehiscence of the

pancreatic anastomosis after a Whipple resection can be managed only by removal of the offending pancreatic remnant (see Ch. 53).

This operation also has two phases: resection and reconstruction, similar to those of the Whipple pancreatoduodenectomy (see Ch. 40). In order to avoid repetition, only those points that differ from the Whipple procedure will be highlighted in the following description.

RESECTION

1. Incision

The transverse upper abdominal approach is carried further to the left, since good exposure of the spleen and pancreatic tail is essential.

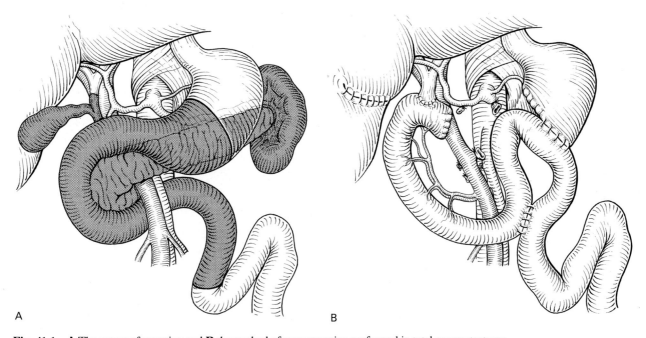

A   B

Fig. 41.1 **A** The extent of resection and **B** the method of reconstruction performed in total pancreatectomy.

2. Exploration

When dealing with carcinoma of the body or tail of the pancreas, particular attention is directed early on to the region of the coeliac axis and its trifurcation. Is the tumour mobile? Are the coeliac lymph nodes obviously involved? If there is any doubt about this, we begin dissection here, entering the lesser sac from above through the lesser omentum. By retracting the liver upwards and the stomach downwards, the upper border of the pancreas is exposed. Coursing along this edge, the common hepatic artery can be palpated. The artery is isolated by a vessel loop and dissected clean of all lymphoid tissue, going from the right towards the coeliac axis and its trifurcation. Here one meets the origin of the splenic artery continuing its course along the upper pancreatic border towards the left (Fig. 41.2). Now one must identify (and spare!) the smaller left gastric artery, also emanating from the coeliac trifurcation. By the end of the operation, the gastric remnant will depend for its blood supply more or less entirely on this vessel.

At this stage, it is opportune to test the mobility of the pancreatic neck over the underlying portal vein. However, if the pancreatic neck cannot be underrun and taped easily, it is wiser to leave this manoeuvre to a later stage, when control of the large retropancreatic veins is greater, and

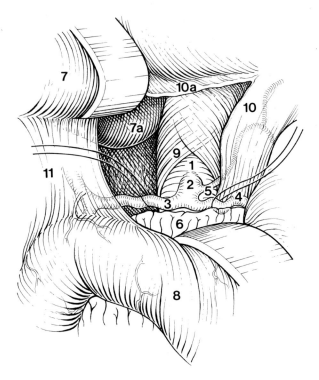

Fig. 41.2 Dissection of the branches of the coeliac axis. 1, Aorta; 2, coeliac axis; 3, hepatic artery; 4, splenic artery; 5, left gastric artery; 6, pancreas; 7, liver (quadrate lobe); 7a, liver (caudate lobe); 8, stomach; 9, right crus of diaphragm; 10, lesser omentum; 10a, cut edge of lesser omentum; 11, hepatoduodenal ligament.

their resection if needed, together with the tumour, can be more safely performed.

If total pancreatectomy is to be proceeded with, the whole of the greater omentum is now freed from the transverse colon and left suspended from the greater gastric curvature.

3, 4. Cholecystectomy, dissection of the hepatoduodenal ligament, and mobilization of the pancreatic neck

These steps are followed as described in Chapter 40.

One additional note of caution should be sounded. It is important to preserve the left gastric or 'coronary' vein, which enters the portal vein from the left (usually near the confluence of the splenic vein). This vein will provide the only venous drainage route from the stomach (apart from fundic veins coursing into the oesophagus) once total pancreatectomy is completed.

Since partial gastrectomy is deferred to a later stage and division of the pancreas is unnecessary, the next step is to mobilize the pancreatic tail and spleen.

5. Mobilization of the pancreatic tail and spleen

In order to reduce blood loss to a minimum during the following dissection, we ligate the splenic artery at its origin, leaving the ligature long for later identification (see Fig. 41.2). Next, the left flexure of the colon is reflected downwards by dividing the splenocolic ligament. With the left hand retracting and lifting the spleen out of its bed towards the right, the diaphragmatic attachments of the spleen are severed. Thus, the space behind the spleen and pancreatic tail is reached. It is now easy to 'dig' the spleen and pancreas out of the retroperitoneum in a loosely areolar and avascular plane (Fig. 41.3). This leaves the left kidney, adrenal gland and left crus of the diaphragm exposed.

The lower border of the pancreas is freed from its avascular connections to the base of the mesocolon. Should a tumour of the pancreatic tail have infiltrated the mesocolon, it is sometimes possible to resect a segment of this together with the tumour, whilst preserving the vascular arcade supplying the transverse colon.

6. Partial gastrectomy

Together with spleen and pancreas, the stomach will have been retracted towards the right. It is now much easier to skeletonize the greater curvature by dividing the short gastric arteries between stomach and spleen, since this can now be done almost in front of the abdominal wall. The greater omentum is also detached from the proximal half of the greater curve, thus leaving it hanging from the distal stomach that will be resected. The lesser curve is

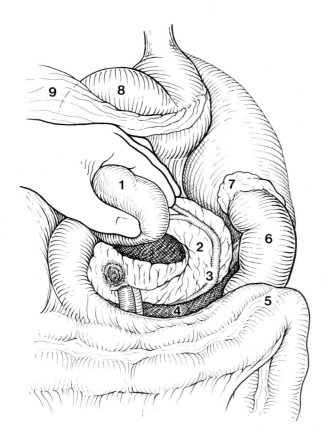

Fig. 41.3 Mobilization of spleen and pancreatic tail from the retroperitoneum. 1, Spleen; 2, pancreatic tail; 3, splenic vein; 4, plane of dissection between pancreas and root of mesocolon; 5, left colonic flexure; 6, left kidney; 7, left adrenal gland; 8, stomach; 9, greater omentum.

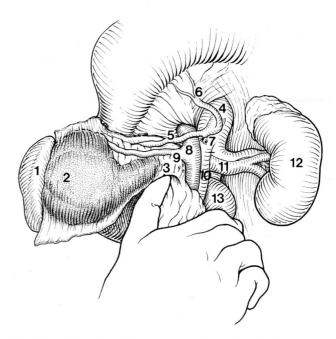

Fig. 41.4 Dissection of the retropancreatic vessels. 1, Spleen; 2, tumour; 3, pancreas; 4, coeliac artery; 5, hepatic artery; 6, left gastric artery; 7, stump of splenic artery; 8, portal vein; 9, splenic vein; 10, superior mesenteric artery; 11, left renal vein; 12, left kidney; 13, jejunum.

then skeletonized up to the level of Latarjet's nerve and the stomach transected with a stapler.

The only difference in technique as compared to step 5 of the Whipple resection (see Ch. 40) is the use of an extra row of seromuscular sutures (3:0 silk) to cover the greater curve, denuded as it is of its serosa. We have experienced subsequent perforation of this part of the stomach, possibly due to ischaemia. While they cannot improve blood supply, the sutures do help to cover the weakest areas and so prevent an ischaemic ulcer from perforating into the abdominal cavity (see Ch. 53).

The importance of preserving the left gastric artery and vein in preventing ischaemia of the gastric remnant cannot be overemphasized.

7. Dissection of the retropancreatic vessels

With the pancreas (and spleen) avulsed towards the right, the large retropancreatic vessels are approached from the left. The splenic vein, adherent to the posterior pancreatic surface is the guide to the portal vein and it is divided flush with its confluence with the superior mesenteric vein (Fig. 41.4). The inferior mesenteric vein is also

divided if it should enter the splenic vein, but it can be spared if it runs into the superior mesenteric more caudally.

At the upper border of the pancreas, the ligature on the splenic artery is located and this large vessel is now divided.

Coming from the left, the superior mesenteric artery is encountered before its accompanying vein. The excellent exposure facilitates an extensive lymph node clearance of the mesenteric root.

Dissection of the vessels running from the portal vein and mesenteric root into the pancreatic head and uncinate process follows the procedure as described in Chapter 40. The same applies to the next step.

8. Division of the jejunum (see Ch. 40)

With the jejunum divided the specimen can be discarded en bloc (Fig. 41.5) leaving the operative site as shown schematically in Figure 41.6.

RECONSTRUCTION

End-to-side hepaticojejunostomy using the closed end of the jejunum, and an end-to-side antecolic gastrojejunostomy with a Braun anastomosis, complete this operation exactly as described in Chapter 40 and shown in Figure 41.1b.

The operative field is drained by two soft silastic tubes, one placed subhepatically near the biliary anastomosis

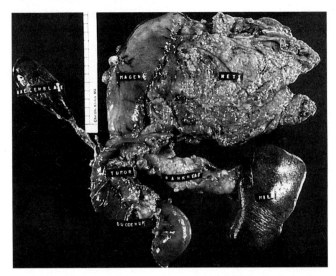

Fig. 41.5 57-year-old man; en bloc specimen following total pancreatectomy for a $pT_2 N_0 M_x$ tumour. The patient is alive and free of recurrence 9 years later. (Reproduced with permission of J B Lippincott and Co, from Trede et al 1990 Annals of Surgery 21: 448)

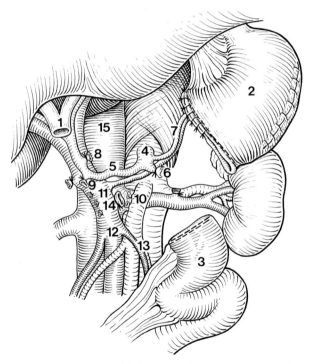

Fig. 41.6 Operative field following total pancreatectomy. 1, Common hepatic duct; 2, stomach; 3, jejunum; 4, coeliac axis; 5, common hepatic artery; 6, stump of splenic artery; 7, left gastric artery and vein; 8, right gastric artery (stump); 9, gastroduodenal artery (stump); 10, superior mesenteric artery with stumps of posterior pancreatoduodenal arteries; 11, portal vein; 12, superior mesenteric vein; 13, inferior mesenteric vein; 14, stump of splenic vein; 15, inferior vena cava.

and one in the left hypochondrium. Due to the large retroperitoneal wound and extensive lymph node dissection, more fluid is usually drained following total than after partial pancreatoduodenectomy (see also Ch. 53).

POSTOPERATIVE CARE

Postoperative care differs from that following conventional pancreatoduodenectomy in just one respect: the patient requires insulin (and later on, pancreatic enzyme substitution).

We used to monitor blood sugar and insulin requirements by attaching the patient to a computerized artificial-β-cell ('Biostator'). Difficulties with keeping the two intravenous lines open and working for more than a few days and nights, have led to the return to simpler and equally effective 2-hourly monitoring of blood sugar on the surgical intensive care unit. For the first 48 hours, the patient receives intravenous fluids and alimentation, including 750 ml 50% glucose per 24 hours. Simultaneously, about 100 i.u. of human insulin (diluted in 5% human albumin) are administered over 24 hours via an intravenous drip. With this regimen, the blood sugar level of a 70 kg patient is kept fairly constant between 100 and 200 mg% (5.6–11.2 mmol/l).

Sips of tea are allowed as soon as peristalsis recommences. After the 3rd postoperative day, light nourishment (soup, yoghurt etc) is permitted. Intravenous alimentation is reduced stepwise and insulin administered intravenously according to the blood sugar levels. On the 5th day, a light diet is begun. The intravenous line remains in place for another 2 days in case it is needed. At the same time, a long-acting insulin (16–24 i.u. Depot H insulin) is given in the morning, boosted by a second dose, as required, in the evening. Hypoglycaemia is feared more than a transient rise of the blood sugar above 200 mg% (11.2 mmol/l).

The patient learns to monitor his own blood sugar under normal exercise and food intake by means of a portable apparatus while still in hospital. In contrast to patients who undergo pancreatectomy for complicated alcoholic pancreatitis, these cancer patients, if they survive total pancreatectomy for any length of time, cope satisfactorily with their diabetic state. The average insulin requirements are no more than 20–28 i.u. per day, administered by the 'Pen-injection' technique.

Exocrine insufficiency is more easily controlled by regular substitution with pancreatic enzyme preparations that must contain sufficient active lipase, (e.g. Creon, two capsules with each of three meals).

42. Vascular problems and techniques associated with pancreatectomy and regional pancreatectomy

M. Trede

The following groups of vascular problems may confront the surgeon embarking upon pancreatectomy: congenital vascular anomalies, arteriosclerotic vascular stenosis or occlusion, vascular infiltration or compression by disease and iatrogenic vascular injuries.

CONGENITAL VASCULAR ANOMALIES

The main variations in blood supply as they affect pancreatic resection are described in Chapter 2. Since it is impossible to memorize all of these (Michels 1953) and since preoperative angiography can be misleading (Trede et al 1990), the surgeon must proceed with caution and at least be aware of the possibilities.

This means that no structure should be divided before it has been clearly identified. Nowhere is this axiom of greater importance than during dissection of the hepato-duodenal ligament, particularly to the right of the portal vein and common bile duct. The author has come across accessory right hepatic arteries in this location on two occasions, when the preoperative arteriography gave no hint of such an anomaly.

Even if angiography points to an accessory or replaced right or common hepatic artery arising from the superior mesenteric (as it does in some 26% of patients), it will give little information as to whether this vessel runs behind, through or even in front of the pancreatic head. Whereas the retropancreatic course is commonest, on occasions a replaced right hepatic artery can run in front of the pancreatic neck (Bodner & Poisel 1977) (Fig. 42.1). Whenever an accessory right hepatic artery runs through a tumorous pancreatic head, it will have to be sacrificed en bloc with the tumour and, as a rule, this can be done with impunity.

Case report: In the course of a difficult total pancreatectomy performed in 1973 for severe chronic pancreatitis (with fever, marasmus, intractable pain and diabetes), an accessory right hepatic artery was divided, leading to temporary cyanosis of the right lobe. Since the artery was only 2 mm in diameter and there was brisk back-bleeding from the hepatic stump, no repair

was attempted. Apart from a transient rise in transaminase levels, postoperative recovery was uneventful and a subsequent angiogram clearly demonstrated collateral vessels perfusing the distal branches of the severed artery (Fig. 42.2A, B).

Indeed Michels has cited 26 possible collateral pathways of blood supply to the liver (Michels 1953). These are 'possible' and at best 'probable' routes that should not be relied upon too heavily when a replaced, i.e. totally aberrant, hepatic artery is damaged (Crist et al 1987, Lansing et al 1972). If this happens accidentally or deliberately (because of tumour infiltration of the vessel), revascularization can be performed by anastomosis of the hepatic arterial stump to one of the branches of the coeliac axis (Rong & Sindelar 1987).

The anomalous course of an hepatic artery has been known to cause compression of the portal vein and so suggest inoperability on the preoperative angiogram. In the case shown in Figure 42.3, the tumour itself played no part in this compression and turned out to be easily resectable.

ARTERIOSCLEROTIC VASCULAR STENOSIS OR OCCLUSION

Obstruction of the coeliac axis is found in between 10 and 50% of patients undergoing abdominal arteriography (Szilagyi et al 1972). Its clinical significance is questionable, particularly when arteriosclerotic stenosis develops slowly and therefore leaves time for an adequate collateral blood supply to develop and reach the upper abdominal organs, especially the liver. However, this collateral pathway, via the pancreatoduodenal arcades, would have to be abruptly divided during pancreatoduodenectomy (Fig. 42.4).

The fear of potential ischaemia of the liver and pancreatic tail (possibly leading to disruption of the pancreato-jejunostomy) has led some surgeons to revascularize the branches of the coeliac trunk, following the Whipple operation (Fig. 42.5A, B). Thompson et al (1981) anastomosed the proximal segment of the divided splenic artery

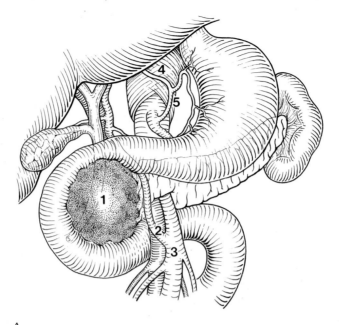

A

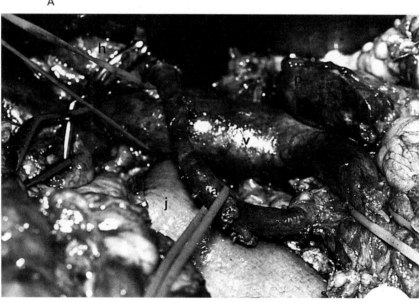

B

Fig. 42.1   68-year-old man. **A** Operative sketch of carcinoma of the pancreatic head (1) with a replaced right hepatic artery (2) arising form the superior mesenteric artery (3), running in front of the pancreatic neck to the hepatoduodenal ligament. (Note that the left hepatic artery (4) branches off the left gastric (5)). **B** Operative site after removal of specimen; a, mobilized aberrant right hepatic artery; v, portal vein; P, pancreatic remnant; h, hepatic duct (clamped by bull dog clamp); j, proximal jejunum.

to the superior mesenteric, relying on the short gastric vessels to perfuse the spleen and pancreatic tail. Miyata et al achieved a similar result by means of an aortohepatic saphenous vein graft (Miyata et al 1988).

In our first such case (in 1973), we thought we had solved the problem of 'coeliac compression' by simply dividing the arcuate ligament at the end of a pancreato-duodenectomy (Fortner & Watson 1981). The patient

did well. However, eight further cases with impressive angiographic evidence of coeliac occlusion did equally well without any attempt at reconstruction (Trede 1985). In each case, preliminary clamping, prior to division of the gastroduodenal artery, demonstrated some residual and reassuring pulsation in the hepatic artery (during palpation and flow measurement).

Although revascularization as shown in Figure 42.5 may

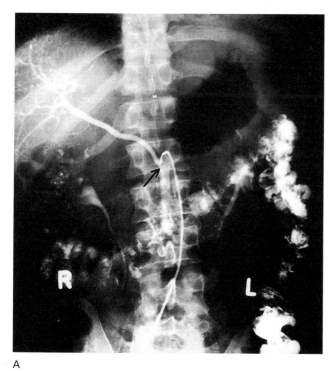

A

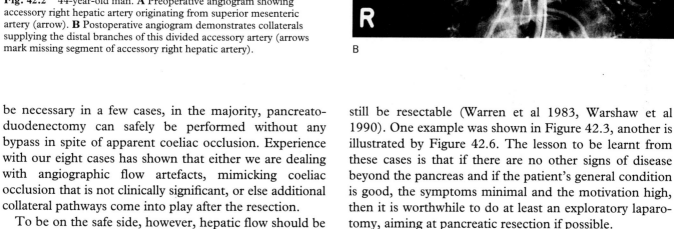

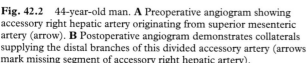

B

Fig. 42.2 44-year-old man. **A** Preoperative angiogram showing accessory right hepatic artery originating from superior mesenteric artery (arrow). **B** Postoperative angiogram demonstrates collaterals supplying the distal branches of this divided accessory artery (arrows mark missing segment of accessory right hepatic artery).

be necessary in a few cases, in the majority, pancreato-duodenectomy can safely be performed without any bypass in spite of apparent coeliac occlusion. Experience with our eight cases has shown that either we are dealing with angiographic flow artefacts, mimicking coeliac occlusion that is not clinically significant, or else additional collateral pathways come into play after the resection.

To be on the safe side, however, hepatic flow should be monitored (perhaps with a sterile Doppler probe) following preliminary occlusion of the gastroduodenal artery.

VASCULAR INFILTRATION OR COMPRESSION CAUSED BY THE DISEASE

As discussed in Chapters 9 and 37, overt tumour infiltration of the large retropancreatic arteries and veins, usually accompanied by severe backache (Mannell 1986), spells inoperability. However, there are exceptions to this rule.

First, in spite of angiographic stenosis the tumour may

still be resectable (Warren et al 1983, Warshaw et al 1990). One example was shown in Figure 42.3, another is illustrated by Figure 42.6. The lesson to be learnt from these cases is that if there are no other signs of disease beyond the pancreas and if the patient's general condition is good, the symptoms minimal and the motivation high, then it is worthwhile to do at least an exploratory laparotomy, aiming at pancreatic resection if possible.

Secondly, there are cases with tumour infiltration of the retropancreatic veins that are missed on the preoperative angiogram (Appleton et al 1989). They may even be missed by the probing retropancreatic finger (see Fig. 40.4), if the tumour comes from a posterolateral direction. Thus, venous involvement may not be discovered until late in the procedure and too late for retreat. The surgeon now has two options: he can dissect the tumour off the vein as far as possible. This means that tumour will inevitably be left behind so that the resection will be only palliative (R_2 resection). Alternatively he can remove the involved segment of vein along with the pancreas. Unfortunately, most of these resections will also turn out to be

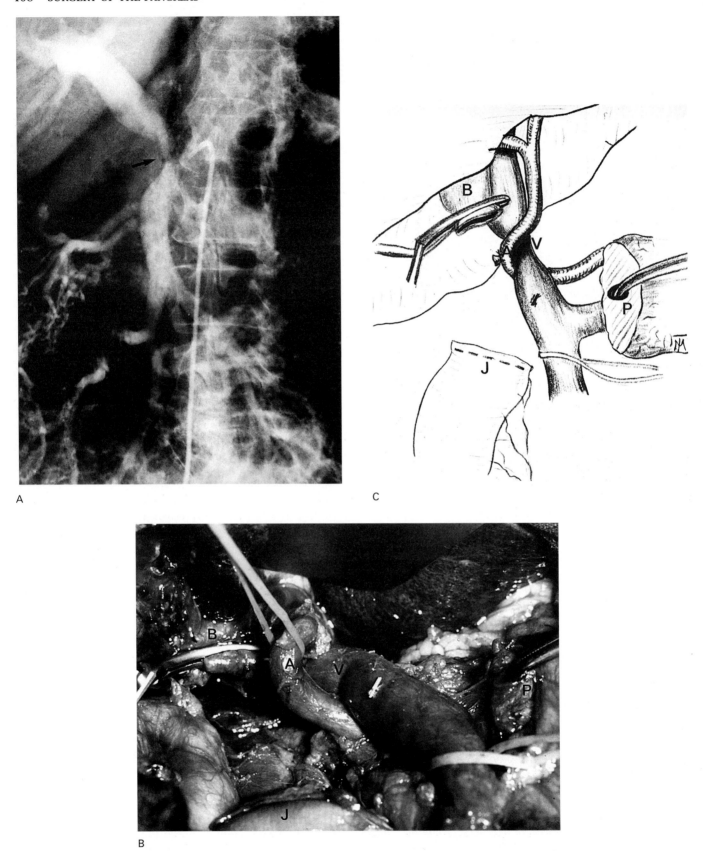

A

B

C

Fig. 42.3   72-year-old woman. **A** Carcinoma of the head of the pancreas with obstructive jaundice. Preoperative angiography of superior mesenteric and portal veins shows severe stenosis (arrow) indicative of tumour infiltration and inoperability. **B and C** Operative site and sketch showing that stenosis of portal vein (V) was merely caused by an unusual coiling of the hepatic artery (A); B, dilated common hepatic duct; P pancreatic remnant; J, stapled proximal end of jejunum. (Reproduced with permission of J B Lippincott Co, Philadelphia, from Trede et al 1990 Annals of Surgery 211: 447–458.)

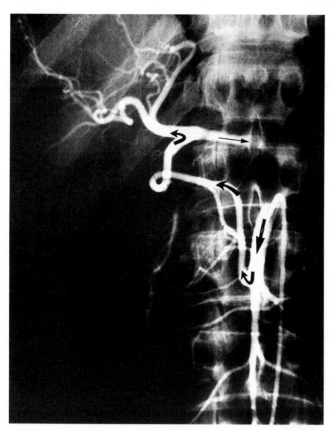

Fig. 42.4 45-year-old man; selective superior mesenteric arteriogram showing coeliac artery occlusion and perfusion of the hepatic arteries via the pancreatoduodenal arcades. (Reproduced with permission of C V Mosby Co, from Trede 1985 Surgery 97: 28–35).

palliative (R_1 resection). That is why these variants of regional pancreatectomy (see Table 38.1) are not performed as planned operations, but rather as the best way out of an impasse.

As in all vascular procedures, the first step is to obtain complete haemostatic control over the vessel to be resected. If the area of infiltration is small, it may be possible to underrun the portal vein with an atraumatic vascular clamp and to excise the involved venous segment, together with the tumour in the pancreatic head. The defect is easily oversewn (with 6:0 monofilament resorbable suture) without interruption of blood flow or excessive narrowing of the vein (Fig. 42.7).

If the area of involvement is more extensive, haemostatic control should preferably be obtained before the neck of the pancreas is taped or even transected. This is achieved by passing a vessel loop around the portal vein above the pancreas and another around the superior mesenteric vein at the inferior pancreatic border. The pancreas is now divided very carefully until the scalpel blade reaches the portal vein behind it. The specimen is held and portal venous flow is controlled by the surgeon's left hand as shown in Figure 40.8. At this stage, it is usually possible to retract the pancreatic body gently towards the left so as to expose the splenic vein behind. This, too, is now taped as is the inferior mesenteric vein, if encountered (Fig. 42.8).

Now, all the veins named are occluded by atraumatic vascular clamps and the involved segment is excised

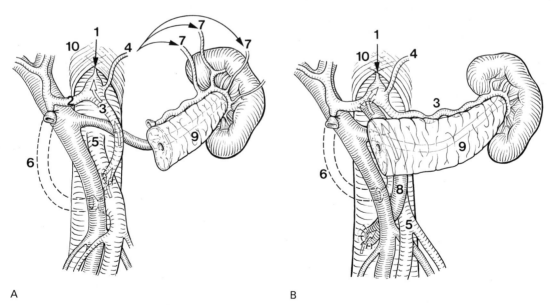

A   B

Fig. 42.5 Coeliac axis occlusion. **A** Revascularization by means of a spleno-mesenteric anastomosis (after Thompson et al 1981). **B** Revascularization by means of an aortohepatic saphenous vein bypass (after Miyata, 1985). 1, Coeliac axis occlusion; 2, hepatic artery; 3, splenic artery; 4, left gastric artery; 5, superior mesenteric artery; 6, resected pancreatoduodenal collaterals; 7, short gastric arteries; 8, aortohepatic saphenous vein graft; 9, pancreatic remnant; 10, arcuate ligament. Arrows show direction of blood flow after revascularization.

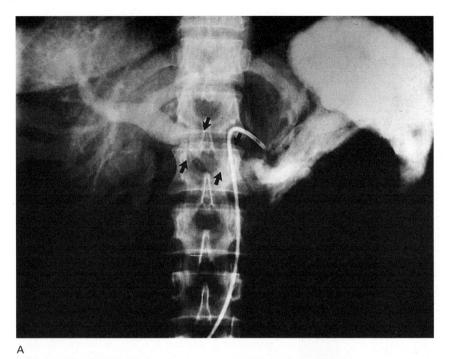

A

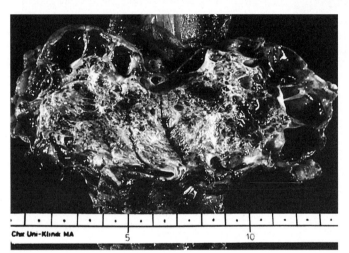

B

Fig. 42.6 50-year-old woman. **A** Venous phase of preoperative coeliac arteriography shows severe obstruction of the portal vein in a patient with a palpable epigastric mass. The patient's surprisingly good physical condition persuaded us to attempt resection. **B** Operative specimen following pancreatoduodenectomy which removed a large cystadenocarcinoma that had merely compressed, but not infiltrated the portal vein. (Reproduced with permission of C V Mosby Co, from Trede 1985 Surgery 97: 28–35).

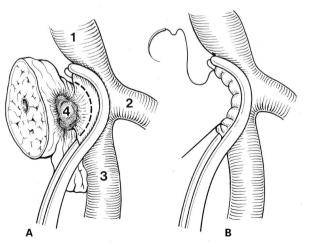

A   B

Fig. 42.7 **A** Tangential resection of a small segment of portal vein adherent to a pancreatic head tumour. **B** Closure of the small venous defect with 6:0 suture. 1, Portal vein; 2, splenic vein; 3, superior mesenteric vein; 4, tumour infiltrating venous adventitia.

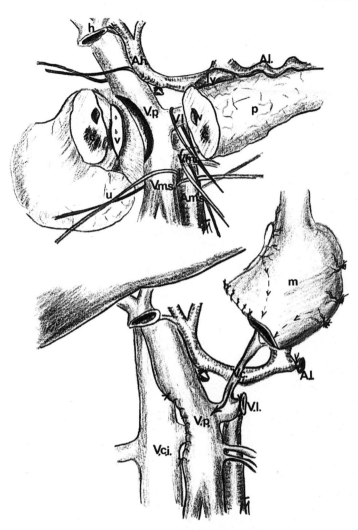

Fig. 42.8 63-year-old female patient. Above: operative sketch showing infiltration of portal vein (V.p.) by cancer (c), necessitating tangential resection of a segment of vein (v) along with total pancreatectomy. Below: operative site before biliodigestive reconstruction. h, Common hepatic duct; A.h., hepatic artery; ly, lymph node along neck of pancreas; A.l., splenic artery; p, pancreas; u, uncinate process; V.ms, superior mesenteric vein; V.mi, inferior mesenteric vein; A.ms, superior mesenteric artery; m, stomach; V.c.i, inferior vena cava. (Reproduced with permission of J B Lippincott Co, from Trede et al 1990 Annals of Surgery 211: 447–458).

tangentially. The defect can be covered with a pTFE patch or simply oversewn (Fig. 42.8). Although portal occlusion time rarely exceeds 15 minutes, mesenteric congestion can be considerable. This can be minimized by also taping and clamping the mesenteric arterial inflow, i. e. the superior mesenteric artery.

Sometimes, the extent of tumour infiltration requires complete resection of a venous segment. In this case, defects of up to 3–4 cm can be bridged by mobilization of the mesenteric root and a tension-free end-to-end anastomosis (Fig. 42.9).

If more extensive resection is required or the mesenteric root is fixed, perhaps by the scars of previous operations, then some sort of interposition is resorted to. For this, we prefer 10 mm ring-enforced pTFE tubing (Fig. 42.10). (Though perhaps preferable for biological reasons, the use of a composite autologous vein graft of adequate calibre is too cumbersome in actual practice.)

A final way out of the dilemma of bridging a large portal venous defect is to drain the transected end of the superior mesenteric vein into the inferior vena cava, as originally suggested by McDermott (1952). Following pancreatoduodenectomy, this mesocaval shunt is simple to perform, since vena cava and mesenteric vein lie close together without any intervening tissue (Fig. 42.11). Although this shunt is tolerated surprisingly well for a time (Marchal 1971), it should be used only as a last resort for obvious reasons relating to liver function and encephalopathy.

When tumour involves the hepatic and/or superior mesenteric arteries, the limits of resectability are reached. The author has replaced both these arteries but once. This particular patient with an otherwise irresectable pancreatic carcinoma succumbed after 8 days following thrombosis of the mesenteric arterial graft. This was the one fatality in 33 vascular reconstructions in connection with pancreatectomy (Table 42.1).

Table 42.1 Vascular procedures in 439 pancreatic resections undertaken in the Surgical Clinic, University of Mannheim (1.10.1972–1.1.1992); 37 times out of 'oncological' necessity, 3 times due to iatrogenic vascular injury

Number of patients		40
Portal vein resection	Tangential	28
	Segmental	8
Portal vein reconstruction	Simple suture	28
	End-to-end anastomosis	5
	Interposition	2
	Mesentericocaval shunt	1
Mesenterical arterial reconstruction	End-to-end suture	1
	Interposition	2
Hepatic arterial reconstruction	Operative median, and hospital mortality	1
	Died since discharge (median survival, 12 months)	29
	Still alive (1 Patient with $T_3 N_1$ carcinoma, 13 years free of recurrence)	8

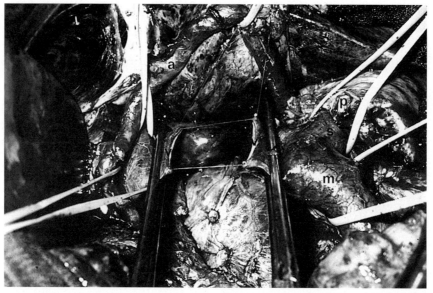

A

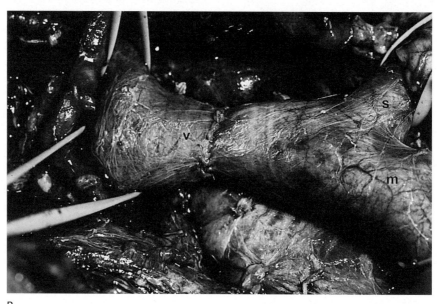

B

Fig. 42.9   47-year-old man. **A** Preoperative site after pancreatoduodenectomy and resection of a segment of the portal vein (v). m, superior mesenteric vein; s, splenic vein; p, pancreatic remnant; a, hepatic artery. **B** End-to-end anastomosis of the portal vein.

IATROGENIC VASCULAR INJURIES

Venous bleeding in the course of pancreatectomy can be voluminous, particularly from the retropancreatic veins. As with similar situations elsewhere, the safest control is obtained by local pressure (see Fig. 40.8), patience and judicious suction before applying vascular clamps. Venous tears can usually be oversewn with 6:0 prolene. But the damage may be so severe that an interposition graft is required to bridge the defect.

The most endangered arteries are the hepatic and its branches as well as the superior mesenteric artery. Hepatic arterial anomalies that are pertinent to pancreatectomy occur in 26% of patients (Michels 1953) and, of course, these are particularly prone to damage, as discussed above. If the hepatic artery is accidentally divided, the damage can best be repaired by means of a tension-free side-to-side anastomosis. This is facilitated by mobilization of the

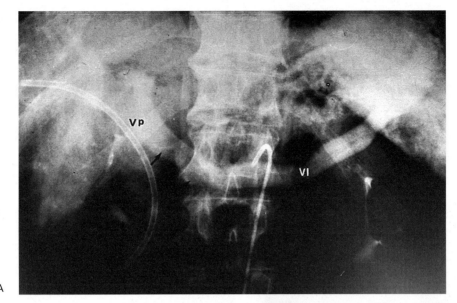

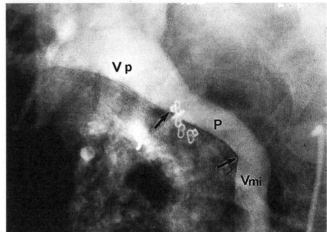

Fig. 42.10   56-year-old man. **A** Preoperative portogram showing only minimal tumour infiltration (arrows). Vp, Portal vein; Vl, splenic vein. **B** Postoperative angiogram with a 5 cm length of 10 mm pTFE ring-enforced prosthesis (P). Vmi, Superior mesenteric vein.

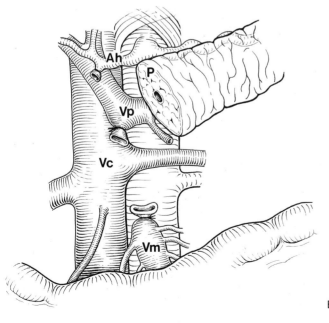

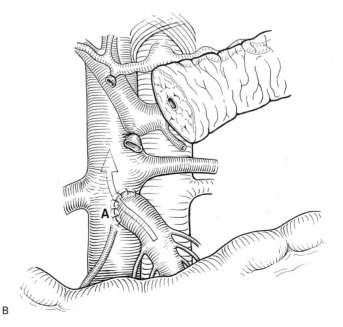

Fig. 42.11   60-year-old man. **A** Defect left by resection of superior mesenteric vein could not be bridged due to fixation of mesenteric root by adhesions. **B** A mesocaval shunt serves to drain mesenteric venous blood. A.h, Hepatic artery; P, pancreatic remnant; V.p, portal vein; V.c, inferior vena cava; V.m, superior mesenteric vein; A, mesocaval anastomosis.

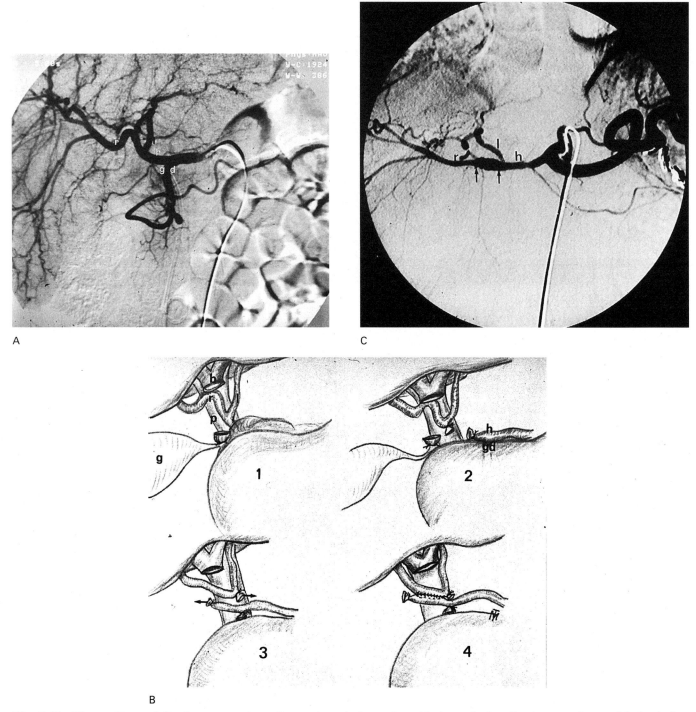

Fig. 42.12 55-year-old man. **A** Routine pre-operative coeliac arteriography in a patient with obstructive jaundice due to carcinoma of the head of the pancreas. **B** Sketch of dissection of hepatoduodenal ligament; 1, Before, and 2, after inadvertent division of common hepatic artery; 3, mobilization of proximal common hepatic artery after division of gastroduodenal artery; 4, tension-free side-to-side anastomosis. **C** Post-operative angiography showing patent anastomosis (arrows). r, Right hepatic artery; l, left hepatic artery; h, common hepatic artery; gd, gastroduodenal artery; p, portal vein; b, hepatic duct; g, gallbladder.

proximal common hepatic artery once its main branch, the gastroduodenal, has been divided (Fig. 42.12).

The superior mesenteric artery is in jeopardy during the dissection of retropancreatic vessels (Studley & Williamson 1992). Traction on the pancreatic specimen to the right may pull this artery from under the accompanying vein as shown in Figure 40.8. In over 400 pancreatectomies, damage was done twice by clamps placed too close to the right margin of the superior mesenteric artery. Repair was successful once by end-to-

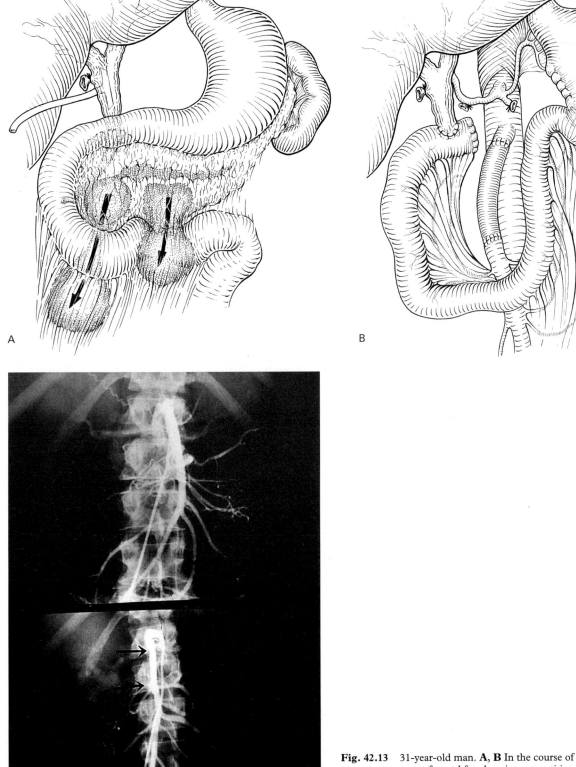

Fig. 42.13   31-year-old man. **A, B** In the course of total pancreatectomy performed for chronic pancreatitis, complicated by obstructive jaundice (relieved by cholecystectomy and T-drain 3 weeks previously) and cysts penetrating into the mesenteric root, a segment of the superior mesenteric artery was inadvertently 'resected' and then replaced by a 5 cm saphenous vein graft. **C** Preoperative, and **D** postoperative arteriography demonstrating the patent graft (between arrows).

end suture and once by means of a saphenous vein interposition graft (Fig. 42.13). The final lesson taught by these cases is that the surgeon who ventures into the field of pancreatectomy for cancer will profit greatly by a good training in vascular surgery.

REFERENCES

Appleton G V N, Bathurst N C G, Virjee J, Cooper M J, Williamson R C N 1989 The value of angiography in the surgical management of pancreatic disease. Annals of the Royal College of Surgeons of England 71: 92–96

Bodner E, Poisel S 1977 Varietäten der Leberarterien und deren Bedeutung für die Duodenokephalopankreatektomie. Chirurgische Praxis 22: 599–605

Crist D W, Sitzmann J V, Cameron J L 1987 Improved hospital morbidity, mortality, and survival after the Whipple procedure. Annals of Surgery 206: 358–373

Fortner J G, Watson R C 1981 Median arcuate ligament obstruction of celiac axis and pancreatic cancer. Annals of Surgery 194: 698–700

Lansing P B, Blalock J B, Ochsner J L 1972 Pancreatoduodenectomy: a retrospective review 1949 to 1969. American Surgeon 38: 79–86

Mannell A, van Heerden J A, Weiland L H, Ilstrup D M 1971 Factors influencing survival after resection for ductal adenocarcinoma of the pancreas. Annals of Surgery 203: 403–407

Mannell A, Weiland L H, Van Heerden J A, Ilstrup D M 1986 Factors influencing survival after resection for ductal adenocarcinoma of the pancreas. Annals of Surgery 203: 403–407

Marchal M M G, Balmes M, Vergues J, Grynfelt E 1971 Les problèmes vasculaires en rapport avec la chirurgie d'exerese pancrèatique. Montpelier Chirurgie 17:408–427

McDermott Jr W V 1952 A one-stage pancreatoduodenectomy with resection of the portal vein for carcinoma of the pancreas. Annals of Surgery 136: 1012–1018

Michels N A 1953 Collateral arterial pathways to the liver after ligation of the hepatic artery and removal of the celiac axis. Cancer 6: 708–724

Miyata M, Takao T, Okuda A, Sasako Y, Sunada S 1988 Pancreatoduodenectomy for periampullary cancer associated with celiac occlusion: a case report. Surgery 103: 261–263

Rong G H, Sindelar W F 1987 Aberrant peripancreatic arterial anatomy. Considerations in performing pancreatectomy for malignant neoplasms. American Surgeon 12: 726–729

Studley J G N, Williamson R C N 1992 Injury to the superior mesenteric artery during pancreatectomy for chronic pancreatitis. Annals of the Royal College of Surgeons of England 74: 35–39

Szilagyi D E, Rian R L, Elliot J P, Smith R F 1972 The celiac artery compression syndrome: does it exist? Surgery 72: 849–863

Thompson N W, Eckhauser F E, Talpos G, Cho K J 1981 Pancreaticoduodenectomy and celiac occlusive disease. Annals of Surgery 193: 399–406

Trede M 1985 The surgical treatment of pancreatic carcinoma. Surgery 97: 28–35

Trede M, Schwall G, Saeger H D 1990 Survival after pancreatoduodenectomy. 118 consecutive resections without an operative mortality. Annals of Surgery 211: 447–458

Warren K W, Christophi C, Armendariz R, Basu S 1983 Current trends in the diagnosis and treatment of carcinoma of the pancreas. American Journal of Surgery 145: 813–818

Warshaw A L, Zhuo-yun G V, Wittenberg J et al 1990 Pre-operative staging and assessment of resectability of pancreatic cancer. Archives of Surgery 125: 230–233

43. Left hemipancreatectomy

M. Trede

The chief indications for resection of the body and tail of the pancreas, including the spleen, are summarized in Table 43.1. Resection for benign lesions is dealt with in the appropriate chapters.

Hemipancreatectomy from the left for malignant disease is being performed more frequently with the advent of modern imaging methods. It may be well worthwhile, if a gastric carcinoma involving the greater curvature is firmly adherent to the pancreas. Gastrectomy and hemipancreatectomy is then the best technical solution of the problem, even if histological examination only rarely confirms actual tumour infiltration of the pancreas.

The resections of cystadenocarcinoma or islet cell carcinoma are also rewarding procedures, even in the presence of metastases, since long-term survival, if not cure, is possible.

Ductal adenocarcinoma of the body or tail of the pancreas is also being discovered at earlier stages, due to the increasing use of ultrasound in patients with vague upper abdominal pain. But even if such tumours are increasingly found to be resectable, they seldom are curable (Nordback et al 1992).

Case report: A 78-year-old woman presented with upper abdominal pain and minimal weight loss. Her general practitioner using sonography found a suspicious lesion in the pancreas, which was confirmed on CT and localized by means of endoscopic retrograde cholangiopancreatography (ERCP) (Fig. 43.1). At operation, a small (3 cm) tumour, confined to the pancreas, was removed by left pancreatectomy. Histology

confirmed an adenocarcinoma, however, with invasion of perineural lymphatics ($pT_2 N_1 M_x$–G3). Two years later, the patient is up and about with few symptoms from multiple pulmonary metastases, due to a mammary carcinoma that had been treated by mastectomy 5 years previously.

Although preservation of the spleen in left-sided pancreatic resections has been propagated recently by several authors (Cooper & Williamson 1985, Warshaw 1988, Richardson & Scott-Conner 1989), this seems inappropriate when dealing with malignant tumours.

TECHNIQUE

The technique of left hemipancreatectomy is divided into four steps.

1. Incision. A left subcostal incision is carried over to the right of the midline, if resectability has been confirmed.

2. Exploration. As usual, hepatic and peritoneal metastases are looked for first. Attention is then directed especially to lymph nodes of the coeliac axis, the splenic hilum and the mesenteric root.

Wide skeletonization of the gastrocolic ligament between the gastroepiploic vessels above and the transverse colon below, opens the lesser sac and provides optimal exposure of the whole of the body and tail of the pancreas.

Exposure and dissection begins at the trifurcation of the coeliac axis at the upper border of the pancreas. With the stomach retracted upwards and the transverse colon downwards, the hepatic artery is freed from the superior margin of the pancreas (Fig. 43.2; see also Fig. 41.2). This artery is then followed towards the left until it merges with the origin of the splenic artery from the coeliac axis. The splenic artery is now tied to reduce vascularity of the organs to be removed.

Now the neck of the pancreas is freed from the underlying portal vein and taped, thus marking the subsequent plane of resection (Fig 43.2). In tumours of the pancreatic tail that are resectable, this manoeuvre should be easy. If it is not, then the case is not suitable for a left

Table 43.1 Indications for left hemipancreatectomy

Benign lesions	Trauma
	Chronic pancreatitis
	Pseudocysts
	Tumours: cystadenoma, apudoma etc.
Malignant lesions	Islet cell carcinoma
	Cystadenocarcinoma
	Ductal adenocarcinoma
	Gastric or colon carcinoma (infiltrating pancreatic tail)

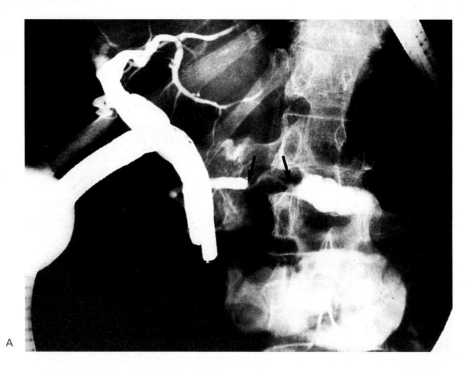

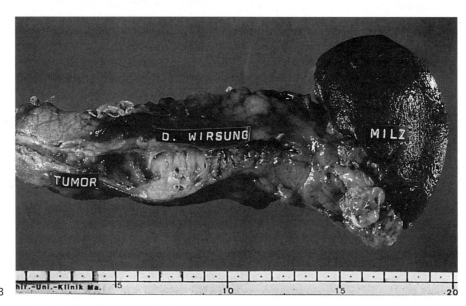

Fig. 43.1 78-year-old female patient. **A** Endoscopic retrograde cholangiopancreatography (ERCP) demonstrates severe stenosis of the pancreatic duct caused by a tumour of the pancreatic body. Note prestenotic dilatation of the pancreatic duct. **B** Operative specimen following left hemipancreatectomy (and splenectomy) in the same patient. Note normal pancreas to the (anatomical) right of the tumour (3cm) and the marked prestenotic dilatation of the duct of Wirsung.

hemipancreatectomy and preparation for a total resection must be made.

3. Mobilization of the pancreatic tail and spleen. This step is identical to that described in Chapter 41 (see Fig. 41.3).

The spleen is easily freed from the greater curvature of the stomach by dividing the short gastric vessels between ligatures. With the spleen retracted well up and to the right, this step can be performed almost in front of the abdominal wall.

4. Dissection of the retropancreatic vessels and division of the pancreas. Again, this resembles step 7

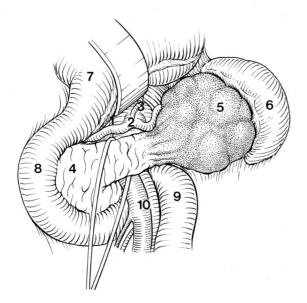

Fig. 43.2 Dissection of the branches of the coeliac axis. 1, Hepatic artery; 2, splenic artery; 3, left gastric artery; 4, pancreas; 5, tumour of pancreatic tail; 6, spleen; 7, stomach; 8, duodenum; 9, jejunum; 10, mesenteric vein and artery.

of total pancreatectomy as described in Chapter 41 (see Fig. 41.4). However, with the splenic artery and vein divided, dissection stops somewhere to the right of the portal vein.

The specimen is now retained solely by the neck of the pancreas (Fig. 43.3). This is divided with a scalpel, at least some 3 cm clear of the tumour, and the specimen is removed.

Two technical points should be noted. First, the incision should be fashioned so that the cut surface of the pancreatic head resembles a 'fish-mouth' and can therefore be closed without tension. Secondly beware of carrying the line of resection too far towards the right, where the terminal bile duct is running within the pancreatic head (Fig. 43.3).

Before closing the transected pancreas, one must ensure that drainage of the duct towards and through the papilla is unimpeded. There are three ways to do this:

- usually the preoperative ERCP provides proof of patency
- if not, the duct may be threaded with a fine balloon catheter, the tip of which would be felt within the duodenal lumen
- finally, as a last resort, a retrograde pancreaticogram may have to be done on the table (Desa & Williamson 1990).

If the duct is patent, it is closed by a single figure-of-eight suture (3:0 silk) and the cut surface is closed by figure-of-eight mattress sutures with 3:0 silk (Fig. 43.4).

The closed pancreatic stump can then either be 'buried' in the retroperitoneum with a few sutures, or it may be covered by a portion of omentum or mesocolon. In any case, a soft silastic drain, which traverses the pancreatic and splenic bed, is placed close to the pancreas and brought out through a stab wound in the left flank.

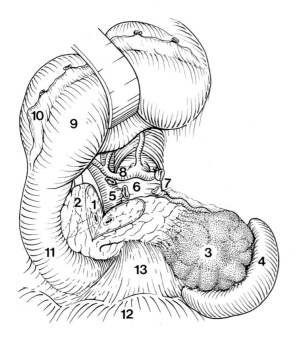

Fig. 43.3 Transection of the pancreatic neck. 1, Pancreatic neck (and duct) being divided; 2, common bile duct; 3, tumour; 4, spleen; 5, portal vein; 6, stump of splenic vein; 7, stump of splenic artery; 8, hepatic artery; 9, stomach; 10, divided omentum attached to greater gastric curvature; 11, duodenum; 12, transverse colon; 13, mesocolon.

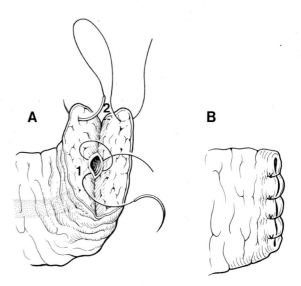

Fig. 43.4 **A** 1, Pancreatic duct (within the 'fish-mouth' trough of cut surface) is closed by a figure-of-eight suture (3:0 silk); 2, The transected surface of the pancreas is closed by interrupted sutures (3:0 silk). **B** The closed pancreatic stump.

If there is any doubt about duct patency, the transsected end of the pancreas has to be anastomosed to a Roux-en-Y loop of jejunum. For this, we prefer the end-to-end invaginating pancreatojejunostomy as described in Chapter 40.

REFERENCES

Cooper M J, Williamson R C N 1985 Conservative pancreatectomy .British Journal of Surgery 72: 801–803

Desa L A, Williamson R C N 1990 On-table pancreatography: importance in planning operative strategy. British Journal of Surgery 77: 1145–1150

Nordback I H, Hruban R H, Boitnott J K, Pitt H A, Cameron J L 1992 Carcinoma of the body and tail of the pancreas. American Journal of Surgery 164: 26–31

Richardson D Q, Scott-Conner C E H 1989 Distal pancreatectomy with and without splenectomy. A comparative study. American Surgeon 55: 21–25

Warshaw A L 1988 Conservation of the spleen with distal pancreatectomy. Archives of Surgery 123: 550–553

44. Palliative management by endoscopic procedures

B. C. Manegold

This chapter considers the use of peroral endoluminal endoscopic procedures for the diagnosis and treatment of pancreatic carcinoma. The laparoscopic approach (diagnostic for the assessment of peritoneal, serosal or subserosal carcinomatosis, and therapeutic for cholecystojejunal bypass and other procedures) is not considered.

ACCESS

First of all, there must be free access to the papilla of Vater. This access may be impeded by unrelated conditions, such as previous total or partial gastrectomy and gastroenterostomy for gastric outlet obstruction, or by tumour-related disorders, such as duodenal compression by extraluminal malignant growth, and papillary or periampullary oedema caused by carcinomatous lymphangiomatosis.

Once the papilla has been reached, its orifice has to be cannulated. This may be rendered impossible because of non-identification of the stoma; by its position in the base of a diverticulum; by intraduodenal bulging of the prepapillary common bile duct (choledochocoele), or by duodenal stenosis which interferes with vision and manoeuvring.

Cannulation of the orifice may readily succeed for 1–3 mm and endoscopic retrograde cholangiopancreatography (ERCP) may seem to have been achieved, but the injected contrast material pours off retrogradely without any opacification of a duct. This problem may be due to a carcinoma arising in the pancreatic duct just behind the papilla, or to a periampullary tumour obstructing both the biliary and pancreatic duct systems. But this must not be taken as clear evidence of pathology. Even with normal papillary, prepapillary and peripapillary structures, the tip of the cannula may be captured in intrapapillary mucosal folds so that the injected contrast material has no other escape and has to flow back into the duodenum. Enforced manoeuvres may perforate the mucosal layer and result in peripapillary contrast extravasation, an appearance often misdiagnosed as malignant necrosis.

DIAGNOSTIC ERCP

The completeness of ERCP is readily assessed on the screen. A normal ERP (endoscopic retrograde pancreatogram) does not include the presence of pancreatic malignancy in the tail, body or even in the head of the gland, and a normal ERC (endoscopic retrograde cholangiogram) does not rule out pancreatic neoplasia. Stenosis of the common bile duct at ERC is far from an unequivocal sign of malignancy. Usually a pancreatic carcinoma, encircling the lower third of the common bile duct, causes a concentric smooth stenosis, sometimes displacing the axis to the lateral or medial side according to the location of the bulk of the tumour. The stenosis is often so tight, that the narrowed area is not visible on the monitor, even if an obviously dilated prestenotic biliary tract is demonstrated. Stenosis of the confluence of the hepatic ducts by lymph node metastasis can be the only sign at ERCP of a tumour of the pancreatic tail, while stenosis of the common bile duct may stem from a tumour in the pancreatic head that originates from Santorini's duct. In this case, the remainder of the pancreatic duct may appear quite normal and opacified throughout its length and side branches.

Pancreatic carcinoma usually develops from the epithelium of the main pancreatic duct and should be detected from its very early stages by the demonstration of ductal irregularities, stenoses, prestenotic dilatations or obstructions at retrograde pancreatography. Unfortunately, few patients have symptoms in the earliest stages of pancreatic duct carcinoma that would justify ERCP. Furthermore, the broad indication for diagnostic ERCP has to be balanced by the invasive nature of the procedure, by its costs, by its possible complications such as necrotizing pancreatitis, and its mortality rate of 0.01%. Nevertheless, when pancreatic carcinoma is suspected clinically, ERCP is of immense diagnostic value and should always be performed. ERCP in this context aims to visualize both the pancreatic and the common bile duct; however, in the event that the pancreatic duct shows unequivocal signs of malignancy, we do not proceed to delineate the biliary system in unjaundiced patients (see below).

The rate of success of ERCP in 532 consecutive patients, presenting to the University Surgical Clinic at Mannheim, with clinically suspected pancreatic carcinoma from July 1986–December 1989 was 93% (Table 44.1); a total of 3596 ERCPs were performed in the same period. The high rate (30%) of incomplete or absent filling of the pancreatic duct reflects the fact that in 88 cases the pancreatic duct system failed to fill at some point in its course, a finding interpreted as a possible sign of malignancy. Other reasons were malignancy of the ampulla and insufficient pressure for injection (21 cases); pancreas divisum (7 cases); extravasation of dye (2 cases); bleeding from the papilla (1 case); presence of contrast material in the bowel from a previous barium meal (2 cases); faults with the X-ray apparatus (1 case), and failure to opacify the pancreatic duct despite successful ERCP (35 cases). In 39 cases (7%) the papilla could not be cannulated.

ENDOSCOPIC DIAGNOSIS AND HISTOLOGICAL PROOF

The final endoscopic diagnosis in 532 of our patients, with clinically suspected pancreatic tumours, who underwent ERCP was malignant tumour in 308 cases (pancreatic 283, biliary 25), benign lesions in 167 cases and indeterminate findings in 57 cases. Histological or cytological proof of malignancy in the 308 patients diagnosed by ERCP was established in only 157 cases (51%) (Table 44.2). Pretreatment histological proof was attempted only in those relatively rare cases (15 patients in this series) where the tumour had macroscopically invaded the gastric, duodenal or prepapillary mucosa. Blind transpapillary endocanalicular biopsy or brush cytology was undertaken in only two cases because of the possible risk of bleeding and pancreatitis, while percutaneous fine-needle biopsy was performed in only five cases because of the risk of peritoneal or retroperitoneal dissemination of malignant cells. In 13 patients, malignancy was confirmed subsequently by histological investigation of obstructing material harvested from an extracted prosthesis. In all 120 remaining patients, malignancy was confirmed by laparotomy or autopsy.

The great majority of the 151 patients suspected of having pancreatic carcinoma in the absence of histological/cytological proof were, from the outset, not regarded as candidates for laparotomy. Imaging procedures (ERCP in conjunction with ultrasonography and CT) appeared to be so conclusive that it was decided to avoid further invasive manoeuvres designed to secure histological proof. Therapy in such cases was strictly symptomatic, including analgesics for pain and transpapillary biliary drainage for jaundice and pruritis.

ENDOSCOPIC SPHINCTEROTOMY (EST) AND TRANSPAPILLARY BILIARY DRAINAGE

Endoscopic treatment of pancreatic carcinoma is limited to the relief of jaundice and pruritis. Papillotomy may be sufficient in otherwise inoperable patients with circumscribed prepapillary tumours which obstruct the bile duct so that it bulges like a choledochocoele into the duodenum. Transpapillary biliary drainage procedures are more suitable for stenosis of the common bile duct. Sphincterotomy and transpapillary biliary drainage are performed as part of the first (diagnostic) ERCP if biliary obstruction and jaundice are present, regardless of operability and the patient's age. Confirmation of operability and tumour staging are the objectives of further assessment. We justify this attitude by the possible, and not insignificant, risk of inducing septic cholangitis by injecting contrast material into an obstructed bile duct.

The drainage catheter used preferentially for transpapillary drainage is a slightly curved French 9.6 plastic tube (Surgimed), 12 or 14 cm in length with two side flaps at the ends to restrict movement, and no side holes (to avoid turbulence and premature clogging). The catheter is stiffened by a guide catheter, and is introduced via the 3.2 mm instrumental channel of an Olympus duodenoscope (TJF-20) with the aid of a pushing catheter. Intravenous premedication with 7.5–10 mg of diazepam for sedation and 1 mg glucagon for duodenal relaxation is usually sufficient. Pulse rate, blood pressure and PaO_2 are monitored throughout the procedure. The catheter is inserted under X-ray control with the patient in the prone position.

Table 44.1 Rate of visualization of pancreatic and biliary ducts, in 532 patients undergoing endoscopic retrograde cholangiopancreatography (ERCP), on suspicion of pancreatic carcinoma, in the University Surgical Clinic, Mannheim. (ERP, endoscopic retrograde pancreatography; ERC, endoscopic retrograde cholangiography.)

ERP	n (%)	ERC	n (%)
ERP complete	336 (63)	ERC complete	392 (74)
ERP partial	122 (23)	ERC partial	35 (6)
ERP negative (ERC positive)	35 (7)	ERC negative (ERP positive)	66 (13)
Papilla not cannulated	39 (7)	Papilla not cannulated	39 (7)
Total	532 (100)	Total	532 (100)

Table 44.2 Success in obtaining histological/cytological proof of malignancy in 308 patients diagnosed as having malignancy at ERCP

	Number of patients
Histological/cytological proof from:	
Pancreatectomy (partial/total)	53
Palliative bypass operation (bilioenteric and/or gastroenteric)	38
Exploratory laparotomy	26
Duodenal, gastric biopsy	17
Biopsy/brush cytology from the pancreatic/ common bile duct	2
Percutaneous fine-needle biopsy	5
Material from obstructed drainage catheters (transpapillary biliary drainage)	13
Autopsy	3
Total proven	157
No histological/cytological proof	151
Total	308

Table 44.3 Reasons for unsuccessful transpapillary biliary drainage in 68 patients, out of 252 (ERC, endoscopic retrograde cholangiography; ERP, endoscopic retrograde pancreatography)

	Number of patients
ERC not successful (ERP succeeded)	29
Negotiation of stenosis impossible	20
Selective biliary cannulation impossible	11
Extravasation of contrast material	3
Uncooperative patient	3
Duodenal perforation	1
Metastatic occlusion of hepaticojejunostomy	1
Total	68

The new self-expanding metallic (Wallstent) endoprosthesis has an internal diameter of 1 cm when fully expanded and is currently the subject of a prospective trial in patients with malignant biliary obstruction. It is hoped that stent occlusion by biliary sludge will be less troublesome than is the case with conventional plastic catheters. Studies are also underway to assess whether providing such metallic stents with an outer plastic coat will further reduce the problem of stent occlusion by preventing the ingrowth of tumour between the interstices of the metallic stent.

Results of transpapillary drainage

Transpapillary biliary drainage was indicated in 252 of our patients, the age group of this series being 35–92 years. It succeeded in 184 patients (73%), while in 68 cases (27%) the transpapillary endoscopic insertion of a stenting tube was not possible (Table 44.3).

Transpapillary insertion of a drainage catheter may be particularly difficult in patients with tumours immediately behind the papilla and in those with tumours at the hepatic duct confluence. Prepapillary stenoses prevent passage of the guide-wire, particularly when they are close to the papilla and when there is mucosal oedema, and the guide-wire then frequently proves difficult to manoeuvre. Central biliary stenoses can be difficult to negotiate if resistance is sufficient to withstand the pushing force, so allowing the catheter to become bowed in the elastic post-stenotic common bile duct. Pretreatment by bouginage or pneumatic dilatation may prove helpful, or a combined approach (see below, and Chapter 46) may also be useful.

Definitive diagnosis and treatment following drainage

After successful insertion of the drainage catheter, the jaundiced patient is considered for definitive diagnosis and treatment. All transpapillary inserted endoprostheses will obstruct with time, because of retrograde passage of food particles and accretion of biliary sludge or malignant cells. The median time of unimpaired function is about 3–4 months; exceptionally such catheters may function for 18 months (Table 44.4). Preoperative transpapillary biliary drainage buys time for further specific investigation after which it may be decided that no further procedures are indicated. In this case, transpapillary drainage becomes the definitive treatment and repeated insertion of drainage catheters may be needed until death.

The life expectancy of patients with pancreatic carcinoma depends on the stage of the tumour and the influence of therapeutic procedures. Patients with the best expectations are those whose tumour is confined to the pancreas and totally removed by partial or total

Table 44.4 Further treatment after successful transpapillary biliary drainage (TPBD) for pancreatic carcinoma

Treatment	Number of patients
Transpapillary biliary drainage, no further treatment	92
Exploratory laparotomy (+ splanchnicectomy 1)	3
Pancreatectomy (partial/total)	28
Palliative bypass operation (bilioenteric and/or gastroenteric)	26
Repeated transpapillary biliary drainage	32
Percutaneous transhepatic biliary drainage	3
Total	184

Table 44.5 Life expectancy of 249 patients with pancreatic carcinoma, in relation to therapeutic procedure undertaken. TPBD, transpapillary biliary drainage; PTBD, percutaneous transhepatic biliary drainage

Treatment	Number of patients	Days
Pancreatic resection (partial, total)	40	614
Bypass operation(bilioenteric and/or gastroenteric)	30	243
TPBD successful	122	262
TPBD bypass operation	24	220
TPBD not successful; bypass operation	11	222
TPBD unsuccessful; PTBD instituted	18	157
TPBD unsuccessful, no further therapy	4	67
Total	249	

pancreatectomy. Little hope can be given to those in whom transpapillary biliary drainage does not succeed and where further intervention is deemed inappropriate (Table 44.5).

Complications

Complications of transpapillary biliary drainage were seen in 28 of our 252 cases. The common bile duct may be perforated by the guide-wire within, beneath or above the stenotic area. Creation of a false passage may be suspected and is confirmed by injection of contrast material through a cannula threaded up over the guide-wire. The correct intraluminal position has to be achieved by repeated probing manoeuvres. If not successful, transpapillary drainage has to be abandoned in favour of percutaneous transhepatic biliary drainage or a combined procedure (see Ch. 45) in which the radiologist first introduces a transhepatic catheter, through which a guide-wire is steered into the duodenum. The endoscopist can then grasp the guide-wire and pull it through the instrumentation channel of the endoscope. The guide-wire can then be used to insert an endoprosthesis by the endoscopic route. The combination (or 'rendezvous') procedure is used sparingly, but may avoid the need to insert a prosthesis transhepatically and obviate the need for a large transhepatic track.

ENDOSCOPIC ULTRASONOGRAPHY

Transgastric and transduodenal ultrasonography provide excellent close-up visualization of the entire pancreas, distal biliary tract and regional lymph nodes (see Chapter 11). Correct tumour-staging is achievable in up to 92% of cases. Wirsung's duct with its side branches and all structures which may be affected by pancreatic diseases can be visualized and duct diameter can be measured. For detection of small pancreatic tumours, below a diameter of 20 mm, endoscopic ultrasonography has proved to have the highest rate of success of all imaging procedures.

However, the histological nature of the mass (e.g. cancer, sarcoma or insulinoma) cannot be determined from the ultrasonic image. Proof or exclusion of carcinoma in cases of chronic pancreatitis is also difficult.

TRANSPAPILLARY PANCREATICOSCOPY

The newly developed miniscope, 200 mm in length and 0.5 mm outside diameter, is passed down the instrument channel of a conventional side-viewing duodenoscope, and inserted via an overtube passed through the papilla, to allow inspection of the whole length of the pancreatic duct. There is no need for papillotomy. Ductal lesions can be inspected and biopsies can be taken under X-ray control. This new technique, especially when used in combination with staining procedures may improve diagnostic reliability decisively when dealing with pancreatic duct lesions. This in combination with endoscopic ultrasonography will be an important step towards the better diagnosis of early pancreatic carcinoma.

ADDITIONAL ENDOSCOPIC THERAPEUTIC PROCEDURES

Transpapillary drainage of the obstructed pancreatic duct, using quite similar catheters and almost the same implantation technique as transpapillary biliary drainage, has been advocated as a means of reducing pancreatic pain and improving the nutritional status of patients with pancreatic disease. The benefit of this approach in malignant pancreatic disease is as yet inconclusive.

CONCLUSION

ERCP and its associated procedures have had a decisive impact in the diagnosis and palliation of pancreatic carcinoma. ERCP should not be delayed when there is any clinical suspicion of pancreatic carcinoma. Transpapillary biliary drainage is a minimally invasive procedure which occupies leading position in the list of palliative therapeutic methods available. Now, after a long period of relative stasis in fibreoptic endoscopic development, endoscopic ultrasound and pancreaticoscopy with miniscopes may give new hope in the earlier diagnosis of pancreatic carcinoma.

45. Palliative management with percutaneous and rendezvous techniques

W. R. Jaschke   B. C. Manegold

INTRODUCTION

Percutaneous transhepatic biliary drainage (PTBD) was first described by Molnar and Stockum in 1974, but did not gain wide acceptance in the medical community until the beginning of the 1980s (Molnar & Stockum 1974, Hoevels et al 1978, Ring et al 1978, Ferrucci et al 1980, Mueller et al 1982). Initial attempts at PTBD were designed to reduce the rate of bleeding and bile leakage quite frequently encountered after percutaneous transhepatic cholangiography (PTC) (Ring et al 1979). The increased risk of surgery reported in the presence of jaundice (Blamey et al 1983) provided additional stimulus toward refining the technique of PTBD and broadening the scope of its application (Feduska et al 1971, Classen et al 1984).

The introduction of transpapillary endoscopic biliary drainage did not eliminate the need for transhepatic drainage procedures since technical failures are not uncommon (Huitbregtse & Tytgat 1982, Classen et al 1984, Huitbregtse 1984, Deviere & Cremer 1990). Also, a common complication of failed transpapillary drainage, acute cholangitis, necessitates immediate relief of obstruction. This is readily achieved using the transhepatic approach in most cases (Kadir et al 1982). Thus, transhepatic and transpapillary biliary drainage should be viewed as complementary rather than as competitive techniques.

Over the years, transhepatic biliary drainage has become a safe and reliable procedure in most of the larger medical centres around the world (Mueller et al 1982, Norlander et al 1982, Stambuck et al 1983, Carrasco et al 1984, Mueller et al 1985, Wittich et al 1985, Lammer & Neumayer 1986, Günther et al 1988). The increasing number of patients referred for PTBD at our institution reflects this development (Fig. 45.1). It is now well accepted that primarily non-surgical techniques should be used to palliate symptoms of obstructive jaundice caused by malignant disease (Shepard et al 1988, Sirinek & Levine 1989). Thus, surgeons involved in treatment of

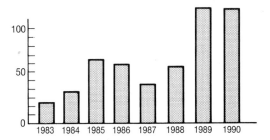

Fig. 45.1 Number of patients referred annually for percutaneous transhepatic biliary drainage (PTBD) between 1983 and 1990 at Mannheim Clinic

patients in this situation should know of the different techniques which are currently available.

METHODOLOGY

Patient preparation

Prior to PTBD, a thorough diagnostic work-up is mandatory. This should include a high quality cholangiogram demonstrating the site of the obstruction, as well as other imaging procedures demonstrating the nature and extent of the underlying disease. The access to the biliary tree can be planned accordingly. In addition, the type of drainage procedure can be tailored to the patient's specific anatomical pattern and prognosis.

Coagulation factors should be checked and, if necessary, corrected. Informed consent is obtained the day before the procedure. The patient is asked to avoid any solid food after midnight, but is free to drink until 4 hours before the procedure.

The patient should receive his regular medication and, if necessary, additional medication in order to relieve anxiety. A venous line is inserted on the day of the procedure to administer fluids, sedatives and analgesics. Antibiotics are not routinely given in our institution. In case of cholangitis, i.v. mezlocillin is administered (3 × 2 g per day). If necessary the antibiotic therapy is modified once

487

an infecting organism has been identified. The skin is washed and disinfected so that a sterile percutaneous puncture can be performed.

Transhepatic catheterization of the biliary tree and duodenum

Two different percutaneous puncture sites provide a safe access route to the biliary tree (Healy & Schroy 1953, Jaques et al 1982, Coons 1990). The right intercostal approach allows for puncturing the ducts of segments 7 or 8. The left hepatic duct or the duct draining segment 1 or segment 4 is entered using a subxiphoid puncture site in the epigastric triangle.

The needle is inserted under fluoroscopic or ultrasonographic guidance. Sometimes, both imaging methods are required to select the best route for intubation of the biliary system. In order to avoid acute angles between catheter track and bile duct, several punctures may be necessary until an appropriate duct has been entered. The risk of bleeding can be minimized by selecting a peripheral segment of the biliary ductal system.

A skinny needle (22 G) or a sheathed needle (16 G) can be used for puncture (Coons 1990). Usually, the needle tip is directed towards the right 10th intercostal space, regardless of the cutaneous entry point. The 16 G needle allows for aspiration of fluids and its position can be easily checked by aspirating blood or bile. Once a bile duct has been entered, a curved guide-wire is inserted and manipulated into the extrahepatic biliary-tree. The sheath is then pushed over the guide-wire. Since a rigid 0.035 inch guide-wire can be passed through the sheath, it can be readily replaced by a drainage catheter. The rather large outer diameter of the needle implies, however, a higher risk of complications, especially if several punctures are required for cannulation of a suitable bile duct.

The skinny needle is less traumatic but aspiration of fluids is difficult, and, very often, impossible. The position of the needle tip is, therefore, controlled by frequent injections of small amounts of contrast material. Once a bile duct has been entered, a soft 0.018 inch steerable guide-wire is passed through the needle (Cope 1982). After a stable position has been achieved, the needle is removed and a coaxial catheter system is passed over the wire. After removal of the 0.018 inch guide-wire and the inner catheter, a 0.035 inch guide-wire can be inserted for catheterization of the extrahepatic bile ducts.

After successful catheterization of the common duct, a guide-wire is negotiated through the tumour stenosis into the duodenum. If this fails initially, temporary external drainage is established. After a couple of days, the biliary system is sufficiently decompressed and passage of the guide wire into the duodenum is more easily accomplish-ed. A multi-side-hole drainage catheter can then be inserted for antegrade biliary drainage.

Technique of long-term biliary drainage

There are several options for permanent PTBD (Coons 1990). The most appropriate method depends upon the extent and location of the lesion, the clinical status and prognosis of the patient as well as the expertise within an institution.

External drainage

This procedure is easy to perform since it requires only intubation of a central bile duct without cannulation of the duodenum (Fig. 45.2). Frequently patients suffer, however, from dehydration and loss of potassium (Mueller et al 1982, Taber et al 1982, Günther et al 1988). Thus, in our opinion external drainage is unsuitable for long-term palliation.

External-internal drainage

External-internal drainage provides a physiological antegrade bile flow. Multi-side-hole catheters with an inner

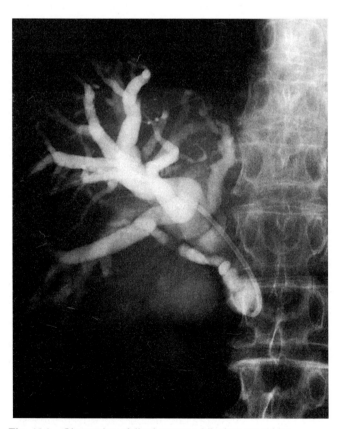

Fig. 45.2 Obstruction of distal common bile duct caused by unresectable pancreatic carcinoma. A pigtail catheter was inserted from a right intercostal approach.

lumen of at least 2 mm have to be used for decompression of the biliary tree (Ring et al 1979). Regular flushing of the catheter prevents occlusion by bile incrustation. If the internal limb is clogged, the catheter can be easily removed over a guide-wire and replaced by a new tube. In order to avoid complications associated with catheter occlusion, catheters should be exchanged on a regular basis, for example every 2 months. This procedure is performed on an outpatient basis. Thus, the patient has to return to the hospital several times. This is one of the major drawbacks of long-term catheter drainage. In addition, inflammatory reactions at the puncture site and recurrent cholangitis are frequently observed in these patients (Pollock et al 1979, Mueller et al 1982, Wittich et al 1985, Hamlin et al 1986, Günther et al 1988). Patient discomfort due to pain during respiration is another disturbing problem (Mueller et al 1982, Wittich et al 1985, Hamlin et al 1986, Günther et al 1988).

Internal drainage using biliary endoprostheses

This is another recognized option for palliative treatment of inoperable malignant biliary stenosis (Hoevels & Ihse 1979, Dooly et al 1984, Lammer & Neumayer 1986, Dick et al 1987, McLean & Burke 1989). Endoprostheses achieve satisfactory drainage of bile into the bowel without the above-mentioned physical and psychological problems associated with drainage catheters. One of the major drawbacks of biliary endoprostheses is the difficulty of replacing or exchanging them when they become occluded (Dooly et al 1984, Mendez et al 1984, Lammer & Neumayer 1986, Jackson et al 1990, Lee et al 1990). In addition, long-term drainage necessitates the use of an endoprosthesis with an inner lumen of approximately 3 mm or larger (Lammer & Neumayer 1986, Lammer et al 1986). Thus, insertion is an invasive procedure implying discomfort for the patient and a higher risk of bleeding.

Biliary endoprostheses: materials. Several types of biliary endoprostheses are currently available for the treatment of biliary strictures. Endoprostheses made of plastic materials are most commonly used. The plastic materials differ in terms of flexibility, wall thickness and biocompatibility (Lammer et al 1986). The term biocompatibility includes surface interaction with the surrounding tissue and with bile. Bile incrustations are mainly a problem of surface chemistry rather than of fluid dynamics. For example, in vitro experiments showed that Teflon had an incrustation rate 4 times higher than polyurethane (Lammer et al 1986).

It is generally accepted that migration of the endoprosthesis can be prevented by choosing an appropriate length of the endoprosthesis, for example approximately 20 cm (Hoevels & Ihse 1979, Mueller et al 1985,

Lammer & Neumayer 1986, Dick et al 1987, Günther et al 1988, Coons 1990, Jackson et al 1990). Anchoring mechanisms are another solution to the problem (Huitbregtse 1982). However, placement and removal of such an endoprosthesis is more difficult and implies a higher risk of tissue trauma.

Perforation of the bowel wall can be avoided by correct placement of endoprostheses i.e. the tip of the endoprosthesis should be centred within the bowel lumen and should not distort the bowel wall (Gould et al 1988). An atraumatic tip such as the pigtail configuration can also eliminate the problem of wall perforation. However, dislocation due to bowel movements is much more frequently encountered. In our hands, slightly curved 10 French endoprostheses, with a cylindrically shaped tip, proved to be safe and effective devices for biliary drainage (Dick et al 1987, Coons 1990). This particular type of endoprosthesis is manufactured from highly flexible polyurethane with a satisfactory biocompatibility.

Metallic mesh endoprostheses, commonly referred to as biliary stents, represent the newest development (Carrasco et al 1985, Strecker et al 1988, Alvarado et al 1989, Huitbregtse et al 1989, Schatz 1989, Coons 1990, Adam et al 1991, Jaschke et al 1992). These stents are inserted in the biliary system in a collapsed state using small caliber catheters. After expansion their diameter increases from approximately 8 Fr (2.6 mm) to 24 Fr or even 30 Fr (8–10 mm). Due to their thin-walled construction biliary stents provide a larger inner diameter than comparable plastic endoprostheses. The wire struts cover approximately 15% of the mucosal surface. Thus, surface–bile interactions are minimized. Tumour growth into the lumen is, however, more likely than with plastic endoprostheses. Due to their self-anchoring mechanism migration does not occur. The papillary function can, therefore, be preserved in patients with mid-duct or hilar obstructions without increasing the risk of stent migration. For the same reasons, stents are extremely well suited for patients with tumour stenosis at an enterobiliary anastomosis.

Currently, two different types of stents are available, namely balloon expandable and self expanding stents (Table 45.1). Also, the various stents differ in terms of flexibility. In our institution only flexible stents are used.

Technique of placement. Placement of plastic endoprostheses is a procedure with three stages. First, percutaneous transhepatic drainage is established (Fig. 45.3A). Whenever possible, the stenosis is crossed during this procedure so that the tip of the drainage catheter lies within the duodenum. Then, the transhepatic tract is dilated to an appropriate diameter for placement of the endoprosthesis. This is usually accomplished by exchanging the drainage catheter after 2 or 3 days. Typically, a 7 Fr catheter is used initially and a 9 Fr catheter replaces this catheter after a couple of days. After another 2 or 3 days, a 10 Fr endoprosthesis can be easily inserted

Table 45.1   Characteristics of currently available metallic stents

Type	Mechanism of expansion	Flexibility	Shortening during expansion	Pressure resistance
Gianturco	Self-expanding	Rigid	Minimal	High
Palmaz	Balloon expansion	Rigid	Minimal	High
Strecker	Balloon expansion	High	Minimal	Low
Medinvent	Self-expanding	High	30–50% of total length	Intermediate

transhepatically with patient discomfort at an acceptable level and without the risk of tissue trauma (Fig. 45.3B).

Transhepatic placement of large bore endoprostheses (>14 Fr) requires additional exchanges of catheters which is time-consuming and implies a higher risk of bleeding. Therefore, large bore endoprostheses are usually inserted in a combined endoscopic-transhepatic procedure ('rendezvous' manoeuvre, Brambs et al 1986). After transhepatic catheterization of the duodenum, biliary drainage is instituted for 2 or 3 days. Then the drainage catheter is removed over a 300 cm long guide-wire which is extracted transorally by the use of an endoscope (Fig. 45.4A). A large bore endoprosthesis is then pushed via the transoral end of the guide-wire over the biliary stenosis into the biliary tree (Fig. 45.4B, C).

The whole procedure requires two medical teams and necessitates transhepatic catheterization as well as transoral insertion of an endoscope into the duodenum. Thus, scheduling of the implantation of the endoprosthesis is naturally more difficult. The patient may be spared a second procedure, but the discomfort of the first procedure is considerably greater. For these reasons, the rendezvous manoeuvre is rarely performed in our institution.

Prior to placement of a metallic stent, internal-external drainage is also established for 2 or 3 days as described above. A 23 cm long catheter introduction sheath, with an appropriate inner diameter, is introduced into the biliary system over an Amplatz Extra Stiff Exchange Guide Wire (BSIC or Cook Co). The sheath is positioned

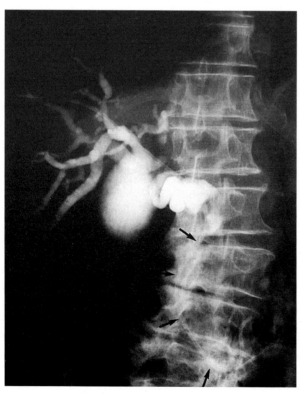

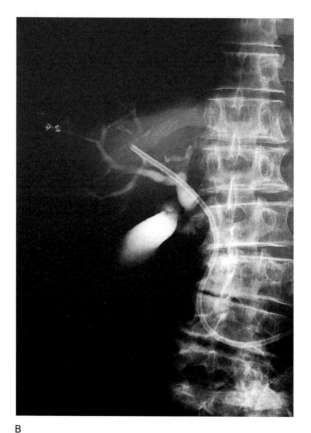

A

B

Fig. 45.3   Percutaneous cholangiogram in a patient with metastatic disease from gastric carcinoma. **A** The tip of the internal-external drainage catheter (arrows) is located in the duodenum. **B** Some days later, after removal of the drainage catheter a 20 cm long 10 Fr plastic endoprosthesis was positioned, providing bile flow across the tumour stenosis.

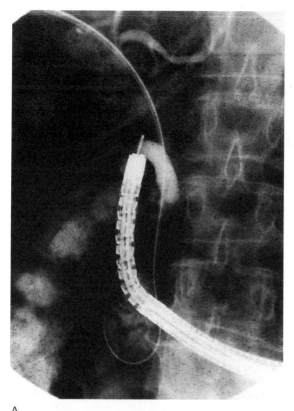

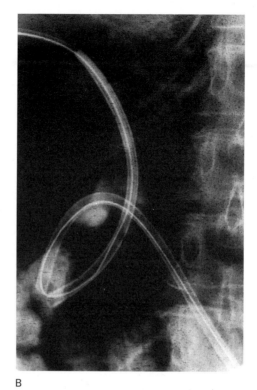

A

B

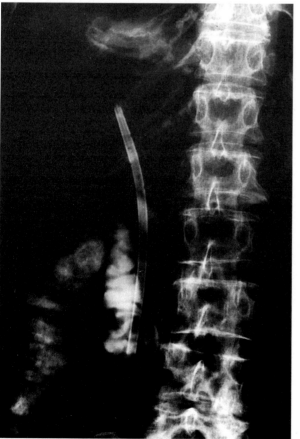

C

Fig. 45.4 Patient with carcinoma of the common bile duct. **A** A guide-wire was delivered through a transhepatic catheter sheath into the duodenal bulb. The endoscopist grasped the guide-wire in the duodenal bulb and extracted the guide-wire transorally. **B** A large bore plastic endoprosthesis was passed over the guide-wire through the papilla and the obstruction using a plastic pusher. **C** Final radiograph after positioning of the large bore endoprosthesis.

proximally to the biliary stenosis and a balloon catheter, with a 7 mm balloon of appropriate length, inserted for dilatation. After successful dilatation of the stenosis, the catheter is removed and the catheter carrying a stent of appropriate length is inserted into the sheath. Under fluoroscopic control the stent is carefully advanced into the stenosed segment of the bile duct. After accurate positioning, the stent is deployed either by inflating the balloon up to a pressure of 8 bar or by releasing the self-expanding metallic mesh (Strecker et al 1988, Adam et al 1991, Jaschke et al 1992). After expansion, the catheter is carefully removed in order to avoid displacement of the stent (Fig. 45.5A–C). If necessary additional stents can be placed overlapping each other.

RESULTS AND COMPLICATIONS

Patients considered for transhepatic biliary drainage can be divided into two groups: those requiring temporary drainage to improve their condition before surgery, and those requiring permanent intubation for palliation.

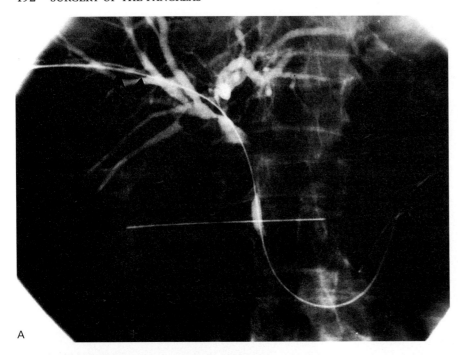

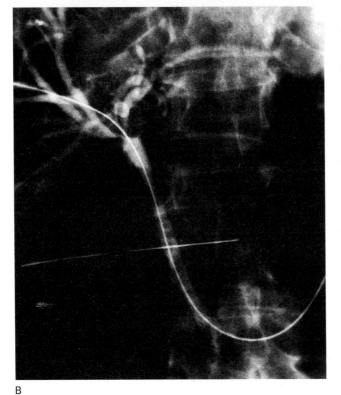

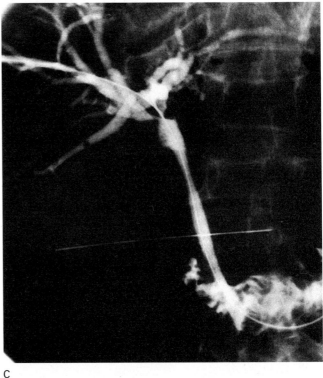

Fig. 45.5   Patient with metastatic disease from gastric carcinoma. **A** Arrows mark distal tip of catheter sheath inserted for stent placement. A guide-wire crosses the lesion obstructing the common bile duct. **B** A metallic biliary endoprosthesis was inserted reaching from hepatic bifurcation to the duodenum. **C** Adequate flow of contrast material through the endoprosthesis into the duodenum indicating a good result.

Temporary biliary drainage

The utility of percutaneous transhepatic biliary drainage (PTBD) as a preoperative measure to relieve symptoms of jaundice has been controversial (Denning et al 1981, Norlander et al 1982, Stambuck et al 1983, Gobien et al 1984, Gouma & Moody 1984, Gundry et al 1984, Passariello et al 1985, Trede & Schwall 1985). Although two studies concluded that PTBD led to a reduction in operative mortality and morbidity (Denning et al 1981, Gobien et al 1984), several other reports have challenged this view (Stambuck et al 1983, Gouma & Moody 1984, Gundry et al 1984, Sirinek & Levine 1989). The major criticism is that the morbidity of PTBD may offset the therapeutic benefit of the procedure (Stambuck 1983, Gouma & Moody 1984). This issue has not, however, been completely resolved since the morbidity added by transhepatic biliary drainage depends largely on the experience of the operator and the type of procedure. Thus, PTBD remains an option for preoperative biliary decompression, but it should not be used indiscriminately.

Permanent biliary drainage

PTBD is reserved for patients in whom endoscopic drainage fails and who are in a poor clinical state with an expected survival of just a few months (Tables 45.2, 45.3). In a retrospective analysis at our institution we found that the mean survival time is approximately 4 months and that only 5% of our patients survive more than 12 months. This is in agreement with other reports (Table 45.3) (Gobien et al 1984, Cohan et al 1986, Lammer & Neumayer 1986, Günther et al 1988). For example, Lammer & Neumayer (1986) reported a mean survival time of 5 months. The same authors state that only 8% of their patients were still alive after 1 year.

The mean survival time of patients with unresectable pancreatic carcinoma is well within this range (Feduska et al 1971). Only a minority of patients with inoperable pancreatic carcinoma survive longer than 1 year. The short survival time has to be considered when selecting the type of drainage procedure for these patients. Hospitalization for palliative treatment should be as short as possible. Patient discomfort caused by the procedure and the drainage device should also be minimized. Since the time of incrustation for plastic endoprostheses ranges from 20 to 35 weeks (Lammer et al 1986), we believe that internal drainage is the most appropriate form of palliative treatment for patients with unresectable pancreatic carcinoma. Several reports in the literature support this view (Huitbregtse & Tygat 1982, Mueller et al 1985, Lammer & Neumayer 1986, Dick et al 1987, Günther et al 1988, McLean & Burke 1989).

In a restrospective analysis of 109 patients, including 35 patients with pancreatic carcinoma, we found that approximately 20% of our patients required reintervention due to clogging of the 10 Fr endoprosthesis. Occlusion during the first 30 days after implantation was not observed in this series. The percentage of delayed

Table 45.2 Reasons for failure of endoscopic biliary drainage in 139 out of 604 cases. (Data collected at the Department of Endoscopy, Mannheim Hospital, University of Heidelberg, 1982–1987)

Duodenal stenosis	17
Cannulation of papilla impossible	57
Passage through duct stenosis impossible	60
Bleeding and other causes	5
Total	139 (23%)

Table 45.3 Long term prognosis after palliative treatment of malignant biliary stenosis

Authors	Number of patients	Mean duration of survival (weeks)
Gobien et al 1984	34	20
Cohan et al 1986	105	11
Lammer et al 1986	162	20
Günther et al 1988	24	18
Jaschke et al 1989*	168	13

* Unpublished data

occlusions is considerably higher than in the series reported by Lammer & Neumayer (1986), but lies within the range of the series reported by Mueller et al (1985). Lammer & Neumayer and Mueller et al used endoprostheses with an outer diameter of 9–14 Fr. Organic fibres from duodenal contents and bile ingredients are usually found in the obstructed lumen of the endoprosthesis (Groen et al 1987). Thus, it appears to be reasonable to assume that enterobiliary reflux, probably in combination with bacterial contamination of the plastic foreign body, is the leading cause for obstruction. Presently, there is no study proving that large bore endoprostheses are less prone to clogging than the widely used 10 Fr endoprosthesis.

Migration is another problem associated with the use of plastic endoprostheses. This occurred in approximately 3–6% of patients in two large series (Mueller et al 1985, Lammer & Neumayer 1986). We encountered this problem in less than 2% of our patient population.

Patients with endoprosthetic dysfunction can be managed either endoscopically or transhepatically. In most cases, when transpapillary cannulation of the bile duct failed initially, the occluded endoprosthesis can be removed and replaced endoscopically. If endoscopy is impossible due to duodenal stenosis or previous gastric surgery we insert another endoprosthesis transhepatically, without necessarily removing the occluded prosthesis.

Most of the above-mentioned problems should potentially be overcome by using metallic stents. However, initial reports did not confirm this expectation (Dick et al 1989, Irving et al 1989, Gillams et al 1990). For example, an early clinical trial with the Wallstent in 45 patients showed a rate of reobstruction of 42%, although this may have been related to the unfavourable patient population (Gillams et al 1990). In another more recent study with 41 patients the occlusion rate was only 7% (Adam et al 1991). Obstruction was due to progressive tumour growth above or below the stent. The median survival in the studied group of patients was 105 days. These favourable results are supported by data reported by Neuhaus et al (1990). The Gianturco-Stent was used by Coons and others for relief of benign and malignant biliary stenosis (Coons 1989, Irving et al 1989). The frequency of reocclusion varied between 10 and 50% (Coons 1989, Irving et al 1989). The poorer results were achieved in patients with malignant disease. At Mannheim, a preliminary study performed with the Strecker-Stent in 30 patients showed reocclusion in three of 22 patients (Strecker et al 1988, Jaschke et al 1992). All three patients suffered from unresectable pancreatic carcinoma. Occlusions were due to tumour growth through the wire mesh into the lumen. Thus, at present we caution against the use of metallic stents in this particular group of patients. Coated stents may solve this problem in the near future (Alvarado et al 1989). None of the patients with a malignant anastomotic stricture after a Whipple procedure demonstrated, however, invasion of the stent by tumour growth. Thus, implantation of metallic stents appears to be justified in this particular subgroup of patients.

Complications

Tables 45.4 and 45.5 give an overview of the complications associated with catheter drainage and placement of biliary endoprosthesis (Classen et al 1984). Infection is one of the major problems associated with non-surgical biliary drainage (Pollock et al 1979; Mueller et al 1982, 1985, Nilsson et al 1983, Classen et al 1984, Cohan et al 1986, Hamlin et al 1986, Hoevels 1986, Lammer & Neumayer 1986, Szabo et al 1987, Günther et al 1988). Procedure-related infective episodes have been reported with a frequency ranging from 21 to 47% (Classen et al 1984, Cohan et al 1986, Szabo et al 1987, Günther et al 1988). Cholangitis is even more frequent in patients on long-term drainage (Classen et al 1984), the rate varying from 32 to 64% (Classen et al 1984, Cohan et al 1986, Szabo et al 1987). As mentioned before, the rate of infection is considerably higher in patients with drainage catheters than in patients with endoprostheses or stents (Classen et al 1984, Cohan et al 1986, Szabo et al 1987). Blenkharn et al (1984) demonstrated that the frequency

Table 45.4 Complications of catheter drainage out of 2471 cases. (Data collected by Riemann et al, see Classen et al 1984)

Complication	Number of cases	% of total
Major		
Bile leakage/biliary peritonitis	49	2.0
Sepsis	42	1.7
Haemobilia	41	1.6
Haemorrhage	39	1.6
Abscess + other	12	0.5
Total	183	7.4
Minor		
Catheter displacement	164	6.6
Cholangitis	146	5.9
Hypotension	33	1.3
Hyponatraemia + others	32	1.3
Total	375	15.2
Fatal outcome (death due to procedure-related complications)	35	1.4

Table 45.5 Complications associated with placement of biliary plastic endoprosthesis, out of 493 cases. (Data collected by Riemann et al, see Classen et al 1984)

	Number of cases	% of total
Major complications	47	9.5
Minor complications	103	20.8
Death due to procedure-related complications	7	1.4

of bacteraemia can be diminished by an antiseptic barrier and use of a closed drainage system. Although contamination by environmental flora is an important factor in these patients, the most important cause in the pathogenesis of cholangitis is inadequate bile drainage. This may be due to malfunction of the drainage system or due to multiple duct obstruction.

Haemorrhage including haemobilia is another common problem of PTBD (Hoevels & Nilsson 1980, Classen et al 1984, Hoevels 1986). Clinically significant blood loss is, however, rarely observed. In large series, significant bleeding occurred in less than 2% of all patients (Classen et al 1984, Mueller et al 1985, Hoevels 1986, Lammer & Neumayer 1986). Biliary peritonitis is another dangerous complication which has to be expected in approximately 1–2% of patients (Classen et al 1984, Mueller et al 1985, Hoevels 1986, Lammer & Neumayer 1986). Acute duodenal perforation is mostly related to technical failures or to use of an inadequate type of endoprosthesis. Delayed perforations rarely cause clinical symptoms. Thus, the vast majority of perforations remain undetected. Death due to procedure-related complications is reported with a frequency of 0.8–3.2% (Classen et al 1984, Mueller et al 1985, Hoevels 1986, Lammer & Neumayer 1986).

Whenever possible, complications should be managed percutaneously since surgical procedures have a very high mortality rate in these terminally ill patients. Bleeding from arterial or portal venous branches is effectively controlled by embolization in most cases (Rosen & Rothberg 1982). CT-guided drainage is the method of choice for patients with bile leaks and abscesses (Lambiase 1991).

REFERENCES

Adam A, Chetty N, Roddie M, Yeung E, Benjamin I S 1991 Self-expandable stainless steel endoprostheses for treatment of malignant bile duct obstruction. American Journal of Radiology 156:321–325

Alvarado R, Palmaz J C, Garcia O J, Tio F O, Rees C R 1989 Evaluation of polymer-coated balloon-expandable stents in bile ducts. Radiology 170:975–978

Blamey S L, Fearon K C H, Gilmour W H et al 1983 Prediction of risk in biliary surgery. British Journal of Surgery 70:535–538

Blenkharn J I, McPherson G A D, Blumgart L H 1984 Septic complications of percutaneous transhepatic biliary drainage. Evaluation of a new closed drainage system. American Journal of Surgery 147:318–321

Brambs H J, Billmann P, Pausch J, Holstgege A, Salm R 1986 Non-surgical biliary drainage: endoscopic conversion of percutaneous transhepatic into endoprosthetic drainage. Endoscopy 18:52–54

Carrasco C H, Zornoza J, Bechtel W J 1984 Malignant biliary obstruction: complications of percutaneous biliary drainage. Radiology 152:343–346

Carrasco C H, Wallace S, Charnsangaval C, Richli W, Wright K C, Fanning T, Gianturco C 1985 Expandable biliary endoprosthesis: an experimental study. American Journal of Radiology 145:1279–1281

Classen M, Geenen J, Kawai K 1984 Non-surgical biliary drainage. Sringer-Verlag, Berlin

Cohan R H, Illescas F F, Saeed M, Perlmutt L M, Braun S D, Newman G E, Dunnick N R 1986 Infectious complications of percutaneous biliary drainage. Investigations in Radiology 21:705–706

Coons H G 1989 Self-expanding stainless steel biliary stents. Radiology 170:979–983

Coons H G 1990 Biliary intervention – technique and devices (commentary). Cardiovascular Interventional Radiology 13:211–216

Cope C 1982 Conversion from small (0.018 inch) to large (0.038 inch) guide wire in percutaneous drainage procedures. American Journal of Radiology 138:170–171

Denning D A, Ellison E C, Carey L C 1981 Preoperative percutaneous transhepatic biliary decompression lowers operative morbidity in patients with obstructive jaundice. American Journal of Surgery 141:61–63

Deviere J, Cremer M 1990 Endoscopic approach to malignant biliary obstruction (review and commentary). Cardiovascular Interventional Radiology 13(4):223–230

Dick R, Platts A, Gilford J, Reddy K, Irving D 1987 The Carey-Coons percutaneous biliary endoprosthesis: a three center experience in 87 patients. Clinical Radiology 38:175–178

Dick R, Gillams A, Dooley J S Hobbs K E F 1989 Stainless steel mesh stents for biliary strictures. Journal of Interventional Radiology 4:95–98

Dooly J S, Dick P, Kirk R M, Hobbs K E F 1984 Percutaneous transhepatic endoprosthesis for bile duct obstruction. Complications and results. Gastroenterology 86:605–609

Feduska N J, Dent T L, Lindauer S M 1971 Results of palliative operations for carcinoma of the pancreas. Archives of Surgery 103:330–334

Ferrucci J T, Müller P R, Harbin W P 1980 Percutaneous transhepatic biliary drainage. Radiology 135:1–13

Gillams A, Dick R, Dooley J S, Wallsten H, El-Din A 1990 Self-expandable stainless steel braided endoprosthesis for biliary strictures. Radiology 174:137–140

Gobien R P, Stanley J H, Soucek C D, Anderson M C, Vujic I, Gobien B S 1984 Routine preoperative biliary drainage: effect on management of obstructive jaundice. Radiology 152:353–356

Gould J, Train J S, Dan S J, Mitty H A 1988 Duodenal perforation as a delayed complication of placement of biliary endoprosthesis. Radiology 167:467–469

Gouma D J, Moody F G 1984 Preoperative percutaneous transhepatic drainage: use or abuse? Surgical Gastroenterology 3:74–80

Groen A K, Out T, Huitbregtse K, Delzenne B, Hoek F J, Tytgat G N J 1987 Characterization of the contents of occluded biliary endoprosthesis. Endoscopy 19:57–59

Gundry S R, Strodel W E, Kol J A, Eckhauser F E, Thompson N W 1984 Efficacy of preoperative biliary tract decompression in patients with obstructive jaundice. Archives of Surgery 119:703–708

Günther R W, Schild H, Thelen M 1988 Percutaneous biliary drainage: experience with 311 procedures (review article). Cardiovascular Interventional Radiology 11:65–71

Hamlin J A, Friedman M, Stein M G, Bray J F 1986 Percutaneous biliary drainage: complications of 118 consecutive catheterizations. Radiology 158:199–202

Healy J E, Schroy P C 1953 Anatomy of the bile ducts within the human liver. Archives of Surgery 66:599–616

Hoevels J 1986 Complications of percutaneous transhepatic biliary drainage. Annals of Radiology 29(2):148–150

Hoevels J, Ihse I 1979 Percutaneous transhepatic insertion of a permanent endoprosthesis in obstructive lesions of the extrahepatic bile ducts. Gastrointestinal Radiology 4:367–377

Hoevels J, Nilsson U 1980 Intrahepatic vascular lesions following nonsurgical percutaneous transhepatic bile duct intubation. Gastrointestinal Radiology 5:127–137

Hoevels J, Lunderquist A, Ihse I 1978 Percutaneous transhepatic intubation of bile ducts for combined internal-external drainage in preoperative and palliative treatment of obstructive jaundice. Gastrointestinal Radiology 3:23–31

Huitbregtse K 1984 Endoscopic biliary and pancreatic drainage. Thieme Verlag, Stuttgart

Huitbregtse K, Tytgat G N 1982 Palliative treatment of obstructive jaundice by transpapillary introduction of large bore bile duct endoprosthesis. Gut 23:371–375

Huitbregtse K, Cheng J, Coene P P L O, Fockens P, Tytgat G N J 1989 Endoscopic placement of expandable metal stents for biliary strictures. Endoscopy 21:280–282

Irving J D, Adam A, Dick R, Dondelinger R F, Lungerquist A, Roche A 1989 Gianturco expandable metallic biliary stents: results of a European clinical trial. Radiology 172:321–326

Jackson J E, Roddie M E, Yeung E Y C, Benjamin I S, Adam A 1990 Biliary endoprosthesis dysfunction in patients with malignant hilar tumors: successful treatment by percutaneous replacement of the stent. American Journal of Radiology 155:391–395

Jaques P F, Mandell V F, Delany D J, Nath P H 1982 Percutaneous transhepatic biliary drainage: advantages of left lobe subxiphoid approach. Radiology 145:534–536

Jaschke W, Klose K J, Strecker E P 1992 A new balloon expandable tantalum stent (Strecker-Stent™) for the biliary system: preliminary experience. Cardiovascular Interventional Radiology 15:356–359

Kadir S, Baassiri A, Barth K H, Kaufman S L, Cameron J L, White Jr R I 1982 Percutaneous biliary drainage in the management of biliary sepsis. American Journal of Radiology 138:25–29

Lambiase R E 1991 Percutaneous abscess and fluid drainage: a critical review. Cardiovascular Interventional Radiology 14:143–157

Lammer J, Neumayer K 1986 Biliary drainage endoprostheses: experience with 201 placements. Radiology 159:625–629

Lammer J, Stöffler G, Petek W W, Höfler H 1986 In vitro long term perfusion of different materials for biliary endoprostheses. Investigations in Radiology 21:329–331

Lee M J, Mueller P R, Saini S, Morrison M C, Brink J A, Hahn P F 1990 Occlusion of biliary endoprosthesis: presentation and management. Radiology 176:531–543

McLean G, Burke D R 1989 Role of endoprostheses in the management of malignant biliary obstruction. Radiology 170:961–967

Mendez G, Russel E, LePage J R, Guerra J J, Posniak R A, Trefler M 1984 Abandonment of endoprosthesis drainage technique in malignant biliary obstruction. American Journal of Radiology 143:617–622

Molnar W, Stockum A E 1974 Relief of obstructive jaundice through percutaneous transhepatic catheter – a new therapeutic method. American Journal of Radiology 122:356–367

Mueller P R, van Sonnenberg E, Ferrucci J T 1982 Percutaneous biliary drainage: technical and catheter related problems in 200 procedures. American Journal of Radiology 138:17–23

Mueller P R, Ferrucci J T, Teplick S K, van Sonnenberg E, Haskin P H, Butch R J, Papanicolaou N 1985 Biliary stent endoprosthesis: analysis of complications in 113 patients. Radiology 156: 637–639

Neuhaus H, Hagenmüller F, Griebel M, Rotter M, Classen M 1990 Endoskopische und perkutane Implantation selbstexpandierender Endoprothesen bei biliären Stenosen. Deutsche Medizinische Wochenschrift 115:1299–1306

Nilsson U, Evander A, Ihse I, Lunderquist A, Mocibob A 1983 Percutaneous transhepatic cholangiography and drainage: risks and complications. Acta Radiologica 24:433–439

Norlander A, Kalin B, Sunbald R 1982 Effect of percutaneous transhepatic drainage upon liver function and postoperative mortality. Surgery Obstetrics and Gynecology 155:161–166

Passariello R, Pavone P, Rossi P, Simonetti G, Mondini C, Lasagni R P, Manella P, Gazzaniga G M, Paolini R M, Feltrin V, Roversi R, Mallarini G 1985 Percutaneous biliary drainage in neoplastic jaundice: statistical data from a computerized multicenter investigation. Acta Radiologica 26:681–688

Pollock T W, Ring E J, Oleaga J A, Freiman D B, Mullen J L, Rosato

E F 1979 Percutaneous decompression of benign and malignant
biliary obstruction. Archives of Surgery 114:148–151

Ring E J, Oleaga J A, Freiman D B, Husted J W, Lunderquist A 1978
Therapeutic applications of catheter cholangiography. Radiology
128:333–338

Ring E J, Husted J W, Oleaga J A, Freiman D B 1979 A multihole
catheter for maintaining long term percutaneous antegrade biliary
drainage. Radiology 132:752–754

Rosen R J, Rothberg M 1982 Transhepatic embolization of hepatic
artery pseudoaneurysm following biliary drainage. Radiology
145:532–533

Schatz R A 1989 A view of vascular stents. Circulation 79:445–457

Shepard H A, Royle G, Ross A P R 1988 Endoscopic biliary
endoprothesis in the palliation of malignant obstruction of the distal
common bile duct: a randomized trial. British Journal of Surgery
75:1166–1169

Sirinek K R, Levine B A 1989 Percutaneous transhepatic
cholangiography and biliary decompression. Archives of Surgery
124:885–888

Stambuck E C, Pitt H A, Pias S O, Mann L L, Lois J F, Gomas A S
1983 Percutaneous transhepatic drainage – risks and benefits.
Archives of Surgery 118:1388–1394

Strecker E P, Berg G, Schneider B, Freudenberg N, Weber H, Wolf
R D 1988 A new vascular balloon-expandable prosthesis:
experimental studies and first clinical results. Journal of Interventional
Radiology 3:59–65

Szabo S, Mendelson M H, Bruckner H W, Hirschman S Z 1987
Infections associated with transhepatic biliary drainage devices.
American Journal of Medicine 82:921–926

Taber D S, Stoehlein J R, Zornoza J 1982 Hypotension and high
volume biliary excretion following external percutaneous transhepatic
biliary drainage (work in progress). Radiology 145:639–640

Trede M, Schwall G 1985 Nutzen und Risiko präoperativer
Gallendrainage aus chirurgischer Sicht. Deutsche Medizinische
Wochenschrift 110:556–560

Wittich G R, van Sonnenberg E, Simone J F 1985 Results and
complications of percutaneous biliary drainage. Seminars in
Interventional Radiology 2(1):473–489

46. Surgical palliation of pancreatic and periampullary tumours

P. C. Bornman   J. E. J. Krige

INTRODUCTION

The treatment of carcinoma of the pancreas is almost entirely palliative. Only 10–20% of tumours will be resectable at the time of diagnosis and even in these patients, survival beyond 5 years can be anticipated in no more than 10% (Warshaw 1984). Tumours of the body and tail are hardly ever resectable and are never curable (Moossa & Levin 1981). Overall survival is measured in months (median 4–5 months) and actual 5-year survival figures have been estimated to be only 0.4% (Gudjonsson et al 1978, Gudjonsson 1987). These gloomy survival statistics have remained unchanged, and with the alarming increase in its incidence, cancer of the pancreas has become one of the most important oncological challenges in developed countries (Williamson 1988).

The complexity of palliative treatment of pancreatic carcinoma is generally underestimated. There are several facets in the management of these patients that require careful judgement and expertise if appropriate palliative treatment is to be selected. More than 50% of patients are over the age of 70 years (Fentiman et al 1990) and they often have associated medical illnesses. Additional risk factors such as jaundice and poor nutritional status further compound management decisions. Although the mortality for palliative operations has improved considerably in specialized centres in recent years, morbidity figures have remained high (Dunn 1987). Unfortunately this is still often related to poor selection and intraoperative errors of judgement.

Decision-making in the palliative treatment of carcinoma of the pancreas has become more complex. Treatment options have broadened with the advent of non-operative stenting, and this has increased the demand for accurate staging, the need to establish tissue diagnosis and the need for more careful consideration of risk factors.

PREOPERATIVE ASSESSMENT

Tumour staging

Clinical evaluation and use of preoperative diagnostic tests have been covered in detail in Section 2. In the selection of appropriate palliative treatment, three categories of patients should ideally be identified: those with extensive metastatic disease; those with locally advanced disease, and those with potentially resectable lesions.

It is important to identify patients with metastatic disease and a short life expectancy. Unnecessary laparotomy, in which patients are explored only to find diffuse metastases precluding a bypass procedure is unacceptable and is still all too common. In a collected series of 2840 patients undergoing surgery for carcinoma of the pancreas, no fewer than 833 (29%) had laparotomy only (Table 46.1). The diagnosis of advanced disease is apparent when patients present with overt clinical metastases such as a Virchow–Troissier node, ascites, a palpable abdominal mass or an enlarged nodular liver. In such patients, active treatment should be withdrawn when these findings are supported by ultrasonography and confirmed by positive cytology.

In patients without clinically overt metastases the United States Tumor Study Group (Kalser et al 1985) have gone some way to identify those with advanced disease and a short life expectancy. Non-jaundiced patients who presented with pain from tumours originating in the body or tail of the pancreas had extensive disease with a poor prognosis.

An important finding in this study was that the performance status of patients, as determined by the Eastern Cooperative Oncology Group classification, was a reliable predictor of outcome in all stages of the disease. In this classification, patients with a status of 0 are fully ambulatory and symptom-free; status 1 means fully ambulatory, but with symptoms; status 2 patients are those who must stay in bed less than 50% of the day; status 3 patients are in bed more than 50% of the day, and status 5 patients are confined to bed all day. In patients with advanced disease, those with a performance status of 2 or 3 had a median survival of only 8 weeks.

The presence of liver and distant metastases portends a high postoperative mortality (Feduska et al 1971, Gillen &

Table 46.1   Operative procedures for pancreatic carcinoma

Author	Date	Period of study	Total operation	Laparotomy		Bypass		Resection	
				n	%	n	%	n	%
Feduska et al	1971	1959–70	98	22	22	60	61	16	16
Brooks & Culebras	1976	1964–70	79	25	31	39	44	20	25
Gudjonsson et al	1978	1960–71	84	34	40	49	58	1	1.2
Moossa et al	1979	1970–77	157	74	47	31	20	52	33
Brooks et al	1981	1974–78	92	21	19	53	48	18	16
Van Stiegmann et al*	1981	1975–79	107	29	27	62	58	3	3
Thompson & Walker	1983	1969–78	139	39	28	98	70	2	0.14
Kümmerle & Rückert	1984	1964–82	714	218	30	322	45	174	24
Trede	1985	1973–84	353	78	22	216	61	59	17
Matsumo & Sato*	1986	1960–85	272	84	31	105	39	45	18
Gillen & Peel	1986	1977–82	44	11	25	33	75	0	0
Gudjonsson*	1987	1972–81	165	54	33	97	59	8	5
Dunn*	1987	1960–82	190	69	36	99	52	22	12
Pedrazzoli et al	1987	1962–83	305	71	23	186	61	48	16
De Roos et al	1990	1979–88	41	4	10	28	68	9	22
Total			2840	833	29	1478	52	477	17

*Other procedures described are not included

Peel 1986) and short survival (Bonnel et al 1984). 'Real time' ultrasonography and the new generation of CT scanners have increased the diagnostic yield of metastatic disease, and cytological confirmation can usually be obtained by fine-needle aspiration. However, only two-thirds of liver nodules are visible on CT (Ward et al 1983) and the false negative rate increases substantially with tumours less than 2 cm in size (Warshaw et al 1990). In one study (Warshaw et al 1986), no fewer than 40% of small liver and peritoneal metastases detected on peritoneoscopy had been missed on CT, magnetic resonance imaging (MRI) and angiography. On the other hand it must be stressed that small benign haemangiomas and simple cysts of the liver may mimic metastatic disease, so that histological confirmation is essential before considering withdrawing active treatment.

Another subgroup of patients who should be identified before embarking on palliative treatment are those with locally advanced disease in whom the extent of tumour precludes a biliary decompression operation. Although few data are available with which to address this particular aspect, a large tumour bulk, the absence of a distended gallbladder on ultrasonography (Eyre-Brook et al 1983), and encroachment of the tumour on the confluence of the left and right hepatic ducts, best shown on CT or endoscopic retrograde cholangiopancreatography (ERCP), are useful indicators. In such patients non-operative stenting is more appropriate, thus avoiding unnecessary surgery.

The differentiation between resectable ('curable') and unresectable tumours remains problematic, despite the plethora of modern imaging techniques. A number of studies have evaluated the size of the tumour as a predictor of resectability. Nix and colleagues (1984) found that tumours <3 cm in diameter were always resectable while those >8 cm were seldom removable. However, size is not always a reliable indicator of resectability. In a study by Mackie et al (1979) some tumours as large as 6.5 cm were resectable while some lesions 2.5 cm in size were unresectable. A similar experience has been reported by others (Cubilla et al 1978, Hemmingsson et al 1982, de Roos et al 1990). The discrepancies in various series comparing tumour size and resectability may be due to factors such as differing criteria for resectability, overestimating tumour size due to associated inflammatory changes, and early infiltration of vital structures by small tumours. Other indices of unresectability such as gross nodal involvement and extrapancreatic extension on CT scan can be misleading (Wittenberg et al 1984), even in expert hands (Freeny et al 1988, Ross et al 1988). The role of angiography in the staging of pancreatic carcinoma has not been fully defined. In some series angiography has yielded disappointing results in predicting resectability (Mackie et al 1979, Warshaw et al 1990). The early enthusiasm for its use (Freeny & Ball 1978, Ferrucci & Wittenberg 1980, Levin et al 1980, Stanley et al 1980) has been tempered by the invasive nature of the procedure, coupled with the reluctance of many to accept angiography as the final arbiter in determining resectability in the presence of favourable CT scan findings.

The extent to which patients should be investigated before embarking on treatment will be determined largely by the strengths of imaging methods, availability of non-operative stenting facilities, financial constraints and the philosophy of treatment at any given institution. Those with a nihilistic approach would limit their preoperative investigation to a minimum, arguing that it is seldom justified to spend an excessive amount of health care money and time on staging a tumour with a dismal prognosis. Others, however, would pursue complex evaluation algorithms, including peritoneoscopy and angiography (Warshaw & Swanson 1988). For most, the standard diagnostic tests, including ultrasonography or CT and ERCP or percutaneous transhepatic cholangiography (PTC), will suffice in formulating rational treatment strategies.

Risk factors

Apart from associated medical illnesses, there are specific risk factors which need to be considered in patients with carcinoma of the pancreas when surgery is contemplated. These include hyperbilirubinaemia, malignancy and malnutrition, factors which may result in serious complications such as renal failure, coagulation disorders, gastrointestinal haemorrhage, sepsis and delayed wound healing.

Renal failure

Renal impairment remains a common complication of biliary obstruction. About two-thirds of patients have a fall in glomerular filtration rate (Bailey 1976, Cahill 1983) despite taking the necessary preoperative precautions, and one in 10 patients will develop frank renal failure (Pain et al 1985). The risk seems to correlate with the depth of jaundice (Dawson 1965a) and is a major cause of postoperative mortality (Williams et al 1960, Dixon et al 1983). The pathogenesis of renal failure in patients with obstructive jaundice is complex. Several mechanisms have been implicated including: hypovolaemia (Williams et al 1960), hyperbilirubinaemia with increased susceptibility to anoxic renal damage (Dawson 1964, 1968) and bile salt toxicity (Aoyagi & Lowenstein 1968). In recent years the endotoxin hypothesis has enjoyed much attention. Studies in animals (Cavanagh et al 1970, Wardle & Wright 1970, Bailey 1976) and man (Bailey 1976, Wilkinson et al 1976, Cahill 1983, Pain & Bailey 1987) have consistently shown a high incidence of endotoxaemia when obstructive jaundice is complicated by renal failure.

The current view on the mechanism of renal failure is that the absence of bile salts from the bowel leads to increased absorption of gut-derived endotoxin with consequent portal endotoxaemia. The study by Cahill (1983) suggests that the prevention of endotoxin absorption by bile salts is more likely to be due to a direct effect on the lipopolysaccharide molecule (Shands & Chun 1980) rather than the inhibitory effect of bacterial proliferation in the gut. Depressed Kupffer cell function in jaundiced patients allows endotoxins to enter the systemic circulation (Bradfield 1974) causing renal vasoconstriction (Cavanagh et al 1970), redistribution of blood flow away from the cortex, (Bomzon & Kew 1978) intravascular coagulation with fibrin deposition (Morrison & Ulevitch 1978, Allison et al 1979) and cortical necrosis. The mechanism of redistribution of blood flow in the kidney is complex (Wait & Kahng 1989). Both catecholamines (Bloom et al

1976) and prostaglandins (Zambraski & Dunn 1984) have been implicated in these pathophysiological disturbances.

Haemorrhage

Coagulation disorders due mostly to disseminated intravascular coagulation (Kunz et al 1974, Wardle 1974, Hunt et al 1982), and the increased tendency to gastric erosions (Armstrong et al 1984a, Dixon et al 1984) constitute major risk factors in patients undergoing interventional procedures and surgery. The incidence of postoperative bleeding varies from 6–21% (Pitt et al 1981, Hunt et al 1982, Dixon et al 1983, Blamey et al 1983) and the risk seems to increase with bilirubin levels exceeding 100 μmol/l (Blamey et al 1983), raised fibrin degradation products (Hunt 1980) and endotoxaemia (Wardle 1974, Hunt 1980, Hunt et al 1982). Patients who bleed from the gastrointestinal tract have a prohibitive mortality with figures of 33% (Pitt et al 1981) and 48% (Dixon et al 1983) being reported.

Sepsis

Despite the recommended use of prophylactic antibiotics (Meiyer et al, 1990) sepsis is still responsible for most of the postoperative morbidity and mortality. Several factors increase the susceptibility to sepsis. These include: impaired Kupffer cell function caused by endotoxaemia (Wardle & Wright 1970, Bradfield 1974); depression of specific (Roughneen et al 1986, Thompson et al 1990) and non-specific cellular immunity (Roughneen et al 1987) and associated malnutrition; malignancy and impaired renal function. Although bile is usually sterile in patients with carcinoma of the pancreas (Ishikawa et al 1980), sepsis may be introduced by interventional procedures such as ERCP and PTC, unless early surgical or non-operative decompression is instituted.

Wound healing

Delay in fibroblast migration (Lee 1972) and lowered prolylhydroxylase levels demonstrated in a number of studies reflect reduced collagen synthesis essential for tissue tensile strength (Than-Than et al 1974, Grande et al 1990). The impaired healing, however, is not only due to hyperbilirubinaemia. The biochemical changes are more marked (Irvin et al 1978, Grande et al 1990) and the incidence of wound dehiscence and incisional hernias is appreciably higher in patients with malignant rather than benign biliary obstruction. Grande et al (1990) also found that after biliary decompression, contrasting with benign conditions, skin prolylhydroxylase activity did not return to normal in malignant conditions. This suggests that additional factors such as malnutrition and postoperative sepsis play a more important role than hyperbilirubinaemia per se in impaired wound healing (Armstrong et al 1984b).

Predictors of morbidity and mortality

The evaluation of the effectiveness of preoperative biliary drainage, and the development of non-operative stenting as an alternative to palliative bypass operations, have stimulated a number of studies to identify risk factors that might influence prognosis and management (Table 46.2).

Pitt et al (1981), evaluated 15 potential risk factors in 155 patients undergoing biliary tract surgery. They found that three clinical and seven laboratory parameters were associated with an increased mortality. Using eight of these risk factors a simple scoring system could be formulated where the mortality increased progressively with an increasing number of risk factors (Table 46.2). This study also showed that renal failure, upper gastro-intestinal haemorrhage and intra-abdominal abscesses were associated with a significantly increased mortality. In order to limit the number of risk factors several authors have used multivariate analyses to identify independent risk factors (Blamey et al 1983, Dixon et al 1983, Bonnel et al 1984). The risk factors which emerged from these studies were malignancy, haematocrit <30%, albumin <30 g/l, creatinine >130 μmol/l, blood urea nitrogen (BUN) ≥20 mg/l, and bilirubin >200 μmol/l (Table 46.2).

Other workers have utilized computerized formulae to predict morbidity and mortality. Little (1987) calculated two formulae; a K value which reflected bilirubin clearance, and a mortality index (Table 46.3). Both formulae accurately predicted mortality which facilitated the clinical management and timing of surgical intervention. Buzby and colleagues (1980) working on the premise that malnutrition is an important prognostic factor in malignancy, formulated a linear predictive prognostic nutritional index (PNI). This index incorporated albumin, triceps skinfold measurement, serum transferrin and cutaneous delayed hypersensitivity (Table 46.4). The value of this formula, however, was limited by its low specificity in predicting intermediate and high-risk patients.

While jaundice was the common denominator in the foregoing studies, the patients in the population were suffering from a wide spectrum of conditions. With the exception of that of Bonnel et al (1984), the studies included a large proportion of patients with benign disease. There were also differences in the magnitude of the operative procedures, ranging from simple surgery for gallstone disease to major resections for biliary malignancies. The only study evaluating risk factors in a homogeneous group of patients with carcinoma of the pancreas comes from Padua, Italy (Pedrazolli et al 1987). The study included 126 patients undergoing bypass surgery and 48 resections. The order of stepwise discriminant values for complications and mortality in the bypass group, was weight loss (% usual weight), duration of jaundice, total blood protein levels, and the age of the patient. These four variables correctly predicted the outcome in 88% of patients who underwent bypass surgery. For those who underwent resection procedures the order of importance of

Table 46.2 Risk factors in biliary obstruction. In the Pitt et al scoring system, mortality related to the number of risk factors is: 0–2 = 0%, 3 = 4%, 4 = 7%, 5 = 44%, 6 = 67%, 8 = 100%

	Risk factors		% Mortality	
	Univariate analysis	Independent risk factors	Present	Absent
Pitt et al (1981)	Malignancy		20.0	3.5
	Age >60 years		16.2	1.2
	Albumin <30 g/l		41.2	3.2
	haematocrit <30%		43.8	3.8
	White blood cells >10 000/mm^3		18.4	3.0
	Total bilirubin 171 μmol/l		23.3	4.2
	Alkaline phosphatase > 100 i.u./l		15.5	1.3
	Creatinine >130 μmol/l		20.8	5.6
Dixon et al (1983)	Haematocrit <30%	Multiple logistic regression	40.9	2.3
	Total bilirubin >200 μmol/l	Multiple logistic regression	23.5	3.7
	Malignancy	Multiple logistic regression	26.1	3.7
Blamey et al (1983)	Age >60 years		32.6	12.5
	Haematocrit <30%		55.5	20.2
	White blood cells >10 000/mm^3		44.4	14.5
	Albumin <30 g/l	Linear discriminant analysis	61.1	14.1
	Creatinine >130 μmol/l	Linear discriminant analysis	100.0	13.9
Bonnel et al (1984)	Albumin <30 g/l	Multivariate logistic regression	28	13
	Haematocrit <30%		35	17
	Blood urea nitrogen (BUN) ≥20 mg/l	Multivariate logistic regression	43	14
	Creatinine >130 μmol/l		39	16
	Liver metastases		31	17
	Bilirubin >171 μmol/l		24	13

Table 46.3   Prediction of morbidity and mortality. Little (1987) calculated a 'K' value which reflected bilirubin clearance and a mortality index

$$K\ value = (0.0294 \times cholangitis\ score) - (0.002 \times ALT) + (0.0001 \times bilirubin) - (0.0343 \times sex) - 0.0769$$

$$Mortality\ index = (0.0016 \times creatinine) - (0.0227 \times albumin) + (0.0641 \times cholangitis\ score) + 0.6935$$

K value > −0.04 and mortality index >0.4 were associated with significantly higher mortality

Cholangitis score	Units
0 = afebrile	ALT (alanine aminotransferase) i.u./l
1 = temperature <37.5°C	Bilirubin µmol/l
2 = temperature >37.5°C	Creatinine µmol/l
3 = temperature >37.5°C and rigors and/or right quadrant pain	Albumin g/l
4 = fever with shock and/or mental obtundation	Sex: male = 1, female = 2

discriminant values was hypoproteinaemia, hyperbilirubinaemia, weight loss, and the patient's age. These correctly predicted outcome in 83% of patients. Unfortunately the use of a small random number of risk factors limited the conclusions from this study.

Despite the limitations of the above studies, cognizance should be taken of simple biochemical parameters, such as a low albumin or haematocrit or a raised creatinine, in the planning and preparation of definitive treatment in patients with malignant biliary obstruction. Hyperbilirubinaemia per se does not seem to constitute an independent risk factor and this may explain why patients with malignant biliary obstruction have not benefited significantly from preoperative biliary drainage.

PREOPERATIVE PREPARATION

In addition to treating associated medical conditions, special attention should be given to those risk factors specifically related to malignant biliary obstruction.

General management

The patient's state of hydration and renal function should be careful assessed. Serum urea and creatinine levels will detect gross renal dysfunction, but ideally a creatinine clearance test is required to identify early renal impairment. The vascular responsiveness to surgical trauma is impaired in patients with obstructive jaundice (Williams et al 1960)

and the risk of hypovolaemia is further increased by general anaesthesia. Adequate rehydration, correction of the haematocrit and initiating diuresis remain the most important measures in the prevention and treatment of renal failure. (Wait & Kahng 1989). The efficacy of mannitol (500 ml of a 10% solution infused over 1–2 hours) prior to, or during, surgery has been established in the prevention of renal failure (Dawson 1964, 1965b), and should be administered when conventional rehydration fails to establish a diuresis. The routine use of mannitol is probably unnecessary and over-enthusiastic administration may lead to hyponatraemia. Non-steroidal anti-inflammatory drugs should be avoided since their inhibitory effect on prostaglandin production may result in a decrease in both renal blood flow and glomerular filtration rate (Zambraski & Dunn 1984).

The administration of one or two doses of vitamin K usually corrects the deficient coagulation factors related to reduced absorption. Additional fresh frozen plasma may be needed in patients with associated liver disease. Disseminated intravascular coagulation requires more intensive therapy with the emphasis on controlling underlying sepsis or endotoxaemia.

A number of methods have been used to control endotoxaemia and its related complications. Preoperative administration of oral bile salts (sodium deoxycholate, 500 mg 8-hourly, for 48 hours preoperatively) prevents systemic endotoxaemia (Bailey 1976, Cahill 1983) and protects against postoperative renal failure (Evans et al

Table 46.4   The prognostic nutritional index of Buzby et al (1980)

$$Prognostic\ nutritional\ index\ (PNI) = 158 - (16.6 \times albumin) - (0.78 \times TSF) - (0.2 \times TFN) - (5.8 \times DH)$$

DH: cutaneous delayed hypersensitivity is reactivity to any of three recall antigens (mumps, streptokinase-streptodornase, candida)
Grade 0 = non-reactive
Grade 1 = <5 mm induration
Grade 2 = >5 mm induration

Units
Albumin g/l
TSF (triceps skinfold) mm
TFN (serum transferrin) mg/100ml

Mortality
Low risk, PNI <40% = 3%
Intermediate risk, PNI 40–49% = 4.3%
High risk, PNI ≥ 50% = 33%

1982, Cahill 1983). Its value, however, has been questioned in one randomized controlled study in humans (Thompson et al 1986). The cyclic polypeptide antibiotics, (polymixin B and colistin) which successfully interact with endotoxin in experimental animals (Ingoldby 1980) do not have a protective effect in man (Ingoldby et al 1984). The use of oral antibiotics to deal with Gram-negative endotoxin-producing organisms should be avoided as destruction of these organisms releases free endotoxin which may then be absorbed (Goto & Nakamura 1980). The use of oral lactulose has also been suggested, but its effect as a protector against endotoxaemia in obstructive jaundice has not been sufficiently investigated in man (Pain et al 1985).

Preoperative systemic antibiotics remain the most effective means of combating the effects of endotoxaemia and the increased susceptibility to sepsis. Antibiotic prophylaxis should be effective against coliforms as well as staphylococci which are frequently responsible for wound infection in malignant biliary obstruction (Keighley et al 1984, Willis et al 1984). A combination of penicillin and an aminoglycoside is commonly used but care should be taken with the latter in patients with renal impairment. The use of a second generation cephalosporin fulfils the same need and has the added advantage of being effective against staphylococci.

Preoperative biliary drainage

The role of preoperative biliary drainage (PBD) in reducing the high morbidity and mortality following surgery in obstructive jaundice has been the subject of intense study (Table 46.5). Although employed as early as 1952 by Carter & Saypol (1952), the reports by Nakayama et al (1978) and Denning et al (1981), led to the widespread use of PBD in malignant biliary obstruction. These studies were supported by other non-randomized studies (Ellison

et al 1984, Gundry et al 1984). However, even in expert hands (McPherson et al 1982) life-threatening complications related to PBD, such as haemorrhage, cholangitis, bile leakage, and fluid and electrolyte disturbance with renal failure, were common and, in most instances, unavoidable. The early enthusiastic reports were soon tempered by four randomized studies (Table 46.5). No significant benefit was shown and the high catheter-related complication rate often delayed definitive treatment, prolonged hospital stay and increased costs (Pitt et al 1985). There were, however, a number of shortcomings in these studies. Some included benign conditions while others had a high proportion of patients with cholangiocarcinoma undergoing major operations (McPherson et al 1984). Several multivariate analyses have shown that hyperbilirubinaemia is not an independent risk factor when limited to malignant biliary obstruction, and it is conceivable that the number of high-risk patients who could have benefited from PBD were too small to show a difference (Bonnel et al 1984). Furthermore in none of these studies was attention given to the correction of malnutrition which is a well recognized risk factor in malignant biliary obstruction.

In one controlled study (Foschi et al 1986), nutritional support as an adjunct to PBD was beneficial in reducing postoperative morbidity and mortality but catheter complications negated any potential benefits. The selection of patients who might benefit from prolonged hyperalimentation remains problematic, considering the doubtful benefit in patients with advanced malignant disease and a short life expectancy.

The routine use of preoperative antibiotics and the careful attention to other supportive measures such as rehydration and correction of anaemia and coagulation defects have to a large extent ameliorated the risks associated with obstructive jaundice. The high complication rate and the delay in definitive treatment have been largely responsible for abandoning the routine use of PBD. Its use

Table 46.5 Studies evaluating preoperative biliary drainage; n is the number of patients, figures in parentheses are percentages

	Biliary drainage			No biliary drainage		
	n	Morbidity (%)	Mortality (%)	n	Morbidity (%)	Mortality (%)
Non-randomized						
Nakayama et al 1977 [†]	49	—	4 (8)	148	—	36 (28)
Denning et al 1981 [†]	25	7 (28)*	4 (16)	32	18 (56)*	8 (25)
Norlander et al 1982 [†]	58	—	8 (14)	65	—	14 (21)
Bonnel et al 1984	79	—	— (9)	32	—	— (11)
Gundry et al 1984	25	2 (8)*	1 (4)*	25	13 (52)*	4 (20)*
Ellison et al 1984						
Palliative	17	3 (18)	1 (6)	10	2 (20)	0
Resections	7	4 (40)*	2 (28)*	10	6 (60)*	2 (28)*
Randomized studies						
Hatfield et al 1982[†]	20	4 (14)	4 (14)	29	4 (15)	4(15)
McPherson et al 1984	27	9 (33)	6 (22)	31	13 (42)	6 (19)
Pitt et al 1985[†]	37	16 (43)	3 (8)	38	20 (53)	2 (5)
Smith et al 1985[†]	15	10 (67)	3 (20)	15	2 (13)	1 (6)

[†] Studies included patients with benign disease. * p <0.05

is now restricted to selected cases with overt cholangitis that is not responding to intensive antibiotic therapy.

Surprisingly, the use of internal stenting which overcomes most of the disadvantages of external biliary drainage has only been studied in animals. In a randomized study in bile duct-ligated rats, Gouma et al (1987) achieved a significant reduction in mortality from 83% (untreated) to 25% with internal stenting, compared to an insignificant reduction to 63% with external drainage. The increasing use of endoscopic stenting as a definitive form of treatment in high-risk patients with advanced disease may explain why its application as a preoperative drainage procedure has not gained more widespread acceptance. It is also unlikely that internal stenting will substantially reduce morbidity and mortality in good risk patients with potentially resectable tumours. In this situation most surgeons (and patients) would prefer not to delay the definitive operation.

OBJECTIVES AND CHOICE OF PALLIATIVE TREATMENT

When planning the palliative treatment of carcinoma of the pancreas, it is important to define clearly the primary objectives in the individual patient. Optimal palliation should strive to alleviate symptoms effectively, thereby improving the quality of life and extending the period of useful survival, while minimizing the duration of hospital stay.

Obstructive jaundice is the most common symptom requiring palliation, occurring in 60–70% of patients seeking treatment. There are no controlled studies nor objective assessments to validate the importance of relieving jaundice, but few would argue with the contention that this is usually associated with an improvement in the patient's general performance status. The disappearance of the jaundice, which is a constant reminder to the patient (and his family) of the disease, also improves morale. There is no effective medical treatment for pruritis and it remains the most important indication for biliary drainage. Duodenal obstruction without jaundice is seldom a presenting symptom, and is usually due to advanced tumour originating in the uncinate process or body and neck of the pancreas. Most patients at presentation experience some degree of pain but this often becomes intractable as the disease progresses. The management of pain is often difficult, particularly during the terminal stage of the disease.

The advent of non-operative stenting has widened the scope of palliative treatment. Stenting is now the treatment of choice in poor operative risk patients and those with obvious advanced disease without duodenal obstruction (Cotton 1990). However, among these patients, there is a subgroup in whom active treatment should be withdrawn. These are patients of advanced age and poor performance status, particularly when the jaundice is unassociated with

pruritis and gross ascites is present. On the other hand younger and surgically fit patients with unresectable but localized tumour should be referred for surgery. They are more likely to live longer and the possible advantage of stenting will be gradually eroded by the need for frequent stent replacement and the increased risk of duodenal obstruction (Hatfield 1990).

In elderly but otherwise fit patients without overt metastatic disease the choice between palliative bypass surgery and non-operative stenting is less clear. Four randomized studies have now addressed this question, one using transhepatic stenting and three the endoscopic route (Table 46.6). In the transhepatically-placed endoprosthesis trial, Bornman et al (1986) found no major differences in hospital morbidity and mortality, overall hospitalization time (including readmissions) and survival. Endoscopic stenting is associated with less morbidity and mortality (Speer et al 1987), and the trend in favour of endoscopic stenting over bypass surgery shown in the first two randomized series (Shepherd et al 1988, Anderson et al 1989) was confirmed by a larger Middlesex study (Cotton 1990). While duodenal obstruction was a rare event, frequent clogging of the stents requiring readmission lessened the benefit of the initial shorter hospital stay. In all these studies, survival was similar and when quality of life was assessed in the Aarhus study (Anderson et al 1989) no benefit of one treatment over the other was noted.

From these studies it would appear that while there is little to choose between non-operative treatment and bypass surgery, stenting is preferred for the elderly and those with a short life expectancy, particular when they live close to centres with the necessary expertise. On the other hand it must be stressed that in many parts of the world facilities for stenting are not easily accessible, and bypass surgery remains the usual method of palliation.

PALLIATIVE SURGERY

The surgical options for palliation of carcinoma of the head of the pancreas range from a cholecystojejunostomy, with or without gastrojejunostomy, to a triple bypass. Despite careful preoperative evaluation, the final decision determining operative strategy is made at the time of laparotomy. Selection of the appropriate procedure will depend on:

1. tumour factors, including the presence of diffuse metastases, the size and extent of the primary tumour, proximal bile duct infiltration, cystic duct obstruction and the presence or absence of duodenal involvement
2. anatomical considerations such as previous biliary surgery (e.g. cholecystectomy), obesity, and mobility of the small bowel mesentery.

There remains unfortunately a group of patients with extensive disease, discovered unexpectedly at laparotomy,

Table 46.6   Randomized studies of bypass surgery versus stenting (figures in parentheses are percentages)

	Transhepatic	Endoscopic		
	Bornman et al (1986)	Shepherd et al (1988)	Anderson et al (1989)	Cotton (1990)
Bypass surgery				
No. of patients	25	25	25	103
Morbidity	8 (32)	14 (56)	5 (20)	— (28)*
Mortality	5 (20)	5 (20)	6 (24)	— (17)*
Hospital stay (days)	35	13*	27	—
Survival	15 weeks	124.5 days	100 days	5 months
Duodenal obstruction	3/21	1/4	0	— (1)*
Recurrent jaundice	3/19	0	4 (6)	— (3)*
Stenting				
No. of patients	25	23	25	101
Morbidity	7 (28)	7 (30)	9 (36)	— (10)*
Mortality	2 (8)	2 (9)	5 (20)	— (7)*
Hospital stay (days)	27	8*	26	—
Survival	19 weeks	152 days	84 days	5 months
Duodenal obstruction	0	2 (9)	0	— (6)*
Recurrent jaundice	8/21	7 (30)	7 (28)	— (18)*

*$p < 0.05$

in whom surgical palliation should not be attempted. These are patients with diffuse liver and peritoneal metastases, ascites, or porta hepatis involvement by tumour, factors which preclude safe and effective biliary bypass. Such patients should be referred for postoperative stenting unless gastrojejunostomy is required for duodenal obstruction.

Biliary and duodenal bypass

Surgical options for palliative biliary drainage are the anastomosis of either the gallbladder or bile duct to the jejunum or duodenum. External biliary drainage via a T-tube is unacceptable as it condemns patients to the discomfort and morbidity of an external biliary fistula for the remainder of their life. Drainage into the stomach using a cholecystgastrostomy, originally described by Whipple et al (1935) for preliminary biliary drainage prior to resection, is now of historic interest only.

Cholecystojejunostomy and choledochojejunostomy

Cholecystojejunostomy is still the most widely used method of palliative biliary decompression and has particular appeal in the high-risk patient. Easy access to the gallbladder and the readily available jejunum allow a technically easy and safe anastomosis which can be performed through a small abdominal incision or nowadays, by a laparoscopic approach.

Before selecting the gallbladder for biliary drainage, the surgeon must ensure that the cystic duct is patent and will remain so for a reasonable length of time. A tense distended gallbladder may be due to cystic duct obstruction and does not per se indicate communication with an obstructed common bile duct. The level of the cystic duct entry and its relationship to the obstructing carcinoma is the most

important factor in determining the selection of the gallbladder for biliary drainage. In 10% of patients the cystic duct descends parallel and in close proximity to the bile duct and enters the common bile duct low down (Singh & Reber 1989). Assessment of cystic duct compromise by tumour is notoriously difficult at operation, and the point of entry into the common bile duct may be impossible to define by inspection and palpation. Even careful dissection may not accurately determine the level of entry. Although the cystic duct may be patent at the time of surgery, there is a risk of occlusion by advancing tumour and early recurrent jaundice. It is therefore prudent to demonstrate not only patency of the cystic duct but also an adequate distance from the level of obstruction before embarking upon cholecystojejunostomy. If preoperative endoscopic or percutaneous transhepatic cholangiography are unhelpful, intraoperative cholangiography via the gallbladder may resolve the dilemma. No clear guidelines exist for the safe distance between anastomosis and tumour but a 2–3 cm gap seems reasonable (Singh & Reber 1989). If the cystic duct is not patent or entry is close to the obstructing tumour, the common bile duct should be used for decompression (Fig. 46.1).

The indiscriminate use of the gallbladder may have been responsible for the poor results reported in some studies. In the past some surgeons have proceeded to laparotomy without the benefit of preoperative cholangiography (Ubhi & Doran 1986). In an analysis of 600 patients who underwent biliary bypass (Table 46.7), 93 of 400 patients (23%) developed recurrent jaundice after cholecystojejunostomy compared to 14 of 200 patients (7%) after choledochojejunostomy. Ubhi & Doran (1986) reported an alarming 67% incidence of recurrent jaundice due to malignant occlusion of the cystic duct, compared to a significantly lower recurrence rate (17%) in patients who

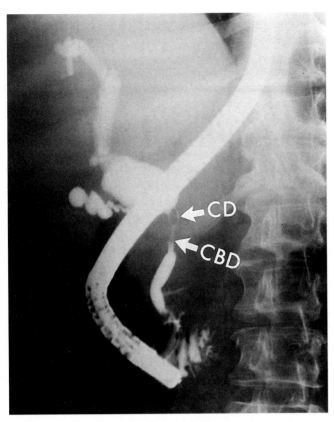

Fig. 46.1 Endoscopic retrograde cholangiogram showing common bile duct (CBD) and cystic and duct (CD) obstruction.

rate for jaundice after the two procedures was similar (13.5% vs. 13.1%).

In a prospective controlled trial assessing the efficacy of biliary enteric bypass (duodenum or jejunum) in non-calculous proximal biliary obstruction, Sarfeh et al (1988) found that cholecystenterostomy was significantly quicker to perform and was associated with less blood loss than choledochoenterostomy. In the 31 patients randomized, seven bypasses failed after use of the gallbladder and only two after using the bile duct (*p* < 0.04). Prior to death 47% of cholecystoenterostomies failed. Sarfeh concluded that choledochoenterostomy was a significantly more effective method of palliation and should be the procedure of choice. On the basis of these data, many authors have preferred the routine use of the common bile duct for palliative biliary drainage. Unfortunately in all these reports, including the only prospective randomized study (Sarfeh et al 1988), no uniform cholangiographic evaluation of cystic duct patency was obtained, nor is any explanation offered regarding the selection of patients or choice of biliary drainage.

In evaluating over 60 published series Sarr and Cameron (1984) did not find any clear advantage of choledo-chojejunostomy over cholecystojejunostomy in either operative mortality (16 vs. 20%) or survival (6.5 vs. 5.3 months). It is likely that the injudicious use of the gallbladder is largely reponsible for the poor results and for cholecystojejunostomy falling into disrepute as a palliative drainage procedure. Nevertheless, we continue to advocate the operation provided that cystic duct patency has been demonstrated. When prolonged survival is anticipated, common duct drainage is preferable.

Roux-en-Y and loop-jejunostomy

Because of the perception that the Roux-en-Y loop may be more difficult to perform and adds a further anastomosis to the procedure, some have argued against its use for palliation. On the other hand there is support for the use of Roux-en-Y loop on the basis of reduced reflux of intestinal contents which may lead to cholangitis (Singh &

had a bypass to the bile duct. Blievernicht et al (1980) reported persistent jaundice in six of 87 patients after cholecystojejunostomy while in seven additional patients jaundice recurred within 2–15 months of the initial procedure. The Brisbane group (Gough & Mumme 1984) reported failure of palliation in 14 of 53 patients when the gallbladder was used. In seven patients jaundice was not relieved and, in another seven, recurrent jaundice and cholangitis developed. In the UCLA experience, Singh et al (1990) found that biochemical jaundice cleared in only 42% of patients after cholecystojejunostomy, and in 32% of those who had a choledochojejunostomy. The recurrence

Table 46.7 Incidence of recurrent jaundice after palliative bypass using the common duct or gallbladder. Figures in parentheses are percentages

Author	Year	Total number of patients	Recurrent jaundice	
			Common duct (%)	Gallbladder (%)
Blievernicht et al	1980	108	0/21 (0)	13/87 (15)
Ross & Jonas	1980	55	0/9 (0)	3/46 (7)
Brooks et al	1981	34	1/10 (10)	0/24 (0)
Gough & Mumme	1984	66	0/13 (0)	14/53 (26)
Schouten	1986	41	1/23 (4)	5/18 (27)
Ubhi & Doran	1986	78	2/12 (17)	42/66 (67)
Potts et al	1990	84	2/52 (8)	6/23 (19)
Singh et al	1990	134	8/60 (13)	10/74 (14)
Total		600	14/200 (7)	93/400 (23)

Reber 1990). Sarr & Cameron (1984) found advantage of a Roux-en-Y over a simple loop cholecystojejunostomy in an analysis of 1100 patients. A Roux-en-Y anastomosis is preferable in selected patients when obesity or a large tumour mass make it difficult for the bowel to reach the porta hepatis without tension.

Cholecystoduodenostomy and choledochoduodenostomy

The duodenum has not been recommended for use in biliary decompression in malignant disease, as it has been for benign biliary obstruction, because of possible later encroachment by tumour. This concern has been confirmed by the UCLA group who found that jaundice persisted in one-third of patients when a choledochoduodenostomy, was used and in a further one-third of patients, jaundice recurred (Singh et al 1990). Proctor & Mauro (1990) reported a similar experience. The only support for cholecystoduodenostomy comes from the Cleveland Clinic group who reported a lower complication rate and superior efficacy compared to other drainage procedures (Potts et al 1990). While we concede that choledochoduodenostomy may be effective in selected patients, this procedure should be avoided in patients with a large mass or close proximity of the tumour to the first part of the duodenum.

Duodenal obstruction

Duodenal obstruction unassociated with jaundice is an uncommon initial presentation in pancreatic carcinoma and occurs in less than 5% of patients. This presentation usually signals advanced disease originating in the body or uncinate process of the pancreas with obstruction involving the third and fourth part of the duodenum. In contrast, duodenal involvement is more common in patients who present with jaundice and up to 30% will have evidence of mechanical obstruction of the second part of the duodenum. In addition there are some who have nausea and vomiting due to functional obstruction without evidence of duodenal involvement. Even in asymptomatic patients evidence of delayed emptying has been demonstrated on solid-phase gastric emptying studies (Barkin et al 1986). In patients who initially do not have symptoms of obstruction, the incidence increases progressively with prolonged survival (Gudjonsson 1987).

In patients with clinically overt gastric outlet obstruction the need for a gastrojejunostomy is clear. A bypass procedure is also indicated in the asymptomatic patient in whom there is evidence of duodenal infiltration or displacement by tumour on endoscopy, barium meal or at laparotomy. In the absence of incipient obstruction, the role of a prophylactic gastrojejunostomy remains controversial. Those in support of gastrojejunostomy cite the substantial incidence of later duodenal obstruction which may require

a second operation at a stage when further surgery is undesirable (Sarr & Cameron 1982). The argument against routine gastrojejunostomy centres around the added morbidity of a longer procedure and a further anastomosis, and potential stomal malfunction including impaired emptying, bile reflux or stomal ulceration. While both views have merit, the available data are insufficient to support a specific dogmatic approach.

Two major reviews have shown that 13–24% of patients undergoing palliative biliary bypass alone will eventually require reoperation for duodenal obstruction (Sarr & Cameron 1982, Gudjonsson 1987). In our review of 1452 patients in 24 reports published between 1980 and 1990, 17% of patients developed duodenal obstruction (Table 46.8). This incidence increases substantially the longer patients live. In the Yale–New Haven series, 47% of 1-year survivors developed duodenal obstruction and needed reoperation (Gudjonsson 1987).

Series documenting the incidence of subsequent duodenal obstruction may be misleading. The inclusion criteria are often not clearly defined and the high incidence reported in some studies may reflect poor selection. When a policy of selective gastric bypass was followed on the basis of operative assessment, in two Cape Town series (Bornman et al 1986, Van Stiegmann et al 1981) and one study from Sydney (Huang & Little 1987), the incidence of subsequent gastric outlet obstruction was 0%, 7% and 7% respectively.

Table 46.8 Incidence of duodenal obstruction after biliary bypass alone

Author	Year	Number of patients	% Requiring subsequent gastrojejunostomy
Appleqvist et al	1983	68	3
van Heerden et al	1980	76	6
Lee	1984	66	8
Parker & Postlethwaite	1985	55	9
Potts et al	1990	67	10
Brooks et al	1981	41	10
Schantz et al	1984	57	11
Rosenberg et al	1985	140	13
La Ferla & Murray	1987	62	13
Ross & Jonas	1980	44	14
Sarr et al	1981	53	15
Thompson & Walker	1983	96	16
Herter et al	1980	113	16
Nardi	1984	55	16
Wongsuwanporn & Basse	1983	40	18
Gough & Mumme	1984	29	21
Gudjonsson	1987	54	24
Singh et al	1990	80	25
Eastman & Kune	1980	31	26
Meinke et al	1983	105	30
Piorkowski et al	1982	42	38
Blievernicht et al	1980	34	38
Ubhi & Doran	1986	25	44
Bungay et al	1980	19	47
Total		1425	17

The argument against prophylactic gastrojejunostomy because of added morbidity and mortality has also not been substantiated. In a collected series of over 1100 patients the operative mortality (13 vs. 14%) and survival (5.6 vs. 6.4 months) were similar when compared to biliary bypass alone (Sarr & Cameron 1984). The perception that gastrojejunostomy in pancreatic cancer is often associated with stomal malfunction, including delayed emptying and bile reflux originates from a few dissenting reports (Doberneck & Berndt 1987, Weaver et al 1987). Weaver et al (1987) argue that effective palliation is rarely achieved in symptomatic patients with or without impingement on the duodenum. In their experience, 90% of patients had a poor outcome and they suggest that vomiting is in itself a harbinger of outcome failure. They indicated that a gastrojejunostomy does not facilitate, and may sometimes impair, gastric emptying and that patients without duodenal obstruction are not benefited by its gratuitous addition. These poor results do not, however, reflect the general experience and it is possible that most failures of gastrojejunostomy represent functional hold-up due to advanced disease.

We advocate a flexible approach when considering the need for duodenal bypass (Van Stiegmann et al 1981, Bornman et al 1986). Those patients with obvious duodenal involvement or encroachment by tumour should undergo gastrojejunostomy while bypass is avoided in those with advanced disease without overt evidence of duodenal obstruction. When longer survival is anticipated in patients with less extensive disease an argument can be made for a prophylactic gastrojejunostomy.

Despite careful perioperative care, palliative bypass surgery has a distressingly high morbidity and mortality. Several studies indicate that one-third of patients die in hospital following palliative bypass (Schouten 1986, Sonnenfeld et al 1986, Ubhi & Doran 1986). Doubt persists as to whether these unduly high figures represent a property intrinsic to the presence of risk factors associated with malignant biliary obstruction and associated medical illnesses in the elderly, or simply poor selection and inappropriate surgery.

Operative techniques

Cholecystojejunostomy. An intraoperative cholangiography via the gallbladder should be performed when patency of the cystic duct has not been confirmed on preoperative investigations. The gallbladder is then emptied using a trochar suction to facilitate construction of the anastomosis. The most mobile proximal loop of jejunum is selected and passed through the right transverse meso-colon. The apex of the jejunal loop is positioned alongside the gallbladder. The gallbladder and adjacent jejunum are opened along the length of the proposed stoma (about 5 cm) and a continuous single layer full-thickness suture

(3:0 synthetic monofilament) is inserted (Fig. 46.2). A locking stitch prevents narrowing of the stoma and minimizes the risk of bile leakage. An enteroanastomosis is probably superfluous (Sarr & Cameron 1984).

Hepaticojejunostomy. When the bile duct is selected for drainage, a Roux-en-Y 40 cm loop is preferable to an intact jejunal loop, especially when a large tumour mass is present. The additional length and easier handling of the single loop permit a technically easier high side-to-side hepaticojejunostomy. The gallbladder should be removed to facilitate construction of the common hepatic duct anastomosis, and to prevent the possible later complications of cystic duct obstruction (e.g. cholecystitis). A longitudinal or oblique choledochotomy allows for an easy and adequate anastomosis using the standard method for high biliary-enteric anastomosis (Fig. 46.3). The Roux-en-Y jejunal loop is prepared in the standard fashion and passed to the subhepatic space through the right transverse meso-colon. A row of interrupted sutures is first placed through the anterior wall of the bile duct to avoid overlapping by pouting jejunal mucosa. The advantage of this technique is improved exposure for the accurate placement of all sutures. With the jejunum and bile duct apposed, the posterior layers are inserted and then tied on the inside. The anterior row is then completed using the previously placed sutures.

Gastrojejunostomy. When required, an antecolic gastrojejunostomy is preferable, to lessen the possibility of subsequent infiltration by tumour. The debate about whether this anastomosis should be sited proximal or distal to the biliary anastomosis is unresolved. The risk of stomal

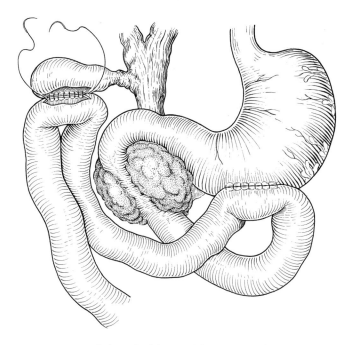

Fig. 46.2 Antecolic isoperistaltic gastrojejunostomy and cholecystojejunostomy.

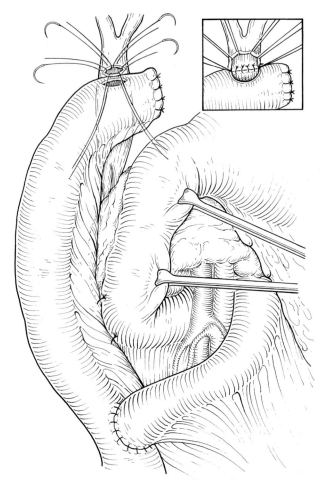

Fig. 46.3   Side-to-side Roux-en-Y hepaticojejunostomy. Inset: placement of sutures before tying facilitates an accurate mucosa-to-mucosa anastomosis.

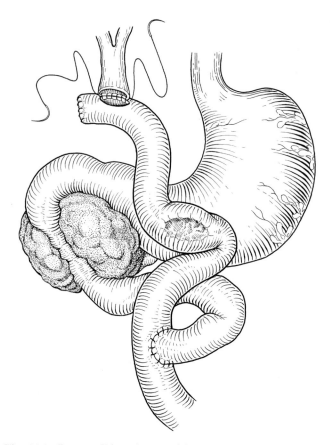

Fig. 46.4   Roux-en-Y hepaticogastrojejunostomy.

ulceration in the former and the development of troublesome bile reflux in the latter, have been overemphasized. The sequence of anastomoses should be determined instead by anatomical convenience rather than possible adverse pathophysiological considerations. Since the risk of stomal ulceration is negligible with a proximal gastrojejunostomy (Sarr & Cameron 1984), we prefer this arrangement to avoid the occasional problem of bile reflux encountered with a distal gastrojejunostomy. On the other hand, when a Roux-en-Y loop is used for the biliary decompression, the same limb can be used for a gastrojejunostomy when required (Fig. 46.4).

Resection for palliation

One of the arguments in favour of resection is that although cure is seldom achieved, removal of the tumour bulk provides better palliation and survival than bypass surgery. Such views are difficult to substantiate as most patients undergoing resection have less extensive disease than those undergoing palliative bypass operations. No controlled data are available and it is unlikely that such studies will ever be mounted because of the lack of sufficient numbers and biased views of surgeons who would not deny their patients with potentially resectable tumours the glimmer of hope for a cure. The most widely quoted studies by Crile (1970) and Shapiro (1975) comparing bypass surgery with resection for comparable localized tumours to the head of the pancreas concluded in favour of bypass surgery. Morbidity and mortality was lower after bypass surgery and survival figures were equivalent. Lund et al (1968) came to a similar conclusion and in the series reported by Hertzberg (1974), patients who had bypass surgery survived longer than those who underwent resection. In contrast both Mongé (1967) and Hermreck et al (1974) found that resection provided longer palliation and survival than bypass, in patients with small carcinomas of the head of the pancreas.

The major consideration in the choice between resection and bypass surgery centres around operative morbidity and in particular mortality of the two procedures. With the increasing number of specialized units, mortality figures of below 5% are now frequently reported (Crist et al 1987, Trede 1987). Therefore the argument that resection for carcinoma should not be undertaken if the operative mortality exceeds the 5-year survival has largely fallen away.

Most resections start with the intention of cure, only to find unexpected spread beyond the pancreatic capsule and/or lymph node involvement. The decision to perform a palliative resection can only be made by an experienced pancreatic surgeon, who is qualified to make the critical judgement of the risk/benefit ratio of such a radical procedure (Carter 1990). It remains unacceptable to carry out a resection operation when it is clear from the beginning that macroscopic clearance of tumour cannot be safely achieved.

PAIN RELIEF

Although pain is a common presenting symptom with carcinoma of the pancreas, occurring in about 50% of patients (Singh & Reber 1989), it is seldom severe at the onset and can usually be controlled by non-narcotic analgesics. The severity of pain often intensifies with disease progression and may become the most difficult and demoralizing symptom requiring palliation during the terminal stages of the disease. Many patients will require large doses of opiates which in itself interferes with their quality of life. Pain is mostly due to local tumour infiltration rather than duct or bowel obstruction. Biliary and gastric bypass seldom afford pain relief (Flanigan & Kraft 1978, Singh & Reber 1989) and the reputed benefit of pancreatic duct drainage advocated by some (Catell 1947, Gallitano et al 1968) is no longer justified considering the additional risk involved.

Chemical splanchnicectomy, either at the time of surgery (Bridenbaugh et al 1964, Copping et al 1969, Flanigan & Kraft 1978, Gardner & Solomon 1984) or percutaneously under radiological control, is now being increasingly advocated for pain relief. In a study by Flanigan & Kraft (1978) using intraoperative phenol injections of the coeliac plexus, 28 of 32 patients experienced pain relief for most of their remaining survival. This was significantly better than the four of 19 historic controls, who underwent bypass surgery alone. Gardner & Solomon (1984) using a similar technique found that 30 of 37 patients experienced relief of pain and in 26 (70%) this persisted until death. The accurate delivery of intraoperative chemical splanchnicectomy may be hampered by tumour bulk and in this situation better results can be achieved by a percutaneous technique using either biplanar X-ray screening (Gorbitz & Leavens 1971) or CT scanning (Moore et al 1982, Filshie et al 1983). Leung et al (1983) have achieved similar results to surgical splanchnicectomy by the injection of 25ml of 75% alcohol under radiological control. Of 13 cancer patients 11 had complete relief initially, and seven remained free of pain at the time of death. Similar results were reported by Jones and Gough (1977) and from a group in Italy (Ventafridda et al 1990). Apart from transient postural hypotension, chemical splanchnicectomy is generally a safe procedure.

Although rare, nerve root pain and more serious lower limb weakness or loss of bladder and anal sphincter function have been reported (Leung et al 1983).

Regrettably, pain control is often neglected. A wide range of analgesics is now available and should be prescribed according to a set protocol. In larger centres early consultation with a pain clinic is often helpful, particularly with regard to the timing of chemical splanchnicectomy. The more liberal use of intraoperative chemical splanchnicectomy in patients who present with pain has merit and surgeons should familiarize themselves with this technique which does not add much to the operating time. The method used by Flanigan & Kraft (1978) allows easy and safe access to the coeliac plexus and splanchnic nerves. The lesser omentum is opened between the lesser curve of the stomach and the liver and the abdominal aorta is identified between the index and middle finger above the superior border of the pancreas. Using a 20 or 50 ml syringe and a long 18-gauge needle, 40 ml of 5% phenol in almond oil or 75% alcohol is injected retroperitoneally on each side and in front of the aorta. Repeated aspiration is necessary to avoid the possibility of intravascular injection.

SUMMARY

The palliative treatment of carcinoma of the pancreas has become more complex with the plethora of imaging techniques available for diagnosis and staging and the alternative option of non-operating stenting. Treatment is no longer the exclusive domain of the surgeon and patients are being increasingly referred to radiologists and endoscopists in the hope of achieving safer and simpler palliation. This conservative trend has come as no surprise, considering the short life expectancy and the poor results often associated with surgical palliation in this disease. The fragmentation of treatment has raised concern that some patients may receive inappropriate treatment, particularly those with possibly resectable tumours and those in whom the diagnosis cannot be confirmed histologically.

There is now a pressing need for the multidisciplinary approach to patients with carcinoma of the pancreas. The issue no longer is whether surgery or stenting is better, but rather which procedure is best for the individual patient. Close consultation at an early stage between the referring physician, surgeon, endoscopist and radiologist is essential to plan appropriate diagnostic and treatment strategies. Intervention must be governed by clearly defined objectives for palliation based on risk factors, staging and severity of symptoms. Patients and their family require careful counselling and it is important to resist the temptation of trying to accommodate unrealistic expectations.

In competent hands, non-operative stenting is now the method of palliation of choice in elderly high-risk patients and those with advanced disease. The lack of expertise outside referral centres has, however, limited its widespread application. Stent blockage, and its attendant complications requiring readmission to hospital, remain a major stumbling block especially in patients who live longer. Although it is not always possible to predict prolonged survival, operative bypass is the preferred treatment in the surgically fit patient, when appropriate and technically feasible.

REFERENCES

Allison M E M, Prentice C R M, Kennedy A C, Blumgart L H 1979 Renal function and other factors in obstructive jaundice. British Journal of Surgery 66: 392–397.

Anderson J R, Sorenson S M, Kruse A, Rokkjaer M, Matzan P 1989 Randomised trial of endoscopic endoprosthesis versus operative bypass in malignant obstructive jaundice. Gut 30:1132–1135

Aoyagi T, Lowenstein L M 1968 The effect of bile acids and renal ischaemia on renal function. Journal of Laboratory and Clinical Medicine 71: 689–692

Appelqvist P, Viren M, Minkkinen J, Kajanti M, Kostiainen S, Rissanen P 1983 Operative finding, treatment and prognosis of carcinoma of the pancreas: an analysis of 267 cases. Journal of Surgical Oncology 23: 143–150

Armstrong C P, Dixon J M, Taylor T V, Davis G C 1984a Surgical experience of deeply jaundiced patients with bile duct obstruction. British Journal of Surgery 71: 234–238

Armstrong C P, Dixon J M, Duffy S W, Elton R A, Davies G C 1984b Wound healing in obstructive jaundice. British Journal of Surgery 71: 267–270

Bailey M E 1976 Endotoxin, bile salts and renal function in obstructive jaundice. British Journal of Surgery 63: 774–778

Barkin J S, Goldberg R I, Sfakianakis G N, Levi J 1986 Pancreatic carcinoma is associated with delayed gastric emptying. Digestive Diseases and Sciences 31: 265–267

Blamey S L, Fearson K C H, Gilmour W H, Osborne D H, Carter D C 1983 Prediction of risk in biliary surgery. British Journal of Surgery 70: 535–538

Blievernicht S W, Neifeld J P, Terz J J, Lawrence W L 1980 The role of prophylactic gastrojejunostomy for unresectable periampullary carcinoma. Surgery, Gynecology and Obstetrics 151:794–796

Bloom D, Bomzon L, Rosendorff C et al 1976 Renal blood flow in obstructive jaundice: an experimental study in baboons. Clinical and Experimental Pharmacology and Physiology 3: 461–472

Bomzon L, Kew M C 1978 Renal blood flow in obstructive jaundice: the baboon as an experimental model. In: Epstein M (ed): The kidney in liver disease. New York, Elsevier p 167–183

Bonnel D, Ferrucci J T, Muller P R, Lacaine F, Peterson H F 1984 Surgical and radiological decompression in malignant biliary obstruction: A retrospective study using multivariate risk factor analysis. Radiology 152:347–351

Bornman P C, Harries-Jones E P, Tobias R, van Stiegmann G, Terblanche J 1986 Prospective controlled trial of transhepatic biliary endoprosthesis versus bypass surgery for incurable carcinoma of head of pancreas. Lancet 1:69–71

Bradfield J W B 1974 Control of spillover: the importance of Kupffer cell function in clinical medicine. Lancet 2:883–886

Bridenbaugh L D, Moore D C, Campbell D D 1964 Management of upper abdominal cancer pain: Treatment with coeliac plexus block with alcohol. Journal of the American Medical Association 190:877–890

Brooks J R, Culebras J M 1976 Cancer of the pancreas. Palliative operation, Whipple procedure or total pancreatectomy. American Journal of Surgery 131: 516–520

Brooks D C, Osteen R T, Gray E B, Steele G D, Wilson R E 1981 Evaluation of palliative procedures for pancreatic cancer. American Journal of Surgery 141: 430–433

Bungay K, Dennistone S, Hunt P S 1980 Duodenal obstruction and carcinoma of the head of the pancreas. Medical Journal of Australia 2:150–151

Buzby G P, Mullen J L, Matthews D C, Hobbs C L, Rosato E F 1980 Prognostic nutritional index in gastrointestinal surgery. American Journal of Surgery 139:160–167

Cahill C J 1983 Prevention of post-operative renal failure in patients with obstructive jaundice – the role of bile salts. British Journal of Surgery 70:590–595

Carter D C 1990 Cancer of the pancreas. Gut 31:494–496

Carter R F, Saypol M G 1952 Trans-abdominal cholangiography. Journal of the American Medical Association 148:253–255

Cattell R B 1947 Anastomosis of the duct of Wirsung. Surgical Clinics of North America 27:636–643

Cavanagh D, Rao P S, Sutton D M C, Dev Bhagat B, Bachmann F 1970 Pathophysiology of endotoxin shock in the primate. American Journal of Obstetrics Gynecology 108:705–722

Copping J, Willix R, Kraft R 1969 Palliative chemical splanchnicectomy. Archives of Surgery 98:418–420

Cotton P B 1990 Management of malignant bile duct obstruction. Journal of Gastroenterology and Hepatology Suppl. 1:63–77

Crile G 1970 The advantages of bypass operations over radical pancreatoduodenectomy in the treatment of pancreatic carcinoma. Surgery, Gynecology and Obstetrics 130:1049–1053

Crist D W, Sitzmann J V, Cameron J L 1987 Improved hospital morbidity, mortality and survival after the Whipple procedure. Annals of Surgery 206:358–365

Cubilla A L, Fitzgerald P J, Fortner J G 1978 Pancreas cancer-duct cell adenocarcinoma: survival in relation to site, size, stage and type of therapy. Journal of Surgical Oncology 10: 465–482

Dawson J L 1964 Jaundice and anoxic renal damage: protective effect of mannitol. British Medical Journal 1:810–811

Dawson J L 1965a The incidence of postoperative renal failure in obstructive jaundice. British Journal of Surgery 52:633–665

Dawson J L 1965b Post-operative renal function in obstructive jaundice: effect of a mannitol diuresis. British Medical Journal 1:82–86

Dawson J L 1968 Acute postoperative renal failure in obstructive jaundice. Annals of the Royal College of Surgeons of England 42: 163–181

Denning D A, Ellison E C, Carey L C 1981 Preoperative percutaneous transhepatic biliary decompression lowers operative morbidity in patients with obstructive jaundice. American Journal of Surgery 141:61–65

De Roos W K, Welvaart K, Bloem J L, Hermans J 1990 Assessment of resectability of carcinoma of the pancreatic head by ultrasonography and computed tomography. A retrospective analysis. European Journal of Surgical Oncology 16:411–416

Dixon J M, Armstrong C P, Duffy S W, Davies G C 1983 Factors affecting morbidity and mortality after surgery for obstructive jaundice. A review of 373 patients. Gut 24:845–852

Dixon J M, Armstrong C P, Duffy S W, Elton R A, Davies G C 1984 Upper gastrointestinal bleeding: A significant complication after surgery for relief of obstructive jaundice. Annals of Surgery 199:271–275

Doberneck R C, Berndt G A 1987 Delayed gastric emptying after palliative gastrojejunostomy for carcinoma of the pancreas. Archives of Surgery 122:827–829

Dunn E 1987 The impact of technology and improved perioperative management upon survival from carcinoma of the pancreas. Surgery, Gynecology and Obstetrics 164:237–244

Eastman M C, Kune G A 1980 The objectives of palliative surgery in pancreas cancer: a retrospective study of 73 cases. Australian and New Zealand Journal of Surgery 50:462–464

Ellison E C, van Aman M E, Carey L C 1984 Preoperative transhepatic biliary decompression in pancreatic and periampullary cancer. World Journal of Surgery 8:862–871

Evans H J R, Torrealba V, Hudd C, Knight M 1982 The effect of pre-operative bile salt administration on postoperative renal function in patients with obstructive jaundice. British Journal of Surgery 69:706–708

Eyre-Brooke I A, Ross B, Johnson A G 1983 Should surgeons operate on the evidence of ultrasound alone in jaundiced patients? British Journal of Surgery 70:587–589

Feduska N J, Dent T L, Lindenauer S M 1971 Results of palliative operations for carcinoma of the pancreas. Archives of Surgery 103:330–334

Fentiman I S, Tirelli U, Monfardini S, Schneider M, Festen J, Cognetti F, Aapro M S 1990 Cancer in the elderly: why so badly treated? Lancet 1:1020–1022

Ferrucci J T, Wittenberg J 1980 A comprehensive approach for diagnosing pancreatic disease. Radiology 136:255–256

Filshie J, Golding S, Robbie D S, Husband J E 1983 Unilateral computerised tomography guided coeliac plexus block: a technique for pain relief. Anaesthesia 38: 498–503

Flanigan D P, Kraft R O 1978 Continuing experience with palliative chemical splanchnicectomy. Archives of Surgery 113:509–511

Foschi D, Cavagna G, Callioni F, Morandi E, Rovati V 1986 Hyperalimentation of jaundiced patients on percutaneous transhepatic biliary drainage. British Journal of Surgery 73:716–719

Freeny P C, Ball T J 1978 Evaluation of endoscopic retrograde cholangiopancreatography and angiography in the diagnosis of pancreatic carcinoma. American Journal of Roentgenology 130:683–691

Freeny P C, Marks W M, Ryan J A Traverso L W 1988. Pancreatic ductal adenocarcinoma: Diagnosis and staging with dynamic CT. Radiology 166:125–133

Gallitano A, Fransen H, Martin R G 1968 Carcinoma of the pancreas Cancer 22:939–944

Gardner A M N, Solomon G 1984 Relief of the pain of unresectable carcinoma of pancreas by chemical splanchnicectomy during laparotomy. Annals of the Royal College of Surgeons of England 66:409–411

Gillen P, Peel ALG 1986 Failure to improve survival by improved diagnostic techniques in patients with malignant jaundice. British Journal of Surgery 74:631–633

Gorbitz C, Leavens M E 1971 Alcohol block of the celiac plexus for control of upper abdominal pain caused by cancer and pancreatitis. Journal of Neurosurgery 34:575–579

Goto H, Nakamura S 1980 Liberation of endotoxin from *Escherichia coli* by addition of antibiotics. Japanese Journal of Experimental Medicine 50:35–43

Gouma D J, Coelho J C U, Schlegel J F, Li Y F, Moody F G 1987 The effect of preoperative internal and external biliary drainage on mortality of jaundiced rats. Archives of Surgery 122:731–734

Gough I R, Mumme G 1984 Biliary and duodenal bypass for carcinoma of the head of the pancreas. Journal of Surgical Oncology 26:282–284

Grande L, Garcia-Valdecasas J S, Fuster J, Visa J, Pera C 1990 Obstructive jaundice and wound healing. British Journal of Surgery 77:440–442

Gudjonsson B 1987 Cancer of the pancreas: 50 years experience. Cancer 60:2284–2303

Gudjonsson B, Livstone E M, Spiro H M 1978 Cancer of the pancreas; diagnostic accuracy and survival statistics. Cancer 42:2494–2506

Gundry S R, Strodel W E, Knol J A, Eckhauser F E, Thompson W 1984 Efficacy of preoperative biliary tract decompression in patients with obstructive jaundice. Surgery, Gynecology and Obstetrics 119:703–708

Hatfield A R W 1990 Palliation of malignant biliary obstruction – surgery or stent? Gut 31:1339–1340

Hatfield A R W, Tobias R, Terblanche J et al 1982 Preoperative external biliary drainage in obstructive jaundice. Lancet 2:896–899

Hemmingsson A, Jacobson G, Lindgren P G, Lönnerholm T, Lörelius L E, Nordgren C E 1982 Radiologic assessment of resectability of carcinoma of the head of the pancreas. Acta Radiologica 23:127–130

Hermreck A S, Thomas C Y, Friesen S R 1974 Importance of pathologic staging in the surgical management of adenocarcinoma of the exocrine pancreas. American Journal of Surgery 127:653–657

Herter F P, Cooperman A M, Ahlborn T N, Antinori C 1980 Surgical experience with pancreatic and periampullary cancer. Annals of Surgery 195:274–281

Hertzberg J 1974 Pancreaticoduodenal resection and bypass operation in patients with carcinoma of the head of the pancreas, ampulla, and distal end of the common duct. Acta Chirurgica Scandinavica 140:523–527

Huang J F, Little J M 1987 Malignant jaundice. Australian and New Zealand Journal of Surgery 57:905–908

Hunt D R 1980 The identification of risk factors and their application to the management of obstructive jaundice. Australian and New Journal of Medicine 50:476–480

Hunt D R, Allison M E M, Prentice C R M, Blumgart L H 1982 Endotoxaemia, disturbance of coagulation and obstructive jaundice. American Journal of Surgery 144:325–329

Ingoldby C J H 1980 The value of polymixin B in endotoxaemia due to experimental obstructive jaundice and mesenteric ischaemia. British Journal of Surgery 67:565–567

Ingoldby C J, McPherson G A D, Blumgart L A 1984 Endotoxaemia in obstructive jaundice. Effect of polymixin B. American Journal of Surgery 147:766–771

Irvin T T, Vassilakis J S, Chattopanhyay D K, Greaney M G 1978 Abdominal wound healing in jaundiced patients. British Journal of Surgery 65:521–522

Ishikawa Y, Oshi I, Miyoni M et al 1980 Percutaneous transhepatic drainage: experience in 100 cases. Journal of Clinical Gastroenterology 2:305–314

Jones J, Gough D 1977 Coeliac plexus block with alcohol for relief of upper abdominal pain due to cancer. Annals of the Royal College of Surgeons of England 59:46–49

Kalser M H, Barkin J, MacIntyre J M 1985 Pancreatic cancer: Assessment of prognosis by clinical presentation. Cancer 56:397–402

Keighley M R, Razay G, Fitzgerald M G 1984 Influence of diabetes on mortality and morbidity following operations for obstructive jaundice. Annals of the Royal College of Surgeons of England 66:49–51

Kümmerle F, Rückert K 1984 Surgical treatment of pancreatic cancer. World Journal of Surgery 8:889–894

Kunz F, Amor H, Hortnagl G, Weiser F, Folzknecht F, Braustein H 1974 Disseminierte intravasculare Gerinnung und letale Makrothrombosierung bei einem Patienten unt Gallenwegskarzinom. Deutsche Medizinische Wochenschrift 99:2643–2647

La Ferla G, Murray W R 1987 Carcinoma of the head of the pancreas: bypass surgery in unresectable disease. British Journal of Surgery 74:212–213

Lee M 1972 The effect of obstructive jaundice on the migration of reticulo-endothelial cells and fibroblasts into early experimental granulomata. British Journal of Surgery 59:875–877

Lee Y N 1984 Surgery for carcinoma of the pancreas and periampullary structures: complications of resectional and palliative procedures. Journal of Surgical Oncology 27:280–285

Leung J W C, Bowen-Wright M, Aveling W, Shorvon P J, Cotton P B 1983 Coeliac plexus block for pain in pancreatic cancer and chronic pancreatitis. British Journal of Surgery 70:730–732

Levin D C, Wilson R, Abrams H L 1980 The changing role of pancreatic arteriography in the era of computed tomography. Radiology 136:245–249

Little J M 1987 A prospective evaluation of computerized estimates of risk in the management of obstructive jaundice. Surgery 102:473–476

Lund F 1968 Carcinoma of the pancreas. Palliative or radical surgery? Acta Chirurgica Scandinavica 134:461–465

Mackie C R, Dhorajiwala J, Blackstone M O, Bowie J, Moossa A R 1979 Value of new diagnostic aids in relation to the disease process in pancreatic cancer. Lancet 2:385–389

Mackie C R, Lu C T, Noble H G, Cooper M J, Collins P, Block G E, Moossa A R 1979 Prospective evaluation of angiography in the diagnosis and management of patients suspected of having pancreatic cancer. Annals of Surgery 189:11–17

McPherson G A D, Benjamin I S, Habib N A, Bowley I B, Blumgart L H 1982 Percutaneous transhepatic drainage in obstructive jaundice: advantages and problems. British Journal of Surgery 69:261–264

McPherson G A D, Benjamin I S, Hodgson H J F, Bowley N B, Allison D J, Blumgart L H 1984 Pre-operative percutaneous transhepatic biliary drainage: the results of a controlled trial. British Journal of Surgery 71:371–375

Matsumo S, Sato T 1986 Surgical treatment of cancer of the pancreas: Experiences in 272 patients. American Journal of Surgery 152:499–503

Meinke W B, Twomey P L, Guernsey J M, Frey C F, Higgins G, Keehn R 1983 Gastric outlet obstruction after palliative surgery for cancer of head of pancreas. Archives of Surgery 118:550–553

Meiyer W S, Schmitz P I M, Jeckel J 1990 Meta-analysis of randomised, controlled clinical trials of antibiotic prophylaxis in biliary tract surgery. British Journal of Surgery 77:283–290

Mongé J J 1967 Survival of patients with small carcinomas of the head of the pancreas. Biliary–intestinal bypass vs pancreatoduodenectomy. Annals of Surgery 166:908–912

Moore D C, Bush W H, Burnett L 1982 An improved technique for coeliac plexus block may be more theoretical than real. Anaesthesiology 57:347–348

Moossa A R, Levin B 1981 The diagnosis of 'early' pancreatic cancer: The University of Chicago experience. Cancer 47:1688–1697

Moossa A R, Lewis M H, Mackie C 1979 Surgical treatment of pancreatic cancer. Mayo Clinic Proceedings 54:468–474

Morrison D C, Ulevitch R J 1978 The effects of bacterial endotoxins on most medication systems. American Journal of Pathology 93:525–618

Nakayama T, Ikeda A, Okuda K 1978 Percutaneous transhepatic drainage of the biliary tract. Technique and results in 104 cases. Gastroenterology 74:554–559

Nardi G 1984 Pancreatic cancer and palliative gastroenterostomy. American Journal of Surgery 147:839–840

Nix G A J J, Schmitz P I M, Wilson J H P, van Blankenstein M, Groeneveld C F M, Hofwijk R 1984 Carcinoma of the head of the pancreas: Therapeutic implications of endoscopic retrograde cholangiopancreatography findings. Gastroenterology 87:37–43

Norlander A, Kalin B, Sundblad R 1982 Effect of percutaneous transhepatic drainage upon liver function and post operative mortality. Surgery, Gynecology and Obstetrics 155:161–166

Pain J A, Bailey M E 1987 Measurement of operative plasma endotoxin levels in jaundiced and non-jaundiced patients. European Surgical Research 19:207–216

Pain J A, Cahill C J, Bailey M E 1985 Preoperative complications in obstructive jaundice: therapeutic considerations. British Journal of Surgery 72:942–945

Parker G A, Postlethwaite R W 1985 The continuing problem of carcinoma of the pancreas. Journal of Surgical Oncology 28:36–38

Pedrazzoli S, Bonadimani B, Sperti C, Cappellazzo F, Piccoli A, Militello C 1987 Forecast of surgical risk in pancreatic cancer. American Journal of Surgery 153:374–377

Piorkowski R J, Blievernicht S W, Lawrence W, Madariaga J, Horsly J S, Neifeld P J, Terz J J 1982 Pancreatic and periampullary carcinoma: experience with 200 patients over a 12 year period. American Journal of Surgery 143:189–193

Pitt H A, Cameron J L, Postier R G, Gadacz T R 1981 Factors affecting mortality in biliary tract surgery. American Journal of Surgery 141:66–72

Pitt H A, Gomes A S, Louis J F, Mann L L, Deutsch L S, Longmire W P 1985 Does pre-operative percutaneous biliary drainage reduce operative risk or increase hospital cost? Annals of Surgery 201:545–553

Potts J R, Broughan T A, Herman R E 1990 Palliative operations for pancreatic carcinoma. American Journal of Surgery 159:72–78

Proctor H J, Mauro M 1990 Biliary diversion for pancreatic carcinoma: matching the methods and the patient. American Journal of Surgery 159:67–71

Rosenberg J M, Welch J P, Macaulay W P 1985 Cancer of the head of the pancreas: an institutional review with emphasis on surgical therapy. Journal of Surgical Oncology 28:217–221

Ross H, Jonas R A 1980 The results of surgery for carcinoma of the pancreas. Australian and New Zealand Journal of Surgery 50:454–458

Ross C B, Sharp K W, Kaufman A J, Andrews T, Williams L F 1988 Efficacy of computerized tomography in the preoperative staging of pancreatic carcinoma. American Journal of Surgery 54:221–226

Roughneen P T, Gouma D J, Kulkarni A D, Fanslow W F, Rowlands B J 1986 Impaired specific cell-mediated immunity in experimental biliary obstruction and its reversibility by internal biliary drainage. Journal of Surgical Research 41:113–125

Roughneen P T, Drath D B, Kulkarni A D, Rowlands B J 1987 Impaired non-specific cellular immunity in experimental cholestasis. Annals of Surgery 206: 578–582

Sarfeh I J, Rypins E B, Jakowatz J G, Juler G L 1988 A prospective randomized clinical investigation of cholecystoenterostomy and choledochoenterostomy. American Journal of Surgery 155:411–414

Sarr M G, Cameron J L 1982 Surgical management of unresectable carcinoma of the pancreas. Surgery 91:123–133

Sarr M G, Cameron J L 1984 Surgical palliation of unresectable carcinoma of the pancreas. World Journal of Surgery 8:906–918

Sarr M G, Gladen H E, van Heerden J A 1981 Role of gastroenterostomy in patients with unresectable carcinoma of the pancreas. Surgery, Gynecology and Obstetrics 152:597–600

Schantz S P, Schickler W, Evans T K, Coffey R J 1984 Palliative gastroenterostomy for pancreatic cancer. American Journal of Surgery 147:793–796

Schouten J T 1986 Operative therapy for pancreatic carcinoma. American Journal of Surgery 151:626–630

Shands Jr J W, Chun P W 1980 The dispersion of gram negative lipopolysaccharide by deoxycholate. Journal of Biological Chemistry 255:1221–1226

Shapiro T M 1975 Adenocarcinoma of the pancreas: a statistical analysis of biliary bypass vs. Whipples resection in good risk patients. Annals of Surgery 12:715–721

Shepherd H A, Royle G, Ross A P R, Diba A, Arthur M, Colin-Jones D 1988 Endoscopic biliary endoprosthesis in the palliation of malignant obstruction of the distal common bile duct: a randomized trial. British Journal of Surgery 75:1166–1168

Singh S M, Reber H A 1990 Surgical palliation for pancreatic cancer. Surgical Clinics of North America 63:599–611

Singh S M, Longmire W P, Reber H A 1990 Surgical palliation of pancreatic cancer. Annals of Surgery 212:132–139

Smith R C, Pooley M, George C R P, Faithful G 1985 Preoperative percutaneous transhepatic internal drainage in obstructive jaundice: a randomized controlled trial examining renal function. Surgery 97:641–648

Sonnenfeld T, Nyberg B, Perbeck L 1986 The effect of palliative biliodigestive operations for unresectable pancreatic cancer. Acta Chirurgica Scandinavica (Suppl) 530:47–50

Speer A G, Cotton P B, Russell R C G et al 1987 Randomised trial of endoscopic versus percutaneous stent insertion in malignant obstructive jaundice Lancet 1:57–62

Stanley R J, Sagel S J, Evans R G 1980 The impact of new imaging methods on pancreatic arteriography. Radiology 136:251–253

Than Than, McGee J O, Sokhi G S, Patrick R S, Blumgart L H 1974 Skin prolylhydroxylase in patients with obstructive jaundice. Lancet 2:807–808

Thompson J F, Walker C J 1983 The management of pancreatic carcinoma: a review of 173 cases. Australian and New Zealand Journal of Surgery 53:25–30

Thompson J N, Cohen J, Blenkharn J I, McConnell J S, Barr J, Blumgart L H 1986 A randomized clinical trial of oral ursodeoxycholic acid in obstructive jaundice. British Journal of Surgery 73:634–636

Thompson R L E, Hoper M, Diamond T, Rowlands B J 1990 Development and reversibility of T lymphocyte dysfunction in experimental obstructive jaundice. British Journal of Surgery 77:1229–1232

Trede M 1975 The surgical treatment of pancreatic carcinoma. Surgery 97:28–35

Trede M 1987 Treatment of pancreatic carcinoma: the surgeon's dilemma. British Journal of Surgery 74:79–80

Ubhi C S, Doran J 1986 Palliation for carcinoma of head of pancreas. Annals of the Royal College of Surgeons of England 68:158–162

Van Heerden J A, Heath P M, Alden C R 1980. Biliary bypass for ductal adenocarcinoma of the pancreas: Mayo Clinic experience 1970–1975. Mayo Clinic Proceedings 55:537–540

Van Stiegmann G, Bornman P C, Terblanche J 1981 Carcinoma of the pancreas at Groote Schuur Hospital, 1975–1979. South African Medical Journal 60:97–99

Ventafridda G V, Caraceni A T, Sbanotto A M, Barletta L, de Conno F 1990 Pain treatment in cancer of the pancreas. European Journal of Surgical Oncology 169:1–6

Wait R B, Kahng K U 1989 Renal failure complicating obstructive jaundice. American Journal of Surgery 157:256–263

Ward E M, Stephens D H, Sheedy P R 1983 Computed tomography characteristics of pancreatic carcinoma: An analysis of 100 cases. Radiographics 3:547–565

Wardle E N 1974 Fibrinogen in liver disease. Archives of Surgery 109:741–746

Wardle E N, Wright N A 1970 Endotoxin and acute renal failure associated with obstructive jaundice. British Medical Journal 4:472–474

Warshaw A L 1984 Progress in pancreatic cancer. World Journal of Surgery 8:801–802

Warshaw A L, Swanson R S 1988 Pancreatic cancer in 1988: Possibilities and probabilities. Annals of Surgery 208:531–533

Warshaw A L, Tepper J E, Shipley W U 1986 Laparoscopy in the staging and planning of therapy for pancreatic carcinoma. American Journal of Surgery 151:76–80

Warshaw A L, Zhuo-yun G U, Wittenberg J, Waltman A C 1990 Preoperative staging and assessment of resectability of pancreatic cancer. Archives of Surgery 125:230–233

Weaver D W, Wiencek R G, Bouwman D L, Walt A J 1987 Gastrojejunostomy: is it helpful for patients with pancreatic cancer? Surgery 102:608–613

Whipple A O, Parsons W B, Mullins C R 1935 Treatment of carcinoma of the ampulla of Vater. Annals of Surgery 102:763–779

Wilkinson S P, Moodie H, Stamatakis J D, Kakkar V V, Williams R 1976 Endotoxaemia and renal failure in cirrhosis and obstructive jaundice: British Medical Journal 2:1415–1418

Williams R D, Elliott D W, Zollinger R M 1960 The effect of hypotension in obstructive jaundice. Archives of Surgery 81:182–188

Williamson R C N 1988 Pancreatic cancer: the greatest oncological challenge. British Medical Journal 296:445–446

Willis R G, Lawson W C, Hoare E M, Kingstone R D, Sykes P A 1984 Are bile bacteria relevant to septic complications after biliary surgery? British Journal of Surgery 71:845–849

Wittenberg J, Ferrucci J T, Warshaw A L 1984. Contribution of computer tomography to patients with pancreatic adenocarcinoma. World Journal of Surgery 8:831–838

Wongsuwanporn T, Basse E 1983 Palliative surgical treatment of sixty-eight patients with carcinoma of the head of the pancreas. Surgery, Gynecology and Obstetrics 156:73–75

Zambraski E J, Dunn M J 1984 Importance of renal prostaglandins in control of renal function after chronic ligation of the common bile duct in dogs. Journal of Laboratory and Clinical Medicine 103:549–559

47. Chemotherapy and radiotherapy in the treatment of pancreatic cancer

J. Jeekel

INTRODUCTION

Cancer of the pancreas is a silent and rather unknown disease: silent with regard to symptoms because its position gives rise to complications only at a relatively late stage of the disease; unknown because most physicians do not see many patients with pancreatic cancer. Patients do not live long once the diagnosis is established, and this may explain the fatalistic approach towards the disease. Yet cancer of the pancreas occurs frequently in the Western world and is the fourth leading cause of death from cancer.

Surgical resection is the only known curative treatment, as it is for many cancers, but can only play a role in a small percentage of cases. In the majority of patients the disease has spread beyond surgical curative options by the time of presentation. In these cases, other forms of treatment should be considered. Probably the best way to improve the results of surgical treatment of pancreatic cancer is to develop and apply additional non-surgical treatment. This should be considered when there is microscopic and macroscopic extension of the tumour beyond its primary location in the pancreas. Microscopic dissemination is in fact present in most cases of resectable cancer of the pancreas, and adjuvant treatment must be considered in these patients. The same philosophy applies to the peroperative spill of tumour cells which may lead to intra-abdominal recurrence. Treatment may also be considered for locally advanced unresectable tumour without the presence of metastases. Finally, recurrence of tumour may sometimes be amenable to treatment. Unfortunately, most patients fall into one of these categories. In some 75% of the cases the tumour is unresectable or metastases are present. The median survival time in such patients varies from 3–10 months. Even if the tumour is resectable, metastases still develop in around 95% of cases. Surgical treatment is only advantageous in a small percentage of all patients with pancreatic cancer, prolonging life in less than half and achieving cure in 0–5% of the patients. A better life expectancy might be provided if other treatment modalities could be added to the surgical arsenal or used to replace surgery.

DIAGNOSTIC PROCEDURES

It is of great importance to establish accurately the nature of the disease before treatment is commenced. Unnecessary laparotomy should be avoided, particularly in patients with metastatic disease. Chest X-ray and an ultrasound investigation of the abdomen by an experienced radiologist are often sufficient to establish the stage of the disease. The more expensive CT scan (and magnetic resonance imaging, MRI) will not usually add further knowledge. Ultrasound-guided biopsies are not mandatory as they may give false negative information, a problem encountered with small early carcinomas (e.g. in villous adenoma) as well as with larger tumours. Resectability cannot be easily established by diagnostic procedures. Exact measurement of the size of the tumours is not possible because concurrent pancreatitis affecting the surrounding tissue may mimic tumour tissue. An angiogram may be helpful and demonstrate ingrowth of cancer in vascular structures but is far from infallible (see Ch. 37). If no metastases have been demonstrated, a laparotomy should be performed to establish resectability. A biopsy should always be taken at laparotomy to establish the nature of the disease.

TREATMENT IN PATIENTS WITH DISTANT METASTASES

Surgery should be avoided in the presence of distant metastases, because operative mortality in these patients is relatively high. If surgery is not contemplated, histological confirmation of metastases by ultrasound-guided puncture is mandatory.

Generally there is no place for active treatment in patients with distant metastases. Pancreatic cancer is a fast-spreading disease with a short life expectancy. Median survival time in patients with distant metastases is 3–4 months. In these last few months of life there is only place for the treatment of symptoms and alleviation of discomfort. Chemotherapy may be considered in patients who are in relatively good condition but only when it is part of a

515

coordinated prospective study. Surgical relief of obstructive disease should be avoided. The operative mortality of gastroenterostomy or choledochojejunostomy in these patients is high, in most series between 6 and 24% (Morrow et al 1984). In addition, a gastroenterostomy in pancreatic cancer is often not functional for weeks to months. An endoprothesis in the bile duct is, at this stage of the disease, a good alternative to bypass surgery (Laméris et al 1987).

Metastatic pancreatic disease may in some cases progress slowly, particularly in the case of endocrine tumours (Eriksson et al 1990).

TREATMENT OF UNRESECTABLE PANCREATIC TUMOURS

Resectability can only be fully assessed by laparotomy, performed by an experienced surgeon. Even then, accurate assessment is not always possible. Invasion of surrounding tissue may be caused by inflammatory cells and this can only be distinguished by pathological examination of an excised specimen, which obviously is not a realistic option in these cases. If concomitant metastases cannot be found at laparotomy, the local extent of the tumour should be carefully determined. In its typical anatomical position the pancreas is intimately associated with the duodenum, small bowel mesentery, superior mesenteric vein and artery, and the portal vein. Tumour infiltration in these structures may occur at an early stage, without manifest distant metastases. At this stage of the disease it is often not possible to assess accurately whether one is confronted by pancreatic or periampullary cancer. Neither is it possible to assess the exact nature of infiltration in surrounding tissue. Other forms of locally invasive digestive tract cancer, such as colon or gastric cancer, can often be treated by adequate en bloc resection (Papachristou et al 1981, Kroneman et al 1991). Distant metastases may not have developed in such cases, and this may also be the case in pancreatic cancer.

Radiotherapy

Unfortunately, such en bloc resection is usually not possible in locally invasive pancreatic cancer. Yet, treatment should be considered, as a chance for cure may exist in the absence of distant metastases. Unresectable localized pancreatic cancer without manifest distant metastases may be treated by local radiotherapy combined with 5-fluorouracil therapy. The value of this combined treatment has been described in a study conducted by the Gastrointestinal Tumor Study Group (GITSG) (Moertel et al 1981). Histological diagnosis of the cancer should be obtained in all cases. Therapy now consists of 50 Gy external beam radiation to the upper abdomen, concomitant with intravenous 5-fluorouracil (375 mg/m^2), given as a bolus injection on each of the first 4 days of each treatment course of 25 Gy radiation. Median survival of 9–12 months may be obtained, which compares favourably to a median survival time of 3–4 months when no treatment is given (Jeekel & Treurniet-Donker, 1991). Long-term survival of more than 5 years can be obtained in a few cases (Treurniet-Donker 1990). Toxicity of the treatment with radiotherapy and 5-fluorouracil is low.

Intraoperative radiotherapy and combined treatment using radioactive iodine-125 implantation, external beam radiation and chemotherapy have also been studied (Nishimura et al 1984, Mohiuddin et al 1988). Morbidity is higher after this form of treatment. Operative mortality was 7% after combined modality treatment, but median survival was high (12.5 months) and the 2-year survival was 22% (Mohiuddin et al 1988).

Efforts to improve survival further may be extended to the performance of second-look laparotomy in selected cases. Radiation and 5-fluorouracil therapy may reduce the process to the extent that resection of the tumour may be reconsidered. It has indeed been possible to perform Whipple's resection after radiotherapy of locally unresectable tumours (Pilepich & Miller 1980, Jeekel & Treurniet-Donker, 1991) and survival of more than 5 years has been achieved in some of these patients.

Hormonal therapy

Hormonal therapy has also been used in unresectable pancreatic cancer. A prospective randomized trial was performed in Norway to assess the effect of tamoxifen therapy in 176 cases of unresectable cancer of pancreas and papilla of Vater (Bakkevold et al 1990). A beneficial effect of tamoxifen on survival was not noted, although survival was significantly better in one subgroup of women with stage III (any T, $N_1 M_0$) disease.

One other prospective randomized controlled trial was performed with tamoxifen and cyproterone acetate treatment in pancreatic carcinoma (Keating et al 1989). The median survival of patients receiving tamoxifen (5.25 months) or cyproterone acetate treatment (4.25 months) was significantly different from that of patients receiving no treatment (3 months).

Chemotherapy

Chemotherapy has given disappointing results in pancreatic cancer. In one controlled trial, survival was significantly prolonged after treatment with 5-fluorouracil, cyclophosphamide, methotrexate, vincristine and mitomycin (Mallinson et al 1980). Yet only one patient lived longer than 2 years and side-effects were severe. Furthermore, the nature of the tumour was not histologically confirmed in more than one-third of the patients. The beneficial effect of chemotherapy could not be confirmed in another randomized trial in which the above mentioned regimen was compared to 5-fluorouracil and combined 5-fluorouracil, doxorubicin and cisplatin. Median survivals of all treatment groups were short, varying from 3.5 to 4.5 months (Cullinan et al 1990). In one other randomized trial, no survival benefit was observed after treatment with 5-fluorouracil plus CCNU (lomustine) versus no treatment in controls, median survival being 3 and 4 months respectively (Frey et al 1981).

Immunotherapy

Immunotherapy with monoclonal antibody has been studied recently. It has been demonstrated that monoclonal antibodies can bind to pancreatic tumour tissue (Bosslet et al 1990). Tumour regression and stable disease up to 40 weeks, was noted after treatment with murine monoclonal antibody (M_0 Ab BW 494) (Schulz et al 1988).

ADJUVANT TREATMENT OF RESECTABLE PANCREATIC CANCER

After resection with curative intention, the 1-year survival rate is only 50–60% and 5-year survival rates range from zero to 15%. The question may be raised as to whether surgical resection should be used as the only treatment in pancreatic cancer. Metastases occur at an early stage of the disease, predominantly at a local and regional level. Distant metastases in lung and liver are seldom seen without local or intra-abdominal tumour spread. It is reasonable to assume that locoregional spread is an important and early pathway for pancreatic cancer cells. Intraoperative and postoperative treatment may be directed towards possible micrometastases in such locoregional situations.

Adjuvant treatment has been given in pancreatic cancer either as hormonal therapy, chemotherapy, radiotherapy in combination with chemotherapy, or immunotherapy. One randomized trial has been performed with combined therapy of radiation and 5-fluorouracil treatment after Whipple resection (GTSG 1987). Radiotherapy consisted of two courses of 20 Gy, and 5-fluorouracil was given concomitantly and during the 2 following years. The 2-year survival rate was 43% in the group of 21 patients receiving adjuvant treatment, significantly higher than the 2-year survival rate of 18% in the untreated control group. After 5 years, 19% of the treated group were still alive and 4% of the controls. These results look promising, but patient accrual took many years and the number of patients was small. An EORTC (European Organization for Research and Treatment of Cancer) study was started in Rotterdam in 1990 to study the effect of radiotherapy and 5-fluorouracil after Whipple resection.

Adjuvant chemotherapy with 5-fluorouracil, adriamycin and mitomycin (FAM) has been studied in a non-ran-

domized fashion in patients with adenocarcinoma of the periampullary region and head of the pancreas. Treatment was not well tolerated and did not prolong survival (Splinter et al 1989).

Adjuvant chemotherapy after resection for pancreatic cancer has also been studied recently in a randomized trial in Norway. The preliminary results indicate that FAM-chemotherapy led to a median survival of 23 months in 31 patients vs. 11 months in 30 controls, and further data are awaited with interest. In a recent report, passive immunotherapy using the murine monoclonal antibody (M_0 Ab BW 494/32) failed to show significant benefit in patients who had undergone Whipple resection (Büchler et al 1991).

TREATMENT OF RECURRENT DISEASE

Although pancreatic cancer is a rapidly metastasing process, it is confined to the upper abdomen in the early stages of the disease. The incidence of locoregional recurrence varies between 50 and 67% (Tepper et al 1976, Rokuema et al 1985), and local recurrence may occur without distant metastases. Local recurrence has been attributed to the presence of multifocal cancer within the pancreas (van Heerden et al 1981) or to microscopic cancer infiltration of regional lymphatic vessels, nerves or connective tissue (Nagai et al 1986). Total or regional pancreatectomy has therefore been recommended by some. Although the evidence in favour of total pancreatectomy is conflicting (see Ch. 38), Ishiwaka et al (1988) report a significant decrease in cumulative death rate from local recurrence when an extended dissection was performed.

Treatment of locoregional recurrence should also be considered. In one study of 34 patients with such recurrence, 1-year survival was 22% when no distant metastases were present and treatment was given if this was possible. However, surgical resection of tumour recurrence was feasible in only a few cases although it was followed by survival of up to 74 months (Menke-Pluymers et al, 1992).

OPTIONS FOR IMPROVED SURVIVAL

Survival in pancreatic cancer could be improved if a few rules could be adopted. In the first place the tumour should be diagnosed at an early stage whenever possible. Early cancer may be present in villous adenomas in the pancreatic duct or at the papilla of Vater. Endoscopic biopsies of villous tumours give a false negative diagnosis in more than half of cases (Ryan et al 1986), and the pathologist requires the entire tumour if malignancy is to be excluded. Surgery in the presence of metastatic disease should be avoided as it has a high operative mortality. In patients with resectable cancers, careful operative technique should be directed towards radicality and avoidance of local spillage. Preoperative use of blood transfusions is avoided if at all possible, because a potential effect on metastatic growth has been shown experimentally (Jeekel et al 1982), and postulated in the case of a number of malignancies (Blumberg & Heal 1989). Survival in pancreatic cancer could be improved from the outset by avoiding operative mortality. Experienced surgeons should now be able to limit operative mortality to well under 10% and in many cases to beneath 5%. Adjuvant treatment with radiotherapy and chemotherapy may prolong survival, but the value of these treatments has still to be firmly established and the results of phase III trials are awaited.

Irresectability of a pancreatic cancer is difficult to define and the judgement should be only made by experienced pancreatic surgeons. In the case of locally advanced pancreatic carcinoma without metastases, treatment with radiotherapy and 5-fluorouracil may prolong survival and in a few cases lead to cure. During second-look laparotomy, a resection may appear to be possible. This means that the presence and operability of every pancreatic tumour should be established at laparotomy by an experienced surgeon, unless metastases have been demonstrated preoperatively. Treatment in the event of local tumour recurrence should be considered and can occasionally lead to long-term survival.

REFERENCES

Bakkevold K E, Pettersen A, Arnesjo B et al 1990 Tamoxifen therapy in unresectable adenocarcinoma of the pancreas and the papilla of Vater. British Journal of Surgery 77:725–730

Blumberg N, Heal J M 1989 Transfusion and host defenses against cancer recurrence and infection. Transfusion 29:236–245

Bosslet J, Keweloh H-C, Hermentin P et al 1990 Percolation and binding of monoclonal antibody BW494 to pancreatic carcinoma tissues. British Journal of Cancer 62:37–39

Büchler M, Friess H, Schultheiss K H et al 1991 A randomised controlled trial of adjuvant immunotherapy (murine monoclonal antibody 494/32) in resectable pancreatic cancer. Cancer 68:1507–1512

Cullinan S, Moertel C G, Wieand H S et al 1990 A phase III trial on the therapy of advanced pancreatic carcinoma. Cancer 65:2207–2212

Eriksson B, Skogseid B, Lundqvist G et al 1990 Medical treatment and long-term survival in a prospective study of 84 patients with endocrine pancreatic tumors. Cancer 65:1883–1890

Frey C, Twomey P, Keehn R et al 1981 Randomized study of 5-FU and CCNU in pancreatic cancer. Cancer 47:27

Gastrointestinal Tumor Study Group 1987 Further evidence of effective adjuvant combined radiation and chemotherapy. Cancer 59:2006–2010

Ishiwaka O, Ohigashi H, Sasaki Y et al 1988 Practical usefulness of lymphatic and connective tissue clearance for carcinoma of the pancreas head. Ann Surg 1988; 208:215–220

Jeekel J, Eggermont A, Heystek G et al 1982 Inhibition of tumor growth by blood transfusions in the rat. European Surgical Research 14:549–554

Jeekel J, Treurniet-Donker A D 1991 Treatment perspectives in locally advanced unresectable pancreas cancer. British Journal of Surgery 78:1332–1334

Keating J J, Johnson P J, Cochrane A M G et al 1989 A prospective randomised controlled trial of tamoxifen and cyproterone acetate in pancreatic carcinoma. British Journal of Cancer 60:789–792

Kroneman H, Castelein A, Jeekel J 1991 En bloc resection of colon carcinoma adherent to other organs: an efficacious treatment? Dis Colon Rectum 34:780–783

Laméris J S, Stoker J, Dees J et al 1987 Non-surgical palliative treatment of patients with malignant biliary obstruction – the place of endoscopic and percutaneous drainage. Clinical Radiology 38:603–608

Mallinson C N, Rake M O, Cocking J B et al 1980 Chemotherapy in pancreatic cancer: results of a controlled, prospective, randomised, multicentre trial. British Medical Journal 281:1589–1591

Menke-Pluymers M B E, Klinkenbijl J H G, Tjioe M et al 1992 Treatment of locoregional recurrence after intentional curative resection of pancreatic cancer. Hepato-Gastroenterology 39:429–432

Moertel C G, Frytak S, Hahn R G et al 1981 Therapy of locally unresectable pancreatic carcinoma. Cancer 48:1705–1710

Mohiuddin M, Cantor R J, Biermann W et al 1988 Combined modality treatment of localized unresectable adenocarcinoma of the pancreas. International Journal of Radiation Oncology 14:79–84

Morrow M, Hilaris B, Brennan M F 1984 Comparison of conventional surgical resection, Radioactive implantation and bypass procedures for exocrine carcinoma of the pancreas 1975–1980. Annals of Surgery 199:1–5

Nagai H, Kuroda A, Morioka Y 1986 Lymphatic and local spread of T1 and T2 pancreatic cancer. Annals of Surgery 204:65–71

Nishimura A, Nakano M, Otsu H et al 1984 Intraoperative radiotherapy for advanced carcinoma of the pancreas. Cancer 54:2375–2384

Papachristou D N, Shiu M H 1981 Management by en bloc multiple organ resecton of carcinoma of the stomach invading adjacent organs. Surgery, Gynecology and Obstetrics 152:483–487

Pilepich M V, Miller H H 1980 Preoperative irradiation in carcinoma of the pancreas. Cancer 46:1945–1949

Roukema J A, Zoetmulder F A N, Herman J M M 1985 Is there still a place for Whipple's operation? Netherlands Journal of Surgery 37:79–82

Ryan D P, Schapiro R H, Washaw A L 1986 Villous tumors of the duodenum. Annals of Surgery 203:301–306

Schulz G, Büchler M, Muhrer K H 1988 Immunotherapy of pancreatic cancer with monoclonal antibody BW 494. International Journal of Cancer 2:89–94

Splinter T A W, Obertop H, Kok T C et al 1989 Adjuvant chemotherapy after resection of adenocarcinoma of the periampullary region and the head of the pancreas. Journal of Cancer Research and Clinical Oncology 115:200–202

Tepper J, Nardi G, Suit H 1976 Carcinoma of the pancreas. Cancer 37:1519–1524

Treurniet-Donker A D, van Mierlo M J M, van Putten W L J 1990 Localized unresectable pancreatic cancer. International Journal of Radiation Oncology 18:59–62

Van Heerden J A, ReMine W H, Weiland L H et al 1981 Total pancreatectomy for ductal adenocarcinoma of the pancreas. American Journal of Surgery 142:308–311

Endocrine tumours of the pancreas

48. Endocrine tumours of the pancreas: clinical picture, diagnosis and therapy

W. Creutzfeldt   R. Arnold

GENERAL ASPECTS

In 1927 Wilder et al established that an endocrine tumour of the pancreas can cause clinical hypoglycaemia. Since their report, the attribute 'functional' or 'non-functional' has been added to the so-called endocrine pancreatic tumours. For nearly 30 years an endocrine pancreatic tumour was regarded as functional only if hypoglycaemia had been observed.

The spectrum of functioning endocrine tumours of the pancreas was broadened by the description in 1955 by Zollinger and Ellison of ulcerogenic tumours and, in 1958, by the recognition by Verner and Morrison of diarrheogenic tumours of the pancreas. The glucagonoma syndrome was defined in 1974 by Mallinson et al. The existence of clinical syndromes related to pancreatic tumours which produce pancreatic polypeptide, somatostatin, and neurotensin is still being debated.

Prevalence

The clinical prevalence of symptomatic endocrine tumours of the pancreas, i.e. those leading to hypoglycaemia, gastric acid hypersecretion, dermatitis necroticans, or diarrhoea, is extremely low at less than 1 per 100 000 population (Schein et al 1973). On the other hand, the prevalence of endocrine tumours in unselected necropsy specimens is much higher, between 0.5 and 1.5% (Becker 1971, Grimelius et al 1975). However, the absence of gross clinical symptoms does not exclude hormone production by a pancreatic tumour. The rate of hormone secretion of endocrine tumours varies greatly and is not related to their size. The threshold for the appearance of clinical symptoms possibly also varies individually, and elevated hormone levels may be compensated by regulatory hypersecretion of other hormones. Thus, a subclinical state may last for years, and even decades, because the growth of non-metastatic endocrine tumours is usually extremely slow. The use of modern methods such as radioimmunological estimation of numerous peptide hormones in the blood and tissue staining by immunocytochemical methods, will doubtless result in the detection of more functioning neuroendocrine tumours of the pancreas. Still, it is doubtful whether many more patients with clinical symptoms related to such tumours will eventually be detected, because most of the lesions function below the threshold of clinical expression.

Origin

Morphologists usually call neuroendocrine tumours of the gastroenteropancreatic system 'islet cell tumours'. This name implies that they originated from the islets of Langerhans; however, this has not been proven. Ductular structures are regularly found in these tumours (Heitz et al 1982, Creutzfeldt 1985), and the tumours can produce hormones that normally are not found in the adult human pancreas (i.e. gastrin), or are found only in neural tissue (i.e. vasoactive intestinal polylpeptide, VIP). Also, multiple hormone production by endocrine pancreatic tumours has been recognized as a characteristic phenomenon (Heitz et al 1982, Creutzfeldt 1985). The production of multiple and frequently even ectopic peptides of neuronal or epithelial origin by the same tumour has been interpreted as dedifferentiation of the tumour cells and as an indication of their origin from immature stem cells (Creutzfeldt 1975). Ontogenetically, such stem cells bud from the ductular system. The close relationship between cells of the 'helle Zellen System' of Feyrter or the 'APUD system' of Pearse and endocrine tumours of the pancreas, has been proved by the immunocytochemical demonstration of neurone specific enolase (Tapja et al 1981, Lloyd et al 1984), chromogranin A (Lloyd et al 1984, Wiedemann et al 1988, Wiedemann & Huttner 1989), and synaptophysin (Gould et al 1987, Wiedemann et al 1988, Wiedemann & Huttner 1989) in all of them.

Classification

A categorization of the endocrine tumours of the pancreas

should be based on the hormone levels estimated in blood and tumour tissue and on the immunocytochemical analysis of adequately fixed tissue. The tumour is named after the identified hormone. If more than one hormone is produced, the tumour is called after the hormone responsible for the clinical symptoms.

Table 48.1 lists the endocrine pancreatic tumours producing clinical syndromes in the order of their historical recognition, which is identical to the frequency of their occurrence. Clinical syndromes related to pancreatic polypeptide- and neurotensin-producing tumours have not been established with certainty. Also listed are the characteristic features of the tumours. If no clinical symptom prevails, the tumour is called 'non-functioning endocrine tumour'. Frequently, such tumours contain multiple hormones which are not released into the circulation ('multiple hormone-producing tumours'). If multiple tumours are found that produce different hormones, the entity is named the multiple endocrine neoplasia (MEN) or multiple endocrine adenomatosis (MEA) syndrome which may occur sporadically or as a familial disease. As mentioned before, many endocrine pancreatic tumours are, in fact, functioning, but do so below the threshold of clinical expression. In these cases classification is made retrospectively by the pathologist. In our own experience consisting of more than 150 endocrine tumours of the pancreas producing clinical symptoms, about 68% were insulinomas, 24% were gastrinomas, and 4% each were VIPomas and glucagonomas (Creutzfeldt 1985). A similar distribution has been observed in other large series (Heitz 1984).

Endocrine tumours of the pancreas are almost evenly distributed throughout the gland (Ellison & Wilson 1964, Stefanini et al 1974, Burkhardt & Mitschke 1974). Multiple tumours are found rarely in the case of insulinomas and frequently in the case of gastrinomas.

Histological features

Most pathologists agree that the diagnosis of a benign or malignant tumour cannot be made on histological grounds (Heitz et al 1982, Creutzfeldt 1985) and has to be based on the observation of gross invasion or metastases into lymph nodes or the liver. Persistence of elevated serum hormone levels after tumour extirpation is indicative of metastases overlooked during surgery. In this situation, the finding of frequent secretion of the alpha chain of glycoprotein hormones by malignant endocrine pancreatic tumours (Kahn et al 1977) is of considerable interest. Immunocytochemically, chorionic gonadotropin (CG) α-immunoreactive cells were present in 75% of functioning malignant endocrine pancreatic tumours but not in benign functioning or non-functioning ones. More recently, it was shown that the α-subunit of human (h)CG is a valuable serum marker in patients with gastrinoma, although not specific for malignancy (McCarthy et al 1977, Bardram et al 1988).

The growth pattern of the tumours (trabecular or gyriform; rosette-like or glandular; medullary or solid) has no diagnostic significance regarding hormone production. Also, the numerous histochemical reactions applied to

Table 48.1 Classification and features of endocrine tumours of the pancreas and their clinical syndromes. The very rare pancreatic carcinoma with ectopic hormone production (ACTH, corticotropin-releasing factor (CRF), growth hormone-releasing factor (GHRF)) are not included

Name (synonym)	Clinical symptoms	Hormone responsible	Other hormones frequently produced	Rate of malignancy	Extrapancreatic localization
Insulinoma (insulin-producing tumour)	Fasting hypoglycaemia	Insulin	Pancreatic polypeptide, glucagon	10%	1% (stomach, duodenum, Meckel's diverticulum, mesentery)
Gastrinoma (gastrin-producing tumour; ulcerogenic tumour)	Gastric hypersecretion; recurrent ulcer disease, steatorrhoea (diarrhoea): Zollinger-Ellison syndrome	Gastrin	Insulin, pancreatic polypeptide, glucagon, ACTH	>90%	Frequent (20% duodenum, 1% gastric antrum)
VIPoma (Vasoactive intestinal polypeptide) (VIP)-producing tumour; diarrhoegoenic tumour; Verner-Morrison syndrome; pancreatic cholera)	Watery diarrhoea; hypokalaemia, gastric hyposecretion	VIP	Pancreatic polypeptide, glucagon	75%	Frequent (neuroblastoma or ganglioneuroma of any localization)
Glucagonoma (glucagon-producing tumour)	Necrolytic, migratory erythema; diabetes mellitus; anaemia	Glucagon	Pancreatic polypeptide, somatostatin, insulin	50%	Rare
Somatostatinoma (somatostatin-producing tumour)	Diabetes mellitus; steatorrhoea; cholelithiasis; gastric hyposecretion	Somatostatin	Pancreatic polypeptide, insulin, calcitonin	50%	Frequent (duodenum)

endocrine tumours do not allow differentiation. The only reliable method is immunocytochemistry, i.e. staining with antibodies directed specifically against the different gastrointestinal hormones. A prerequisite for positive immunochemical staining is some residual intracellular hormone storage. Completely dedifferentiated tumour cells contain very little hormone activity and, therefore, cannot be stained with immunochemical methods. This happens often with metastatic endocrine tumours of high grade malignancy. In these cases, the diagnosis has to be based on the elevated plasma hormone levels, and possibly the hormone concentration in tumour extracts.

Ultrastructural analysis of the type of secretory granules can also help in establishing the diagnosis of an endocrine pancreatic tumour. A certain percentage of insulinomas, gastrinomas, glucagonomas, and somatostatinomas contain tumour cells whose secretory granules have the same structure as found in normal B, G, A, PP, and D cells. However, they may additionally contain or even be exclusively composed of atypical (non-diagnostic) secretory granules or agranular cells. Thus, in the ultrastructural analysis of tumour tissue, only a positive finding is of diagnostic help.

Pathophysiology

The mechanism of hormone overproduction by endocrine tumours, i.e. the inappropriate hormone release responsible for the endocrine disease, is still debated. It is best explained by uncontrolled release of the hormone owing to defective storage capacity or inability of the tumour cell to turn off hormone secretion. Failure to store the hormone properly in the secretory granules is reflected by a decreased number of secretory granules in the majority of tumour cells and decreased hormone content of the tumour tissue when compared with normal hormone-producing cells (Creutzfeldt et al 1973, 1975, 1980).

In a certain percentage of the endocrine tumour syndromes listed in Table 48.1, no tumour was found at surgery and hyperplasia of the pancreatic islets was regarded as the cause of the disease. The existence of an endocrine disease without pancreatic tumour has been established only for neonatal or infantile hyperinsulinaemic hypoglycaemia. The existence of 'nesidioblastosis' in adults is not established (Nauck & Creutzfeldt 1991); at best it is 'exceedingly rare' (Goosens et al 1991). Morphometry has not revealed an increase of total endocrine cell mass or a specific cell type (Albers et al 1989). Therefore, it is not justified (except in neonatal hyperinsulinaemic hypoglycaemia) to perform partial or subtotal pancreatectomy in order to eliminate 'diffuse islet cell hyperplasia' if no tumour is found. Endocrine tumours may be small, hidden in the head of the pancreas or the duodenal wall, or may even be ectopic.

Diagnosis and localization

There are no general markers for the endocrine pancreatic tumours. Plasma levels for pancreatic polypeptide have been reported to be increased in half of the patients with a variety of pancreatic endocrine tumours (Polak et al 1976). However, this has not proved to be of great diagnostic help (Floyd et al 1977) except in family studies of patients with the multiple endocrine neoplasia syndrome (Friesen 1982).

If a pancreatic endocrine tumour syndrome is under clinical consideration, the diagnosis must be based on the demonstration of inappropriately high serum levels of the secretory product concerned, both fasting and after stimulation. Sensitive and specific radioimmunoassays of the different pancreatic and gut hormones are now available and their application will be discussed later.

When the diagnosis of an endocrine pancreatic tumour has been made, the therapeutic strategy (surgical, anti-tumour therapy, anti-hormone therapy) depends on the exact localization of the tumour and the presence or absence of metastases, regardless of which hormone(s) the tumour produces. The whole spectrum of modern imaging methods may be applied (sonography, computed tomography (CT), nuclear magnetic resonance (NMR), angiography, somatostatin receptor scintigraphy) to localize the primary tumour and (possibly) any metastases.

However, it must be appreciated that present imaging methods cannot visualize pancreatic tumours with a diameter below 10 mm. For instance only in two-thirds of 170 patients with an insulinoma could the tumour be demonstrated by angiography (Stefanini et al 1974a). CT and ultrasonography are positive in less than 20% of cases (Dunnick et al 1980). The sensitivity of somatostatin receptor scintigraphy for detection of small pancreatic endocrine tumours (Lamberts et al 1990a) has still to be established. The technique of operative sonography employing an ultrasonic transducer directly within the abdomen at operation (Sigel et al 1983, Galiber et al 1988) has greatly improved in the last years, and allows operative intervention if the diagnosis of an endocrine pancreatic tumour has been established by endocrinological methods, even if the tumour has not been visualized by preoperative imaging methods.

We do not recommend percutaneous transhepatic portal and pancreatic vein catheterization and hormone estimation in the collected blood samples (Ingemansson et al 1975, Turner et al 1978, Glaser et al 1981, Doppman et al 1981). This method is technically difficult and needs great skill. The results are not reliable (Daggett et al 1981) and can, at the most, regionalize but not localize the tumour. The experienced surgeon is able to palpate the tumour at operation with a high degree of probability when the diagnosis has been soundly made by adequate endocrinological methods (Daggett et al 1981). In addition, intraoperative sonography is now an established method of tumour localization.

Extirpation of the primary endocrine pancreatic tumour is not indicated in the presence of metastases. Hence, a major diagnostic goal is exclusion of metastatic disease. Autonomous hormone release, decreased suppressibility of hormone secretion, and increased percentage of prohormone levels are more pronounced in malignant than in benign endocrine pancreatic tumours. There is an overlap of the secretory pattern between these two groups, however, and differentiation is impossible on the grounds of endocrine tests. As shown in Table 48.1, the probability of metastatic disease is low with insulinoma (<10%), very high with gastrinoma (>90%), and intermediate with VIPoma, glucagonoma, and somatostatinoma. Successful surgical treatment is more likely, therefore, in cases of insulinoma than in cases of gastrinoma, in which the search for metastases should be more extensive. More recently, a scintigraphic method has been developed using indium-labelled octreotide for visualizing endocrine tumours and their metastases (Lamberts et al 1990a, b). Since most benign and many malignant endocrine tumours possess somatostatin receptors (Reubi et al 1987), this method can be used for documentation of metastatic disease (Fig. 48.1). According to present experience this method allows the localization of endocrine tumours and their metastases in more than 70% of patients (Lamberts et al 1990a). In addition, a positive scintigram may indicate the possibility of response to octreotide treatment.

Therapeutic principles

If at all possible, an endocrine pancreatic tumour should be surgically extirpated. Medical treatment is indicated in the preoperative phase, during the necessary diagnostic

procedures, to improve the general state of the patient when this is poor, and in cases of inoperable tumour.

If no metastasis is demonstrated by the available imaging methods, laparotomy is indicated even though the primary tumour has not been localized. As a rule, the surgeon will find the tumour by gross inspection of the mobilized pancreas and all adjacent structures, or by an ultrasonic device that allows sonographic mapping of the pancreas and neighbouring tissue. If no tumour is found, blind resection of the pancreas is not indicated.

Palliative treatment can be divided into measures directed against the tumour (its hormone secretion or its growth) and against the effect of the hormone on the target organ. With the development of the long-acting somatostatin analogue, octreotide, effective antisecretory treatment has become possible for hormone-secreting tumours and should always be tried for symptomatic treatment, if operative measures or cytostatic treatment are not indicated.

Malignant pancreatic endocrine tumours have a slow growth rate. Therefore, excision of an easily resectable tumour mass should always be considered because this will reduce elevated plasma hormone levels and improve the clinical symptoms related to them. Long-lasting clinical remissions may be induced by palliative surgery. Owing to their common cellular origin, the different tumours respond to the same cytostatic drugs (especially streptozotocin) and their highly vascularized liver metastases to arterial embolization.

Cytostatic treatment

The small number of malignant endocrine pancreatic tumours observed even in large centres makes evaluation of different cytostatic drugs difficult. The standard cytostatic

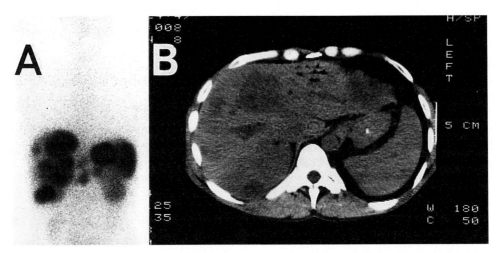

Fig. 48.1 Demonstration of multiple metastases in the right and left lobe of the liver by **A** indium-labelled octreotide (Octreoscan 111), and **B** by CT scan, in a patient with a non-functioning metastasized endocrine tumour. The primary, located in the head of the pancreas, was resected several years before the appearance of metastases.

drugs have not been investigated in controlled studies. Streptozotocin, an antibiotic derived from *Streptomyces achromogenes*, is closely related to the nitrosourea derivatives BCNU and CCNU and has a cytostatic effect on the islet B cells of several species. This has been widely used since 1967 for the treatment of endocrine pancreatic tumours. For example, Broder and Carter, reporting in 1973 on 52 patients found that the average survival in treated patients was 30 months as compared with 10 months in untreated patients. The most frequent side effects of streptozotocin are nausea and vomiting (>80%) and mild, usually reversible, renal tubular damage (30%).

These favourable results have been confirmed and extended in a controlled multicentre study of 84 patients with endocrine pancreatic tumours of which only 50% were functioning (Moertel et al 1980). Half of the patients received streptozotocin alone, the other half streptozotocin plus fluorouracil. The combination had advantages over streptozotocin alone in terms of overall rate of response (33 vs. 12%). Treatment with the combination also yielded a survival advantage over treatment with streptozotocin alone. The gastrointestinal toxic effects (nausea, vomiting) and the renal toxicity were equal with both therapeutic regimens, while reversible bone marrow depression occurred only with the combination therapy (75% of the cases).

Any other form of cytostatic treatment must be regarded as experimental and should be used only after combined treatment with streptozotocin and fluorouracil has failed. The therapeutic scheme is as follows (Moertel et al 1980):

1. Streptozotocin, 500 mg/m^2 of body surface, is given daily for 5 consecutive days concurrently with fluorouracil, 400 mg/m^2 of body surface by rapid i.v. injection. Phenothiazine is given to prevent and treat nausea and vomiting. More recently we have used ondansetrone successfully against the sometimes severe nausea.

2. Courses of therapy are repeated every 6 weeks if tumour size has decreased or remained stable. Treatment is monitored by determinations of leukocyte and platelet counts and by renal and liver tests.

3. Initiation of subsequent courses is deferred to allow complete recovery from any haematological or renal toxic effects that may develop.

4. In case of complete clinical, endocrinological, and morphological remission, treatment can be interrupted.

The question of a preferential response of certain types of endocrine tumours to streptozotocin, or to combined treatment with 5-fluorouracil, cannot yet be answered because the number of treated patients with different endocrine pancreatic tumours is still small. However, from a review of other reports and from personal experience with 40 patients it can be concluded that VIPomas and insulinomas respond best, and gastrinomas (and carcinoids) respond least to this form of cytostatic treatment. Because of the unsatisfactory results in the treatment of metastatic gastrinoma, a new protocol involving streptozotocin, 5-fluorouracil, and doxorubicin has been inaugurated. We have used this scheme for more than 5 years, under cardiological control, in about 25 patients with functioning and non-functioning endocrine gastrointestinal tumours and have achieved partial remission in half of them. The major side-effects were nausea in all and nephrotoxicity in one patient. This therapeutic scheme is as follows (Jensen et al 1983b):

- Day 1: Streptozotocin 1.5 g/ml, 5-fluorouracil 600 mg/m^2, doxorubicin 40 mg/m^2
- Day 8: Streptozotocin 1.5 mg/m^2, 5-fluorouracil 600 mg/m^2
- Repetition every 4 weeks.

Ondansetrone is given to prevent nausea. Therapy with other cytostatic drugs (mithramycin, L-asparaginase) cannot be recommended because the respective case reports are anecdotal. Effective cytostatic treatment of endocrine gut tumours has been reported with dacarbazine (DTIC); nine of 11 patients were considered to have benefitted from treatment, with the most remarkable remissions occurring in five cases of glucagonoma (Kessinger et al 1983).

Tumour remission has been observed in single but well-documented cases of endocrine gastrointestinal tumours after daily subcutaneous injections with interferon alpha (IFNα) (Öberg et al 1983, Hanssen et al 1989, Öberg & Eriksson 1989, Creutzfeldt et al 1991) or with the somatostatin analogue octreotide (Kvols et al 1986, 1987, Creutzfeldt et al 1991).

The mechanism of action of these substances is poorly understood. However, the lack of serious side-effects justifies their use in patients with metastatic disease, regardless of the presence of symptoms due to hormone hypersecretion. Several reports have shown that patients have stable tumour size during long-term IFNα or octreotide treatment despite progressive disease before treatment.

The recommended dose for recombinant IFNα is 2×10^6 i.u./m^2 daily and for octreotide it is 3×200 μg, s.c. daily. The octreotide dose can be increased to 3×500 μg. The treatment result has to be assessed by imaging methods every 4 months. Side-effects of IFNα are initially flu-like symptoms and fever and, rarely, bone marrow suppression, mental depression, and hypothyroidism. Octreotide may induce mild steatorrhoea and as a consequence of sluggish gallbladder emptying, cholesterol gallstones. The latter were asymptomatic in our patients and dissolved with combined therapy of ursodeoxycholic acid and chenodeoxycholic acid within 3–4 months.

Arterial embolization

Endocrine tumours with liver metastases have been successfully treated by hepatic artery embolization (Allison et al 1977, Carrasco et al 1983, Clouse et al 1983). The effect of this procedure on tumour growth and hormone production can be dramatic, and long-lasting remissions may occur without major complications. In one case, a recurrent pancreatic insulinoma was successfully treated by arterial embolization (Moore et al 1982). We have performed hepatic artery embolization with prolamine (Ethibloc) in four patients with insulinoma and liver metastases who had ceased to respond to cytostatic treatment. Previously we had observed a patient with metastatic insulinoma, who had not responded to streptozotocin, in whom remission for 18 months followed hepatic artery ligation. Remissions after hepatic arterial embolization last between 10 and 30 months. We do believe, therefore, that arterial embolization is indicated in endocrine pancreatic tumours with liver metastases when conventional treatment with cytostatic drugs is or has become ineffective, and operative tumour debulking too risky.

INSULINOMA

Insulin-secreting tumours leading to hypoglycaemia are by far the most frequent endocrine tumours of the pancreas (about 70–80% of clinically symptomatic cases). Exact prevalence data with respect to insulinomas in the general population are not available. Several authors give the annual incidence of diagnosed insulinomas as one case per million persons (Kavlie & White 1972, Watson et al 1989) which may be an underestimate.

Pathology and pathophysiology

Insulinomas are mostly solitary tumours and are evenly distributed throughout the pancreas. The size of the tumour at the time of diagnosis varies considerably and is not related to the severity of clinical symptoms (Howard et al 1950). The smallest insulinoma producing clinical symptoms (and fasting insulin plasma levels >100 µg/ml) in our experience weighed 0.5 g, the largest 25 g (metastases excluded). Multiple tumours are found in about 10% of cases, mostly in association with multiple endocrine adenomatosis, type I (Service et al 1976). Metastatic disease develops in 5–10% of cases (Howard et al 1950). Ectopic localization occurs in less than 1% of cases at places known for pancreatic heterotopia (stomach, duodenum, Meckel's diverticulum, bile ducts, omentum) (Elfving & Hästbacka 1965). In our own series of 90 insulinomas, the only ectopic insulinoma was situated in the mesentery.

Insulinoma cells contain less insulin than do normal B cells. However, the insulin concentration in the tumours is mostly higher than in the surrounding pancreas, of which only 1% is islet tissue (Creutzfeldt et al 1973, Hayashi et al 1977). The tumour cells also contain fewer secretory granules than normal B cells. Ultrastructurally, atypical secretory granules and virtually agranular cells are frequent. The percentage of proinsulin in the tumours is higher than in the normal pancreas. Furthermore, a higher proinsulin percentage than in the normal population has been estimated in the serum of insulinoma patients (Creutzfeldt et al 1973, Hayashi et al 1977). These findings have been interpreted as indicative of a decreased storage capacity of the tumour cells leading to inappropriate insulin release, i.e. insulin secretion at normal or even abnormally low blood glucose levels. The clinical consequence is fasting hypoglycaemia.

Based on the ultrastructural appearance of secretory granules, four types of insulinomas have been defined (Creutzfeldt et al 1973, Fig. 48.2):

1. only typical beta granules present
2. typical as well as atypical granules present
3. only atypical granules present
4. virtually agranular insulinomas.

The characteristics that form the basis of this classification, in general predict the tumour insulin content, the relative proportion of proinsulin, the staining with aldehyde-thionine, and also the clinical response to diazoxide (Creutzfeldt et al 1973). This implies that atypical granules contain less insulin than typical ones, and that processing of proinsulin to insulin and C-peptide is mainly performed by enzymes contained in mature beta-granules. Furthermore, suppression of insulin secretion by somatostatin and diazoxide can be predicted if typical beta-granules are present, whereas no response is seen in patients with predominantly atypical or virtually absent granules (Creutzfeldt et al 1973, Nauck et al 1990).

Clinical aspects

Insulinomas are found in all age groups but mostly in the third to fifth decade of life and only rarely in small children.

Hypoglycaemia induces rather non-specific symptoms that are related to an adrenergic reaction and to neuroglycopenia. Despite the fact that these adrenergic and neuroglycopenic symptoms are well known, the diagnosis of fasting hypoglycaemia in an insulinoma patient is usually made relatively late in the course of the disease.

The most frequently experienced adrenergic symptoms are weakness, sweating, tremulousness, tachycardia, and hunger. The neuroglycopenic symptoms vary from mild fatigue, mental dullness, headache, dizziness, and blurring of vision to severe symptoms with abnormal behaviour, disorientation, seizures, and episodic unconsciousness. The most important clue is the relation of the symptoms to periods of food deprivation or to muscular exercise, with relief obtained by ingestion of food. In the majority of cases,

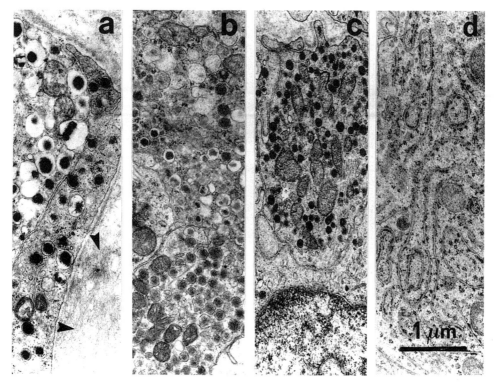

Fig. 48.2 Ultrastructural appearance of insulinomas: **a** Type I insulinoma, only typical beta granules; **b** Type II insulinoma, both typical and atypical secretory granules present; **c** Type III insulinoma, only atypical secretory granules present; **d** Type IV insulinoma, containing virtually no secretory granules. The arrows in **a** indicate an area with fibrillar amyloid deposits. (From Nauck et al 1990, with permission)

hypoglycaemic attacks occur sporadically at first with symptom-free intervals of weeks or months. This favours an erroneous diagnosis. In most insulinoma patients, neuro-glycopenia-related symptoms have been present for several years before the correct diagnosis was made (Frerichs & Creutzfeldt 1976). In such cases, hypoglycaemia is often compensated for by increased carbohydrate intake with progressive weight increase and obesity. In some patients, late diagnosis results in permanent brain damage with mental retardation.

Diagnosis and differential diagnosis

Considering the normal variation, fasting plasma levels of insulin need not be elevated in insulinoma patients in absolute terms (Fig. 48.3). This is also true for C-peptide, the second product of proinsulin conversion, and to a lesser degree for proinsulin plasma concentrations (Fig. 48.3). However, the biochemical diagnosis of insulinoma can be made with absolute certainly by applying provocative tests. As already noted, the clue to diagnosis is the close relation of the hypoglycaemic episodes to the fasting state and their relief by food intake. If a low blood glucose level is found during such an episode, Whipple's triad is fulfilled. A low blood glucose level is usually defined as less than 2.2 mmol/l (40 mg/dl) during the fasting state. The list of diseases that may result in hypoglycaemia is long. However,

the relation of the episodes to food deprivation and the relief by food ingestion are consistent with fasting hypo-glycaemia, reducing this list of diagnostic possibilities considerably (Fajans & Floyd 1976). This can be documented by performing the most important diagnostic test, that is prolonged fasting under strict supervision with concomitant estimations of serum glucose. Within 24 hours, 75% of the patients with insulinoma will have blood glucose levels <2.2 mmol/l and adrenergic or neuro-glycopenic symptoms; by 48 hours 98%, and by 72 hours virtually all of them will be hypoglycaemic (Schein et al 1973, Service et al 1976, Frerichs & Creutzfeldt 1976).

If exogenous insulin injection in the diabetic is excluded, only few causes for fasting hypoglycaemia have to be considered, i.e. alcohol, drugs, liver disease, endocrine deficiencies, insulin-producing tumours, and other large tumours. Each of these conditions will eventually show hypoglycaemic symptoms during prolonged fasting. However, only in the insulinoma patient will the hypoglycaemia occur with an inappropriate but not necessarily absolute elevation of the serum insulin level. Therefore, serum levels of immunoreactive insulin (IRI) must be estimated during prolonged fasting together with the blood glucose levels every 3–4 hours. Insulin values at the time point of discontinuation of starvation need not be higher than normal fasting insulin values (although they usually are), but they are inappropriately high for the prevailing plasma

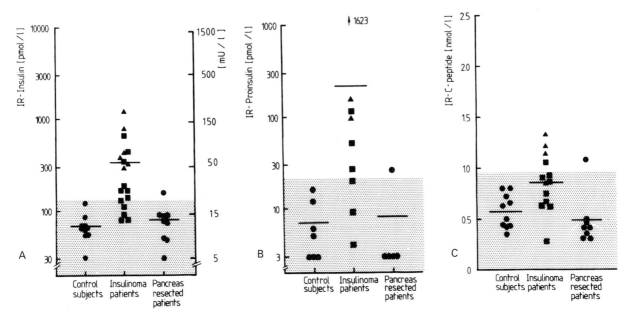

Fig. 48.3 Fasting values of: **A** IR-insulin, **B** IR-proinsulin, and **C** IR-C-peptide; for control patients whose thorough examination excluded an insulinoma, ●; insulinoma patients, benign ■; malignant insulinoma patients ▲ and; patients in whom a benign insulinoma had been successfully removed, ●. Bars indicate the mean value for the respective group of patients. Shaded areas are means ± SD for all patients without an insulin-producing tumour (normal range). Note the logarithmic scales for IR-insulin and IR-proinsulin. (From Nauck M, Creutzfeldt W 1991, with permission)

glucose concentration. The inappropriateness can be demonstrated by mathematically deriving the insulin-to-glucose ratio (Fajans & Floyd 1976, Turner et al 1971). A value of 0.3 (insulin concentration, mU/l, divided by glucose concentration, mg/dl), equivalent to a molar ratio of 38×10^{-6} (insulin concentration, pmol/l, divided by glucose concentration, mmol/l) is usually thought to represent the upper limit of normal. However, variations between laboratories make it necessary to define the normal range by taking into account the specific methodology used. In our laboratory a value of 20 pmol/mmol best separated patients with (n = 15) and without (n = 17) insulinoma (Nauck & Creutzfeldt 1991).

Based on the assumption that at plasma glucose concentrations of below 1.7 mmol/l (30 mg/dl) normal pancreatic B cells do not secrete appreciable amounts of insulin, an 'amended' insulin-to-glucose ratio has been suggested (calculated by subtracting 1.7 mmol/l (30 mg/dl) from the prevailing plasma glucose concentration) to improve diagnostic accuracy. In the literature, the upper limit of normal is a molar ratio of 63×10^{-6} (insulin concentration, pmol/l divided by glucose concentration, mmol/l, − 1.7 mmol/l), equivalent to 0.5 mU/l × dl/mg (insulin concentration, mU/l, divided by glucose concentration, mg/dl, − 30 mg/dl) (Fajans & Floyd 1976, Turner et al 1971). In our series an amended (molar) insulin-to-glucose ratio of 39×10^{-6} (equivalent to 0.31 mU/l × dl/mg) allows a complete separation of patients with and without insulinoma (Fig. 48.4).

While no other test is as simple and safe, and at the same

time as specific and sensitive, as prolonged fasting with glucose and IRI estimation, stimulatory and suppressive tests may be needed on rare occasions.

For stimulation of insulin secretion, tolbutamide, leucine, glucagon, or calcium, have been used (Frerichs & Creutzfeldt 1976). However, none of these tests is diagnostic in more than 70% of cases (Schein et al 1973, Fajans & Floyd 1976, Service et al 1976, Frerichs & Creutzfeldt 1980). The same is true for the use of suppression tests. They are based on the assumption that insulin secretion by an insulinoma is autonomous, i.e. does not decrease if the blood glucose level falls. To achieve this, blood glucose levels are lowered by injecting regular insulin, and thereafter plasma levels of C-peptide are estimated. Since insulin and C-peptide are secreted in equimolar amounts by the normal B cell and the insulinoma cell, a fall of C-peptide levels indicates suppressibility of insulin secretion and excludes an insulinoma (Turner & Heding 1977). The disadvantage of this test is again the necessity to provoke hypoglycaemia.

In order to avoid hypoglycaemia provoked by insulin administration, euglycaemic clamp experiments with infusions of exogenous insulin have been performed (Reynolds et al 1984, Gin et al 1988). Under conditions that allowed the detection of an intact feedback regulation in normal controls and obese subjects, no reduction in circulating C-peptide was observed in insulinoma patients during the maintenance of exogenous hyperinsulinaemia. IR-proinsulin also declined in normal and obese subjects, but not in insulinoma patients. The number of patients with insulinoma investigated until now is too small to

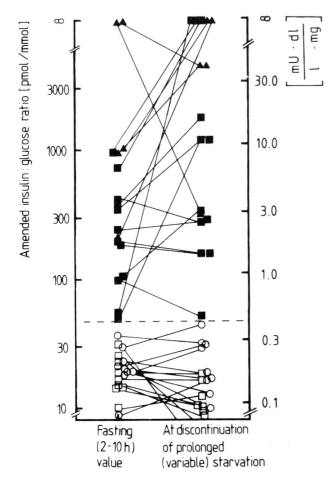

Fig. 48.4 'Amended' insulin-to-glucose ratios before breakfast (after a period of 2–10 hours without food intake, repeated measurements on 2–7 successive days, symbols on the left), and at the time of discontinuation of prolonged starvation (symbols on the right) because of sustained hypoglycaemia in insulinoma patients, or after 48 hours in control patients. Patients with benign insulinoma, ■; patients with malignant insulinoma, ▲; patients in whom an insulinoma could be excluded, ○; patients with previous successful surgical removal of a benign insulinoma, □. The dotted line completely separates the results of patients with and without insulin-producing tumour. (From Nauck M, Creutzfeldt W 1991, with permission)

allow an evaluation of the specificity of this elaborate test, in comparison to the much simpler prolonged fasting. So far, we have investigated eight insulinoma patients and observed no significant reduction of C-peptide levels during the hyperinsulinaemic clamp.

It has been suggested that steady-state glucose infusion rates, necessary to maintain a predetermined euglycaemic plasma glucose level, can be used in order to demonstrate the biological activity of elevated fasting plasma insulin concentrations in insulinoma patients. More recent studies in a larger number of patients and control subjects, however, have demonstrated a high degree of overlap between patients with and without insulinoma (Nauck et al 1990). This test, therefore, does not reach the high diagnostic accuracy of prolonged starvation. During these euglycaemic clamp tests somatostatin or diazoxide have also usually

been infused in order to evaluate whether the plasma insulin levels of insulinoma patients can be suppressed by these substances as in normal subjects.

It has been suggested that non-suppressibility of endocrine tumours is a sign of malignancy. However, this is not the case with insulinomas. We have seen patients with metastatic insulinoma and well-suppressible insulin secretion as well as patients with non-suppressible benign insulinoma. On the other hand, the functional behaviour of the insulinomas correlates well with their ultrastructure; non-suppressible tumours are virtually agranular, whereas suppressible tumours contain numerous secretory granules. Thus, a different degree of suppressibility reflects a different degree of functional dedifferentiation but not necessarily malignancy (Creutzfeldt et al 1973, Berger et al 1983, Nauck & Creutzfeldt 1991).

The presence of fasting hyperinsulinaemia excludes all forms of fasting hypoglycaemia except factitious hypoglycaemia due to self-administration of insulin or an insulin-releasing oral hypoglycaemic agent. Personal experience with several such patients has taught us to be very careful if fasting hypoglycaemia occurs in patients from the medical community or in relatives of diabetics (Creutzfeldt & Frerichs 1969, Siegel et al 1987). All the tests previously discussed can become positive after insulin administration except for elevated C-peptide levels during fasting or after stimulation. After ingestion of an insulin-releasing agent, however, even the C-peptide levels are elevated. In such instances, the correct diagnosis can be made only by screening the serum for the presence of hypoglycaemic drugs. The ratio of patients with proven factitious hypoglycaemia (diabetics excluded) to patients with proven insulinoma in our institution is 1:10. This psychoneurotic entity should always be considered before surgical treatment is advised.

Treatment

If symptoms of hypoglycaemia occur during the diagnostic phase, counteracting treatment in the form of oral or parenteral glucose is employed until the symptoms resolve. Some authors recommend the subcutaneous injection of 1 mg glucagon. Superiority of glucagon over glucose, however, has not been shown.

After the biochemical diagnosis of an insulinoma has been made and metastatic disease is excluded, surgical exploration is indicated. The pancreas is mobilized and the tumour removed by enucleation or partial resection of the pancreas. The mortality of operative treatment for benign insulinoma is reported as ranging from 4.5 to 13% (Stefanini et al 1974a). Postoperatively, blood glucose levels usually rise and may remain elevated for several days, especially if glucose-containing infusions are given. No insulin is needed in most of the cases if glucose-free electrolyte solutions are administered. Permanent diabetes is a very rare sequel when the insulinoma has only been enucleated or when only a small portion of the pancreas has been resected together with the insulinoma. Only one of our 90 patients became diabetic after operation and required permanent insulin treatment. Since idiopathic diabetes has a general prevalence rate of 1.5%, it is possible that the diabetes in this patient and in other similar cases may not be related to the removal of the insulinoma.

In the uncommon case in which a tumour is not found despite applying modern equipment for intraoperative ultrasonography, blind pancreatic resection is not advised as pointed out earlier. The patient should then undergo intraoperative portal-venous sampling with IRI estimation. If the tumour still cannot be identified, conservative treatment with antisecretory drugs is advised with repetition of the diagnostic procedures after 1–2 years (Glaser et al 1981).

Antisecretory therapy. This is indicated in the pre-operative phase and when operation is contraindicated because of advanced age or poor physical condition, and in the case of metastatic disease. A series of drugs have been shown to inhibit insulin secretion from normal B cells and insulinoma cells (Frerichs & Track 1974). Of these, only diazoxide has proved to be sufficiently effective to prevent fasting hypoglycaemia in most insulinoma patients. In as much as this non-diuretic benzothiadiazine has antihypertensive potency and induces water and sodium retention, it should be combined with a diuretic thiazide. Diazoxide inhibits the release of secretory granules from the normal B cells and the insulinoma cells. Therefore, it is ineffective or only minimally effective in insulinomas containing agranular tumour cells (Creutzfeldt et al 1973). Diaxozide tablets are given two to three times daily. The necessary dosage, determined individually on the basis of tolerance and effectiveness, may range from as little as 25 mg twice daily to as much as 200 mg three times daily. Side-effects, especially with higher doses, include anorexia, vomiting, hyperuricaemia, water and sodium retention, bone marrow depression, cardiomyopathy with cardiac arrhythmia, and hirsutism in females. Patients on diazoxide need permanent medical supervision.

The long-acting somatostatin analogue octreotide may be tried in inoperable patients with hyperinsulinaemic hypoglycaemia, due to an insulinoma, who do not tolerate diazoxide. The effect is variable because this peptide also suppresses glucagon and growth hormone secretion and, therefore, may worsen hypoglycaemia (Nauck & Creutzfeldt 1991).

In patients with metastatic insulinoma, cytostatic treatment and ultimately arterial embolization are indicated, as discussed earlier. The slow growth characteristic of malignant insulinomas makes the results of antisecretory and anti-tumour treatment rewarding. Such agents not only prolong life but also significantly improve the quality of life. Operative tumour debulking should always be considered. It may lead to long-lasting palliation.

GASTRINOMA (ZOLLINGER–ELLISON SYNDROME)

Although endocrine pancreatic tumours in patients with severe ulcer disease had been reported earlier (Seiler & Zinninger 1946, Forty & Barrett 1952), Zollinger and Ellison must be credited with establishing the concept in 1955 of a hormone-producing tumour responsible for the clinical syndrome that now bears their names (Zollinger–Ellison or ZE syndrome).

Pathology

Gastrinomas are situated within the pancreas in 60–80% of the cases, within the duodenal wall in 10–25%, and in the stomach or an extraintestinal site (such as the omentum, the ovary, and the biliary system) in less than 5% (Ellison & Wilson 1964 Weichert & Roth 1971, Bernades et al 1972, Wolfe et al 1982). In contrast to insulinomas, multiple pancreatic tumours are frequently observed in patients with gastrinomas. In most cases, the additional tumours are incidental findings at surgery and appear on immunohistological study to be either insulinomas, glucagonomas, pancreatic polypeptide-producing tumours, or even tumours without any hormone production (Arnold et al 1977).

In 15–26% of patients with the ZE syndrome, additional tumours of extrapancreatic endocrine glands have been described (Ellison & Wilson 1964, Jensen et al 1983b, Way et al 1968, Bonfils & Bader 1970). In these circumstances, the gastrinomas are but part of the multiple endocrine neoplasia syndrome, type I (MEN I). Hyperparathyroidism is the commonest coexistent endocrine abnormality.

Epidemiology

The most complete data concerning the prevalence of the ZE syndrome stem from Denmark. In the period 1972 to 1978, with a total population in Denmark of approximately 5 million people, approximately 50 patients were given a diagnosis of ZE syndrome. This would fix the incidence at 1.5 per 1 million population per year (Stadil & Stage 1979).

Pathophysiology

The basic mechanism responsible for the clinical and pathological alterations that characterize the ZE syndrome is hypergastrinaemia arising from inability of the tumour cells to store newly-synthesized hormones. This is substantiated by the remarkably low gastrin content found in most gastrinomas (Creutzfeldt et al 1975). Secretin, calcium, glucagon, and even food intake induce considerable release into the circulation. In healthy subjects and in duodenal ulcer patients, immunoreactive serum gastrin consists of at least four major but different molecular forms. Each of the different components exists in two different forms, with tyrosine in position 12 being sulphated or non-sulphated (Rehfeld 1974). In the fasting state, gastrin-34 is twice as abundant in the serum as gastrin-17, whereas both components increase to a similar extent after a meal (Lamers et al 1982). In the ZE syndrome, gastrin-34 or gastrin-17 may be the predominant gastrin component in serum and tumour tissue; the percentage distribution of the main gastrin components in the serum and in tumour extracts differs from one gastrinoma patient to the next. No obvious relationship appears to exist between the distribution of gastrin components in tumour tissue and sera of individual ZE patients (Creutzfeldt et al 1975, Dockray et al 1975).

The hypergastrinaemia induces a marked increase in basal acid secretion (Fig. 48.5) and the trophic action of gastrin (Johnson & Guthrie 1976, Hansen et al 1976) results in an increased number of fundic parietal cells and the endocrine ECL cells, and in an increase of the mucosal thickness in most ZE patients. This increase is reflected in visible hypertrophy of the fundic mucosal folds.

Peptic ulcers result from the marked gastric acid hypersecretion. Diarrhoea and steatorrhoea are also related to the gastric acid hypersecretion as shown by the fact that they may be completely abolished by continuous gastric acid aspiration, total gastrectomy, or treatment with H_2-receptor blockers (Delen et al 1964, Singleton et al 1965, McCarthy et al 1977), or proton pump inhibitors (McArthur et al 1985, Maton et al 1989). Whether acid-induced damage to the intestinal mucosal architecture, inactivation of pancreatic enzymes, precipitation of bile acids, or fluid overloading are responsible for the diarrhoea is unknown. Food intake markedly reduces postprandial

acid secretion and gastric emptying in ZE patients, opposite findings to those in duodenal ulcer patients (Malagelada 1978, 1980). This may explain why malabsorption is an inconstant finding and why steatorrhoea is absent or mild in most ZE patients. In contrast, in the interdigestive state, gastric acid release into the gut may overcome the absorptive capacity of the bowel and induce watery diarrhoea in the early morning.

Clinical aspects

The ZE syndrome is a disease of middle age. The age at onset of symptoms is greatest between the third and the fifth decades of life (Ellison & Wilson 1964); only 15 of 800 cases were in children less than 16 years of age (Wilson et al 1971). The ratio of men to women is 3:2 (Ellison & Wilson 1964).

The predominant symptoms of patients with the ZE syndrome are abdominal pain, ulcer disease, vomiting, and diarhoea, all of which result from the pathophysiological events listed in Figure 48.5.

Recurrence rate of ulcers is much higher in gastrinoma patients than in patients with idiopathic peptic ulcer disease, and the same pertains to the frequency of complications, such as bleeding, perforation, and reflux oesophagitis.

Earlier diagnosis, stemming from liberal use of serum gastrin assay in recent years and better understanding of the disease process, has led to reduction in the frequency of virulent ulcer disease (Deveney et al 1978) and a change in the clinical picture originally described by Zollinger & Ellison (1955). For example, unusual location of peptic ulcer in the distal duodenum or jejunum, previously

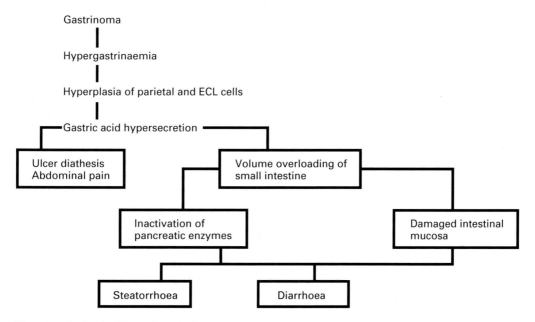

Fig. 48.5 Pathophysiology of the Zollinger–Ellison syndrome

occurring in up to 25% of patients (Ellison & Wilson 1964), is today a rather unusual finding in gastrinoma. Even the absence of peptic ulceration has been observed in up to 10% of patients with a proven gastrinoma. Surprisingly, dysphagia and pyrosis are not predominant symptoms in the early stages of the disease; the reported occurrence rates of these symptoms range from 0 to 7% (Jensen et al 1983) but increase with the duration of the disease to 19% (Ranfman et al 1983).

Associated endocrine abnormalities exist in up to 25% of gastrinoma patients (Ellison & Wilson 1964, Bonfils & Bader 1970, Jensen et al 1983). They result from the presence of multiple hormones produced by either the same tumour or coexisting pancreatic tumours, or are due to Wermer's syndrome (MEN type I) as the primary underlying disease. Hypercalcaemia caused by hyperparathyroidism is the most common clinically apparent abnormality accompanying the ZE syndrome. Mostly, the involvement of other endocrine glands is documented only by elevated blood hormone levels and not by clinical symptoms. For instance, in our own series, we found elevated urine corticosteroid concentrations in 11 of 19 Z E patients, but overt Cushing's syndrome in only two of these patients. More recently, ECL cell carcinoids of the fundic mucosa of the stomach have been described in patients with the ZE syndrome, if the gastrinoma was part of a MEN I syndrome (Solcia et al 1990).

Diagnosis and differential diagnosis

The presence of the ZE syndrome should be considered in cases of severe chronic peptic ulceration, particularly if the ulcer disease persists despite adequate treatment, or if there is ulcer recurrence after vagotomy and antrectomy. Accompanying diarrhoea is a further important hint. A gastrinoma can be identified or excluded with high accuracy by assaying gastric acid secretion and serum gastrin. Additional diagnostic steps depend on the results of these basic investigations.

Other conditions with similar clinical features, elevated serum gastrin levels, and increased gastric acid secretion have to be ruled out. They include patients in whom some antral mucosa has been left after Billroth II gastric resection; patients who have undergone small bowel resection, and patients with gastric outlet obstruction due to duodenal or pyloric ulceration. In contrast to findings in pigs (Schöön et al 1981), gastric distension does not appreciably increase serum gastrin in man; serum gastrin levels in patients with gastric outlet obstruction are either within normal range or only slightly elevated, and return to normal after gastric emptying. Both gastric acid secretion and serum gastrin levels are markedly elevated in patients with an excluded antrum (Korman et al 1972, Arnold et al 1976), but serum gastrin does not increase in response to secretin. Endoscopic biopsy of the excluded mucosa with immunohistological demonstration of G cells will provide confirmatory evidence of remnant antral mucosa.

Exaggerated basal and postprandial gastrin release, with normalization of circulating serum gastrin levels after antrectomy, characterizes antral G cell hyperfunction and antral G cell hyperplasia (Cowley et al 1973). The misleading terms 'Zollinger–Ellison syndrome type I' (Polak et al 1972) and 'pseudo-Zollinger–Ellison syndrome' (Friesen & Tomita, 1981) have been used for this entity. Since the volume density of antral G cells has been found to be both increased (Ganguli et al 1974, Keuppens et al 1980) and normal (Lamers et al 1978a), and since an increased antral G cell density can occur in hypergastrinaemic ulcer patients without gastrinoma as well as in healthy subjects, the term 'antral G cell hyperfunction' seems more appropriate. Serum gastrin in these subjects does not respond to secretin with an exaggerated increase.

Basal serum gastrin levels of patients with gastrinoma and antral G cell hyperfunction observed by us until 1982 are shown in Figure 48.6. As may be seen, the basal serum

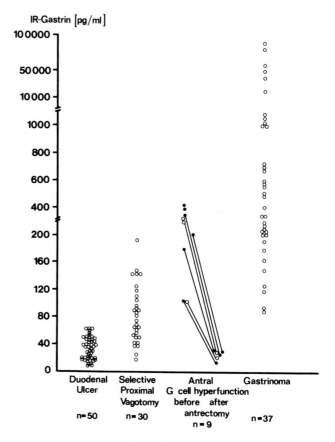

Fig. 48.6 Fasting serum levels of immunoreactive gastrin in patients with hypergastrinaemia and gastric hypersecretion, in comparison with patients with duodenal ulcer and patients after proximal vagotomy. Six patients with G-cell hyperfunction had been vagotomized before without effect •—•. (From Creutzfeldt W 1982 Scandinavian Journal of Gastroenterology (Suppl) 77:7–20, reproduced with permission).

gastrin levels of most gastrinoma patients exceed by far those of patients with antral G cell hyperfunction. However, one-third of the patients with proven gastrinoma have basal serum gastrin levels in the upper range of those of patients with duodenal ulcer disease, and equal to those of patients following selective proximal vagotomy or with antral G cell hyperfunction.

Basal acid secretion >15 mmol/hour in patients with an intact stomach, or >5 mmol/hour in patients after partial antrectomy, and a ratio of basal to pentagastrin-stimulated acid secretion >0.6 have been claimed to be highly suggestive of ZE syndrome (Ellison & Wilson 1964, Aoyagi & Summerskill 1966). These values are rarely achieved by duodenal ulcer patients without gastric outlet obstruction. Basal acid secretion in patients with antral G cell hyperfunction rarely reaches the high acid output found in most gastrinoma patients.

Special diagnostic tests

Elevated basal serum gastrin levels in the presence of gastric acid hypersecretion may be due not only to gastrinoma, but also to antral G cell hyperfunction or to an excluded antrum after Billroth II gastrectomy. Provocative tests have been recommended for differentiation. These tests are based on the observation that agents, such as calcium ions and theophylline, and peptides, such as secretin, glucagon and bombesin, stimulate gastrin secretion from gastrinoma cells to a much greater extent than from antral G cells. The diagnostic gain from the use of the different provocative agents is limited because of a considerable overlap between gastrinoma patients and duodenal ulcer patients with slightly elevated serum gastrin levels.

Of all proposed secretagogues, the gastrin response to secretin is of the greatest diagnostic significance. A substantial increase of serum gastrin within 2–10 minutes after i.v. secretin is highly suggestive of a gastrinoma (Isenberg et al 1972, Deveney et al 1977, Lamers & van Tongeren 1977). However, lack of response to secretin does not exclude this disorder. In up to 10% of patients with proven gastrinoma, no significant increase, and even a decrease, of serum gastrin may occur (Deveney et al 1977, Stage et al 1978, Jensen et al 1983a).

Some controversy exists regarding the extent of serum gastrin elevation indicative of gastrinoma. An increase of more than 50% of basal (Lamers et al 1978), of more than 100% of basal (Creutzfeldt et al 1975), and of more than 110 pg/ml of basal (Deveney et al 1977) have all been proposed as criteria. Our procedure is as follows: after an overnight fast, 75 KU secretin (natural porcine from the Karolinska Institute, Stockholm, or synthetic from Hoechst, Frankfurt) is given i.v. Samples of blood are taken before as well as 2, 5, 10, and 15 minutes after the secretin administration. A 'positive' test is an increase in serum gastrin of more than 100 pg/ml from basal, 2–5 minutes after secretin

injection. Stimulatory tests using glucagon, calcium, or bombesin are less sensitive.

The serum gastrin response to a test meal is not specific for antral G cell hyperfunction; serum gastrin also increases after feeding in some gastrinoma patients (Creutzfeldt et al 1975, Lamers & van Tongeren 1977, 115) and even in antrectomized patients (Creutzfeldt et al 1975). Serum gastrin response to a defined test meal should be investigated only in patients with a negative secretin test as described.

Localization

The occurrence in about 20% of cases of duodenal gastrinomas, and the better prognosis of these tumours after resection (Malagelada et al 1983), calls for careful radiological and endoscopic investigation of the duodenal wall in all patients with hypergastrinaemia and gastric hypersecretion. Duodenal gastrinomas may be easily found by duodenoscopy (Fig. 48.7). In addition, all modern imaging techniques have to be applied (see p. 523).

Treatment

Medical

The initial approach in the management of a patient with a gastrinoma is to attempt to control the gastric acid hypersecretion through antisecretory drugs. This may be achieved with H_2-receptor blocking agents (cimetidine, ranitidine, famotidine) (Malagelada et al 1983, Howard et al 1985). The acid-reducing effect of these H_2-blockers may be augmented and prolonged by concomitant administration of anticholinergics (Crane et al 1979, Mignon et al 1980). The antimuscarinic pirenzipine has been shown to be as effective in this regard as its classic precursors but with much smaller anticholinergic side-effects.

Some patients respond sufficiently to this scheme (Table 48.2). The dose of H_2-receptor blocking agent must be individually titrated to ensure that the basal acid output immediately before the next dose does not exceed 5 mmol/hour (Bonfils et al 1981). Doses of 0.4–1 g of cimetidine, or 0.15–0.3 g of ranitidine, 4 times daily, alone, or in combination with 50 mg of pirenzipine, 3 times daily, are generally necessary to achieve adequate suppression of acid secretion. Such high doses of H_2-receptor blocking agents can induce impotence and gynaecomastia (Jensen et al 1983a, Howard et al 1985).

A new class of antisecretory agents, the substituted benzimidazoles which act as inhibitors of the K^+-H^+-ATPase of the parietal cell are now the treatment of choice for patients with the ZE syndrome (Lamers et al 1984, McArthur et al 1985, Maton et al 1989). Table 48.3 demonstrates the long-lasting effect of omeprazole on acid secretion.

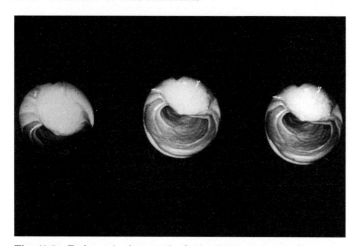

Fig. 48.7 Endoscopic photograph of a duodenal gastrinoma. Serum gastrin levels normalized after duodenopancreatectomy (Whipple's procedure) and there has been complete clinical remission for the years the patient has been followed-up.

Table 48.2 Effect on gastric acid secretion of the combination of ranitidine and pirenzipine and of vagotomy in a patient with gastrinoma (D.F.) (serum gastrin 250 pg/ml)

Treatment	Basal volume (ml/60 min)	Basal acid output (mmol/60 min)
None	555	52.7
5 x 150 mg ranitidine + 2 x 25 mg pirenzepine	76	4.0
Vagotomy	186	22.0

Surgical

Tumour resection should be tried in all cases, if metastases have been excluded. Normalization of serum gastrin levels used to be rare (<10%) after resection of a primary pancreatic gastrinoma (Jensen et al 1983) and more frequent (20–38%) after resection of primary duodenal gastrinoma (Hofmann et al 1973, Bonfils et al 1981, Malagelada et al 1983). However, with earlier diagnosis and better methods of localization, the rate of cured patients has been raised to 33% (Vogel et al 1987). As emphasized earlier, blind pancreatic resection is not advised should no tumour be found. In these cases, and also if metastases are found, selective proximal vagotomy may be considered because this procedure facilitates control of acid secretion by H_2-blocking agents (Richardson et al 1979).

Total gastrectomy was the procedure of choice in the ZE syndrome before H_2-blocking agents and omeprazole became available. It still serves as a possible alternative to medical therapy if patients are not compliant. Treatment of metastatic disease with cytostatic drugs or arterial embolization is indicated only if significant growth of the metastases is documented. Gastrinomas respond poorly to cytostatic treatment and partial remission is reported after combined treatment with streptozotocin, 5-fluorouracil

and adriamycin in 40% of cases without prolongation of life (von Schrenk et al 1988). Octreotide may be tried for inhibition of tumour growth but remission is rare.

DIARRHOEGENIC TUMOUR: PANCREATIC CHOLERA; WATERY DIARRHOEA-HYPOKALAEMIA-HYPOCHLORHYDRIA (WDHH) SYNDROME; VERNER-MORRISON SYNDROME; VIPOMA

Verner & Morrison in 1958, described a patient with an islet cell tumour who had severe refractory diarrhoea and hypokalaemia and who died of renal failure. It was later shown that this syndrome results from exaggerated release of vasoactive intestinal polypeptide (VIP) from either an endocrine pancreatic tumour or a ganglioneuroblastoma.

Pathology and pathophysiology

About 50% of the tumours causing the syndrome of so-called pancreatic cholera are malignant and 80% are situated in the pancreas. In 10–20% of cases, extra-pancreatic tumours (oat cell carcinoma, ganglioneuroma, ganglioneuroblastoma) account for the syndrome (Verner & Morrison 1974). Hyperplasia of pancreatic islets has been described in the presence of diarrhoegenic tumours, but this has not been documented by morphometry. 'Islet hyperplasia' has also been noted in the absence of a tumour, but in such instances the tumour may have been overlooked or situated at an extrapancreatic site.

Most of the tumours contain vasoactive intestinal polypeptide (VIP) and other peptides, most frequently pancreatic polypeptide and glucagon (Heitz et al 1982). It is now agreed, however, that VIP is the hormone causing the syndrome. Prostaglandins and calcitonin could contribute to the diarrhoea and cause hypochlorhydria. Pancreatic polypeptide, however, has never been shown in pharmacological studies to produce excessive diarrhoea. Moreover, many patients with other types of endocrine pancreatic tumours have high plasma levels of pancreatic polypeptide and yet are free of diarrhoea. Tumours producing only pancreatic polypeptide (PP) have never been demonstrated to induce diarrhoea or any specific clinical syndrome (Tomita et al 1991). On the other hand, the frequent secretion of PP by different endocrine tumours of the gut (28% in insulinomas, 31% in gastrinomas, 58% in glucagonomas, 74% in VIPomas) (Tomita et al 1991) make PP an interesting marker for endocrine pancreatic tumours.

VIP, first isolated from porcine gut (Said & Mutt 1970), is exclusively localized in nerve fibres but not in epithelial cells. Not only may it be extracted from the tumours in patients with the watery diarrhoea syndrome, but greatly elevated VIP plasma levels may also be observed in such patients (Said & Faloona 1975, Bloom

Table 48.3 Effect of omeprazole on gastric acid secretion in two antrectomized patients (Billroth II procedure) with gastrinoma. In both patients the ulcers healed 3–6 weeks after starting treatment

	Basal volume (ml/60 min)	Basal acid output (mmol/60 min)
Patient E. T.		
(Serum gastrin 64 700 pg/ml)		
Before treatment (omeprazole 60 mg once in the morning)	168	16.5
Day 2, before dose	47	1.5
Day 8, before dose	57	2.6
Day 45, before dose	62	1.7
Patient D. Sch.		
(Serum gastrin 440 pg/ml)		
Before treatment (omeprazole 60 mg)	330	23.1
Day 2, before dose	38	0.8
Day 8, before dose	140	3.1
Omeprazole 80 mg		
Day 22, before dose	74	1.9

& Polak 1976). VIP stimulates small intestinal secretion, reduces jejunal water, sodium, potassium, and chloride absorption, and increases the negative potential difference between the jejunal lumen and plasma. At high VIP levels, a net chloride secretion occurs resulting in increased negative potential difference and passive secretion of sodium and potassium (Krejs et al 1980). The underlying cellular mechanism for these events is activation of mucosal adenylate cyclase causing a rise in intracellular cAMP levels. In addition, VIP stimulates pancreatic bicarbonate secretion, relaxes the gallbladder, increases the hepatic output of glucose, and causes vasodilatation.

Clinical aspects

The disease is characterized by excessive watery diarrhoea with fluid loss of up to 6–8 litres per 24 hours. The stool, sometimes resembles dilute tea, is rich in electrolytes, and the loss of potassium may exceed 300 mmol/L. This potassium loss explains the hypokalaemia and acidosis that is invariably present during attacks of diarrhoea. Weight loss, dehydration, abdominal cramps, and confusion are commonly seen. Basal hypo- or achlorhydria and diabetes mellitus are both present in 50% of patients. Haemoconcentration may occur, giving rise to thromboembolic complications. A total of 20% of patients suffer from either patchy erythematous or urticarial attacks. Hypercalcaemia is another frequent finding (50% of patients). Despite hypercalcaemia, some patients have episodes of tetany. The tetanic attacks may result from hypomagnesaemia, which is found in 10% of patients.

The disease tends to fluctuate as part of its natural course with intervening episodes of clinical improvement (Krejs 1987).

Diagnosis and differential diagnosis

Diagnosis is confirmed by the demonstration of an elevated plasma VIP level. Since VIP is rapidly degraded by proteolytic enzymes, aprotinin (1000 kallikrein inhibitor units per ml blood) should be added, and after centrifugation the plasma should be frozen, within 15–30 minutes after blood sampling, to −30° C until assay. Alternatively, the plasma may be lyophilized and then transported to a reference laboratory. Demonstration of a reduced gastric acid secretion would support the diagnosis but by itself has no specificity.

With respect to efforts to localize the tumour, it should be kept in mind that VIPomas are situated at extrapancreatic sites in 20% of patients; in children, for instance, as a ganglioneuroblastoma (Said & Faloona 1975). Also, a Verner-Morrison-like syndrome has been reported to occur without any endocrine pancreatic tumour and without elevated plasma levels of VIP and other potential diarrhoegenic hormones. The term 'pseudo-Verner-Morrison syndrome' has been proposed for these patients, in some of whom pancreatic islet cell hyperplasia was observed at necropsy or after total pancreatectomy (Bloom & Polak 1976). In none of these cases, however, has a diarrhoegenic hormone been found immunohistologically or by extraction. In our experience with several cases considered to be instances of 'pseudo-Verner-Morrison syndrome', the diarrhoea proved to be factitious owing to laxative abuse. Blind pancreatic resection in patients without elevated plasma levels of VIP, therefore, is unwise.

Treatment

Treatment initially is symptomatic and consists of replacement of fluid (5 litres or more per day) and electrolytes. This may be supported by antihormone therapy in the form of glucocorticoids (50–100 mg prednisone daily). The i.v. infusion of somatostatin (100–250 µg/hour), or s.c. injection of 50–100 µg of octreotide (somatostatin) every

8 hours, have a dramatic effect on the diarrhoea and the fluid and electrolyte loss. This gives sufficient time to improve the metabolic situation, localize the tumour, exclude metastases, and develop an adequate therapeutic strategy. If a single tumour has been identified and localized, surgical resection should be carried out. In patients with metastatic disease, cytostatic treatment with streptozotocin and 5-fluorouracil is rewarding. The remission rate is higher than 90%. Figure 48.8 depicts the long-lasting remission of a patient with liver metastases after this type of treatment.

Immediately after administration of streptozotocin, diarrhoea and plasma VIP may increase dramatically for several days, necessitating replacement of large amounts of fluid and electrolytes (Fig. 48.9). VIP levels closely parallel the reduction in diarrhoea. The availability of the long-acting somatostatin analogue octreotide offers a very

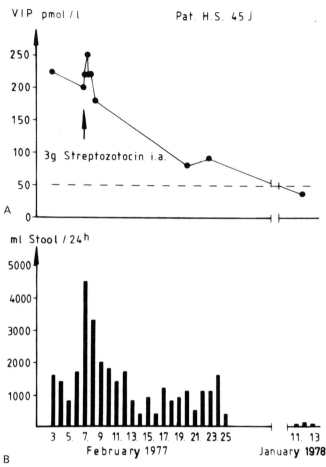

Fig. 48.9   Effects of 3 g of streptozotocin injected into the hepatic artery of a patient with liver metastasis from a VIPoma. **A** Plasma levels of vasoactive intestinal peptide (VIP); normal VIP levels are indicated by the dotted line. **B** Stool volume. The patient had a complete remission (including remission of insulin-dependent diabetes mellitus) for 2 years.

successful symptomatic therapeutic alternative (Rushone et al 1982, Krejs 1987). Patients with metastatic VIPoma can be kept asymptomatic for years with octreotide (3 x 100–500 µg s.c. daily). In single patients even tumour regression has been reported (Santangelo et al 1985, Kraezlin et al 1985).

In patients who do not respond to chemotherapy, hepatic artery embolization or surgical reduction of tumour mass (debulking) should be considered.

Prognosis

Prognosis varies with the stage of disease at the time of diagnosis. In those who are diagnosed at a very late stage with metastases, thromboembolic complications due to excessive dehydration often determine the course of the disease. In general, modern treatments (surgical resection, chemotherapy, and symptomatic treatment with octreotide) have greatly improved prognosis.

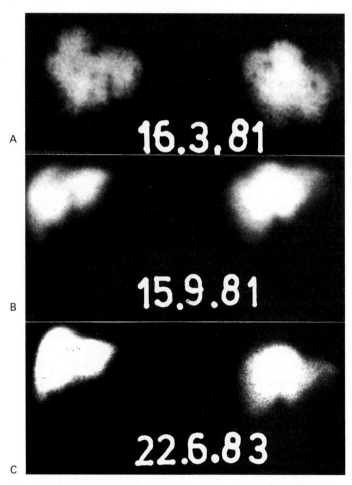

Fig. 48.8   **A** Technetium scintigram in a patient with the watery diarrhoea syndrome and liver metastases 5 years after resection of a VIPoma. **B** At 6 months. 2 years after cytostatic treatment with streptozotocin and 5-fluorouracil. Clinical and anatomical remission persisted for 5 years and responded to a second chemotherapy (streptozotocin, 5-fluorouracil and doxorubicin) for another 2 years. When watery diarrhoea started again, diffuse liver metastases were demonstrated. Therefore in 1990, daily injections of 100 µg octreotide s.c. were started. The patient remains asymptomatic.

GLUCAGONOMA

These tumours are classified into subtypes according to their clinical manifestations:

- Those which are associated with the typical 'glucagonoma syndrome' (skin disease, diabetes mellitus, weight loss, and anaemia).
- Those which are not associated with a clear clinical syndrome. They may or may not give rise to diabetes mellitus; occur frequently in association with other pancreatic endocrine tumours, and, in MEN I, are incidental postmortem findings in elderly patients (Ruttman et al 1980).

Glucagonomas associated with the 'glucagonoma syndrome' are rare. To date, less than 200 cases exhibiting the full syndrome have been reported. The mean age of diagnosis is around 55 years. The sex ratio is about 2:1 (Bloom & Polak 1987). In the last 20 years we have seen more than 200 patients with gastroenteropancreatic endocrine tumours, but only two with glucagonoma syndrome. Both had metastatic disease. No epidemiological data are available concerning the frequency of glucagonomas without a clinical syndrome. However, silent glucagonomas seem to be most frequent in MEN I.

Pathology and pathophysiology

Tumours giving rise to the typical glucagonoma syndrome have been found as single pancreatic neoplasms, sometimes of considerable size, evenly distributed throughout the whole pancreas (Ruttman et al 1980, Stacpoole 1981). The rate of malignancy is high; by the time the diagnosis is established 50–62% of the lesions have already metastasized. Glucagonomas not associated with the classic syndrome may also be found as an isolated malignant pancreatic tumour. They may occur in association with other pancreatic endocrine tumours (insulinoma, gastrinoma), especially in MEN I. As already noted, they may additionally appear as an incidental finding at necropsy in elderly patients.

The pathophysiology of the glucagonoma syndrome is traceable to the catabolic action of glucagon. Hyperglycaemia results from increased hepatic glycogenolysis and gluconeogenesis. Ketonaemia rarely develops because increased circulating insulin levels prevent excess lipolysis and maintain normal free fatty acid concentration (Boden et al 1978). The skin rash, described by Wilkinson (1973) as necrolytic migratory erythema, shows histologically superficial epidermal spongiosis and necrosis, with subcorneal and mid-epidermal clefts and bullae, fusiform keratinocytes with pyknotic nuclei, and mononuclear inflammatory infiltrates but rarely mononuclear acantholysis (Barber & Hamer 1976). These skin changes are definitely linked to the glucagon-producing tumour, since they disappear after excision of the glucagonoma, or improve during cytostatic or somatostatin therapy. Similar skin lesions have been observed in a patient under long-term exogenous glucagon administration (Barber & Hamer 1976). Zinc deficiency has been discussed.

Panhypoaminoacidaemia is a uniform finding and has been suggested as the initiator of the skin rash, inasmuch as administration of amino acids induces prompt remission of the rash while the levels of amino acids increase in the plasma. Glucagon physiologically stimulates hepatic uptake and utilization of certain amino acids. Conversely, acute or chronic glucagon deficiency leads to an increase of plasma amino acids (Fitzpatrick et al 1977, Boden et al 1979). The anaemia of the glucagonoma syndrome has likewise been hypothetically related to the hypoaminoacidaemia.

Gel filtration programs, obtained from immunoreactive glucagon studies in plasma and tumour samples of patients with the glucagonoma syndrome, have demonstrated that the tumour mainly contains material corresponding to true glucagon; large molecular weight substances have been found only inconsistently (Holst 1983). These larger components were predominant in most plasma samples from tumour patients, but were also found in normal subjects. Thus, gel filtration profiles do not distinguish patients with glucagonomas from normal and are of no greater value than simple radioimmunological estimation of plasma levels (Holst 1983).

Clinical aspects

Diabetes mellitus was the predominant symptom in 90% of cases in one reported series of 84 glucagonomas. Further symptoms included skin rash, often accompanied by stomatitis and nail changes (64%), weight loss (56%), anaemia (44%), hypoaminoacidaemia (26%), diarrhoea (15%), abdominal pain (14%), venous disorders (13%), nausea or vomiting (8.3%), anorexia (6%), and constipation (3.6%).

The skin lesions are undoubtedly the most specific symptom of the disease but are often initially misdiagnosed (Stacpoole 1981). The lesions frequently begin around the perineum and on the thighs. They appear initially as erythematous areas and later become raised and develop superficial central blisters that rupture to leave crusts. In areas exposed to friction, such as the groins and feet, there may be a weeping surface. The lesions tend to heal in the centre while the edges display red crusting which spreads in an annular or figurate outline. Healing is commonly associated with hyperpigmentation. The whole sequence usually takes 7–14 days to complete (Mallinson et al 1974). For unknown reasons the lesions characteristically remit and relapse, making the assessment of therapeutic measures difficult (Bloom & Polak 1987). A representative picture of these skin lesions is depicted in Figure 48.10.

The anaemia is usually normochromic and normocytic and does not respond to iron, vitamin B12, or folate. The venous changes do not appear to be associated with any special kind of coagulopathy. Neuropsychiatric disturbances have been observed in some patients, including dementia, optic atrophy, nystagmus, dysarthria, ataxia, and abnormal reflexes. These alterations tend to improve after chemotherapy.

Diagnosis

Diagnosis is based on the presence of the typical clinical features, fortified by the demonstration of elevated plasma glucagon levels, a pancreatic tumour, and possibly liver metastases. Glucose has been shown to cause a paradoxical rise, a fall, or no change in circulating glucagon levels (Stacpoole 1981). As in normal subjects, tumour glucagon can in most patients be stimulated by arginine (Lamers et al 1978) and tolbutamide (Stacpoole 1981). Analysis of the

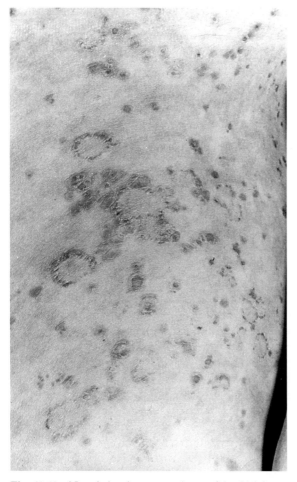

Fig. 48.10 Necrolytic migratory erythema of the thigh in a patient with the glucagonoma syndrome. Depicted are early changes which later spread out and developed into complete necrosis of the skin.

plasma amino acids can be helpful. However, this determination is difficult and from a practical point of view not essential. Nor does plasma fractionation for different molecular forms of glucagon contribute to the diagnosis or evaluation of the prognosis (Holst 1983).

Treatment

Of great importance for the choice of treatment is localization of the primary tumour and detection of any metastases. Tumour resection should be attempted, but the size of the tumour and its tendency to metastasize often defeat the surgical effort. In most cases, surgery should be the primary therapeutic approach followed by tumour embolization or chemotherapy, as discussed earlier in considering the general principles of management. Chemotherapy may have dramatic effects on the clinical syndrome and tumour size, however, recurrence is the rule (Bloom & Polak 1987). Our two patients responded to the combination of streptozotocin, 5-fluorouracil and doxorubicin for 6–12 months. Dacarbazine (DTIC) has been described to be especially effective in glucagonoma patients (Kessinger et al 1983). Octreotide (3 x 100–200 µg s.c. daily) lowers the plasma glucagon levels and improves the skin rash, the anaemia, and the general state of the patients (Bloom & Polak 1987). Due to incomplete glucagon suppression and simultaneous suppression of insulin secretion, diabetes mellitus may deteriorate and insulin treatment is then needed. Tumour regression caused by octreotide has not been described in patients with the glucagonoma syndrome. The skin lesions may be temporarily improved by the systemic administration of amino acids, and respond also to oral and local zinc supplementation.

SOMATOSTATINOMA

The existence of a somatostatinoma syndrome has been postulated by the presence of an endocrine tumour with somatostatin-producing cells, and a constellation of clinical features that include diabetes mellitus, dyspepsia, steatorrhoea, diarrhoea, achlorhydria, and cholelithiasis (Ganda et al 1977, Larsson et al 1977). Since the clinical features of the postulated syndrome are non-specific and are commonly found in patients without any endocrine tumour, it has been questioned whether this syndrome really exists (Stacpoole et al 1983).

Pathology and pathophysiology

Only some 80 patients with somatostatinomas have been described to date (Krejs et al 1979, Kaneko et al 1983, Schusdziarra et al 1983, Stacpoole et al 1983, Dayal & Ganda 1991). In addition to somatostatin-producing cells most of the tumours contained such hormones as calcitonin, cortisol, VIP, prostaglandin E_2, pancreatic polypeptide, and gastrin. The symptoms and other features observed in patients with a somatostatin-producing tumour could be explained by the inhibiting action of somatostatin on acid secretion, gastric emptying, gastrointestinal hormone activity, absorption of carbohydrates, amino acids, and fat from the intestine, contractility of the gallbladder, and volume, bicarbonate, and enzyme secretion of the pancreas. This contention is supported by the finding of markedly elevated levels of somatostatin as well as large molecular weight substances in the plasma of patients with a somatostatinoma.

However, only 30% of these 80 cases showed the clinical picture of the 'somatostatinoma syndrome', had tumours located in the pancreas, and had elevated plasma levels of somatostatin. The remaining 70% had lesions located in the duodenal mucosa and these were frequently associated with von Recklinghausen's neurofibromatosis, MEN-Type II syndrome, phaeochromocytoma or carcinoids elsewhere (Dayal & Ganda 1991). The patients with these so-called type B (duodenal) somatostatinomas had neither characteristic clinical symptoms nor elevated somatostatin plasma levels (Kaneko et al 1983, Dayal & Ganda 1991). Therefore, they may be classified as clinically silent somatostatinomas.

Both, type A (pancreatic) and type B (duodenal) somatostatinomas are nearly always malignant tumours that invade tissues locally at their site of origin and metastasize widely (Dayal & Ganda 1991).

Not all patients with a somatostatin-producing tumour reveal the full clinical picture of the 'somatostatinoma syndrome' originally described in 1977 (Ganda et al 1977, Larsson et al 1977) and associated with mild diabetes mellitus, abdominal pain, steatorrhoea, vomiting, hypochlorhydria or achlorhydria, and anaemia. The most frequent symptom is epigastric pain, which may in some instances be related to cholelithiasis.

Patients with a somatostatinoma also may have symptoms that do not relate to excessive somatostatin production, such as, for example, tachycardia, flushing, hypertension, hypokalaemia, alkalosis, or hypoglycaemia. Thus, the clinical features in the majority of patients are non-specific. The duodenal (type B) somatostatinomas usually present with local symptoms such as epigastric pain, nausea, vomiting, signs of intestinal obstruction or gastrointestinal bleeding and jaundice (Dayal & Ganda 1991).

Diagnosis

Because of the non-specific nature of the clinical manifestations, the diagnosis of a somatostatinoma has not yet been established preoperatively. Rather, the tumours have been detected by chance by imaging methods, by endoscopy, or even during laparotomy for cholecystectomy.

Estimation of plasma levels of somatostatin may be helpful in patients with suspicious symptoms in the presence of a pancreatic or duodenal tumour. Somatostatin release by the tumour may be stimulated by tolbutamide (Stacpoole et al 1983), but whether this can serve as a provocative test of diagnostic relevance cannot be answered at present.

Treatment

Treatment is similar to that of other endocrine tumours. If metastases have been excluded, the tumour should be resected. Antihormone therapy is not known, except for control of diabetes if present. Antitumour therapy of the type outlined in the earlier discussion of this subject may be tried. Experience is still limited.

MULTIPLE ENDOCRINE NEOPLASIA (MEN) AND MULTIPLE ENDOCRINE ADENOMATOSIS (MEA)

Multiple endocrine tumours in different organs, first described by Erdheim in 1903, has become recognized as a hereditary disorder, probably inherited as an autosomal dominant trait (Ballard et al 1964, Wermer 1974). Several subtypes can be distinguished with occasional overlap even within the same family:

1. Type I (Wermer's syndrome) is characterized by endocrine tumours involving the parathyroid glands, the pancreas, and the pituitary; the thyroid, the adrenal cortex and the thymus are rarely involved, and additional bronchial and intestinal carcinoids, lipomas, brown fat tumours, gastric polyps, and Schwannomas have been observed.

2. Type IIa (or II) (Sipple's syndrome) consists of hyperparathyroidism, phaeochromocytoma, and medullary carcinoma of the thyroid.

3. Type IIb (or III) includes mucosal neuromas (thickened lips/facies), intestinal ganglioneuromatosis leading to megacolon and constipation, hyperplastic corneal nerves, a Marfan-like habitus, and rarely, hyperparathyroidism in addition to medullary carcinoma of the thyroid and phaeochromocytoma.

The different syndromes have been described in detail in recent reviews (Lamers et al 1978b, Eberle & Grün 1981, DeLellis 1991). Discussion here will only deal with endocrine pancreatic tumours associated with MEN type I. Recent studies indicate that a single inherited locus on chromosome 11, band q13, is responsible for the development of MEN I and that the development of pancreatic and parathyroid tumours involves similar allelic deletions on chromosome 11 (Larsson et al 1988, Friedman et al 1989, Thakker et al 1989, DeLellis 1991).

Endocrine pancreatic tumours (gastrinomas, glucagonomas, pancreatic polypeptide-producing tumours (PPomas), and insulinomas) have been described in up to 60% of patients with MEN type I. Non-insulin-producing tumours predominate. The tumours are frequently multiple with as many as 15 glucagonomas having been found in a single asymptomatic patient. Peptic ulcer disease due to a gastrinoma is present in half of the patients.

Since the endocrine tumours of MEN I syndrome are benign, operative intervention is indicated only if hormone secretion or its sequelae cannot be controlled by medical treatment, i.e. in case of hyperparathyroidism due to adenomas of the parathyroids, or of hyperinsulinaemic hypoglycaemia due to insulinoma. Gastric hypersecretion as a consequence of gastrinoma, can be successfully treated by H_2-receptor blockers or proton pump inhibitors, and hyperprolactinaemia by dopamine agonists.

A study of the frequency of associated endocrinopathies in 109 relatives of 10 patients with proven gastrinoma (Lamers et al 1978b) showed that six patients had blood relatives with endocrinopathies. In 69% of these the endocrinopathies were symptomless. Hyperparathyroidism was diagnosed in 30 members of the six families, gastrinomas in 15, and insulin-producing tumours in eight. Eight relatives had pituitary tumours. Thus, patients with endocrine pancreatic tumours should be carefully investigated for additional endocrinopathies. Estimations of serum levels of calcium, phosphate, parathormone, prolactin, growth hormone, and ACTH performed at regular intervals may help to uncover an underlying MEN I syndrome.

NON-FUNCTIONING ENDOCRINE TUMOURS

An immunocytochemical analysis (Heitz et al 1982) of 125 endocrine pancreatic tumours established that 30 were 'non-secreting', inasmuch as no elevated serum hormone levels could be detected by radioimmunoassay and no clinical syndrome was present. These tumours contained varying amounts of insulin, glucagon, somatostatin, and pancreatic polypeptide (PP), but in four no hormone could be demonstrated. Another 10 patients with tumours described as pancreatic polypeptide-producing tumours also did not suffer from a hormonally induced syndrome, although serum PP levels were found to be significantly elevated. Of these 40 endocrine tumours without a manifest clinical syndrome, 15 were classified as malignant on the basis of development of metastases. The relative frequency of non-functioning tumours found in this collection may not be representative but demonstrates that these silent endocrine tumours do occur in appreciable number. They are clinically apparent because their growth produces a mass and their endocrine nature is in general a surprise finding by the pathologist.

In a later publication, the same group have reported a collection of 365 pancreatic endocrine tumours (Klöppel & Heitz 1988), of which 36.4% were non-functioning locally symptomatic tumours. Of these 64% were malignant. Similar figures are given in a recent review article on 132 cases from one centre (Solcia et al 1991): 29.5% were non-functioning and clinically silent, and of these 45% were malignant.

As mentioned above, when systematically searched for, clinically silent pancreatic endocrine tumours have been detected in 0.3–1.5% of unselected autopsies (Warren 1926, Spencer 1955, Becker 1971, Grimelius et al 1975). These tumours were mostly small (less than 1 cm), well encapsulated and found in elderly patients (mean age around 70 years). They have no clinical relevance. Conversely, given their high malignancy rate of more than 60%, non-functioning locally symptomatic tumours should undergo biopsy and surgical treatment (Solcia et al 1991).

If surgical resection is not possible, antitumour measures may be tried, following the principles already outlined for functioning endocrine pancreatic tumours, i.e. cytostatic treatment and hepatic arterial embolization. However, these measures are indicated only if there is progressive tumour growth.

REFERENCES

Albers N, Löhr M, Bogner U, Loy V, Klöppel G 1989 Nesidioblastosis of the pancreas in an adult with persistent hyperinsulinemic hypoglycemia. American Journal of Clinical Pathology 91:336–340

Allison D J, Modlin I M, Jenkins W J 1977 Treatment of carcinoid liver metastases by hepatic artery embolization. Lancet 2:1323–1325

Aoyagi T, Summerskill W H J 1966 Gastric secretion with ulcerogenic islet tumors. Importance of basal acid output. Archives of Internal Medicine 117:667–672

Arnold R, Creutzfeldt W, Peiper H J 1976 Befunde beim Antrumrest nach Billroth-II Operation ('excluded antrum') – ein Beitrag zur Differentialdiagnose des Rezidivulkus mit Hypergastrinämie. Verhandlungen de Deutschen Gesellschaft für innere Medizin 82:1002–1006

Arnold R, Creutzfeldt C, Creutzfeldt W 1977 Multiple hormone production of endocrine tumors of the gastrointestinal tract. In: James V H T (ed.) Endocrinology. Excerpta Medica Amsterdam, Oxford, vol 2, p 448–452

Ballard H S, Frame B, Hartsock R J 1964 Familial multiple endocrine adenoma-peptic ulcer complex. Medicine 43:481–516

Barber S G, Hamer J D 1976 Skin rash in patients receiving glucagon. Lancet 2:1138

Bardram L, Agner T, Hagen C 1988 Levels of α-subunits of gonadotropins can be increased in Zollinger–Ellison syndrome, both in patients with malignant tumours and with apparently benign disease. Acta Endocrinologica (Copenhagen) 118:135–141

Becker V 1971 Pathologisch-anatomische Aspekte dei endokrin wirksamen Tumoren. Langenbecks Archiv Klinische Chirurgie 88:426-437

Bernades P, Bonnefond A, Bonfils S 1972 Syndrome de Zollinger–Ellison avec tumeurs endocrines carcinoiides insulaires de siège vesiculaire primitif. Archive Français Maladies Appareil Digestif 61:759–766

Berger M, Bordi C, Cüppers H J, Berchtold P, Gries F A, Müntefering H, Sailer R, Zimmermann H, Orci L 1983 Functional and morphological characterization of human insulinomas. Diabetes 32:921–931

Bloom S R, Polak J M 1976 VIP measurement in distinguishing Verner–Morrison syndrome and pseudo Verner–Morrison syndrome. Clinical Endocrinology 5:223–228

Bloom S R, Polak J M 1987 Glucagonoma syndrome. American Journal of Medicine 82 (Suppl 5B):25–35

Boden G, Wilson R M, Owen O E 1978 Effects of chronic glucagon excess on hepatic metabolism. Diabetes 27:643–648

Boden G, Rezvani I, Master R W, Trapp V, Schwartz M, Owen O E 1979 Glucagon deficiency causes hyperaminoacidemia. Clinical Research 27:482A

Bonfils S, Bader J P 1970 The diagnosis of Zollinger–Ellison syndrome with special reference to the multiple endocrine adenomas. In: Jerzy-Glass B G, (ed.) Progress in Gastroenterology. Grune and Stratton, New York vol 2, p 332–355

Bonfils S, Landor J H, Mignon M, Hervoir P 1981 Results of surgical management in 92 consecutive patients with Zollinger–Ellison syndrome. Annals of Surgery 194:692–697

Broder L E, Carter S K 1973 Pancreatic islet cell carcinoma. II. Results of therapy with streptozotocin in 52 patients. Annals of Internal Medicine 79:108–118

Burkhardt A, Mitschke H 1974 Zur pathologischen Anatomie des Verner–Morrison-Syndroms. Virchows Archiv Pathologie Anatomie 364:145-163

Carrasco C E, Chuang V P, Wallace S 1983 Apudomas metastatic to the liver: treatment by hepatic artery embolization. Radiology 149:79–83

Clouse M E, Lee R G L, Duszlak E J, Lokich J J, Trey C, Alday M R, Yoburn D C, Diamond J, Crosson A W, Costello O 1983 Peripheral hepatic artery embolization for primary and secondary hepatic neoplasms. Radiology 147:407–411

Cowley D J, Dymock I W, Boyes B E, Wilson R Y, Stagg B H, Lewin M R, Polak J M, Pearse A G E 1973 Zollinger–Ellison syndrome type 1: clinical and pathological correlations in a case. Gut 14:25–29

Crane S A, Summers R W, Heeringa W G 1979 Long-term cimetidine and anticholinergic therapy in patients with gastrinoma. American Journal of Surgery 138:446–550

Creutzfeldt W 1975 Pancreatic endocrine tumors – the riddle of their origin and hormone secretion. Israeli Journal of Medical Science 11:762–776

Creutzfeldt W 1985 Endocrine tumors of the pancreas. In: Arquilla E, Volk B W, (eds) The diabetic pancreas, 2nd edn. Plenum, New York

Creutzfeldt W, Frerichs H 1969 Factitious hypoglycaemia. Its importance in the differential diagnosis of hyperinsulinism. German Medical Monthly 14:421–426

Creutzfeldt W, Arnold R, Creutzfeldt C, Deuticke U, Frerichs H, Track N S 1973 Biochemical and morphological investigations of 30 human insulinomas. Diabetologia 9:217–231

Creutzfeldt W, Arnold R, Creutzfeldt C, Track N S 1975 Pathomorphologic, biochemical and diagnostic aspects of gastrinoma (Zollinger–Ellison syndrome). Human Pathology 6:47–76

Creutzfeldt W, Arnold R, Creutzfeldt C, Frerichs H 1980 Induction of hormone-producing pancreatic tumors in the rat. In: Andreani D, Lefebvre P J, Marks V (eds) Current views on hypoglycaemia and glucagon. Academic Press, London, p 205–221

Creutzfeldt W, Bartsch H H, Jacubaschke U, Stöckmann F 1991 Treatment of gastrointestinal endocrine tumours with interferon-α and octreotide. Acta Oncologica; 30:529–535

Daggett P R, Goodburn E A, Kurtz A B, Le Quesne L P, Morris D V, Nabarro J D N, Raphael M J 1981 Is preoperative localisation of insulinomas necessary? Lancet 1:483–486

Dayal Y, Ganda O P 1991 Somatostatin-producing tumors. In: Dayal Y (ed.) Endocrine pathology of the gut and pancreas. CRC Press, Boston p 241–277

Delen J, Tytgat H, van Goidsenhoven G E 1964 Diarrhea associated with pancreatic islet cell tumors. American Journal of Digestive Diseases 9:97–108

DeLellis R A 1991 The multiple endocrine neoplasia syndromes. In: Dayal Y (ed.) Endocrine pathology of the gut and pancreas. CRC Press, Boston p 305–317

Deveney L W, Deveney K S, Jaffe B M, Jones R S, Way L W. 1977 Use of calcium and secretin in the diagnosis of gastrinoma (Zollinger–Ellison syndrome). Annals of Internal Medicine 87:680–686

Deveney L W, Deveney K S, Way L W 1978 The Zollinger–Ellison syndrome – 23 years later. Annals of Surgery 188:384–393

Dockray G J, Walsh J H, Passaro E 1975 Relative abundance of big and little gastrin in the tumors and blood of patients with the Zollinger–Ellison syndrome. Gut 16:353–358

Doppman J L, Brennan M F, Dunnick N R, Kahn C R, Gorden P 1981 The role of pancreatic venous sampling in the localization of occult insulinomas. Radiology 138:557–662

Dunnick N R, Longt Jr J A, Krudy A, Shawker T H, Doppman J L 1980 Localizing insulinomas with combined radiographic methods. American Journal of Radiology 135:747–752

Eberle F, Grün R 1981 Multiple endocrine neoplasia, type I (MEN I). Ergebnisse innere Medizin und Kinderheil Kunde 46:75–150

Elfving G, Hästbacka J 1965 Pancreatic heterotopia and its clinical importance. Acta Chirurgica Scandinavica 130:593–602

Ellison E H, Wilson S D 1964 The Zollinger–Ellison syndrome: reappraisal and evaluation of 260 registered cases. Annals of Surgery 160:512–530

Erdheim H 1903 Zur normalen und pathologischen Histologie der Glandula thyreoidea, parathyreoidea und Hypophysis. Beitrage Pathologische Anatomic und Allgemeine Pathologic 33:158–236

Fajans S S, Floyd J C 1976 Fasting hypoglycemia in adults. New England Journal of Medicine 294:766–772

Fitzpatrick G F, Meguid M M, Gitlitz P H, Brennan M F 1977 Glucagon infusion in normal man: effects on 3-methyl-histidine excretion and plasma amino acids. Metabolism 26:477–501

Floyd Jr J C, Fajans S S, Pek S, Chance R E 1977 A newly recognized pancreatic polypeptide: plasma levels in health and disease. Recent Progress in Hormone Research 33:519–570

Forty R, Barrett G M 1952 Peptic ulceration of third part of duodenum associated with islet cell tumors. British Journal of Surgery 40:60–64

Frerichs H, Creutzfeldt W 1976 Hypoglycaemia. 1. Insulin secreting tumors. Clinics in Endocrinology and Metabolism 5:747–767

Frerichs H, Creutzfeldt W 1980 Glucose-calcium infusion test for the diagnosis of insulinoma. In: Andreani D, Lefebvre P J, Marks V (eds) Current views on hypoglycemia and glucagon. Academic Press, London, p 259–267

Frerichs H, Track N S 1974 Pharmacotherapy of hormone-secreting tumours. Clinical Gastroenterology 3:721–732

Friedman E, Sakaguchi K, Bale A E et al 1989 Clonality of parathyroid tumors in familial multiple endocrine neoplasia type I. New England Journal of Medicine 312:213–218

Friesen S R 1982 Tumors of the endocrine pancreas. New England Journal of Medicine 306:580–590

Friesen S R, Tomita T 1981 Pseudo-Zollinger–Ellison syndrome: hypergastrinemia, hyperchlorhydria without tumor. Annals of Surgery 194:481–493

Galiber A K, Reading C C, Charboneau J W, Sheedy P F, Lames E M, Gorman B, Grant C S, van Heerden J A, Telander R L 1988 Localization of pancreatic insulinoma: comparison of pre- and intraoperative US with CT and angiography. Radiology 166:405–408

Ganda O P, Weir G C, Soeldner J S, Legg M A, Chick W L, Patel Y C, Ebeid A M, Gabbay K H, Reichlin S 1977 'Somatostatinoma': a somatostatin-containing tumor of the endocrine pancreas. New England Journal of Medicine 296:963–967

Ganguli P C, Polak J M, Pearse A G E, Elder J B, Hegarty M 1974 Antral-gastrin-cell hyperplasia in peptic ulcer disease. Lancet 1:583–586

Gin H, Erny P, Perissat J, Doutre L P, Aubertin J 1988 Artificial pancreas in the diagnosis and treatment of insulinoma: a report of five cases. British Journal of Surgery 75:584

Glaser B, Valtysson G, Fajans S S, Vinik A I, Cho K, Thompson N 1981 Gastrointestinal pancreatic hormone concentrations in the portal venous system of nine patients with organic hyperinsulinism. Metabolism 30:1001–1010

Goosens A, Heitz P, Klöppel G 1991 Pancreatic endocrine cells and their non-neoplastic proliferations. In: Dayal Y (ed.) Endocrine pathology of the gut and pancreas. CRC Press, Boston, p 69–104

Gould V E, Wiedemann B, Lee I, Schwechheimer K, Dworniczak B D,

Radosevich J A, Moll R, Franke W W 1987 Synaptophysin expression in neuroendocrine neoplasms as determined by immunochemistry. American Journal of Pathology 126:243–257

Grimelius L, Hultquist G T, Stenkvist B 1975 Cytological differentiation of asymptomatic pancreatic islet cell tumors in autopsy material. Virchows Archiv Pathologie Anatomie 365:275–288

Hansen O H, Pedersen T, Larson J K, Rehfeld J F 1976 Effect of gastrin on gastric mucosal cell proliferation in man. Gut 17:536–541

Hanssen L E, Schrumpf E, Kolbenstvedt A N, Tausjo J, Dolva L O 1989 Recombinant α-2 interferon with or without hepatic artery embolization in the treatment of midgut carcinoid tumours – A preliminary report. Acta Oncologica 28:439–443

Hayashi M, Floyd J C, Pek S, Fajans S S 1977 Insulin, proinsulin, glucagon and gastrin in pancreatic tumors and in plasma of patients with organic hyperinsulinism. Journal of Clinical Endocrinology and Metabolism 44:681–694

Heitz P U 1984 Pancreatic endocrine tumors. In: Klöppel G, Heitz P U (eds) Pathology of the pancreas. Churchill Livingstone, Edinburgh

Heitz P U, Kasper M, Polak J M, Klöppel G 1982 Pancreatic endocrine tumors: immunocytochemical analysis of 125 tumors. Human Pathology 13:261–271

Heitz P U, Kasper M, Klöppel G, Polak J M, Vaitukaitis J L 1983 Glycoprotein-hormone alpha-chain production by pancreatic endocrine tumors: a specific marker for malignancy. Cancer 51:277–282

Hofmann J W, Fox P S, Wilson S D 1973 Duodenal wall tumors and the Zollinger–Ellison syndrome: surgical management. Archives of Surgery 107:334–339

Holst J J 1983 Molecular heterogeneity of glucagon in normal subjects and in patients with glucagon-producing tumors. Diabetologia 24:359–365

Holst J J, Helland S, Ingemannson S, Bang Pedersen N, von Schenck H 1979 Functional studies in patients with the glucagonoma syndrome. Diabetologia 17:151–156

Howard J M, Moss N H, Rhoads J E 1950 Hyperinsulinism and islet cell tumors of the pancreas. With 398 recorded tumors. International Abstracts Surgery 90:417–455

Howard J M, Chremos A N, Collen M J, McArthur K E, Cherner J A, Maton P N, Ciarleglio C A, Cornelius M J, Gardner J D 1985 Famotidine, a new potent, long-acting histamine H$_2$ receptor antagonist: comparison with cimetidine and ranitidine in the treatment of Zollinger–Ellison syndrome. Gastroenterology 88:1026–1033

Ingemansson S, Lunderquist A, Lövdahl R, Tibbin S 1975 Portal and pancreatic vein characterization with radioimmunologic determination of insulin. Surgery, Gynecology and Obstetrics 141:705–711

Isenberg J I, Walsh J H, Passaro Jr E 1972 Unusual effect of secretion on serum gastrin, serum calcium, and gastric acid secretion in a patient with suspected Zollinger–Ellison syndrome. Gastroenterology 62:626–631

Jensen R T, Collen M J, Pandol S J, Allende H D, Raufmann J P, Bissonette B M, Duncan W C, Durgin P L, Gillin J C, Gardner J D 1983a Cimetidine-induced impotence and breast changes in patients with gastric hypersecretory states. New England Journal of Medicine 308:883–887

Jensen R T, Gardner J D, Raufmann J P, Pandol S J, Doppman J L, Collen M J 1983b Zollinger–Ellison syndrome: current concepts and management. Annals of Internal Medicine 98:59–75

Johnson L R, Guthrie P D 1976 Stimulation of DNA synthesis by big and little gastrin (G-34 and G-17). Gastroenterology 71:599–602

Kahn C R, Rosen S W, Weintraub B D, Fajans S S, Gorden P 1977 Ectopic production of chorionic gonadotropin and its subunits by islet-cell tumors. New England Journal of Medicine 297:565–569

Kaneko H, Toshima T, Kobayashi H, Kitazawa M, Ito S, Iwanaga T, Kusumoto Y, Fujita T, Nitta H 1983 Duodenal somatostatinoma. Immunohistopathology and review of literature. Acta Pathologica Japonica 33:153–158

Kavlie H, White T T 1972 Pancreatic islet beta cell tumors and hyperplasia: experience in 14 Seattle hospitals. Annals of Surgery 175:326–335

Kessinger A, Foley J F, Lemon H M 1983 Therapy of malignant APUD cell tumors. Cancer 51:790–794

Keuppens F, Willems G, de Graef J, Woussen-Colle M C 1980 Antral gastrin cell hyperplasia in patients with peptic ulcer. Annals of Surgery 191:276–281

Klöppel G, Heitz P U 1988 Pancreatic endocrine tumors. Pathology Research and Practice 183:155–168

Korman M G, Scott D F, Hansky J, Wilson H 1972 Hypergastrinemia due to excluded antrum: a proposed method for differentiation from Zollinger–Ellison syndrome. Australian and New Zealand Journal of Medicine 3:266–271

Kraezlin M E, Ch'ng J L C, Wood S M, Carr D H, Bloom S R 1985 Long-term treatment of a VIPoma with somatostatin analogue resulting in remission of symptoms and possible shrinkage of metastases. Gastroenterology 88:185–187

Krejs G J 1987 VIPoma syndrome. American Journal of Medicine 82 (Suppl. 5B):37–47

Krejs G J, Orci L, Conlon M, Ravazzola M, Davis G R, Raskin P, Collins S M, McCarthy D M, Baetens D, Rubenstein A, Aldor T A M, Unger R H 1979 Somatostatinoma syndrome: biochemical, morphologic and clinical features. New England Journal of Medicine 301:285–292

Krejs G J, Fordtran J S, Bloom S R, Fahrenkrug J, Schaffalitzky de Muckadell O B, Fischer J E, Humphrey C S, O'Dorisio T M, Said S I, Walsh J H, Shulkes A A 1980 Effect of VIP infusion on water and ion transport in the human jejunum. Gastroenterology 78:722–727

Kvols L K, Moertel C G, O'Connell M J, Schutt A J, Rubin L, Hahn R G 1986 Treatment of the malignant carcinoid syndrome: Evaluation of a long-acting somatostatin analogue. New England Journal of Medicine 315:663–666

Kvols L K, Buck M, Moertel C G et al 1987 Treatment of metastatic islet cell carcinoma with a somatostatin analogue (SMS 201-996). Annals of Internal Medicine 107:162–168

Lamberts S W J, Hofland L J, van Koetsveld P M, Reubi J-C, Bruining H A, Bakker W H, Krenning E P 1990a Parallel in vivo and in vitro detection of functional somatostatin receptors in human endocrine pancreatic tumors: Consequences with regard to diagnosis, localization, and therapy. Journal of Clinical and Endocrinological Metabolism 71:566–574

Lamberts S W J, Bakker W H, Reubi J C, Krenning E P 1990b Somatostatin-receptor in the localisation of endocrine tumours. New England Journal of Medicine 323:1246–1249

Lamers C B H, van Tongeren J H M 1977 Comparative study of the value of the calcium, secretin, and meal stimulated increase in serum gastrin to the diagnosis of the Zollinger–Ellison syndrome. Gut 18:128–134

Lamers C B H, Ruland C M, Joosten H J M, Verkoogen H C M, van Tongeren J H M, Rehfeld J F 1978a Hypergastrinemia of antral origin in duodenal ulcer. Digestive Diseases 23:998–1002

Lamers C B, Stadil F, van Tongeren J H 1978b Prevalence of endocrine abnormalities in patients with the Zollinger–Ellison syndrome and in their families. American Journal of Medicine 64:607–612

Lamers C B, Walsh J H, Jansen J B, Harrison A R, Ippoliti A F, van Tongeren J H 1982 Evidence that gastrin 34 is preferentially released from the human duodenum. Gastroenterology 83:233–239

Lamers C B H W, Lind T, Morberg S, Jansen J B M J, Olbe L 1984 Omeprazole in Zollinger–Ellison syndrome. New England Journal of Medicine 310:758–761

Larsson L I, Hirsch M A, Holst J J, Ingemansson S, Kuhl C, Lindkaer Jensen S, Lundquist G, Rehfeld J F, Schwartz T W 1977 Pancreatic somatostatinoma: clinical features and physical implications. Lancet 1:666–668

Larsson C, Skogseid B, Oberg K, Nakamura Y, Nordenkjold M 1988 Multiple endocrine neoplasia maps to chromosome 11 and is lost in insulinoma. Nature 332:85–87

Lloyd R V, Mervak T, Schmidt K, Warner T F C S, Wilson B S 1984 Immunohistochemical detection of chromogranin and neuron specific enolase in pancreatic endocrine neoplasms. American Journal of Surgical Pathology 8:607–614

McArthur K E, Collen M J, Maton P N, Cherner J A, Howard J M, Ciarleglio C A, Cornelius M J, Jensen R T, Gardner J D 1985 Omeprazole: effective, convenient therapy for Zollinger–Ellison syndrome. Gastroenterology 88:939–944

McCarthy D M, Weintraub B D, Rosen S W 1974 Subunits of human chorionic gonadotropin in malignant gastrinoma. Gastroenterology 76:1198(A)

McCarthy D M, Olinger E J, May R J, Long B W, Gardner J D 1977 H$_2$-histamine receptor blocking agents in the Zollinger–Ellison syndrome: experience in serum cases and implications for long-term therapy. Annals of Internal Medicine 87:668–675

Malagelada J R 1978 Pathophysiological responses to meals in the Zollinger–Ellison syndrome. 1. Paradoxical postprandial inhibition of gastrin secretion. Gut 19:284–289

Malagelada J R 1980 Pathophysiological responses to meals in the Zollinger–Ellison syndrome. 2. Gastric emptying and its effect on duodenal function. Gut 21:98–104

Malagelada J R, Edis A J, Adson M A, van Heerden J A, Go V L M 1983 Medical and surgical options in the management of patients with gastrinoma. Gastroenterology 84:1524–1532

Mallinson C N, Bloom S R, Warin A P, Salmon P R, Cox B 1974 A glucagonoma syndrome. Lancet 2:1–5

Maton P N, Vinayek R, Frucht H, McArthur K A, Miller L S, Saeed Z A, Gardner J D, Jensen R T 1986 Long-term efficacy and safety of omeprazole in patients with Zollinger–Ellison syndrome: a prospective study. Gastroenterology 97:827–836

Mignon M, Vallot T, Galmische J P, Dupas J L, Bonfils S 1980 Interest of a combined antisecretory treatment, cimetidine and pirenzepin, in the management of severe forms of Zollinger–Ellison syndrome. Digestion 20:56–61

Moertel C G, Hanley J A, Johnson L A 1980 Streptozocin alone compared with streptozocin plus fluorouracil in the treatment of advanced islet-cell carcinoma. New England Journal of Medicine 303:1189–1194

Moore T J, Peterson L M, Harrington D P, Smith R J 1982 Successful arterial embolization of an insulinoma. Journal of the American Medical Association JAMA 248:1353–1355

Nauck M, Creutzfeldt W 1991 Insulin-producing tumors and the insulinoma syndrome. In: Dayal Y (ed.) Endocrine pathology of the gut and pancreas. CRC Press, Boston, p 195–225

Nauck M, Stöckmann F, Creutzfeldt W 1990 Evaluation of a euglycaemic clamp procedure as a diagnostic test in insulinoma patients. European Journal of Clinical Investigation 20:15–28

Öberg K, Eriksson B 1989 Medical treatment of neuroendocrine gut and pancreatic tumors. Acta Oncologica 28:425–431

Öberg K, Funa K, Alm G 1983 Effects of leucocyte interferon on clinical symptoms and hormone levels in patients with midgut carcinoid tumors and carcinoid syndrome. New England Journal of Medicine 309:129–132

Polak J M, Stagg B, Pearse A G E 1972 Two types of Zollinger–Ellison syndrome: immunofluorescent, cytochemical, and ultrastructural studies of the antral and pancreatic gastrin cells in different clinical states. Gut 13:501–512

Polak J M, Bloom S R, Adrian T E, Heitz P, Bryant M G, Pearse A G E 1976 Pancreatic polypeptide in insulinomas, gastrinomas, vipomas and glucagonomas. Lancet 1:328–330

Raufmann J P, Collins S M, Pandol S J, Korman L Y, Collen M S, Cornelius M J, Feld M K, McCarthy D M, Gardner J D, Jensen R T 1983 Reliability of symptoms in assessing control of gastric acid secretion in patients with Zollinger–Ellison syndrome. Gastroenterology 84:108–113

Rehfeld J F 1974 What is gastrin? A progress report on the heterogeneity of gastrin in serum and tissue. Digestion 11:397–405

Reynolds J H, Kaminsky N I, Schade D S, Eaton R P 1984 Use of a computerized glucose clamp technique to diagnose an insulinoma. Annals of Internal Medicine 101:648–649

Reubi J L, Häcki W H, Lamberts S W J 1987 Hormone-producing gatrointestinal tumours contain a high density of somatostatin receptors. Journal of Clinical and Endocrinological Metabolism 65:1127–1134

Richardson C T, Feldmann M, McClelland R N, Dickeman R M, Kumpuris D, Fordtran J S 1979 Effect of vagotomy in Zollinger–Ellison syndrome. Gastroenterology 77:682–686

Rushone A, Rene E, Chayvialle J A, Bonin N, Pignal F, Kremer M, Bonfils S, Rambaud J C 1982 Effect of somatostatin on diarrhea and on small intestine water and electrolyte transport in a patient with pancreatic cholera. Digestive Diseases and Sciences 27:459–466

Ruttman E, Klöppel G, Bommer G, Kiehn M, Heitz P U 1980 Pancreatic glucagoma with and without syndrome. Virchows Archiv Pathologie Anatomie 388:51–67

Said S I, Mutt V 1970 Polypeptide with broad biological activity; isolation from small intestine. Science 169:1217–1218

Said S I, Faloona G R 1975 Elevated plasma and tissue levels of vasoactive intestinal polypeptide in the watery-diarrhea syndrome due to pancreatic, bronchogenic and other tumors. New England Journal of Medicine 293:155–160

Santangelo W C, O'Dorisio T M, Kim J G, Severino G, Krejs G J 1985 Effect of synthetic somatostatin analogue on intestinal water and ion transport in pancreatic cholera syndrome. Annals of Internal Medicine 103:363–367

Schein P S, De Lellis R A, Kahn C R, Gordon P, Kraft A R 1973 Islet cell tumors. Current concepts and management. Annals International Medicine 79:239–257

Schöön I M, Lundqvist G, Rehfeld J F, Olbe L 1981 A study of the effect of antral distension on gastric acid secretion in man. Digestion 21:57–64

Schusdziarra V, Grube D, Seifert H, Galle J, Etzrodt H, Beischer W, Haferkamp O, Pfeiffer E F 1983 Somatostatinoma syndrome. Clinical, morphological and metabolic features and therapeutic aspects. Klinische Wochenschrift 61:681–689

Seiler S, Zinninger M M 1946 Massive islet cell tumor of pancreas without hypoglycaemia. Surgery Gynecology and Obstetrics 82:301–305

Service F J, Dale A J D, Elveback L R, Jiang N S 1976 Insulinoma: clinical and diagnostic features in 60 consecutive cases. Mayo Clinic Proceedings 51:417–429

Siegel E G, Mayer G, Nauck M, Creutzfeldt W 1987 Hypoglycaemia facticia durch Sulfonylharnstoff-Einnahme. Deutsche Medizinische Wochenschrift 112:1575–1579

Sigel B, Duarte B, Coelho J C U, Nyhus L M, Baker R J, Machi J 1983 Localization of insulinomas of the pancreas at operation by real-time ultrasound scanning. Surgery, Gynecology and Obstetrics 156:145–147

Singleton J W, Kern Jr F, Waddell W K 1965 Diarrhea and pancreatic islet cell tumor: report of a case with a severe jejunal mucosal lesion. Gastroenterology 49:197–208

Solcia E, Capella C, Fioca R, Rindi G, Rosai J 1990 Gastric argyrophil carcinoidosis in patients with Zollinger–Ellison syndrome due to type 1 multiple endocrine neoplasia. American Journal of Surgical Pathology 14(6):503–513

Solcia E, Sessa F, Rindi G, Bonato M, Capella C 1991 Pancreatic endocrine tumors: general concepts; nonfunctioning tumors and tumors with uncommon function. In: Dayal Y (ed.) Endocrine pathology of the gut and pancreas. CRC Press, Boston 105–131

Spencer H 1955 Pancreatic islet-cell adenomata. Journal of Pathology and Bacteriology 69:259–267

Stacpoole P W 1981 The glucagonoma syndrome: clinical features, diagnosis, and treatment. Endocrine Review 2:347–361

Stacpoole P W, Kasselberg A G, Berelowitz M, Chey W Y 1983 Somatostatinoma syndrome: does a clinical entity exist? Acta Endocrinologica 102:80–87

Stadil F, Stage J G 1979 The Zollinger–Ellison syndrome. Clinics in Endocrinology and Metabolism 8:433–446

Stage J G, Stadil F, Rehfeld J F, Fahrenkrug J, Schaffalitzky de Muckadell O B 1978 Secretin and the Zollinger–Ellison syndrome: reliability of secretin tests and pathogenetic role of secretin. Scandinavian Journal of Gastroenterology 13:501–511

Stefanini P, Carboni M, Patrassi N 1974a Surgical treatment and prognosis of insulinoma. Clinical Gastroenterology 3:697–719

Stefanini P, Carboni M, Patrassi N, Basoli A 1974b Beta islet-cell tumors of the pancreas: results of a statistical study on 1067 cases collected. Surgery 75:597–609

Tapja F J, Polak J M, Barbosa A J A, Bloom S R, Marangos P J, Dermody C, Pearse A G E 1981 Neurone-specific enolase is produced by neuroendocrine tumors. Lancet 1:808–811

Thakker R V, Bouloux P, Wooding C et al 1989 Association of parathyroid tumors in multiple endocrine neoplasia type 1 with loss of alleles on chromosome 11. New England Journal of Medicine 321:218–224

Tomita T, Friesen S R, Pollock H G 1991 PP-producing tumors (PPomas). In: Dayal Y (ed.) Endocrine pathology of the gut and pancreas. CRC Press, Boston p 279–304

Turner R C, Heding L G 1977 Plasma proinsulin, C-peptide and insulin in diagnostic suppression test for insulinomas. Diabetologia 13:571–577

Turner R C, Oakley N W, Nabarro J D N 1971 Control of basal insulin secretion with special reference to the diagnosis of insulinomas. British Medical Journal of Medicine 2:132–135

Turner R C, Lee E C G, Morris P J, Lee E G G, Harris E A 1978 Localization of insulinomas. Lancet 1:515–518

Verner J V, Morrison A B 1958 Islet-cell tumor and a syndrome of refractory watery diarrhea and hypokalemia. American Journal of Medicine 25:374–380

Verner J V, Morrison A B 1974 Non-B islet tumours and the syndrome of watery diarrhoea, hypokalaemia and hypochlorhydria. Clinical Gastroenterology 3:595–608

Vogel S B, Wolfe M M, McGuigan J E, Hawkins Jr I F, Howard R J, Woodward E R 1987 Localization and resection of gastrinoma in Zollinger–Ellison syndrome. Annals of Surgery 205:550–556

von Schrenck T, Howard J M, Doppman J L, Norton J A, Maton P N, Smith F P, Vinayek R, Frucht H, Wank S A, Gardner J D, Jensen R T 1988 Prospective study of chemotherapy in patients with metastatic gastrinoma. Gastroenterology 94:1326–1334

Warren S 1926 Adenomas of the islands of Langerhans. American Journal of Pathology 2:335–340

Watson R G P, Johnston C F, O'Hare M M T, Anderson J R, Wilson B G, Collins J S A, Sloan J M, Buchanan K D 1989 The frequency of gastrointestinal endocrine tumours in a well-defined population – Northern Ireland 1970-1985. Quarterly Journal of Medicine 72:647–657

Way L, Goldman L, Dumphy J E 1968 Zollinger–Ellison syndrome. An analysis of 25 cases. American Journal of Surgery 116:293-299

Weichert R F, Roth L M 1971 Carcinoid-islet cell tumors of the duodenum. Report on twenty-one cases. American Journal of Surgery 121:195–205

Wermer P 1974 Genetic aspects of adenomatosis of endocrine glands. American Journal of Medicine 16:363–371

Wiedemann B, Waldherr R, Buhr H, Hille A, Rosa P, Huttner W B 1988 Identification of gastroenteropancreatic neuroendocrine cells in normal and neoplastic human tissue with antibodies against synaptophysin, chromogranin A, secretogranin I (chromogranin B), and secretogranin II. Gastroenterology 95:1364–1374

Wiedemann B, Huttner W B 1989 Synaptophysin and chromogranins/secretogranins – widespread constituents of distinct types of neuroendocrine vesicles and new tools in tumor diagnosis. Virchows [Pathol Anat] Archiv B Cell Pathology 58:95–121

Wilder R M, Allan F N, Power M H, Robertson H Z E 1927 Carcinoma of islands of pancreas hyperinsulinism and hypoglycemia. Journal of the American Medical Association 89:348–355

Wilkinson D S 1973 Necrolytic migratory erythema with carcinoma of the pancreas. Transactions of St John's Hospital Dermatological Society 59:244–250

Wilson S D, Schulte W J, Meade R C 1971 Longevity studies following total gastrectomy in children with the Zollinger–Ellison syndrome. Archives of Surgery 103:108–115

Wolfe M M, Alexander R W, McGuigan J E 1982 Extrapancreatic, extraintestinal gastrinoma. Effective treatment by surgery. New England Journal of Medicine 306:1533–1536

Zollinger R M, Ellison E H 1955 Primary peptic ulcerations of the jejunum associated with islet cell tumors of the pancreas. Annals of Surgery 142:709–726

49. Islet cell tumours of the pancreas

J. A. van Heerden   G. B. Thompson

In 1869, a medical student in Berlin worked on his inaugural thesis in which he, for the first time, differentiated between pancreatic islet and acinar tissue. The student's name was Paul Langerhans a name which is immortalized today by the islets which bear his name.

Little could this young student foretell what was to follow this fundamental study. The ubiquitous and seemingly totipotent cells of the islets have stimulated research workers and clinicians as an increasing number of syndromes have been elucidated, syndromes secondary to the production of various polypeptides by the many different cells within the islets. In addition, since the advent of computerized tomography in the mid-seventies, an increasing number of 'pancreatic incidentalomas' are being found which have minimal or no obvious endocrine function, emphasizing that all pancreatic islet cell tumours, be they benign or malignant, may be clinically functioning or non-functioning.

Today, approximately a dozen syndromes are identified with abnormalities of the islets of Langerhans:

1. Insulinoma (insulin)
2. Gastrinoma (gastrin) Zollinger–Ellison syndrome
3. Watery diarrhoea hypokalaemia achlorhydria (WDHA) syndrome, (vasoactive intestinal polypeptide) Verner–Morrison syndrome
4. Glucagonoma (glucagon)
5. Somatostatinoma (somatostatin)
6. CCKoma (cholecystokinin)
7. Ectopic adrenocorticotrophic hormone (ACTH) syndrome
8. Hyperpigmentation syndrome (melanocyte stimulating hormone)
9. Ectopic hyperparathyroidism (parathyroid hormone-like substance)
10. Carcinoid syndrome (5-hydroxytryptamine)
11. Pancreatic polypeptidoma (pancreatic polypeptide), PPoma
12. Growth hormone-releasing factor secreting tumours (GRFomas)

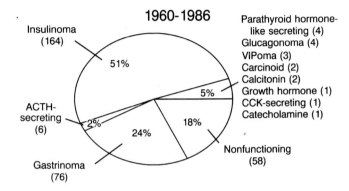

Fig. 49.1 Distribution of islet cell tumours in 322 patients treated at the Mayo Clinic, 1960–1986. CCK, cholecystokinin; VIP, vasoactive intestinal polypeptide.

13. Questionable:
    – neurotensin-secreting tumours
    – calcitonin-secreting tumours

With the exception of insulinomas and gastrinomas, these tumours are encountered so infrequently that most recorded literature takes the form of single case reports. The breakdown of a large series of such patients from the Mayo Clinic is seen in Figure 49.1. It might be anticipated that the steady identification of the many polypeptide hormones arising from the islet cells of the pancreas would result in fewer non-functioning tumours being identified. This, however, is not the case (Fig. 49.2) and the recent increase in the reported number of non-functioning tumours is most likely due to the current availability and widespread use of abdominal computerized tomography.

PATHOPHYSIOLOGY AND PATHOGENESIS

It was A G E Pearse who first proposed the amine precursor uptake and decarboxylation (APUD) concept (Pearse et al 1966). He noted that endocrine cells throughout the body had similar cytochemical and ultrastructural

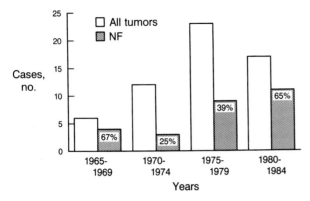

Fig. 49.2 Proportion of non-functioning (NF) islet cell tumours at the Mayo Clinic, 1965–1984.

characteristics and that they shared the ability to take up amine precursors, decarboxylate them and produce various bioactive peptides and amines. He postulated that these cells were of neuroectodermal origin, arising from neural crest tissue (Mozell et al 1990). This concept has of late come into some disfavour and recent evidence (Pictet et al 1976, Fontaine et al 1977, Sidhu 1979, Pfluger et al 1981, Stevens & Moore 1983, Oleesky et al 1990) has suggested that pancreatic endocrine cells may well have an endodermal origin (Creutzfeldt 1985, Le Douarin 1988).

In 1954, Wermer, whose name serves as the eponym for the MEN I syndrome, reported a family in which five members had evidence of involvement of one or more endocrine glands (Wermer 1954). The MEN I locus is known to be on chromosome 11 and loss of one constitutional allele has been described in two brothers with insulinomas and MEN I (Larsson et al 1988). According to the two-mutation model, (Knudson 1971) development of neoplasia requires two separate mutational events at the involved alleles.

When part of a hereditary syndrome, the first mutation is present in the inherited germ cell line and the second mutation occurs later in the somatic cell. When not inherited, both these events occur at the somatic level, explaining their sporadic nature. In the MEN I syndrome, it may be that the locus identified on chromosome eleven, codes for onco-suppressor genes that, when lost, result in endocrine neoplasia and pancreatic endocrine tumours. (Spandidos & Andenan 1989, Mozell et al 1990).

All of the tumours to be discussed vary with regard to their hormone production, size, location, age, distribution, sex distribution, malignant (and metastatic) potential, and prognosis. The morbidity associated with these tumours more often than not relates to the hormonal sequelae and less often to the tumour burden (Mozell et al 1990).

There is a striking histological similarity between pancreatic endocrine tumours. These tumours are com-

posed of very uniform cells within a vascular stroma. The cells coalesce into trabecular, acinar or solid patterns. There is poor correlation between histological pattern and hormone production (Mukai et al 1982). Anaplastic forms and unusual features with clear cells, oncocytes or mucin production can make it difficult to recognize a small percentage of endocrine tumours in routinely stained sections (Rosai 1989). Immunostains for neurone specific enolase and chromogranin A appear to be relatively sensitive markers for pancreatic endocrine tumours that can be used to make this difficult distinction. Thompson et al (1984) have reported the most detailed histological and immunohistochemical study of the pancreas in the MEN I syndrome to date. In all 14 non-tumorous pancreatic segments studied, diffuse islet cell hyperplasia and micro-adenomatosis were seen. Nesidioblastosis or islet cell proliferation arising from exocrine ducts was demonstrated in all but one specimen. Grossly visible tumours were present in 13 or 14 patients, of which seven were multiple. Two patients had duodenal, in addition to pancreatic, tumours. Most of the tumours were less than 2 cm in maximum diameter, and four patients had single metastatically involved peripancreatic lymph nodes. Hormonal hetergeneity was demonstrated immunohistochemically in 71% of tumours studied. Every tumour stained positive for neurone specific enolase. MEN patients have diffuse islet cell involvement whereas sporadic cases are most often associated with a solitary primary pancreatic neoplasm. Because endocrine tumours have such benign histology the diagnosis of malignancy rests primarily on the demonstration of either local invasion, metastatic lymph node involvement, or distant metastases. Pancreatic endocrine tumours typically metastasize to regional lymph nodes and to the liver. Involvement of bone and other systems is much less common.

Nucleic acid methods utilizing in situ hybridization may in future help in the differential diagnosis of pancreatic endocrine tumours (Hamid et al 1989). Electron microscopy demonstrates secretory granules of the neuroendocrine type among nearly all pancreatic endocrine tumours. Specific granules of the alpha and beta cell type can be differentiated ultrastructurally in patients with insulinomas and glucagonomas (Liu et al 1985).

The differentiation of specific tumour type can be achieved by the demonstration of excessive circulating levels of peptide by radioimmunoassay, as well as by peptide identification in tumour sections utilizing immunohistochemical staining. It must, however, be realized that while tissue sections may stain positively for the hormone produced, they may also stain weakly or not at all for some hormones that are produced and secreted rapidly, or they may stain positively for other hormones that are not clinically detectable. In the last instance, the hormone may be produced but not secreted in sufficient levels to allow clinical detection (Thompson et al 1989b).

Production of multiple peptides is well recognized. This may occur from the outset or develop in a metachronous fashion. It is thought that the dedifferentiation of the tumour cell may result in loss of post-transcriptional and post-translational controls of peptide production resulting in peptide excess (Bordelon-Riser et al 1979 Kahn et al 1981).

Numerous circulating markers can now be measured including insulin, gastrin, glucagon, VIP, somatostatin, pancreatic polypeptide, adrenocorticotrophic hormone (ACTH), gastric inhibitory polypeptide (GIP), cholecystokinin (CCK) melanocyte stimulating hormone (MSH) and parathyroid hormone-related protein. Provocative testing is rarely necessary, but is most useful in patients suspected of having the Zollinger–Ellison syndrome (secretin challenge test). The ability to measure C-peptide levels allows differentiation between endogenous and exogenous (factitious) hyperinsulinism. High proinsulin levels are often associated with malignant insulinomas. Alpha human chorionic gonadotrophin (hCG), never detected in benign pancreatic endocrine tumours, is present in 23–52% of malignant pancreatic endocrine tumours (Mozell et al 1990).

Primary hyperparathyroidism is seen in almost all MEN I patients, usually by the end of the third decade of life. The presence of pancreatic islet cell tumours tends to occur 10–15 years later. These are most commonly gastrin-producing tumours, followed by insulin-producing tumours. Rare islet cell tumours producing glucagon, somatostatin, pancreatic polypeptide and VIP have, however, all been described in this syndrome. Pituitary tumours occur in about 10–30% of patients. These are most commonly prolactin-producing adenomas which may or may not cause optic chiasmal pressure symptoms. Pituitary tumours producing growth hormone, ACTH, MSH, FSH and TSH have all been well documented. In a suspected MEN patient, one must selectively screen for these specific peptides (van Heerden et al 1990).

The histological, immunocytochemical, ultrastructural and peptide hormone assay data taken in conjunction with clinical presentation and localizing methods has given us a better understanding of the endocrine pancreatic tumours. There are still many unanswered questions for the decades ahead, but a firm foundation has been established upon which future generations can build.

From a clinical standpoint, there are four important questions which need to be addressed when dealing with any islet cell tumour.

Is there abnormal endocrine production or is the tumour clinically non-functioning?

Approximately two-thirds of islet cell tumours encountered are non-functioning. However, when such tumours are removed, immunohistochemical staining is invariably positive for one or more of the polypeptide hormones produced by the islets. Although hormonal overactivity may not be clinically evident, it is difficult teleologically to imagine a tumour arising from the islets of Langerhans that does not produce one or more hormones.

Is the tumour benign or malignant?

The importance of this question, with its obvious prognostic and therapeutic implications, varies between syndromes and is based on the demonstration of neoplastic tissue at a distant site, since histological verification of malignancy in islet cell tumours, as in most endocrine tumours, is notoriously difficult.

If functioning, is the tumour a sporadic occurrence or a manifestation of multiple endocrine neoplasia type I (men I)?

The incidence of this association ranges from 10 to 30%. Besides the importance of screening the patient and his/her family for other endocrinopathies, the hallmark of the pathology in the pancreas should be remembered, namely multiplicity of tumours and diffuse islet cell dysplasia. The therapuetic implications are self-evident.

What is the age of the patient?

This question revolves around endogenous hyperinsulinism. In the adult, the cause of the hyperinsulinism is almost invariably (in more than 90% of cases) a single, benign, islet cell adenoma. In the neonate, however, the aetiology is that of diffuse islet cell adenomatosis (Telander 1989), (nesidioblastosis), an entity in the neonate which is thought to be morphologically normal, although physiologically overactive. The treatment thus varies from simple and safe adenoma enucleation in the adult, to near-total (95%+) pancreatectomy in the neonate.

DISTRIBUTION

A most practical contribution regarding the anatomical distribution of these tumours has been made by Howard & Passaro (1989). They have grouped pancreatic islet cell tumours into cluster I (gastrinomas, PPomas, somatostatinomas) and cluster II (insulinomas, glucagonomas) tumours. They noted that 75% of cluster I tumours occur to the right of the superior mesenteric vessels while 75% of cluster II tumours occur to the left. They suggested that this distribution is roughly equal to the volume density of the insulin-secreting (beta), glucagon-secreting (alpha), and pancreatic polypeptide-secreting cells. There is, however, a disparity between the anatomical location and volume distribution of somatostatinomas and the somatostatin-secreting (delta) cells.

INSULINOMA

Although Nicholls (1902) was the first to describe a pancreatic islet cell tumour in 1902, it was Wilder and his associates (1927) who first associated excessive insulin production with an islet cell tumour. It is of historical interest that the patient was an orthopaedic surgeon with a metastatic islet-cell carcinoma. Extracts from tissue removed from this patient's liver (by Dr C W Mayo) produced profound hypoglycaemia when injected into a rabbit. Two quotations from this patient's referring physician's letter are noteworthy:

A year ago he noticed that he would develop a tremor, sweating and nervousness after going without food or after severe exertion. He discovered that taking sugar would prevent the occurrence of these attacks.

and

On one occasion, the patient had been operating later than usual and, being overtaken by weariness, was soon mentally confused and collapsed in a stupor – but he was able to swallow an eggnog – and in a few minutes was completely revived.

These quotations accurately describe the now well-known Whipple's triad.

Diagnosis

As the above quotations emphasize, the clinical presentation of these patients can be both bizarre and atypical. This presentation and the rarity of the entity (1:1.25 million of the population of the USA) (Kavlie & White 1972) most often lead to either a delay in the diagnosis or more seriously, an incorrect diagnosis. Before the diagnosis of hyperinsulinism is confirmed, many patients have been incorrectly labelled as alcoholics, drug addicts, epileptics, or psychotics. Patients have been involved in automobile accidents during spells of hypoglycaemia, have been dismissed from their employment for bizarre behaviour, have been jailed for drunkenness, and at times, have been admitted to mental institutions. The patients themselves may realize that food intake prevents neuroglycopaenic symptoms and therefore tend to eat often and at unusual times, such as in the middle of the night. The diagnosis, once thought of, is confirmed by the following assessment.

1. Demonstration of Whipple's triad, which consists of
a. the signs and symptoms of hypoglycaemia
b. serum glucose levels of less than 2.8 mmol/l (50 mg/dl), and
c. the prompt relief of symptoms by the administration of glucose.

This demonstration is ideally accomplished in the hospital setting with a controlled fast.

2. Documentation of hyperinsulinaemia at the time of hypoglycaemia. It is important to stress that in approximately one-third of patients, insulin levels may be normal after fasting but will still be inappropriate (>6μU/dl), a situation analogous to normal range but inappropriate levels of parathyroid hormone in patients with hypercalcaemia due to primary hyperparathyroidism.

3. If further diagnostic confirmation is needed, or if there is any question regarding possible factitious hypoglycaemia, C-peptide levels should be measured. If C-peptide levels are elevated, the diagnosis of endogenous hyperinsulinism is assured.

This diagnostic approach has proved to be highly accurate. Although some have expressed enthusiasm for insulin: glucose ratios, provocation testing using either calcium or tolbutamide, or the C-peptide suppression test, such tests are seldom required in current practice. (Edis et al 1976, Service et al 1976, Kaplan et al 1979, 1987).

Localization

Insulinomas are highly vascular tumours that have a characteristic blush on selective angiography. For a long time this has been the gold standard in localization, with sensitivity rates of approximately 80%. There are many alternative methods of localization and each is championed by its proponents. The most common methods, with the ranges of reported success rates, are depicted in Table 49.1. To this list should be added magnetic resonance imaging (MRI), intraoperative ultrasonography and surgical palpation of the pancreas. It has long been recognized that surgical palpation is the most accurate method of localization, and that all of the other methods are of importance principally in the reoperative situation where the changes resulting from the previous operation decrease the sensitivity of surgical palpation. Daggett et al (1981) asked the crucial question almost a decade ago; 'Is preoperative localization of insulinomas necessary?'. They thought not.

It is our opinion that localizing studies in patients with insulinoma are overdone and are not cost-effective. Recognizing that surgical palpation is indeed the best method of localization and that intraoperative ultrasonography is both non-invasive and has a high specificity, the schema in Figure 49.3 might be suggested in the previously unoperated patient. A bonus of intraoperative ultrasonography is the identification of the pancreatic duct, the common bile duct, and the splenic vein. Knowledge regard-

Table 49.1 Methods of localization of insulinoma

Test	% Success rate
Selective angiography	29–90
Computerized tomography	12–60
Preoperative ultrasonography	17–65
Selective venous sampling	25–85

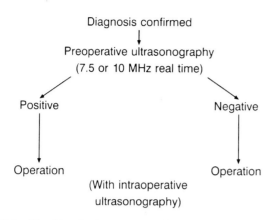

Diagnosis confirmed

↓

Preoperative ultrasonography
(7.5 or 10 MHz real time)

Positive   Negative

↓   ↓

Operation   Operation

(With intraoperative
ultrasonography)

Fig. 49.3 Algorithm for the treatment of insulinoma.

ing the relationship of these structures to the insulinoma may contribute to safer enucleation or to the decision to undertake pancreatic resection (Fig. 49.4), thus reducing postoperative morbidity.

In the reoperative situation the surgeon needs as much localization data as possible. Once again, though, the philosophy should be to start with low-cost non-invasive technology (ultrasonography) before proceeding to the selective use of more expensive and more invasive procedures (angiography, selective venous sampling, MRI).

Pathology

In approximately 90% of patients, the lesions are solitary benign adenomas, of which some 80% are 1.5 cm or less

in diameter. In slightly less than 10% of patients, the source of abnormal insulin secretion is an islet cell carcinoma or multiple adenomas which may or may not be associated with MEN I. Such multiple tumours tend to be distributed equally throughout the pancreas, although Howard & Passaro (1989) have suggested that 75% will be located to the left of the superior mesenteric vessels.

Treatment

It is well accepted that the optimal treatment of insulinomas is surgical excision. This philosophy is aided by the nature of the pancreas, which, despite its rather poor surgical reputation lends itself to excellent surgical exposure, inspection and palpation throughout its length (Figs. 49.5, 49.6). In the majority of patients, this can be accomplished by 'simple' enucleation of a benign adenoma. The safety of adenoma enucleation is enhanced by knowledge of its relationship to the main pancreatic duct, information provided by intraoperative ultrasonography. We recommend the routine use of intraoperative ultrasonography even if the tumour is readily found by palpation. Close proximity to the pancreatic duct may suggest to the surgeon that distal pancreatectomy may be safer than enucleation. The technique of enucleation varies from surgeon to surgeon but is aided by the use of electrocautery, small haemoclips, and on appropriate occasions, the Cavitron ultrasonic aspirator (CUSA). The latter, which has gained popularity in hepatic surgery, 'melts' the pancreas, without disruption of the small intrapancreatic vessels which can then be

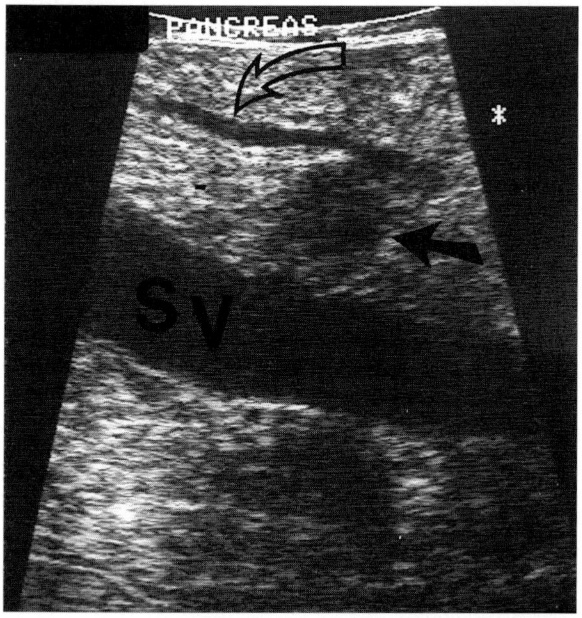

Fig. 49.4 Small part (10 megaHertz) longitudinal ultrasound of the pancreas demonstrating the close relationship between the pancreatic duct (open arrow) and an islet cell adenoma (solid arrow); SV, splenic vein.

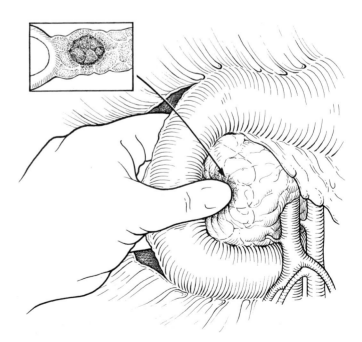

Fig. 49.5 Palpation of the head of the pancreas and duodenum following Kocherization.

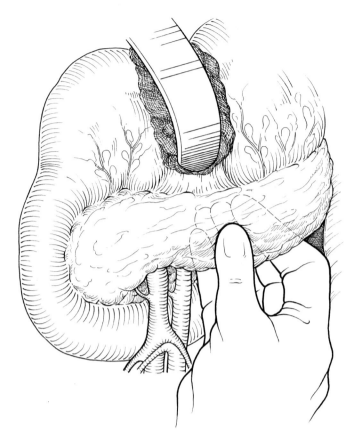

Fig. 49.6 Palpation of the body and tail of the pancreas after mobilization of the pancreas.

controlled with haemoclips, leading to a tidier and more pleasing dissection. Enucleation is possible for tumours located in any portion of the pancreas, the uncinate process included. On extremely rare occasions the surgeon has to resort to a more radical resection such as radical pancreatoduodenectomy or even more rarely, total pancreatectomy. The majority of these pancreatic resections are reserved for patients with larger malignant tumours.

When a tumour is not found at exploration, the question of whether to proceed to 'blind distal pancreatectomy' always arises. Since the likelihood of failing to cure the hyperinsulinism is at least 50% with this procedure, it should not be undertaken lightly, and in our view is to be condemned. Fortunately, this situation is now rare and will become increasingly so with more frequent use of intraoperative ultrasonography.

Despite meticulous surgical techniques and routine pancreatic drainage, morbidity follows enucleation or resection in 10–15% of patients. This morbidity is often secondary to a pancreatic leak and may result in pancreatitis, pancreatic fistulae, or subphrenic abscess formation. Although there are no prospective controlled trial data to confirm its use, an increasing number of surgeons (Williams et al 1989), including our group, now routinely

administer octreotide acetate (Sandostatin) in a dose of 150 μg subcutaneously three times a day starting immediately preoperatively. It is our impression that the pancreatic leak rate may have decreased since the introduction of this practice.

Mortality rates following operation range from 0% (Edis et al 1976) to 6% (Proye 1987). To date, there has not been an operative death at the Mayo Clinic since Dr Charles Mayo's first patient died a few weeks postoperatively of uncontrollable hypoglycaemia, in 1927.

Malignant insulinoma

The long-term survival following excision of a benign insulinoma should approach that of the normal population. This is not so for the 5–10% of patients with malignant tumours. However, these patients fare considerably better than patients with malignancy of the exocrine pancreas and can survive for prolonged periods despite the presence of metastases (Table 49.2).

Symptomatic control and increased survival in patients with malignant insulinomas is aided by the judicious use of diazoxide, somatostatin and hepatic debulking procedures (Nagorney et al 1983) in appropriate circumstances. In exceptional circumstances, hepatic transplantation has been employed (Makowka et al 1989) although the value of this radical approach remains uncertain.

The chemotherapeutic agent of choice in patients with metastatic disease is streptozotocin, a cytotoxic agent directed at pancreatic beta cells. Response rates (usually reported as suppression of hyperinsulinaemia) range from 30 to 60% and may be enhanced by the addition of 5-fluorouracil (Stefanini et al 1974, Moertel et al 1980).

Intraoperative glucose monitoring

Figure 49.7 depicts a typical response of the serum glucose to tumour excision. This response (>1.2 mmol/l (20mg/dl) rise) not only reassures the surgeon that no further tumours remain, but helps the anaesthetist to prevent the serum glucose falling to unduly low levels. Because of the ease of obtaining rapid glucose levels, intra-

Table 49.2 Malignant insulinomas: long-term results. (Mayo Clinic 1965–1985)

Procedure	Metastases	Result	Duration of follow-up (months)
Biopsy	+	Well	105
Distal pancreatectomy	+	Well	60
Biopsy	+	Died	2
Distal pancreatectomy	−	Well	156
Distal pancreatectomy	+	Died	72
Distal pancreatectomy	+	Died	48
Whipple procedure	−	Died	60
Biopsy	+	Died	39

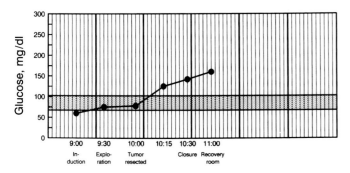

Fig. 49.7 Graphic record of intraoperative glucose monitoring.

operative glucose monitoring should be encouraged. A suggested practice is to stop all glucose intake for approximately 4–6 hours prior to exploration and to refrain from administering any glucose-containing solution for 24 hours postoperatively. In our recent series of 30 consecutive patients, the serum glucose rebounded promptly (within 20 minutes) in all patients following removal of the insulinoma, a rebound which can be most reassuring to the operating team.

Hyperinsulinism in MEN I

Pancreatic tumours are present in 50–80% of patients with MEN I although only 5–10% of patients with insulinomas belong to MEN I families. In this rare but challenging group of patients, the pancreatic pathology is characterized by diffuse, small adenomas (few of which are radiologically visible) and by diffusely dysplastic islet cell tissue. Radical removal of the pancreas (95%+ subtotal pancreatectomy) is the surgical treatment of choice and persisting symptoms are controlled by life-long administration of octreotide acetate (Rasbach et al 1985).

ZOLLINGER–ELLISON SYNDROME (ZES)

Gastrinoma is the most common of the islet cell tumours and the syndrome associated with its presence was initially described in 1955 by Zollinger and Ellison in a classical article entitled 'Primary peptic ulceration of the jejunum associated with islet cell tumours of the pancreas' (Zollinger & Ellison 1955). These pioneers postulated that an ulcerogenic humoral factor (? glucagon) was being secreted by the pancreas and was the cause of the peptic ulceration, but it was Gregory et al (1960) who first isolated a gastrin-like substance from a pancreatic tumour in a patient with the syndrome. In the early days of the elucidation of the ZES, the suggestion was that all patients should be treated by removal of the end or target organ, that is by total gastrectomy. This philosophy has certainly changed a great deal in the ensuing 35 years.

Approximately one-third of patients with the Zollinger–Ellison syndrome have MEN I. As would be anticipated, patients with this rare but important association have multicentric pathology, are younger than those with sporadic gastrinoma at the time of diagnosis, and have a higher percentage of benign tumours (about 70%) than sporadic gastrinoma patients (about 40%) (Mallinson et al 1974, Zollinger 1985).

Diagnosis

The presentation of ZES has changed. Before the syndrome became more widely recognized, patients most often presented with the ravages of severe peptic ulceration, such as perforation or haemorrhage. Today, many patients are recognized with mild peptic ulcer disease, with no peptic ulcer disease (diarrhoea only), with duodenitis alone, or with severe peptic oesophagitis. Although a high index of suspicion is the best aid to diagnosis, ZES should be suspected when any of the following features are present, either singly or in combination:

- peptic ulcer disease at a young age
- virulent peptic ulcer disease
- peptic ulcer disease in unusual sites, such as the third part of the duodenum or jejunum
- marginal ulcer after an operation for peptic ulcer disease
- unexplained diarrhoea
- parathyroid or pituitary pathology
- family history of endocrinopathy.

The diagnosis of ZES is confirmed by the demonstration of hypergastrinaemia and concurrent gastric hyperacidity. The clinician should recall that there are causes other than ZES for this combination, the most common being chronic renal failure, the short bowel syndrome, gastric outlet obstruction, and rarely, a retained gastric antrum following Billroth II gastrectomy or antral G-cell hyperplasia.

Gastric hyperacidity is a less reliable finding than hypergastrinaemia since there is a 10–15% overlap between the basal levels of gastric acid in the ZES and type ordinaire duodenal ulceration. Basal acid output (BAO) exceeding 15 mmol/hour should alert the investigator to the diagnosis of ZES; the ratio of this basal level to the maximal output (MAO) achieved after pentagastrin stimulation is even more suggestive and a ratio of 0.6 or more strongly supports the diagnosis.

The advent of a sensitive radioimmunoassay for gastrin has been a great aid in the diagnosis and evaluation of hypergastrinaemia. Approximately 40% of patients with the ZES have levels below 500 pg/ml but a level above this is almost diagnostic. A provocative secretin test (patients with ZES secrete gastrin in response to secretin or calcium infusion) is most valuable in the assessment of patients with low levels of serum gastrin (below 500 pg/ml), and in separating ZES patients from those with antral G-cell hyperplasia or a retained gastric antrum (Table 49.3).

After an injection of 2 i.u./kg of secretin or 15 mg/kg of calcium, a rise in serum gastrin of 200 pg/ml or greater is considered to be a positive response and diagnostic of ZES. The calcium test has essentially been abandoned due to the high incidence of nausea in acutely hyper-calcaemic patients. Its use might still be entertained in those patients with a high index of suspicion for ZES and who have a negative secretin test; this would be extremely rare. Levels of serum gastrin above 1000 pg/ml should lead one to suspect the presence of metastatic gastrinoma.

Location and localization

In 1984, Stabile et al (1984) described the gastrinoma triangle (confluence of the cystic duct and common bile duct superiorly, junction of the second and third parts of the duodenum inferiorly, and the junction of the neck and body of the pancreas medially) and suggested that 80–90% of gastrinomas will be found within this triangle. This is indeed the case and of particular importance is the increasing recognition that a high percentage of gastrinomas will be found, not in the pancreas, but in the duodenal wall immediately beneath the mucosa. These duodenal 'carcinoid gastrinomas' are usually quite small (4–6 mm) but can be readily detected by their firmness to palpation of the duodenum after thorough Kocherization ('millet seed feel') (Thompson et al 1989b) (Fig. 49.8).

Preoperative attempts to localize gastrinomas are un-successful in 30–50% of patients. Norton et al (1986) prospectively evaluated various preoperative localizing methods and pointed out the limitations of techniques such as selective angiography, selective venous sampling, preoperative ultrasonography, computerized tomography and magnetic resonance imaging (Table 49.4). We and most other investigators have been frustrated in our attempts to localize gastrinomas prior to operation.

A recent test developed by Imamura et al (1987) is worth noting. These investigators have localized gastri-nomas which were not radiologically visible, by the selec-tive intra-arterial secretin injection (SASI test) which results in a prompt (within 40 seconds) rise in gastrin levels in patients with small tumours. This work should be

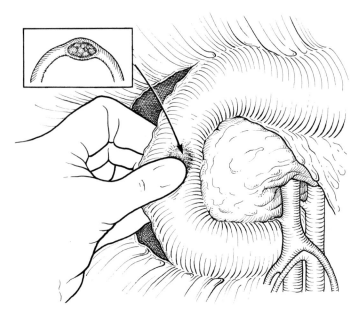

Fig. 49.8   Palpation of the duodenum in the Zollinger–Ellison syndrome.

followed closely and has already been duplicated by others (Rosato et al 1990).

Palpation of the pancreas, the duodenum, and the meticulous search for peripancreatic primary or metastatic gastrinomas remains the mainstay of localization of these tumours, most of which are 1.0 cm or less in diameter. To this surgical armamentarium, intraoperative ultraso-nography should now be added and should be under-taken routinely during the surgical exploration of patients with ZES (Norton et al 1988).

Since 50–60% of patients with ZES have malignant tumours we recommend that all patients should initially undergo abdominal computerized tomography, searching in particular for metastatic disease. If this investigation is negative, ultrasonography (using a 7.5 or 10 megaHertz real-time microview system) should be the next step. If both investigations are negative, we advocate proceeding to abdominal exploration, paying particular attention to the gastrinoma triangle and the use of intraoperative ultrasonography. In our opinion, the more invasive local-izing tests such as selective angiography (with or without the SASI test) and selective venous sampling should be reserved for those patients who have undergone a pre-viously unsuccessful exploration in search of a gastri-noma. Such tests may be particularly useful if partial pancreatic resection has been performed previously.

A localizing method that is sometimes lost sight of, given the available technology, is palpation of the pan-creas and surrounding structures by an experienced human hand. It is our opinion that manual palpation, coupled with intraoperative real-time ultrasonography, is

Table 49.3   Response of serum gastrin to secretin infusion and a protein meal

	Secretin	Protein
Zollinger–Ellison syndrome	↑↑	0
G–cell hyperplasia	0	↑↑
Retained antrum	↓	0
Duodenal ulcer	0	↑↑

Table 49.4 Results of localization in Zollinger–Ellison syndrome (ZES) (52 patients). Figures are percentages

	Ultrasound	Infusion computerized tomography	Selective angiography	Combined
Sensitivity	21	40	60	70
Specificity	92	100	100	92
Positive predictive value	80	100	100	93
Negative predictive value	44	50	60	67

today the most accurate method for the localization of pancreatic endocrine tumours.

Treatment

The treatment of this rare syndrome remains controversial. The controversy exists because we now have powerful acid-reducing agents (e.g. omeprazole) and islet cell secretion inhibitors (somatostatin and its analogues), and because of the association of ZES with MEN I in which the pathology is diffuse and multicentric. These considerations, coupled with a rate of malignancy of around 60%, has created a number of opposing treatment camps. The suggested approaches to current management include:

1. resection of the tumour with debulking of metastatic disease
2. removal of the end-organ by total gastrectomy
3. reduction of gastric acid secretion (e.g. H_2-blockade, omeprazole)
4. reduction of islet cell secretion (octreotide acetate).

Proponents of surgery feel that medical therapy denies the patient a chance for cure and ignores the fact that many of the causative tumours are malignant. Medical enthusiasts point to the efficacy of the currently available medications and to the bad reputation of both pancreatic resection and total gastrectomy. They also remind the surgical community that the surgical cure rate for ZES is at present only some 30% (Vogel et al 1987). This high failure rate can be attributed to three principal factors:

1. inability to find the tumour
2. metastatic disease, and
3. multiple tumours (MEN I).

Dr James Thompson, a long-time student of this syndrome, has succinctly stated his solution to the dilemma (Thompson 1989):

There are problems with either medical or surgical approaches. Medical therapy is posited on a life-long commitment to rigid schedules of pill-taking . . . . We believe that any patient with a gastrinoma should be operated on for the chance of removing a malignant tumour and saving his life . . . . I truly cannot understand how anyone could fail to recommend operation for the tumour.

What then should be the recommendation? There is no doubt that gastric acid secretion and pancreatic islet cell secretion can be 'turned off' by medical means. This approach does, however, deny a chance for cure (albeit low) and ignores the potentially malignant nature of the causative tumour. There is also no argument that the pathology in MEN I patients is multiple and that, with rare exceptions, the only surgical attack (on the pancreas) of any value in this group is total pancreatectomy. There is also little argument that surgical debulking should be reserved for a small group of patients only, namely those with seemingly solitary, large, and perhaps locally symptomatic metastases. Based on these statements, we suggest adoption of the algorithm outlined in Figure 49.9.

It will be noted that neither proximal gastric vagotomy (PGV) or total gastrectomy has a place in this schema. It is our opinion that PGV has not been of much benefit to these patients and has complicated subsequent gastrectomy if this becomes necessary. Total gastrectomy, the treatment initially suggested by Zollinger and Ellison in 1955, should today be reserved for those patients in whom no tumour is found at exploration, or for patients with any variant of the ZES who for a variety of reasons (lack of tolerance to, or efficacy of medication, or probable lack of compliance, and cost) are not considered to be candidates for medical therapy.

ZES and MEN I

This complex subgroup of patients deserves special consideration. Since most of these patients will already have primary hyperparathyroidism, this should be treated initially. Correction of the hypercalcaemic state is particularly important since it is possible that this will reduce both the serum gastrin levels and the acid output of the stomach.

From the standpoint of pancreatic surgery, consideration should be given to the fact that the pathology is usually multiple and that more benign tumours (about 70%) are encountered in the MEN I population than in patients with sporadic gastrinoma. There are a number of therapeutic alternatives in this subgroup of patients and each has its proponents. The options include the following:

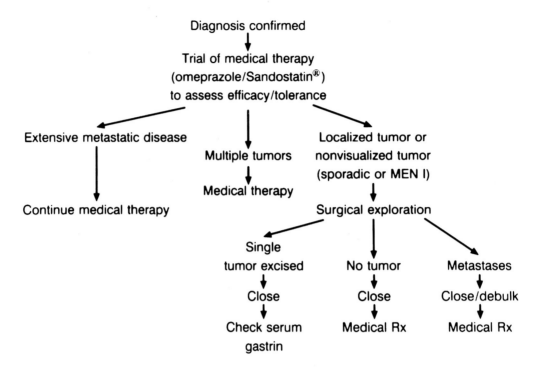

Fig. 49.9 Zollinger–Ellison syndrome: therapeutic algorithm.

1. none of these patients should be explored and all should be treated medically
2. all should be explored, or
3. exploration is warranted only if localized disease is suggested by the preoperative studies.

Thompson and his colleagues (1989a) from the University of Michigan, have renewed their enthusiasm for surgical exploration in selected patients with ZES/MEN I. With percutaneous transhepatic portal venous sampling they were able to identify two patterns of gastrin secretion; diffuse secretion from multiple pancreatic sites and localized or regional secretion.

They identified six patients from the latter group who have had gastrinoma excision without gastrectomy or pancreatic resection, and who now have had normal basal serum gastrin values for periods of 5 months to 12 years following operation. This experience, from recognized leaders in this field, who had previously reported poor results from gastrinoma excision in MEN I patients, is intriguing and deserves careful consideration.

An equally noteworthy recent contribution to this field has been made by Pipeleers-Marichal and colleagues (1990) who reported eight patients with ZES in MEN I, all of whom had duodenal gastrinomas. Of particular interest in this report were the observations that: three patients had solitary tumours: immunocytochemical analysis revealed gastrin-positivity in all duodenal gastrinomas but in none of seven pancreatic 'gastrinomas' similarly studied, and there was a return to normogastrinaemia in four of six patients whose duodenal gastrinomas were removed.

These fascinating data may provide an explanation for the difficulty encountered in attempting to treat hypergastrinaemia in MEN I by the removal of pancreatic tumours. Another consideration is the contention that total pancreatectomy should be considered the treatment of choice in families who have displayed a virulent history of pancreatic malignancy leading to death, as recently emphasized by Tisell et al (1988).

In their review of the newer medical and surgical approaches to gastrinomas, Howard & Passaro (1989) concluded that: 'On the basis of these recent advances, the optimal treatment of gastrinoma is surgical excision for cure'. Multiple endocrine neoplasia type I remains an obstacle to achievement of this ideal. Exploration in carefully selected patients now seems to be the treatment of choice, with the mainstay of therapy being either long-term somatostatin or omeprazole.

GLUCAGONOMA

Glucagonomas are rare tumours. A patient with a malignant islet cell tumour, and signs and symptoms compatible with what we would now call the glucagonoma syndrome was first reported in 1942 (Becker et al 1942). McGavran et al (1966) described a similar patient in the 1960s, and histochemical analysis of the causal neoplasm revealed a glucagon-secreting alpha cell tumour. The classic syndrome however, as we know it today, was not fully appreciated until Mallinson et al (1974), described nine patients with the glucagonoma symdrome in 1974. Glucagonomas rank below gastrinomas and insulinomas in terms of frequency (Mozell et al 1990). Women patients appear to outnumber men with a frequency two to three to one (Bloom & Polak 1987). The mean age at diagnosis is 52 years (range 20–73 years) (Leichter 1980). Although glucagonomas have been associated with the MEN I syndrome (Warner et al 1983), this is a rare occurrence.

Unlike their gastrin and insulin secreting counterparts, glucagonomas tend to be large (range 3–35cm) (Holst 1985). Over 80% of glucagonomas are malignant and over half have evidence of metastatic disease at the time of diagnosis (Leichter 1980). Multiplicity of primary tumours is rare and metastases are most often found, as one might expect, in the liver and regional lymph nodes. Glucagonomas rarely, if ever, have an extrapancreatic origin (Gleeson et al 1971). Close to 90% of these tumours are found within the body and tail of the pancreas, a distribution which coincides with the normal alpha cell distribution within the pancreas (Leichter 1980). Glucagonomas show no specific histological characteristics other than those shared by endocrine tumours (Bloom & Polak 1987) and mitotic figures and nuclear atypia are rare (Warner et al 1983). Immunostaining tends to be positive for glucagon-containing granules but these cells may also stain for other peptides, most frequently, pancreatic polypeptide (Warner et al 1983). Electron microscopy typically reveals variable numbers of secretory granules; the cells of benign tumours are fully granulated while malignant tumours have few such granules (Bloom & Polak 1987).

Glucagon is stored and released by the pancreas in response to hypoglycaemia or stress (Mozell et al 1990). It is a potent stimulator of gluconeogenesis, glycogenolysis and ketogenesis. It also inhibits glycolysis and lipogenesis. It is the exaggeration of these effects that leads to the biochemical and clinical features of the glucagonoma syndrome (Mozell et al 1990).

The most common manifestation of the glucagonoma syndrome is some degree of glucose intolerance, this occurs in over 80% of patients (Leichter 1980). Because the glucose intolerance is rarely of great clinical significance, patients will often go undiagnosed for many years until the effects of metastatic disease become apparent, or the patient develops the necrotizing skin rash characteristic of the glucagonoma syndrome (Fig. 49.10). This necrolytic migratory erythema occurs in approximately two-thirds of patients with the glucagonoma syndrome (Leichter 1980). The association of this rash with the clinical finding of glucose intolerance strongly suggests the presence of a glucagonoma. The rash begins most frequently in intertriginous areas and in the skin around the mouth, vagina or anus (Kahan et al 1977), but it eventually involves the trunk, thighs, extremities and face. The rash begins as erythematous patches that spread annularly or serpiginously to become confluent. The erythematous plaques become raised and develop central bullae that slough leaving necrotic centres and serous crusts. Healing takes place in 2–3 weeks, leaving behind hyperpigmented sites. The process is chronic, recurrent, and migratory (Mozell et al 1990). The rash is attributed to the hypoaminoacidaemia that results from the profound catabolic effects of glucagon. Interestingly, intravenous administration of amino acids has been shown to resolve this dermatitis (Naets & Gans 1980).

A normochromic, normocytic anaemia occurs in about 85% of patients with the glucagonoma syndrome (Leichter 1980), and may be related to glucagon's ability to depress erythropoiesis (Naets & Gans 1980).

Stomatitis, glossitis and chronic vulvovaginitis are also seen with this syndrome (Leichter 1980). Weight loss can be quite severe and may be explained by excessive lipolysis and gluconeogenesis. Both muscular and visceral protein stores are significantly diminished (Naets & Gans 1980).

Deep venous thrombosis and thromboembolism are quite common in patients with the glucagonoma syndrome. The exact aetiology of this is not clear but fatal pulmonary embolism is a common cause of death (Bloom & Polak 1987). Long-term anticoagulant therapy is commonly required to prevent such lethal events.

Diarrhoea occurs in a small number of patients with the glucagonoma syndrome (Mozell et al 1990). Glucagonomas, like many functional endocrine tumours, produce and secrete other peptides, some of which may enhance intestinal motility (Polak et al 1976).

Because most of the clinical findings in patients with the glucagonoma syndrome are non-specific, it is not until the cutaneous manifestations appear that the diagnosis is considered. This delay is probably responsible for the high rate of metastatic spread and attainment of large tumour size prior to clinical detection. Although a skin biopsy may be diagnostic, it is the finding of hyperglucagonaemia that is usually confirmatory. Normal glucagon values range from 25 to 250 pg/ml (Mallinson et al 1974). Although glucagon levels can be elevated in patients with renal failure, cirrhosis, hepatic failure, or severe stress, the level rarely exceeds 500 pg/ml. In patients with the glucagonoma syndrome, the level is often above 1000 pg/ml. A secretin challenge test will yield a paradoxical rise in glucagon secretion in patients with the glucagonoma syndrome, (Mallinson et al 1974) but this test is rarely, if ever, necessary.

Since glucagonomas are usually very large and solitary, CT is a very accurate and sensitive method for localizing these tumours. Angiography and percutaneous transhepatic venous sampling (Ingemansson et al 1977, Wawrukiewicz et al 1982, Bloom & Polak 1987) can be helpful in localizing smaller tumours not detected by computerized tomography, but are rarely required.

Surgical removal of the primary tumour before it has metastasized offers the only chance for cure. However, for

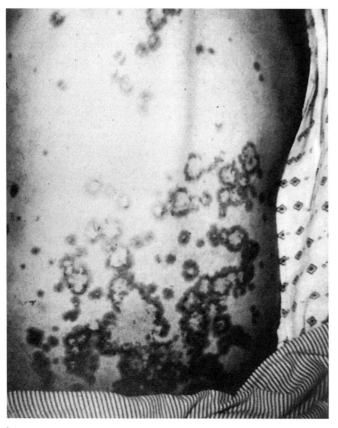

A

reasons previously discussed, the surgical cure rate is low and only 30% of cases were cured in one series (Higgins et al 1979). With surgical removal, the clinical manifestations rapidly abate, unless an extensive pancreatic resection leaves the patient with persistently abnormal glucose metabolism from reduction of the beta cell mass. As with other endocrine tumours of the pancreas, small solitary tumours can sometimes be enucleated although more often than not, given their large size and location, distal pancreatectomy or near total pancreatectomy is required. Even if there is metastatic tumour, radical excision or debulking should be considered because of the tumour's slow growth and the profoundly debilitating effects of excess glucagon secretion. Debulking may result in prolonged remission (Higgins et al 1979, Moertel et al 1982). Significant symptomatic improvement has also been achieved in patients with the use of long-acting somatostatin analogue (Kahn et al 1977, Boden et al 1986, Santangelo et al 1986, Woltering et al 1988). Other treatments, including systemic chemotherapy, with streptozotocin, 5-fluorouracil, DTIC, Adriamycin and Chlorzoticin given singly or in various combinations, have been used with response rates of up to 33% (Moertel et al 1980, Moertel et al 1982, Kessinger et al 1983, Kvols & Buck 1987, Reyes-Govea et al 1989). Hepatic artery embolization followed by intra-arterial chemotherapy or systemic chemotherapy for the treatment of functioning hepatic metastases, has also been used with variable degrees of success (Ajani et al 1988).

It is extremely important, prior to surgery, to bring these patients into the best possible condition. The pre-operative use of hyperalimentation, long-acting somato-

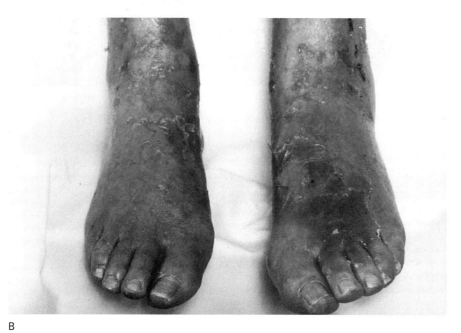

B

Fig. 49.10 Necrotizing migratory erythema of **A** the back, and **B** the feet in a patient with glucagonoma syndrome. This figure is reproduced in colour in the plated section at the front of the volume.

statin analogue and anticoagulants may greatly improve the underlying catabolic state and lessen the risk of fatal perioperative embolic complications (Mozell et al 1990).

VERNER–MORRISON SYNDROME (VIPOMA SYNDROME)

The VIPoma syndrome is again very rare with only 200 cases reported in the literature (Friesen 1987). It is characterized by the combination of watery diarrhoea, hypokalaemia, and achlorhydria, and for this reason is sometimes referred to as the WDHA syndrome. Verner and Morrison first described this syndrome in 1958. It was not however, until 1970, (Said & Mutt 1970) that vasoactive intestinal peptide (VIP), was first isolated from bovine intestine. VIP causes smooth muscle relaxation, stimulation of small intestinal secretion and inhibition of gastric acid secretion (Mozell et al 1990). There is still significant controversy as to whether or not VIP acts alone or in combination with other substances to produce the clinical manifestations of the syndrome. Levels of histidine isoleucine, a potent stimulator of small intestinal secretion (Anaganostides et al 1984), are elevated in patients with the VIPoma syndrome. Prostaglandin E has also been suggested as the primary secretagogue in these patients (Jaffe & Condon 1976).

The VIPoma syndrome typically occurs in middle-aged adults, although 10% of patients are under the age of 10. Of the tumours, 85% are located in the pancreas, while the remaining 15% have the VIPoma syndrome associated with ganglioneuromas (Dorney et al 1984). The location of 75% of VIPomas is the body and tail of the pancreas, 50% are malignant and over half of these have metastasized to liver or regional lymph nodes at the time of diagnosis (Mozell et al 1990). Of the neural tumours, 90% are benign. Approximately 4% of patients with the VIPoma syndrome have the MEN I syndrome. The vast majority of the tumours are solitary, ranging in size from 2 to 6 cm. Islet cell hyperplasia has also been described in association with the VIPoma syndrome (Mozell et al 1990).

VIP is widely distributed throughout the gastrointestinal tract and the nervous system. In the pancreas, it is found in conjunction with the nerve cells and pancreatic D1 cells (Polak et al 1974). VIP has several potential physiological roles. For example, it may facilitate peristalsis, stimulate pancreatic fluid and bicarbonate secretion, and inhibit solute absorption while stimulating water and ion secretion by the intestine (Mozell et al 1990).

The pathophysiological effects of raised levels of VIP and other peptides give rise to the VIPoma syndrome. The predominant symptom is a profuse secretory diarrhoea with over 70% of patients producing 3 litres of stool or more per day (Krejs 1987). Diarrhoea is typically episodic and usually explosive and has been characterized

as thin and tea-coloured (Mozell et al 1990). Abdominal cramping, weakness and hypotension result, along with severe electrolyte imbalance and metabolic acidosis. A total of 75% of patients are either hypochlorhydric or achlorhydric. Other findings less commonly seen include flushing, glucose intolerance, hypophosphataemia, hypercalcaemia and nephrolithiasis. Death usually results from dehydration and severe electrolyte abnormalities leading to cardiac rhythm disturbances or renal failure (Mozell et al 1990). Diagnosis of the VIPoma syndrome is made by confirming the presence of a secretory diarrhoea. Stool cultures should be performed to rule out infectious causes and a 48–72 hour fast should be instituted to rule out osmotic causes such as lactose intolerance. The Zollinger–Ellison syndrome is characterized by a low gastric pH and by an ulcer diathesis, in contrast to the situation affecting patients with the VIPoma syndrome. Nasogastric drainage will ablate the diarrhoea seen in ZES patients but will not affect the diarrhoea experienced in the VIPoma syndrome. The somatostatinoma syndrome typically yields steatorrhoea while the carcinoid syndrome is characterized by increased levels of urinary 5-HIAA. The best diagnostic test, however, is to measure the fasting VIP level; with VIPoma mean levels of 1000 pg/ml are typical. VIP secretion may be episodic, so that repeated measurements can be necessary (Mozell et al 1990).

CT scanning has been found to be the most reliable localizing method; angiography (Inamoto et al 1980) and portal venous sampling less so. Ultrasonography may play a role intraoperatively.

The treatment of choice is surgical removal of the offending tumour. Small solitary tumours can be treated by enucleation or distal pancreatectomy. Because 75% of these tumours are located in the body and tail of the pancreas, blind subtotal pancreatectomy can be considered in patients with tumours too small to localize. Before adopting this approach however, both adrenal glands as well as the abdominal midline should be carefully examined from the diaphragm to the bladder. Like glucagonomas, metastatic tumours may respond to debulking, even if this is only palliative (Nagorney et al 1983). Preoperative stabilization of the patient is extremely important. This includes adequate hydration with correction of electrolyte and acid–base abnormalities. Prednisone may help to control the diarrhoea. Indomethacin, because of its inhibitory effect on prostaglandin synthesis, may also be of benefit in decreasing stool volume. Sandostatin, the long-acting somatostatin analogue, has been the most promising agent used in the management of these patients and in over 70% of cases it decreases circulating VIP levels, decreases stool volume, and reverses many of the metabolic and electrolyte abnormalities (Rosato et al 1990).

Chemotherapy may be of some benefit. Streptozotocin has produced a 50% response rate (Moertel et al 1980), and combination with 5-fluorouracil may increase the response rate further (Moertel et al 1980). Intrahepatic arterial infusion with streptozotocin may also be of some benefit (Kahn et al 1975). More recently, the use of interferon has been considered in the management of VIPoma patients (Moertel et al 1980).

RARER ISLET CELL TUMOURS

Somatostatinoma

Ganda et al (1977) and Larsson et al (1977) first reported patients with somatostatinomas in 1977. The syndrome is characterized by steatorrhoea, diabetes mellitus, hypochlorhydria and cholelithiasis. Somatostatin, when first identified in 1968 (Krulich et al 1968), was shown to inhibit growth hormone secretion. Since that time, somatostatin has been localized not only to the hypothalamus, but also to the pancreatic D cell, stomach, duodenum and small intestine (Polak et al 1975). It is now known to be a universal inhibitor of peptide release (Mozel et al 1990).

Less than 50 cases of somatostatinoma have been reported in the literature. The mean age of onset is 51 years, and the sex distribution is equal (Mozell et al 1990). The tumours tend to be large and solitary. Two-thirds of these tumours occur in the pancreas and two-thirds of these are found in the pancreatic head. Other primary sites include the duodenum, the ampulla of Vater and the small bowel. Most of these tumours are malignant. They may rarely be associated with other familial endocrinopathies (Kelly 1983, Harris et al 1987).

Somatostatin has significant inhibitory effects (direct and indirect) on a variety of gastroenteropancreatic peptides, and appears to play a pivotal role in the maintenance of nutrient homeostasis (Mozell et al 1990).

All of the clinical findings in the somatostatinoma syndrome can be explained on the basis of inhibition of peptide secretion secondary to somatostatin excess. Diabetes mellitus is secondary to suppression of insulin secretion, hypochlorhydria is secondary to suppression of gastrin and gastric acid secretion, and steatorrhoea is secondary to decreased pancreatic exocrine secretion and impaired fat absorption. Gallstones are common and are probably due to suppression of cholecystokinin secretion, and perhaps to inhibition of biliary motility by somatostatin (Mozell et al 1990). The constellation of symptoms, along with elevated circulating somatostatin levels, confirms the diagnosis. Tolbutamide may be used to provoke somatostatin release in these patients. Because of the large size of these tumours, CT and ultrasonography are very sensitive localizing methods. The surgical management is similar to that described for glucagonomas and VIPomas. However, with the predominance of somatostatinomas in the head of the pancreas, a Whipple pro-

cedure may be necessary. Again, debulking a large primary, or debulking hepatic metastases, may give effective palliation of symptoms for prolonged periods. Streptozotocin and 5-fluorouracil and Adriamycin have achieved a variable response in advanced cases (Mozell et al 1990).

Pancreatic polypeptidoma

Only a few cases of pancreatic polypeptidoma have been reported in the literature. Most are malignant and metastases are common. The vast majority arise in the pancreatic head. Pancreatic polypeptide inhibits both pancreatic and biliary secretions, and its physiological role may be to conserve bile and pancreatic enzymes between meals (Adrian et al 1981, Tomita et al 1983). Pancreatic polypeptidomas are often clinically silent and many feel that pancreatic polypeptide is best considered to be a marker for other functional endocrine tumours, as it is often co-secreted with the principal hormone. Pure pancreatic polypeptide-secreting and -staining tumours have however been described in association with a rash and diarrhoea (Choksi et al 1988). Treatment is surgical and consists of palliative debulking; intravenous chemotherapy and somatostatin therapy may play supportive roles.

Other rare functional endocrine tumours include those that secrete a PTH-like substance (hypercalcaemia), ACTH (Cushing's syndrome), serotonin (carcinoid syndrome), cholecystokinin (CCK, diarrhoea), neurotensin, GIP, GHRH (acromegaly) and MSH (Morzell et al 1990).

Islet cell carcinoma

Although reference has been made to the malignant potential of various functioning pancreatic endocrine tumours, it should be noted that nearly half of all islet cell carcinomas are clinically non-functioning (Prinz et al 1983, Dial et al 1985, Friesen 1987). Between 1965 and 1984, 58 patients have been treated surgically at the Mayo Clinic for islet cell carcinoma. Of these patients 46% had non-functioning tumours and 54% had functioning tumours (19% gastrinomas, 14% insulinomas, 7% glucagonomas, 5% vipomas and 9% miscellaneous) (Thompson et al 1988). During recent years, an increasing proportion of functioning tumours has been reported (Broder & Carter 1973, Gould 1977, Kent et al 1981). This has resulted from our increased recognition of known syndromes, as well as our increased ability to detect hormones in previously unrecognized syndromes. Over 90% of non-functioning tumours are malignant and they are most often localized to the pancreatic head. In our series, the large size of islet cell carcinomas was reflected in the fact that computed tomography localized the tumours in over 96% of cases (Thompson et al 1988).

Potentially curative operations were performed in only 15 (26%) of our patients with islet cell carcinoma, and two-thirds of these resections were performed in patients with non-functioning tumours (Thompson et al 1988). Curative resection was most often possible in patients with malignant insulinomas (38%) and least likely in patients with malignant gastrinomas (9%). Despite our low surgical cure rate, worthwhile symptomatic improvement following surgical intervention was achieved in patients undergoing potentially curative and non-curative procedures. Among those patients undergoing a potentially curative operation, 90% had significant symptomatic improvement for a mean duration of 84 months (range, 10–206 months). Even though the vast majority of patients underwent a non-curative procedure, 51% of these still achieved significant symptomatic improvement following operation, for a mean duration of 39 months (range, 1–116 months). Patients with non-functioning malignant islet cell tumours and malignant insulinomas appeared to benefit least from palliative surgical procedures (symptomatic improvement 20–25%).

Surgical debulking is of obvious benefit in patients with hormonally active tumours but can even be of benefit in patients with non-functioning tumours, for the relief of pain and bleeding, and the correction of left-sided portal hypertension following splenic vein thrombosis (Legaspi & Brennan, 1988). Of our patients who received chemotherapy for symptomatic disease (25%), there was a 52% response rate for a mean duration of 27 months. Streptozotocin and 5-fluorouracil in combination were the most effective agents used (Thompson et al 1988).

There were four patients with malignant islet cell tumours and the MEN I syndrome in our series. Two patients had the Zollinger–Ellison syndrome, one had multiple insulinomas, and one had a solitary, malignant non-functioning tumour. All four had demonstrable parathyroid hyperplasia, two had pituitary adenomas and two had jejunal carcinoid tumours. With a mean follow-up of 5 years, two patients were alive without biochemical or radiological evidence of disease, one being a patient who underwent pancreatic resection of a solitary nonfunctioning tumour, while the other underwent near-total pancreatic resection for hyperinsulinism. The two ZE syndrome patients had demonstrable disease but were without symptoms on medical treatment at the time of follow-up. Despite the fact that these patients have dysplastic islets and multiple tumours throughout the gland, they appear to live in harmony with their tumours and often do well for long periods. In general, the tumours are slow-growing and associated with a long life expectancy from the time of diagnosis. Death results from local growth, metastatic disease and the sequelae of uncontrolled hormonal production. Although potentially curative resections are rare, long-term survival is frequently possible. Palliative debulking, both of primary and metastatic deposits, intravenous and hepatic intra-arterial chemotherapy, hepatic artery embolization, medical therapy (e.g. long-acting somatostatin analogue, omeprazole, H_2-blockers), and total gastrectomy for ZE patients, may all play important roles in the long-term management and palliation of selected patients with malignant indolent islet cell tumours.

SUMMARY

Islet cell tumours will continue to fascinate and intrigue many disciplines in the field of medicine. New syndromes will be elucidated as new peptide hormones are discovered. DNA and RNA probes are being developed which can detect messenger RNA specific for both the peptide hormones being secreted and their protein precursors. Coupled with this technology, chromosomal mapping may allow early identification of patients who are likely to develop manifestations of the multiple endocrine neoplasia syndromes. The future is exciting.

REFERENCES

Adrian T, Greenburg G, Bloom S 1981 Actions of pancreatic polypeptide in man. In: Bloom S R, Polak J M (eds) Gut hormones, 2nd edn. Churchill Livingstone, New York, p 206–221

Ajani J A, Carrasco C H, Charnsangavej C, Samaan N A, Levin B, Wallace S 1988 Islet cell tumors metastatic to the liver: Effective palliation by sequential hepatic artery embolization. Annals of Internal Medicine 108:340–344

Anaganostides A A, Christofides N D, Tatemoto K, Chadwick V S, Bloom S R 1984 Peptide histidine isoleucine: A secretagogue in human jejunum. Gut 25:381–385

Becker S W, Kahn D, Rothman S 1942 Cutaneous manifestations of internal malignant tumors. Archives of Dermatological Syphilis 45:1069–1080

Bloom S R, Polak J M 1987 Glucagonoma syndrome. American Journal of Medicine 82:25–36

Boden G, Ryan I G, Eisenschmid B L, Shelmet J J, Owen O E 1986 Treatment of inoperable glucagonoma with the long-acting somatostatin analog SMS 201-995. New England Journal of Medicine 315:1686–1689

Bordelon-Riser M E, Siciliano M J, Kohler R O 1979 Necessity for two human chromosomes for human chorionic gonadotropin production in human-mouse hybrids. Somatic Cell Genetics 5:597–613

Broder L E, Carter S K 1973 Pancreatic islet cell carcinoma: Clinical features of 52 patients. Annals of Internal Medicine 79:101–107

Choksi U A, Sellin R V, Hickey R C, Samaan N A 1988 An unusual skin rash associated with a pancreatic polypeptide-producing tumor. Annals of Internal Medicine 108:64–65

Creutzfeldt W 1985 Endocrine tumors of the pancreas. In: Volk B W, Arquilla E R (eds): The diabetic pancreas, 2nd end. Plenum, New York, p 543–586

Daggett R R, Kurtz A B, Morris D V, Goodburn E A, LeQuesne L P, Nabarro J D N 1981 Is preoperative localization of insulinomas necessary? Lancet 1:483–486

Dial P F, Braasch J W, Rossi R L, Lee A K, Jin G L 1985 Management of nonfunctioning islet cell tumors of the pancreas. Surgical Clinics of North America 65:291–299

Dorney S F, Kamath K R, Shulkes A A, Middleton A W 1984 Watery diarrhoea and a vasoactive intestinal peptide secreting ganglioneuroma. Medical Journal of Australia 140:97–99

Eckhauser F E, Cheung P S, Vinik A I, Stroden W E, Lloyd R V, Thompson N W 1986 Nonfunctioning malignant neuroendocrine tumors of the pancreas. Surgery 100:978–988

Edis A J, McIlrath D C, van Heerden J A et al 1976 Insulinoma – Current diagnosis and surgical management. Current Problems in Surgery 13:1–45

Fontaine J, LeLievre C, Le Douarin N M 1977 What is the developmental fate of the neural crest cells which migrate into the pancreas in the avian embryo? General and Comparative Endocrinology 33:394–404

Friesen S R 1987 Update on the diagnosis and treatment of rare neuroendocrine tumors. Surgical Clinics of North America 67:379–393

Ganda O P, Weir G C, Soeldner J S et al 1977 'Somatostatinoma': A somatostatin-containing tumor of the endocrine pancreas. New England Journal of Medicine 296:963–967

Gleeson M R, Bloom S R, Polak J M, Henry K, Dowling R H 1971 Endocrine tumor in kidney affecting small bowel structure, mortality and absorptive function. Gut 12:773–782

Gould V E 1977 Neuroendocrinomas and neuroendocrine carcinomas: APUD cell system neoplasms and their aberrant secretory activities. Pathology Annual 2:33–62

Gregory R A, Tracy H J, French J M, Sircus W 1960 Extraction of a gastrin-like substance from a pancreatic tumour in a case of Zollinger–Ellison syndrome. Lancet 1:1045–1048

Hamid Q A, Bishop A E, Springall D R et al 1989 Detection of human probombesin mRNA in neuroendocrine (small cell) carcinoma of the lung: In situ hybridization with cRNA probe. Cancer 63:266–271

Harris G J, Tio F, Cruz Jr A B 1987 Somatostatinoma: A case report and review of the literature. Journal of Surgical Oncology 36:8–16

Higgins G A, Recant L, Fischman A B 1979 The glucagonoma syndrome: Surgically curable diabetes. American Journal of Surgery 137:142–148

Holst J J 1985 Glucagon-producing tumors. Contemporary Issues in Gastroenterology 5:57–84

Howard T J, Passaro Jr E 1989 Gastrinoma – New medical and surgical approaches. Surgical Clinics of North America 69:667–681

Howard T J, Stabile B E, Zinner M J, Chang S, Bhagavan B S, Passaro Jr E 1990 Anatomic distribution of pancreatic endocrine tumors. American Journal of Surgery 159:258–264

Imamura M, Minematsu S, Suzuki T et al 1987 Usefulness of selective arterial secretin injection test for localization of gastrinoma in the Zollinger–Ellison syndrome. Annals of Surgery 205:230–239

Inamoto K, Yoshino F, Nakao N, Kawanaka M 1980 Angiographic diagnosis of a pancreatic islet tumor in a patient with the WDHA syndrome. Gastrointestinal Radiology 5:259–261

Ingemansson S, Holst J, Larsson L–I, Lunderquist A 1977 Localization of glucagonomas by pancreatic vein catheterization and glucagon assay. Surgery, Gynecology and Obstetrics 145:509–516

Jaffe B M, Condon S 1976 Prostaglandins E and F in endocrine diarrheagenic syndromes. Annals of Surgery 184:516–524

Kahan R S, Perez-Figaredo R A, Neimanis A 1977 Necrolytic migratory erythema: Distinctive dermatosis of the glucagonoma syndrome. Archives of Dermatology 113:792–797

Kahn C R, Levy A G, Gardner J D, Miller J V, Gorden P, Schein P S 1975 Pancreatic cholera: Beneficial effect of treatment with Streptozotocin. New England Journal of Medicine 292:941–945

Kahn C R, Rosen S W, Weintraub B D, Fajans S S, Gorden P 1977 Ectopic production of chorionic gonadotropin and its subunits by islet cell tumors. A specific marker for malignancy. New England Journal of Medicine 297:565–569

Kahn C R, Bhathena S J, Recant L, Rivier J 1981 Use of somatostatin and somatostatin analog in a patient with a glucagonoma. Journal of Clinical Endocrinology and Metabolism 53:543–549

Kaplan E L, Rubenstein A H, Evans R, Lee C H, Klementschitsch P 1979 Calcium infusion: A new provocative test for insulinomas. Annals of Surgery 190:501–507

Kaplan E L, Arganini M, Kang S J 1987 Diagnosis and treatment of hypoglycemic disorders. Surgical Clinics of North American 67:395–410

Kavlie H, White T T 1972 Pancreatic islet beta cell tumors and hyperplasia: Experience in 14 Seattle hospitals. Annals of Surgery 175:326–335

Kelly T R 1983 Pancreatic somatostatinoma. American Journal of Surgery 146:671–673

Kent R B III, van Heerden J A, Weiland L H 1981 Nonfunctioning islet cell tumors. Annals of Surgery 193:185–190

Kessinger A, Foley J F, Lemon H M 1983 Therapy of malignant APUD cell tumors: Effectiveness of DTIC. Cancer 51:790–794

Knudson Jr A G 1971 Mutation and cancer: Statistical study of retinoblastoma. Proceedings of the National Academy of Science USA 68:820–823

Krejs G 1987 VIPoma syndrome. American Journal of Medicine 82:37–48

Krulich L, Dhariwal A P S, McCann S M 1968 Stimulatory and inhibitory effects of purified hypothalamic extracts on growth hormone release from rat pituitary in vitro. Endocrinology 83:783–790

Kvols L K, Buck M 1987 Chemotherapy of metastatic carcinoid and islet cell tumors. American Journal of Medicine 82:77–83

Larsson C, Skogseid B, Oberg K, Nakamura Y, Nordenskjold M 1988 Multiple endocrine neoplasia type I gene maps to chromosome 11 and is lost in insulinoma. Nature 332:85–87

Larsson L-I, Hirsch M A, Holst JJ et al 1977 Pancreatic somatostatinoma: Clinical features and physiologic implications. Lancet 1:666–668

LeDouarin N M 1988 On the origin of pancreatic endocrine cells. Cell 53:169–171

Legaspi A, Brennan M F 1988 Management of islet cell carcinoma. Surgery 104:1018–1023

Leichter S B 1980 Clinical and metabolic aspects of glucagonoma. Medicine 59:100–113

Liu T-H, Tseng H-C, Zhu Y, Zhong S-X, Chen J, Cui Q-C 1985 Insulinoma: An immunocytochemical and morphologic analysis of 95 cases. Cancer 56:1420–1429

McCarthy D M, Jensen R T 1985 Zollinger Ellison syndrome – Current issues. Contemporary Issues in Gastroenterology 5:25–55

McGavran M H, Unger R H, Recant L, Polk H C, Kilo C, Levin M E 1966 A glucagon-secreting alpha-cell carcinoma of the pancreas. New England Journal of Medicine 274:1408–1413

Makowka L, Tzakis A G, Mazzaferro V et al 1989 Transplantation of the liver for metastatic endocrine tumors of the intestine and pancreas. Surgery, Gynecology and Obstetrics 1168:107–111

Mallinson C N, Bloom S R, Warin A P, Salmon P R, Cox B 1974 A glucagonoma syndrome. Lancet 2:1–5

Moertel C G, Hanley J A, Johnson L A 1980 Streptozotocin alone compared to streptozotocin and fluorouracil in the treatment of advanced islet cell carcinoma. New England Journal of Medicine 303:1189–1194

Moertel C G, Lavin P T, Hahn R G 1982 Phase II trial of doxorubicin treatment for advanced islet cell carcinoma. Cancer Treatment Report 66:1567–1569

Montenegro F, Lawrence G D, Macon W, Pass C 1980 Metastatic glucagonoma. Improvement after surgical debulking. American Journal of Surgery 139:424–427

Mozell E, Stenzel P, Wolterine E A, Rösch J, O'Dorisio T M 1990 Functional endocrine tumors of the pancreas: Clinical presentation, diagnosis and treatment. Current Problems in Surgery 27:309–386

Mukai K, Grotting J C, Greider M H, Rosai J 1982 Islet retrospective study of 77 pancreatic endocrine tumors using the immunoperoxidase method. American Journal of Surgical Pathology 6:387–399

Naets J P, Gans M 1980 Inhibitory effect of glucagon on erythropoiesis. Blood 55:997–1002

Nagorney D M, Bloom S R, Polak J M, Blumgart L H 1983 Resolution of recurrent Verner–Morrison Syndrome by resection of metastatic VIPoma. Surgery 93:348–353

Nicholls A 1902 Simple adenoma of the pancreas arising from an islet of Langerhans. Journal of Medical Research 8:385–395

Norton J A, Kahn C R, Schiebinger R, Gorschboth C, Brennan M F 1979 Amino acid deficiency and the skin rash associated with glucagonoma. Annals of Internal Medicine 91:213–215

Norton J A, Doppmann J L, Collen M J et al 1986 Prospective study of gastrinoma localization and resection in patients with Zollinger–Ellison syndrome. Annals of Surgery 204:468–479

Norton J A, Cromack D T, Shawker T H et al 1988 Intraoperative ultrasonic localization of islet cell tumors: A prospective comparison to palpation. Annals of Surgery 207:160–168

Oleesky S, Bailey I, Samolse E, Bilkus D 1990 A fibrosarcoma with hypoglycaemia and high serum-insulin level. Lancet 1:378

Pearse A G E 1966 5-hydroxytryptophan uptake by dog thyroid 'C' cells and its possible significance in polypeptide hormone production. Nature 211:598–600

Pfluger K-H, Gramse M, Gropp C, Havemann K 1981 Ectopic ACTH production with autoantibody formation in a patient with acute myeloblastic leukemia. New England Journal of Medicine 305:1632–1636

Pictet R L, Rall L B, Phelps P, Rutter W J 1976 The neural crest and the origin of the insulin-producing and other gastrointestinal hormone-producing cells. Science 191:191–192

Pipeleers-Marichal M, Somers G, Willems G et al 1990 Gastrinomas in the duodenums of patients with multiple endocrine neoplasia type 1 and the Zollinger–Ellison syndrome. New England Journal of Medicine 322:723–727

Polak J M, Pearse A G E, Garaud J-C, Bloom S R 1974 Cellular localization of vasoactive intestinal peptide in the mammalian and avian gastrointestinal tract. Gut 15:720–724

Polak J M, Pearse A G E, Grimelius L, Bloom S R 1975 Growth hormone release-inhibiting hormone in gastrointestinal and pancreatic D cells. Lancet 1:1220–1222

Polak J M, Adrian T E, Bryant M G, Bloom S R, Heitz P H, Pearse A G E 1976 Pancreatic polypeptide in insulinomas, gastrinomas, VIPomas and glucagonomas. Lancet 1:328–330

Prinz R A, Badrinath K, Chejfec G, Freeark R J, Greenlec H B 1983 'Nonfunctioning' islet cell carcinoma of the pancreas. American Surgeon 49:345–349

Proye C 1987 Surgical strategy in insulinoma of adults: Clinical review. Acta Chirurgica Scandinavica 153:481–491

Rasbach D A, van Heerden J A, Telander R L, Grant C S, Carney J A 1985 Surgical management of hyperinsulinism in the multiple endocrine neoplasia type I syndrome. Archives of Surgery 120:584–589

Reyes-Govea J, Holm A, Aldrete J S 1989 Response of glucagonomas to surgical excision and chemotherapy: Report of two cases and review of the literature. American Surgeon 55:523–527

Rosai J 1989 Ackerman's Surgical Pathology Vol 1, 7th edn. Mosby, St Louis, p 770–779

Rosato F E, Bonn J, Shapiro M, Barbot D J, Furnary A M, Gardiner G A 1990 Selective arterial stimulation of secretin in localization of gastrinomas. Surgery, Gynecology and Obstetrics 171:196–200

Ruskone A, Rene E, Chayvialle J A et al 1982 Effect of somatostatin on small bowel water and electrolyte transport in a patient with pancreatic cholera. Digestive Diseases and Sciences 27:459–466

Said S I, Mutt V 1970 Polypeptide with broad biological activity: Isolation from small intestine. Science 169:1217–1218

Santangelo W C, Unger R H, Orci L, Dueno M I, Popma J J, Krejs G J 1986 Somatostatin analog-induced remission of necrolytic migratory erythema without changes in plasma glucagon concentration. Pancreas 1:464–469

Service F J, Dale A J D, Elveback L R, Jiang N-S 1976 Insulinoma – Clinical and diagnostic features of 60 consecutive cases. Mayo Clinic Proceedings 51:417–429

Sidhu G S 1979 The endodermal origin of digestive and respiratory tract APUD cells: Histopathologic evidence and review of the literature. American Journal of Pathology 96:5–20

Spandidos D A, Anderson M L M 1989 Oncogenes and onco-suppressor genes: Their involvement in cancer. Journal of Pathology 157:1–10

Stabile B E, Morrow D J, Passaro Jr E 1984 The gastrinoma triangle: Operative indications. American Journal of Surgery 147:25–31

Stefanini P, Carboni M, Patrassi N, Basoli A 1974 Beta-islet cell tumors of the pancreas: Results of a study on 1067 cases. Surgery 75:597–609

Stevens R E, Moore G E 1983 Inadequacy of APUD concept in explaining production of peptide hormones by tumours. Lancet 1:118–119

Telander R L 1989 Neonatal hypoglycemia. In: van Heerden JA (ed) Common problems in endocrine surgery. Year Book, Chicago, p 301–306

Thompson G B, van Heerden J A, Grant C S, Carney J A, Ilstrup D M 1988 Islet cell carcinomas of the pancreas: A twenty-year experience. Surgery 104:1011–1017

Thompson J C 1989 Management of patients with the Zollinger–Ellison syndrome. In: van Heerden J A (ed) Common problems in endocrine surgery. Year Book, Chicago, p 290–295

Thompson N W, Lloyd R V, Nishiyama R H et al 1984 MEN I pancreas: A histological and immunohistochemical study. World Journal of Surgery 8:561–574

Thompson N W, Bondeson A-G, Bondeson L, Vinik A 1989a The surgical treatment of gastrinoma in MEN I syndrome patients. Surgery 106:1081–1086

Thompson N W, Vinik A I, Eckhauser F E 1989b Microgastrinomas of the duodenum: A cause for failed operations for the Zollinger–Ellison syndrome. Annals of Surgery 209:396–404

Tisell L E, Ahlman H, Jansson S, Grimelius L 1988 Total pancreatectomy in the MEN I syndrome. British Journal of Surgery 75:154–157

Tomita T, Fiersen S R, Kimmel J R, Doull V, Pollock H G 1983 Pancreatic polypeptide secreting islet cell tumor: A study of 3 cases. American Journal of Pathology 113:134–142

Van Heerden J A, Thompson G B 1991 The Zollinger–Ellison syndrome. In: Landor J, Nyhus, L M (eds) Problems in General Surgery vol 7. J B Lippincott, Philadelphia p 550–563

Verner J V, Morrison A B 1958 Islet cell tumor and a syndrome of refractory watery diarrhea and hypokalemia. American Journal of Medicine 25:374–380

Vogel S B, Wolfe M M, McGuigan E J, Hawkins Jr I F, Howard R J, Woodward E R 1987 Localization and resection of gastrinomas in Zollinger–Ellison syndrome. Annals of Surgery 205:550–556

Warner T F C S, Block M, Hafiz G, Mack E, Lloyd R V, Bloom S R 1983 Glucagonomas: Ultrastructure and immunocytochemistry. Cancer 51:1091–1096

Wawrukiewicz A S, Rosch J, Keller F S, Lieberman D A 1982 Glucagonoma and its angiographic diagnosis. Cardiovascular and Interventional Radiology 5:318–324

Wermer P 1954 Genetic aspects of adenomatosis of endocrine glands. American Journal of Surgery 16:363–371

Wilder R M, Allan F N, Power M H, Robertson H E 1927 Carcinoma of the islets of the pancreas: Hyperinsulinism and hypoglycemia. Journal of the American Medical Association 89:348–355

Williams S T, Woltering E A, O'Dorisio T M, Fletcher W S 1989 Effect of octreotide acetate on pancreatic exocrine function. American Journal of Surgery 157:459–462

Woltering E A, Mozell E J, O'Dorisio T M, Fletcher W S, Howe B 1988 Suppression of primary and secondary peptides with somatostatin analog in the therapy of functional endocrine tumors. Surgery, Gynecology and Obstetrics 167:453–462

Zollinger R M 1985 Gastrinoma: Factors influencing prognosis. Surgery 97:49–54

Zollinger R M, Ellison E H 1955 Primary peptic ulceration of the jejunum associated with islet cell tumors of the pancreas. Annals of Surgery 142:709–728

Injuries to the pancreas

50. Injuries to the pancreas

C. F. Frey   J. W. Wardell

INTRODUCTION

Historical background

Pancreatic injury from blunt or penetrating abdominal trauma is relatively uncommon, with early studies reporting an incidence of pancreatic injury of 1–2% (Cullota et al 1956, Graham et al 1978a, Glancy 1989). More recent studies, however, report an incidence of 3–4% in patients with abdominal trauma (Berni et al 1982, Glancy 1989). The apparent increase in pancreatic trauma may be attributable to more frequent high speed motor vehicle accidents, changes in motor vehicle safety equipment and an increasing use of knives and guns in violent civil crime. While relatively infrequent, these injuries can have devastating consequences, with combined morbidity and mortality rates approaching 100% for untreated pancreatic injuries. (Bach & Frey 1971, Lucas 1977, Nilsson et al 1986, Leppaniemi et al 1988).

The first reported case of blunt pancreatic trauma was published by Travers in the 1827 Lancet. He reported on an intoxicated woman who was struck in the chest and abdomen by a stage coach wheel and was brought to St. Thomas' Hospital where she succumbed within hours of her injury. At autopsy she was found to have a transverse tear of the pancreas as well as an hepatic laceration. The cause of death was attributable to intraabdominal haemorrhage from the associated hepatic injury.

The earliest report of penetrating pancreatic trauma and the first report of pancreatic resection for trauma is credited to Kleberg by Otis in 1876 (who edited a report on the American Civil War: 'Medical and surgical history of the War of Rebellion (1861–1865)'). Kleberg described in 1868, a 60-year-old soldier who was attacked by thieves and was stabbed in the abdomen. He was found to have a herniation of the pancreas through the stab wound. This was ligated and resected. The patient had an uncomplicated course and was subsequently discharged.

Otis reported on five other patients with penetrating pancreatic injuries, with a mortality rate of 80%. The only survivor underwent ligation and excision of damaged pancreatic tissue. The other four patients had survived long delays between injury and definitive hospitalization (the shortest of which was one-and-a-half days) only to expire from the late complications, peritonitis and haemorrhage, which in three cases were due to associated injuries to liver, stomach or splenic vessels.

While the significance of an intact pancreatic duct was not fully appreciated by Otis, he described two patients who had, at autopsy, a ball (bullet) lodged in the pancreas. In both cases, the main pancreatic duct was intact and the gland was without evidence of pancreatic inflammation or necrosis. Both patients, in fact, died of associated injuries. Otis then went on to quote several surgical treatises and textbooks of surgery which outline the problems and importance of diagnosing pancreatic injury, the consequences of not doing so, and what constitutes a significant pancreatic injury. These concepts have only recently been reaffirmed and generally recognized as valid almost 150 years after the original publication. Bell states in *A System of Surgery* (Volume V, published in 1787):

As the pancreas lies deeply covered with the other viscera, wounds of it can seldom be discovered; but as a division of the duct of this gland will prevent the secretion which it affords from being carried to the bowels, this may, be interrupting or impeding digestion, do much injury to the constitution; and as the liquor will be effused into the cavity of the abdomen, it may thus be productive of collections, the removal of which may ultimately require the assistance of surgery.

Gooch, writing in *Chirugical Works* (Vol. 1, p. 99, 1752) declares that:

Wounds of the pancreas are to be concluded mortal if its duct or blood vessels are injured, whence the succus pancreaticus or blood may be discharged into the cavity of the abdomen and there putrefying, cause inevitable death.

Mikulicz in 1903 was able to identify 45 cases of pancreatic trauma reported in the literature up to that time. He found an overall mortality of 60%; all 20 patients who did not undergo surgery died, while of the 25 who underwent surgical treatment, seven died giving a morality rate

565

of 28%. Mikulicz recommended thorough abdominal exploration through a midline incision, suture of the pancreas where needed for haemostasis, and drainage in all cases.

Little progress was made in either the recognition or management of pancreatic injuries during World War I. Treatment was largely non-operative with Mikulicz's remaining recommendations unheeded. Of five patients reported by the British with pancreatic injuries, only one survived, a mortality rate similar to that reported for the American Civil War.

Poole's World War II report on the Second Auxiliary Surgical Group in 1944 and 1945 recorded 62 pancreatic injuries associated with a 56% mortality. The importance of associated injuries as factors contributing to mortality received appropriate emphasis, as only one of the 62 patients was noted to have an isolated pancreatic injury. Of the 35 deaths, 13 were associated with major vascular injury. The mortality rose progressively from 33% with one associated viscus injury, to 50% with two viscera, to 60% with three viscera and to 100% with four viscera injured in addition to the pancreas.

During the Korean conflict, the mortality rate in nine patients with pancreatic injuries was reduced to 22%, according to Sako et al (1955), reporting the experiences of the surgical research team of the US Army Medical Services Graduate School. The report provides no evidence of any enhanced awareness of the appropriate operative management of the injuries. The decreasing mortality of pancreatic injury, as well as of other injury, was attributed to improvements in supportive care (including resuscitation, fluid replacement and antibiotics) and in the management of associated injuries.

A major step in improved diagnosis of pancreatic injury, was the observation by Elman et al in 1929 that the serum amylase became elevated in some pancreatic injuries if the pancreatic duct was injured or obstructed. This observation was later confirmed by McCorkle & Goldman in 1942 and reaffirmed the following year in a report by Naffziger and McCorkle.

Walton, in 1923, recommended pancreatic resection of the portion of the pancreas distal to the fracture and oversewing the proximal end of the pancreas as the safest form of management of injuries to the body and tail of the pancreas in which the pancreatic duct had been severed. Whipple, in 1946, reported his techniques for duodenal resection with total or partial pancreatectomy. Although not originally proposed for traumatic injuries to the duodenum and pancreas, this operation has proved valuable in dealing with complicated combined injuries of these organs. The report by Kerry & Glas in 1962 emphasized the significance of injury to the major ductal system of the pancreas through clinical and laboratory investigations, and has become a landmark in establishing appropriate operative management of patients with complex pancreatic injuries and associated injuries to the duodenum and common bile duct.

Mechanisms and nature of pancreatic injury

The pancreas, a retroperitoneal organ, is relatively well protected by the spinal column and paraspinous muscles posteriorly and the abdominal viscera anteriorly. This accounts for its relatively infrequent rate of injury. The pancreas is usually injured by direct laceration in penetrating trauma or is fractured over the spinal column in cases of blunt trauma. The location of fracture in cases of blunt trauma is dependent on the vector of force, the pancreatic head, neck or body and tail being injured respectively by forces directed obliquely right, centrally, or obliquely left.

The magnitude of force required for pancreatic injury in blunt trauma or the path of the lacerating agent in penetrating trauma make associated organ injury likely. Table 50.1 lists the wounding agent and associated intraabdominal injuries in 28 series reporting on 2351 patients with traumatic pancreatic or combined pancreaticoduodenal injuries. Penetrating trauma accounted for 69% and blunt trauma for 31% of the injuries. Associated injuries were reported to the liver (26%), colon or small bowel (25%), duodenum (24%), major vessels (25%), stomach (19%), spleen (12%), kidney (10%), and biliary tree (3%). In addition to the pancreatic injury, there were an average of 1.4 associated intra-abdominal injuries per patient. This does not include maxillofacial, CNS, thoracic or skeletal traumatic injuries so that the actual number of associated injuries per patient is higher, particularly in blunt trauma. Approximately 90% of patients with pancreatic trauma will have one or more associated injuries.

Mortality rates for pancreatic or combined pancreaticoduodenal injuries range from zero to 32%. The lowest rates are generally reported for isolated distal pancreatic injuries with progressively higher rates for more complex injuries and those with associated injuries. Table 50.2 relates mortality by wounding agent and average mortality in 18 reported series of pancreatic and combined pancreaticoduodenal injuries. Shotgun injuries carry the highest mortality followed by gunshot wounds, blunt trauma, and stab wounds.

The majority of deaths occur from associated injuries. Haemorrhage occurring intraoperatively, or exsanguination from coagulation disorders within the first 48 hours post injury, account for over two-thirds of the fatalities (Table 50.3). Abscess and other septic complications account for approximately 16% of the deaths, many of these a result of shock or injury to colon or small bowel, while multiple system/organ failure (perhaps secondary to prolonged infection or shock) and miscellaneous causes account for the remainder. The actual percentage of

Table 50.1 Injuries associated with pancreatic trauma. CBD/GB, common bile duct/gallbladder; Colon/SB, colon/small bowel; P, penetrating injury; B, blunt injury, NS, not stated

Author	Injury	No. of patients	Major vascular	Liver	Stomach	Spleen	Duodenum	CBD/GB	Kidney	Colon/SB
Glancy	P	544	164	259	178	159	79	34	129	192
(1989)*	B	272								
Bass et al (1988)	B	26	—	2	—	2	1	—	1	—
Whalen et al	P	100	16	48	44	15	69	8	14	19
(1987)†	B	26								
Feliciano et al	P	104	33	60	43	—	129	—	35	82
(1987)	B	25								
Nowak et al	P	39	10	20	26	12	13	3	7	25
(1986)	B	3								
Wynn et al (1985)†	NS	57	3	17	12	15	6	—	10	17
Jones (1985)	P	362	190	—	—	—	91	—	—	101
	B	138								
Sims et al (1984)	P	37	—	23	—	10	14	—	—	17
	B	7								
Moore & Moore	P	19	11	17	—	—	—	7	—	12
(1984)†	B	15								
Sorenson et al (1985)	P	41	10	17	19	—	6	3	6	19
Nilsson et al	P	2	1	3	3	7	—	—	1	—
(1986)	B	27								
Leppaniemi et al	P	32	13	18	—	—	—	—	—	—
(1988)	B	11								
Wisner et al	P	44	—	—	—	—	19	—	—	—
(1990)	B	47								
Ivatury et al	P	107	50	37	42	19	21	4	15	29
(1990)			(25 deaths)	(13 deaths)	(8 deaths)	(6 deaths)	(8 deaths)		(7 deaths)	(8 deaths)
Fabian et al	P	42	11	19	21	12	7	—	—	15
(1990)	B	17								
Fitzgibbons et al	P	44	9	23	23	9	7	—	15	16
(1982)	B	12								
Mansour et al	P	37	43	29	17	5	88	13	—	37
(1989)	B	25								
Wilkinson	P	12	2	11	11	17	—	—	—	4
(1989)	B	27								
Combined	P	16	12	14	6	5	15	2	6	8
series	B	38								
Total		2355	578	617	445	287	565	74	239	593

* This review excludes patients reported in the other series listed below.
† These reports also include combined pancreaticoduodenal injuries.

deaths directly attributable to the pancreatic injury range from 6 to 10%.

Factors influencing overall mortality rates include degree of preoperative shock, number of associated injuries, and the location and complexity of pancreatic injury. Several series have shown that mortality rates increase seven- to eight-fold in patients with pancreatic injuries who present with a systolic blood pressure of less than 90 mmHg. (Anderson et al 1974, Graham et al 1978a, Jones 1978) Glancy (1989) quotes a mortality rate of 2.5% for patients with 0–1 associated injuries, 13.6% with 2–3 associated injuries and 29.6% with 4 or more associated injuries. Mortality rates of 21.9, 17.7, and 9.8% have been estimated for injuries occurring in the head, body and tail of the pancreas respectively. (Baker et al 1963, Jones & Shires 1971, Jones 1978, Stone et al 1981).

Morbidity associated with pancreatic trauma occurs in 20–40% of patients (Bach & Frey 1971, Graham et al 1978a, Sims et al 1984, Jones 1985, Smego et al 1985). The majority of these consist of wound infections, intra-abdominal abscess or pulmonary difficulties. Morbidity directly associated with the pancreatic injury occurs in approximately 8–10% of the patients. Complications attributable to the pancreatic injury include fistula, pseudocyst, pancreatic abscess, pancreatitis, haemorrhagic or necrotizing pancreatitis, delayed pancreatic haemorrhage, sepsis secondary to infected pancreatic abscess or pseudocyst, and in rare cases, diabetes or exocrine pancreatic insufficiency following pancreatic resection.

SURGICAL ANATOMY

The surgical anatomy of the pancreas is described in detail in Chapter 2. The abundant blood supply of the

Table 50.2 Wounding agent and mortality after pancreatic injury. % mortality rates shown in parentheses; (?), mortality rates or number of deaths not stated.

Author	Penetrating	Stab	Gunshot	Shotgun	Blunt	% Overall mortality
Glancy (1989)*	548 (19.0)	74 (5.4)	291 (7.9)	56 (39.3)	271 (26.6)	21.5
Bass et al (1988)	—	—	—	—	26 (?)	—
McKone et al (1988)	1 (0)	—	—	—	4 (0)	0
Lausten et al (1988)	2	—	—	—	2 (0)	0
Whalen et al (1987)†	100 (?)	—	—	—	26 (?)	—
Feliciano et al (1987)	104 (?)	15 (?)	82 (?)	7 (?)	25 (?)	29.5
Keeling et al (1987)	—	—	—	—	9 (11.1)	11.1
Nowak et al (1986)	39 (20.5)	2 (0)	34 (23.5)	3 (0)	3 (66.7)	23.8
Wynn et al (1985)†	35 (?)	14 (?)	20 (?)	1 (?)	49 (?)	17.5
Jones (1985)	362 (22)	76 (5)	252 (22)	34 (56)	138 (19)	21.2
Sims et al (1984)	37 (10.8)	7 (?)	30 (?)	—	7 (28.6)	13.6
Moore & Moore (1984)†	19 (10.5)	1 (0)	16 (6.3)	2 (50)	15 (13.3)	11.8
Sorenson et al (1985)	41 (14.5)	13 (?)	25 (?)	3 (66.7)	—	14.5
Oreskovich & Carrico (1984)	10 (0)	0	7 (0)	3 (0)	—	0
Nilsson et al 1986	2 (?)	—	—	—	27 (?)	21.0
Leppaniemi et al (1988)	32 (7)	—	—	—	11 (45)	16.3
Wisner et al (1990)	44	21	19	4	47	9
Ivatury et al (1990)	107 (32)	32 (21)	69 (34.6%)	—	—	32
Total	1483	255	845	113	660	

* This review excludes patients in the other series listed below.

† This report includes combined pancreaticoduodenal injuries.

pancreas and its intimate association with major vessels (Fig. 50.1) explains the high incidence of associated vascular injury when the organ is damaged.

Injury to the pancreatic ductal system anywhere in its course through the pancreas or duodenum sets the stage for pancreatic ductal obstruction or extravasation with all their attendant complications, such as pancreatitis, pancreatic fistulas, pancreatic pseudocysts, and pancreatic abscess. In our opinion, the key to successful management of pancreatic trauma is the recognition and appropriate management of pancreatic ductal injury following control of more immediately life-threatening associated injuries.

DIAGNOSIS AND MANAGEMENT OF PANCREATIC INJURY

Preoperative evaluation

The majority of patients with pancreatic injury will have associated intra-abdominal injuries which may mandate

Table 50.3 Cause of death following pancreatic injury

Author	Haemorrhage associated injuries	Pancreatic injury, abscess and sepsis	Organ failure	Miscellaneous	Not specified
Graham et al (1978a)	47	8	11	6	—
Whalen et al (1987)†	11	4	—	—	—
Feliciano et al (1987)	22	9	7	—	—
Keeling et al (1987)	1	—	—	—	—
Nowak et al (1986)	8	1	—	1	—
Wynn et al (1985)†	5	3	1	1	—
Jones (1985)	68	16	—	2	18
Sims et al (1984)	3	2	1	—	—
Moore & Moore (1984)†	2	1	—	—	—
Sorenson et al (1985)	4	—	—	—	2
Leppaniemi et al (1988)	7	1	—	—	—
Smego et al (1985)	12	2	0	7	—
Wisner et al 1990	6	—	1	1	—
Ivatury et al (1990)	27	6	0	0	—
Total	217 (72.1%)	47 (15.6%)	25 (8.3%)	12 (4%)	—

† These reports also include combined pancreaticoduodenal injuries.

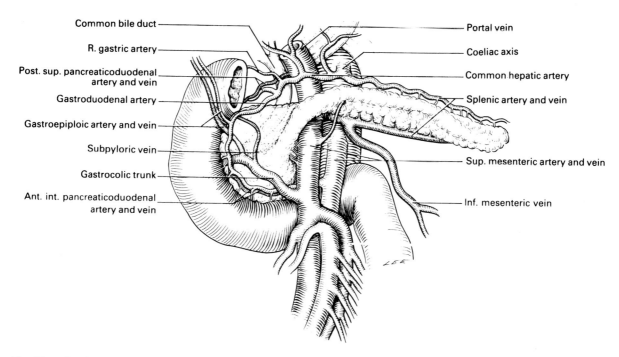

Fig. 50.1 Surgical anatomy of the pancreas. (From Frey F, Bodai B The surgical management of pancreaticoduodenal trauma. In: Rob & Smith's Operative surgery: Alimentary tract and abdominal wall, 4th edn, by permission of the publishers, Butterworth & Co (Publishers) Ltd. ©)

emergency abdominal exploration (Table 50.1). Indications for immediate laparotomy include hypotension, declining serial haematocrits, positive peritoneal lavage, evidence of peritoneal irritation on physical examination or inability to rule out abdominal injury by other means prior to other prolonged surgical procedures.

At our institution, all cases of abdominal trauma with documented peritoneal penetration are explored, although some institutions prefer a policy of observation and selective exploration in the absence of other immediate indications for laparotomy. As pointed out earlier, the cause of death in the majority of patients with fatal pancreatic trauma is haemorrhage, sepsis secondary to bowel injury, or prolonged shock. Rapid correction of these conditions is the key to survival in patients with severe combined injuries.

If a patient has an indication for immediate laparotomy, no time should be wasted performing diagnostic tests to evaluate pancreatic or duodenal injury. Airway patency and adequacy of ventilation must be assured, followed by a cursory physical examination to identify other immediately correctable life-threatening conditions. Adequate venous access is obtained and resuscitation begun immediately. A urinary bladder catheter and nasogastric tube are inserted and blood withdrawn for typing, cross-matching and appropriate haematological and biochemical studies. A chest X-ray and, in cases of gross haematuria or penetrating injuries in proximity to the kidney, a single shot IVP should complete the radiological work-up. While these activities are underway, a more detailed physical examination from head to toe completes the preoperative evaluation. Any less severe injuries identified at this stage, can be evaluated postoperatively once injuries forming an immediate threat to life have been controlled.

Operative management

The patient should be taken to the operating room and readied for surgery with complete preparation of the torso from clavicle to pubis and bedsheet to bedsheet, so permitting dependent flank drainage if this proves necessary.

The incision used routinely is a midline abdominal one. When there is tenderness in the upper abdomen, and the most likely source is in this region, the initial incision should extend at least from the xiphoid to umbilicus. It should then be extended well below the umbilicus once the presence of injury or reasonable probability of injury has been verified.

The small intestine is withdrawn promptly to permit thorough abdominal exploration with inspection of the retroperitoneum. All blood and clots should be rapidly evacuated. Any injury not causing catastrophic bleeding should be isolated temporarily with packs to avoid missing more major sources of haemorrhage.

Control of major haemorrhage and the closure of hollow viscus injuries (to limit bacterial contamination), have the highest priority. Once injury to intra-abdominal structures has been excluded or high priority injuries have been dealt with, attention should be directed toward the retroperitoneum and the duodenum and pancreas. Since injuries of these structures rarely produce catastrophic haemorrhage in themselves, they do not have high priority in the initial exploration. (Sheldon et al 1970, Stigall & Dorsey 1989). The sites of injury in duodenum and pancreas, from collected reviews of pancreatic and duodenal injuries, are shown in Figure 50.2.

The initial exploration of the free peritoneal cavity with the small bowel withdrawn permits inspection of the inferior aspect of the base of the mesocolon from the ligament of Treitz outward to the left. Injury to the pancreatic ductal system is suspected whenever retroperitoneal hemorrhage can be seen through the base of the mesocolon or gastrohepatic mesentery. Sometimes it is possible to visualize a ductal injury in penetrating trauma or appreciate that the duct must be fractured if the pancreas is more than half transected. A severely macerated gland or one which has a central perforation should be assumed to have a ductal injury until this is ruled out by pancreatography or operative exploration (Gougeon et al 1976). In most patients, the pancreatic substance can be inspected along its inferior surface, and injury to the body and tail ruled out relatively firmly. Attention can next be directed toward the gastrohepatic ligament, as in thin patients, the upper portion of the body and tail can often be visualized through the gastrohepatic ligament; once again, haemorrhage seen through the gastrohepatic ligament suggests the possibility of pancreatic injury.

Attention should next be directed toward the duodenum, mobilizing the colon downward and, if necessary, sweeping the mesocolon down with sponges. The hepatic flexure of the colon should be mobilized when there is any reason to suspect injury to the duodenum or the head of the pancreas. By severing the lateral attachments of the hepatic flexure of the colon, the entire mesocolon can be mobilized downward to permit inspection of the anterior and lateral surface of the first, second, and third portion of the duodenum. Evidence of haemorrhage in the duodenum or behind it requires mobilization of the duodenum by severing its lateral attachments (Kocher manoeuvre). These attachments should be cut from the foramen of Winslow round to the fourth portion of the duodenum. This permits the entire duodenum to be mobilized upward so that its posterior surface can be inspected and palpated.

It also permits evaluation of the head of the pancreas. If there is even a small haematoma in the head of the pancreas, bimanual palpation should be carried out to determine whether there is loss of substance or pulpefaction of the head. This finding is associated with the possibility of injury to major pancreatic ducts. The fourth portion of the duodenum can be inspected from the area of the ligament of Treitz. The absence of haemorrhage around this ligament makes injury to the fourth portion of the duodenum unlikely. If there is any suggestion of injury, the entire right colon and small bowel mesentery can be mobilized, and swung upwards and medially to expose the entire sweep of the duodenum (Cattell & Braasch 1960). When there is any reason to suspect injury to the body and tail of the pancreas or when there is evidence of trauma to the head of the pancreas, the lesser sac should be opened and the entire pancreas exposed. This is best done by ligating two to three arcades outside the gastric epiploic vessels in a relatively avascular area of the gastroeploic omentum and coming down on the pancreas through the lesser sac. Once the lesser sac is entered in the right place, the entire body and tail of the pancreas are open to view.

If there is evidence of haemorrhage in the retroperitoneum, the entire transverse colon should be separated from the omentum to permit direct inspection of the entire anterior surface of the pancreas. Ecchymosis in the area of the neck, body, or tail of the pancreas requires exploration. Bimanual palpation is another method for evaluating a pancreatic injury. This is best done by sweeping the mesocolon downward, separating it from the inferior surface of the pancreas or by opening the mesocolon at its junction with the retroperitoneum inferiorly. The latter manoeuvre, unless done carefully, risks injuring the colonic arcade that provides collateral blood flow from the middle colic artery to the left colic artery. Once the colon and the mesentery have been separated from the body and tail of the pancreas, the distal pancreas can be rotated superiorly along its length without having

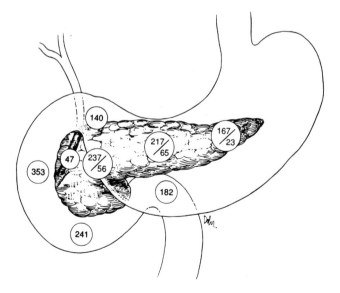

Fig. 50.2 Location of injury to the pancreas and duodenum in collected reviews. Each circle shows the number of injuries in that location over the number of deaths. Injuries to the pancreas (larger circles) should be considered separately from injuries of the duodenum or bile duct (small circles). (From Blaisdell & Trunkey 1982 Trauma management. Thieme Medical Publishers Inc, New York. Reprinted with permission.)

to mobilize the spleen. The posterior aspect of the gland can be visualized and the body and of the tail of the pancreas can be palpated bimanually. Loss of integrity of pancreatic substance provides indirect evidence of ductal injury.

An alternative method of exploration for those with experience of pancreatic injury is accomplished by duodenotomy and retrograde pancreatography through the papilla of Vater using a Fogarty irrigating catheter. The pancreatic duct can also be intubated by incising the tail of the pancreas and using the Fogarty irrigating catheter to perform a pancreatogram.

The importance of assessing ductal integrity and planning an appropriate operation as emphasized in the 1960s and 1970s (Kerry & Glas 1962, Bach & Frey 1971), was confirmed recently by Berni et al (1982) who, by the use of intraoperative pancreaticography, sharply reduced the morbidity of pancreas-related complications. The liberal use of intraoperative pancreatography has also been supported by Ivatury et al (1985) who noted few complications resulting from duodenotomy and no instances of duodenal fistulization. However, a less invasive and superior technique, if the patient is stable, is preoperative or intraoperative endoscopic retrograde cholangiopancreatography (ERCP) in order to assess the integrity of the major pancreatic duct (Hayward et al 1989).

Absence of any haemorrhage over the pancreas and duodenum makes injury very unlikely. The only exception is the possibility of injury to the posterior aspect of the duodenum, although this is most unlikely if palpation of the duodenum does not reveal induration, crepitus or bile staining nor, on inspection, the slightest trace of ecchymosis. Small, ecchymotic lesions, however, demand definitive evaluation, since injuries to the pancreas and duodenum are easily missed (Cleveland & Waddell 1963, Bach & Frey 1971).

Intramural haematomas and lacerations of the duodenum are relatively easily recognized, the former by severe ecchymosis and induration of the duodenum on mobilization (Stone et al 1962, Janson & Stockinger 1975). The consequences of such injury may be difficult to evaluate if the time between injury and operation is short. If 4 or 5 hours have passed and there is no evidence of duodenal obstruction, intramural haematomas can be left intact. (Janson & Stockinger 1975). If preoperatively, obstruction is suggested by biliary drainage from the nasogastric tube or X-ray studies, the serosa should be opened through the main area of the induration and the submucosal haematoma evacuated (Janson & Stockinger 1975).

The pancreas is the most difficult of all abdominal organs to evaluate. In the dog, the pancreas can be pounded with a hammer, squeezed and macerated, its substance and capsule lacerated, yet no serious injury results as long as the main pancreatic duct remains intact (Kerry & Glas 1962). The human pancreas also appears to have sur-

prising resistance to injury. Conversely, a seemingly minor injury may result in disruption or obstruction of a brittle main pancreatic duct, resulting in leakage of pancreatic juice sometimes causing acute pancreatitis and if untreated, pancreatic pseudocysts, fistulas, ascites, abscesses, sepsis, or chronic pancreatitis (Wilson et al 1967, Fraser 1969, Bach & Frey 1971, Steele et al 1973, Grosfeld & Cooney 1975, Balasegaram & Lumpur 1976, Frey et al 1976, Heitsch et al 1976, Karl & Chandler 1977, Jones 1978, Stigall & Dorsey 1989).

For all practical purposes, if the major pancreatic ductal system is intact, the pancreatic injury, be it capsular tear, haematoma, or laceration is not significant. Any leakage of pancreatic fluid from a tributary duct will resolve spontaneously, usually in less than 4–6 weeks, if drainage is instituted. Haematomas of the pancreas and capsular injuries, if encountered at operation, should be drained. If the pancreatic ductal system is disrupted it is essential that the injury is recognized and treated appropriately to prevent mortality and serious morbidity.

A great clinical challenge is posed by the diagnosis of pancreatic injury in patients with minimal associated abdominal injuries or isolated pancreatic trauma. Classically, with injuries to the retroperitoneal pancreas or duodenum, abdominal discomfort may be out of proportion to the abdominal findings and the patient usually has abdominal tenderness and no bowel sounds. The protected position of the pancreas and duodenum does not result in peritoneal irritation as severe as that seen with more common intra-abdominal injuries, as the extravasated blood, gut contents and enzymes are initially contained retroperitoneally. Unless the surgeon has a high index of suspicion, these injuries may not be recognized immediately.

The typical blunt trauma resulting in pancreatic injury is a blow to the abdomen. Most commonly this is due to impalement of a driver of a motor vehicle on the steering wheel (Jones 1978, DeMars et al 1979, Snyder et al 1980, Nilsson et al 1986). History of such a severe blow to the upper abdomen should lead to the suspicion that pancreatic or duodenal injury may exist. In children, bicycle handlebar injuries or falls against an object are the most common cause of pancreatic and duodenal injuries other than being a passenger in an automobile involved in an accident (Martin et al 1968, Pollock 1974, Jones 1978, DeMars et al 1979, Pokorny et al 1986, Bass et al 1988). Tenderness in the region of these organs should suggest the possibility of pancreatic or duodenal injury.

In blunt trauma, the direction of the impinging force relative to the vertebral column is the key determinant of injury location. If the force is sufficient, fracture of the pancreas or duodenum may result, the steering wheel compressing the organ between the abdominal wall and the unyielding spinal column. The spinal column is like the hub of a wheel around which the pancreas is wrapped. If the patient has his left side between the steering wheel and vertebral column, the tail of the pancreas will be injured; if his right side is forward, then the head of the pancreas and duodenum are at risk; if he is struck in the mid-epigastric region, the neck of the pancreas may be divided over the mesenteric vessels. The major pancreatic duct is a more rigid, brittle structure than the vessels, the capsule, and pancreatic parenchyma. Often the duct is fractured in the absence of appreciable haemorrhage or capsular disruption, a fact which must be appreciated if significant injury is not to be overlooked at operation (Fig. 50.3). If the main duct is fractured, the injury is significant owing to the leakage of enzymes which will result from ductal obstruction and laceration, and owing to the sequelae which include pancreatic fistula, pseudocysts, and pancreatitis. If the main duct is intact, pancreatic injury is not significant. Extravasation of pancreatic secretion from tributary ducts or obstruction of tributary ducts causes self-limited fistula or pancreatitis.

The duodenum may be ruptured if compression of the abdominal wall by the impinging force traps its distal portion against the vertebral column while the pylorus is shut, so creating a closed loop while the duodenum is full of fluid (Cocke & Meyer 1964, DeMars et al 1979). This type of closed loop injury leads to extravasation of digestive enzymes into the retroperitoneum and the associated severe symptoms mean that it is usually suspected and diagnosed. However, when the duodenum is crushed against the vertebral column, the non-viable crushed wall can remain intact for hours, or even days, until it is digested by a combination of gastric juice and pancreatic enzymes. In such instances, initial abdominal findings may be minimal.

A less common problem is intramural haematoma of the duodenal lumen. The vomiting of bile or gastric juice following epigastric trauma should lead to the suspicion of the possibility of duodenal obstruction. (Janson & Stockinger 1975). This is particularly likely if there is very little associated abdominal distension. If there is a question of intramural duodenal haematoma, a gastrointestinal

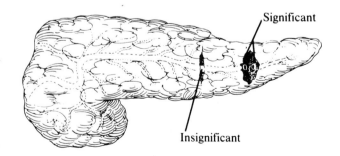

Fig. 50.3 Significant pancreatic ductal injury involves disruption of duct continuity whereas insignificant injury does not. (From Blaisdell & Trunkey 1982 Trauma Management. Thieme Medical Publishers, Inc, New York. Reprinted by permission.)

series, with soluble radio-opaque material demonstrating the characteristic inverted fir-tree sign due to swelling of the plicae of the duodenal mucosa, will lead to the diagnosis (Janson & Stockinger 1975).

Injury to the pancreas resulting from blunt trauma should be suspected when there is tenderness over its anatomical distribution. Pancreatic injury is often associated with ileus and very frequently the serum amylase and lipase are elevated. This does not provide any clues as to the magnitude of pancreatic injury and is not specific for the pancreas; any upper gastrointestinal enteric perforation may release pancreatic enzymes in the free peritoneal cavity and their absorption by the abdominal lymphatics will result in elevation of the serum enzymes. Mild trauma that is of no clinical significance may, on occasion, be associated with amylase elevations (Moretz et al 1975).

Patients with isolated duodenal or pancreatic compression injuries are often haemodynamically stable and sometimes may initially have no abnormal abdominal finding (Bach & Frey 1971, Snyder et al 1980). Diagnostic peritoneal lavage may well be normal (returns should also be checked for elevated amylase level) because of the retroperitoneal position of the pancreas and posterior aspect of the duodenum, or because a necrotic duodenal wall initially remains intact. In such patients, where there is no immediate indication for operation, the serum amylase or urine amylase is a very useful means of monitoring progress (Wilson et al 1967, Bach & Frey 1971, Babb & Harmon 1976). If the serum or urine amylase increases progressively, on the basis of serial determinations every 3–4 hours, or remains elevated, then the duodenum and pancreas should be examined at operation in the absence of other indications for laparotomy. If an initially elevated serum amylase declines and there is no other indication for operation, none should be undertaken. A single amylase determination should not be used as a basis for deciding whether a patient does or does not need an operation (Moretz et al 1975). In many patients with total disruption of the pancreatic ductal system, the serum amylase will not become elevated until 24–48 hours after injury (Bach & Frey 1971). Serum amylase levels may rise more with ductal injuries of the head and body than with injuries of the tail (Wilson et al 1967). This is understandable as serum amylase is a measure of ductal obstruction. The more proximal the fracture of the duct to the duodenum, the more gland there is secreting behind the obstruction or ductal disruption. The amylase behind an obstructed duct diffuses into the interstices of the gland and may be absorbed and returned to venous stream by the pancreatic capillaries and lymphatics, or if the secretions pour into the abdominal cavity, the amylase will be picked up by the abdominal lymphatics and returned to the venous circulation, raising serum amylase levels. Similarly, it is not surprising that the serum amylase may remain normal when the tail of the gland has been shot away. First, there is no proximal obstruction, so that pancreatic juice in the uninjured body and head continues to flow into the duodenum. Secondly, with the tail shot away, there are no viable acinar cells left to produce pancreatic secretions.

Radiological aids in evaluation

Computed tomography (CT) has proved valuable in the evaluation and diagnosis of abdominal injuries. It is particularly valuable in the diagnosis of hepatic, splenic and renal injuries with a reported sensitivity of approximately 95% for injuries to these organs. (Meredith & Trunkey 1988). However, it is less sensitive in the evaluation of pancreatic injuries. The combined results of series involving 502 patients undergoing abdominal CT scanning to evaluate trauma, revealed that 20 of 23 pancreatic injuries were correctly diagnosed, for a sensitivity of 87%, and nine patients incorrectly diagnosed as having pancreatic injury for a specificity of 98% (Jeffrey et al 1983, Cook et al 1986, Peitzman et al 1986). Of particular concern is that the three missed pancreatic injuries involved complete pancreatic transection, the most serious form of injury.

Findings on CT scan suggestive of pancreatic injury include changes in peripancreatic fat, particularly of the mesentery and peripancreatic fat, thickening of the anterior renal fascia, parenchymal disruption, and oedema surrounding the mesenteric vessels. Factors leading to falsely positive CT scans include unopacified bowel, fluid within the lesser sac, peripancreatic haematoma secondary to splenic or renal injury, and artefacts secondary to nasogastric tubes. To improve the accuracy of CT evaluation of the pancreas, maximum bowel opacification should be achieved, nasogastric tubes withdrawn to the distal oesophagus, patient motion minimized, and dynamic CT scanning employed with bolus i.v. contrast administration and 5 mm scan segments of the pancreas. Furthermore, repeat CT scanning 24–48 hours later may reveal CT evidence of pancreatic injury not seen on the original scans, as many of the CT findings of pancreatic trauma are caused by peripancreatic inflammation, which is minimal early after injury (Jeffrey et al 1983, Cook et al 1986, Peitzman et al 1986).

CT evaluation of the pancreas may be particularly poor in children and patients with a paucity of peripancreatic fat. In these cases, ultrasonography may be useful, although in general, it is inferior in evaluating traumatic pancreatic injury until the sequelae such as pancreatic pseudocyst, have developed (Jeffrey et al 1986, Gorenstein et al 1987, Van Steenbergen et al 1987).

While computed tomography and ultrasonography can play an important role in the evaluation of intra-abdominal and retroperitoneal traumatic injuries, the fact that their sensitivity in diagnosis is less than 100% must always be considered. The absence of radiographic evidence of injury should never delay abdominal exploration if the clinical course of the patients warrants exploration.

Endoscopic retrograde cholangiopancreatography (ERCP) has proved extremely valuable in the evaluation of pancreatic injury. The first report of its use in this context was by Vallon et al (1979) who evaluated 11 patients, with injuries preceding ERCP by 6 weeks to 15 years. ERCP was particularly valuable in defining the nature of ductal injury and in planning surgical correction in these patients with complications due to delayed recognition of ductal injury. Six of the 11 patients had undergone previous laparotomy with failure to diagnose or manage pancreatic ductal injuries adequately.

Subsequent reports have described the use of ERCP in similar settings (Belohlavek et al 1978, Taxier et al 1980, Bozymski et al 1981, Hall et al 1986). More recently, however, several authors have reported the use of ERCP immediately following trauma when pancreatic injury is suspected (LaRaja et al 1986, Barkin et al 1988, Hayward et al 1989, Whittwell et al 1989). Barkin et al (1988) reported 14 patients who were evaluated by peritoneal lavage, CT scanning and ERCP within 72 hours of injury. Two of the seven patients undergoing lavage had abnormal results; both were explored and neither had significant injuries. Of five patients with negative peritoneal lavage, two were found to have significant pancreatic injury at surgery, one with ductal rupture documented preoperatively by ERCP. Abdominal CT scanning correctly diagnosed all cases of parenchymal pancreatic injury but ductal abnormalities were missed in two of the three patients with CT scans interpreted as normal. ERCP successfully demonstrated all cases of ductal injury. No complications of ERCP were noted although one patient required repeat ERCP because of an inadequate initial study.

ERCP is at present the most sensitive non-operative method of evaluating pancreatic ductal trauma. Preoperative ERCP obviates the need for the time-consuming and often difficult operative cannulation of the papilla via duodenotomy, or the technically challenging cannulation of the small, non-dilated, distal duct via transection of the pancreatic tail. However, ERCP may be technically more difficult in trauma patients as many of them will be unable to assume the decubitus position so that the study has to be performed in the more difficult supine position. Approximately 1% of patients undergoing ERCP will develop post ERCP pancreatitis.

Other limitations of ERCP are that it gives no information about pancreatic parenchymal injuries. While less severe than injuries associated with ductal disruption, many of these injuries require operative debridement and drainage to prevent the formation of pancreatic abscess. ERCP alone cannot predict which patients with minor pancreatic injury can be managed non-operatively (Sugawa & Lucas 1988). Additionally, ERCP requires that the patient is haemodynamically stable and gives little information about other possible associated injuries. As many patients with pancreatic trauma have associated injuries and are haemodynamically unstable, only a minority are candidates for early ERCP.

LaRaja et al (1986) reported intraoperative use of ERCP to evaluate pancreatic ductal injury in a case of penetrating pancreatic trauma. Intraoperative ERCP may be useful where major pancreatic injury is suspected and associated injuries can be rapidly controlled, and the patient can be stabilized to a sufficient degree to allow its safe performance.

In summary, we feel that if pancreatic injury is suspected in a patient who is sufficiently stable, and there is no other immediate indication for laparotomy, the patient should undergo ERCP to ascertain whether pancreatic ductal rupture has occurred and if so, to define its anatomical location, prior to surgical repair. If no evidence of ductal injury is seen on ERCP, the patient may be managed selectively, with CT scanning delayed for 24–48 hours. Patients with evidence of pancreatic necrosis on CT scan should undergo exploration, debridement, and drainage of any pancreatic parenchymal injuries. Peripancreatic fluid collections seen on CT scanning may be followed with ultrasonography or CT, or may be drained percutaneously under radiological guidance. If ERCP is not available, all patients in whom pancreatic injury is suspected should undergo operative exploration without delay. Any patient with clinical deterioration or evidence of sepsis should undergo exploratory laparotomy regardless of the results of prior diagnostic studies. In the final analysis, the diagnosis of pancreatic injury rests on a high index of suspicion leading to laparotomy. Whether the injury is due to blunt or penetrating trauma, there is no substitute for careful exploration of the abdomen.

Table 50.4 Classification of pancreatic injury by various authors

Lucas (1977)	Class I Contusion, peripheral laceration, intact ductal system	Class II Distal laceration, transection, disruption suspected ductal disruption, no duodenal injury	Class III Proximal laceration, transection, disruption, no duodenal injury	Class IV Severe combined pancreaticoduodenal disruption
Smego et al (1985)	Grade I Contusion and/or small volume haematoma surrounding the pancreas with an intact capsule and no parenchymal disruption	Grade II Parenchymal lacerations without major duct injury	Grade III Ductal laceration, >50% thickness gland disruption	Grade IV Severe crush injury
Moore et al (1981)	Grade I Tangential injury	Grade II Through and through injury with intact ductal system	Grade III Major debridement or distal duct injury	Grade IV Proximal duct injury	Grade V Injuries requiring pancreatico-duodenectomy
Jurkovich & Carrico (1990)	Type I Contusion, haematoma, peripheral laceration	Type II Distal transection, distal injury with duct disruption	Type III Proximal transection or injury with probable duct disruption	Type IV Combined severe pancreaticoduodenal injury	
Booth & Flint (1990)	Class I Simple contusion (superficial) with minimal parenchymal injury. No haematoma or capsule disruption and no question of ductal involvement. Small haematoma permissible	Class II More extensive contusion. Capsule disruption lacerations of the parenchyma <50% thickness. No visible evidence of ductal disruption.	Class III Documented or strong clinical evidence of ductal disruption. (1) complete transection of pancreas, (2) laceration >75% of gland thickness, (3) central gland perforation, (4) region of severe maceration	Class IV Severe crush injury with areas of devitalized tissue, frequently with duodenal involvement	
Frey & Araida (1991)	Category I Haematoma, contusion, or capsular tear	Category II Injury associated with fracture or disruption of the major duct in the body or tail of pancreas	Category III Disruption of the major pancreatic duct in the head of the pancreas	Category IV Disruption of the major duct in the head of the pancreas associated with injury to the duodenum and/or common bile duct	

CLASSIFICATION OF PANCREATIC INJURIES

Direct comparison of morbidity and mortality rates of pancreatic and combined pancreaticoduodenal injuries between institutions has been complicated by a lack of uniform classification of injury severity. Numerous authors have suggested various classification schemes for pancreatic, duodenal, and combined pancreaticoduodenal trauma and some of these are listed in Tables 50.4 and 50.5. As can be seen, the classifications vary considerably in complexity and completeness. Such classification schemes centre around key features of pancreatic and duodenal injury, including ductal injury and its location, associated common bile duct or ampullary injury, degree of duodenal disruption, delay in surgical treatment and presence of severe combined pancreaticoduodenal injury.

The morbidity and mortality associated with combined pancreaticoduodenal injuries is not additive of those associated with isolated pancreatic or duodenal injuries. The intimate anatomical relationships of the duodenum and pancreas, their shared blood supply and the joined pancreatic and biliary ductal drainage system, suggest that an integrated classification scheme should be adopted. Such a system would be useful not only for comparison of

treatment methods but may also assist in the assessment and management by providing a systematic means of defining treatment priorities.

The classification system we propose is described in Table 50.6. Minor injuries to the pancreas include capsular damage, and minor injuries to the substance of the gland with its associated minor bleeding. Minor duodenal injuries include contusion, haematoma, and injuries which do not result in contamination by luminal contents. Moderately severe injuries to the pancreas consist of injuries where ductal disruption involves the pancreas to the left of the superior mesenteric vessels. Moderate duodenal injuries include those with full thickness injuries with contamination by luminal contents. Severe pancreatic injuries consist of those with major pancreatic ductal injury to the right of the superior mesenteric vessels or which involve the intrapancreatic common bile duct. Severe duodenal injuries include those with >75% circumferential disruption or full thickness injury with associated extrapancreatic common bile duct injury.

Combined pancreaticoduodenal injuries are graded by increasing severity of combinations of the pancreatic or duodenal injuries. The severity of each injury can be

Table 50.5 Classification of duodenal and combined pancreaticoduodenal injuries by various authors

Lucas (1977)	Class I Serosal tear, contusion or intramural haematoma, no pancreatic injury	Class II Complete perforation; no pancreatic injury	Class III Duodenal contusion or perforation; pancreatic contusion, or small peripheral laceration	Class IV Combined pancreaticoduodenal disruption (severe)	
Jurkovich & Carrico (1990)	Type I Seromuscular tear, haematoma (intramural), contusion	Type II Full thickness laceration	Type III Any duodenal injury combined with a Type I pancreatic injury	Type IV Severe combined pancreaticoduodenal injury	
Frey & Araida (1991)	Category I Duodenal haematoma or contusion	Category II Full thickness, duodenal penetration	Category III Major duodenal injury >75% circumferential defect	Category IV Major duodenal injury involving the common bile duct, with/without major pancreatic duct injury	

Combined pancreaticoduodenal injuries

Moore & Moore (1984)	Grade I Partial thickness injuries of both pancreas and duodenum with minimal tissue damage, and without pancreaticoduodenal injury	Grade II Full thickness defects of either pancreas or duodenum amenable to repair or resection	Grade III Full thickness disruption of both pancreas and duodenum amenable to resection or repair	Grade IV Grade II or III with one or more of the following: (1) major pancreatic duct injury that was not resected, (2) duodenal injury to the 1st or 2nd portion >75% circumference, (3) associated common bile duct injury, (4) >24 hours delay from injury to operation	
Mansour et al (1989)	Grade I Partial thickness, duodenal injury, injury to pancreas without ductal injury	Grade II Full thickness duodenal injury, injury to pancreas without ductal injury	Grade III Full thickness duodenal injury, pancreatic ductal injury in body or tail	Grade IV Grade III injury with proximal pancreatic duct injury, duodenal injury involving the second portion of duodenum, duodenal defect >75% circumference, common bile duct injury or >24 hours delay from injury to operation	Grade V Massive devascularizing injury to the pancreatic head and duodenum

Table 50.6 Classification of pancreatic injury proposed by Frey and Wardell

Pancreatic injury
Class I   Capsule damage, minor gland substance damage (P$_1$)
Class II   Body or tail pancreatic duct transection, partial or complete (P$_2$)
Class III   Major duct injury involving the head of the pancreas or intrapancreatic common bile duct (P$_3$)

Duodenal injury
Class I   Contusion, haematoma, or partial thickness injury (D$_1$)
Class II   Full thickness duodenal injury (D$_2$)
Class III   Full thickness duodenal injury with greater than 75% circumference injury; or full thickness duodenal injury with injury to the extrapancreatic common bile duct (D$_3$)

Combined pancreaticoduodenal injuries
Type I   P$_1$ D$_1$, P$_2$D$_1$ or D$_2$ P$_1$
Type II   D$_2$P$_2$
Type III   D$_3$ P$_{1-2}$ or P$_3$ D$_{1-2}$
Type IV   D$_3$P$_3$

Note
If surgery is delayed >24 hours after injury, classification should be subclassified as delayed (D) for purposes of comparison of equivalent injuries and expected higher incidence of morbidity and mortality

increased by the designation (D) if surgical treatment is delayed beyond 24 hours.

PRINCIPLES OF MANAGEMENT OF PANCREATIC AND COMBINED PANCREATICODUODENAL INJURIES

Rationale for choice of operation

The aim of operation in duodenal and pancreatic trauma, which may occur independently, together, or in association with common duct injury, should be reconstitution of enteric and ductal integrity and preservation of function. However, the first priority must be to save life and, in a haemodynamically unstable patient with severe associated injuries to major vessels, definitive therapy of the pancreatic or duodenal injury may have to be delayed in order to shorten operating time.

Some useful concepts in the management of pancreatic trauma are as follows:

1. At operation, the diagnosis and management of pancreatic and duodenal injuries should be deferred in patients with multiple injuries until haemorrhage from major vessels and damaged viscera has been controlled. This recommendation is based on the knowledge that the single most frequent cause of death in pancreatic and duodenal injury is haemorrhage and shock from associated injuries (Table 50.3). Most of these deaths occur within 48 hours of injury (Halgrimson et al 1969, Anderson et al 1973, Chambers et al 1975, Balasegarem & Lumpur 1976, Heyse-Moore 1976, Graham et al 1979, Sims et al 1984, Ivatury et al 1985, Smego et al 1985, Sorenson et al 1986, Feliciano et al 1987).

2. Definitive management of isolated pancreatic injuries requires recognition of ductal injury and, in general, either resection of the distal segment if this is less than 50–60% of the gland, or drainage of the distal segment if it exceeds 60–70% of the gland by means of a Roux-en-Y limb of jejunum. The pancreaticojejunostomy should be an end-to-side mucosa to mucosa anastomosis (Cattell 1948). While most patients do not become diabetic unless 80% or more of the gland is resected, an occasional patient may do so with what is judged to be a smaller resection (Frey et al 1976). One has no way of knowing whether these patients were prediabetic, but it seems prudent, particularly in the young, to allow some margin of error for the surgeon's estimate of what constitutes an 80% resection in a particular gland. When a gland lacks an uncinate process there is a marked decrease in the volume of the head of the pancreas. The surgeon may not recognize this congenital variation and assume that resection through the neck is removing 60–65% of the gland when it is more likely that 70–80% is being removed.

While definitive treatment of the pancreatic injury is an important goal, the first priority is to save the patient's life and in the event that the patient's condition is precarious and operative time needs to be minimized, pancreatic ductal disruption can be managed by sump drainage (Jordan et al 1969, Sturm et al 1973, Jones 1978). Creation of a controlled fistula will prevent collections forming which might culminate in pseudocyst or abscess formation.

3. Most duodenal injuries (85%) can be managed by debridement and simple closure (Stone et al 1962, Snyder et al 1980, Kashuk et al 1982, Martin et al 1983). However, the few patients with 75% circumferential crush injuries, large lacerations with loss of tissue, or devascularization of a large segment of duodenum require an operative solution tailored to the anatomy of the injury (Snyder et al 1980). No one form of repair is suitable for all duodenal injuries and the trauma surgeon must be familiar with the various options available, as will be discussed (Stone et al 1962, Morton & Jordan 1968, Corley et al 1975, DeMars et al 1979, Snyder et al 1980).

4. If the common duct and duodenum have been damaged in association with a pancreatic ductal disruption, there is the potential for major morbidity from the devastation created by uncontrolled loss of gastric, duodenal, pancreatic, and biliary secretions, which may lead to fluid and electrolyte disorders, dehydration, digestion of skin, intra-abdominal collections, abscesses and sepsis. Therefore, it is desirable that intestinal and ductal integrity are established by pancreaticoduodenectomy. If the patient is judged to be unable to tolerate pancreaticoduodenectomy (Freeak et al 1965, Salyer & McClelland 1967, Brawley et al 1968, Halgrimson et al 1969, Gibbs et al 1970, Bach & Frey 1971, Nance & DeLoach 1971, Anderson et al 1973, Owens & Wolfman 1973, Lowe et al 1977, Jones 1978, Whalen et al 1987, Wisner et al 1990), then diversionary drainage separating the secretions should be implemented.

INJURIES LIMITED TO THE PANCREAS

Class I injuries

Minor pancreatic contusions and capsular lacerations account for 60% of all pancreatic injuries and minor parenchymal lacerations without ductal injury account for a further 20% of all pancreatic injuries (Jurkovich & Carrico 1990).

Management of these Class I injuries should be directed at obtaining haemostasis, debridement of devitalized tissue, and adequate drainage. No attempt should be made to repair capsular injury, as closure of the capsule over minor ductal injuries may result in pseudocyst formation. Minor ductal injuries, if adequately drained, will form controlled pancreatic fistulae, the majority of which will close spontaneously over a period of days. Care must be taken when suturing parenchymal injuries to limit the depth of the suturing to prevent iatrogenic major pancreatic duct injury or ligation. Such injuries may result in pancreatic fistula, pseudocyst, or chronic pancreatitis.

Drainage can be accomplished by a number of means. Soft silastic sump drains provide reliable drainage and minimize the risk of drain erosion. Closed suction drains minimize contamination, but may fail to drain extensive injuries adequately, allowing pancreatic autodigestion to occur and particulate matter to accumulate. Penrose drains, used extensively at our institution, can provide adequate drainage, but must be positioned dependently (preferably through the flank below the twelfth rib) and brought through the abdominal wall through a generous 5–8 cm incision for adequate drainage to occur. The pancreatic drainage can be collected with a colostomy appliance to allow accurate quantification, minimize skin excoriation and reduce the likelihood of external contamination. Postoperative drain management is discussed later in this chapter.

Class II injuries

The junction of the neck and body of the pancreas is the most common site of injury (Fig. 50.2). The portion of pancreas distal to the neck constitutes about 60–65% of the mass of the pancreas and can be resected with little immediate or late morbidity from pancreatic exocrine or endocrine insufficiency (Fig. 50.4) (Wittingen & Frey 1974, Frey et al 1976). Distal pancreatic resection is therefore the treatment of choice for any injury involving the neck, body, or tail of the pancreas (Fig. 50.5).

The pancreas is most often resected with the spleen. Short gastric vessels are divided and the attachments between the splenic flexure of the colon and the spleen are severed. The spleen and tail of the pancreas are mobilized and rotated to the right, the splenic artery is divided as it joins the body of the pancreas, and the pancreas is transected at the point of the laceration. Interrupted, interlocking mattress sutures of 2:0 silk on an atraumatic needle has been our standard method of closing the cut end of the pancreas. However, stapling, using the larger 4.5 mm staples, has also been effective in our experience. The main pancreatic duct, if identified, is ligated separately. If the patient is unstable, time should not be spent searching for the main duct which is only 1–2 mm in diameter in the normal pancreas. In isolated injuries of the body and tail, it is usually possible to preserve the spleen by ligating and dividing the branches of the splenic vein and artery to the tail of the pancreas. The importance of the spleen in immunity and prevention of the overwhelming postsplenectomy sepsis syndrome, particularly in children, is now well recognized (Scher et al 1985). Resection of the tail of the pancreas with splenic preservation in trauma (Robey et al 1982) is usually more easily accomplished than when it is performed for chronic pancreatitis. Pachter et al (1989) reported that it was possible to preserve the spleen in nine consecutive patients with pancreatic injuries requiring distal pancreatectomy. Over an 8-year-period we have been able to preserve the spleen in 44% of 32 patients undergoing distal pancreatectomy; of the 18 patients undergoing distal pancrea-

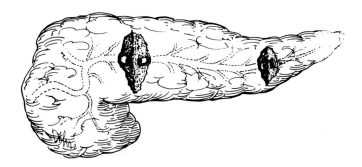

Fig. 50.4 Lesions readily amenable to treatment by distal pancreatic resection. (From Blaisdell & Trunkey 1982 Trauma management. Thieme Medical Publishers, Inc, New York. Reprinted by permission.)

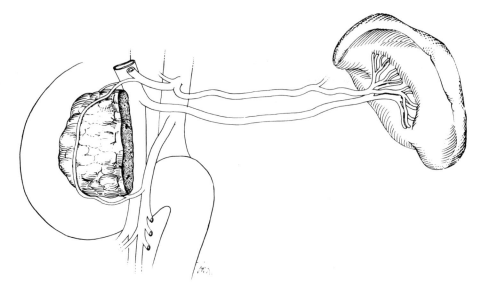

Fig. 50.5 An example of extensive (80%) distal pancreatic resection with preservation of the spleen and its blood supply. Preservation of the splenic vein is critical; as the dissection can be difficult, splenic preservation is indicated only in good-risk patients with isolated pancreatic injury. (From Blaisdell & Trunkey 1982 Trauma management. Thieme Medical Publishers, Inc, New York. Reprinted by permission.)

tectomy and splenectomy, eight had major injuries to the spleen itself (Wisner et al 1990).

However, it should be kept in mind that in adult trauma patients, concern over postsplenectomy sepsis does not justify preserving the spleen if the patient is haemodynamically unstable, requires blood transfusions in attempts to preserve the spleen, or has major associated injuries (Luna & Dellinger 1987). Beal & Spisso (1988) calculated that hepatitis from blood transfusion would result in 87 deaths out of 31 000 patients transfused, vs. eight deaths from postsplenectomy sepsis out of 31 000 patients undergoing splenectomy.

Class III injuries

In injuries involving the main pancreatic duct in the head of the gland, 80–95% distal pancreatectomy can be carried out. However, because of the high incidence of pancreatic endocrine and exocrine insufficiency, 80–95% resection should be avoided unless the patient is unstable, already diabetic, and when a longer operation might jeopardize survival. For the proximal pancreatic ductal fractures, the preferred option is to oversew the proximal severed end of pancreas with interlocking mattress sutures of 2:0 silk and then to anastomose the distal pancreas end-to-side into a Roux-en-Y limb of jejunum using a mucosa-to-mucosa anastomosis (Fig. 50.6). We do not recommend placing a Roux-en-Y limb blindly over fresh lacerations and stellate fractures in lieu of a duct-to-jejunal mucosal anastomosis nor do we recommend trying to drain the proximal portion of the pancreas into the

Roux-en-Y limb as well as the distal segment in a T-type anastomosis. Draining the proximal pancreas with a Roux-en-Y limb is unnecessary and may compromise the

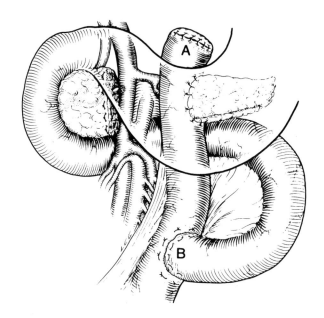

Fig. 50.6 The proximal severed end of the pancreas is oversewn with interlocking mattress sutures of 2:0 silk in addition to individual ligation of the main pancreatic duct. Alternatively, a stapling device may be used to achieve the same end. A Roux-en-Y jejunal limb should not be placed blindly over fresh lacerations and stellate lesions in lieu of a duct-to-jejunal anastomosis. (From Frey F, Bodai B, The surgical management of pancreaticoduodenal trauma. In: Rob & Smith's Operative surgery: Alimentary tract and abdominal wall, 4th edn, by permission of the publishers, Butterworth & Co (Publishers) Ltd. ©.)

anatomosis of the distal segment of pancreas to the Roux-en-Y limb. There is the additional risk of gastrointestinal contamination from two suture lines rather than one. If the duodenum and common bile duct are intact, pancreaticoduodenectomy is not indicated for injury to the main pancreatic duct in the head of the gland. Very occasionally, in the patient in whom there has been minimal trauma to the adjacent pancreatic tissue, primary repair of the fractured duct may be considered (Freeark et al 1965, Martin et al 1968).

ISOLATED DUODENAL INJURIES IN THE ABSENCE OF INJURY TO THE PANCREAS OR COMMON BILE DUCT

The site and presence of duodenal injury may be identified at operation by tracing the missile track or noting the site of active bleeding or haematoma, or by bile staining or crepitation of surrounding tissues. Blunt injuries are more often extensive than those due to penetrating trauma (46% vs. 7%), extensive being defined as involvement of more than 75% of the circumference of the duodenal wall (Snyder et al 1980) (Fig. 50.7). Fortunately, in most patients with penetrating duodenal injury which is not extensive, local debridement and duodenal closure in two layers will suffice (Stone et al 1962, Snyder et al 1980). Closure of the duodenum should be performed without tension. This may be accomplished by closing the duodenum transversely or in a vertical direction (Kraus & Gordon 1974). The mortality associated with duodenotomy is high but is attributable to the condition that prompted duodenotomy (Hutchinson 1971). In larger defects, application of a serosal patch may be helpful.

There is controversy over whether tube duodenostomy or gastrostomy is beneficial in these injuries (Stone et al 1962, Lucas & Ledgerwood 1975, Snyder et al 1980). Neither Kashuk et al (1982) nor Martin et al (1983) employ tube duodenostomy, and Kashuk et al support the use of feeding jejunostomy.

More extensive duodenal wounds require segmental resection or Roux-en-Y duodenojejunostomy (Fig. 50.8). Segmental resection and end-to-end anastomosis with standard two layer closure is indicated in circumferential crush injuries. This can be accomplished in all parts of the duodenum. To avoid injury to the common duct and ampulla, the distal bile duct can be intubated with a Bakes dilator which is passed into the duodenum and kept there during the resection and anastomosis. If a large segment of duodenum has been devitalized and segmental resection performed, it may not be possible to mobilize enough duodenum for end-to-end duodenostomy. This problem, particularly if the duodenal injury is distal to the ampulla, lends itself to Roux-en-Y duodenojejunostomy (Fig. 50.9). The jejunum is divided 20 cm distal to the ligament of Treitz, and the distal limb is

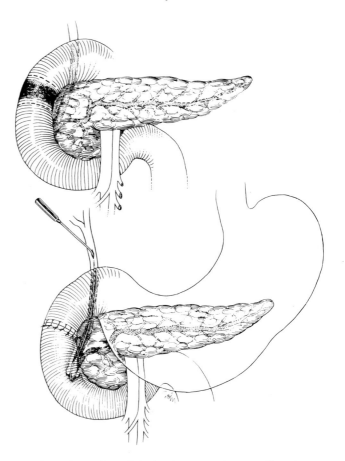

Fig. 50.7 Lacerations of the duodenum may be treated by primary suture or by resection and reanastomosis, if there is segmental circumferential injury. (From Blaisdell & Trunkey 1982 Trauma management. Thieme Medical Publishers, Inc, New York. Reprinted by permission.)

advanced and anastomosed end-to-side to the proximal duodenum. The proximal jejunum is anastomosed end-to-side 30 cm distal to the duodenojejunostomy. The distal duodenum can be oversewn.

Side-to-end duodenojejunostomy has limited applicability except for injuries of the third part of the duodenum along its antimesenteric border (see Fig. 50.9). Occasionally patching of the duodenum by Roux-en-Y duodenojejunostomy in useful.

Diverticulization procedure

Patients having more than one duodenal perforation, loss of more than 75% of the duodenal circumference which could compromise the lumen, injury from a high velocity missile, delay in operation leading to peritonitis, oedema, and infection, or compromise of the blood supply may benefit from the diverticulization procedure. This procedure converts a lateral fistula, should it develop, into an end fistula (Fig. 50.10). As described by Berne et al (1968) the procedure included a gastrojejunostomy and

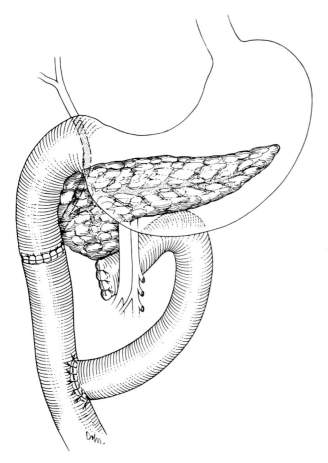

Fig. 50.8   Distal duodenal injuries may be treated by resection and duodenal-jejunal anastomosis. (From Blaisdell & Trunkey 1982 Trauma management. Thieme Medical Publishers, Inc, New York. Reprinted by permission.)

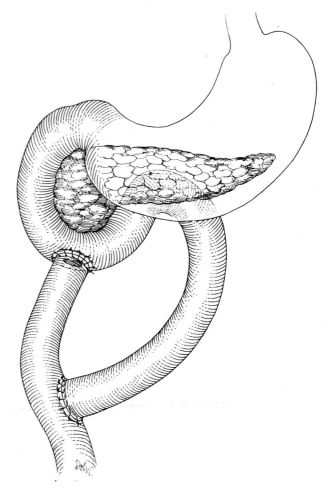

Fig. 50.9   In rare instances, localized injuries may be treated by jejunal patch or Roux-en-Y duodenal anastomosis as shown here. (From Blaisdell & Trunkey 1982 Trauma management. Thieme Medical Publishers, Inc, New York. Reprinted by permission.)

tube duodenostomy, T-tube biliary drainage, and oversewing the duodenal lacerations. Mortality associated with its use was reported to be 16% (Berne et al 1974). The modified diverticulization or pylorus exclusion procedure described by Graham et al (1979) is now widely used. The stomach is opened at the site for a gastro-jejunostomy and the pylorus oversewn through the opening (Fig. 50.10). Mortality associated with the Graham diverticulization in severely injured patients in recent reports ranges from 4 to 15% (Kashuk et al 1982, Martin et al 1983).

We do not recommend diverticulization in patients having associated disruption of the duct of Wirsung in the head of the pancreas, and/or transection of the common bile duct, unless it is accompanied by other operative manoeuvres to deal with the divided bile duct or pancreatic duct. These problems are not addressed by diverticulization. There is no substitute for pancreaticoduodenectomy in patients with combined injures of the main pancreatic duct, common bile duct, and duodenum.

COMBINED PANCREATICODUODENAL INJURIES

Except under unusual circumstances, neither 80–95% distal pancreatectomy nor pancreaticoduodenectomy is indicated.

Segmental resection and end-to-end repair of the duodenum is often possible even in the second portion of the duodenum close to the papilla of Vater. A Fogarty irrigation catheter may be employed to intubate the papilla through the duodenal wound and obtain an on-table pancreaticogram to ascertain the integrity of the pancreatic duct. If the duct is injured in the head of the gland, a Roux-en-Y jejunal limb may be used to drain the distal pancreas. The proximal end of the pancreas is oversewn (Fig. 50.11).

When the duodenum is extensively lacerated, but repair is still possible, though tenuous, and the pancreatic duct is transected in the head of the pancreas, the surgeon

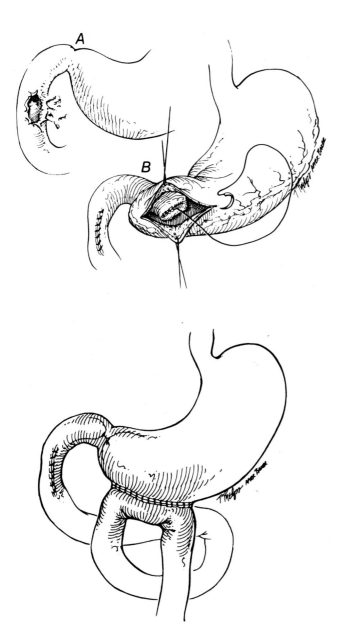

Fig. 50.10 Graham and Mattox technique for management of major duodenal injury. (From Frey F, Bodai B, The surgical management of pancreaticoduodenal trauma. In: Rob & Smith's Operative surgery: Alimentary tract and abdominal wall, 4th edn, by permission of the publishers, Butterworth & Co (Publishers) Ltd. ©.)

is faced with a dilemma. There is no truly ideal operation that deals with both a major duodenal injury and major pancreatic duct injury. The surgeon must weigh the risk of a less extensive procedure, such as duodenal exclusion or diverticulization (which does not adequately deal with the major pancreatic duct fracture as Jones (1978) has noted) against that of pancreaticoduodenectomy, which does deal with the problem but has the disadvantage of requiring a biliary anastomosis when none is required by the injury.

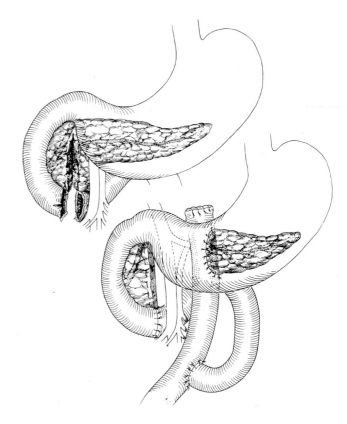

Fig. 50.11 Combined duodenal pancreatic distal injury is treated by resection of the body of the gland, repairing the duodenum and draining the distal pancreas into a Roux-en-Y jejunal limb. (From Blaisdell & Trunkey 1982 Trauma management. Thieme Medical Publishers, Inc, New York. Reprinted by permission.)

Duodenal diverticulization as described by Berne et al (1968) is effective in the management of duodenal laceration, as it diverts gastric and biliary secretions from the duodenum. Likewise, temporary pyloric exclusion, as described by Graham and colleagues (1978), which includes closing the pylorus with absorbable suture is an effective method for dealing with major duodenal injury. However, neither of these operations allows management of associated major ductal injury of the pancreas except by Penrose or sump drainage. Therefore, we remain sceptical about whether pyloric exclusion or diverticulization of the duodenum has a major role in the management of a combined major duodenal injury and major pancreatic duct fracture; neither operation addresses the problem of major pancreatic ductal disruption.

Injuries in which the major pancreatic duct remains intact are not associated with serious sequelae, and should not be considered significant. Patients whose duodenal wound was treated definitively but in whom injury to the major pancreatic duct was treated by suction, may require reoperation if the fistula from the distal pancreas has not closed within 3–4 months.

COMBINED DUODENAL AND BILIARY TRACT INJURIES

These serious injuries fortunately comprise only about 5% of all duodenal injuries (Martin et al 1983). In patients with injury to the duodenum and common duct, it may be possible to perform duodenal closure and end-to-side choledochojejunostomy using a Roux-en-Y limb of jejunum, after injury to the major pancreatic duct has been ruled out by retrograde pancreaticogram (Fig. 50.12). Rarely, avulsion of the papilla occurs in association with duodenal injury. This injury has also been treated by closure of the duodenum, and anastomosis of the papilla of Vater end-to-side to a Roux-en-Y jejunal limb. However, combined duodenal and biliary tract injuries usually requires pancreaticoduodenectomy if the duodenal injury is major (Fish & Johnson 1965, Lee et al 1976) and is justified in patients with this serious injury. Pancreaticoduodenectomy for trauma carries a 30% mortality, but with other forms of treatment, the mortality is closer to 100% (Kerry & Glas 1962, Thompson & Hinshow 1966, Yeo & McNamara 1973, Lowe et al 1977,

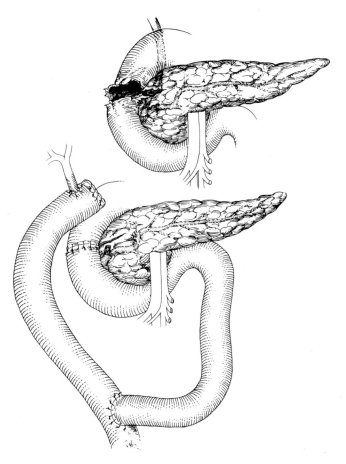

Fig. 50.12 Combined duodenal and biliary injury can be treated by duodenal repair and choledochojejunostomy using a Roux-en-Y limb. (From Blaisdell & Trunkey 1982 Trauma management. Thieme Medical Publishers, Inc, New York. Reprinted by permission.)

Jones 1978, Wisner et al 1990). The common duct is usually of normal calibre and not as easy to anastomose to a loop of bowel as is the obstructed duct associated with pancreatic tumour or chronic pancreatitis. Cholecysto-jejunostomy, ligation of the injured common bile duct below the cystic duct, and diverticulization is an option in these circumstances. Unfortunately, this cholecysto-jejunostomy has a failure rate approaching 40% at 1 year when performed for conditions such as chronic pancreatitis and there is no reason to believe the failure rate would be different when performed for trauma (Yellin & Rossoff 1975, Aranha et al 1984). Therefore, it should only be considered in patients who are too unstable for pancreaticoduodenectomy. Pancreaticoduodenectomy should be carried out when indicated and whenever the patient's condition permits. While the antrum and pylorus of the stomach is frequently resected in pancreaticoduodenectomy for cancer, it is not necessary in trauma (Traverso & Longmire 1978).

As much common duct as possible should be preserved by carrying its dissection behind the duodenum before dividing it. The pancreatic head is mobilized carefully from the portal vein and the gastroduodenal artery is ligated as it passes under the duodenum. The uncinate process can then be mobilized from the mesenteric vessels after the mesocolon has been retracted downward and separated from the body of the pancreas; it is then divided at the site of the fracture. During dissection of the uncinate, careful attention must be paid to the possibility that the right hepatic, accessory hepatic, or common hepatic artery arises from the superior mesenteric artery and traverses the uncinate process. The splenic vein is preserved at its junction with the superior mesenteric vein. In freeing the distal segment of pancreas from the splenic vein, numerous small veins entering the pancreas directly from the splenic vein need to be divided and ligated. After removal of the head and uncinate, the distal end of the pancreas is anastomosed end-to-side to the Roux-en-Y jejunal limb (duct-to-jejunal mucosa-serosa) with 4 : 0 or 5 : 0 prolene sutures. An end-to-side anastomosis between the common duct and the jejunal limb can then be performed some 10–15 cm distal to the pancreatic anastomosis, using a precise two-layered anastomosis; 20–30 cm further distally, an end-to-side gastrojejunostomy or pylorojejunostomy is carried out (Fig. 50.13).

COMBINED DUODENAL, COMMON BILE DUCT, AND MAJOR PANCREATIC DUCTAL INJURIES

Combined duodenal, common bile duct, and major pancreatic ductal injuries of the head of the pancreas (Fig. 50.14) are fatal if treated by drainage alone and are best managed by pancreaticoduodenectomy as recommended by Kerry & Glas (1962) and others (Baker et al 1963, Freeark et al 1965, Freeark et al 1966, Thompson &

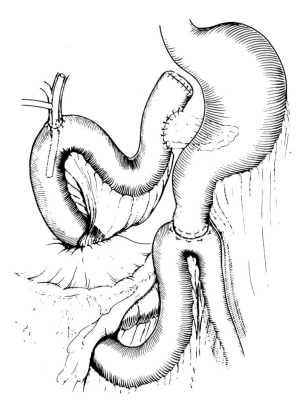

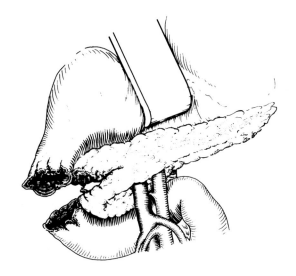

Fig. 50.14 An injury to the duodenum, the common bile duct, and the major pancreatic duct is illustrated. Such injuries are fatal if treated by drainage alone and are best managed by pancreaticoduodenectomy. Pancreaticoduodenectomy following trauma is associated with a mortality rate of 30%. (From Frey F, Budai B, The surgical management of pancreaticoduodenal trauma. In: Rub & Smith's operative surgery: Alimentary tract and abdominal wall, 4th edn, by permission of the publishers, Butterworth & Co (Publishers) Ltd ©.)

Fig. 50.13 If the distal common duct has been injured there may be insufficient space to insert a T-tube between the anastomosis and the junction of the left and right hepatic ducts. In such instances, a Robinson catheter with extra holes placed within it may be inserted retrograde through the anastomosis from the jejunal limb. Finally, an antecolic two-layer duodenojejunostomy consisting of an inner continuous layer of 3 : 0 polyglactin 910 and an outer layer of inverting Lembert sutures of 3 : 0 silk completes the reconstruction. We do not use drains in the region of the pancreaticojejunostomy. A Penrose drain is placed near the choledochojejunostomy. This is brought out through a separate stab incision, as is the T-tube or Robinson catheter from the common bile duct.

McFarland 1969, Halgrimson et al 1969, Salyer & McClelland 1967, Gibbs et al 1970, Bach & Frey 1971, Nance & DeLoach 1971, Anderson et al 1973, Lowe et al 1977, Jones 1978, Kashuk et al 1982, Martin et al 1983, Oreskovich & Carrico 1984, Feliciano et al 1987). The role of pancreaticoduodenectomy in trauma to the pancreatic head and duodenum continues to be controversial largely because the precise nature of the injury to the pancreatic head is often uncertain i.e. it is not known whether the main pancreatic duct is intact, severed, or partially disrupted (Jones 1985, Feliciano et al 1987, Ivatury et al 1990). One would expect quite different outcomes and complications depending on the nature of the ductal injury and its treatment. Some reports do not mention whether the common bile duct was also injured in patients subjected to pancreaticoduodenectomy. Mortality associated with pancreaticoduodenectomy is attributable to the nature of the injury, the condition of the patient, and the skill of the operator, and one centre has reported no deaths in 10 consecutive patients undergoing pancreaticoduodenectomy for this combined injury (Oreskovich & Carrico 1984).

The most severe combined injuries are also associated with severe injuries to the liver and major vessels, and it may be necessary to resort to a series of exteriorization procedures until the patient is stable enough to restore ductal and enteric continuity (Owens & Wolfman 1973, Wynn et al 1985).

POSTOPERATIVE CARE

In patients with pancreatic injuries, the gastrointestinal tract is kept at rest until the ileus has subsided. For major pancreatic injuries, we maintain nasogastric suction to avoid acid entering the duodenum with the resulting call to bicarbonate secretion by the pancreas. For duodenal injuries we also keep the gastrointestinal tract decompressed by nasogastric tube and maintain an infusion of intravenous fluids. If there is any evidence of complications, as manifest by severe ileus or infection, intravenous hyperalimentation is initiated on the 4th or 5th postoperative day. If duodenal diverticulization or pancreaticoduodenectomy has been performed, hyperalimentation may be started as soon as the patient is haemodynamically stable.

If, at the time of original surgery, a feeding jejunostomy tube has been inserted, tube feeding can be instituted after resolution of ileus. If the initial tube feedings are well tolerated, the volume and concentration of the feed can be increased until caloric needs are met by this means. In cases of pancreatic injury, it may be preferable to use a low-fat, higher pH feed than normal to minimize pancreatic stimulation and lower the volume and enzyme concentration of pancreatic secretions (Cogbill et al 1982, Kellum et al 1988). If attempts at tube feeding are unsuccessful, intravenous hyperalimentation should not be delayed, as maintenance of adequate nutrition is essential for recovery.

If after 5–7 days the patient is well, nasogastric suction is discontinued and oral intake is commenced cautiously. When oral intake is adequate and reliably maintained, tube feeding or intravenous alimentation can be discontinued.

The possibility of infection should be anticipated, particularly in penetrating injuries. Preoperative prophylactic antibiotics are administered routinely and it is our practice to give gentamicin or ceftizoxime and metronidazole preoperatively and continue the course for 2–5 days according to the patient's postoperative course.

Timing of drain removal is dictated by the clinical course and the volume and composition of drainage. If drainage has ceased by the 4th or 5th day or none has developed, the drains can be removed. In general, drains should not be removed until the volume recovered is less than 25–50 ml/day and the clinical course is stable. Drainage amylase levels should be measured and some have used them as a guide to withdrawal of the drains. However, we found that drain amylase concentrations of less than 100 000 units/l at 1 week gave little guide to the development of postoperative complications, e.g., persistence of drainage (fistula) pseudocyst or abscess formation (Wisner et al 1990). However, in three patients with drain amylase values greater than 100 000 units/l, complications (fistula or abscess) developed. Although our experience in patients with drain amylase values of this magnitude is small, we recommend caution in withdrawing drains in such a situation. Persistent drainage of greater than 25–50 ml/day or drainage amylase levels over 100 000 units/l 1 week post injury should prompt further investigation with abdominal CT scanning with vascular enhancement or, preferably, if the patient's clinical condition permits, ERCP, to exclude pancreatic ductal injury or necrosis. High drain output may be secondary to traumatic lymphatic disruption and in the absence of significant pancreatic injury will be self-limited. Persistently high pancreatic drainage without major ductal injury on ERCP can be managed by bowel rest, total parenteral nutrition, H_2 antagonists and somatostatin analogues (Prinz et al 1988). The majority of these pancreatic fistulae will close spontaneously within 4–6 weeks and drains are left in place during this time.

PAEDIATRIC PANCREATIC TRAUMA

Blunt trauma is the cause of 90% of intra-abdominal injuries in children. The pancreas is the fourth most commonly injured intra-abdominal organ in trauma in this age group after the spleen, kidney, and liver (Salonen & Aarnio 1985). Currently CT scanning is the diagnostic test of choice in evaluating blunt paediatric abdominal trauma (Kuhn & Berger 1981). CT scanning has the advantages of allowing relatively quick, non-invasive assessment of intra-abdominal and retroperitoneal organs and detection of intraperitoneal and retroperitoneal fluid (haematomas). Exploratory laparotomy is performed less frequently following trauma in children than adults and many hepatic, renal or splenic injuries may be managed non-operatively in this age group.

The principles of pancreatic trauma, its pathophysiology, consequences and management, as discussed in this chapter, are no different in children. Prompt recognition and appropriate management of significant pancreatic injuries remain the key to minimizing morbidity and mortality (Vane et al 1989). Smith et al (1988) found that early diagnosis of major childhood pancreatic injuries and prompt surgical management decreased the length of hospital stay by approximately one-half and that there were minimal complications associated with surgical intervention.

CT scanning in paediatric trauma appears to be reliable in the diagnosis of injury to the three most commonly injured organs, namely the spleen, kidney and liver. However, its accuracy in early detection of pancreatic injury in children is disputed. Bass et al (1988) evaluated seven of 26 children with suspected pancreatic trauma by CT scanning and documented pancreatic injury in all seven. Injuries diagnosed included complete gland transection and laceration, and pancreatitis and pancreatic pseudocysts were revealed in some cases. The interval between injury and CT scanning was not specified and while delay in CT scanning increases the sensitivity of diagnosis it also increases the morbidity associated with the pancreatic injury. This is supported by reports from Ivancev and Kullendorff (1983) who documented late pancreatic injury in both of their two patients undergoing CT scanning (both of whom had traumatic pseudocysts), and by a study by Jeffrey et al (1983) where acute pancreatic injury was diagnosed correctly by CT scanning in only eight of 10 patients while long-standing pancreatic injury (pseudocysts) was correctly diagnosed in all three patients.

Other authors have expressed reservations about the accuracy of pancreatic evaluation by CT scanning in children. Haftel et al (1988) reported on 90 children with blunt abdominal trauma who had abdominal CT scans. The scan suggested minor pancreatic injury in six patients, but laparotomy revealed one false positive and one false negative diagnosis of pancreatic injury. One child with CT evidence of traumatic pancreatitis went on to develop pancreatic pseudocysts which required internal drainage approximately 2 months after injury. Peitzman et al (1986) found that abdominal CT scanning failed to diagnose one of three acute pancreatic injuries while

Cook et al (1986) reported false positive CT diagnosis of pancreatic injury in seven of 77 children studied, a 9% false positive rate. Smith et al (1988) failed to diagnose pancreatic injury by CT scan in all six children studied. Injuries confirmed at laparotomy included four complete gland transections and two cases of pancreatic contusion. A retrospective review by Melone & Schwartz (1991) at our institution revealed that CT scanning correctly diagnosed pancreatic trauma in only one of six children undergoing abdominal CT scanning, for a sensitivity of 17%. Injuries confirmed at laparotomy included gland transection in two, contusion in two, and presumed traumatic pancreatitis in two patients. Five further children underwent exploration on the basis of clinical examination and/or rising serum amylase levels without undergoing abdominal CT scanning, and three cases of gland transection and two cases of pancreatic contusion were diagnosed and treated.

The use of serum amylase levels to diagnose pancreatic trauma in children must, as in adults, be interpreted with caution. Elevations of serum amylase of non-pancreatic origin may occur in closed head injury, maxillofacial injury, bowel injury, and shock. Hyperamylasaemia, secondary to alcohol, drug use, or pancreatitis preceding acute injury, is rare but elevations can follow other significant injuries such as rupture of a hollow viscus. It follows that all children with hyperamylasaemia should be carefully evaluated even if other diagnostic studies appear normal.

Retrospective studies of hyperamylasaemia and pancreatic injury in childhood show a variability in the sensitivity of amylase measurement as a means of detecting pancreatic injury which ranges from 75 to 100% (Eichelberger et al 1982, Gorenstein et al 1987, Smith et al 1988, Grosfeld et al 1989). The study by Smith et al (1988) classified pancreatic injury as minor (minor contusion or laceration that required no specific treatment) or major (injuries which would result in pseudocyst formation) and found that the initial serum amylase value did not distinguish between the two. Progressive rise in serum amylase values suggested major pancreatic injury, although statistical significance could not be demonstrated because of the small number of patients.

Review of our institution's experience with paediatric pancreatic trauma shows that of 11 children with pancreatic injury, nine presented with amylase values greater than 200 u/l (normal <100 u/l) in contrast to elevations of greater than 200 u/l in only four of the 85 children suffering blunt trauma without pancreatic injury. Five of the 11 children with pancreatic injury had complete or partial transection and in this group mean serum amylase was 604 ± 101 u/l, whereas in four children with pancreatic contusion, the value was 205 ± 65 u/l. Absence of a twofold or greater elevation in admission serum amylase had a 95% predictive value in excluding pancreatic injury whereas a twofold or greater elevation in serum amylase had an 81% value in predicting pancreatic injury. Threefold, or greater, amylase elevation was 100% sensitive and 93% specific for the detection of pancreatic transection (Melone & Schwartz 1991).

Treatment of pancreatic injuries in children should follow the guidelines outlined earlier with some exceptions. Children may tolerate pancreatic injuries and their sequelae better than adults (Ford et al 1990) and traumatic pancreatic pseudocysts, the most frequent complications in this age group (38–48% in some series), resolve spontaneously in 25–60% of cases (Gorenstein et al 1987, Bass et al 1988, Ford et al 1990).

The higher incidence of traumatic pseudocyst formation in childhood reflects the non-operative approach to paediatric trauma in general. Because of the difficulties of diagnosing pancreatic injury, many of these children will be observed. Furthermore a higher percentage of children will have relatively isolated pancreatic injuries compared with adults, and immediate indications for laparotomy will not exist. In one study, 50% of the traumatic pseudocysts in children were due to bicycle handlebar injuries (Ford et al 1990). Abdominal CT scanning may reveal solid organ injury but it may be decided to follow these patients with serial haematocrits and defer exploratory laparotomy. Without prompt treatment, unrecognized minor or major pancreatic ductal injuries may result in pseudocyst formation.

While many of these pseudocysts resolve with non-operative therapy, complications occur in as many as 25% of cases (Ford et al 1990). Percutaneous pseudocyst drainage under CT or ultrasound guidance has been reported to be effective in children in up to 100% of cases (Gorenstein et al 1987, Bass et al 1988, Jaffe et al 1989). Pseudocysts which fail to resolve with percutaneous drainage or which become infected require operative intervention, with internal or external drainage or pancreatic resection. Delayed operation for pancreatic injury may carry a higher incidence of complications, including iatrogenic splenic injury requiring splenectomy, than early operative intervention (Smith et al 1988). We suggest that if conservative management of traumatic pancreatic injuries is to be considered in children, ERCP should be carried out if at all possible (Hall et al 1986, Cotton & Laaje 1982). This would allow early recognition of major ductal injury, not likely to resolve without operative intervention, and minimize the morbidity and length of hospitalization. When operative intervention is required, efforts should be made to preserve pancreatic substance by internal drainage whenever possible. To prevent postsplenectomy sepsis, more common in children than adults, all efforts should be made to preserve the spleen when distal pancreatectomy or pseudocyst drainage is required.

COMPLICATIONS OF PANCREATIC TRAUMA

Complications associated with pancreatic trauma include pancreatic fistula, pseudocyst, pancreatic abscess, acute or chronic pancreatitis, intra-abdominal abscess and wound infections as well as the pulmonary, cardiovascular, metabolic, renal and septic complications associated with severe trauma. The majority of these complications are not directly related to pancreatic injury but are secondary to haemorrhagic shock or other associated injuries. Intra-abdominal abscesses and wound infections are most often related to associated bowel injury while multiple organ system failure and overwhelming sepsis may be secondary to profound tissue injury and prolonged shock (Stone et al 1962, Wilson et al 1967, Thompson & McFarland 1969, Sturm et al 1973, Heitsch et al 1976, Karl & Chandle 1977, Jones 1978, Whalen et al 1987, Wisner et al 1990).

Pancreatic fistulas have been reported in 3–35% of patients with pancreatic injury and are the most common complication associated with pancreatic injury (Whalen et al 1987). These close spontaneously with time in the majority of cases. However, if major duct injury is present, a chronic fistula may develop and require surgical intervention if conservative management fails (see above). Pseudocysts which follow pancreatic injury are essentially contained pancreatic fistulas, and are usually the result of inadequate drainage of pancreatic injury or failure to recognize major ductal injury. Pseudocysts may be managed by percutaneous drainage under ultrasound or CT guidance if they are a result of minor injury; if major ductal injury is present, internal drainage or pancreatic resection may be necessary. ERCP may allow differentiation between pseudocysts amenable to percutaneous management and those which require surgical intervention. Traumatic pseudocysts, particularly in children, may resolve spontaneously with time. Some pseudocysts may become secondarily infected resulting in pancreatic abscess or fluid collections, and if poorly contained may result in pancreatic ascites. Recognition and management of major ductal injuries and adequate drainage of minor injuries will decrease the incidence of post traumatic pseudocysts.

Pancreatic necrosis may result from secondary infection of devitalized pancreatic tissue and autodigestion from uncontrolled pancreatic drainage. Infected pancreatic necrosis does not respond well to percutaneous drainage and requires operative debridement of all necrotic tissue and external drainage or lavage and appropriate antibiotic therapy. Infected collections consisting principally of fluid may be treated by percutaneous or open drainage. Complications of infection may be prevented by adequate initial debridement of devitalized pancreatic tissue and external drainage. Pancreatic infection is reported to occur in 2–3% of pancreatic injuries (Graham et al 1978a, Cogbill et al 1982, Jones 1985).

Acute pancreatitis develops in up to 13% of patients following surgery for pancreatic injury (Stone et al 1981, Cogbill et al 1982). This may be manifested by a delayed rise in serum amylase and epigastric abdominal pain, and will usually resolve spontaneously with pancreatic rest. However, haemorrhagic or necrotizing pancreatitis can develop after pancreatic injury and results in extensive necrosis and haemorrhage from pancreatic autodigestion. This complication has been reported in less than 2% of patients undergoing surgery for pancreatic trauma, but early recognition and aggressive treatment is necessary for survival. The initial manifestation may be the development of bloody pancreatic drainage or rapidly developing shock, declining haematocrit and increased abdominal pain. Treatment consists of prompt aggressive debridement and drainage. Haemorrhagic pancreatitis in these circumstances has a mortality rate of up to 80% (Graham et al 1978a, Jones 1985). Chronic pancreatitis may develop secondary to ductal stricture, fibrosis or stricture of a ductal-enteric anastomosis. Revision of the ductal-enteric anastomosis or pancreatic drainage surgery may be necessary to deal with pain, and exocrine and endocrine replacement therapy may be necessary in some patients.

REFERENCES

Anderson C B, Weisz D, Rodger M R, Tucker G L 1973 Combined pancreaticoduodenal trauma. American Journal of Surgery 125:530

Anderson C B, Connors J P, Majia D C, Wise L 1974 Drainage methods in the treatment of pancreatic injuries. Surgery, Gynecology and Obstetrics 135:587

Aranha G V, Prinz R A, Freeark R J, Greenlee H B 1984 The spectrum of biliary tract obstruction from chronic pancreatitis. Archives of Surgery 119:595

Babb J, Harmon H 1976 Diagnosis and management of pancreatic trauma. American Surgeon 42:390

Bach R D, Frey C F 1971 Diagnosis and treatment of pancreatic trauma. American Journal of Surgery 121:20

Baker R J, Dippel W F, Freeark R J, Strohl E L 1963 The surgical significance of trauma to the pancreas. Archives of Surgery 86:1038

Balasegarem M, Lumpur K 1976 Surgical management of pancreatic trauma. American Journal of Surgery 131:536

Barkin J S, Ferstenberg R M, Panullo W, Manten H D, Davis R C 1988 Endoscopic retrograde cholangiopancreatography in pancreatic trauma. Gastrointestinal Endoscopy 34:102

Bass J, DiLorenzo M, Desjardins J G, Grignon A, Ouimet A 1988 Blunt pancreatic injuries in children: the role of percutaneous external drainage on the treatment of pancreatic pseudocysts. Journal of Pediatric Surgery 23:721

Beal S L, Spisso J 1988 The risk of splenorrhaphy. Archives of Surgery 123:1158

Belohlavek D, Merkle P, Probst M 1978 Identification of traumatic rupture of the pancreatic duct by endoscopic retrograde pancreatography. Gastrointestinal Endoscopy 24 255

Berne C J, Donovan A J, Hagen W E 1968 Combined duodenal pancreatic trauma. The role of end-to-side gastrojejunostomy. Archives of Surgery 96:712

Berne C J, Donovan A J, White E J, Yellin A E 1974 Duodenal 'diverticulization' for duodenal and pancreatic injury. American Journal of Surgery 127:503

Berni G A, Bandyk D F, Oreskovich M R, Carrico C J 1982 Role of intraoperative pancreatography in patients with injury to the pancreas. American Journal of Surgery 143:602

Booth F V, Flint L M 1990 Pancreatico-duodenal trauma. In Border J R (ed) Blunt multiple trauma. Marcel Dekker, New York and Basel, Ch 36: p 497

Bozymski E M, Orlando R C, Holt III J W 1981 Traumatic disruption of the pancreatic duct demonstrated by endoscopic retrograde pancreatography. Journal of Trauma 21:244

Brawley R K, Cameron J L, Zuidema G D 1968 Severe upper abdominal injury treated by pancreaticoduodenectomy. Surgery, Gynecology and Obstetrics 126:516

Cattell R B 1948 A technique for pancreatoduodenal resection. Surgical Clinics of North America 28:761

Cattell R B, Braasch J W 1960 A technique for exposure of the third and fourth portions of the duodenum. Surgery, Gynecology and Obstetrics 111:378

Chambers R T, Norton L, Hinchey J E 1975 Massive right upper quadrant intra-abdominal injury requiring pancreaticoduodenectomy and partial hepatectomy. Journal of Trauma 15: 714

Chapman W C, Morris Jr J A 1989 Diagnosis and management of blunt pancreatic injury. Journal of the Tennessee Medical Association 82:2

Cleveland H C, Waddell W R 1963 Retroperitoneal rupture of the duodenum due to nonpenetrating trauma. Surgical Clinics of North America 43 413

Cocke Jr W M, Meyer K K 1964 Retroperitoneal duodenal rupture. Proposed mechanism, review of literature and report of a case. America Journal of Surgery 108:834

Cogbill T H, Moore E E, Kashuk J L 1982 Changing trends in the management of pancreatic trauma. Archives of Surgery 117:722

Cook D E, Walsh J W, Vick C W, Brewer W H 1986 Upper abdominal trauma: pitfalls in CT diagnosis. Radiology 159:65

Corley R D, Norcross W J, Shoemaker W C 1975 Traumatic injuries to the duodenum: a report of 98 patients. Annals of Surgery 181:92

Cotton P B, Laaje N J 1982 Endoscopic retrograde cholangiopancreatography in children. Archives of Diseases in Children 57:131

Culotta R J, Howard J M, Jorand Jr G L 1956 Traumatic injuries to the pancreas. Surgery 40:320

DeMars J J, Bubrick M P, Hitchcock C R 1979 Duodenal perforation in blunt abdominal trauma. Surgery 86:632

DeVries J E, Eeftinck Schattenkerk M, Eggink W F, Bruining H A, Obertop H, Van Der Slikke W, Van Houten H 1984 Treatment of pancreatic injuries. Netherlands Journal of Surgery 36:13

Dodds W J, Taylor A J, Erickson S J, Lawson T L 1990 Traumatic fracture of the pancreas: CT characteristics. Journal of Computer Assisted Tomography 14:375

Eichelberger M R, Hoelzer D J, Koup C E 1982 Acute pancreatitis: The difficulties of diagnosis and therapy. Journal of Pediatric Surgery 17(3):244

Elman R, Arneson N, Graham E A 1929 Value of blood amylase estimations in the diagnosis of pancreatic disease. Archives of Surgery 19:943

Fabian T C, Kudsk K A, Croce M A, Payne L W, Mangiante E C, Voeller G R, Britt L G 1990 Superiority of closed suction drainage for pancreatic trauma. Annals of Surgery 211:724

Feliciano D V, Martin T D, Cruse P A, Graham J M, Burch J M, Mattox K L, Bitondo C D, Jordan Jr G L 1987 Management of combined pancreatoduodenal injuries. Annals of Surgery 205:673

Fish J C, Johnson G L 1965 Rupture of duodenum following blunt trauma: Report of a case with avulsion of papilla of Vater. Annals of Surgery 162:917

Fitzgibbons T J, Yellin A E, Maruyama M M, Donovan A J 1982 Management of the transected pancreas following distal pancreatectomy. Surgery, Gynecology and Obstetrics 154:225

Ford E G, Hardin Jr W D, Mahour G H, Woolley M M 1990 Pseudocysts of the pancreas in children. American Surgeon 56:384

Fraser G C 1969 Handlebar injury of the pancreas. Journal of Pediatric Surgery 4:216

Freeark R J, Kane J M, Folk F A, Baker R J 1965 Traumatic disruption of the head of the pancreas. Archives of Surgery 91:5

Freeark R J, Corley R D, Norcross W J, Baker R J 1966 Unusual aspects of pancreatoduodenal trauma. Journal of Trauma 6:482

Friend P J, Jamieson N V, MacFarline R 1985. Blunt pancreatic injury: two case reports and a review of the literature. British Journal of Accident Surgery 16:391

Frey C F, Araida T 1991 Trauma to the pancreas and duodenum. In Blaisdell F W, Trunkey D D (eds) Trauma management. Vol I, Abdominal trauma, Thieme-Stratton, New York, Ch 6

Frey C F, Child C G, Fry W 1976 Pancreatectomy for chronic pancreatic. Annals of Surgery 184:403

Gibbs B F, Crow J L, Rupnik E J 1970 Pancreatoduodenectomy for blunt pancreatoduodenal injury. Journal of Trauma 10:702

Glancy K E 1989 Review of pancreatic trauma. Western Journal of Medicine 151:45

Gorenstein A, O'Halpin D, Wesson D W, Daneman A, Filler R M 1987 Blunt injury to the pancreas in children: Selective management based on ultrasound. Journal of Pediatric Surgery 22:1110

Gougeon F W, Legros C, Archambault A, Bessette G, Bastien E 1976 Pancreatic trauma: A new diagnostic approach. American Journal of Surgery 132:400

Graham J M, Mattox K L, Jordan Jr G L 1978a Traumatic injuries of the pancreas. American Journal of Surgery 136: 744

Graham J M, Pokorny W J, Mattox K L, Jordan G L 1978b Surgical management of acute pancreatic injuries in children. Journal of Pediatric Surgery 13: 693

Graham J M, Mattox K L, Vaughan G D, Jordan Jr G L 1979 Combined pancreaticoduodenal injuries. Journal of Trauma 19: 340

Grosfeld J L, Cooney D R 1975 Pancreatic and gastrointestinal trauma in children. Pediatric Clinics of North America 22: 365

Grosfeld J L, Rescorla F J, West K W, Vane D W 1989 Gastrointestinal injuries in childhood: Analysis of 53 patients. Journal of Pediatric Surgery 24:580

Haftel A J, Lev R, Mahour G H, Senac M, Shar S I A 1988 Abdominal CT scanning in pediatric blunt trauma. Annals of Emergency Medicine 684

Halgrimson C G, Trimble C, Gale S, Waddell W R 1969 Pancreaticoduodenectomy for traumatic lesions. American Journal of Surgery 118:877

Hall R I, Lavell M I, Venables C W 1986 Use of ERCP to identify the site of traumatic injuries of the main pancreatic duct in children. British Journal of Surgery 73:411

Hayward S R, Lucas C E, Sugawa C, Ledgerwood A M 1989 Emergent endoscopic retrograde cholangiopancreatography: A highly specific test for acute pancreatic trauma. Archives of Surgery 124:745

Heimansohn D A, Canal D F, McCarthy M C, Yaw P B, Madura J A, Broadie T A 1990 The role of pancreaticoduodenectomy in the management of traumatic injuries to the pancreas and duodenum. American Surgeon 56:511

Heiss F W, Shea J A 1978 Association of pancreatitis and variant ductal anatomy, dominant drainage of the duct of Santorini. American Journal of Gastroenterology 70:158

Heitsch R C, Knutson C O, Fulton R L, Jones C E 1976 Delineation of critical factors in the treatment of pancreatic trauma. Surgery 80:523

Heyse-Moore G H 1976 Blunt pancreatic and pancreaticoduodenal trauma. British Journal of Surgery 63:226

Hutchinson W B 1971 Duodenotomy. American Journal of Surgery 122:777

Ivancev K, Kullendorff C M 1983 Value of computed tomography in traumatic pancreatitis in children. Acta Radiological Diagnostica 24:441

Ivatury R R, Gaudino J, Ascer E, Nallathambi M, Ramirez-Schon G, Stahl W M 1985 Treatment of penetrating duodenal injuries: primary repair vs. repair with decompressive enterostomy/serosal patch. Journal of Trauma 25:337

Ivatury R R, Nallathambi M, Rao P, Stahl W M 1990 Penetrating pancreatic injuries: analysis of 103 consecutive cases. American Surgeon 56:90

Jaffe R B, Arata J A, Matlak M E 1989 Percutaneous drainage of traumatic pancreatic pseudocysts in children. American Journal of Radiology 152:591

Janson K L, Stockinger F 1975 Duodenal hematoma. American Journal of Surgery 129: 304

Jeffrey R B, Federle M P, Crass R A 1983 Computed tomography of pancreatic trauma. Radiology 147: 491

Jeffrey R B, Laing F C, Wing V W 1986 Ultrasound in acute pancreatic trauma. Gastrointestinal Radiology 11: 44

Jones R C 1978 Management of pancreatic trauma. Annals of Surgery 187: 555

Jones R C 1985 Management of pancreatic trauma. American Journal of Surgery 150: 698

Jones R C, Shires G T 1971 Pancreatic trauma. Archives of Surgery 102: 424

Jordan G L, Overton R, Werschky L R 1969 Traumatic transection of the pancreas. Southern Medicine Journal 62:90

Jurkovich G J, Carrico C J 1990 Pancreatic trauma. Surgical Clinics of North American 70(3):575

Karl H W, Chandler J G 1977 Mortality and morbidity of pancreatic injury. American Journal of Surgery 134:549

Kashuk J L, Moore E E, Cogbill T H 1982 Management of the intermediate severity duodenal injury. Surgery 92:758

Keeling P, Calthorpe D, Lane B, Collins P G 1987 Blunt injury of the neck of the pancreas: a report of nine patients. Injury 18: 93

Kellum J M, Holland G F, McNeil P 1988 Traumatic pancreatic cutaneous fistula: Comparison of enteral and parenteral feedings. Journal of Trauma 28:700

Kerry R L, Glas W W 1962 Traumatic injuries of the pancreas and duodenum. Archives of Surgery 85:813

Kraus M, Gordon R E 1974 Alternate techniques of duodenotomy. Surgery, Gynecology and Obstetrics 139:417

Kuhn J P, Berger P E 1981 Computer tomography in the evaluation of blunt abdominal trauma in children. Radiologic Clinics of North America 19:503

LaRaja R D, Lobbato V J, Cassaro S, Reddy S S 1986 Intraoperative endoscopic retrograde cholangiopancreatography (ERCP) in penetrating trauma of the pancreas. Journal of Trauma 26:1146

Laustsen J, Jensen K E, Bach-Nielsen P 1988 Closed pancreatic transection treated by Roux-en-Y anastomosis. Injury 19: 42

Lee D, Zacher J, Vogel T T 1976 Primary repair in transection of duodenum with avulsion of the common duct. Archives of Surgery 111:592

Leppaniemi A, Haapiainen R, Kiviluoto T, Lempinen M 1988 Pancreatic trauma: acute and late manifestations. British Journal of Surgery 75:165

Lowe R J, Saletta J D, Moss G S 1977 Pancreatoduodenectomy for penetrating pancreatic trauma. Journal of Trauma 17:732

Lucas C E 1977 Diagnosis and treatment of pancreatic and duodenal injury. Surgical Clinics of North America 57:49

Lucas C E, Ledgerwood A M 1975 Factors influencing outcome after blunt duodenal injury. Journal of Trauma 15:839

Luna G K, Dellinger E P 1987 Nonoperative observation therapy for splenic injuries: a safe therapeutic option? American Journal of Surgery 153:462

McCorkle H, Goldman L 1942 The clinical significance of the serum amylase test in the diagnosis of acute pancreatitis. Surgery, Gynecology and Obstetrics 74:439

McKone T K, Bursch L R, Scholten D J 1988 Pancreaticoduodenectomy for trauma: a life-saving procedure. American Surgeon 54:361

Mansour M A, Moore J B, Moore E E, Moore F A 1989 Conservative management of combined pancreatoduodenal injuries. American Journal of Surgery 158:531

Martin L W, Henderson B M, Welsh N 1968 Disruption of the head of the pancreas caused by blunt trauma in children: a report of two cases treated with primary repair of the pancreatic duct. Surgery 63:697

Martin T D, Feliciano D V, Mattox K L, Jordan Jr G L 1983 Severe duodenal injuries. Archives of Surgery 118:631

Melone J, Schwartz M 1991 Pancreatic trauma in children; diagnostic value of physical examination, serum amylase and computerized tomography. In preparation

Meredith J W, Trunkey D D 1988 CT scanning in acute abdominal injuries. Surgical Clinics of North America 68:255

Michels N A 1951 The hepatic, cystic and retroduodenal arteries and their relation to the biliary ducts. Annals of Surgery 133:503

Mikulicz-Radeckii J 1903 Surgery of the pancreas. Annals of Surgery 38:1

Moore E E, Dunn E L, Moore J B, Thompson J S 1981 Penetrating abdominal trauma index. Journal of Trauma 21:439

Moore J B, Moore E E 1984 Changing trends in the management of combined pancreatoduodenal injuries. World Journal of Surgery 8:791

Moretz J A III, Campbell D P, Parker D E, William G R 1975 Significance of serum amylase in evaluating pancreatic trauma. American Journal of Surgery 130:739

Morton J R, Jordon Jr G L 1968 Traumatic duodenal injuries. Review of 131 cases. Journal of Trauma 8:127

Naffziger H C, McCorkle H J 1943 The recognition and management of acute trauma of the pancreas, with particular reference to the use of the serum amylase test. Annals of Surgery 118:594

Nance F C, DeLoach D H 1971 Pancreaticoduodenectomy following abdominal trauma. Journal of Trauma 11:577

Nilsson E, Norrby S, Skullman S, Sjodahl R 1986 Pancreatic trauma in a defined population. Acta Chirurgica Scandinavica 152:647

Nowak M M, Baringer D C, Ponsky J L 1986 Pancreatic injuries. Effectiveness of debridement and drainage for nontransecting injuries. American Surgeon 52:599

Oreskovich M R, Carrico C J 1984 Pancreaticoduodenectomy for trauma: a viable option? American Journal of Surgery 147:618

Otis G A (ed) 1876. Penetrating wounds of the abdomen; surgical history. In: The medical and surgical history of the War of the Rebellion (1861–1865). Prepared under the direction of Surgeon General J.K. Barnes. Government Printing Office, Washington DC, vol 2, ch 4, p 158–161

Owens M P, Wolfman Jr E F 1973 Pancreatic trauma: management and presentation of a new technique. Surgery 73:881

Pachter H L, Hofstetter S R, Liang H G, Hoballah J 1989 Traumatic injuries to the pancreas: the role of distal pancreatectomy with splenic preservation. Journal of Trauma 29:1352

Peitzman A B, Makaroun M S, Slasky S, Ritter R 1986 Prospective study of computed tomography in initial management of blunt abdominal trauma. Journal of Trauma 26:585

Pokorny W J, Brandt M L, Harberg F J 1986 Major duodenal injuries in children: diagnosis, operative management, and outcome. Journal of Pediatric Surgery 21:613

Pollock A V 1974 Pancreatic trauma and idiopathic retroperitoneal fibrosis: a long term follow up study of 4 patients. British Journal of Surgery 61:112

Poole L H Wounds of the pancreas (62 casualties). Surgical history of World War II, Office of the Surgeon General Government Printing Office, Washington DC, ch 22

Prinz R A, Pickleman J, Hoffman J P 1988 Treatment of pancreatic cutaneous fistulas with a somatostatin analog. American Journal of Surgery 155:36

Robey E, Mullen J T, Schwab C W 1982 Blunt transection of the pancreas treated by distal pancreatectomy, splenic salvage, and hyperalimentation. Annals of Surgery 196:695

Sako Y et al 1955 A survey of evacuation, resuscitation, and mortality in a forward surgical hospital. Surgery 37:602

Salonen I S, Aarnio P 1985 Treatment of acute pancreatic injuries in childhood. Annales Chirurgiae et Gynaecologiae 74:167

Salyer K, McClelland R N 1967 Pancreatoduodenectomy for trauma. Archives of Surgery 95:636

Scher K, Scott-Connor C, Jones C W, Wroczynski A F 1985 Methods of splenic preservation and their effect on clearance of pneumococcal bacteremia. Annals of Surgery 202:595

Sheldon G F, Cohn L H, Blaisdell F W 1970 Surgical treatment of pancreatic trauma. Journal of Trauma 10:795

Sims E H, Mandal A K, Schlater T, Fleming A W, Lou M A 1984 Factors affecting outcome in pancreatic trauma. Journal of Trauma 24:125

Smego D R, Richardson J D, Flint L M 1985 Determinants of outcome in pancreatic trauma. Journal of Trauma 25:771

Smith S D, Nakayama D K, Gantt N, Lloyd D, Rower M I 1988 Pancreatic injuries in childhood due to blunt trauma. Journal of Pediatric Surgery 23:610

Snyder W H, Weigelt J A, Watkins W L, Beitz D S 1980 The surgical management of duodenal trauma. Archives of Surgery 115:422

Sorensen V J, Obeid F N, Horst H M, Bivins B A 1986 Penetrating pancreatic injuries 1978–1983. American Surgeon 52: 354

Steele M, Sheldon G F, Blaisdell F W 1973 Pancreatic injuries. Archives of Surgery 106:544

Stigall K E, Dorsey J S 1989 Transection of the first portion of jejunum from blast injury in accidental discharge of (2.75-inch aircraft) rocket from an F-15. Military Medicine 154:431

Stone H H, Stowers K B, Shippey S H 1962 Injuries to the pancreas. Archives of Surgery 85:525

Stone H H, Fabian T L, Santiani B, Turkleson M L 1981 Experience in the management of pancreatic trauma. Journal of Trauma 21:257

Sturm J T, Quattlebaum F W, Mowlem A, Perry Jr J F 1973 Patterns of injury requiring pancreaticoduodenectomy. Surgery, Gynecology and Obstetrics 137:629

Sugawa C, Lucas C E 1988 The case for preoperative and intraoperative ERCP in pancreatic trauma. Gastrointestinal Endoscopy 34:145

Taxier M, Sivak Jr M V, Cooperman A M, Sullivan Jr B H 1980 Endoscopic retrograde pancreatography in the evaluation of trauma to the pancreas. Surgery, Gynecology and Obstetrics 150:65

Thompson Jr R J, Hinshow D B 1966 Pancreatic trauma: review of 87 cases. Annals of Surgery 163:153

Thompson R G, McFarland J B 1969 Traumatic rupture of the pancreas with complications. British Journal of Surgery 56:117

Travers B 1827 Rupture of the pancreas. Lancet 12:384

Traverso L W, Longmire Jr W P 1978 Preservation of the pylorus during pancreaticoduodenectomy. Surgery, Gynecology and Obstetrics 146:959

Vallon A G, Lees W R, Cotton P B 1979 Grey-scale ultrasonography and endoscopic pancreatography after pancreatic trauma. British Journal of Surgery 66:169

Vane D W, Grosfeld J L, West K W, Rescorla F J 1989 Pancreatic disorders in infancy and childhood: Experience with 92 cases. Journal of Pediatric Surgery 24:771

Van Steenbergen W, Samain H, Pouillon M, Van Roost W, Marchal G, Baert A, Penninckx F, Kerremans R, DeGrotte J 1987 Transection of the pancreas demonstrated by ultrasound and computed tomography. Gastrointestinal Radiology 12:128

Walker M L 1986 Management of pancreatic trauma: Concepts and controversy. Journal of the National Medical Association 78:1177

Walton A J 1923 A Textbook of the surgical dyspepsia. E Arnold, London, 1923

Whalen G F, Robbs J V, Baker L W 1987 Injuries of the pancreas and duodenum: results of a conservative approach. South African Journal of Surgery 25:15

Whipple A O 1946 Observations on radical surgery for lesions of the pancreas. Surgery, Gynecology and Obstetrics 82:808

Whittwell A E, Gomez G A, Byers P, Kreis Jr D J, Manten H, Casillas V J 1989 Blunt pancreatic trauma: prospective evaluation of early endoscopic retrograde pancreatography. Southern Medical Journal 82:586

Wilkinson A E 1989 Injuries of the pancreas. Suid-Afrikaanse Tydskrif Vir Chirurgie 27:67

Wilson R F, Tagett J P, Pucelik J P, Walt A J 1967 Pancreatic trauma. Journal of Trauma 7:643

Wisner D H, Wold R L, Frey C F 1990 Diagnosis and treatment of pancreatic injuries: An analysis of management principles. Archives of Surgery 125:1109

Wittingen J, Frey C F 1974 Islet concentration in the head, body, tail and uncinate process of the pancreas. Annals of Surgery 179:412

Wynn M, Hill D M, Miller D R, Waxaman K, Eisner M E, Gazzaniga A B 1985 Management of pancreatic and duodenal trauma. American Journal of Surgery 150:327

Yellin N E, Rosoff L 1975 Pancreatoduodenectomy for combined pancreatoduodenal injuries. Archives of Surgery 110:1117

Yeo C K, McNamara J 1973 Retroperitoneal rupture of duodenum with complicating gas gangrene. Archives of Surgery 106:856

Pancreatic transplantation

51. Pancreatic transplantation

K. L. Brayman   D. E. R. Sutherland   J. S. Najarian

INTRODUCTION

The goal of pancreas transplantation is to restore nor-moglycaemia in diabetic recipients by providing functioning beta cells. Restoring euglycaemia should prevent, or halt the progression of, vascular complications that arise from disordered glucose metabolism; it should thus prevent the ocular, nervous, renal, and other organ dysfunction that occurs in over 50% of diabetic individuals (Tchobroutsky 1978, Hanssen et al 1986). No current method of administering exogenous insulin can produce consistent euglycaemia over a period of several years. To achieve this, functioning beta cells must be provided (Sutherland et al 1980, Rajotte 1989, Tzakis et al 1990, Scharp et al 1991). Clinically, the best way to do so is with an immediately vascularized pancreas transplant (Kelly et al 1967, Lillehei et al 1976, Gliedman et al 1978, Sutherland et al 1981, Pozza et al 1983, Ostman et al 1989, Robertson et al 1989). A technically successful whole or segmental pancreas graft establishes a euglycaemic, insulin-independent state in almost all recipients. By mid-1991, over 3000 pancreas transplants at over 150 institutions worldwide had been reported to the International Pancreas Transplant Registry (Sutherland et al 1991a, c, d). The frequency of pancreas transplantation has increased in recent years, as the results have improved. Over 600 cases were reported to the Registry for 1990 alone. Over half of these procedures have been performed in the United States; several centres have published the results of their individual experience (Sutherland et al 1984a, 1988, 1989a, LaRocca et al 1987, Illner et al 1987, Tyden et al 1987, Cosimi et al 1988, Sollinger et al 1988, Wright et al 1989, Schulak et al 1990).

In uraemic type I diabetic patients, transplantation of immediately vascularized cadaver pancreas grafts has been done either at the same time as, or after, kidney transplantation. Inducing and maintaining immunosuppression following transplantation requires multiple anti-rejection drugs to prevent or reverse rejection of both grafts. Thus, when considering a pancreas transplant, the potential for serious side-effects (e.g. infection, malignancy) from these drugs must be weighed against the problems associated with the alternatives, i.e. dialysis to treat uraemia and insulin to treat diabetes.

In nonuraemic type I diabetic patients, isolated pancreas transplantation has also been done in an attempt to prevent the progression of complications of chronic hyperglycaemia or to improve a poor quality of life secondary to hyperlabile diabetes (Sutherland et al 1988, 1991b). In this group, the problems of immunosuppression and the risk of infection and malignancy must be weighed against the severe problems of diabetes alone. Patients who have undergone transplantation are almost unanimous in saying that independence from insulin markedly improved their quality of life (Zehrer & Cross 1990, 1991).

INDICATIONS AND COSTS

Reasons for the slow development of pancreas transplantation have included technical problems with the operation itself and immunosuppressive side-effects. Currently, pancreas transplantation is restricted to patients who already have, or are prone to develop, complications of diabetes that are more serious than the side-effects of immunosuppression. For this reason, most pancreas transplants have been done in diabetic patients who have already developed end-stage renal failure and also require a kidney transplant. In these patients, immunosuppressive drugs are mandatory, so the only risk, now low, attached to the pancreas transplant is surgical. However, diabetic patients with emerging complications, albeit not yet end-stage, are also candidates, as are those who have extreme difficulty with diabetic control which seriously interferes with day-to-day activities.

Studies of pancreas transplant recipients have shown that diabetic nephropathy does not recur in their transplanted kidneys and that progression of diabetic nephropathy is halted in their native kidneys if the pancreas transplant is done early enough (Bohman et al 1985, 1987, Bilous et al 1987, 1989). Neuropathy also improves

593

(Solders et al 1987, Kennedy et al 1990, Navarro et al 1990) and there may be long-term stabilization of diabetic retinopathy (Ulbig et al 1987, Ramsay et al 1988). These benefits, in addition to the improved quality of life (no more need for dietary regulation and insulin injections), have led to an ever-increasing number of pancreas transplants.

Table 51.1 shows the pancreas transplant recipient categories and selection criteria established by the University of Minnesota Pancreas Transplant Evaluation Committee. Type I diabetic uraemic candidates for cadaver donor kidney transplants should almost always be considered for a simultaneous pancreas transplant. Immunosuppressive management will be no different from that of a kidney transplant alone, and the surgical risk of adding the pancreas is low. Coronary artery disease, if any, should be corrected before pancreas or kidney transplantation. Similarly, diabetic patients with previous kidney transplants, from either related or cadaver donors, can be considered for a subsequent pancreas transplant. Again, the only added risk is surgical, since the immunosuppressive risks have already been assumed. The indications for pancreas transplantation to the third category – non-uraemic diabetic, non-kidney transplant patients – are still being defined (University of Michigan 1988, Sutherland et al 1988). Those with diabetes so labile that day-to-day living is difficult can be considered for this reason alone. In their case, the immunosuppressive risks are clearly being substituted for the risks of insulin administration. Other indications for pancreas transplantation in non-uraemic diabetic, non-kidney transplant patients include progressive secondary complications, particularly early nephropathy. A beneficial effect on existing retinopathy is not seen for several years after a pancreas transplant, so it may not be justified for retinopathy alone. A pancreas transplant favourably affects neuropathy, but a transplant candidate's actual or predicted neuropathic disability must be sufficient to justify the immunosuppressive risks.

In patients with early diabetic nephropathy, micro- or macroalbuminuria indicates renal disease at a stage where progression is inevitable if they remain diabetic (Viberti et al 1982). Although controlling hypertension may slow the progression, either dialysis or kidney transplantation will ultimately be required if a pancreas transplant is not done. In early diabetic nephropathy, the lesions are such that progression may be halted if the diabetes is corrected by a pancreas transplant. If the pancreas transplant prevents progression of nephropathy, the patient has the double benefit of not needing insulin and not developing uraemia (which would then require dialysis or a kidney transplant). In addition, associated or emerging secondary complications of other organ systems may also be thwarted.

The pancreas transplant costs are comparable to those for a kidney transplant. For patients already undergoing a kidney transplant, simultaneously adding a new pancreas increases their hospitalization cost in the USA by about $20 000. The cost of procuring a pancreas averages $15 000. Thus, the total increased expense for a pancreas transplant done simultaneously with a kidney transplant is $35 000. For recipients of a pancreas transplant alone, the average cost of hospitalization is $60 000; immunosuppressive drugs add a few thousand dollars per year. Obviously, it is more expensive to treat diabetes with a pancreas transplant than with insulin injections. But transplantation is certainly worthwhile if the complications of diabetes are prevented or ameliorated; complications that in themselves may be even more expensive to treat.

Table 51.1 University of Minnesota pancreas transplant recipient categories and selection criteria (Mauer et al 1984)

I. Uraemic diabetic patients – simultaneous kidney and pancreas transplant (SPK)	Most candidates for a new kidney are also candidates for a new pancreas. Screening for coronary artery disease and any corrective measures (e.g. angioplasty, bypass) should be done pretransplant. If there is no living kidney donor, a simultaneous kidney–pancreas transplant from a cadaver donor is the treatment of choice.
II. Previous kidney transplant (functioning) – subsequent pancreas transplant (PAK)	This is an option for diabetic patients who have undergone a successful living related or cadaver donor kidney transplant.
III. Non-uraemic diabetic, non-kidney transplant patients – pancreas transplant alone (PTA)	a. Patients with such severe difficulty with diabetes control that day-to-day quality of life is poor on exogenous insulin are considered for this reason alone; so far, recipients in this category are few to number.
	b. Patients with early but progressive secondary diabetic complications, that are predicted to be more serious than the potential side-effects of immunosuppression, are considered, whether or not they have day-to-day diabetes control problems; most nonuraemic pancreas recipients are in this category.

	Such patients usually have retinopathy and neuropathy, as well as early nephropathy characterized by:
	 – Albuminuria
	 – Diabetic lesions on kidney biopsy
	  Mesangium 20–40% of glomerular volume (< 20% is normal; > 40% is severe nephropathy) (Mauer et al 1984)
	  Creatinine clearance > 70 ml/min, cyclosporine will be tolerated

SURGICAL TECHNIQUE

Pancreas procurement

The general criteria for selecting cadaver pancreas donors are similar to those for liver, renal, or thoracic organ donors (Brayman et al 1990). A history of type I diabetes mellitus is an absolute contraindication. Relapsing acute pancreatitis and chronic pancreatitis are relative contraindications. In our experience, examining the pancreas at the time of procurement is worthwhile, to confirm the presence or absence of chronic disease. Hyperglycaemia occurring after brain death is not a contraindication; this metabolic abnormality is often a consequence of intravenous glucose administration or an insulin-resistant state that develops after severe head trauma. Serum amylase levels have not prove helpful in evaluating prospective donors. Exploration at the time of laparotomy is often the best, or only, way to confirm the suitability of a given pancreas.

The success of pancreas transplantation is greatly influenced by the expertise of the surgical team. Experienced transplant surgeons in the United States and Europe routinely procure both the liver and the pancreas from the same donor. The operation is done by the same team (Marsh et al 1989). The controversy as to whether both the pancreas and the liver can be procured from a given donor has been resolved; neither the liver nor the pancreas suffers from combined liver–pancreas procurement (Dunn et al 1991).

The standard multiorgan procurement is used in most situations. The brain-dead donor is placed in the supine position, paralysed with a neuromuscular blocking agent. A midline laparotomy incision in made, and extended upwards to join the midline thoracic incision and downwards to the pubis. In organ donors who are obese or large, a cruciate incision is made in the abdominal wall at the level of the umbilicus and carried laterally to the midaxillary line. The four flaps of abdominal wall are then retracted. This incision allows better exposure of the left upper quadrant and facilitates dissection of the pancreas. Before the sternal incision is completed and the thoracic cage and abdominal wall retracted, the falciform ligament is divided to avoid injuring the liver.

The distal aorta and vena cava are first isolated and encircled with umbilical tapes, to prepare for cannulation and perfusion if the donor becomes haemodynamically unstable. After a systematic abdominal exploration to rule out intra-abdominal pathology, the upper abdomen and the blood supply to the liver are evaluated (Fig. 51.1A). Arterial anomalies in the blood supply to the liver are common and may influence whether the pancreas can be procured. Priority is always given to the liver in such situations. If an aberrant left hepatic artery (coming off either the coeliac axis, left gastric artery, or aorta) is not found, the gastrohepatic ligament is divided and the left

triangular ligament is incised. This mobilizes the left lateral segment of the liver and improves access to the supracoeliac aorta and the gastro-oesophageal junction. If an aberrant right hepatic artery coming off the superior mesenteric artery is found, a decision needs to be made; is the procuring surgeon capable of undertaking the dissection to isolate the superior mesenteric artery and dissect the right hepatic artery off the inferior and posterior aspects of the pancreatic head and body? Some pancreas transplant surgeons consider this anomaly to be a contraindication to combined liver–pancreas procurement.

Once the decision is made to procure the pancreas and the liver, the gastrocolic ligament is divided from the pylorus to the uppermost reaches of the greater curvature of the stomach. This facilitates exposure of the anterior surface of the pancreas through the lesser sac. The lieno-colic ligament is incised. The transverse colon is completely mobilized from hepatic to splenic flexure, so that the pancreas may be adequately dissected from the surrounding retroperitoneal structures. Excessive manipulation of the pancreas proper must be avoided. The peripancreatic tissue is ligated and divided in a manner that does not encroach on the pancreatic parenchyma. Short gastric vessels are ligated and divided to the level of the gastro-oesophageal junction. Adhesions between the posterior aspect of the stomach and the anterior surface of the pancreas are sharply incised. The left gastric vessels are ligated and divided close to the stomach, to preserve the blood supply to the liver via the coeliac axis. The stomach is thus completely mobilized. The nasogastric tube, placed before laparotomy, is advanced into the duodenum and 300 ml of amphotericin/antibiotic solution is instilled into the duodenal segment. The tube is then pulled back into the stomach. A GIA stapler is used to divide the stomach and the duodenum just distal to the pylorus. The stomach, entirely free of attachments, is then allowed to fall back into the left subdiaphragmatic area to facilitate dissection of the distal pancreas. Alternatively, the nasogastric tube is pulled back into the oesophagus prior to firing a TA55 stapler twice across the distal oesophagus, which is then divided with removal of the entire stomach. The supracoeliac aorta is then exposed by dividing the diaphragmatic crura with electrocautery. The aorta superior to the coeliac axis is encircled with an umbilical tape.

The pancreaticoduodenal allograft is further mobilized by dividing the lienophrenic ligament. Blunt and sharp dissection is used to free the pancreas from its posterior attachments to the left kidney and the left adrenal gland. Peripancreatic lymphatic tissue should be ligated. The spleen remains in continuity with the pancreas throughout the dissection, and serves as a useful handle when manipulating the pancreas graft (Fig. 51.1B, C). The inferior mesenteric vein is usually ligated and divided at this time. Portal vein access for in situ flush of the portal

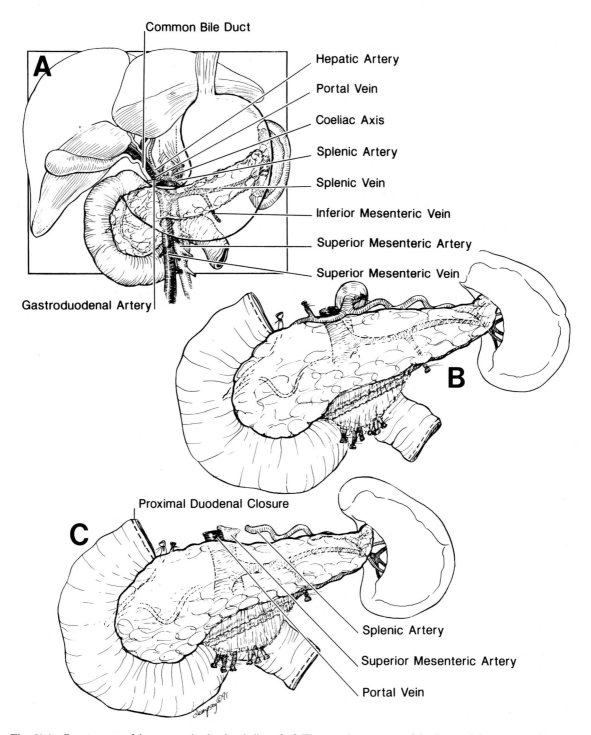

Common Bile Duct

Hepatic Artery

Portal Vein

Coeliac Axis

Splenic Artery

Splenic Vein

Inferior Mesenteric Vein

Superior Mesenteric Artery

Superior Mesenteric Vein

Gastroduodenal Artery

Proximal Duodenal Closure

Splenic Artery

Superior Mesenteric Artery

Portal Vein

Fig. 51.1   Procurement of the pancreaticoduodenal allograft. **A** The vascular anatomy of the liver and the pancreas. Note the gastroduodenal artery, which is divided during simultaneous procurement of the liver and the pancreas, but not the pancreas alone. **B** The pancreaticoduodenal allograft after procurement (non-liver donor). The proximal duodenum has been divided with the GIA stapler. The mesentery to the small intestine inferior to the inferior border of the pancreas has also been ligated and divided, after placement of two parallel rows of TA90 staples. **C** The pancreaticoduodenal allograft after procurement from a donor whose liver was also procured. Note the splenic and superior mesenteric arteries, which require ex vivo reconstruction.

system can be obtained through the inferior mesentric vein. If the proximal vein stump is left·long enough (3–4 cm), cannulation can readily be achieved even if the vein has been divided.

The diaphragmatic crura and the coeliac ganglion and lymphatics are further divided to expose the coeliac axis, superior mesenteric and splenic arteries. On the right side, the infrahepatic inferior vena cava is exposed and encircled above the level of the left and right renal veins to facilitate dividing the inferior vena cava after the in situ flush. It is not necessary to dissect the renal hilar structures in the multiorgan procedure; to do so risks injury to the renal vasculature.

Attention is then directed to the hepatoduodenal ligament. The portal vein, hepatic artery, and common bile duct are dissected free of surrounding lymphatic tissue. The lymphatics on the pancreas side are ligated using 4:0 silk. The gastroduodenal artery is identified, ligated, and divided in the liver–pancreas donor (Fig. 51.1C), but it is preserved if only the pancreas, and not the liver, is procured (Fig. 51.1B). The common bile duct is ligated distally as it enters the pancreas and divided proximal to the ligature. The fundus of the gallbladder is opened and the gallbladder and biliary ductal system are flushed with normal saline solution. A Kocher manoeuvre is performed, and the head of the pancreas is mobilized. The hepatic artery is traced proximal to the coeliac axis and freed of surrounding lymphatic tissue. Vasospasm in the hepatic artery must be prevented. The splenic artery is identified and dissected free of surrounding peripancreatic tissue for a distance of 1–2 cm. After the portal triad is completely dissected, the patient is systemically heparinized (70 units/kg).

The thoracic organ procurement team is allowed to finish dissecting the thoracic organs and to prepare the heart and lung for perfusion and procurement. The jejunum at the level of the ligament of Treitz is divided with the GIA stapler. The distal abdominal aorta is ligated at the level of the aortic bifurcation. A perfusion cannula is inserted into the aorta below the level of the inferior mesenteric artery (which was previously ligated and divided, during the initial aortic dissection). The aortic cannula tip must not be advanced superior to the take-off of the renal arteries. The cannula is secured in place with an umbilical tape or 1:0 silk suture. In coordination with the thoracic organ procurement team, the liver–pancreas procurement surgeons clamps the supracoeliac aorta while the thoracic team clamp the proximal thoracic aorta. The portal vein is divided (about 1 cm cephalad to the superior margin of the pancreatic parenchyma), and the in situ arterial flush is begun. The moment that in situ flushing is begun, the suprahepatic vein cava is divided by the liver–pancreas procurement surgeons. The venous return is vented into the right chest and removed by suction. The liver is also flushed through the open end of the

portal vein. About 1000 ml of (University of Wisconsin) UW preservation solution is delivered through the portal vein and 2000 ml through the aorta. The liver and the pancreas are topically cooled. Excessive flushing of the intra-abdominal organs, especially the pancreas, must be avoided. The pancreas and the liver can be separated in situ or ex vivo.

For combined liver–pancreas donation, the coeliac axis usually remains with the hepatic artery. The splenic artery is divided about 0.5 cm beyond its takeoff from the coeliac trunk. The stump of the proximal splenic artery is suture-ligated. The distal splenic artery, since it commonly retracts, is tagged with a through-and-through suture of 7:0 prolene. The aorta is incised laterally on the left side above the level of the coeliac axis. The aortotomy is carried inferiorly. The renal arteries must not be injured when the aortic patch, including the takeoff of the coeliac axis and the superior mesentric artery, is procured. The liver is dissected free of its remaining attachments by dividing the inferior vena cava above the renal veins, by separating the origins of the coeliac axis and the superior mesenteric artery, and by ligating the right adrenal vein. The liver is carefully removed, inspected, and packaged on the back table.

Attention is directed back to the pancreas. The blood supply to the small intestine, which also courses through the pancreas parenchyma, must be divided inferiorly to the inferior pancreatic border. This can be done before, during, or after the in situ flush. The mesenteric axis can be ligated with individual 0 silk sutures. Alternatively, the peritoneum can be incised, a TA90 stapler fired twice across this tissue, and the tissue divided distal to both parallel staple lines. After the pancreas dissection is completed, the pancreas is carefully removed and inspected on the back table (Fig. 51.1B, C). At this time, the midportion of the antimesenteric border of the duodenum or the distal duodenal staple line may be opened carefully (the former if a hand-sewn duodenocystostomy will be performed, the latter for stapled duodenocystostomy). The duodenal segment is reflushed to remove residual bile or duodenal contents.

Vascular extension grafts are always procured from the cadaver donor. Long segments of the common, internal, and external iliac arteries and veins are carefully dissected free of surrounding tissue, then removed and packaged with the pancreaticoduodenal graft. The graft is stored in UW solution at 4°C and transported for transplantation. The kidneys are removed en bloc in the standard fashion.

Preparation of the donor pancreas

During the dissection and preparation of the recipient vessels and bladder, a second team of surgeons may prepare the pancreas graft on a separate back table (Fig. 51.2). The distal duodenal segment is recannulated and

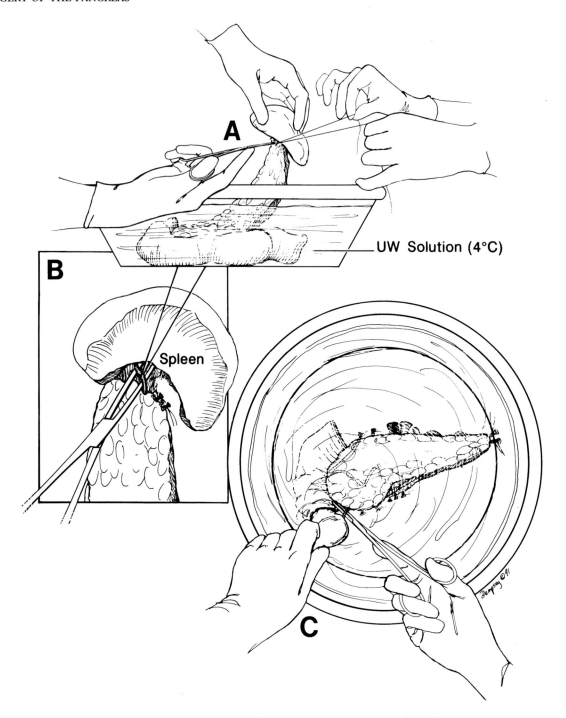

Fig. 51.2   Ex vivo preparation of the pancreaticoduodenal allograft I: Splenectomy and the distal duodenal segment.
A The spleen is removed ex vivo at 4°C with the pancreaticoduodenal allograft immersed in University of Wisconsin
(UW) preservation solution. **B** The splenic hilar vessels are ligated close to the spleen to avoid injury to the tail of the
pancreas. **C** The distal limb of the duodenal segment of the pancreaticoduodenal allograft is shortened to minimize
bicarbonate loss, a problem with the bladder drainage technique. The divided tissue on the pancreatic and duodenal
sides has been ligated to prevent troublesome bleeding after revascularization.

the duodenum flushed a second time with cold UW
solution to remove residual duodenal contents. The
pancreaticoduodenal graft is then placed in a sterile steel
basin and submerged in cold UW solution. The spleen is
removed first, and the splenic hilar vessels are ligated with

2:0 silk suture. The tail of the pancreas must not be injured
during this dissection (Fig. 51.2B).

Excess distal duodenum is removed from the pancreaticoduodenal graft by carefully mobilizing the distal
duodenal segment (Fig. 51.2C). The blood vessels between

the pancreas and the duodenum are dissected and ligated using 4:0 silk suture. The distal duodenum is mobilized to an area about 3 cm distal to the papilla of Vater. Peripancreatic lymphatic tissue that had not been ligated previously is identified and ligated at this time. Proximal duodenal mobilization is rarely necessary. The proximal duodenal closure, accomplished at the time of procurement with the GIA stapler, is reinforced with a running non-absorbable 4:0 prolene suture. A third layer of interrupted 4:0 prolene sutures is inserted to invert the entire suture line (Fig. 51.3). If the mesenteric axis was divided with the TA90 stapler, this staple line is overrun with 2 rows of running 3:0 prolene sutures to ensure haemostasis.

The vascular reconstruction is usually the last ex vivo work to be done on the pancreas graft before transplantation. The splenic and superior mesenteric arteries are identified and prepared for transplantation by carefully removing surrounding lymphatic or ganglion tissue. An arterial extension Y graft is used frequently (Fig.

51.4). The external iliac artery of the extension graft is anastomosed first to the superior mesenteric artery of the graft in end-to-end fashion using running 6:0 prolene sutures. The internal iliac artery of the extension graft is then anastomosed end-to-end to the splenic artery of the graft using 6:0 or 7:0 prolene sutures. The splenic artery can be quite fragile, so intimal dissection must be avoided. The splenic artery of the pancreas graft can be also anastomosed end-to-side to the superior mesenteric artery (7:0 prolene sutures) if sufficient length on both arteries is available. If the liver was not procured or if the liver team allowed the coeliac axis to remain with the pancreas graft, a patch of aorta, including the origins of the coeliac axis and the superior mesenteric artery, is available for anastomosis directly to the recipient's vessels (Fig. 51.4). No vascular reconstruction is necessary in this circumstance. A portal vein extension graft is rarely necessary, but can be done at this time by anastomosing the donor external iliac vein to the portal vein using 6:0 or 7:0 prolene sutures.

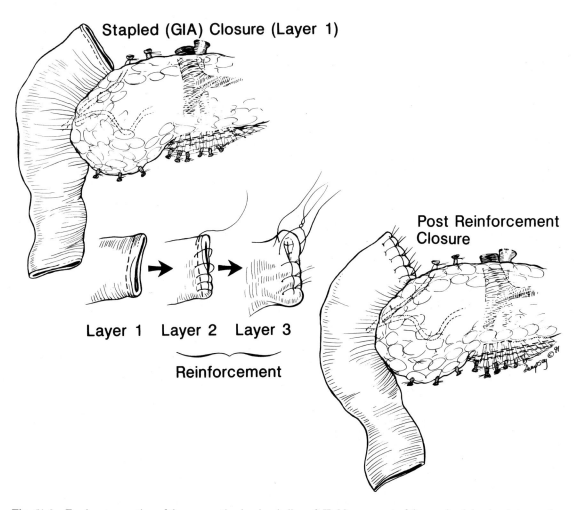

Fig. 51.3 Ex vivo preparation of the pancreaticoduodenal allograft II: Management of the proximal duodenal stump. A three-layered closure is secure. The first layer is completed in the donor at the time of procurement (GIA staple line). Layers two and three (reinforcement layers) are performed ex vivo before transplantation. (See text for details.)

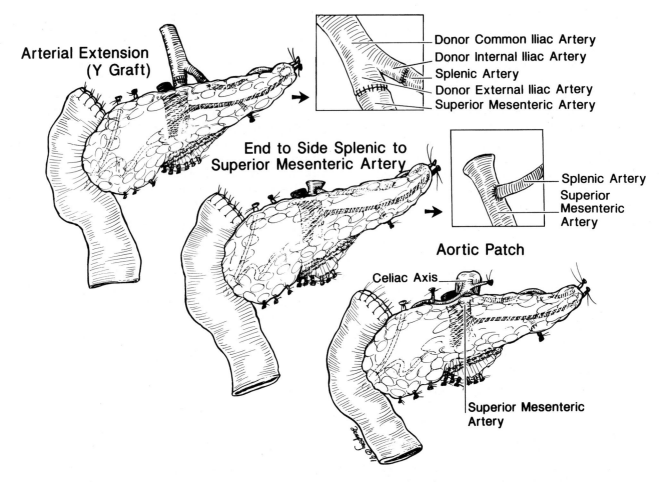

Fig. 51.4 Ex vivo preparation of the pancreaticoduodenal allograft III: Revascularization. An arterial extension (Y graft) is commonly used to revascularize the splenic and superior mesenteric arteries of the pancreas. (See Fig. 51.1C.) Alternatively, an end-to-side splenic to superior mesenteric artery reconstruction (no Y-graft required) can be done if adequate length and mobility of the arteries can be achieved. The aortic patch (including the coeliac and superior mesenteric arteries) of a pancreas procured from a non-liver donor requires no vascular reconstruction.

Transplant procedure

A number of important issues related to surgical technique have been, or currently are being, evaluated by pancreas transplant centres, both in the United States and abroad. Technical considerations that remain under review include:

- Must the entire pancreas be transplanted, or is a segmental graft sufficient to normalize glucose metabolism?
- Should the pancreatic duct be obliterated with a polymer (and the exocrine secretions ablated), and will this affect long-term graft endocrine function?
- Should the pancreatic exocrine secretions be retained, and if so, should they be drained externally or internally?
- For internal drainage, should the exocrine secretions be drained into the gut or into the bladder (the latter so that urinary amylase can be monitored to permit earlier diagnosis of rejection)?
- Does the use of the duodenum along with the pancreas affect long-term graft function and/or patient survival?
- Should the pancreaticoduodenal graft be placed within the peritoneal cavity or in the retroperitoneum?
- Is simultaneous pancreas–kidney transplantation beneficial or detrimental to long-term kidney and/or pancreas graft function?

Most transplant centres in the United States currently use the bladder drainage technique to manage the pancreas graft exocrine secretions. Adding a pancreaticoduodenal transplant has no apparent detrimental effect on long-term function of a kidney allograft (Morel et al 1991c). Most surgeons place both the kidney and the pancreas grafts within the peritoneal cavity through a midline incision. Bladder drainage has been associated with higher actuarial graft survival rates than intestinal drainage or duct injection (according to analysis of data from the International Pancreas Transplant Registry) (Sutherland et al 1991c, d). Technical failure seems to be least likely in the bladder drainage group.

Draining exocrine pancreatic secretions into the urinary tract was first described by Gliedman and colleagues (1973) who reported five patients who underwent pancreatic grafting with anastomosis of the donor pancreatic duct to the recipient's ureter. The modification of bladder drainage was introduced in 1983 by Sollinger and colleagues at the University of Wisconsin who anastomosed a button of duodenum surrounding the papilla of Vater to the bladder (Sollinger et al 1983, 1984). This technique was subsequently modified by Ngheim and Corry at the University of Iowa to include a segment of duodenum (Ngheim et al 1986) and was adopted at the University of Minnesota in 1984. Today, a duodenal segment of about 10 cm in length is anastomosed side-to-side to the bladder, using either a hand-sewn or EEA-stapled technique (described below).

Recipient operation

The recipient is anaesthetized and a central venous line is placed for measurement of central venous pressure. An arterial line and/or a Swan-Ganz catheter may also be used for more invasive haemodynamic monitoring. A midline abdominal incision is made from an area midway between the xiphoid process and umbilicus, and carried inferiorly to an area 3 cm superior to the pubis. Carrying the skin and fascial incision to the pubis should be avoided, since a number of lower abdominal wound infections occur when the incision is carried to the pubis. The right common, internal, and external iliac arteries and veins and the ureter are mobilized (Fig. 51.5A). Major lymphatics are ligated, even though the transplant is performed within the peritoneal cavity. The caecum is mobilized to allow ureteral and vessel exposure and comfortable placement of the pancreaticoduodenal graft. A self-retaining retractor is useful. The hypogastric artery is preserved, but all posterior branches of the common and external iliac veins are ligated and divided, including the internal iliac vein (Fig. 51.5A). The iliac vein, from the vena cava to the inguinal ligament, is completely mobilized. The portal vein of the pancreaticoduodenal graft should be extremely short, to prevent kinking and possible venous thrombosis. Mobilizing the iliac vein thus helps to complete the venous anastomosis, and also prevents tension, as well as possible laceration and anastomotic disruption of the venous anastomosis while the subsequent arterial anastomosis is completed. A venous interposition graft is never needed when the iliac vein is adequately mobilized.

The bladder is mobilized by dividing its lateral peritoneal attachments. In female recipients, it is often necessary to divide the suspensory ligaments and the ovarian vein of the right ovary; this allows the right tube and ovary to fall into the pelvis and facilitates approximation of the graft duodenum and the bladder. Crystalloid replacement is kept to a minimum while the recipient vessels are dissected; this

prevents overhydration and oedema of the graft after blood flow is restored, especially in dialysis-dependent recipients.

Before the iliac artery and vein are clamped, the recipient is systemically heparinized (70 units/kg). The ureter is placed medial to the arterial anastomosis, which is medial and superior to the venous anastomosis (Fig. 51.5A, B, C). First, the venous anastomosis is undertaken, using running 6:0 prolene sutures (Fig. 51.5B). A fine suture technique with multiple small suture bites is preferred, to prevent narrowing of the venous anastomosis. Next, the arterial anastomosis is performed, also using 6:0 prolene sutures, and using either the aortic patch (composed of the coeliac axis and superior mesenteric artery) or the common iliac artery of the vascular Y graft extension (this revascularizes the splenic and superior mesenteric arteries), or the superior mesenteric if the splenic artery was anastomosed to it (Fig. 51.5C). While the arterial anastomosis is being completed, 25 g of mannitol are administered to the recipient.

The venous clamps are removed. If the integrity of the venous anastomosis is adequate, the arterial clamps are removed (hypogastric, then common iliac, then external iliac). Arterial bleeding sites are identified and carefully controlled using 5:0 and 6:0 prolene sutures; the pancreatic parenchyma must not be injured. The entire pancreas is inspected. When haemostasis is judged to be adequate, retractors are removed from the abdominal cavity; this prevents pressure on the distal vena cava and subsequent impairment of venous outflow from the graft. After revascularization, the duodenum is cultured (aerobic, anaerobic, and fungal culture).

Pancreaticoduodenocystostomy is done using either a hand-sewn or an EEA-stapled technique (Fig. 51.6). For the hand-sewn anastomosis, a horizontal cystotomy is made on the posterosuperior aspect of the bladder, and a two-layer anastomosis in constructed between the bladder and the duodenum. Absorbable 4:0 sutures (Maxon) inserted in a simple running manner are used for the inner layer. Non-absorbable 4:0 prolene sutures are used for the outer layer of interrupted seromuscular Lembert sutures. If the distal duodenal segment is still open, it is closed using a TA55 or 90 stapler. The staple line is oversewn and subsequently inverted with an interrupted layer of 4:0 prolene sutures, as described above for the proximal duodenal closure (Fig. 51.3).

For the stapled pancreaticoduodenocystostomy, the duodenum is sized. A circular EEA stapler (25, 27, or 29 mm in diameter with the anvil removed) is inserted into the open distal end of the duodenum and then passed gently toward the proximal duodenum (Fig. 51.6A). The rod projecting from within the ring of staples is pushed through the wall of the duodenum opposite the papilla; electrocautery facilitates this procedure. The bladder, previously mobilized by dividing its lateral peritoneal attachments, is opened anteriorly (Fig. 51.6A). The

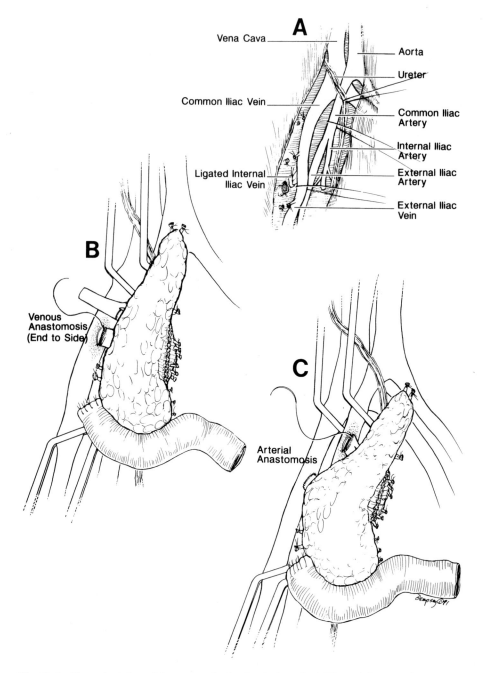

Fig. 51.5 Transplantation of the pancreaticoduodenal allograft. **A** The recipient vessels are prepared. Note that all deep branches of the common and external iliac veins are ligated and divided. The vein is brought lateral to the artery. The ureter is mobilized and brought medial to the artery. **B** The venous anastomosis is done end-to-side, with the portal vein of the pancreas graft anastomosed to the proximal external or distal common iliac vein. **C** The arterial anastomosis is done after the venous anastomosis and placed superior to the venous anastomosis. The recipient's common iliac artery is frequently used as the site for the arterial anastomosis.

duodenum of the pancreas graft and the bladder must be approximated without tension. The rod of the EEA the stapler is then pushed through the posterosuperior wall of the bladder under direct vision (facilitated by the electrocautery). The anvil is attached to the stapler from within the bladder, and stapler is closed and fired. The anvil is removed and the staple rings examined for com-

pleteness. The circular stapler is removed from the distal aspect of the duodenal segment. To facilitate haemostasis and secure the stapled duodenocystostomy, continuous 4:0 Maxon sutures are used to overrun the completed duodenocystostomy circular staple line from within the bladder (Fig. 51.6B). The distal duodenal segment is closed in three layers, as described above for the hand-sewn

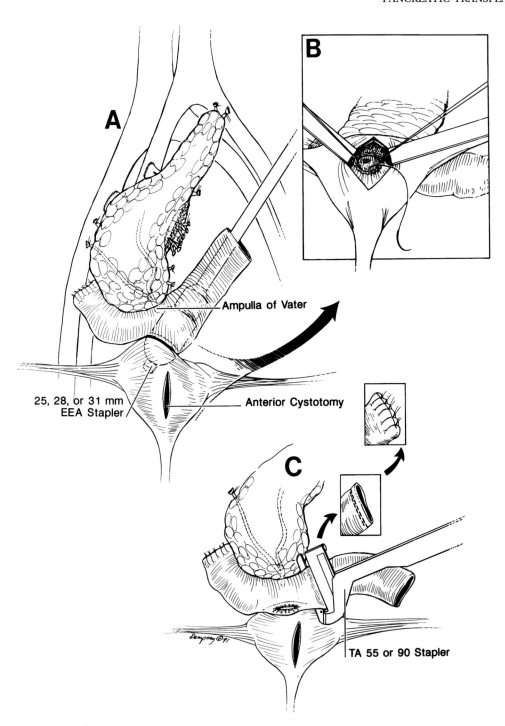

Fig. 51.6 Managment of the pancreatic exocrine secretions: The stapled duodenocystostomy. **A** A 25, 28, or 31mm EEA stapler is passed proximally through the open end of the distal duodenal segment to an area opposite the ampulla. A cystotomy is made on the anterosuperior aspect of the bladder to facilitate exposure and placement of the anvil of the EEA stapler. The anastomosis is done between the antimesenteric border of the duodenum and the posterosuperior aspect of the bladder. **B** The EEA staple line is reinforced with a whip stitch of 4:0 absorbable sutures (PDS or Maxon) to facilitate haemostasis and ensure a watertight closure. **C** The distal duodenal segment is closed with a TA 55 or 90 stapler. Excess distal duodenum is removed. The TA stapler places a parallel row of staples. The distal duodenal segment closure is reinforced in two layers, similar to the proximal duodenal reinforcement shown in Figure 51.3.

duodenocystostomy (Fig. 51.6C). The anterior cystotomy is closed following irrigation of the Foley catheter.

If a combined kidney and pancreas transplant is done, the kidney is usually transplanted after the pancreas, unless the preservation time of the pancreas was extremely short, or the recipient has a history of problems, with volume overload. The kidney is transplanted to the left iliac fossa, using an intraperitoneal approach. The vascular anastomoses are done to the external iliac artery and vein distal to the mesentery of the sigmoid colon. The sigmoid colon is retracted medially to provide exposure to complete the vascular anastomosis. The arterial blood supply or venous return from the pancreas must not be impeded during this retraction. A standard Litch (for the hand-sewn duodenocystostomy) of Leadbetter–Politano ureteroneocystostomy (for the stapled duodenocystostomy) is performed (Fig. 51.7A–D). After the ureteroneocystostomy is completed, the Foley catheter

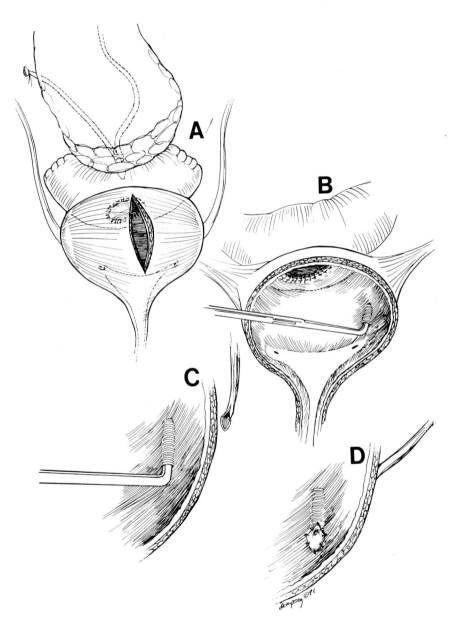

Fig. 51.7 The ureteroneocystostomy. For simultaneous pancreas–kidney grafts where the stapler was used for the duodenocystostomy, a Leadbetter–Politano ureteroneocystostomy is done through the anterior cystotomy. The ureter is placed lateral and inferior to the duodenocystostomy and superior to the trigone and the native ureteral orifice. (For the hand-sewn duodenocystostomy, a Litch ureteroneocystostomy is done.) **A** The completed duodenocystostomy as seen through the open anterior cystotomy. **B** Creation of the submucosal tunnel for the Leadbetter–Politano ureteroneocystostomy. **C** The ureter being brought in apposition to the bladder. **D** The completed Leadbetter–Politano ureteroneocystotomy.

is irrigated and the bladder is closed in three layers using running 4:0 Maxon sutures for the mucosal and submucosal layers and interrupted 4:0 Maxon sutures for the seromuscular layer. After the kidney transplant and the bladder closure (Fig. 51.8), the abdomen is copiously irrigated with an antibiotic (Keflin, 1 g/1000 ml saline) and amphotericin irrigation solution (10 mg/1000 ml of water). The fascia of the abdominal wall is closed with interrupted sutures and the skin closed with clips. No intraperitoneal or wound drains are used. A Foley catheter is left in the bladder (through the urethra) for at least 7 days.

For pancreas recipients who already have a functioning renal transplant on the right side, we place the pancreaticoduodenal graft on the opposite side (Fig. 51.9). We do not interrupt blood flow to the kidney when placing the pancreas graft. The vessels of the graft are anastomosed to the common iliac artery and vein proximal to the mesentery of the sigmoid colon. Caution should be used when mobilizing the left common iliac vein proximal to the mesentery of the sigmoid colon. After the pancreas is revascularized, the duodenocystostomy is done as described above (Fig. 51.6). The transplant ureter must be avoided while the bladder is being mobilized and subsequently closed in pancreas-after-kidney-transplant procedures.

RESULTS

Current patient and graft survival rates for pancreas transplantation are now similar to those achieved with transplantation of other solid organs. As of May 1991, 3100 pancreas transplants had been reported to the International Pancreas Transplant Registry (Sutherland et al 1991c, d). The most recent Registry data analysis, in

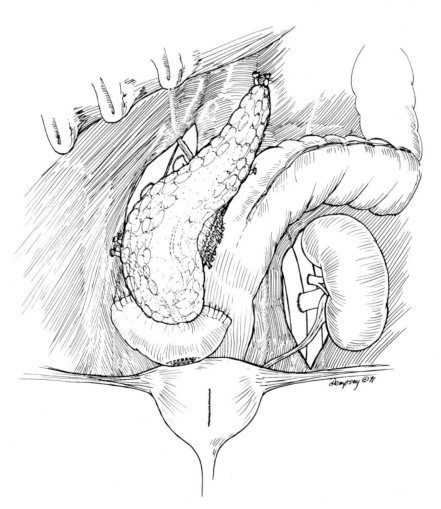

Fig. 51.8 The completed simultaneous pancreaticoduodenal and renal allografts in situ. The renal allograft is placed intraperitoneally, and the vascular anastomoses are placed distal to the mesentery of the sigmoid colon. This facilitates percutaneous biopsy of the intraperitoneal kidney by minimizing intervening large and small bowel between the abdominal wall and the kidney. (See text for details.)

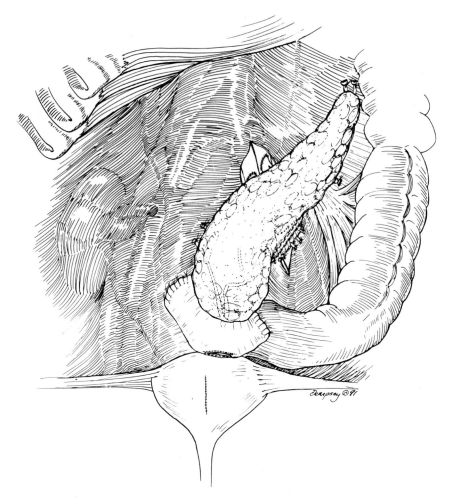

Fig. 51.9 The pancreaticoduodenal allograft performed on the left side. If the patient has undergone a previous renal transplant on the right side, the pancreaticoduodenal allograft is best placed on the left side. The vascular anastomoses are placed proximal to the mesentery of the sigmoid colon. This permits a more comfortable lie for the pancreas after the duodenocystostomy is completed.

October 1990, showed 2871 pancreas transplants (2703 primary, 168 regrafts). Recipient and pancreas graft survival rates continue to improve with time. In five consecutive eras, 1-year patient survival rates were 41, 71, 79, 86 and 91% respectively (Fig. 51.10A), and 1-year graft survival rates were 5, 21, 40, 52 and 68% respectively (Fig. 51.10B) ($P \leq 0.002$ for all comparisons after 1977). For 1347 primary pancreas transplants reported during 1988–1990, the 1-year graft functional survival rate was 70% and the 1-year patient survival rate was 91%. Multiple variables may affect outcome after pancreas transplantation. These include exocrine secretion (duct) management technique, recipient category (i.e. simultaneous pancreas and kidney transplantation (SPK), pancreas after kidney (PAK), or pancreas alone (PTA)), duration of preservation time, and preservation solution. Diagnosis of pancreas rejection remains problematic, especially for PTA recipients, since a simultaneously transplanted kidney is not available in their case to allow host antidonor immune reactivity to be monitored.

In general, the use of triple or quadruple immunosuppressive regimens (Sollinger et al 1987), a decreasing incidence of technical failure in transplantation of both non-urinary (Tyden et al 1987) and urinary drained pancreas grafts (13% for 1988–1990 cases vs. 23% for 1986–1987 cases, Burke et al 1988), and monitoring of renal allograft function when the kidney comes from the same donor as the pancreas (LaRocca et al 1987, Illner et al 1987, Tyden et al 1987, Sollinger et al 1988, Cosimi et al 1988, Wright et al 1989, Sutherland et al 1989a, Schulak et al 1990) have been associated with a dramatic improvement in results. SPK transplants are now a routine in uraemic diabetic patients at many institutions, and the functional survival rate of the pancreas is nearly the same as that of the kidney for US cases (Sutherland et al 1991a, c, d).

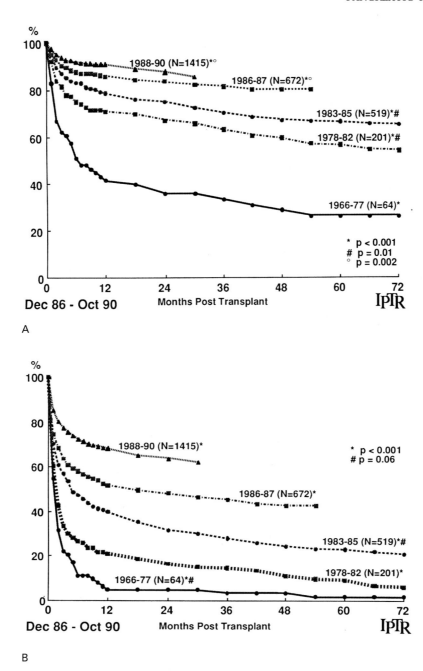

Fig. 51.10 A Recipient survival rates and **B** graft functional (insulin-independent) survival rates for pancreas transplants done throughout the world and reported to the International Pancreas Transplant Registry in 5 consecutive eras since 1966.

Since 1 October 1987, it has been mandatory for all US institutions performing organ transplants to report demographic and outcome information to organ transplant registries maintained under the auspices of the Scientific Studies Committee of the United Network for Organ Sharing (UNOS). UNOS operates the Organ Procurement and Transplant Network, under contract with the US Department of Health and Human Services. Between 1 October 1987 and 30 September 1990, 1021 pancreas transplants were reported to the UNOS Registry, 515 of which were done in 1990. The number of pancreas transplants in the US has increased by about 50% in each recent 12-month period since October 1987. The patient and graft functional survival (defined as insulin independence) rates for all U.S. cases in recent eras are shown in Figure 51.11. For the most recent era, 1-year patient and graft functional survival rates were 92% and 72%, respectively.

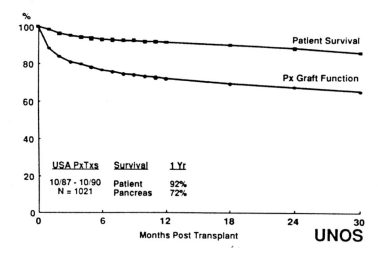

Fig. 51.11   Recipient and pancreas graft functional survival rates for all US pancreas transplants reported to the UNOS Registry (between 1 October 1987 and 21 October 1990).

Duct management technique

The worldwide functional graft survival rate curves for pancreas grafts transplanted with bladder drainage (BD), duct injection (DI) or intestinal drainage (ID), are shown in Figure 51.12. The most frequently used technique, bladder drainage, was associated with a significantly higher graft functional survival rate than either DI or ID. Bladder drainage had a lower technical failure rate (14%) than DI (25%) or ID (23%). Even for technically successful cases, 1-year graft functional survival rates were significantly higher for BD (75%, 1354 cases) than for DI (72%, 242 cases) or ID (66%, 133 cases).

The overwhelming majority (980 cases, or 96%) of pancreas transplants done between 1 October 1987 and

30 September 1990 in the US used the bladder drainage technique; only 33 used ID. In contrast, only half of the non-US cases reported during this era used BD (249 cases); DI (183 cases) was more popular than ID (48 cases) for non-US transplants.

An analysis of bladder drainage cases in the US showed 1-year patient and graft survival rates of 92 and 71%, respectively. For non-US BD cases, the 1-year graft survival rate was 62%. The 1-year functional graft survival rates for technically successful BD cases (n = 877) in the US. was 81% as opposed to 73% for comparable non-US cases (n = 214). The technical failure rate for US BD cases was 11% while for non-US cases it was 14%.

With intestinal drainage, the 1-year patient and graft

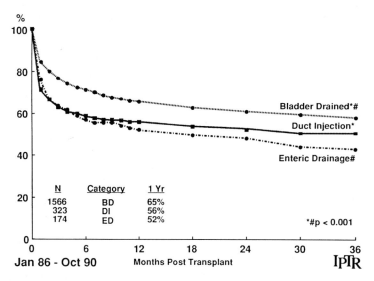

Fig. 51.12   Pancreas graft functional (insulin-independent) survival rates worldwide according to duct management categories for cases reported to the International Registry between 1986 and 1990.

survival rates in the US were 90 and 67%, respectively. For non-US intestinal drainage pancreas transplants, the 1-year graft survival rate was 39%, and not significantly different. For technically successful ID pancreas transplants, the 1-year functional graft survival rate was 80% for US cases (n = 28) and 47% for non-US cases (n = 40). The technical failure rate for ID pancreas transplants was 15% in the US as opposed to 17% for non-US cases.

With duct injection, the 1-year graft survival rate in non-US cases was 58% for all cases and 77% for technically successful cases (n = 135). There were no US cases for comparison. The technical failure rate for non-US duct injection pancreas transplants was 26%.

Recipient categories

As shown in Figure 51.13, the majority (82%) of pancreas grafts transplanted in the US between 1 October

1987 and 30 September 1990 were done simultaneously with a kidney transplant. In most of the remaining cases, the pancreas was transplanted after a kidney, but some were pancreas transplants alone in non-uraemic, non-kidney transplant recipients. In all three categories, 1-year patient survival rates were 92% (Fig. 51.13A). However, 1-year graft survival rates in the US (Fig. 51.13B), were significantly higher in the SPK (77%) than the PAK (52%) and the PTA (54%) groups. For technically successful cases, 1-year graft survival rates were 86% for SPK (n = 746), 62% for PAK (n = 98), and 59% for PTA (n = 62). The corresponding technical failure rates were 10, 12, and 13% respectively. Two simultaneous pancreas–liver–kidney (SPK) transplants and three simultaneous pancreas–liver transplants (PLT, non-cluster) have been reported to the UNOS Registry.

The overall US results with SPK transplants during the first 3 years of the UNOS Registry are excellent (Fig. 51.14). Uraemic diabetic recipients of a double transplant

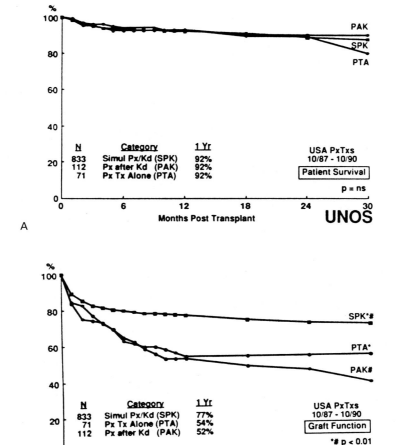

Fig. 51.13 A Recipient survival rates and **B** graft functional survival rates by recipient category (SPK vs. PTA vs. PAK) for US cases reported to the UNOS Registry between 1 October 1987 and 21 October 1990.

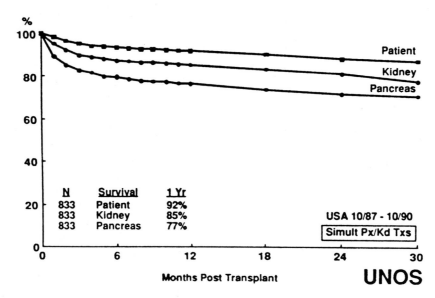

Fig. 51.14   Patient, kidney, and pancreas graft survival rates for simultaneous pancreas–kidney recipients for US cases reported to the UNOS Registry between 1 October 1987 and 21 October 1990.

have a 92% probability of being alive, an 85% probability of being dialysis-free, and a 77% probability of being insulin-independent at 1 year. During the second year, the probability of losing their life or either graft was no more than 5%.

A slightly higher percentage (86%) of non-US cases reported during the same interval were SPK transplants (n = 417); the rest were PAK (n = 25) and PTA (n = 37). For non-US cases, 1-year patient survival rates were 88% for SPK, 88% for PAK, and 93% for PTA and 1-year graft survival rates were 63, 15 and 26% respectively, results which were significantly worse than those achieved in the US. For technically successful non-US cases, 1-year graft survival rates were 75% for SPK (n = 349), 20% for PAK (n = 19), and 53% for PTA (n = 20). The corresponding technical failure rates for non-US cases were 14, 24 and 46% respectively. Differences in graft survival between US and non-US cases for PAK and PTA groups can be attributed to the higher technical failure rate for non-US cases.

Preservation solution

Most (81%) pancreas grafts transplanted in the US in the 3 years up to 21 October 1990 were preserved by cold storage in UW solution (Table 51. 2). Use of UW solution was associated with higher 1-year graft survival rates than either Collins or plasma-based solution, but the differences were not statistically significant (Table 51.2).

For non-US pancreas transplants during the same era, UW was used in only half the cases and Collins solution was much more popular outside the US (Table 51.2). The graft survival rates with UW solution were significantly higher for US than non-US cases, both for all cases and technically successful cases. Thus, the generally higher graft survival rates in the US cases is not explained by the more frequent use of UW solution.

Preservation time

The duration of pancreas graft preservation had little influence on outcome (Table 51.3), and does not explain

Table 51.2   Influence of preservation solution on results of pancreatic transplantation (1.10.1987 – 21.10.1990)

| | | All cases | | Technically successful cases | |
Solution	n	% 1-year graft survival rate	% Technical Failure	n	% 1-year graft survival rate
US					
University of Wisconsin (UW)	830	74	10	747	82
Collins	89	69	12	78	77
Plasma-based	88	62	14	76	72
Non-US					
University of Wisconsin	243	59	18	200	73
Collins	207	60	22	161	76
Others	32	34	11	25	78

Table 51.3 Influence of preservation time on results of pancreatic transplantation (1.10.1987–30.9.1990)

Preservation time (hours)	n	All cases			Technically successful cases	
		% 1 year graft survival rate	% Technical failure		n	% 1 year graft survival rate
US						
< 12	439	72	12		386	82
12–24	422	72	9		383	79
24–30	42	72	7		42	78
> 30	8	50	12		7	57
Unknown	98	79	—		—	87
Non-US						
< 12	412	57	19		333	71
12–24	49	62	18		40	80
Unknown	21	—	—		—	—

the higher overall graft survival rates in the US. Indeed, preservation times have tended to be much longer in the US, where preservation for up to 30 hours is not a limiting factor in pancreas transplantation. This is probably true for non-US cases in which the pancreas was stored in UW solution, but preservation times over 24 hours have not been tested outside the US. Almost all pancreas transplants in non-US centres have been undertaken with grafts preserved for less than 12 hours (Table 51.3) but the survival rate of 57% was significantly inferior to that recorded in US cases.

Diagnosis and treatment of rejection episodes

Early diagnosis of pancreas graft rejection has been more difficult in nonuraemic, diabetic, non-kidney transplant recipients than in uraemic recipients of a simultaneous pancreas–kidney transplant from the same donor. In SPK recipients, kidney graft function serves as an early marker of rejection at a time when the process may be subclinical. The bladder drainage technique allows rejection episodes to be diagnosed early, especially in PTA recipients. Urinary amylase activity is a direct reflection of graft exocrine function, and during rejection episodes declines before hyperglycaemia occurs (Prieto et al 1987a). Measurement of serum anodal trypsinogen (Marks et al 1990) and serial observation of urinary cytology (Radio et al 1991) after bladder drainage pancreas transplants may also help to diagnose rejection early. Rejection episodes can usually be reversed if treatment is initiated when urine amylase decreases, while treatment after hyperglycaemia has occurred is much less successful (Prieto et al 1987b). When in doubt, rejection in a bladder drainage pancreas graft can be confirmed by a transcystoscopic biopsy (Perkins et al 1990, Brayman et al 1991).

Pancreas transplant alone in non-uraemic diabetics

Only one centre, the University of Minnesota, has a large experience with pancreas transplants alone in patients without end-stage diabetic nephropathy. More than 160 such procedures (out of 400) have been undertaken. Initially, pancreas-only transplants had a high rate of graft loss from irreversible rejection, particularly in the non-bladder-drained cases (Sutherland et al 1984a). The bladder drainage technique was adopted along with a quadruple immunosuppression regimen similar to that used by other groups (Sollinger et al 1987). With bladder drainage, the rejection loss rate was lowered (Sutherland et al 1988). Anti-rejection treatment was initiated before there was a change in blood sugar levels, and was based on a decline in urine amylase (Prieto et al 1987a, b). However, even with bladder drainage, the functional survival rate of pancreas-only transplants was initially less than that of SPK transplants (Gruessner et al 1990).

Analysis of the experience with pancreas-only transplants at the University of Minnesota indicated that the results were significantly better in recipients of grafts from donors mismatched for 0 or 1 than for 2 DR antigens (So et al 1990). Quadruple immunosuppression, in use since 1984 (Sutherland et al 1984a), was then modified to include 14 days rather than 7 days of antilymphocyte globulin for induction immunosuppression. Maintenance immunosuppression (cyclosporine, azathioprine, and prednisone) was continued. Rejection episodes, formerly treated on the basis of a greater than 50% decline in urine amylase from baseline, have since 1988 been treated on the basis of a greater than 25% decline. Transcystoscopic pancreas and duodenal allograft biopsies have also been used, following the lead of the Mayo Clinic (Perkins et al 1990, Brayman et al 1991). With these changes in protocol, 1-year pancreas graft survival rate for bladder drainage PTA cases (n = 39) was 61%, and for PAK cases (n = 34) it was 58% in the era 1988–1990. Patient survival rates at 1 year for these cases were 95 and 93% respectively. Thus, it appears that by deliberate matching for HLA-DR antigens, use of antilymphocyte globulin for induction immunosuppression, and early treatment of rejection episodes, pancreas graft survival rates approaching those achieved with simultaneous pancreas–kidney transplants are also possible in patients receiving pancreas-only transplants.

One method of achieving good HLA matches is to transplant segmental pancreas grafts from living related donors (Sutherland et al 1984b). The largest experience with living related pancreas transplants is at the University of Minnesota, where more than 70 have been performed in a 10-year period (Sutherland et al 1991e). The criteria which relatives have to fulfil before becoming a hemi-pancreas donor include normal fasting and postprandial glucose levels, a normal oral glucose tolerance test, and an age which is more than 10 years older than the age of onset of diabetes in the recipient; in addition the recipient must have had diabetes for at least 10 years. When these demographic criteria are met, family members are not at any higher risk than the general population of developing diabetes in the future (Barbosa et al 1977, Kendall et al 1989, 1990).

Patients who developed cytotoxic antibodies (from previous blood transfusions, transplants, or pregnancies) rarely have negative crossmatches to cadaver donors, but often have a negative crossmatch to a closely matched family member. In these situations, a living-related donor may be the only practical way of achieving a pancreas transplant. The incidence of rejection episodes is also much lower for transplants from related donors than from cadaver donors, and even methods other than bladder drainage can be applied with a relatively high success rate for pancreas-only grafts in this specific situation (Sutherland et al 1991d, e, Morel et al 1991a).

Kidney graft survival in SPK recipients

Kidney graft survival rates in SPK recipients were determined for cases reported to the Registry between 1 October 1987 and 30 September 1990. The 1-year kidney graft survival rate was 85% for all US SPK transplants (all duct management techniques) during this period (Fig. 51.14). Where the pancreas failed for technical reasons, the 1-year kidney graft survival rate was 69% (n = 86); where the procedure was technically successful it was 88% (n = 747). Interestingly, the kidney and pancreas graft survival rates were exactly the same in the technically successful cases, a finding consistent with the hypothesis that the risk of immunological failure is similar for both organs in recipients of double transplants.

For non-US SPK cases during the same era, the 1-year kidney graft survival rate was 78% for all cases, falling to 69% when the pancreas graft failed for technical reasons (n = 68) and remaining at 79% when the procedure was technically successful (n = 349).

Metabolic consequences of a pancreas transplant

It has been well documented that successful pancreas transplantation normalizes levels of fasting glucose and glycosylated haemoglobin (Cosimi et al 1988, Sutherland et al 1989a, Morel et al 1991b). The metabolic consequences of a pancreas graft with systemic venous drainage on beta cell function has been evaluated by examining insulin and C-peptide responses to intravenous glucose and intravenous arginine (Diem et al 1990a). Basal insulin levels are elevated in pancreas graft recipients, compared with age-and sex-matched controls or non-diabetic kidney recipients on similar immunosuppression. Acute insulin responses to intravenous glucose were approximately two to three times greater than in control subjects and about 50% higher than in non-diabetic kidney recipients. However, integrated acute C-peptide responses to glucose were not statistically different when comparing pancreas recipients with kidney recipients and with control subjects. Similar insulin and C-peptide results were obtained with both intravenous glucose and intravenous arginine. Recipients of pancreas allografts with systemic venous drainage have elevated basal and stimulated insulin levels. These alterations are primarily due to alterations of first-pass hepatic insulin clearance, although insulin resistance secondary to immunosuppression (including prednisone) probably played a role. To avoid hyperinsulinaemia and its possible long-term adverse consequences, transplantation of pancreas allografts into sites with portal rather than systemic venous drainage may be considered (Land et al 1987, Secchi et al 1987, Ostman et al 1989, Osei et al 1990).

Glucagon, catecholamine, and pancreatic polypeptide secretion in pancreas recipients has also been examined (Diem et al 1990b). Successful pancreas transplantation results in improvement of glucose recovery after insulin-induced hypoglycaemia. Basal glucagon levels were also significantly higher in pancreas transplant recipients, compared with type I diabetic patients not receiving a pancreas graft and with normal subjects. Glucagon responses to insulin-induced hypoglycaemia were significantly greater in the pancreas recipients, compared with control subjects. No differences were observed in epinephrine and pancreatic polypeptide responses to hypoglycaemia. Type I diabetic recipients of pancreas grafts demonstrated significant improvement in glucose recovery after hypoglycaemia, and this was associated with improved glucagon secretion. The lack of improvement in pancreatic polypeptide secretion was interpreted as evidence that the allograft remained denervated after transplantation. An earlier series reported post-transplant, but not pretransplant, data for hormonal responses to insulin-induced hypoglycaemia (Bosi et al 1988). Given the improved counterregulation of hypoglycaemia, pancreas transplants should be considered for type I diabetic patients who are at risk for severe episodes of insulin-induced hypoglycaemia and who are unable to control their disease with diet, altered insulin dosages, or exogenous glucagon injections.

Course of secondary diabetic complications in pancreas transplant recipients

Interpreting data regarding the course of secondary complications after pancreas transplantation is difficult. In SPK recipients, uraemia and diabetes are corrected at the same time. Uraemic diabetic patients who receive only a kidney transplant are a necessary control group when determining the effect that restoring euglycaemia has on the course of retinopathy and neuropathy. Pre- and post-transplant studies in patients who are not uraemic at the time of pancreas transplantation can also provide useful information but interpretation is difficult unless control groups of non-pancreas transplant patients, or patients with early failed transplants, are also studied.

Neuropathy

The Stockholm group reported only minimal improvement in neuropathy at 1 year in diabetic SPK recipients. No difference was observed when the results were compared to uraemic diabetic recipients of kidney transplants alone (Solders et al 1987). Since all of the Stockholm patients were uraemic with extremely advanced neuropathy before transplantation, these observations must be interpreted with caution. Further deterioration could hardly have occurred, making it difficult to discern any effect that pancreas transplantation could have had on halting the progress of diabetic neuropathy.

In contrast, a follow-up of diabetic nonuraemic PTA recipients at the University of Minnesota showed statistically significant improvement in nerve conduction velocities after 1 year (Sutherland et al 1988). In a subsequent study, evoked muscle and nerve action potentials and amplitudes remained stable or improved in patients who maintained long-term pancreas graft function, but the amplitudes continued to decrease in pancreas transplants recipients whose grafts failed early (Kennedy et al 1990). An index (deviation from the normal mean expressed in standard deviations) of neuropathy was calculated for motor (average of eight separate nerve conduction velocities), sensory (average of five nerve conduction velocities), and autonomic (mean of two cardiorespiratory reflex tests) function. In recipients studied before and or after a successful pancreas transplant, the motor nerve index gradually improved, and sensory and autonomic indices stabilized. Patients who were not transplanted or who had early graft failure, within 3 months, showed a decline in all three parameters. Three years after baseline testing, there were significant differences between the two groups for the indices of motor and sensory nerve function. Thus, it appears that restoring

a normoglycaemic state by a functioning pancreas transplant can halt the progression of diabetic polyneuropathy.

Mortality rates in patients with either severe peripheral neuropathy or severe autonomic neuropathy have been analysed (Navarro et al 1990). In those who were not transplanted or whose transplant failed, mortality at 5 years was nearly 40%. In those with successful transplants, it was less than 20%, and the difference was statistically significant (Fig. 51.15A, B).

Retinopathy

Improvement in retinopathy in uraemic diabetic patients after a successful SPK transplant has been reported, but the studies have been poorly controlled (Ulbig et al 1987). In the Minnesota series, PTA recipients were nouuraemic at baseline (Ramsay et al 1989). Patients with successful pancreas transplants (continuous function for >1 year) were studied over a 5-year period and compared with those whose grafts failed early (< 3 months). The probability of progression to a higher grade of retinopathy during the first 3 years post-transplant was 30% in both groups. After 3 years, however, retinopathy stablized in patients with successful transplants but continued to deteriorate in those with failed grafts. At 5 years, the cumulative percentage of patients with failed grafts who had advanced to a more severe state of retinopathy was 55%, compared with 30% in the successfully transplanted group. For diabetic patients with advanced retinopathy, a successful pancreas transplant will not immediately change the course of retinopathy. However, retinopathy may ultimately be stabilized by persistent normoglycaemia.

Nephropathy

In patients undergoing SPK transplants, recurrence of diabetic nephropathy in the transplanted kidney is generally prevented as long as the pancreas continues to function. In some cases, pancreas transplants have been performed several years after a kidney transplant, allowing study of the effect of hyperglycaemia followed by euglycaemia on progression of any recurrent diabetic nephropathy which may have developed.

Microscopic lesions of diabetic nephropathy commonly appear in kidneys transplanted to diabetic patients who do not undergo a pancreas transplant (Mauer et al 1983). The ability of a pancreas transplant to prevent such lesions is suggested by follow-up biopsies in cases from Stockholm (Bohman et al 1985, 1987). Glomerular mesangial volumes (GMV) and glomerular basement membrane (GBM) widths in renal allograft biopsies, taken after transplantation in diabetic recipients of a kidney alone, were compared with biopsies from kidneys

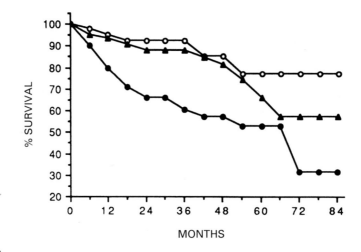

A

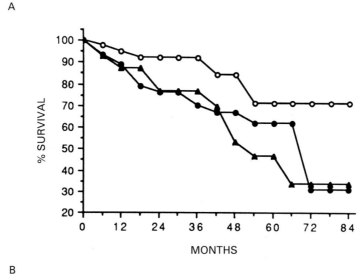

B

Fig. 51.15 **A** Survival curves for diabetic patients with abnormalities in cardiorespiratory reflex tests whohad functioning pancreas transplants (○) failed pancreas transplants (●), or no pancreas transplant (▲). **B** Survival curves for diabetic patients with abnormalities in nerve conduction studies who had functioning pancreas transplants (○), failed pancreas transplants (●), or no pancreas transplant (▲). (From Navarro et al 1990 Diabetes 39:802–806, with permission.)

transplanted simultaneously with successful pancreas grafts. Lesions of diabetic nephropathy were present in most kidneys transplanted in diabetic patients who did not undergo a pancreas transplant, but were completely absent in recipients of successful pancreas transplants. GMV were smaller in recipients of pancreas transplants than in those who received a kidney alone. GMB thickness was above the normal range (Steffes et al 1983) in biopsies obtained more then 27 months post transplant in diabetic recipients of kidney transplants alone. In contrast, GBM width was within the normal range in all kidney biopsies from non-diabetic recipients or from diabetic recipients of a pancreas transplanted simultaneously with the kidney.

The Minnesota group has found that a pancreas transplant after a kidney transplant can halt the progression of lesions that evolved in the renal graft before the pancreas transplant (Bilous et al 1989). In kidneys biopsied an average of 8 years after transplantation, the mean GMV was significantly less in those who had a successful pancreas transplant (within an average of 4 years after the kidney transplant) than in those who did not.

Restoring normoglycaemia with a pancreas transplant also appears to influence the course of pre-existing lesions of diabetic nephropathy in the native kidneys of non-uraemic, diabetic patients without end-stage renal disease. In a preliminary report from the University of Minnesota (Bilous et al 1987), native kidneys were biopsied in seven nonuraemic recipients with early to moderately advanced diabetic nephropathy (albuminuria was present in all; mean creatinine clearance was 90 ± 20 ml/min) before and 2 or more years after a successful pancreas transplant. Mean GMV was significantly reduced post-transplant, compared with pretransplant biopsies. These observations are consistent with the hypothesis that restoring normoglycaemia after a pancreas transplant may prevent or halt progression of early but established diabetic nephropathy. Interestingly, despite the improved morphological findings, the mean creatinine clearance of the pancreas transplant patients was less at 2 years (60 ± 14 ml/min) than at baseline (90 ± 15 ml/min). The nephrotoxic effect of cyclosporine may explain this apparent paradox. An initial decline in creatinine clearance induced by cyclosporine in non-uremic, non-kidney recipients of pancreas transplants is usually not followed by further deterioration in renal function (DeFrancisco et al 1988). A few PTA recipients have become uraemic in spite of a functioning pancreas graft. In general, these patients had an uneventful kidney transplant a year or more after the pancreas graft (Sutherland et al 1988, Sutherland et al 1989a, Morel et al 1991c, Stevens et al 1991). Nonetheless, in most non-uraemic diabetic PTA recipients, serum creatinine and creatinine clearance values at 1–5 years post-transplant are no different from 6 months post-transplant.

In summary, in all three categories of diabetic pancreas graft recipients (those with a simultaneous kidney, those transplanted with a kidney before the pancreas, and those with a pancreas transplant alone), histological observations indicate that restoring euglycaemia prevents or halts the progression of diabetic nephropathy. Whether this benefit offsets the nephrotoxic effect of cyclosporine in the third category (non-uraemic, diabetic non-kidney transplant recipient) is a critical question. This question, of course, could be addressed if a non-nephrotoxic immunosuppressant can be developed, which is as effective as cyclosporine in preventing rejection.

Recurrence of autoimmune diabetes in the pancreas graft

Selective beta cell destruction in type I diabetes mellitus is a consequence of a chronic autoimmune process (Eisenbarth 1986). Theoretically, the beta cells of a transplanted pancreas may be susceptible to the autoimmune process. The relative contribution of disparities in the major histocompatibility complex locus between donor and recipient to the process of recurrent autoimmune beta cell destruction is not yet completely defined. Importantly, recurrence of autoimmune diabetes in segmental pancreas transplants from non-diabetic donors to their diabetic identical twin can be prevented by adequate immunosuppression (Sutherland et al 1984c, Sibley et al 1985). Recipients of pancreas transplants from identical twin donors immunosuppressed with low dose azathioprine and/or cyclosporine enjoy freedom from disease recurrence (Sutherland et al 1989b). Moreover, immuno-suppressive regimens in diabetic recipients of cadaver pancreas grafts have generally been more potent than appears to be necessary to prevent autoimmune disease recurrence in the twin pancreas transplant cases. Thus, as long as generalized immunosuppression is adequate to prevent rejection of a pancreas graft, disease recurrence ('isletitis' with selective beta cell destruction) should be prevented (Sibley & Sutherland 1987).

QUALITY OF LIFE

The quality of life of 131 pancreas transplant recipients was studied 1–11 years post-transplant by Zehrer and Gross (1990, 1991) at the University of Minnesota. Patients with a functioning graft (n = 65) described their current quality of life and rated their health significantly more favourably than those with a non-functioning graft. For example, of patients with a functioning graft, 68% expressed overall satisfaction with their life, 89% felt healthier since their transplant, and 78% reported that they could care for themselves and undertake their routine daily activities. In contrast, of patients with a non-functioning graft, only 48% expressed overall satisfaction with their life, 25% felt healthier since their transplant, and 56% reported that they could care for themselves and undertake their routine daily activities. Regardless of graft function, most patients were comfortable with their decision to have the transplant and most recipients with a functioning graft reported that they would have another transplant if their graft failed.

CONCLUSIONS

The results of pancreas transplantation have improved with time and do not appear to have reached a plateau. In the US, graft survival rates are now similar to those of other organ transplants, particularly when the pancreas is grafted simultaneously with a kidney. There is room for improvement in the results of pancreas-only transplants given that even in the US, where most of these transplants are done, little more than 50% result in insulin independence at 1 year. However, the US results since 1987 indicate that more than 75% of uraemic recipients of simultaneous pancreas and kidney grafts can expect to be insulin-independent as well as dialysis-free more than 1 year post-transplant. Successful pancreas transplantation may not restore all diabetic patients to normal health and function, but recipients report a significantly better quality of life than those who remain diabetic.

Young uraemic diabetic candidates for cadaver donor kidney transplants should almost always be considered for a simultaneous pancreas transplant. Immunosuppressive management is essentially no different from when a kidney transplant alone is performed, and the surgical risk of adding the pancreas is low.

Diabetic patients with nephropathy who have received previous kidney transplants, from either related or cadaver donors, can receive a subsequent pancreas transplant. In our view, the optimal approach with uraemic diabetic patients is to perform a living donor kidney graft, and then transplant a pancreas graft, usually from a cadaver donor. There is a shortage of kidneys, and the long-term functional graft survival rates of kidneys from a living related donor are superior to those from a cadaver.

Non-uraemic, diabetic, non-kidney transplant patients have more stringent criteria (University of Michigan Pancreas Transplant Evaluation Committee 1988). Patients with labile diabetes and glycaemic excursions so extreme that day-to-day living is difficult can be considered for a transplant for this reason alone. Some patients in this category have diabetes secondary to total pancreatectomy (Gruessner et al 1991). The immunosuppressive risks are clearly being substituted for the risks of insulin administration in such patients. In nonuraemic diabetic patients who have undergone a pancreas transplant, prospective studies of quality of life generally indicate an improvement (Nakache et al 1989, Voruganti & Sells 1989, Zehrer & Gross 1990, 1991, Corry & Zehr 1990). This is consistent with studies demonstrating that patients who receive a kidney also usually have a higher quality of life than those who are not transplanted and remain on dialysis.

Another reason for pancreas transplantation in non-uraemic, diabetic non-kidney transplant patients is to prevent progression of secondary complications. Retinopathy by itself is generally not an indication, since a beneficial effect on this complication of pancreas transplantation alone is delayed, or not seen at all (Ramsay et al 1988). Neuropathy improves or stabilizes after pancreas transplantation (Kennedy et al 1990), but the actual or predicted disability of neuropathy must be sufficient to justify subjecting the patient to the immunosuppressive risks. In patients with improved cardiorespiratory reflexes from severe autoimmune neuropathy, a successful pancreas transplant may actually improve longevity (Navarro et al 1990).

In summary, pancreas transplantation in the general diabetic population, including those who have not yet exhibited secondary complications, awaits the availability of minimal or non-toxic immunosuppression. Specific strategies to suppress a specific immune response in humans (e.g. by bone marrow transplantation) may also help to broaden the guidelines for pancreas recipient selection.

EDITOR'S NOTES ON ISLET TRANSPLANTATION

Transplantation of pancreatic islets offers an attractive alternative to organ grafting as a means of maintaining normoglycaemia in diabetes mellitus and, hopefully, preventing or arresting its vascular complications. Although considerable success has attended the transplantation of islets in syngeneic rodents, success in human islet transplantation has been more elusive. The problems encountered include the difficulty of extracting a sufficiently pure preparation of islets in sufficient numbers; definition of the ideal site for transplantation; need to overcome immune rejection, and failure of long-term function. Human pancreas is more fibrous than its rodent counterpart and extraction of pure islets remains problematic. The last few years have seen significant progress and extraction techniques now involve injection of collagenase into the duct system, gentle mechanical disruption and density gradient centrifugation for purification. The number of islets transplanted can be increased by use of more than one donor. It has been demonstrated that islets can survive in the spleen and beneath the renal capsule as well as in the liver, but the last site is more 'physiological' and is generally preferred. Islets can be injected into the portal vein at laparotomy, injected via the umbilical vein, or injected by the percutaneous transhepatic route.

A limited experience with islet autografts indicates that prolonged survival can be achieved in some patients. The Minneapolis group (Farney et al 1991) injected such islets intraportally in 22 patients undergoing total or near-total pancreatectomy for chronic pancreatitis; nine patients were insulin-independent although three of them later required insulin therapy. In a more recent experience, the same group have shown insulin-independence for up to 7.5 years in five patients undergoing total pancreatectomy for chronic pancreatitis (Pyzdrowski et al 1992). It appears that as few as 265 000 islets may be sufficient to maintain insulin and glucagon secretion and maintain euglycaemia. The cause of delayed islet failure is unknown but it is possible that fibrosis is responsible.

Successful transplantation of islet allografts has proved even more elusive, given the additional immunological problems involved. Of 39 patients with type I diabetes who received adult islet allografts, only six achieved a period of insulin independence (London & Bell 1992). Most of this collected series of patients received their islet allografts with, or after, a kidney transplant, and in most cases the islets were infused into the portal vein at laparotomy. Although survival of such allografts may now extend to some 3 years, the problems of immunological rejection have not been solved. Encouraging experimental approaches include the alteration of immunogenicity by tissue culture before transplantation, treatment with monoclonal antibodies, and genetic engineering to delete the expression of major histocompatibility-complex antigens by the islet cells (Barker & Naji 1992). Alternatively, it may become possible to protect allografts (and even xenografts) from rejection by implanting them within semipermeable microcapsules which allow the passage of glucose, insulin and glucagon, but not immune cells or antibodies. It seems likely that the next few years will bring exciting advances in the management of diabetes mellitus by islet transplantation and that the technique will move from its experimental status into routine clinical practice.

REFERENCES

Barbosa J, King R, Goetz F C et al 1977 Histocompatibility antigens (HLA) in families with juvenile insulin dependent diabetes mellitus. Journal of Clinical Investigation 60: 989–999

Barker C F, Naji A 1992 Perspectives in pancreatic and islet transplantation. New England Journal of Medicine 327: 271–273

Bilous R W, Mauer S M, Sutherland D E R, Steffes M W 1987 Glomerular structure and function following successful pancreas transplantation for insulin-dependent diabetes mellitus. Diabetes 36: 43A

Bilous R W, Mauer S M, Sutherland D E R et al 1989 The effects of pancreas transplantation on the glomerular structure of renal allografts in patients with insulin-dependent diabetes. New England Journal of Medicine 321: 80–85

Bohman S O, Tyden G, Wilczek H 1985 Prevention of kidney graft diabetic nephropathy by pancreas transplantation in man. Diabetes 34: 306

Bohman S O, Wilczek H, Tyden C et al 1987 Recurrent diabetic nephropathy in renal transplants placed in diabetic patients and the protective effect of simultaneous pancreatic transplantation. Transplantation Proceedings 19: 2290–2292

Bosi E, Piatti P M, Secchi A, Monti L D, Traeger J, Dubernard J M, Pozza G 1988 Response of glucagon and insulin secretion to insulin-induced hypoglycemia in type I diabetic recipients after pancreatic transplantation. Diabetes, Nutrition and Metabolism 1: 21–27

Brayman K L, Vianello A, Morel P, Payne W D, Sutherland D E R 1990 The organ donor – Choice, preparation and acquisition. In: Cerra F (ed), Critical care clinics, Vol. 6: Critical care of the transplant patient. W B Saunders, Philadelphia, p 821–839

Brayman K L, Moss A, Morel P, Nakhleh R, Moudry-Munns K, Drangstveit M, Dunn D L, Sutherland D E R 1991 Simultaneous pancreas–kidney and solitary pancreaticoduodenal transplantation using a transcystoscopic biopsy technique. Transplantation Proceedings, in press

Burke G W, Sutherland D E R, Najarian J S 1988 Intra-abdominal fluid collection in pancreas transplant recipients: Bladder versus enteric drainage. Transplantation Proceedings 20: 887–888

Corry R J, Zehr P 1990 Quality of life in diabetic recipients of kidney transplants is better with the addition of the pancreas. Clinical Transplantation 4: 238–242

Cosimi A B, Auchincloss H, Delmonico F et al 1988 Combined kidney and pancreas transplantation in diabetics. Archives of Surgery 123: 621–628

DeFrancisco A M, Mauer S M, Steffes M W, Goetz F C, Najarian J S, Sutherland D E R 1988 The effect of cyclosporine on native renal function in non-uremic diabetic recipients of pancreas transplants. Journal of Diabetic Complications 1: 128–131

Diem P D, Manuir A, Redmon J B, Sutherland D E R, Robertson R P 1990a Systemic drainage of pancreas allografts as independent cause of hyperinsulinemia in type I diabetic recipients. Diabetes 39: 534–540

Diem P, Redmon J B, Abid M, Moran A, Sutherland D E R, Halter J B, Robertson R P 1990b Glucagon, catecholamine and pancreatic polypeptide secretion in type I diabetic recipients of pancreas allografts. Journal of Clinical Investigation 86: 2008–2013

Dunn D L, Morel P, Schlumpf R, Mayoral J L, Gillingham K J, Moudry-Munns K C, Krom R A F, Gruessner R W G, Payne, W D, Sutherland D E R, Najarian J S 1991 Evidence that combined procurement of pancreas and liver grafts does not affect transplant outcome. Transplantation 51: 150–157.

Eisenbarth G S 1986 Type I diabetes mellitus: A chronic autoimmune disease. New England Journal of Medicine 314: 1360–1368

Farney A C, Najarian J S, Nakleh R E et al 1991 Autotransplantation of dispersed pancreatic islet tissue combined with total or near-total pancreatectomy for treatment of chronic pancreatitis. Surgery 110: 427–439

Gliedman M L, Gold M, Whittaker J et al 1973 Pancreatic duct to ureter anastomosis for exocrine drainage in pancreatic transplantation. American Journal of Surgery 125: 245

Gliedman M L, Tellis V A, Soberman R et al 1978 Long-term effects of pancreatic transplant function in patients with advanced juvenile onset diabetes. Diabetes Care 1: 1–9

Gruessner R G, Dunn D L et al 1990 Simultaneous pancreas and kidney transplants versus single kidney transplants and previous kidney transplants in uremic, and single pancreas transplants in non-uremic diabetic patients: Comparison of rejection, morbidity, and long-term outcome. Transplantation Proceedings 22: 622–623

Gruessner R W G, Manivel C, Dunn D L, Sutherland D E R 1991 Pancreaticoduodenal transplantation with enteric drainage following native total pancreatectomy for chronic pancreatitis: A case report. Pancreas 6, in press

Hanssen K F, Dahl-Jorgenson K, Lauritzen J et al 1986 Diabetic control and microvascular complications: The near normoglycemic experience. Diabetologia 10: 677–684

Illner W D, Schleibner S, Abendroth R et al 1987 Recent improvement in clinical pancreas transplantation. Transplantation Proceedings 19: 3870–3871

Kelly W D, Lilleheli R C, Merkel F K, Idezuki Y, Goetz F C 1967 Allotransplantation of the pancreas and duodenum along with the kidney in diabetic nephropathy. Surgery 61: 827

Kendall D M, Sutherland D E R, Goetz F C, Najarian J S 1989 Metabolic effect on hemipancreatectomy in donors: Preoperative prediction of postoperative oral glucose tolerance. Diabetes 38 (Suppl 1): 101–103

Kendall D M, Sutherland D E R Najarian J S, Goetz F C, Robertson R P 1990 Effects of hemi-pancreatectomy on insulin secretion and glucose tolerance in healthy human donors. New England Journal of Medicine 322: 898–903

Kennedy W R, Navarro X, Goetz F C, Sutherland D E R, Najarian J S 1990 The effects of pancreas transplantation on diabetic neuropathy. New England Journal of Medicine 15: 1031–1037

Land W, Landgraf R, Illner W D, Abendroth D, Kampik A, Jensen U, Lenhart F P, Burg D, Hillebrand C, Castro L A, Landgraf-Levis M M C, Frey L, Gokel M Schleibner S, Nusser J, Ulbig M 1987 Clinical pancreatic transplantation using the prolamine duct occlusion technique: The Munich experience. Transplantation Proceedings 19 (Suppl 4): 75–84

LaRocca E, Dubernard J M, Sangeverno R et al 1987 Results of simultaneous pancreatico-renal transplantation. Transplantation Proceedings 19 (Suppl 4): 44–47

Lilleheli R C, Ruiz J O, Acquino C, Goetz F C 1976 Transplantation of the pancreas. Acta Endocrinologica 83 (Suppl 205): 303

London N J M, Bell P F R 1992 Pancreas and islet transplantation. British Journal of Surgery 79: 6–7

Marks W H, Borgstrom A, Sollinger H, Marks C 1990 Serum immunoreactive anodal trypsinogen and urinary amylase as biochemical markers for rejection of clinical whole organ pancreas allografts having exocrine drainage into the urinary bladder. Transplantation 49: 112–115

Marsh C L, Perkins J D, Sutherland D E R, Corry R J, Sterioff S 1989 Combined hepatic and pancreaticoduodenal procurement for transplantation. Surgery, Gynecology and Obstetrics 168: 254–258

Mauer SM, Steffes M W, Connett J et al 1983 Development of lesions in glomerular basement membrane and mesangium after transplantation of normal kidneys to diabetic patients. Diabetes 32: 948–952

Mauer S M, Steffes M W, Ellis E N et al 1984 Structural–functional relationships in diabetic nephropathy. Journal of Clinical Investigation 74: 1145–1155

Morel P, Moudry-Munns K, Najarian J S 1990 Influence of preservation time on outcome of metabolic function of bladder-drained pancreas transplants. Transplantation 49: 294–302

Morel P, Gillingham K J, Moudry-Munns K C, Dunn D L, Najarian J S, Sutherland D E R 1991a Factors influencing pancreas transplantation outcome: Cox proportional hazard regression analysis of a single institution's experience with 357 cases. Transplantation Proceedings 23: 1630–1633

Morel P, Goetz F, Moudry-Munns K C, Freier E, Sutherland D E R 1991b Serial glycosylated hemoglobin levels in diabetic recipients of pancreatic transplants. Annals of Internal Medicine, in press

Morel P, Sutherland D E R, Almond P S, Stoblem F, Matas A J, Najarian J S, Dunn D L 1991c Assessment of renal function in type I diabetic patients after kidney, pancreas or combined kidney–pancreas transplantation, in press

Nakache R, Tyden G, Groth C G 1989 Quality of life in diabetic patients after combined pancreas–kidney or kidney transplantation. Diabetes 38 (Suppl 1): 40–42

Navarro X, Kennedy W R, Loewenson R B, Sutherland D E R 1990 Influence of pancreas transplantation on cardiorespiratory reflexes, nerve conduction, and mortality in diabetes mellitus. Diabetes 39: 802–806

Ngheim D D, Bentel W D, Corry R 1986 Duodenocystostomy for exocrine drainage in total pancreatic transplantation. Transplantation Proceedings 18: 1753

Osei K, Henry M L, O'Dorisio T M, Tesi R J, Sommer B G, Ferguson R M 1990 Physiological and pharmacological stimulation of pancreatic islet hormone secretion in type I diabetic pancreas allograft recipients. Diabetes 39: 1235–1242

Ostman J, Bolinder J, Gunnarsson R, Brattstrom C, Tyden G, Wahren J, Groth C G 1989 Metabolic effects of pancreas transplantation: Effects of pancreas transplantation on metabolic and hormonal profiles in IDDM patients. Diabetes 38 (Suppl 1): 88–93

Perkins J D, Munn S R, Marsh C L, Barr D, Engen D E, Carpenter H A 1990 Safety and efficacy of cystoscopically directed biopsy in pancreas transplantation. Transplantation Proceedings 22: 665

Pozza G, Traeger J, Dubernard J M et al 1983 Endocrine responses of type I (insulin-dependent) diabetic patients following successful transplantation. Diabetologia 24: 244–248

Prieto M, Sutherland D E R, Fernandez-Cruz L, Heil J, Najarian J S 1987a Experimental and clinical experience with urine amylase monitoring for early diagnosis of rejection in pancreas transplantation. Transplantation 43: 71–79

Prieto M, Sutherland D E R, Goetz F C, Rosenberg M, Najarian J S 1987b Pancreas transplant results according to technique of duct management: Bladder versus enteric drainage. Surgery 102: 680–691

Pyzdrowski K L, Kendall D M, Halter J B et al 1992 Preserved insulin secretion and insulin independence in recipients of islet autografts. New England Journal of Medicine 327: 220–226

Radio S J, Stratta R, Taylor R, Miller S, Pirucello S, Linder J 1991 Urine cytologic monitoring for rejection after combined pancreas–kidney transplantation. Transplantation Proceedings (in press)

Rajotte R V 1989 Continued function of pancreatic islets after transplantation in type I diabetes. Lancet 1: 570–572

Ramsay R C, Goetz F C, Sutherland D E R, Mauer S M, Robinson L L, Cantrill H L, Knobloch W H, Najarian J S 1988 Progression of diabetic retinopathy after pancreas transplantation for insulin-dependent diabetes mellitus. New England Journal of Medicine 318: 208–214

Robertson R P, Franklin G, Nelson L 1989 Glucose homeostasis and insulin secretion during chronic treatment with cyclosporin in nondiabetic humans. Diabetes 39 (Suppl 1): 99–100

Scharp D W, Lacy P E, Santiago J V, McCullough C S, Weide L G, Boyle P J, Falqui L, Marchetti P, Ricordi C, Gingerich R L, Jaffe A S, Cryer P E, Hanto D W, Anderson C B, Flye M W 1991 Results of our first nine intraportal islet allografts in type I, insulin-dependent diabetic patients. Transplantation 51: 76–85

Schulak J A, Mayes J T, Hricik D E 1990 Combined kidney and pancreas transplantation: A safe and effective treatment for diabetic nephropathy. Archives of Surgery 125: 881–885

Secchi a, Pontiroli A E, Bosi E, Piatti P M, Tourane J L, Monti L D, Gelet A, Traeger J, Dubernard J M, Pozza G 1987 Effects of arginine and arginine plus somatostatis infusion on insulin release in diabetic patients submitted to pancreas allotransplantation. Diabete et Metabolisme 13: 422–425

Sibley R K, Sutherland D E R 1987 Pancreas transplantation: An immunohistologic and histopathologic examination of 100 grafts. American Journal of Pathology 128: 151–170

Sibley R K, Sutherland D E R, Goetz F, Michael A F 1985 Recurrent diabetes mellitus in the pancreas iso- and allograft. A light and electron microscopic and immunohistochemical analysis of four cases. Laboratory Investigation 53: 132–144

So S K, Minford E, Moudry-Munns K C, Gillingham K, Sutherland D E R 1990 DR matching improves cadaveric pancreas transplant results. Transplantation Proceedings 22: 687–688

Solders G, Gunnarsson R, Persson A, Wilczek H, Tyden G, Groth C G 1987 Effects of combined pancreatic and renal transplantation on diabetic neuropathy: A two year follow-up study. Lancet 2: 1232–1235

Sollinger H W, Glass N R, Belzer F O 1983 Clinical experience with pancreatico-cystostomy for exocrine drainage in pancreas transplantation. Diabetic Nephropathy 2: 23

Sollinger H W, Cook K, Kamps D et al 1984 Clinical and experimental experience with pancreatico-cystostomy for exocrine pancreatic drainage in pancreas transplantation. Transplantation Proceedings 16: 799

Sollinger H W, Stratta R J, Kalayoglu M et al 1987 Pancreas transplantation with pancreaticocystostomy and quadruple immunosuppression. Surgery 102: 674–679

Sollinger H, Stratta R J, D'Alessandro A M et al 1988 Experience with simultaneous pancreas kidney transplantation. Annals of Surgery 208: 475–483

Squifflet J P, Moudry K, Sutherland D E R 1988 Is HLA matching relevant in pancreas transplantation? Transplant International 1: 26–29

Steffes M W, Barbosa J, Basgen J M et al 1983 Quantitative glomerular morphology of the human kidney. Laboratory Investigation 49: 82–86

Stevens R B, Chau C L C, Moudry-Munns K C, Rabkin J M, Schmidt W, Gillingham K, Leone J P, Morel P, Sutherland D E R 1991 Experience with and incidence of kidney transplantation (Tx) after a solitary pancreas (Px) Tx in non- or pre-uremic diabetics. Transplantation Proceedings (in press)

Sutherland D E R 1988 Who should get a pancreas transplant? Diabetes Care 11: 681–685

Sutherland D E R, Matas A J, Goetz F C, Najarian J S 1980 Transplantation of dispersed pancreatic islet tissue in humans, autografts and allografts. Diabetes 29 (1): 31–43

Sutherland D E R, Najarian J S, Greensberg B Z, Senske B J et al 1981 Hormonal and metabolic effects of a pancreatic endocrine graft. Annals of Internal Medicine 95: 537–541

Sutherland D E R, Goetz F C, Najarian J S 1984a 100 pancreas transplants at a single institution. Annals of Surgery 200: 414–440

Sutherland D E R, Goetz F C, Najarian J S 1984b Pancreas transplants from living related donors. Transplantation 38: 674–679

Sutherland D E R, Sibley R, Zhu X-Z, Michael A, Srikanta S, Taub F, Najarian J S, Goetz F 1984c Twin-to-twin pancreas transplantation: Reversal and reenactment of the pathogenesis of type I diabetes. Transactions of the American Association of Physicians XCVII: 80–87

Sutherland D E R, Kendall D M, Moudry K C, Navarro X, Kennedy W R, Ramsay R C, Steffes M W, Mauer S M, Goetz F C, Dunn D L, Najarian J S 1988 Pancreas transplantation in nonuremic, type I diabetic recipients. Surgery 104: 453–464

Sutherland D E R, Dunn D L, Goetz F C et al 1989a A ten year experience with 290 pancreas transplants at a single institution. Annals of Surgery 210: 274–288

Sutherland D E R, Goetz F Z, Sibley R K 1989b Recurrence of disease in pancreas transplantation. Diabetes 38 (Suppl 1): 85–87

Sutherland D E R, Moudry-Munns K C, Gillingham K 1990 Pancreas transplantation: Report from International Registry and preliminary analysis of US results from new United Network for Organ Sharing (UNOS) Registry. In: Terasaki P I (ed) Clinical transplants – 1989. Regents University of California, p 19–43

Sutherland D E R, Gillingham K, Moudry-Munns K C 1991a Pancreas transplantation: Report on United States (US) results from United

Network for Organ Sharing (UNOS) Registry with comparison to non-US results from International Registry report on clinical pancreas transplantation. In: Terasaki P (ed) Clinical Transplants – 1990. Regents University of California, p 29–39

Sutherland D E R, Moudry-Munns K C, Gillingham K, Najarian J S, Dunn D L 1991b Solitary pancreas transplantation: Alone in nonuremic and after a kidney in uremic diabetic patients. Transplant Proceedings 23: 1637–1639

Sutherland D E R, Gillingham K, Moudry-Munns Kay 1991c Results of pancreas transplantation in the United States for 1987–90 from the United Network for Organ Sharing (UNOS) Registry with comparison to 1984–87 results. Clinical Transplantation, 5, in press

Sutherland D E R, Gillingham K, Moudry-Munns K 1991d Pancreas transplantation: Report on United States (US) results from United Network for Organ Sharing (UNOS) registry with comparison to non-US results form International Registry. In: Terasaki P I (ed) Clinical transplants – 1991, UCLA Tissue Typing Laboratory, Los Angeles, California, in press

Sutherland D E R, Goetz F C, Kendall D M, Robertson R P, Seaquist E, Gillingham K, Moudry-Munns K C, Najarian J S 1991e Medical risks and benefit of pancreas transplants from living related donors. Ethics, justice, and commerce in organ replacement therapy, Congress book. Springer-Verlag, Heidelberg, in press

Tchobroutsky G 1978 Relation of diabetes control to development of microvascular complications. Diabetologia 15: 143–152

Terashita G Y, Cook J D 1987 Original disease of the recipient. In: Terasaki P I (ed) Clinical transplants – 1987. UCLA Tissue Typing Laboratory, Los Angeles, p 373–379

Tyden G, Brattstrom C, Lundgren G et al 1987 Improved results in pancreatic transplantation by avoidance of nonimmunological graft failures. Transplantation 43: 674–676

Tzakis A G, Ricordi C, Alejandro R et al 1990 Pancreatic islet transplantation after upper abdominal exenteration and liver replacement. Lancet 336: 402–405

Ulbig N, Kampick A, Landgraf R et al 1987 The influence of combined pancreatic and renal transplantation on advanced diabetic retinopathy. Transplantation Proceedings 19: 3554–3556

University of Michigan Pancreas Transplant Evaluation Committe 1988 Pancreas Transplantation as treatment of IDDM: Proposed candidate evaluation before end stage diabetic nephropathy. Diabetes Care 11: 669–675

Viberti G C, Hill R D, Jarre H R J et al 1982 Microalbuminuria as a predictor of clinical diabetic nephropathy. Lancet 1: 1430–1432

Voruganti L M P, Sells R A 1989 Quality of life of diabetic patients after combined pancreatic renal transplantation. Clinical Transplantation 3: 78–82

Wahlberg J A, Lowe R, Landegaard L et al 1987 72 hour preservation of the canine pancreas. Transplantation 43: 5–7

Wright F H, Smith J L, Ames S A et al 1989 Function of pancreas allografts more than one year following transplantation. Archives of Surgery 124: 796–800

Zehrer C, Cross C 1990 Quality of life after pancreas transplantation. Diabetes Care 13: 539–541

Zehrer C, Cross C 1991 Quality of life of pancreas transplant recipient. Diabetologia (in press)

Pancreatic surgery: anaesthesia and complications

52. Anaesthesia in pancreatic surgery

K. van Ackern   D. M. Albrecht

Pancreatectomy remains one of the most challenging abdominal operations for both surgeon and anaesthetist. Successful perioperative management demands a co-ordinated interdisciplinary approach to deal with the complex and diverse problems that can be encountered in the various forms of pancreatic disease. For example, the patient with acute necrotizing pancreatitis may be so ill that intensive care treatment is needed from the outset to deal with shock, sepsis and multiorgan failure (Jones & Linhardt 1982), while the preoperative medical management of cachexia, diabetes or alcohol abuse may be critical to the outcome in patients coming to surgery with chronic pancreatitis (Lerut et al 1984). The anaesthetist has a key role in pre-, intra- and postoperative care, in maintaining homeostasis, in coordinating the activities of physicians and surgeons, and in the prevention and management of complications which may follow the unavoidable surgical trauma to what is often an already damaged organ.

This review will discuss the role of the anaesthetist before, during and after pancreatic surgery, and is based on our experience in the Mannheim Surgical Clinic where approximately two-thirds of patients undergoing such surgery have neoplastic disease (Trede & Schwall 1988).

PREOPERATIVE CARE

Patients with acute necrotizing pancreatitis and those who have suffered multiple injuries with associated major pancreatic trauma require particularly close preoperative supervision by the anaesthetist. Such patients frequently have sepsis in association with shock, and their intensive management must be continued in the operating theatre (Ranson 1988, 1990). The timing of pancreatic surgery is often dictated by a rapid deterioration in the patient's general condition and little time may be available for preoperative preparation. The primary goal of management in these circumstances is to optimize homeostasis by adjustment of fluid and electrolyte balance, aiming to maintain an adequate intravascular volume according to the patient's cardiac function and age. As blood volume cannot be measured clinically, the adequacy of resuscitation must be estimated indirectly by regular clinical examination, calculation of fluid balance, measurement of hourly urine output and central venous pressure determinations. Fluid requirements are notoriously difficult to determine in patients with severe acute pancreatitis, and widespread increases in vascular endothelial permeability may result in major deficits by the time operation is undertaken (Maier & Carrico 1986). Restriction of fluid intake in such patients does not prevent the development of interstitial oedema and, indeed, is contraindicated. The vascular permeability to water, protein and even cellular elements is increased by the toxic effects of the acute pancreatitis and by the translocation of bacteria from the paralysed gut. Large volumes of fluid may therefore be needed to maintain intravascular volume, and the time that this fluid remains within the vascular compartment is determined by its oncotic pressure and the molecular size of its constituents, by vascular permeability, and by the hydrostatic pressure relationships within the microcirculation. It cannot be overemphasized that only an adequate intravascular volume permits normotension and a cardiac output sufficient for the increased peripheral needs in acute pancreatitis. The peripheral perfusion of all organs, including the diseased pancreas itself, depends directly on restitution and maintenance of the intravascular volume.

Type of fluid used in replacement

The type of fluid that should be used in replacement has been discussed by many authors (Sturm et al 1982, Brückner et al 1985, Albrecht et al 1986). The suspected increase in interstitial oedema, which in the lungs results in the adult respiratory distress syndrome (ARDS), is not associated with a particular type of solution. Thus, colloidal solutions of dextrans or hydroxyethyl starch do not appear to be associated with detrimental accumulation of extravascular lung water in the early stages of widespread permeability impairment. Even large amounts of crystalloid solution can be given without increasing pulmonary

623

interstitial oedema, as long as filling pressure is monitored (Hein et al 1988, Zadrobilek et al 1989). Adequate volume replacement in these patients may mean infusion of up to 15 litres in 24 hours. It is obvious that such large amounts of fluid can only be given as a combination of colloid and crystalloid solutions. There are no experimental or pharmacological data to support the use of any particular colloid solution. The patient's protein requirements must be determined on an individual basis by the results of laboratory data, remembering that these patients often have reduced hepatic function. The decision to replace intravascular proteins by fresh frozen plasma or albumin also depends on laboratory results. Although replacement of serum proteins by fresh frozen plasma can be effective, it is important that its limitations are borne in mind when vascular permeability is severely impaired. The suggestion that levels of the naturally occurring antiprotease α_2-macroglobulin are replenished by fresh frozen plasma (Leese et al 1987) awaits further analysis in controlled clinical situations. Kreimeier and Messmer (1987) have provided experimental evidence of improved organ perfusion after volume replacement with hypertonic–hyperoncotic solutions, but further studies are needed to determine whether this approach will be beneficial before and during pancreatic surgery. They suggest that the improvement in the microcirculation is due to the recruitment of vascular segments following mobilization of interstitial fluid into the intravascular space. Although no studies have yet been performed in patients with acute pancreatitis, there are no contraindications at present to perioperative fluid replacement with such solutions. It is essential not to use excessive amounts of crystalloid alone when permeability is impaired. Studies in dogs have shown that when vascular permeability is severely impaired as a result of shock, volume replacement with crystalloids alone does not increase the extravascular lung water but does reduce oxygen extraction significantly (Albrecht et al 1986). This reflects the generalized increase in interstitial oedema, and the diminished oxygen extraction may have major deleterious effects on sensitive organs, including the pancreas.

Evaluation of the patient

Adequate fluid replacement is the key to balanced macro- and microhaemodynamics and is therefore of central importance not only for pancreatic surgery in critically ill patients but also in the preparation for elective surgery. In the latter situation, vascular permeability is unlikely to be impaired so that fluid replacement raises no special problems provided standard clinical criteria are used and central venous pressure is monitored. Attention must be paid to low levels of plasma protein and to the patient's cardio-respiratory status. The mean age of patients undergoing pancreatic surgery is close to 60 years and many have a long history of disease. Many are cachectic and there may be cardiovascular complications due to associated diseases

such as diabetes mellitus, as is commonly seen in patients with alcoholic chronic pancreatitis. It is essential to identify any cardiomyopathy and cardiac insufficiency before operation so that pre- and perioperative fluid replacement can be adjusted accordingly. If left ventricular function cannot be assessed from arterial and central venous pressure (especially when the patient is being ventilated mechanically and urine output is poor), a Swann–Ganz catheter should be used for intraoperative monitoring. Such problems are most likely to be encountered in patients undergoing major elective pancreatic resections, in those with severe acute pancreatitis and in patients who have suffered major abdominal trauma.

The preoperative optimization of homeostasis in elective pancreatic surgery is the same as for all major elective abdominal operations. In addition to the standard full blood count and blood chemistry, a full coagulation analysis is desirable and must include measurement of the bleeding time and platelet count. Pulmonary function tests (Tisi 1979) are carried out as necessary, but apart from serving as a basis for comparison with postoperative values should complications supervene, they give less information about operability and the risk of complications than they do in thoracic surgery. Parameters such as vital capacity and forced expiratory volume (FEV_1) are of little help unless they are extremely low ($FEV_1 < 1.0$ litre). The ability of individual patients to compensate is difficult to predict, and preoperative analysis of blood gas concentrations under normal room conditions and estimation of resistance to stress by clinical criteria often provide more useful information.

The severity of chronic obstructive airway disease is evaluated and it is important to optimize treatment with β_2-receptor antagonists if they are needed. If possible, all elderly patients and those with pre-existing lung disease should be given preoperative ventilation therapy and training, and if necessary physiotherapy, to loosen secretions. The effort will be amply repaid by a reduced rate of postoperative pulmonary complications.

The preoperative management of patients about to undergo pancreatic surgery must include an adequate explanation by both anaesthetist and surgeon of the nature of the operation and its possible consequences. The patient should be gently prepared for the possibility of a difficult postoperative course and given appropriate emotional support. Full cooperation in the immediate postoperative period and in the long term depends to a large degree on the confidence that the patient has in his doctors and on a sound understanding of the nature of his illness and the limitations that it might place on his life.

PRINCIPLES OF ANAESTHESIA

The principles of anaesthesia in pancreatic surgery are identical to those of anaesthesia in other forms of major abdominal surgery. The general condition of the patient and the expected extent of surgery determine the method of intraoperative monitoring. A central venous catheter allows measurement of filling pressure in relation to right ventricular function and is inserted routinely.

Premedication is given as usual. The need for pre-operative fasting should be no contraindication to oral premedication. Patients who are already suffering from severe pain before operation should have an analgesic added to the premedication. Atropine is not necessary and should be avoided.

Endotracheal intubation and controlled mechanical ventilation are used in all cases. There are absolutely no indications for regional anaesthesia alone in this type of surgery. For optimal control of anaesthesia, especially when extubation is planned on the completion of extensive surgery, 'balanced anaesthesia' (Hartung 1988) is recommended, in which neuromuscular blocking agents are injected intravenously so that lighter levels of anaesthesia can be used. After induction of anaesthesia with a barbiturate, supplemented by an opioid depending on the condition of the patient, basic analgesia and anaesthesia is achieved by inhalation of volatile anaesthetics (Kreimeier & Messmer, 1987). The choice of agent used depends on the preferences and experience of the anaesthetist and on the equipment available. There are no contraindications to the use of the volatile anaesthetics enflurane and isoflurane, but halothane should not be used in view of the alleged risk of liver damage.

The dose of volatile anaesthetic depends on the course of the surgery and, especially in the case of isoflurane, on haemodynamic parameters. The use of 'balanced anaesthesia' with additional opioids (usually fentanyl) keeps the dose of volatile anaesthetics in a range where haemodynamic side-effects are not expected. After intubation, relaxation is achieved with non-depolarizing neuromuscular blocking agents such as vecuronium and pancuronium. For major surgery of predictable duration, pancuronium is usually the drug of choice, provided that the patient does not have renal problems. Monitoring the state of relaxation by a relaxometer facilitates adjustment of the dose of neuromuscular blocking drugs needed during extensive and prolonged surgery.

Use of epidural anaesthesia

The combination of balanced anaesthesia and regional anaesthesia in the form of epidural anaesthesia is our method of choice. Not only does this combination truly deserve the name 'balanced anaesthesia', it also has advantages not confined to the period of the operation itself. There is no doubt that adequate anaesthesia can be achieved for major pancreatic surgery without epidural anaesthesia, and the use of the epidural technique and its associated vasomotor paralysis can make it difficult to assess intravascular volume and the need for fluid replacement. However, the real advantage of combining 'balanced anaesthesia' with epidural anaesthesia becomes apparent when extubation is planned at the end of the operation. After elective pancreatic surgery, extubation can usually be performed on the operating table. There is usually no need for mechanical ventilation. Extubation is contraindicated if there is any doubt about whether the patient can breathe spontaneously and possesses competent laryngeal reflexes (to prevent aspiration and tracheal soiling), if there is pulmonary dysfunction, and if the core temperature is below 35 °C. Maintenance of an adequate ambient temperature throughout surgery, heat mats, and warmed infusion solutions all help to avoid hypothermia. Return of consciousness and pulmonary function depend on the preoperative condition of the patient and on the conduct of general anaesthesia. The prolonged supine position tends to reduce functional residual capacity and this has to be restored as soon as possible after the operation. This can be difficult, especially in high-risk elderly patients who may be unable to cooperate because of residual muscle relaxation and continued anaesthetic effects. Intraoperative epidural anaesthesia is of particular value in such patients in that epidural administration of analgesics allows the total dose of opiates and other anaesthetics to be reduced, thus lightening the depth of anaesthesia and allowing a speedier recovery once surgery has been completed.

Moreover, it has recently been suggested that postoperative homeostasis and pain can also be better controlled by a combination of general anaesthesia with epidural anaesthesia (Tigersted 1990). Neurophysiological and experimental evidence indicates that regional anaesthesia of pain-sensitive C-fibres is more effective than systemic use of opiates (Kehlet 1988, Cousins 1989, Tigersted 1990).

Despite the persuasive arguments in favour of the combination of 'balanced' and epidural anaesthesia, it must be admitted that there are no controlled data to show significant benefits in terms of improved management or reduced mortality (Seeling et al 1986). The complexities of this type of surgery and the wide variation in the patients' preoperative condition make it highly unlikely that such absolute proof will ever be forthcoming. As pointed out above, a combination of 'balanced' general anaesthesia with epidural anaesthesia is our method of choice, and, as in all forms of surgery, the experience of the anaesthetist and surgeon, and their close cooperation are crucial to success.

Epidural anaesthesia is contraindicated in seriously ill patients with necrotizing acute pancreatitis and unstable preoperative haemodynamics. In such cases the method of choice is modified neuroleptic anaesthesia, using low doses of volatile anaesthetics. It is usually not possible to extubate these patients once surgery has been completed, as postoperative organ function is often severely impaired by a combination of factors including sepsis, endotoxaemia and interstitial oedema.

Intraoperative homeostasis

Intraoperative fluid replacement has already been discussed. If unexpected bleeding occurs during operation, transfusion of red cell concentrates and additional fresh frozen plasma is preferred to the use of whole blood. The threshold values of haematocrit (packed cell volume) and haemoglobin concentration are as for other surgical operations and depend on the patient's condition. The use of methods to prevent transfusion of heterologous blood, such as preoperative donation of blood by the patient himself and the use of intraoperative 'cell saving' devices, depends on the condition of the patient and the nature of his disease. Patients with malignant tumours or acute pancreatitis are not suitable candidates for intraoperative cell saving, and in practice preoperative donation has not been widely used in patients awaiting elective surgery. In the small group of patients undergoing total pancreatectomy, maintenance of glucose homeostasis is a potential source of difficulty during and after surgery. Frequent monitoring of blood glucose and serum potassium levels, with appropriate administration of insulin and glucose, is the key to successful management.

POSTOPERATIVE COMPLICATIONS AND MANAGEMENT

The risk of complications after pancreatic surgery is greatly influenced by the quality of preoperative preparation, by meticulous attention to detail by both surgeon and anaesthetist during the operation, and by continuous skilled medical and nursing care in the postoperative period. Patients who are critically ill and in need of continued assisted ventilation will have to be transferred to an intensive care unit on leaving the operating room, but most patients undergoing pancreatic surgery can be managed effectively in a high dependency unit during the early postoperative period.

Adequate provision of analgesia is essential for speedy recovery and early mobilization. The advantages of epidural anaesthesia during operation have already been discussed. If the catheter is maintained in the correct position, it can be used postoperatively to infuse low doses of anaesthetics or opiates, and so provide good pain relief without adverse effects on levels of consciousness or ability to cooperate. It must be stressed that maintenance of epidural anaesthesia requires considerable organizational effort and commitment on the part of the patient's attendants. Failure to provide effective pain relief is usually due to incompetent management rather than a failure of the method itself. In such cases, opiates may have to be given systemically, and in conscious cooperative patients intravenous analgesics can be given 'on demand' by using patient-controlled administration. The question whether epidural anaesthesia improves splanchnic perfusion and so encourages early return of gut motility is still debated. However, there is no doubt that high doses of opiates prolong atony.

The principles governing postoperative fluid replacement are the same as those governing replacement in the preoperative period and during operation. Meticulous monitoring of fluid balance greatly reduces the risk of major haemodynamic disturbances with reduced renal perfusion and the need for sympathomimetic drugs such as dopamine. In patients with previously normal cardiac and renal function, problems due to postoperative fluid overload are unlikely to occur but special care is needed in the elderly and those with pre-existing disease. Opinions vary as to the need for perioperative parenteral nutrition in patients undergoing pancreatic surgery. Care has to be exercised in patients with impaired hepatic and renal function, but in general parenteral nutrition is started as soon as possible after surgery. Maintenance of nutritional intake is particularly important in patients who are already malnourished, and in those with severe acute pancreatitis because of its great metabolic demands. Oral feeding should begin as soon as gastrointestinal motility is restored provided there is no evidence of any exacerbation of acute pancreatitis (Niederau 1991). In some patients who are reluctant to eat, the use of a fine-bore nasoenteric tube may prove helpful, while in patients with necrotizing pancreatitis who are recovering from surgery it may be possible to institute enteric feeding by means of a jejunostomy.

Early recognition of an acute exacerbation or the development of complications such as necrosis or sepsis is of crucial importance in patients with severe necrotizing pancreatitis. Hints of renewed or worsening upsets in capillary permeability may be provided by close supervision of fluid balance, with monitoring of hourly urine output, central venous pressure and pulmonary gas exchange. Impairment of pulmonary gas exchange due to ventilation–perfusion disorders, or the development of interstitial pulmonary oedema, should be regarded as a relatively late complication and as an indication that the initial signs of damaged permeability may have been overlooked. The duration of postoperative supervision obviously depends on the age of the patient, the nature of the underlying disease, and on the type of surgery and its duration. Patients with severe necrotizing pancreatitis and those who have suffered major pancreatic trauma pose particularly difficult management problems and may require intensive care monitoring for prolonged periods.

REFERENCES

Albrecht D M, Dworschak M, Frey L, Hein L G, von Ackern K, Brückner U B 1986 Does the resuscitation modality influence lung water after canine traumatic haemorrhagic shock? European Surgical Research 18 (Suppl. 1):12

Brückner U B, Albrecht D M, Dworschak M, Frey L, Hein L G 1985 Alternative Flüssigkeitstherapie im traumatisch-hämorrhagischen Schock. In: Hohlbach G, Schildberg F W (eds) Klinische und experimentelle Notfallmedizin. 7: Schock in der Notfallmedizin. Lübecker Notfallsymposium 3: Zuckschwerdt Verlag, München, p 193–197

Cousins M J 1989 Acute pain and the injury response, immediate and prolonged effects. Research in Anesthetics 14:162–179

Hartung H-J 1988 Klinische Erfahrungen mit Alfentanyl zur 'balanced anesthesia' bei Oberbauch-Eingriffen. Anaesthesist 37:620–624

Hein L G, Albrecht D M, Dworschak M, Frey L, Brückner U B 1988 Long term observation following traumatic hemorrhagic shock in the dog. A comparison of crystalloid versus colloidal fluids. Circulatory Shock 26:353–364

Jones R T, Linhardt G E 1982 Pathology and pathophysiology of the exocrine pancreas in shock. In: Cowley R A, Trump B F (eds) Pathophysiology of shock, anoxia and ischemia. Williams and Wilkins, Baltimore

Kehlet H 1988 Modification of responses to surgery by neural blockade: clinical implications. In: Cousins M J, Bridenbaugh PO (eds) Neural blockade in clinical anesthesia and management of pain.
J B Lippincott, Philadelphia, p 145–190

Kreimeier U, Messmer K 1987 New perspectives in resuscitation and prevention of multiple organ system failure. In: Baethmann A, Messmer K (eds) Surgical research: recent concepts and results. Springer-Verlag, Berlin, p 39–50

Leese T, Holiday M, Heath D, Hall M W, Bell P R 1987 Multicentre clinical trial of low volume fresh frozen plasma therapy in acute pancreatitis. British Journal of Surgery 74 (19):907–911

Lerut J P, Gianello P R, Otte J P, Kestens P J 1984 Pancreaticoduodenal resection. Surgical experience and evaluation of risk factors in 103 patients. Annals of Surgery 199:432–437

Maier R V, Carrico C J 1986 Developments in the resuscitation of critically ill surgical patients. Advances in Surgery 19:271–328

Niederau C 1991 Parenterale Ernährung bei Pankreatitis. Medizinische Welt 42:811–817

Ranson J H 1988 Prognostication in acute pancreatitis. In: Glazer G, Ranson J H C (eds) Acute pancreatitis. Ballière Tindall, London, p 366–389

Ranson J H 1990 The role of surgery in the management of acute pancreatitis. Annals of Surgery 211 (4):382–393

Seeling W, Ahnefeld F W, Grünert A, Heinrich U, Lotz D, Rosenberg G, Wieser E 1986 Aortofemoraler Bifurkationsbypass – der Einfluss des Anaesthesieverfahrens auf Kreislauf, Atmung, Stoffwechsel, Homöostase und Sauerstofftransport. Anaesthesist 35:80–92

Sturm J A, Oestern H-J, Kaul C J 1982 Volumentherapie bei der Sepsis. Der Einsatz von kristalloiden Lösungen. In: Lawin P, Peter K, Hartenauer U. Infektion – Sepsis - Peritonitis INA Thieme, Stuttgart, vol 37, p 373–404

Tigersted I 1990 Postoperative pain. Current Opinions in Anesthesiology 3:771–776

Tisi G M 1979 Preoperative evaluation of pulmonary function. Validity, indications and benefits. American Review of Respiratory Diseases 119:293–310

Trede M, Schwall G 1988 The complications of pancreatectomy. Annals of Surgery 207:39–47

Zadrobilek E, Hackl W, Sporn P, Steinbereithner K 1989 Effect of large volume replacement with balanced electrolyte solution on extravascular water in surgical patients with sepsis syndrome. Intensive Care Medicine 15(8):505–510

53. The complications of pancreatoduodenectomy and their management

M. Trede   D. C. Carter

Duodenopancreatectomy remains one of the most formidable procedures. Indeed it was given the epithet of 'the Cadillac of abdominal operations' (Baker 1979). However, as this quotation goes on to say: 'it is not really a Cadillac he (the surgeon) is trying to drive, it is a Formula I racing car'! Thus, in a survey of 4622 such operations performed over two decades (1960–1983), the average mortality rate was 17.7% (Jordan 1987).

Although the operative mortality has more recently fallen to acceptable levels (see Table 38.5), morbidity is still high. However, it would seem that surgeons, anaesthetists, radiologists, nurses – the whole team – have learnt to cope more effectively with these complications. Nevertheless, only a few publications address themselves specifically to this important aspect of pancreatic surgery (Mongé et al 1964, Pliam & ReMine 1975, Braasch & Gray 1977, Edis et al 1980, Pichlmayr & Rumpf 1986, Trede & Schwall 1988, Schirmer et al 1991).

Complications are obviously important for three reasons. At the very least they lead to a significant increase in postoperative hospital stay of some 7–9 days (Mongé et al 1964, Braasch & Gray 1977, Edis et al 1980). Furthermore they are the cause of urgent and risky relaparotomy in some 15% of cases (Trede & Schwall 1988, Smith et al 1992), and at worst they are fatal.

Table 53.1 Early surgical complications, relaparotomies and mortality after 439 pancreatectomies at the University Surgical Clinic, Mannheim, 1.10.1972–1.1.1992

Complication	n	Relaparotomy	Mortality
Pancreatic leak	34	19	6
Abdominal pain	5	4	—
Bleeding			
Gastrointestinal	20	8	2
Operating field	7	7	—
Bile fistula	11	5	—
Mesenteric ischaemia	1	—	1
Abscess			
Hepatic	5	2	—
Abdominal	3	2	—
Chylous ascites	6	—	—
Gastric perforation	1	1	—
Jejunal torsion	1	1	—
Total	94	49	9

Complications of pancreatoduodenectomy can be classified into two groups: early and late. And these can be further subdivided into surgical and non-surgical mishaps. These four groups of complications will be discussed one by one.

Table 53.2 Pancreatojejunal leaks following the Whipple operation

Author	Institution	Total no of operations	No of complications		Relaparotomy		Mortality of complications	
			n	%	n	%	n	%
Braasch & Gray (1977)	Lahey Clinic	279	20	7	★	—	4	20
Nakase et al (1977)	Collected Japanese series	824	114	14	★	—	★	—
Edis et al (1980)	Mayo Clinic	124	14	11	★	—	5	36
Papachristou & Fortner (1981)	Sloan Kettering	70	37	53	10	14	13	35
Pichlmayr & Rumpf (1986)	Hanover	49	5	10	★	—	4	80
Grace et al (1986)	UCLA	74	13	18	5	38	1	7
Crist & Cameron (1989)	Johns Hopkins	68	12	18	1[†]	8	0	—
Trede (1992) unpublished data	Mannheim	378	34	9	19	56	6	18

★ No data given; † = 2 years later

Table 53.3 Complications occurring at or around 378 pancreatojejunostomies (University Surgical Clinic, Mannheim 1.10.1972–1.1.1992)

Complication	n	Number of deaths
Anastomotic leak	15	5
Acute pancreatitis	12	1
Pancreatic fistula	7	—
Total	34	6

EARLY SURGICAL COMPLICATIONS

These events usually have their root in some technical problem during the procedure and they manifest themselves before the patient is discharged from hospital. Some of these complications can occur after any abdominal procedure. The ones that typically follow pancreatoduodenectomy are listed in Table 53.1.

1. Complications concerning the pancreatic remnant and its anastomosis

Such complications cover a whole gamut of mishaps from a harmless pancreatic fistula (that might even go undiscovered) to an overt anastomotic leak leading to sepsis, haemorrhage and death. Somewhere in between, not easy to define, and denied by some (Jordan 1987) is acute pancreatitis in the pancreatic remnant.

Experience with these complications from several centres is summarized in Table 53.2. Breakdown of the pancreatojejunal anastomosis is the complication feared most following a Whipple operation. This occurred in 15 out of 378 cases (4%) in the Mannheim experience and 5 of these (33%) were fatal (Table 53.3). With the abdomen open for emergency relaparotomy it is not always easy to distinguish this anastomotic breakdown from acute pancreatitis of the remaining pancreas with peripancreatic necroses. Such an acute postoperative pancreatitis (without a demonstrable leak) was diagnosed 12 times in the Mannheim series while 7 bland pancreatic fistulae closed spontaneously after 2–3 weeks.

Diagnosis

The key to successful treatment of anastomotic leakage is early diagnosis. The clinical signs, elicited by close observation of the patient in the surgical intensive care unit, are often of more value than modern laboratory or imaging procedures. We monitor the patient's pulse rate (looking for tachycardia) and temperature (slight rise), examine his tongue (developing dryness) and abdomen (tenderness where there was none before), and assess his respiration (slight tachypnoea), urinary output (oliguria) and psyche (increasing restlessness). These parameters often give warning that something is amiss before laboratory data become

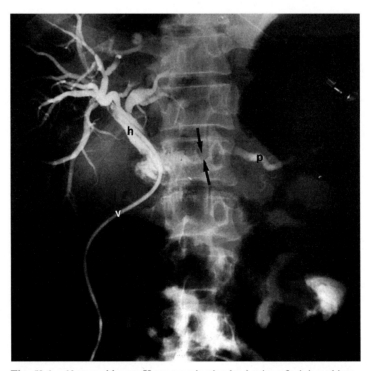

Fig. 53.1 62-year-old man; X-ray examination by Angiografin injected into a Völker drain (V) 12 days after a Whipple resection, demonstrates the hepatic (h) and pancreatic (p) ducts.

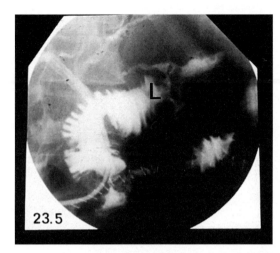 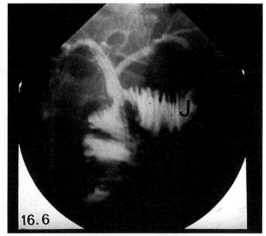

Fig. 53.2 X-ray with contrast medium injected through tube splinting the hepaticojejunostomy. L, leak of contrast medium through the pancreaticojejunostomy; J, the anastomosis has healed 24 days later. (Reprinted with permission of J B Lippincott Company, from Trede and Schwall 1988 Annals of Surgery 207:42.)

abnormal, with a rise in leucocyte count, or creatinine, lactate or amylase concentrations.

Ultrasonography is not very helpful in the first postoperative week, because an atonic gas-bloated gut and 'normal' postoperative fluid collections in the operative field hamper the production of meaningful pictures. However, once postoperative reactions have subsided, ultrasound may help to detect fluid or abscesses related to a pancreatic leak.

Access for direct imaging of the pancreatic anastomosis is provided if a (Völker) drain has been placed in the bilioenteric anastomosis (see Fig. 40.17). Injection of Angiografin-Ultravist into this tube, with the patient lying on his left side, will not only opacify the hepaticojejunostomy, but also the pancreatojejunostomy. Rarely even the pancreatic duct will be delineated (Fig. 53.1). Formerly, this examination was performed routinely some 10 days after pancreatoduodenectomy (Fig. 53.2). This was given up when it became apparent that this retrograde injection caused transient cholangitis in some patients. The method is useful nevertheless, whenever there is suspicion of a leak, although it is by no means immune to false positive or false negative findings.

Case report: 12 days after a Whipple resection in a 61-year-old man for an ampullary carcinoma, gastrografin X-ray through the Völker drain did not demonstrate any leak. (Fig. 53.3).

Nevertheless, ultrasonography and CT scan showed an abscess which was drained percutaneously. The tube was clearly draining a pancreatic fistula which persisted for another 5 weeks.

As a general rule, we warn against relying too heavily on ultrasonography and percutaneous drainage in this particular complication (Pellegrini et al 1989). Although there has never been a controlled trial of this approach, compared to early relaparotomy, we recommend the latter when there is doubt and as long as the patient's general condition permits.

Case report: A 58-year-old obese jaundiced patient had a Whipple procedure performed for a papillary carcinoma. He was restless 10 days later and had a slight rise in temperature with the development of epigastric rigidity. The CT scan showed an oedematous pancreas and ultrasound confirmed the presence of subfascial fluid collection (Fig. 53.4). It was tempting to merely aspirate this percutaneously. However, the clinical signs indicated that something deeper and more serious was going on, and relying on these clinical pointers we found a small anastomotic leak with severe pancreatitis. Removal of the remaining pancreas (completion pancreatectomy) led to the recovery of this patient.

Table 53.4 Treatment of 34 postoperative pancreatic complications (University Surgical Clinic, Mannheim, 1.10.1972–1.1.1992)

| Complication | n | Treatment | | | Deaths (n) |
		Conservative	Drainage	Total pancreatectomy	
Anastomotic leak	15	2	5 (2 deaths)	8 (3 deaths)	5
Acute pancreatitis	12	6 (1 death)	—	6	1
Pancreatic fistula	7	7	—	—	—
Total	34	13 (1 death)	5 (2 deaths)	14 (3 deaths)	6

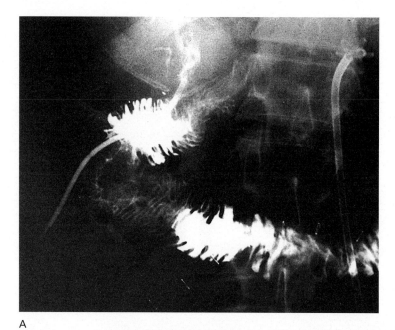

A

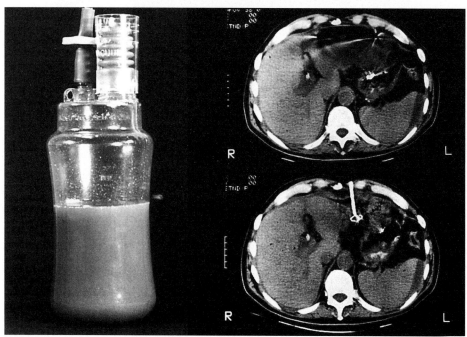

B

Fig. 53.3   61-year-old man 12 days after a Whipple resection for ampullary carcinoma.
A Gastrografin X-ray, and **B** CT scan and drainage (see text).

Treatment

The experience of the Mannheim Clinic (Table 53.4) leaves little doubt that the treatment of a pancreatic leak after a Whipple resection is best individualized. In 15 cases, treatment was entirely conservative, and this group included seven patients with bland pancreatic fistulae that closed spontaneously. In 12 patients thought to have 'acute postoperative pancreatitis' the diagnosis rested mainly on laboratory data (i.e. raised amylase levels). In one of these, the severity of the pancreatitis was misjudged. This patient died 11 days after pancreatoduodenectomy, before it became clear that her acute respiratory distress syndrome (ARDS) was only secondary to the pancreatitis. With a more aggressive approach she might have been saved by a timely 'completion pancreatectomy'.

The lesson learnt from this experience was twofold: first, never rely on the vague diagnosis 'ARDS'; the true

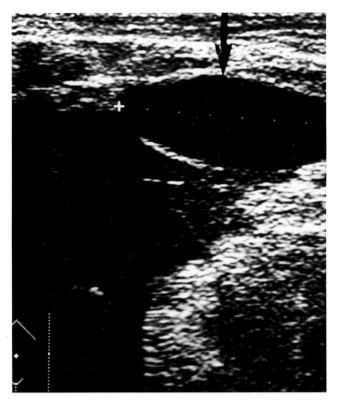

Fig. 53.4 10 days after a Whipple procedure a CT scan showed an oedematous pancreatic remnant. Ultrasonography demonstrated subfascial fluid collection. (Reprinted with permission of J B Lippincott Company, from Trede and Schwall 1988 Annals of Surgery 207:39.)

cause usually lies below the diaphragm and in the surgeon's operative field. Secondly, when in doubt, early reintervention is the safest policy (Smith et al 1992). Adherence to this rule may mean that a few 'unnecessary' relaparotomies are performed in patients with severe postoperative pain but without any intra-abdominal pathology. Fortunately, such reinterventions seldom do any harm.

Operative lavage and reinstitution of drainage is an unsatisfactory solution to the problem of anastomotic leakage, if it arises in the first postoperative week. If the drain placed at the end of the Whipple procedure did not work, another drain placed at relaparotomy is unlikely to do better. However, the general condition of some patients is often so poor that nothing more radical would be tolerated. Thus, two out of five patients treated with lavage and drainage alone in Mannheim succumbed to sepsis following the leak.

In three patients in the Mannheim series a combination of measures, as shown in Figure 53.5, was successful. But these leaks were well localized from the start and it might be argued that here an interventionalist percutaneous approach might have sufficed. However, relying on this policy as a general rule, carries the fatal danger of delaying reoperation for too long (Pellegrini et al 1989, Smith et al 1992).

The radical solution of 'completion pancreatectomy' seemed unavoidable in 14 patients in this series, three of whom succumbed to uncontrollable haemorrhage. Erosion of the ligated stumps of the gastroduodenal or splenic (after total pancreatectomy) arteries by pancreatic juice is indeed one of the most dangerous sequelae of these anastomotic leaks (Braasch & Gray 1977, Herter et al 1982).

However, in 11 of 14 patients 'completion pancreatectomy' was life-saving. Lerut et al (1984) reported success in three out of five such procedures, whereas in the Mayo experience with this emergency four patients were salvaged out of 11 (Smith et al 1992). Everything depends on removing the remaining pancreas early enough, that is before sepsis is generalized.

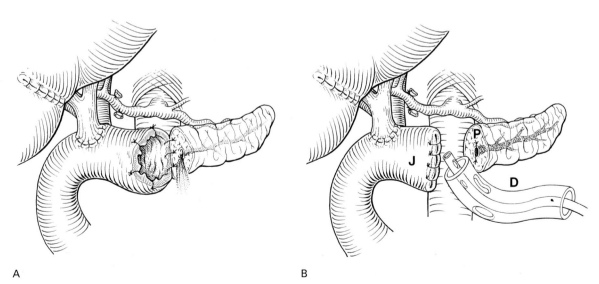

A   B

Fig. 53.5 **A** Breakdown of pancreaticojejunostomy after Whipple procedure. **B** Repair by occlusion of pancreatic duct (P) with Ethibloc, closure of jejunal stump (J), and irrigation-suction drain (D).

Table 53.5 The technical variations of pancreatojejunostomy (intended to prevent leaks)

Method	Authors
Pancreatogastrostomy	Mackie et al (1975), Kapur (1986), Delcore et al (1990), Waugh & Clagett (1946), Telford & Mason (1981), Bradbeer & Johnson (1990), Reding (1988), Icard & Dubois (1988)
End-to-side pancreato-jejunostomy with jejunoplication	Siedeck et al (1985)
2 or 3 separate jejunal loops to separate the pancreatic anastomosis	Schreiber et al (1977), Schopohl et al (1986), Lygidakis & Brummelkamp (1985)
Pancreatic duct drainage	Aston & Longmire (1974), Hall et al (1990), Longmire (1966), Smith (1979), Manabe et al (1986), Porter (1958)
Pancreatic duct ligation	Shiu (1982), Goldsmith et al (1971), Papachristou & Fortner (1981), Aretxabala et al (1991)
Pancreatic duct occlusion (Neoprene, Ethibloc, fibrin)	Gebhardt & Stolte (1978), Di Carlo et al (1989), Kram et al (1991)
Anastomotic coverage with fibrin or collagen	Waclawiczek & Lorenz (1989), Kram et al (1991), Lorenz & Scheele (1990)
Open drainage of pancreatic remnant	Funovics & Wenzl (1987)
Preoperative external radiation	Ishikawa et al (1991)

Prevention

Nowhere would 'prevention be better than cure' than in this particular catastrophe. Although there have been many ingenious suggestions for avoiding pancreatic leaks, there has been only one certain solution to the problem to date, and that is to avoid it altogether by performing total pancreatectomy in the first place. This has indeed been suggested whenever the pancreatic remnant is so friable and the duct so narrow that trouble with the anastomosis would appear inevitable (Smith 1979).

None of the other technical variations aimed at protecting the pancreatojejunal anastomosis has so far proved to be superior to the end-to-end invaginating procedure described in Chapter 40 (see Fig. 40.12) (Table 53.5). It does not seem to matter if additional cover is given by jejunoplication (Siedeck et al 1985), whether the pancreas is anastomosed to the stomach (Waugh & Clagett 1946, Hirano et al 1991) or whether two or three separate Roux-loops are used for the gastric, biliary and pancreatic anastomoses (Schreiber et al 1977). It makes little difference whether the pancreatic duct is drained (Longmire 1966), ligated (Goldsmith et al 1971), occluded (Gebhardt & Stolte 1978), oversewn, or treated with a combination of these methods. In fact, suture ligation of the duct has, if anything, led to a significantly higher rate of leaks, reaching an incidence of up to 70% in some series (Papachristou & Fortner 1981, Grace et al 1986). Even leaving the pancreatic remnant and its duct widely open with a drain placed nearby (Funovics & Wenzl 1987), merely produces the expected refractory fistulae and exocrine insufficiency without any reduction in mortality. Reports on the prophylactic role of a long-acting somatostatin analogue (Büchler et al 1992) await confirmation.

One is left with the conclusion that a meticulous technique is probably more important than the particular type of pancreatic anastomosis employed.

2. Haemorrhagic complications

Bleeding is a close second to anastomostic dehiscence in the list of dangerous postoperative complications. In one early report on 239 pancreatoduodenectomies performed in the Mayo Clinic, 20 patients experienced gastrointestinal haemorrhage (11 associated with pancreatic fistula) and 18 died (Mongé et al 1964). The more recent overall experience from several centres is summarized in Table 53.6. Granted the inadmissibility of comparing these various series, it seems that the incidence of postoperative haemorrhage is around 10% and that it will be fatal in one-third of those afflicted.

One should try to distinguish between gastrointestinal (i.e. intraluminal) bleeding and haemorrhage from the large raw surface of the retroperitoneal operative field. However, the latter often results from erosion of a ligated artery following a pancreatic leak and this may also present as

Table 53.6 Haemorrhagic complications following pancreatoduodenectomy. Operations include Whipple and total pancreatectomies. (ND, no data given)

Author	Institution	Total no of operations	No of complications		Mortality of haemorrhage	
			n	%	n	%
Braasch & Gray (1977)	Lahey Clinic	279	31	11	18	58
Nakase et al (1977)	Collected Japanese series	869	93	11	ND	ND
Edis et al (1980)	Mayo Clinic	162	23	14	9	39
Grace et al (1986)	UCLA	96	12	12.5	4	33
Pichlmayr & Rumpf (1986)	Hannover	62	6	9.6	ND	ND
Crist & Cameron (1989)	Johns Hopkins	88	15	17	ND	ND
Trede (1992) unpublished data	Mannheim	439	27	6	2	7

Table 53.7 Haemorrhagic complications, relaparotomies, and mortalities after 439 pancreatectomies (University Surgical Clinic, Mannheim, 1.10.1972–1.1.1992)

Site of haemorrhage	n	Relaparotomy	Mortality
Gastointestinal	20	8	2
Operative field	7	7	—
Total	27	15	2

haematemesis or melaena (i.e. as an 'intraluminal' bleed) (Brodsky & Turnbull 1991).

The prime cause of both types of haemorrhage is some intraoperative technical fault, notably the suture line that is not really haemostatic or the ligature that slips (see Ch. 42). True coagulation defects are rarely identifiable by laboratory analysis, although there is the impression that patients who present with obstructive jaundice are at greater risk from this complication despite vitamin K substitution (Hunt et al 1982, Dixon et al 1984, Diamond & Rowlands 1991).

Rarely, *preoperative haemorrhage* coming from such causes as a percutaneous biopsy (Grace et al 1986), a transhepatic stent, or the tumour itself leads to a risky emergency pancreatectomy.

Gastrointestinal *haemorrhage* occurred in 20 of 439 patients undergoing pancreatectomy in Mannheim and it originated almost invariably from the gastrojejunal anastomosis (Table 53.7). This was suture line oozing and

never bleeding from a 'stress ulcer'. Routine stress ulcer prophylaxis (with omeprazole) appears to be effective in this context. If there is the slightest suspicion of bleeding (blood in the nasogastric tube, melaena, or a drop in haemoglobin or blood pressure) gastroscopy must be carried out. The presence of a 24-hour endoscopy service (manned by surgeons!) is invaluable. The site of the bleeding is localized and in 12 out of our 20 cases, haemostasis was achieved by endoscopic measures (injection with adrenaline 1:10 000).

In all but one of our remaining eight patients, early relaparotomy with transverse gastrotomy (above the gastrojejunal anastomosis) and an additional suture, stopped the bleeding. The one exception was a jaundiced patient whose postoperative oozing was at first controlled by endoscopy. However, when he bled again and aspirated, relaparotomy came too late to save him. A more aggressive approach with earlier revision might have made all the difference.

A rare combination of mishaps, presenting as a gastrointestinal bleed is illustrated by the following example.

Case report: A 60-year-old man had a palliative biliary bypass (choledochoduodenostomy) performed at another hospital for obstructive jaundice due to carcinoma of the pancreatic head. Four weeks later we performed a Whipple procedure (including portal vein resection with a mesentericocaval anastomosis). On the second postoperative day, he had tachycardia, a dry tongue and epigastric tenderness. The Völker tube placed to splint the biliary anastomosis then began to drain blood. At laparotomy the pancreatic anastomosis was intact. However, the jejunal

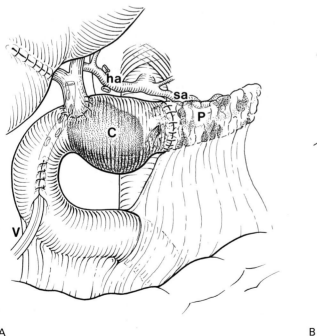
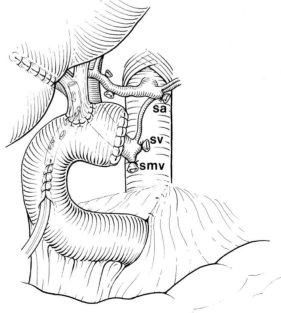

A

B

Fig. 53.6 Diagram showing site of operation two days after Whipple procedure. ha, Hepatic artery; sa, splenic artery; V, Völker drain; C, blood clot; Bl, bleeding from cut surface of pancreas; P, pancreatic remnant with pancreatitis. **B** After removal of remaining pancreas: J, jejunal stump oversewn; sa, stumps of splenic artery, and sv, splenic vein. The superior mesenteric vein (smv) had been anastomosed to the inferior vena cava at the first operation.

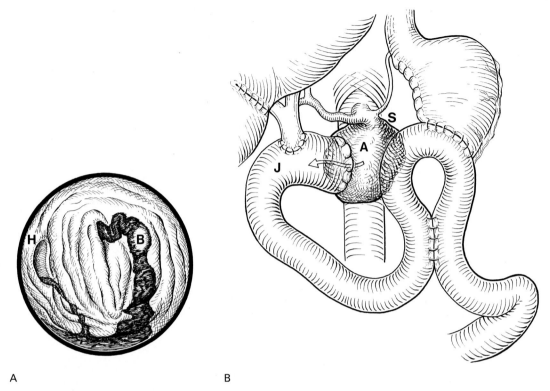

A   B

Fig. 53.7 **A** Diagram of endoscopic view into the proximal jejunal stump following total pancreatectomy. H, Opening of hepaticojejunostomy draining bile; B, blood clot and fresh blood entering the jejunal stump. **B** Situation following total pancreatectomy with false aneurysm (A), arising from ligated splenic artery (S) and penetrating into the jejunal stump (J).

loop draining it was distended and the pancreatic remnant had the mottled appearance of pancreatitis (Fig. 53.6). The explanation for this complication was a spurting bleeding site which we found on the cut surface of the pancreas. Due to a kink in the draining jejunal loop and a large obturating blood clot in that same loop, the blood had no free run-off. The resulting back pressure probably induced the pancreatitis. Again, the solution was completion pancreatectomy and the patient recovered.

Simple *postoperative haemorrhage* from the *operative field* may or may not present with blood loss via the drain, and with or without increasing abdominal pain, tachycardia and drop in haemoglobin levels. If it occurs within the first few postoperative days, early relaparotomy, evacuation of blood and clots, and suture repair can solve the problem.

Later *secondary haemorrhage* from retroperitoneal vessels, possibly due to erosion or infection, occurs 2–3 weeks postoperatively and poses a more difficult problem. This occurred seven times in the Mannheim experience, not counting bleeding in connection with pancreatic leaks. If after an uneventful course, the patient has a rise in temperature, a little abdominal pain and if he also passes blood in his stools, this is the complication to think of and to investigate by immediate endoscopy (Brodsky & Turnbull 1991).

Case report: A 61-year-old obese jaundiced man had a Whipple resection performed for pancreatic carcinoma. Completion pancreatectomy was undertaken 10 days later

because of acute pancreatitis in the remnant. He recovered from both operations and was discharged home 3 weeks later. However, he was readmitted 6 days after that with pyrexia and repeated vomiting of small amounts of blood. The endoscopist located the site of the bleeding by threading the endoscope into the proximal jejunal loop; a trickle of blood was seen clearly coming from the sutured jejunal stump (Fig. 53.7).

At laparotomy a pulsating false aneurysm was found at this point, possibly emanating from the eroded stump of the splenic artery. High clamping of the aorta, exposure of the aneurysm, and suture of the leak stopped the bleeding, and the patient was finally discharged 12 days later.

If bleeding occurs in connection with pancreatic anastomotic dehiscence, the only chance lies in completion pancreatectomy together with suture ligation of the eroded vessel.

Prevention

The prevention of these bleeding complications depends in the first place on meticulous haemostatic technique. Beyond that it is obvious that coagulation defects, particularly in jaundiced patients must be detected and treated in good time, i.e. preoperatively. Although the coagulation factors, even in patients with obstructive jaundice, may appear to be perfectly normal, there is no doubt that in actual practice, these patients are particularly prone to complications involving haemorrhage, infection and anastomotic dehiscence possibly resulting from endotoxaemia

(Trede & Schwall 1988, Greve et al 1990, Diamond & Rowlands 1991). That is why we advocate preoperative drainage of bile into the duodenum, preferably by the endoscopic route, if this can be done safely (see Ch. 37).

There can be no illusion about recovery of all the mitochondrial functions of hepatocytes within the time available (Fraser et al 1989). According to Koyama this takes up to 6 weeks (Koyama et al 1981), far longer than is practicable in most patients, particularly those with pancreatic cancer. However, even a drainage period of 1–2 weeks may reduce postoperative morbidity (Smith et al 1985).

3. Biliary fistula

Biliary fistulae following pancreatectomy are rare and relatively harmless in our experience and that of others (Table 53.8). These fistulae can be divided into true leaks from the hepaticojejunostomy, those due to an overlooked accessory bile duct and those caused by slippage of drains used to splint the bilioenteric anastomosis (Table 53.9).

Such leaks manifest themselves by persistent drainage of bile through the subhepatic drainage tube. If the patient has no symptoms, patience is well worthwhile since more than half of these leaks seal spontaneously within a few days or weeks, provided that there is no distal obstruction.

Symptoms due to undrained bile collections require the insertion of another drain. Nowadays this is usually done percutaneously under ultrasound control. Leakage along a dislodged drain can be demonstrated radiographically and the problem solved by simply removing this tube. Only rarely is a second formal anastomosis required for the rare complication of a persistently leaking accessory bile duct.

4. Miscellaneous complications

There is a long list of non-specific complications that can apply to any other major abdominal operation (see Table 53.1).

Abscesses. Other than those associated with anastomotic leaks, these are rare. They may present as hepatic abscesses, possibly secondary to cholangitis that may indeed be aggravated by preoperative biliary obstruction (Blamey et al 1983). Bacteriological swabs taken routinely at the time of transection of the hepatic duct demonstrate growth of bacteria in about 20% of cases.

Intra-abdominal abscesses are usually found in the right subhepatic or left subdiaphragmatic space; after total pancreatectomy and splenectomy the left side is more often involved. While operative drainage was formerly required in four out of eight abscesses in the Mannheim experience (Trede & Schwall 1988), most of them are now localized by ultrasound and drained percutaneously.

Chylous ascites. This occurs surprisingly rarely, considering the extensive retroperitoneal lymph node clearance that accompanies every pancreatectomy for cancer (Walker 1967, Fortner 1985). This lymphorrhoea can reach alarming proportions with loss of several litres of fluid daily which has to be meticulously replaced parenterally. Fortunately, such drainage ceases spontaneously after a couple of weeks.

Gastrointestinal fistulae. These fistulae, due to dehiscence of the gastrojejunostomy are rare (Braasch & Gray 1977). The authors have observed one leak, however, from an ischaemic perforation of the gastric fundus, following total pancreatectomy with splenectomy. This small area of necrosis, following ligature of the short gastric vessels, was oversewn by another row of seromuscular sutures (see Ch. 41).

Hepatic and mesenteric necrosis. This is usually a fatal complication caused by damage or thrombosis of either the hepatic or superior mesenteric arteries (Waugh & Giberson 1957, Lansing et al 1972, Pliam & ReMine 1975). This has already been discussed in Chapter 42.

A curious combination of complications initiated by jejunal torsion is shown by the following example.

Case report: A 57-year-old jaundiced man had a carcinoma of the pancreatic head removed by a Whipple operation. After an uneventful course he had fever, brief epigastric pain, and dyspnoea on the 7th postoperative day. Since the patient seemed to improve spontaneously, this brief episode was ascribed to a mild basal pneumonia, particularly since a chest X-ray seemed to confirm this.

On the next day a routine CT scan showed curiously dilated loops of bowel in the upper abdomen (Fig. 53.8A). When the patient had another spike of temperature (39°C), it was decided to reoperate. The proximal jejunal loop draining the pancreatic remnant and bile duct was grotesquely dilated and ischaemic

Table 53.8 Biliary fistulae following pancreatoduodenectomy. Operations include Whipple and total pancreatectomies. (ND, no data given)

Author	Institution	Total no of operations	No of complications		Mortality of biliary leak	
			n	%	n	%
Braasch & Gray (1977)	Lahey Clinic	279	38	13.6	4	10.5
Nakase et al (1977)	Collected Japanese series	869	49	6.0	ND	ND
Edis et al (1980)	Mayo Clinic	162	7	4.3	1	14.0
Grace et al (1986)	UCLA	96	3	3.0	ND	ND
Pichlmayr & Rumpf (1986)	Hannover	62	6	9.6	ND	ND
Crist & Cameron (1989)	Johns Hopkins	88	6	7	ND	ND
Trede (1992) unpublished data	Mannheim	439	11	2.5	0	0

Table 53.9   Biliary leakage and its treatment after 439 pancreatectomies (University Surgical Clinic, Mannheim, 1.10.1972–1.1.1992)

Complication	n	Therapy			Mortality
		Conservative	Operative Drainage	Suture	
Hepaticojejunostomy	7	5	2	—	—
Accessory bile duct	2	1	—	1	—
Biliary drainage	2	—	2	—	—
Total	11	6	4	—	—

due to torsion at the Braun jejunostomy (Fig. 53.8B). Again, there was no choice but to convert the Whipple into a total pancreatectomy and to bring up the next loop of jejunum for a new biliary anastomosis (Fig. 53.8C). The patient recovered.

Howard (1990, 1991) observed kinking and obstruction of the jejunal limb between the pancreatojejunostomy and choledochojejunostomy, requiring late reoperation in two cases.

Delayed gastric emptying. This has been discussed in Chapter 38. It can follow any type of gastrectomy, of course, and is not a common complication of the standard Whipple operation. If anything, it seems to afflict the pylorus-preserving variant more frequently (Braasch et al 1986, Warshaw & Torchiana 1985).

Minor degrees of gastric outlet obstruction, demonstrated by gastrografin swallow but not requiring a nasogastric tube for drainage, were seen in eight (2%) of the Mannheim cases. The problem resolved spontaneously after 2–3 weeks with patience, mainly liquid food intake and metoclopramide medication.

EARLY NON-SURGICAL COMPLICATIONS

These postoperative complications are mentioned for the sake of completeness, although none are really specific to pancreatic resection. Nor does their management differ from those following other major operations.

Cardiopulmonary complications. In a series of 1904 pancreatoduodenectomies collected by Jordan, cardiopulmonary complications occurred in 9% of patients (Jordan 1987). In the Mannheim series of over 400 such operations, major cardiopulmonary complications occurred in only 12, leading to death in two. One patient succumbed to aspiration pneumonia and ARDS following total pancreatectomy as well as total gastrectomy for a gastric carcinoma infiltrating the pancreas. The second patient, aged 75 years, died of a myocardial infarct immediately following an otherwise uneventful total pancreatectomy for cancer.

Hepatic insufficiency. This was confined to laboratory findings (rise in transaminase levels) mainly in jaundiced patients, some of whom required several weeks before bilirubin levels returned to normal (Pellegrini et al 1982).

Renal failure. This occurred in earlier series at the rate of some 3% and was fatal in 75% of cases (Mongé et al 1964, Braasch & Gray 1977). Today it still is part of multiorgan failure in severe cases of sepsis or following haemorrhagic shock. However, the so-called 'hepatorenal syndrome' was not encountered once in the Mannheim experience, which included 247 pancreatectomies in jaundiced patients. This is probably the result of preoperative biliary drainage and improved fluid replacement (Wait & Kahng 1989).

LATE SURGICAL SEQUELAE OF PANCREATECTOMY

While there are a number of non-specific late problems such as intestinal obstruction or incisional hernia, the following three complications are directly related to pancreatoduodenectomy.

Marginal ulceration. This was considered to be a common occurrence in patients following pancreatectomy and that is why partial gastrectomy was included as the procedure was developed (Whipple 1942). This did not appear to provide sufficient protection, however, since Scott et al (1980), albeit in a small series, reported stomal ulcers in 36% of patients. In a subsequent series of patients who also had vagotomy no such ulceration was observed. The ulcerogenic potential of total pancreatectomy also led Grant and van Heerden (1979) to recommend truncal vagotomy for these patients, especially if there was a history of peptic ulcer.

However, peptic ulceration has not been a problem in the authors' experience or that reported from other centres more recently (Crist et al 1987, Jordan 1987). Following 439 pancreatectomies for chronic pancreatitis or cancer, 11 patients with marginal ulceration were observed in a long-term follow-up (2.5%) in Mannheim and only four of them required operative treatment of their ulcers. It would appear that vagotomy is not required as part of pancreatoduodenectomy.

Obstructive jaundice. The development of this condition, sometimes several years following pancreatoduodenectomy for cancer, immediately raises the suspicion of recurrence, particularly in the hilum of the liver. Obstruction of the jejunal loop draining the bile duct, as a result of a local recurrence at the mesenteric root may also give

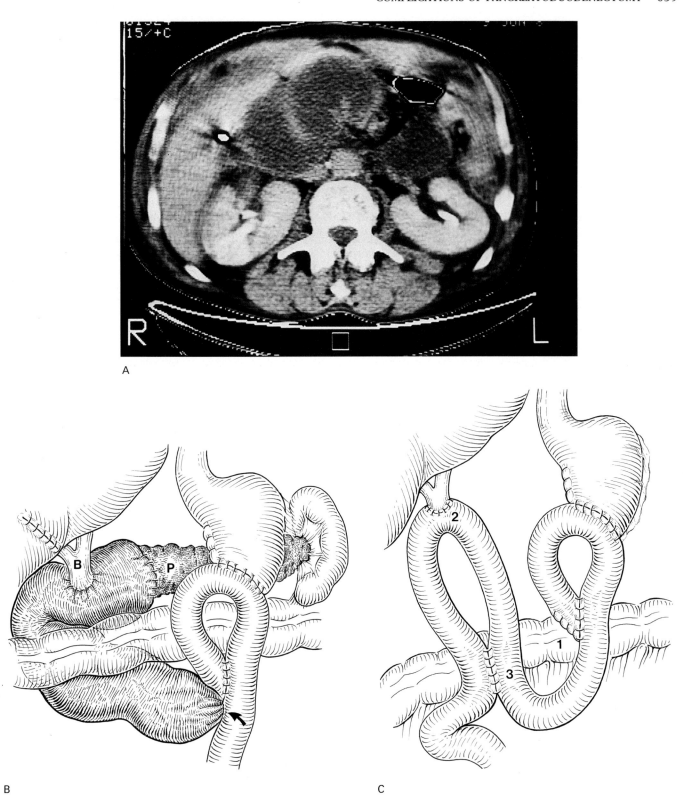

Fig. 53.8 A CT, 8 days after a Whipple procedure showing dilated, oedematous jejunal loop in the immediate subhepatic space. (Reprinted with permission of J B Lippincott Company, from Trede and Schwall 1988 Annals of Surgery 207:45. **B** Diagram of operative site after a Whipple pancreatectomy. Arrow points to torsion of the proximal jejunal loop at the Braun jejunojejunostomy; B, hepaticojejunostomy; P, pancreaticojejunostomy. **C** Operative site after the removal of the offending jejunal loop, remaining pancreas and spleen; 1, oversewn jejunum at site of Braun anastomosis; 2, new hepaticojejunostomy; 3, new Braun jejunojejunostomy.

rise to jaundice. If this happens, temporary palliation can sometimes be achieved by bringing up a second Roux-Y-loop to decompress the first (Fig. 53.9).

Before any patient is given up as inoperable or referred for some palliative drainage procedure, it is worth considering other benign causes for this jaundice (Jordan 1987). Thus, Waugh & Giberson (1957) observed three cases of benign stricture of the bilioenteric anastomosis that were amenable to repair, and the late occurrence of common duct stones, particularly in patients who did not have their gallbladders removed at the time of pancreatectomy has been described (Waugh & Giberson 1957, Jordan 1987). This, and the possible occurrence of acute cholecystitis years after an otherwise successful pancreatoduodenectomy, underscores the importance of including cholecystectomy as part of that operation (Muscroft & Ambrose 1984).

Quite apart from mechanical biliary obstruction, persistent attacks of cholangitis may plague some patients. This may, of course, occur after any bilioenteric anastomosis, particularly if the problem of reflux of intestinal contents has not been adequately solved. We have observed this phenomenon (a brief rise in temperature above 39°C, with rigor but without pain or jaundice) in two patients

following more than 400 such anastomoses. A simple mechanical explanation is malfunction of the Braun jejuno-jejunostomy, which can be demonstrated by an upper gastrointestinal series (Fig. 53.10). If this demonstration of reflux is convincing, then detachment of the jejunal loop from the Braun anastomosis and connecting it to the ileum some 30 cm distally should solve the problem.

Second primary carcinoma. Among late surgical sequelae is the occurrence of a second primary carcinoma in patients who survived pancreatectomy for cancer. Although not a real complication, this occurrence is worth attention, because again the second tumour might be misjudged as an inoperable recurrence (Fig. 53.11).

LATE NON-SURGICAL SEQUELAE OF PANCREATODUODENECTOMY

Standard pancreatoduodenectomy has been under attack as a 'mutilating procedure'. While in most cases of carcinoma this is probably the only solution for the patient, the operation is said to be unnecessarily radical when it comes to treating complicated chronic pancreatitis.

Porter reported a sprue-like condition, which he called 'late post-partial-pancreatectomy syndrome' and which

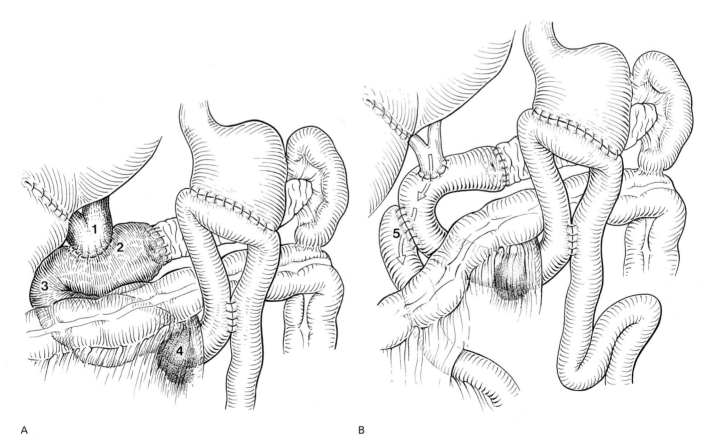

A B

Fig. 53.9 **A** and **B** A 54-year-old man developed local recurrence in the mesenteric root 12 months after pancreatectomy for carcinoma; 1, dilated common hepatic duct; 2, patent hepaticojejunostomy; 3, obstructed jejunal loop; 4, recurrent tumour at mesenteric root; 5, second Roux-Y-loop decompressing the first loop and draining the bile.

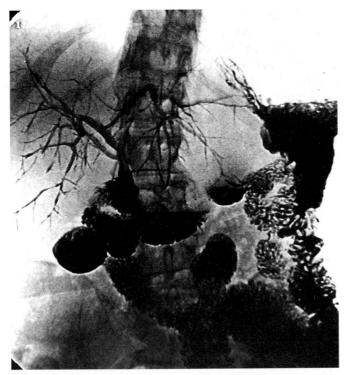

Fig. 53.10 46-year-old man. This upper gastrointestinal roentgenogram 3 years after pancreatoduodenectomy for severe chronic pancreatitis shows reflux into the hepatic ducts. This had caused monthly attacks of cholangitis, which disappeared after detachment of the jejunal loop (from the Braun anastomosis) and its reanastomosis 30 cm distally.

he saw in three of 27 patients following a Whipple resection (Porter 1958). It was assumed that obliteration of the pancreatic duct opening was the cause and the syndrome could be adequately controlled by enzyme substitution.

More recently Beger has criticized the Whipple operation as applied to chronic pancreatitis for destroying the 'entero-insular axis' (by removal of the duodenum) and causing an inordinately high late mortality (Beger & Büchler 1990). Indeed the decision to undertake a Whipple resection should not be made lightly, if any lesser and simpler procedure would be equally effective. But, as discussed in Chapter 26, the operation may well be indicated when severe chronic pancreatitis centred within the pancreatic head causes intractable pain, stenosis of the biliary and pancreatic ducts and possibly of the duodenum.

In the experience of many authors, however, the late functional deficits caused by standard pancreatoduodenectomy do not exceed those of the natural course of the underlying disease, provided the remaining pancreatic body and tail as well as the proximal half of the stomach are relatively normal (Gall 1987, Jordan 1987, Howard 1990), and provided that the patient is disciplined enough to avoid further alcoholic damage to these organs.

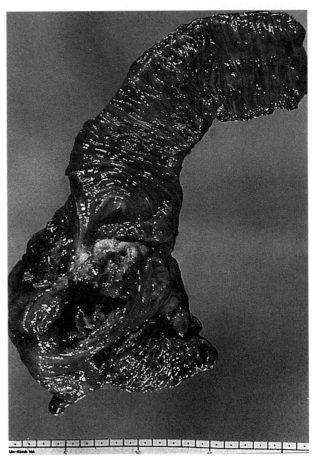

A

Fig. 53.11 69-year-old lady. **A** Specimen following Whipple pancreatoduodenectomy for papillary carcinoma ($T_2N_0M_x$) in November 1983. **B** Operative specimen following right hemicolectomy for a carcinoma of the ascending colon ($T_3N_0M_x$) in July 1991.

B

Table 53.10   Late mortality following pancreatoduodenectomy (for chronic pancreatitis) (Howard 1990)

Author	Institution	Total no of patients	Median follow-up (years)	Mortality n	%
Rossi et al (1987)	Lahey Clinic	73	5	17	23
Gauthier-Benoit & Perissat (1987)	Bordeaux	287	3.8	57	24
Gall (1988)	Erlangen	289	8	55	19
Mannell et al (1988)	Mayo Clinic	10	8	1	10
Howard (1990)	Toledo, Ohio	30	7	0	—
Trede (1992) unpublished data	Mannheim	119	4.8	12	9
Total		808	—	142	17

As shown in Chapter 33, the late results after surgery for chronic pancreatitis depend more on the correct indication than on the particular technique of resection employed. In other words, late mortality and morbidity are related more to continued alcohol abuse than they are to any functional deficits possibly caused by the operation. This is borne out by Table 53.10, which shows that the overall 5-year survival following pancreatoduodenectomy for chronic pancreatitis exceeds 80%.

A more detailed analysis of mortality following pancreatoduodenectomy for chronic pancreatitis in the Mannheim experience is shown in Table 53.11. Seven out of the 12 late deaths were directly or indirectly due to the ravages of alcoholism.

Late exocrine and endocrine function were assessed in 79 patients available for follow-up examination after a median of 4.8 years following pancreatoduodenectomy (Table 53.12).

The management of exocrine insufficiency was seldom a problem with the use of adequate pancreatic enzyme substitution. Perhaps the best criterion of the overall

Table 53.11   Mortality of 119 Whipple operations for chronic pancreatitis (University Surgical Clinic, Mannheim 1.10.1972–1.1.1992)

Operative and hospital mortality	1 (0.8%)
Late mortality (median survival = 32 months)	12 (10%)
Cause of death	
Alcoholism	7
Myocardial infarction	3
Bleeding	1
Unknown	1

Table 53.12   Late functional results following pancreatoduodenectomy (for chronic pancreatitis n = 79). Exocrine function was determined by chymotrypsin and fat in stool, endocrine function by HbAlc, blood glucose and glucagon test

	Exocrine function		Endocrine function	
	n	%	n	%
Preoperative insufficiency	13	16	21	27
Postoperative insufficiency	19	24	10*	12
No insufficiency	47	60	48	61

* Only 5 patients require insulin.

nutritional state is the change in body weight: 61 of the 79 patients had gained weight (median gain 12 kg) following pancreatoduodenectomy. Howard also found that nutrition was significantly better following the Whipple operation (in patients operated upon for severe chronic pancreatitis) than it was preoperatively (Howard 1990).

Endocrine insufficiency after the Whipple operation for chronic pancreatitis affected a minority of patients in the Mannheim experience. Ethibloc occlusion of the (pancreatic) duct, has been reported to increase the incidence of clinical diabetes by 27% (Gall et al 1982). Rumpf and Pichlmayr 1982 found a rise of 9% (from 31% preoperatively to 40% postoperatively).

In summary, it appears that these functional deficits following the Whipple procedure for chronic pancreatitis do not exceed those of the spontaneous course of the disease. As observed by Ammann et al (1984), 5 years after the onset of alcoholic chronic pancreatitis, 50% of the patients manifested both exocrine and endocrine insufficiency.

REFERENCES

Ammann R W, Akovbiantz A, Largadièr F, Schueler G 1984 Course and outcome of chronic pancreatitis. Gastroenterology 86:820–828

Aretxabala de X, Burgos L, Flores P, Nagakawa T, Miyazaki I, Fonseca L 1991 Pancreatojejunostomy. American Surgeon 57:293–294

Aston S J, Longmire Jr W P 1974 Management of the pancreas after pancreaticoduodenectomy. Annals of Surgery 179:322–327

Baker R J 1979 Discussion of Moossa A R. Archives of Surgery 114:502

Beger H G, Büchler M 1990 Duodenum-preserving resection of the head of the pancreas in chronic pancreatitis with inflammatory mass in the head. World Journal of Surgery 14:83–87

Blamey S L, Fearon K C H, Gilmour W H, Osbourne D H, Carter D C 1983 Prediction of risk in biliary surgery. British Journal of Surgery 70:535–538

Braasch J W, Gray B N 1977 Considerations that lower pancreatoduodenectomy mortality. American Journal of Surgery 133:480–484

Braasch J W, Deziel D J, Rossi R L, Watkins Jr E, Winter P F 1986 Pyloric and gastric preserving pancreatic resection. Experience with 87 patients. Annals of Surgery 204:411–418

Bradbeer J W, Johnson C D 1990 Pancreaticogastrostomy after pancreaticoduodenectomy. Annals of the Royal College of Surgeons of England 72:266–269

Brodsky J T, Turnbull A D M 1991 Arterial hemorrhage after pancreaticoduodenectomy. The 'sentinel bleed'. Archives of Surgery 126:1037–1040

Büchler M, Friess H, Klempa I, Hermanek P et al 1992 Role of octreotide in the prevention of postoperative complications following pancreatic resection. American Journal of Surgery 163:125–131

Crist D W, Sitzmann J V, Cameron J L 1987 Improved hospital morbidity, mortality, and survival after the Whipple procedure. Annals of Surgery 206:358–373

Crist D W, Cameron J L 1989 Current status of pancreaticoduodenectomy for periampullary carcinoma. Hepato-gastroenterology 36:478–485

Delcore R, Thomas J H, Pierce G E, Hermreck A S 1990 Pancreatogastrostomy: a safe drainage procedure after pancreaticoduodenectomy. Surgery 108:641–647

Diamond T, Rowlands B J 1991 Review Article: Endotoxaemia in obstructive jaundice. HPB Surgery 4:81–94

Di Carlo V, Chiesa R, Pontiroli A E, Carlucci M, Staudacher C, Zerbi A, Cristallo M, Braga M, Pozza G 1989 Pancreatoduodenectomy with occlusion of the residual stump by Neoprene injection. World Journal of Surgery 13:105–111

Dixon J M, Armstrong C P, Duffy S W, Elton R A, Davies G C 1984 Upper gastrointestinal bleeding. A significant complication after surgery for relief of obstructive jaundice. Annals of Surgery 199:271–275

Edis A J, Kiernan P D, William F T 1980 Attempted curative resection of ductal carcinoma of the pancreas. Reviews of Mayo Clinic experience, 1951–1975. Mayo Clinic Proceedings 55:531–536

Fortner J G 1985 Technique of regional subtotal and total pancreatectomy. American Journal of Surgery 150:593–600

Fraser I A, Shaffer P, Tuttle S V, Lessler M A, Ellison E C, Carey L C 1989 Hepatic recovery after biliary decompression of experimental obstructive jaundice. American Journal of Surgery 158:423–427

Funovics J, Wenzl E 1987 Duodenopancreatectomie: Anastomosierung nicht notwendig. Langenbecks Archiv für Chirurgie 366:613

Gall F P, Gebhardt C, Zirngibl H 1982 Chronic pancreatitis – results in 116 consecutive, partial duodenopancreatectomies combined with pancreatic duct occlusion. Hepato-gastroenterology 29:115

Gall F P 1987 Chronische Pankreatitis: chirurgische Therapie durch Resektionsverfahren. Langenbecks Archiv für Chirurgie 372:363–368

Gall F P 1988 Treatment of chronic pancreatitis. International Hepato-Biliary-Pancreatic Association, Nice

Gauthier-Benoit C, Perissat J 1987 The treatment of chronic pancreatitis. In: 89 ième Congrès de l'Association Française de Chirurgie. Masson, Paris

Gebhardt C, Stolte M 1978 Pankreasgang-Okklusion durch Injektion einer schnellhärtenden Aminosäurenlösung. Experimentelle Studie. Langenbecks Archiv für Chirurgie 346:149–166

Goldsmith H S, Ghosh B C, Huvos A G 1971 Ligation versus implantation of the pancreatic duct after pancreaticoduodenectomy. Surgery, Gynecology and Obstetrics 132:87–92

Grace P A, Pitt H A, Tompkins R K, DenBesten L, Longmire Jr W P 1986 Decreased morbidity and mortality after pancreatoduodenectomy. American Journal of Surgery 151:141–149

Grant C S, van Heerden J A 1979 Anastomotic ulceration following subtotal and total pancreatectomy. Annals of Surgery 190:1–5

Greve J W, Maessen J G, Tiebosch T, Buurman W A, Gouma D J 1990 Prevention of postoperative complications in jaundiced rats. Internal biliary drainage versus oral lactulose. Annals of Surgery 212:221–227

Hall R I, Rhodes M, Isabel-Martinez L, Kelleher J, Venables C W 1990 Pancreatic exocrine function after a sutureless pancreaticojejunostomy following pancreaticoduodenectomy. British Journal of Surgery 77:83–85

Herter F P, Cooperman A M, Ahlborn T N, Antinori C 1982 Surgical experience with pancreatic and periampullary cancer. Annals of Surgery 195:274–281

Hirano T, Miura T, Shimuzu T, Kusano H, Yamaguchi E, Yoshida A, Yoshida K, Shimoyama T, Tomita M, Kawaguchi A, Shiraishi E 1991 Pancreatogastrostomy as a reliable alternative to pancreatojejunostomy in pancreatoduodenectomy. Research in Surgery 3:141–146

Howard J M 1990 Pancreaticoduodenectomy (Whipple resection) in the treatment of chronic pancreatitis: indications, techniques, and results. In: Beger H G, Büchler M, Ditschuneit H, Malfertheiner P (eds) Chronic pancreatitis. Springer-Verlag, Berlin, p 467–480

Howard J M 1991 Efferent limb obstruction after pancreaticojejunostomy. A late cause of pancreatitis following Whipple resection. Archives of Surgery 126:1157–1159

Hunt D R, Allison M E M, Prentice C R M, Blumgart L H 1982 Endotoxaemia disturbance of coagulation and obstructive jaundice. American Journal of Surgery 144:325–329

Icard P, Dubois F 1988 Pancreaticogastrostomy following pancreatoduodenectomy. Annals of Surgery 207:253–256

Ishikawa O, Ohigashi H, Imaoka S, Teshima T, Inoue T, Sasaki Yo, Iwanaga T, Nakaizumi A 1991 Concomitant benefit of preoperative irradiation in preventing pancreas fistula formation after pancreatoduodenectomy. Archives of Surgery 126:885–889

Jordan Jr G L 1987 Pancreatic resection for pancreatic cancer. In: Howard J M, Jordan Jr G L, Reber H A (eds) Surgical diseases of the pancreas, Lea and Febiger, Philadelphia, p 666–714

Kapur B M L 1986 Pancreaticogastrostomy in pancreaticoduodenal resection for ampullary carcinoma: experience in thirty-one cases. Surgery 100:489–493

Koyama K, Takagi Y, Ito K 1981 Experimental and clinical studies on the effect of biliary drainage in obstructive jaundice. American Journal of Surgery 142:293–299

Kram H B, Clark S R, Ocampo H P, Yamaguchi M A, Shoemaker W C 1991 Fibrin glue sealing of pancreatic injuries, resections, and anastomoses. American Journal of Surgery 161:479–482

Lansing P B, Blalock J B, Ochsner J L 1972 Pancreatoduodenectomy: a retrospective review 1949 to 1969. American Surgeon 2:79–86

Lerut J P, Gianello P R, Otte J B, Kestens P J 1984 Pancreaticoduodenal resection. Surgical experience and evaluation of risk factors in 103 patients. Annals of Surgery 199:432–437

Longmire Jr W P 1966 The technique of pancreaticoduodenal resection. Surgery 59:344–352

Lorenz D, Scheele J 1990 Die Anwendung von Kollagen-Vlies (Tachocomb) in der Pankreas-Chirurgie. Zeitschrift für experimentelle Chirurgie, Transplantation und künstliche Organe 23:93–94

Lygidakis N J, Brummelkamp W H 1985 A new approach for the reconstruction of continuity of the alimentary tract after pancreaticoduodenotomy. Surgery, Gynecology and Obstetrics 160:453–458

Mackie J A, Rhoads J E, Park C D 1975 Pancreaticogastrostomy: a further evaluation. Annals of Surgery 181:541–545

Manabe T, Suzuki T, Tobe T 1986 A secured technique for pancreatojejunal anastomosis in pancreaticoduodenectomy. Surgery, Gynecology and Obstetrics 163:379–380

Mannell A, van Heerden J A, Weiland L H, Ilstrup D M 1986 Factors influencing survival after resection for ductal adenocarcinoma of the pancreas. Annals of Surgery 203:403–407

Mannell A, Adson M A, McIlrath D C, Ilstrup D M 1988 Surgical management of chronic pancreatitis: long-term in 141 patients. British Journal of Surgery 75:467

Mongé J J, Judd E S, Gage R P 1964 Radical pancreatoduodenectomy: a 23-year experience with the complications, mortality rate, and survival rate. Annals of Surgery 160:711–722

Muscroft T J, Ambrose N S 1984 Pancreaticoduodenectomy: should the gallbladder be removed routinely? British Journal of Surgery 71:143

Nakase A, Matsumoto Y, Uchida K, Honjo I 1977 Surgical treatment of cancer of the pancreas and the periampullary region: cumulative results in 57 institutions in Japan. Annals of Surgery 185:52–57

Papachristou D N, Fortner J G 1981 Pancreatic fistula complicating pancreatectomy for malignant disease. British Journal of Surgery 68:238–240

Pellegrini C A, Thomas M J, Way L W 1982 Bilirubin and alkaline phosphatase values before and after surgery for biliary obstruction. American Journal of Surgery 143:67–73

Pellegrini C A, Heck C F, Raper S, Way L W 1989 An analysis of the reduced morbidity and mortality rates after pancreaticoduodenectomy. Archives of Surgery 124:778–781

Pichlmayr R, Rumpf K D 1986 Resektionstherapie beim Pankreaskarzinom: Chirurgische Technik, postoperative Komplikationen, Spätergebnisse. In: Beger H G, Bittner R (eds) Das Pankreaskarzinom. Springer-Verlag, Berlin, p 294–303

Pliam M B, ReMine W H 1975 Further evaluation of total pancreatectomy. Archives of Surgery 110:506–512

Porter M R 1958 Carcinoma of the pancreatico-duodenal area. Operability and choice of procedure. Annals of Surgery 148:711–724

Reding R 1988 Pankreasanastomosen. Chirurg 59:820–827

Rossi R L, Rothschild J, Braasch J W et al 1987 Pancreatoduodenectomy in the management of chronic pancreatitis. Archives of Surgery 122:416–420

Rumpf K D, Pichlmayr R 1982 Die chirurgische Behandlung der chronisch-calcifizierenden Pankreatitis. Der Chirurg 53:113

Schirmer W J, Rossi R L, Braasch J W 1991 Common difficulties and complications in pancreatic surgery. Surgical Clinics of North America 71:1391–1417

Schopohl J, Zöckler C E, Draese K 1986 Ein modifiziertes Whipple'sches Operationsverfahren. Der Chirurg 57:517–521

Schreiber H W, Farthmann E H, Eichfuss H P, Kortmann K B 1977 Pankreasresektion, -exstirpation, Reparation durch isoperistaltische Segmentinterposition. Der Chirurg 48:607–612

Scott Jr H W, Dean R H, Parker T, Avant G 1980 The role of vagotomy in pancreaticoduodenectomy. Annals of Surgery 191:688–696

Shiu M H 1982 Resection of pancreas without production of fistula. Surgery, Gynecology and Obstetrics 154:497–500

Siedeck M, Birtel F, Mitrenga I 1985 Pankreasganganastomose und Pankreatojejunoplicatio nach Rechtsresektion. Langenbecks Archiv für Chirurgie 366:610

Smith R 1979 Surgery of cancer of the pancreas. In: Taylor J H, Sarles H (eds) The exocrine pancreas. W B Saunders, London, p 520–535

Smith R C, Pooley M, George C R P, Faithful G R 1985 Preoperative percutaneous transhepatic internal drainage in obstructive jaundice: a randomized, controlled trial examining renal function. Surgery 97:641–647

Smith C D, Sarr M G, van Heerden J A 1992 Completion pancreatectomy following pancreatico-duodenectomy: clinical experience. World Journal of Surgery 16:521–524

Telford G L, Mason G R 1981 Improved technique for pancreaticogastrostomy after pancreaticoduodenectomy. American Journal of Surgery 142:386–387

Trede M, Schwall G 1988 The complications of pancreatectomy. Annals of Surgery 207:39–47

Waclawiczek H W, Lorenz D 1989 Der Schutz der pancreatico-digestiven Anastomose nach Pankreaskopfresektion durch Pankreasgangocclusion mit Fibrin(-kleber). Der Chirurg 60:403–409

Wait R B, Kahng K U 1989 Renal failure complicating obstructive jaundice. American Journal of Surgery 157:256–263

Walker W M 1967 Chylous ascites following pancreatoduodenectomy. Archives of Surgery 95:640–642

Warshaw A L, Torchiana D L 1985 Delayed gastric emptying after pylorus-preserving pancreaticoduodenectomy. Surgery, Gynecology and Obstetrics 160:1–4

Waugh J M, Clagett O T 1946 Resection of the duodenum and head of the pancreas for carcinoma. Surgery 20:224–232

Waugh J M, Giberson R G 1957 Radical resection of the head of the pancreas and of the duodenum for malignant lesions. Some factors in operative technique and preoperative and postoperative care, with an analysis of 85 cases. Surgical Clinics of North America: 965–979

Whipple A O 1942 Present day surgery of the pancreas. New England Journal of Medicine 226:515–526

Index

Abdominal exploration, 141–145
  endoscopic approaches, 145
  intraoperative procedures, 141–158
  Kocher manoeuvre, 143–144, 443, 549
Abdominal trauma, and acute pancreatitis,
  173
Abscess see Pancreatic abscess
ACCR see Amylase: creatinine clearance rate
Acetaldehyde, toxicity mechanisms, 166
Acinar cell carcinoma, 413–414
Acinar cells
  bombesin receptors, 40–41
  proposed secretory pathways,
    normal/abnormal, 178
  secretin receptors, 35, 36
  see also Islet–acinar relationships
Acute pancreatitis, 161–259
  acute interstitial pancreatitis, defined, 163
  acute necrotizing pancreatitis, defined, 163
  aetiology
    age and sex of patients, 194
    lipid metabolism abnormalities, 168–169
    trauma, 586
    see also Acute pancreatitis, models
  alcohol-associated acute pancreatitis,
    165–169
  classification, 161–164
    ULM classification, 233–235
  clinical associations, 165
  clinical features, 194–195
  complications, 245–259
    abscess, 64
    development of chronic pancreatitis, 300
    haemorrhage, 250–252
    intestinal complications, 252–255
    necrosis, 245–248
    pseudocysts, 64, 248–250
    variceal haemorrhage, 250–251
    vascular necrosis, 251–252
  defined, 161–164
  diagnostic assessment, 193–207
    APACHE II score, 205
    grades A–E, 61–63
    peritoneal lavage, 198–199
    severity assessment, 200–205
    see also Acute pancreatitis, imaging
  grading systems
    Glasgow system, 203–204
    Hong Kong system, 204
    Ranson system, 203
  history and examination, 195–196
  imaging
    angiography, 83–85

    barium contrast studies, 53, 199
Acute pancreatitis
  chest radiographs, 199
  computed tomography, 61–66, 200
    complications, 63–66
  endoscopic retrograde
    cholangiopancreatography, 87–89, 173
  plain films, 199
  ultrasonography, 56–58, 199–200
  incidence, 193
  interstitial oedematous pancreatitis,
    233–234
  laboratory assessment, 196–198
    blood tests, 196
    serum amylase, 196–198
    serum lipase, 198
    urinary amylase, 198
  management, historical note, 11–12
  management, non-operative, 209–220
    electrolyte replacement, 210
    intravascular volume management,
      209–210
    limitation of inflammation, 211–213
    measures to interrupt pathophysiology of
      complications, 213–216
    measures to limit inflammation, 211–213
    nutritional support, 210
    peritoneal lavage, 214–215
    respiratory monitoring and support, 210
    supportive and symptomatic treatment,
      209–211
    see also Pain relief
  management, operative, 233–244
    goals, 237
    indications, 235–236
    necrosectomy and peritoneal lavage,
      238–240
    pancreatic resection, contraindications,
      237
    pancreaticoduodenectomy,
      contraindications, 237–238
    percutaneous drainage, 240–241
    timing, algorithm, 235–238
  models
    bile injection, 176
    caerulein model, 177–178
    choline-deficient ethionine-supplemented
      diet model, 176–179, 186
    duodenal ligation, 175–176
    ex vivo isolated perfused canine model,
      178–179
    feline duct obstruction, 176
    ischaemia, 171–172

    non-invasive induction, 176–178
    peritoneal lavage, 183
  mortality
    causes, 215
    rates, 194
  necrotizing pancreatitis, 234
  oral feeding, contraindications, 212
  in pancreatic cancer, 424
  pathogenesis, 165–179, 179–192
    antiproteases, 180
    clotting cascade, 182–183
    complement cascade, 181–182
    interruption of, 213–216
    kininogen cascade, 182
    peritoneal exudate, 215–216
    see also Proteases
  predisposing factors, 165–175
  prognosis, 193–207
    single parameters, 200–203
  treatment see Acute pancreatitis,
    management
  trypsin levels, 320–321
  veins, involvement, CT, 66
Adenoma, benign, enucleation, 549, 550
Age
  ageing patient, malabsorption, 127–130
  and pancreatic changes, 127
  as prognostic factor, 203
AIDS-related pancreatic disorders, 104
Alanine aminotransferase, use in diagnosis,
  226
Albumin, serum levels, prognostic factor, 203
Albumin plugs, alcohol-associated
  pancreatitis, 167–168
Alcohol
  abstinence, 277
  changes in consumption
    and mortality rates, 264
    and risk of chronic pancreatitis, 265
    various countries, 264
  and coffee consumption, in pancreatic
    cancer, 388
  intracellular toxic metabolic actions,
    266–267
  and pancreatic cancer, 388, 400–401
Alcohol-associated pancreatitis, 165–169,
  265–267
  clinical associations, 165–166
  mechanisms of alcohol injury, 166–169
  nutritional factors, 265–266
  pathogenesis, 266–267
    intracellular toxic metabolic actions of
      alcohol, 266–267

Alcohol-associated pancreatitis (contd)
  primary disordered hepatic detoxification,
    267
  primary intraductal obstruction, 266
  vs gallstone-associated pancreatitis,
    225–226
  see also Chronic pancreatitis
Algorithms
  angiography of pancreatic tumours, 427
  diagnostic and therapeutic ERCP of
    tumours, 429
  for operative decision-making in acute
    pancreatitis, 237
  treatment of gastrinoma, 554
  for treatment of insulinoma, 549
Alkaline phosphatase levels, chronic
  pancreatitis, 286
Allergic states, epidemiology of pancreatic
  tumours, 391
Amine precursor uptake and decarboxylation
  (APUD) cells, origin, 546
Ampicillin, interruption of pathogenesis of
  acute pancreatitis, 213
Ampulla of Vater see Papilla of Vater
Amylase, serum, 31, 196–198
  assessment of acute pancreatitis, 196–198
  determinations, 130
  hyperamylasaemia, 104, 196
    associated conditions, 197
    prognosis, 201
    trauma, 585
  macroamylasaemia, 196–197
  sensitivity, 197
Amylase, urinary, 198
  amylase: creatinine clearance rate, 198
Anaemia, glucagonoma syndrome, 555
Anaesthesia in pancreatic surgery, 623–627
  epidural anaesthesia, 625–626
  postoperative care and management,
    626–627
  preoperative care, 623–624
  principles of, 624–626
  replacement fluids, 623–624
Analgesics
  infiltrative techniques, 351–352
  oral
    opioids, 276–277
    stages 1-3, 350–351
    plateau phenomenon, 350
  post surgery, 626
Anatomy of the pancreas, 18–26
Aneurysm, false, 291
Angiography, 81–86, 284
  cystic neoplasms, 95
  indications, 81–82
  pancreatic tumours, 429–430
    algorithm, 427
    predictive value, 429–430
  techniques, 81
Animal models see Acute pancreatitis, models;
  Models
Annular pancreas, 19, 369–371
  aetiology and pathophysiology, 369
  clinical features, 369–370
  developmental anatomy, 369
  incidence and prevalence, 369
  pathology, 446
  treatment, 371
Antacids, interruption of pathogenesis of
  acute pancreatitis, 213–214
Antibiotics
  control of endotoxaemia, 501–502
  interruption of pathogenesis of acute

pancreatitis, 213–214
Anticholinergics, inhibition of pancreatic
  exocrine secretions, 212
Antichymotrypsin, giant cell carcinoma, 408
Anticoagulants, interruption of pathogenesis
  of acute pancreatitis, 214
Antihormone therapy, treatment of endocrine
  tumours, 535–536
Anti-inflammatory agents, in acute
  pancreatitis, 213
Antiproteases
  antitrypsins, 32
  pathogenesis of pancreatitis, 179–180
Antitrypsin, giant cell carcinoma, 408
APACHE II score, assessment of acute
  pancreatitis, 205
Aplasia of the pancreas, 18
Aprotinin
  bovine protease inhibitor, pathogenesis of
    pancreatitis, 212–213
  therapy, 181
APUD see Amine precursor uptake and
  decarboxylation cells
Arteries
  embolization, treatment of endocrine
    tumours, 526
  involvement in acute pancreatitis, CT, 66
Arteritis, erosive, haemorrhage resulting,
  251
Ascites see Pancreatic ascites
Aspartate aminotransferase, use in diagnosis,
  226
Aspirin
  effects, 214
  pain relief, 350
Atropine
  and acute pancreatitis, 167
  and neural control mechanisms of
    pancreatic exocrine secretions, 44
Autodigestion, and safeguards against, 179
Autoimmune disease, causing acute
  pancreatitis, 175
Azaserine, pancreatic tumours, 413
Azathioprine, drug-induced pancreatitis,
  172–173

Barium contrast studies, 52–54
Beger operation, pancreaticojejunostomy, 313
Benzidine, carcinogenicity, 391
Beverages see Coffee; Tea
Bile, bacterial colonization (Escherichia coli),
  224
Bile reflux, 224–225
  bile injection model, 176
  gallstone-associated pancreatitis, 169–170
Biliary cirrhosis, indication for
  pancreaticojejunostomy, 313–314
Biliary disease, and chronic pancreatitis, 269
Biliary endoprostheses, 489–491
  balloon expandable, 489, 490
  causes of obstruction, 493
  complications associated, 494
  endoscopic transpapillary stenting, 306
  materials, 489
  papilla of Vater, 97–98
  placement, 489–490
  self-expanding metallic, 483, 489, 490
  stent wires, 301, 490
Biliary fistula, complication of
  pancreatoduodenectomy (Whipple's),
  633
Biliary tract

atypical epithelium, various sites, 393
biliary–digestive anastomosis, and
  pancreatic tumours, 6–7
bilioenteric bypass, options, 286
bypass surgery, 504–508
common bile duct
  atypical epithelium, 393
  intramural segment variations, 21
  obstruction, 255
  retropancreatic segment variations, 20–21
  stenosis, 285–286
  stones, indication for
    pancreaticojejunostomy, 313–314
  variations, 20
drainage
  endoscopic, 306
  and pancreaticojejunostomy, 313–314
  preoperative biliary drainage, 502–503
  see also Drainage procedures
endoscopic ultrasonography, case studies,
  115–117, 118
inflammation, in acute pancreatitis, 65
injuries, 582
obstruction, 285–286, 427–428
  post surgery, 640
  renal failure, 499
  risk factors, 500–501
  see also Biliary tract, CBD
pancreatic duct, and common bile duct,
  common channel termination, 222
surgery in acute pancreatitis
  deferred, 229
  early, 229
Biopsy see Fine-needle aspiration cytology
Bleeding complications, post surgery,
  634–637
Blood tests
  assessment of acute pancreatitis, 196
  as prognostic factor, 203
Blood transfusion, contraindications in
  pancreatic cancer, 517
Bombesin, properties, 40–41
Bovine protease inhibitors, pathogenesis of
  pancreatitis, 212–213
Brunner's glands, in differential diagnosis,
  405–406
Buprenorphine, 276
n-butyl-2-cyanoacrylate, tissue adhesive, 306

C-peptide levels
  hyperinsulinism
    factitious, 547
    insulinoma, 549
C-reactive protein, and inflammatory
  mediators, 202
CA 19–9, tumour marker, 133–136
Caerulein
  mechanisms of action, 177–178
  model of acute pancreatitis, 177–178
  see also Cholecystokinin
Calcifications, on plain films, 51–52, 53
Calcitonin, inhibition of pancreatic exocrine
  secretions, 212
Calcitonin gene-related peptide, inhibition of
  pancreatic secretion, 42
Calcium
  calcium infusion test, 132
  effect on pancreatic secretion, 41
  serum levels, prognostic factor, 203
Calculi
  development, 300
  duct obstruction, 310–311

Calculi (*contd*)
  endoscopic retrograde
      cholangiopancreatography, 92–93
  treatment, 302–303
  ultrasonography, 56–57
Cambridge–Marseilles classification of
    pancreatitis, 161–164
Camostate, 213
Cancer-associated antigen (CA 19-9), 404,
    426
Canine model, *ex vivo* isolated perfused
    canine model of acute pancreatitis,
    178–179
Canine model of acute pancreatitis, 178–179
Carboxylesterase, 31
Carcinoembryonic antigen (CEA), 404, 426
Carcinogenic substances, and pancreatic
    tumours, 391–392
Carcinoid tumours
  papilla of Vater, 394
  von Recklinghausen's disease, 394
Carcinoma *see* Pancreatic exocrine tumours
Cardiopulmonary complications of surgery,
    638
Catecholamines, neural control mechanisms,
    pancreatic exocrine secretions, 44
Cavitron ultrasonic aspirator (CUSA), 549
CDE diet model *see* Choline-deficient
    ethionine-supplemented diet model
CGRP *see* Calcitonin gene-related peptide
Chemotherapy
  treatment for endocrine tumours, 524–525
  treatment for exocrine tumours, 515–518
Children
  injuries to the pancreas, 584–585
    CT scan, 584–585
  juvenile chronic pancreatitis, 269
  pancreatic exocrine tumours
    epidemiology, 415
    mortality rates, 383–384
  pancreaticojejunostomy, 317
Cholangitis, indication for
    pancreaticojejunostomy, 313–314
Cholecystectomy
  pancreatoduodenectomy (Whipple's),
      447–448
  in total pancreatectomy, 462
  see also Pancreaticojejunostomy
Cholecystoduodenostomy, and pancreatic
    cancer, 506
Cholecystojejunostomy, 286, 504–505, 507
Cholecystokinin
  and acute pancreatitis, 167
  analogue *see* Caerulein
  effects of enzyme supplements, 310
  forms, 29
  function, 38
  historical note, 35–36
  inhibitors, 167
  interaction with secretin, 40
  molecular structure, 36
  monitor peptide, 39
  and pancreatic cancer, 386
  and pancreatic secretion, neural
      mechanisms, 43–44
  receptors, 36
  reducing output, 277
  release
    inhibition, 38–39
    and pancreatic secretion, 37–38
  response of sphincter of Oddi, 34
  secretin–cholecystokinin test, 128
  types, 36

Choledochoduodenostomy
  contraindications, 506
  indications, 286, 506
Choledochojejunostomy, 504–505
Cholelithiasis *see* Gallstones
Choline-deficient ethionine-supplemented
    diet model
  of acute pancreatitis, 176–179, 186
  free radical generation, 186
Chromogranin-A marker, 132, 546
Chronic pancreatitis
  aetiology
    alcohol, 265–267
    biliary disease, 269
    effects of alcohol vs non-alcoholic, 263
    and epidemiology, 263–265
    metabolic disorders, 269
    nutritional deficiency, 267–268
    obstructive pancreatitis, 268
  assessment, preoperative, 283–297
  calcifications
    calcifying vs obstructive, 300
    contributory factors, 267
  chronic obstructive pancreatitis, 268–269
  classification, 161–164, 263
    Marseilles classification, 359
  complications, treatment, 279–280
  defined, 161–164
  diagnosis, 273–275
  differential diagnosis, pancreatic cancer,
      290–292, 294
  grading, imaging methods, 162
  hereditary, 269, 317
    and pancreatic tumours, 39
  history and examination, 273–275, 283
  idiopathic, juvenile and senile forms, 269
  imaging
    angiography, 83–85
    barium contrast studies, 54
    computed tomography, 62–63, 284, 330
    endoscopic interventional techniques,
        299–307
    endoscopic retrograde
        cholangiopancreatography, 89–93, 284
    endoscopic transpapillary stenting,
        306–307
    ultrasonography, 57–58, 283–284
  incidence, major cities, 264
  lymphocytic chronic pancreatitis, 410–411
  management
    complications, 279–280
    conservative management, 273–282
    drainage, stenting, 301–302
    endoscopic interventional techniques,
        299–307
    non-surgical interventional techniques,
        306–307
    pain-relieving procedures, 349–357
      acute exacerbations, 276
      chronic pain, 276–277
      non-surgical treatment, 275–280,
          350–352
    surgery, 352–356
    surgical indications, 285–294
    surgical objectives, 285
    surgical options, 294–295, 352–356
    see also Chronic pancreatitis, surgery
  with metabolic disorders, 269
    hypercalcaemia syndromes, 269
    hyperlipidaemia, 269
  mortality rates, alcohol associations, 264
  nutritional factors, 265–266
    tropical pancreatitis, 267–268

  obstructive vs calcifying, 300
  and pancreatic cancer, 425
  pathogenesis, 263–269
    metabolic disorders, 269
  prognosis, 285
  surgery
    direct and indirect procedures, summary,
        294
    distal pancreatectomy, 321–328
    drainage procedures, 309–319
    historical note, 11–12
    indications, suspicion of pancreatic
        cancer, 290–292
    late results, 359–365
    options, 294–295
    pain-relieving procedures, 352–356
    pancreaticojejunostomy, 309–319
    partial pancreatoduodenectomy,
        329–339
    resection vs drainage, 360–361
    total pancreatoduodenectomy, 339–348
    see also Chronic pancreatitis, management
  tropical pancreatitis, 316–317
  see also Alcohol-associated pancreatitis
Chymotrypsin
  excretion in faeces, 128–129
  NPT-PABA test, 129
  in pathogenesis of pancreatitis, 179
  properties, 179
Chymotrypsinogen, activation, D to O
    conversion, 186
Cigarettes *see* Smoking
Cimetidine, inhibition of gastric acid,
    211–212
Clotting cascade, 182–183
Coagulopathy, 201
Codeine, pain relief, 350
Coeliac arteries (axis), 23
  obstruction, 465–472
Coeliac compression, approaches, 466–469
Coeliac plexus
  block, 341–342, 509
  infiltrative techniques, 351, 509
  neurolysis, 351–352
Coffee consumption, and pancreatic tumours,
    385, 386–388
Colipase, 31
Colon
  'cutoff sign', 51, 52
  obstruction in pancreatitis, 253
Colonic stricture, 286–287
Common bile duct *see* Biliary tract, common
    bile duct
Complement, levels, acute pancreatitis, 202
Complement cascade, 181–183
Computed tomography, 61–72
  acute pancreatitis, 61–62, 200
    assessment of severity, 205
  chronic pancreatitis, 275, 284
    grading, 162
  cystic neoplasms, 95
  injuries to the pancreas, children, 584–585
Congenital anomalies, 18–21, 369–379
  aplasia, 18
  ectopic tissue, 18–19
  see also Annular pancreas; Pancreas divisum
Courvoisier's law, 142
Courvoisier's sign, 425
Cullen's sign, 195
n-butyl-2-cyanoacrylate, tissue adhesive,
    306
Cyanogens, contributory factors in chronic
    pancreatitis, 267–268

Cyproterone acetate, treatment of
    unresectable tumours, 516
Cystic neoplasms
    imaging
        angiography, 85, 95
        computed tomography, 69, 70, 95
        endoscopic retrograde
            cholangiopancreatography, 95–96
        ultrasonography, 95
    premalignancy, 67, 69
    types, 408–410
        cystadenocarcinomas, 408–409
        mucinous cystadenocarcinoma, 409–410
        mucinous cystadenomas (mucinous
            ductal ectasia), 95
        mucinous cystic tumours, 409–410
        papillary cystic tumours, 95
        serous cystadenocarcinomas, 408–409
        serous cystadenoma, 69
Cytochrome oxidase system, oxygen derived
    free radicals, 184
Cytokeratin, differentiation of metastases,
    403
Cytology see Fine-needle aspiration cytology

Dacarbazine, treatment of endocrine gut
    tumours, 525
DAG, enzyme secretion, 36
Desmosomes, 407
Dextran, LMW, 214
Diabetes mellitus
    in pancreatic cancer, 424
    pancreatic transplantation, course of
        secondary complications, 613–615
    and pancreatic tumours, 388–389
    and pancreatoduodenectomy
        partial, 330, 335–336
        total, management, 347
    treatment, 278
Diagnosis
    intraoperative procedures, 141–158
    preoperative procedures, 51–138
    see also Acute pancreatitis; Chronic
        pancreatitis
Diarrhoea, Verner–Morrison syndrome
    (WDHA), 534–536
Diarrhoegenic tumour, 534–536
Diet see Nutrition
Dipipanone hydrochloride, 276
Dipyridamole, effects, 214
Disseminated intravascular coagulation, 499
Doppler imaging, colour, intraoperative
    ultrasonography, 147–151
Drainage procedures
    chronic pancreatitis, 309–319
        drawbacks, 279
    classification, 309
        external drainage, 488
        external–internal drainage, 488–489
        internal drainage using biliary
            endoprostheses, 489–491
        percutaneous transhepatic biliary
            drainage, 487–496
        preoperative biliary drainage, 502–503
    indications, 287
    pancreatic exocrine tumours, 482–484
        complications, 484
        further treatment, 483
    pancreatic tumours, 427–429
    Volker drain removal, 459
    see also Biliary tract, obstruction
Drug-induced pancreatitis, 104, 172–173

Du Val operation, pancreaticojejunostomy,
    311, 361
Ductal carcinoma see Pancreatic exocrine
    tumours
Ductal disease see Pancreatic duct(s)
Duodenal papilla see Ampulla of Vater
Duodenography, hypotonic, 284
Duodenojejunostomy
    annular pancreas, obstruction, 371
    duodenal injuries, 579–580
Duodenopancreatectomy see Pancreatectomy;
    Pancreatoduodenectomy
Duodenum
    arterial supply, 333
    Brunner's glands, in differential diagnosis,
        405–406
    bypass surgery, 504–508
    diverticulization procedure, 579–580, 581
    fluid reflux, gallstone-associated
        pancreatitis, 169–170
    ileus, 52
    injuries, 579–580
    obstruction
        causing acute pancreatitis, 174
        incidence, after biliary bypass, 506
        model of acute pancreatitis, 175–176
        in pancreatic carcinoma, 506–507
        and pancreaticojejunostomy, 314
        surgical options, 286
        see also Annular pancreas
    tumours
        adenomas, in FAP, 393–394
        primary, 394

Echoendoscopy
    instruments, 111–112
    technical data, 113
Ectopic tissue, pancreatic, 18–19
EDTA, phospholipase A-2 inhibitor (CaNa-
    EDTA), 213
Elastase
    activation, 180
    properties, 179–180
Electrolytes, replacement, management of
    acute pancreatitis, 210
Embryology of pancreas, 17–18
    congenital anomalies, 18–21
Encephalomyelopathy, pancreatic, 195
Endocrine markers of malignancy, 132–136
Endoprostheses see Biliary endoprostheses
Endoscopic biliary drainage, 306
Endoscopic cystoduodenostomy, 98–99,
    304–305
Endoscopic cystogastrostomy, 98–99,
    304–305
Endoscopic interventional techniques, chronic
    pancreatitis, 299–307
Endoscopic retrograde cholangiography
    delayed diagnostic, 228
    gallstone-associated pancreatitis, 228
    and sphincterotomy, 227–228
Endoscopic retrograde
        cholangiopancreatography, 87–109,
        309–310
    acute pancreatitis, 87–89, 173
    AIDS-related pancreatic disorders, 104
    before pancreaticojejunostomy, 311–313
    chronic pancreatitis, 89–93, 284
    delayed diagnostic, 228
    grading of chronic pancreatitis, 162
    pancreatic tumours, 93–94, 481–484
        diagnosis and histological proof, 481–482

diagnostic and therapeutic algorithm, 429
    prepapillary tumour, 144
    sphincterotomy and drainage, 482–484
pancreatogram, 303
pseudocysts, 98–99
    and sphincterotomy, 213
total pancreatoduodenectomy, 342
in trauma, 102, 103
Endoscopic therapy
    pancreas divisum, 305
    pseudocysts, 303–305
Endoscopic transpapillary stenting and
    drainage, 306
Endoscopic ultrasonography, 111–119
    instruments, 111–112
        technical data, 113
    interpretation of images, 113–117
        case studies, 115–117
    pancreatic tumours, 94, 484
    technique, 112–113
    see also Ultrasonography
Endotoxaemia
    control methods, 501–502
    Kupffer cells, 499
Endotracheal intubation, 625
Enolase, neuron-specific enolase, 132, 410,
    414, 546
Enterokinase, activation of trypsin within
    pancreatic duct, 32
Enzymes
    in peritoneal lavage fluid exudates, 239
    replacement, after total
        pancreatoduodenectomy, 347
    secretion, 30–32
    supplementation, cholecystokinin effects,
        310
    see also Pancreatic exocrine secretions;
        specific substances and conditions
Epidemiology of pancreatic tumours, 383–397
Erythema
    in glucagonoma, 537–538
    necrotizing migratory erythema, 556
ES see Endoscopic sphincterotomy
Escherichia coli, effect on pancreatic duct, 224
Ethibloc injection, following Whipple
    procedure, 336–337
Ethionine-supplemented diet model, acute
    pancreatitis, 176–179
Exocrine function see Pancreatic exocrine
    function
Extracorporeal shock wave lithotripsy
    (ESWL) see Lithotripsy

Faeces
    chymotrypsin test, 128–129
    faecal fat determination, 129
Familial adenomatous polyposis, risk of
    periampullary tumours, 393–394
Familial pancreatitis, 175
Fat necrosis, abdominal sign on plain films,
    51
Feline duct obstruction model, 176
Fibrinogen levels, 201, 211
    reduction by Ancrod, 214
Fine-needle aspiration cytology
    complications, 123–124, 156–157
    intraoperative FNAC, 154–158
    needle-track seeding, 124, 157
    percutaneous FNAC, 121–125
    results, 155–157
Finnish study, peritoneal lavage vs pancreatic
    drainage, 216

Flank staining, 200
Fluid collections *see* Pseudocysts
Fluid reflux, gallstone-associated pancreatitis, 169–170
Fluid replacement
  postoperative, 626
  preoperative indications, 623–624
  types of fluids, 623–624
5-fluorouracil, 181
  treatment of unresectable tumours, 516, 517, 525
FNAC *see* Fine-needle aspiration cytology
FOY (gabexelate mesilate), 213
Frederickson's familial hyperlipoproteinaemias, 168
Frey procedure, pancreaticojejunostomy, 313

Gabexelate mesilate, studies, 213
Gallstone-associated pancreatitis, 169–170, 221–232
  diagnosis, 225–227
    vs alcohol-associated pancreatitis, 225–226
  endoscopic retrograde cholangiopancreatography sphincterotomy, 213
  incidence, 221
  mortality rates, 222
  pathogenesis, 222–225
  treatment, 227–230
Gallstones
  impaction, 222–224
  and pancreatic cancer, 390
  pathogenesis of chronic pancreatitis, 269
Gardner's syndrome, risk of periampullary tumours, 393
Gastric acid, inhibition, 211–212
Gastric emptying, delayed, 638
Gastric surgery, and pancreatic tumours, 391
Gastric variceal obliteration, 306
Gastrin-releasing peptide
  and cholecystokinin release, 38
  properties, 40–41
  see also Bombesin
Gastrinoma
  clinical features, 531–532
  diagnosis and differential diagnosis, 532–533, 551–52, 557
  duodenal localization, 533
  epidemiology, 530
  location and localization, 552–553
  and MEN-1, 553–554
  with multiple endocrine neoplasia syndromes, 553–554
  pathology, 530
  pathophysiology, 530–531
  transhepatic portal venous sampling, 85
  treatment, 533–534, 553
    algorithm, 554
    medical, 533, 553
    surgical, 534, 553
Gastrointestinal fistula, following surgery, 638
Gastrointestinal involvement in acute pancreatitis, CT, 66
Gastrojejunostomy, 286, 506–508
  mortality, 516
  reconstruction, in pancreatoduodenectomy (Whipple's), 459
German study, peritoneal lavage vs pancreatic drainage, 216
Giant cell carcinoma, of the pancreas, 408, 409

Glasgow system of grading of acute pancreatitis, 203–204
Glucagon
  and acute pancreatitis, 167
  inhibition of pancreatic exocrine secretions, 42, 212
  properties, 555
Glucagonoma, 537–538
  classification, 537
  clinical features, 537–538, 554–555
  pathology and pathophysiology, 537, 555–557
  treatment, 538
Glucose
  intraoperative monitoring, 550
  serum levels, prognostic factor, 203
Glucose intolerance, glucagonoma syndrome, 555
Glutamate oxaloacetic transaminase *see* Aspartate aminotransferase
Glutamyl pyruvate transaminase *see* Alanine aminotransferase
Grading of chronic pancreatitis, imaging methods, 162
Grey–Turner's sign, 195
GRP *see* Gastrin-releasing peptide

H-2 blockers, in gastrinoma, 533–534
Haemofiltration, 216
Haemorrhage *see* Pancreatic haemorrhage
Haemosuccus pancreaticus, 251, 290
Heparin
  dose and use, 210–211
  interruption of pathogenesis of acute pancreatitis, 214
Hepatic arteries
  embolization, treatment of endocrine tumours, 526
  variations, 24, 25, 465, 468, 472
Hepatic necrosis, following surgery, 638
Hepaticojejunostomy
  indications, 286, 507
  reconstruction, pancreatoduodenectomy (Whipple's), 453–459
Hepatoduodenal ligament, and cholecystectomy, pancreatoduodenectomy (Whipple's), 447–449
Hereditary chronic pancreatitis, 269
Heterotopic pancreas, 19, 371
Histological features, pancreatic endocrine tumours, 522–523
History of pancreatic surgery, 3–12
  injuries to the pancreas, 565–566
  landmarks in anatomy/physiology, 4
  landmarks in pathology, 5
  pancreatoduodenectomy (Whipple's), 438
HLA types, and alcohol-associated pancreatitis, 166
Homeostasis, intraoperative, 626
Hong Kong system, grading of acute pancreatitis, 204
Hormonal therapy
  treatment of unresectable tumours, 516
Human epithelial antigen (HEA), 405
Hyperbilirubinaemia, in acute pancreatitis, 255
Hypercalcaemia
  and acute pancreatitis, 173
  effect on pancreatic secretion, 41
Hypercalcaemia syndromes, and chronic pancreatitis, 269

Hyperinsulinaemia
  in insulinoma, 548
  MEN-1, 551
  test, 132
Hyperlipidaemia, 168, 197–198
  and chronic pancreatitis, 269
Hyperlipoproteinaemias, familial, 168
Hyperparathyroidism
  and acute pancreatitis, 173
  pathogenesis of chronic pancreatitis, 269
  primary, in MEN-I patients, 547
Hypoglycaemia, in insulinoma, 526–528, 548
Hypotonic duodenography, 284

Ileus, acute pancreatitis, 195
Imaging methods and grading
  acute pancreatitis, 199–200
  chronic pancreatitis, 162
Imrie's (Glasgow) system, grading of acute pancreatitis, 203–204
Incisions, 141
Inflammation, limitation in acute pancreatitis, 211–213
Inflammatory mediators, and C-reactive protein, 202
Injuries to the duodenum, 579–583
Injuries to the pancreas, 565–589
  classes I, II and III, 577–579
  classification, 576
  complications, 586
  diagnosis and management, 568–576
    pancreatic and pancreaticoduodenal injuries, 576–577
  historical note, 565–566
  with injury to duodenum, 580–581
  with injury to duodenum and biliary tract, 582
  with injury to duodenum, biliary tract and pancreatic duct, 582–583
  mechanisms and nature of injury, 566–567
  paediatric trauma, 584–585
  postoperative care, 583–584
  surgical anatomy, 567–568
Insulin
  antisecretory therapy, 530
  hyperinsulinism test, 132
  immunoreactive (IRI/glucose ratio), 132
  infusion, 345–346
  levels in fasting hypoglycaemia, 526–528
  stimulation tests, 528–529
  see also Islet–acinar relationships
Insulinomas, 548–551
  clinical features, 526–527
  cytology, 122–124
  diagnosis, 548
    and differential diagnosis, 527–529
  imaging and localization
    angiography, 83–85, 548–549
    schema (algorithm), 549
    ultrasonography, 58–60, 548
  metastatic disease, 550
  pathology and pathophysiology, 526
  treatment, 529–530, 549–551
    intraoperative monitoring of glucose, 550–551
    malignancy, 550
  see also Islet cell tumours
Interferon-alpha, treatment of endocrine gut tumours, 525
Interleukin-6, synthesis of CRP, 202
Interstitial oedematous pancreatitis, 233–234

Intestinal complications
  acute pancreatitis, 252–255
    necrosis, 253–255
    obstruction, 252–253
Intraoperative homeostasis, 626
Intraoperative needle aspiration cytology,
    153–158
  fine-needle aspiration cytology, 154–158
Intraoperative ultrasonography, 147–151
  colour Doppler imaging, 147–151
Intrapleural infiltration, contraindications,
    351
Intravascular volume management
  acute pancreatitis, 209–210
  intraoperative homeostasis, 626
Iodine-125 implant, treatment of unresectable
    tumours, 516
IP-3, enzyme secretion, 36
Ischaemia–reperfusion, free radicals, 185
Ischaemic pancreatitis, 170–172
  animal models, 171–172
  clinical experience, 170–171
Islet cell carcinoma, 558–559
Islet cell tumours, 545–561
  clinical questions, 547
  clusters I and II, 547
  distribution (1960-1986, US), 545
  distribution within pancreas, 547
  identifiable syndromes, list, 545
  islet cell carcinoma, 558–559
  pathophysiology and pathogenesis, 545–547
  see also Pancreatic endocrine tumours;
    specific tumours and conditions
Islet cells
  A cells, glucagon production, 42
  calcitonin gene-related peptide, 42
  diagnostic procedures for endocrine
    function, 131
  islet–acinar relationships, 44–45
  PP cells, 41–42
  proliferation (nesidioblastosis), 132, 546
  types, 29

Japan
  incidence of acute pancreatitis, 193
  Japanese system of assessment of acute
    pancreatitis, 204
  Japanese technique in neurotomy, 355
Jaundice
  in acute pancreatitis, 255
  and pancreatic tumours, 424
    recurrence following bypass surgery, 505
Jejunal ulcer, following Whipple procedure,
    336
Jejunum, torsion, 637
Juvenile chronic pancreatitis, 269
  see also Children

Kallikrein kinin system, 182
Ki-ras oncogenes, 'cancer family syndromes',
    392
Kininogen cascade, 182
Kocher manoeuvre
  abdominal exploration, 142–144, 443, 549
  pancreaticojejunostomy, 331, 332
Kupffer cells, function, endotoxaemia, 499
Kwashiorkor, and chronic pancreatitis, 268

Laboratory evaluation of pancreatic function,
    127–138, 285

endocrine tumours, 131–132
  pancreatic carcinoma, 132–136
Lactic dehydrogenase, serum levels,
    prognostic factor, 203
Lactoferrin, as marker, 133
Laparoscopy, preceding abdominal
    exploration, 141–142, 430
Laparotomies
  exploratory, 141–158, 430
  relaparotomies, 631
  see also Abdominal exploration
Laser photodestruction, following endoscopic
    sphincterotomy, 98
Lecithin, role in pancreatitis hydrolysis, 188
Left hemipancreatectomy, 435, 477–480
Left-sided portal hypertension, complication
    of acute pancreatitis, 250–251
Lesser sac see Peritoneal lavage
Leucocyte common antigen (LEA), 410
Leupeptin, 181
Lewis antigens, pancreatic tumours, 404
Lindane, carcinogenicity, 391
Lipase
  lipoprotein lipase activity, PHLA test,
    172–173
  LMW, in acinar cell carcinoma, 414
  role in pancreatitis, 188, 274
  serum, assessment, 198
Lipid metabolism
  abnormalities, aetiology of acute
    pancreatitis, 168–169
  Frederickson's familial
    hyperlipoproteinaemias, 168
Lipolytic enzymes, 31
  lipoprotein lipase activity, PHLA test,
    172–173
Lithotripsy
  electrohydraulic (EHL), 302–303
  extracorporeal shock wave (ESWL),
    302–303
  mechanical, 302
Loxiglumide
  CCK antagonist, 40–41
  and neural control mechanisms of
    pancreatic exocrine secretions, 44
Lundh test, 128
Lycopene, in fruit, protective factor in
    pancreatic cancer, 386
Lymph nodes, metastases, 402
Lymphatic drainage of the pancreas, 25–26
Lymphocytic chronic pancreatitis, 410–411
Lysocompounds, 31
Lysozomal enzymes, 31, 177–178

alpha-2-Macroglobulin
  antiprotease activity, 201
  properties, 180
Magnetic resonance imaging (MRI), 73–75
Malabsorption
  in ageing patient, 127
  causes, 130
  faecal fat determination, 129
  and steatorrhoea, 130
Malignancy, tumour markers, 132–136, 426
Malnutrition see Nutrition
Marseilles classification of pancreatitis,
    161–164
MEN syndromes see Multiple endocrine
    neoplasia syndromes; Pancreatic
    endocrine tumours
Mesenchymal tumours of the pancreas,
    415–416

Mesenteric arteries, 23, 141–143
  iatrogenic injuries, 472–475
Mesenteric necrosis, following surgery, 638
Methaemoglobinaemia, 201
Models
  ex vivo isolated perfused canine model of
    acute pancreatitis, 178–179
  feline duct obstruction model, 176
  ischaemic pancreatitis, 171–172
  see also Acute pancreatitis, models
Morphine
  administration, 276
  stage 3 pancreatitis, 350
Morphine agonists and antagonists, 350
Mucinous cystadenocarcinoma, 409–410
  computed tomography, 70
Mucinous cystic tumours, 409–410
Mucinous ductal ectasia, characteristics, 95
Multiple endocrine adenomatosis, 539–540
Multiple endocrine neoplasia syndromes, 415,
    546–547
  MEN type-1, 539–540, 546–547
    locus, 546
    primary hyperparathyroidism, 547
  with ZES, 553–554

B-naphthylamine, carcinogenicity, 391
Nasogastric suction
  evaluation, 211
  inhibition of pancreatic exocrine secretions,
    211–212
NBT-PABA test, 129
Necrosectomy
  late complications, 241
  and lesser sac lavage, 238–240
  plus other methods, 240
Necrosis, following surgery, 638
Necrotizing migratory erythema, 556
Necrotizing pancreatitis, 234, 245–248
  indicators, 241
  infected necrosis, 246–248
  pancreatic function studies, abnormal
    findings, 241
  sterile necrosis, 245–246
  see also Acute pancreatitis, management;
    Necrosectomy
Needle biopsy see Fine-needle aspiration;
    Intraoperative needle aspiration
Neonates, diffuse islet cell adenomatosis,
    547
Nesidioblasts, origin of islet cell tumours,
    132, 546
Neurolysis, coeliac plexus, 351–352
Neuron-specific enolase, 132, 410, 546
  in acinar cell carcinoma, 414
Neurotensin, properties, 41
Neurotomy, 352–354
  choice of technique, 355–356
  extraperitoneal left splanchnicectomy, 352
  intraperitoneal splanchnicectomy
    left, 353–354
    right, 352–353
  Japanese technique, 355
  pain relief, 509
  results, 356–357
  transhiatal bilateral splanchnicectomy,
    354–355
Nitrosamines, animal models of pancreatic
    cancer, 385, 386
NSE see Neuron-specific enolase
Nutrition
  diet, 277

Nutrition (*contd*)
  in aetiology of pancreatic tumours, 385–386
  fruit as protective factor in pancreatic cancer, 385–386
  micronutrients and pancreatic cancer, 386
  vegetarianism, 385–386
  malnutrition causing acute pancreatitis, 175
  malnutrition-associated pancreatitis, 166
  nutritional deficiency, aetiology of chronic pancreatitis, 267–268
  nutritional support, management of acute pancreatitis, 210
  prognostic nutritional index, 501
  treatment of malnutrition, 277–278

Obstructive pancreatitis, 268
Octreotide
  dose, 525
  indium-labelled, 524
  in insulinoma, 530
  in pancreatic resection, 550
  for pleural effusion, 280
  treatment of endocrine tumours, 535–536
  in VIPoma, 557
Oestrogens, drug-induced pancreatitis, 172–173
Oleic acid injection model (FFA), 185–186
Omental lavage *see* Peritoneal lavage
Omeprazole, effects on gastric acid secretion, 534–535
Oncogenes, Ki-*ras*, 406
Opioids, oral, 276–277
Oral contraception, and drug-induced pancreatitis, 172–173
Oral feeding, contraindications in acute pancreatitis, 212
Oxygen, arterial, as prognostic factor, 203
Oxygen derived free radicals, 166, 183–186
  animal models, 183–184
  'D to O' conversion, 185
  experimental evidence, 185–186
Oxyntomodulin, inhibition of exocrine secretions, 42

p53 tumour suppressor genes, loss, 392
Pain, pancreatic
  characteristics, 194–195
  diminishment with time, 276–277, 294
  indication for operation, 292–294
  neural origin, 349
  in pancreatic cancer, 424
  pattern and periodicity, 273–274
  referral, 349
Pain-relieving procedures
  acute pancreatitis
    drugs, 210
    non-surgical treatment, 210
  chemical splanchnicectomy, 509
  chronic pancreatitis, 273–282, 349–357
    non-surgical treatment, 275–282, 350–352
    surgical treatment, 352–356
  post surgery, 626
  surgical palliation of pancreatic exocrine tumours, 509
Painless pancreatitis, 194–195
Pancreas
  ageing changes, 127

  blood supply, 23–25
    arteries, 23–24
    veins, 24–25
  dimensions, 21
  divisions, 21
  head, dorsal and ventral anlage, 406
  heterotopia, 19, 371
  lymphatic drainage, 25–26
  uncinate process, variations, 22
Pancreas divisum, 19–20, 371–378
  causing acute pancreatitis, 174
  chronic obstructive pancreatitis, 268
  clinical significance, 101
  developmental anatomy, 372–373
  embryology, 99
  endoscopic management, 101–102, 305
    endoscopic retrograde cholangiopancreatography, 99–102
  incidence, 99
  operative technique, 377–378
    stenting, 301–302
  and pathology, 373
  therapeutic outcomes, 374–376
    patient selection, 376–377
Pancreastatin, inhibition of exocrine secretions, 42, 43
Pancreatectomy
  left hemipancreatectomy, 435, 477–480
  pylorus-preserving hemipancreatectomy, 435, 436–438
  regional pancreatectomy, 435
    classification, 435
  total hemipancreatectomy, 435–436, 461–464
  vascular problems and techniques, 465–476
    arteriosclerotic vascular stenosis or occlusion, 465–467
    congenital vascular anomalies, 465
    iatrogenic injuries, 472–475
    vascular infiltration or compression, 467–472
  see also Pancreatectomy, distal, and total; Pancreatoduodenectomy (Whipple's)
Pancreatectomy, distal
  choice of operation, 325
  choice of surgeon, 325
  in chronic pancreatitis, 321–328
  contraindications, 325
  diabetes and steatorrhoea, 322–323
  indications, 325–326, 435
  present status, 324–327
  results, 321–324, 362
    late mortality, 324
    operative mortality, 322
    pain relief, 321–322
  spleen conservation, 326–327
  subtotal resection, 362, 363
  technical considerations, 326–327
  total resection, 363
Pancreatectomy, total
  exploration, 462
  in pancreatic exocrine tumours, 435–436, 461–464
  partial gastrectomy, 462–463
  postoperative care, 464
  resection, 461
    cholecystectomy, 462
  retropancreatic vessels, 463
  see also Pancreatectomy, distal
Pancreatic abscess
  in acute pancreatitis, computed tomography, 64

  complication of necrotizing pancreatitis, 234
  complication of surgery, 637
  on plain films, 51
Pancreatic acinar cell *see* Acinar cell
Pancreatic ascites
  animal models, 183
  complication of surgery, 637
  computed tomography, 64–65
  disruption of pseudocysts, 255
  haemorrhagic, treatment, 239
  internal pancreatic fistulas, 255–256
  management, 288
  treatment, 280
Pancreatic biopsy *see* Fine-needle aspiration; Intraoperative needle aspiration
Pancreatic cancer *see* Insulinoma; Pancreatic endocrine tumours
Pancreatic cholera, 534–536
Pancreatic cyst(s)
  dermoid cysts, 289
  surgery, 288
  see also Pseudocysts
Pancreatic duct(s)
  atypical epithelium, incidence, 393
  chronic pancreatitis, dilatation, intraoperative ultrasonography, 148
  and common bile duct, common channel termination, 222
  congenital anomalies, 19–20
  dimensions, 19
  dual *see* Pancreas divisum
  duct dilatations, 287
  duct of Santorini, 17, 18, 19–20
  duct of Wirsung, 17, 18, 19–20
  effect of bile on, 224–225
  embryology, 17–18
  endoscopic ultrasonography, case studies, 115–117, 118
  epithelial origin of tumours, 401–402
  ex vivo isolated perfused canine model of acute pancreatitis, 178–179
  function, 34–35
  mucosal barrier, 35
  obstruction, 287–288, 310–311
    chronic obstructive pancreatitis, 268
    feline duct obstruction model, 176
    lesions, 174
    partial obstruction plus secretin stimulation model (POSS), 179
    theories, 170
  occlusion, 225
    contraindications, 288
  pancreas divisum, 378
  papillary carcinoma, and intraductal papilloma, 407–408
  pressure measurements, 309–310
  protein deposition, alcohol-associated pancreatitis, 167–168
  small-duct disease, 287
  stenosis/stricture *see* Pancreatic duct(s), obstruction
  stenting, 301–302
  structure, 32–35
  see also Drainage procedures
Pancreatic encephalomyelopathy, 195
Pancreatic endocrine cells, APUD cells, origin, 546
Pancreatic endocrine function
  and pancreatic surgery, 130–131
  tests, 130–131

Pancreatic endocrine tumours, 521–561
  characteristics, 414–415
  classification, 521–522
    WHO, 414–415
  computed tomography, functioning and
      nonfunctioning, 70–72
  diagnosis
    differential diagnosis, 546
    and localization, 523–524
  histological features, 522–523
  histological similarity, 546
  imaging
    angiography, 83–85
    intraoperative ultrasonography, 148–150
    ultrasonography, 58–60
  incidence and prevalence, 414
  laboratory diagnosis, 131–132, 132–136
  list, 522
  multiple endocrine neoplasia syndromes,
      415
  origin, 521
    non-islet cell origin, 132
  pathology, 414–415
  pathophysiology, 523
  prevalence, 521
  treatment, 524–526
    arterial embolization, 526
    cytostatic treatment, 524–525
  see also Islet cell tumours; specific tumours
      and conditions
Pancreatic exocrine function, 29–44
  and cholecystokinin release, 37–38
  components of secretion, 30–34, 127
    electrolytes, 30, 34
    enzymes, 30–31
  ductal secretory mechanisms, 34–35
  and glucagon, 42
  hormonal control, 35–42
  inhibition of secretins, 41–42, 211–213
    attempts, 167
    CGRP, 42
    glucagon, 42
    nasogastric suction, 211–212
    pancreastatin, 42, 43
    pancreatic polypeptide, 41–42
    peptide YY, 42
    somatostatin, 41
  initiation of acute alcohol-associated
      pancreatitis, 166–167
  neural control, 42–44
    atropine, 44
    extrinsic nerve supply, 42–43
    intrinsic nerve supply, 43
    loxiglumide, 44
    mechanisms, 42–44
  and pancreatic surgery, 130
  properties
    electrolytes, 30, 34
    protective mechanisms, 31–32
  stages, 32
  supplements, 464
    treatment of pain, 277
  tests, 127–130
    chymotrypsin test, 128–129
    dual-labelled Schilling test, 130
    faecal fat determination, 129
    Lundh test, 128
    NBT–PABA test, 129
    pancreolauryl test, 129
    secretin–cholecystokinin test, 128
    [C-14] triolein breath test, 129
  see also Enzymes
Pancreatic exocrine tumours

  abdominal exploration, 141–148
  aetiology, 383
  assessment, 423–431
    clinical findings, 424–426
    laboratory findings, 426
  and biliary–digestive anastomosis, 6–7
  case studies, 423–425
  classification, 399–421
    AIP, 400
    Morohoshi's, 400
    UICC, 399, 400, 403
    WHO, 399, 400
  clinical evaluation, 423–431
  diagnosis, 401–406
    algorithms, 427, 429
    characteristic feature, 405–406
    differential diagnosis, 294
    double-duct stenosis, 427, 428
    four criteria, 426
    histomorphological problems, 405–406
    laboratory diagnosis, 132–136
    percutaneous fine-needle aspiration
        cytology, 121–125
    special procedures, 426–430
    suspicion, 290–292
      algorithms, 426–427, 429
    see also Pancreatic exocrine tumours,
        assessment
  epidemiology, 383–397, 399–401
    alcohol consumption, 388
    allergic states, 391
    'cancer family syndromes', 392
    carcinogenic substances, 391–392
    in children, 415
    cholelithiasis, 390–391
    chronic pancreatitis, 390
    consumption of beverages, 386–388
    diabetes, 388–389
    diet, 385–386
    effects of disease, 388–391
    familial chronic pancreatitis, 392
    gastric surgery, 391
    genetic factors, 392
    pernicious anaemia, 389–390
    sex ratio, 400
    smoking, 400–401
  imaging
    angiography, 82, 83–85, 429–430
    barium contrast studies, 54
    computed tomography, 66–67, 68, 93,
        427
    endoscopic retrograde
        cholangiopancreatography, 93–94, 427
    endoscopic ultrasonography, 94, 113–117
      case studies, 115–117
    MRI, 75, 93, 427
    TNM staging, endoscopic
        ultrasonographic criteria, 114
    ultrasonography, 58–60, 93, 427
  immunoreactivity, 404
  incidence, 383–397
    age-standardized, 384
    sex ratio, 384
  metastases
    differentiation, 403
    lymph nodes, 402
    options, 515–518
  mortality rates, 383
    children, 383–384
    predictors, 500–501
  non-functioning, 540
  palliative measures
    endoscopic procedures, 481–485

  percutaneous and rendezvous techniques,
      487–496
  surgical palliation, 497–513
  pathology, 399–421
    acinar cell carcinoma, 413–414
    adenoma, 412–413
    adenomatous hyperplasia, 412–414
    cystic exocrine tumour types, 408–410
    cystadenocarcinomas, 408–409
  cystic tumour types
    imaging, 67–70, 85, 95–96
    mucinous cystic tumours, 409–410
    serous cystadenomas, 408–409
  cytology, 122–124
  ductal carcinoma
    histological and cytological criteria,
        402–404
    immunocytochemistry, 404
  ductal carcinoma variants, 406–408
    adenosquamous carcinoma, 407–408
    carcinoma in situ, 406
    ductal adenocarcinoma, 406–407
    giant cell carcinoma, 408
    intraductal papilloma and papillary
        carcinoma of Wirsung's duct, 407–408
    squamous cell carcinoma, 407–408
  gross features, 401–402
  hyperplasia, 412–413
  immunocytochemistry, 404–405
  infantile pancreatic carcinoma, 415
  'knickerbocker' phenomenon, 402
  location and histogenesis, 402, 404, 406
  lymph node metastasis, 402
  mesenchymal tumours, 415–416
  microglandular adenocarcinomas, 411
  microscopic features, 402–404
  pancreatoblastoma, 415
  small cell carcinoma, 410–411
  solid and cystic tumours, 411–412
  'Stobbe' phenomenon, 403
  ultrastructure, 404
  'permigration problem', 407
  preoperative assessment, 423–431
  staging, and palliation, 497
  surgery
    'activist' approach, 435
    adjuvant treatment, 517
    left hemipancreatectomy, 435, 477–480
    local excision, 434–435
    'nihilist' approach, 433–434
    operative procedures 1959–1988
        compared, 498
    pancreatoduodenectomy (Whipple's),
        438–440, 447–459
    predictors of mortality and morbidity,
        500–501
    pylorus-preserving hemipancreatectomy,
        435, 436–438
    'realistic' approach, 435–440
    regional pancreatectomy, 435
    resectability, two decades, 433
    resection vs bypass, 498, 508–509
    risk factors, 499–500
    surgical options, 433–442
    total hemipancreatectomy, 435–436,
        461–464
    vascular problems and techniques
        associated with pancreatectomy,
        465–476
    Whipple's procedure see
        Pancreatoduodenectomy (Whipple's)
    see also Pancreatectomy
  surgical palliation, 497–513

Pancreatic exocrine tumours (*contd*)
  assessment, 497–501
  non-operative stenting vs bypass surgery,
    503–504
  objectives and choice of treatment, 503
  options, 503–509
  pain relief, 509
  preoperative preparation, 501–503
  summary, 509–510
  survival, increased, options for, 517
  TNM staging, 114
  treatment
    chemotherapy, 515–518
    radiotherapy, 515–518
    recurrent disease, 517
    see also Pancreatic exocrine tumours,
      surgery
  and tropical pancreatitis, 316–317
  tumour markers of malignancy, 132–136,
    426
  types *see* Pancreatic exocrine tumours,
    pathology
Pancreatic fistulas
  causes, 255
    trauma, 586
  endoscopic retrograde
    cholangiopancreatography, 103–104
  external, 280
  internal, 255–256
Pancreatic haemorrhage
  chronic pancreatitis, management, 290
  complication of acute pancreatitis,
    250–252
    left-sided portal hypertension, 250–251
    stress ulceration, 250
    variceal, 250–251
    vascular necrosis, 251–252
  CT, 66
  haemorrhagic complications, post surgery,
    499, 634–637
  herald bleeding, 251
  into pseudocysts, 252
Pancreatic injuries *see* Injuries to the pancreas
Pancreatic islets *see* Islet cells; Islet–acinar
  relationships
Pancreatic juice *see* Pancreatic exocrine
  function
Pancreatic polypeptide
  and chronic pancreatitis, 131
  inhibition of exocrine secretions, 41–42
Pancreatic polypeptide-producing tumours,
  534, 540
Pancreatic polypeptidoma, 558
Pancreatic sphincter *see* Sphincter of Oddi
Pancreatic stones *see* Calculi
Pancreatic surgery
  and pancreatic endocrine function,
    130–131
  and pancreatic exocrine function, 130
Pancreatic transplantation, 593–619
  complications, secondary diabetic, 613–615
  following kidney transplantation, 614
  historical note, 12
  indications and costs, 593–594
  kidney graft survival in pancreas-liver-
    kidney transplants, 612
  metabolic consequences, 612–613
  non-uraemic diabetes mellitus, 611–612
  preservation solutions, compared, 610
  preservation time, 610–611
  recipient categories, 609–610
    pancreas alone (PTA) transplants,
      609–610

    pancreas-liver (PLT) transplants,
      609–610
    pancreas-liver-kidney (SPK) transplants,
      609–610, 612
  recurrence of autoimmune diabetes
    mellitus, 615
  rejection episodes, 611
  results, 605–615
    duct management technique, 608–609
    quality of life, 615
  surgical technique, 595–605
    pancreas procurement, 595–597
    preparation of donor pancreas, 597–599
    recipient operation, 600–605
    technical considerations, 600
Pancreatic trauma *see* Injuries to the
  pancreas
Pancreatic tumours *see* Pancreatic endocrine
  tumours; Pancreatic exocrine tumours
Pancreaticoduodenectomy *see*
  Pancreatoduodenectomy
Pancreaticogastrectomy, and diabetes, 131
Pancreaticogastrostomy, 317
Pancreaticojejunal anastomosis, tumour
  residues, 405
Pancreaticojejunostomy
  Beger operation, 313
  biliary duct drainage, 313–314
  children, 317
  chronic pancreatitis, 309, 311–319
  combined procedures
    Du Val, 311, 361
    Puestow, 334, 361–362
    results, 361–362
    Whipple, 361–362
  distal pancreatectomy, 321–328
  and duodenal obstruction, 314
  end-to-side, with pancreatoduodenectomy,
    partial, 330–333
  Frey procedure, 313
  Kocher manoeuvre, 331, 332
  in management of chronic pancreatitis, 288
  Puestow procedure, reoperation, 334
  pylorus-preserving variant, 330–333
  repeat, 317
  results
    development of cancer, 316
    exocrine/endocrine function, 315–316
    operative mortality, 314, 315
    pain relief, 314–315
    side-to-side, 311, 312
    results, 361, 362
    tropical pancreatitis, 316–317
    Whipple procedure, 314
Pancreaticoscopy, transpapillary, miniscope,
  484
Pancreatitis *see* Acute pancreatitis; Alcohol-
  associated pancreatitis; Chronic
  pancreatitis; Gallstone-associated
  pancreatitis
Pancreatoduodenal arteries, 24–25
Pancreatoduodenal veins, 24–25
Pancreatoduodenectomy
  complications, 629–644
    early non-surgical, 638
    early surgical, 629–638
    late non-surgical sequelae of
      pancreatoduodenectomy, 640–642
    late surgical sequelae of pancreatectomy,
      638–640
  in management of acute pancreatitis,
    237–238
  pylorus-preserving, 330–333

Whipple procedure, *see also*
  Pancreatoduodenectomy (Whipple's)
Pancreatoduodenectomy, partial, 286
  chronic pancreatitis, 329–339
  and diabetes, 131, 330
  with end-to-side pancreaticojejunostomy,
    330–333
  indications, 329–330
  planes I - IV, 330–333
  postoperative care, 334–335
  pylorus-preserving variant, vs Whipple
    procedure, 336–337
  results and discussion, 335–337
  technical considerations, 330–334
  Whipple procedure, 336–337
Pancreatoduodenectomy, total
  chronic pancreatitis, 339–348
  and diabetes management, 347
  duodenum-preserving total
    pancreatectomy, 343–345
  historical note, 339–340
  indications, 340–342
  mortality, 346
  outcome, 346–347
  postoperative care, 345–346
  preparation, 342
  previous distal pancreatectomy, 343
  previous pancreatoduodenectomy, 343
  procedure, choice, 342–343
Pancreatoduodenectomy (Whipple's),
  438–440, 447–459
  5-year survival rate, 439
  Beger variant, 336–337
  complications
    biliary fistula, 634
    general surgical complications,
      637–638
    haemorrhagic, 634–637
    pancreatic remnant and anastomosis,
      629–634
  defined, 447
  diabetes, incidence, 131
  early non-surgical complications, 638
  early surgical complications, 629–638
  historical note, 438
    68 variants in reconstruction, 454–455
  indications, 295, 641
  late non-surgical sequelae of
    pancreatoduodenectomy, 640–642
  late results, 440
  late surgical sequelae, 638–640
  mortality, 438, 642
  outcomes, 293
  pancreaticojejunostomy, 314, 333
  post surgery, exocrine and endocrine
    function, 642
  postoperative care, 459
  technique of reconstruction, 453–459
    gastrojejunostomy, 459
    hepaticojejunostomy, 457–458
    pancreatojejunostomy, 453–457
  technique of resection, 447–453
    cholecystectomy, and dissection of
      hepatoduodenal ligament, 447–449
    dissection of retropancreatic vessels,
      450–452
    division of the jejunum, 453
    division of the pancreas, 450
    incision and exploration, 447
    mobilization of pancreatic neck, 449
    partial gastrectomy, 450
Pancreatoduodenostomy, historical note,
  8–10

Pancreatojejunostomy
  complications, 631
  reconstruction following Whipple's
    procedure, 453–459
Pancreolauryl test, 129
Pancuronium, 625
Papanicalaou procedure, 154
Papilla of Vater
  access, oral route and cannulation, 481
  atypical epithelium, incidence, various sites,
    393
  endoprostheses, 97–98
  ERCP sphincterotomy, 213
  historical note, 7–8
  transpapillary pancreaticoscopy, miniscope,
    484
  variations, 21
  see also Pancreatic ducts
Papillary cystic tumours see Pancreatic
    exocrine tumours, cystic neoplasms
Papillary tumours
  local excision, 443–446
  see also Periampullary (papillary) tumours
Papillotomy see Papilla of Vater
Paracetamol, pain relief, 350
Peptide YY, inhibition of exocrine secretions,
    42
Peptides, multiple, production from islet cells,
    547
Percutaneous fine-needle aspiration cytology,
    121–125
  see also Fine-needle aspiration cytology
Percutaneous transhepatic biliary drainage,
    487–496
  complications, 494
  patient preparation, 487
  permanent drainage, 493–494
    techniques, 488–491
  puncture sites, 488
  temporary drainage, 492–493
  see also Drainage procedures
Percutaneous transhepatic cholangiography,
    77–79
  rendezvous procedure, 77–78
Percutaneous transpapillary biliary drainage,
    484
Periampullary, see Papilla of Vater
Periampullary (papillary) tumours
  adenocarcinoma, prognosis, 96
  aetiology, 392–394
  carcinoid tumours, 394
  carcinoma, TNM staging, endoscopic
    ultrasonography, 114
  carcinoma of Wirsung's duct, and
    intraductal papilloma, 407–408
  defined, 392
  endoscopic retrograde
    cholangiopancreatography, 96–98
  and familial adenomatous polyposis,
    393–394
  intraductal papilloma, and papillary
    carcinoma of Wirsung's duct, 407–408
  lymph node metastases, 402
  primary carcinoid, 96
  surgical palliation, 497–513
  see also Pancreatic exocrine tumours
Peritoneal lavage
  animal models, 216
  clinical trials, 214–216
  diagnostic, 198
    assessment of severity, 203
  Finnish study, 216
  fluid amounts, 239

German study, 216
lesser sac, 238–240
  and necrosectomy, 238–240
models of acute pancreatitis, 183, 215
therapeutic, 181, 183, 214–216, 238
and triple-tube drainage, 238
Periumbilical staining, 200
Pernicious anaemia, and pancreatic exocrine
    tumours, 389–390
PHLA test, lipoprotein lipase activity,
    172–173
Phospholipase A-2, 31
  in acinar cell carcinoma, 414
  in acute pancreatitis, 187–188, 201
  inhibitor (CaNa-EDTA), 213
Physiology of the pancreas, 29–48
  islet–acinar relationships, 44–45
  see also Pancreatic exocrine function
Pituitary tumours, in multiple endocrine
    neoplasia type-1, 547
Plasmapheresis, 216
Pleural effusion
  in acute pancreatitis, 65
  in chronic pancreatitis, 280
  management, 288
Portal hypertension, complication of acute
    pancreatitis, 250–251
Portal vein
  mesocaval shunt, 471
  obstruction, 289–290, 467–471
  reconstruction, 471
  transhepatic sampling, islet cell tumours,
    84–85
  variations, 25
POSS model, partial obstruction plus secretin
    stimulation, 179, 185
Postheparin lipolytic activity test, 172–173
PPoma see Pancreatic polypeptidoma
Prostaglandins, in acute pancreatitis,
    186–187, 213
Proteases, pathogenesis of pancreatitis,
    179–180
  activation, importance, 179, 181
  acute pancreatitis, 179–180
  alpha-1 protease inhibitor, 180
  antiproteases, 179–180, 201
    therapy, 181
  assessment of severity, 201
  bovine protease inhibitors, 212–213
  changes in levels, 180–181
  inhibitor see Proteases, antiproteases
  protease inhibitors, 32
  serine proteases, 30–32
  systemic manifestations, 181
Protein deposition, alcohol-associated
    pancreatitis, 167–168
Pseudoaneurysms
  in acute pancreatitis, 66, 251
  frequency, 251
Pseudocysts
  acute, 248–250
  classification, 234–235
  defined, 248
  diagnosis, 248–250
  endoscopic retrograde
    cholangiopancreatography, 98–99
  endoscopy, treatment, 303–305, 306
  haemorrhage into, 252
  management, 279–280
  Roux loop drainage, 313
  surgery, 288
  treatment, 250
  ultrasonography, 56–57

PTBD see Percutaneous transhepatic biliary
    drainage
Puestow procedure
  pancreaticojejunostomy, 312–313, 361–362
  reoperation, 334
Pylorus-preserving hemipancreatectomy, 435,
    436–438

Radiography, conventional, 51–54
  assessment of severity, 205
  barium contrast studies, 52–54
  plain films, 51–52
Radionuclide scanning, gallstone pancreatitis,
    226
Radiotherapy, treatment for exocrine
    tumours, 515–518
Ranson system, grading of acute pancreatitis,
    203
Regional pancreatectomy, 435
Renal failure, and biliary obstruction, 499
Rendezvous procedure, 484, 487–496
  percutaneous transhepatic cholangiography,
    77–78
Replacement fluids, 623–624
  intraoperative homeostasis, 626
Resection see specific conditions and procedures
Resection, historical note, 10
Respiratory monitoring, management of acute
    pancreatitis, 210
Ribonuclease, serum, 201
Roux-en-Y duodenojejunostomy, 579–580
Roux-en-Y loop
  contraindications, 287, 505
  hepaticogastrojejunostomy, 507–508
  indications, 286, 505–506
  pancreaticojejunostomy, 311
  side-to-side hepaticojejunostomy, 507–508

Sandostatin, in VIPoma, 557
Santorini, duct of
  anatomy and variations, 17–20
  see also Pancreatic duct(s)
Schilling test, 130
Scorpion bites, causing acute pancreatitis, 175
Secretin
  interaction with cholecystokinin, 40
  and pancreatic cancer, 386
  partial obstruction plus secretin stimulation
    model (POSS), 179
  properties, 39–40
  receptors, 35
  release
    inhibition, 40, 211
    stimulation, 40
  secretin challenge test, 547
Secretin–cholecystokinin test, 128
Secretions of the pancreas see Pancreatic
    exocrine function
Selenium, protective factor in pancreatic
    cancer, 386
Senile chronic pancreatitis, 269
Sepsis, postoperative, 499
Serine proteases, 30–32
Serum amylase determinations, 130
Sipple's syndrome, 539–540
Small bowel see Duodenum; Intestine
Small cell carcinoma, of the pancreas,
    410–411
Smoking
  mechanisms of damage, 385
  pancreatic tumours, 400–401

Smoking (*contd*)
    as risk factor for pancreatic cancer,
        384–385, 391
Somatostatin
    and acute pancreatitis, 167
    analogue *see* Octreotide
    inhibition of pancreatic exocrine secretions,
        41, 212
Somatostatinoma, 538–539, 558
    diagnosis, 539
    pathology and pathophysiology, 538–539
Soya flour, trypsin inhibitor and pancreatic
        cancer, 386
Sphincter of Oddi
    alcohol-associated spasm, 167
    function, 33–34
    length, 21
    sphincterotomy, 300–301, 482–484
        and biliary drainage, 482–484
        extraction of calculi, 302–303
        and sphincteroplasty, 317–318
    structure, 33
    variations, 21
Splanchnicectomy *see* Neurotomy
Spleen
    conservation
        distal pancreatectomy, 326–327
        Warshaw's technique, 327
    preservation, pancreatoduodenectomy,
        343
Splenic arteries, 24–25
    embolization, 251–252
Splenic veins, 24
    obstruction, auxiliary techniques, 334
    thrombosis, portal hypertension,
        289–290
Steatorrhoea
    defined, 274
    evaluation, 274
    malabsorption and, 130
    treatment, 278
Stenting
    animal models, 503
    endoscopic transpapillary stenting, 306
    pancreatic duct(s), 301–302
    see also Biliary prostheses
Steroids, as anti-inflammatory agents in acute
        pancreatitis, 213
Stones *see* Calculi; Gallstones
Streptozotocin
    treatment of unresectable tumours, 525,
        536
        response rates, 550
    in VIPoma, 557
Stress ulceration, haemorrhage, complication
        of acute pancreatitis, 250
Superoxide radicals, 184–185
Supraduodenal artery, preservation, 333
Sweden, incidence of acute pancreatitis,
        193

Tamoxifen, treatment of unresectable
        tumours, 516
TAP *see* Trypsinogen activating peptides
Tea drinking, 388
Thyroxine, effect on pancreatic secretion, 41
TI3, nuclear receptors, effect on pancreatic
        secretion, 41
Tissue adhesive (n-butyl-2-cyanoacrylate),
        306
TNM staging, pancreatic carcinoma, 114
Tobacco *see* Smoking
Transpapillary biliary drainage, 482–484, 487
Transpapillary pancreaticoscopy, miniscope,
        484
Transplantation *see* Pancreatic transplantation
Trauma *see* Pancreatic trauma
Treitz, fascia of, 17
    formation, 17–18
[C-14] triolein breath test, 129
Triple bypass, 314
Triple-tube drainage, and peritoneal lavage,
        238
Tropical pancreatitis, 267–268, 316–317
Trousseau's sign, pancreatic tumours, 401
Trypsin
    delayed activation, 31–32
    inhibitors, 32
        giant cell carcinoma, 408
        pancreatitis secretory trypsin inhibitor,
            180
    mesotrypsin, 180
    in pathogenesis of pancreatitis, 179
    properties, 179
Trypsin inhibitor, and pancreatic cancer, 386
Trypsinogen activating peptides, 30, 201
Trypsinogens, 30–31
Tumour markers of malignancy, 132–136,
        426
    CG and hCG, 522
Tumour suppressor genes, p53, loss, 392

Ulceration, haemorrhage, complication of
        acute pancreatitis, 250
ULM classification, acute pancreatitis,
        233–235
Ultrasonography, 55–60
    acute pancreatitis, 56–58, 199–200
    carcinoma, 58–60
    chronic pancreatitis, 57–58, 275, 283–284
        grading, 162
    cystic neoplasms, 95
    gallstone-associated pancreatitis, 226–227
    intraoperative ultrasonography, 147–151
    islet cell tumours, 58–60
    normal pancreas, 55–56
    pancreatic tumours, algorithm, 427
    see also Endoscopic ultrasonography
Urea, serum levels, prognostic factor, 203
Urinary amylase, 198

Variceal haemorrhage, complication of acute
        pancreatitis, 250–251
Vascular problems
    arteriosclerotic vascular stenosis or
        occlusion, 465–467
    congenital vascular anomalies, 465
    iatrogenic injuries, 472–475
    infiltration or compression, in
        pancreatectomy, 467–472
    necrosis, complication of acute pancreatitis,
        251–252
    and techniques, in pancreatectomy,
        465–476
Vasoactive intestinal peptide (VIP)
    and cholecystokinin release, 38
    effects, 557
    see also Verner–Morrison syndrome
Vasopressin, 214
Vegetarianism, in aetiology of pancreatic
        tumours, 385–386
Veins, involvement in acute pancreatitis, CT,
        66
Verner–Morrison syndrome, 534–536,
        557–558
Vimentin, giant cell carcinoma, 408
VIPoma syndrome, 534–536
    see also Verner–Morrison syndrome
Virchow's node, pancreatic tumours, 426
Virchow's ranulae, formation, 407
Vitamin B12, Schilling test, 130
Vitamin K, historical note, 3
Volker drain, 631
    removal, 457
Vomiting, in acute pancreatitis, 195
Von Recklinghausen's disease, carcinoid
        tumours, 394

Warshaw's technique, conservation of the
        spleen, 327
Watery diarrhoea-hypokalaemia-
        hypochlorhydrial (WDHA) syndrome,
        534–536
Weight loss, in pancreatic cancer, 424
Werner's syndrome, 539–540
    see also MEN I syndrome
Whipple's procedure *see*
        Pancreatoduodenectomy
        (Whipple's)
Whipple's triad, 527, 548
Wirsung, duct of *see* Pancreatic duct(s)
Wound healing, postoperative, 499–500

Xanthine oxidase, oxygen derived free
        radicals, 184–185

Zollinger–Ellison syndrome *see* Gastrinoma